AF789944

Lifespan Treatment for Autistic Individuals

Lifespan Treatment for Autistic Individuals

A Guide to Evidence-Based Practices

Edited by
PETER STURMEY
RUSSELL LANG
AND
JAMES K. LUISELLI

OXFORD
UNIVERSITY PRESS

OXFORD
UNIVERSITY PRESS

Oxford University Press is a department of the University of Oxford. It furthers the University's objective of excellence in research, scholarship, and education by publishing worldwide. Oxford is a registered trade mark of Oxford University Press in the UK and in certain other countries.

Published in the United States of America by Oxford University Press
198 Madison Avenue, New York, NY 10016, United States of America.

© Oxford University Press 2025

All rights reserved. No part of this publication may be reproduced, stored in a retrieval system, transmitted, used for text and data mining, or used for training artificial intelligence, in any form or by any means, without the prior permission in writing of Oxford University Press, or as expressly permitted by law, by license or under terms agreed with the appropriate reprographics rights organization. Inquiries concerning reproduction outside the scope of the above should be sent to the Rights Department, Oxford University Press, at the address above.

You must not circulate this work in any other form
and you must impose this same condition on any acquirer.

CIP data is on file at the Library of Congress

ISBN 9780197635841

DOI: 10.1093/oso/9780197635841.001.0001

Printed by Integrated Books International, United States of America

MIX
Paper
FSC FSC® C183721

The manufacturer's authorised representative in the EU for product safety is Oxford University Press España S.A. of El Parque Empresarial San Fernando de Henares, Avenida de Castilla, 2 – 28830 Madrid (www.oup.es/en or product.safety@oup.com). OUP España S.A. also acts as importer into Spain of products made by the manufacturer.

Preface

Autism spectrum disorder (ASD) is a neurodevelopmental disorder associated with significant deficits in adaptive behavior and everyday functioning, which challenges families, service providers, staff, and multidisciplinary professionals. If effective treatments and services are unavailable, significant changes in functioning among persons with ASD are often minimal, caregivers may continue to experience stress and economic hardship, and society will continue to pay for expensive yet ineffective services. The importance of this situation is further highlighted by the very large increase in the prevalence of ASD, which has increased from approximately 4–5/10,000 to approximately 0.9–1.5% (Fombonne, 2020), a trend that is also reflected in both wealthy and developing countries (Salari et al., 2022), as well as in adults with ASD (Brugha et al., 2016). These epidemiological data suggest that the worldwide costs of ASD are very large and are continuing to increase.

Over the last 70 years, outcome research has shifted from unsupported and possibly harmful psychodynamic interventions to a plethora of interventions with varying degrees of support. Further, the status of evidence-based practices (EBPs) continues to shift as new research is reported and new interventions are identified (Steinbrenner et al., 2020) and systematic work on dissemination of EBPs can begin (Sam et al., 2020). Yet, despite the availability of a cadre of EBPs, relatively few autistic individuals receive them, or they are exposed to them and some receive ineffective and even harmful treatments (Jonkman et al., 2022). Further, family members and professionals face a very challenging task in identifying and accessing EBPs due to conflicting and changing evidence, unfounded opinions, and passionate but sometimes incorrect advocacy for certain treatments.

This volume is one of many such handbooks which have been published over the years. It offers updates to the current status of EBPs and ASD, while presenting the information in a standardized format with plain language summaries for ease of access. The chapters are strongly science-based and founded on the best available high-quality empirical research from an international team of highly experienced and skilled research practitioners. The editors express their thanks to all the contributors to these chapters and for the outstanding work they have done for this volume.

We hope that the family members, students, practitioners, and researchers who read these chapters will find inspiration to adopt, disseminate, and continue to refine EDPs for autistic individuals.

References

Brugha, T. S., Spiers, N., Bankart, J., Cooper, S. A., McManus, S., Scott, F. J., ... Tyrer, F. (2016). Epidemiology of autism in adults across age groups and ability levels. *The British Journal of Psychiatry, 209*(6), 498–503.

Fombonne, E. (2020). Epidemiological controversies in autism. *Swiss Archives of Neurology, Psychiatry and Psychotherapy, 171*(1).

Jonkman, K. M., Back, E., Staal, W. G., Benard, L., van der Doelen, D. M., & Begeer, S. (2022). Alternative treatments for autism: Prevalence and predictors. *Research in Autism Spectrum Disorders, 98*, 102046. doi:10.1016/j.rasd.2022.102046

Salari, N., Rasoulpoor, S., Rasoulpoor, S., Shohaimi, S., Jafarpour, S., Abdoli, N., ... Mohammadi, M. (2022). The global prevalence of autism spectrum disorder: A comprehensive systematic review and meta-analysis. *Italian Journal of Pediatrics, 48*(1), 1–16.

Sam, A. M., Cox, A. W., Savage, M. N., Waters, V., & Odom, S. L. (2020). Disseminating information on evidence-based practices for children and youth with autism spectrum disorder: AFIRM. *Journal of Autism and Developmental Disorders, 50*, 1931–1940.

Steinbrenner, J. R., Hume, K., Odom, S. L., Morin, K. L., Nowell, S. W., Tomaszewski, B., ... Savage, M. N. (2020). Evidence-based practices for children, youth, and young adults with autism. FPG Child Development Institute. https://files.eric.ed.gov/fulltext/ED609029.pdf

Contents

Contributors

Suhad S. Abumweis holds a PhD degree in human nutrition from McGill University (Montreal, Canada). She has worked in the Department of Clinical Nutrition and Dietetics at the Hashemite University since 2008. Currently, she is the director of the nutrition and dietetics program at Al Ain University, UAE. Her teaching interests are in nutritional assessment and medical nutrition therapy. She has clinical research experience, particularly in the area of functional foods and lipid metabolism. She has a good knowledge of strengths, limitations, and areas of potential improvement in human nutrition trials. In addition, she is conducting systematic reviews and meta-analysis research on dietary interventions to reduce risk factors for chronic diseases. Dr. Abumweis has published 40 peer-reviewed research articles. Her work has been cited by many regulatory authorities. Her research interests are lipid metabolism, functional foods, nutraceuticals, health claims, evidence-based medical nutrition therapy, systematic reviews, and meta-analysis.

Charlene N. Agnew, PhD, is a researcher and clinician with experience in home, school, and clinic settings and behavior analytic teaching experience in undergraduate and master's programs. She first became interested in behavior analysis as a volunteer for children with autism in Canada while completing her master's degree in counseling psychology. She then moved to New York to pursue doctoral training in both basic and applied research at The Graduate Center, City University of New York (CUNY). After graduation, Dr. Agnew completed her postdoctoral fellowship at Suny Upstate Medical University. She is a guest reviewer for the *Journal of Applied Behavior Analysis*, *Journal of Autism and Developmental Disorders*, and *Behavioral Development.* Dr. Agnew's research interests include mitigation of relapse in treatment programs, including functional communication training. Her clinical interests include treatment of severe problem behavior, trauma therapy, and parent consultation. Dr. Agnew is a Board-Certified Behavior Analyst–Doctoral Level and a licensed behavior analyst in New York State; she is also certified in trauma-focused cognitive-behavioral therapy. She currently lives in New York City, where she works as a clinician.

William H. Ahearn serves as the director of research at the New England Center for Children and as adjunct faculty for the Western New England University's master's and doctoral programs in behavior analysis. Bill's research interests are varied and include peer-reviewed publications on treating pediatric feeding disorders, teaching verbal and social skills, examining implications of the behavioral momentum metaphor, and exploring aspects of autistic behavior. However, his most cited work is on assessing and treating automatically reinforced behavior, specifically, repetitive behavior and restricted interests. Bill and his colleagues have developed a form of redirection referred to as response interruption and redirection (RIRD), which has been identified by the National Clearinghouse on Autism Evidence and Practice (https://ncaep.fpg.unc.edu/) as one of 27 evidence-based practices for treating autism. He has published over 100 papers in a variety of outlets. He currently serves as the editor-in-chief of *Behavioral Interventions.* Bill has provided extensive service throughout his career. He has provided service for BABAT, APBA, BACB®, ABAI, and Autism Speaks. As BABAT's chair of professional practice, Bill organized BABAT's efforts relative to licensure in Massachusetts. After licensure was signed into law, he was appointed as an applied behavior analyst member of the Allied Mental Health and Human Services Professions board in 2013. Subsequently, Bill was appointed chair of this omnibus board by both a Democratic and Republican governor, and at the time of the writing of this chapter, he served as the acting chair of the board.

Ashley N. Anderson worked in direct care as a house parent for adolescents with behavioral issues before earning her master's degree in applied behavior analysis at Auburn University. Currently, she is a doctoral student at Auburn University in the Cognitive and Behavioral Sciences program, where she provides behavior analytic services to adolescents in residential care and their staff. Although her current research includes a mixture of clinical and translational projects, the central theme consists of improving the quality of care for residents and cultivating staff skill sets.

John Augustine is a doctoral student at the University of Missouri–Columbia in the Department of Special Education and a certified special education teacher. John's research examines function-based interventions in applied settings to facilitate and promote inclusion of students with autism or developmental disabilities. This is accomplished through two lines of research, which include (a) the efficacy and social validity of function-based interventions aimed at decreasing challenging or disruptive behavior in educational settings and (b) models to deliver sustainable professional development to increase implementation fidelity of evidence-based behavioral interventions by education personnel, including teachers and paraeducators. John's key aim of research is to develop sustainable and feasible use of evidence-based behavioral interventions in applied settings to serve students with autism and developmental disabilities. John has published peer-reviewed journal articles regarding applied behavior analytic interventions for children with autism spectrum disorders and developmental disabilities.

Lorna Barry is a chartered behavioral psychologist with the Psychological Society of Ireland and Board-Certified Behavior Analyst®. She obtained her MSc in applied behavior analysis from the University of Galway and her PhD in psychology from the University of Limerick, Ireland. Dr. Barry currently works at ASK, a Geneva-based center, focusing on developing programs to promote the social inclusion of individuals diagnosed with special needs.

Rasha R. Baruni is an assistant professor in the Department of Psychology at the University of Manitoba in Canada. She obtained her PhD in applied behavior analysis from the University of South Florida and her MS degree in applied behavior analysis from St. Cloud State University. She has over 15 years of experience providing behavior analytic services to young children and adolescents with autism spectrum disorder in homes, schools, and clinics within Canada, the United States, and the United Arab Emirates. Her research interests include training practitioners to implement evidence-based practices in safety skills, teaching children safety skills, and the assessment and treatment of maladaptive behaviors.

Haifa Batarseh holds her doctor of science degree in occupational therapy/occupational science from Towson University. She has participated in advancing the occupational therapy curriculum at the Hashemite University. Currently, she is an assistant professor in the Department of Physical and Occupational Therapy at the Hashemite University. She held several academic administrative positions such as the assistant dean of the Faculty of Applied Medical Sciences (2017–2018) and assistant dean of the Deanship of Students Affairs (2018–2020), and assistant dean of the Faculty of Applied Medical Sciences (2020–2022) in the Hashemite University, Jordan. Dr. Batarseh has participated in the establishment of Clinical Rehabilitation Sciences Master's program in Jordan, an Erasmus funded project in collaboration with Jordan University of Science and Technology, in addition to the establishment of the Community Base Inclusive Development Diploma program and finally the establishment of the Hashemite University Center for Special Educational and Rehabilitative Services for Clients With Disability. Dr. Batarseh is also a certified sensory integration therapist. She has practiced as an occupational therapist since 1996, specializing in occupational therapy for children and youth. Dr. Batarseh has research interests in occupational therapy for pediatrics; occupational therapy for children and adolescents with autism spectrum disorder; and occupational therapy professional and educational issues and development.

Mark Bellgrove is a professor of cognitive neuroscience at Monash University. His research team investigates the biological foundations of attention, cognitive control, and neurodevelopment using advanced cognitive neuroscience and molecular genomics methodologies. Professor Bellgrove's work has shed light on the genetic and neurochemical underpinnings of attention and cognitive control, with significant contributions to the understanding of attention-deficit/hyperactivity disorder (ADHD). His pioneering studies established links between ADHD risk genes and distinct neurocognitive profiles, shaping the landscape of psychiatric genetics. Recognitions for Bellgrove's accomplishments include awards from prestigious institutions like NARSAD and the Academy of Social Sciences in Australia. In 2021, he was elected as a fellow of the Academy of Social Sciences in Australia (FASSA). Bellgrove's dedication to neurodevelopment extends beyond research; in 2016, he founded the Australian ADHD Professionals Association (AADPA), fostering evidence-based practices for ADHD diagnosis and treatment. Notably, he spearheaded the creation of Australia's evidence-based clinical practice guideline for ADHD, endorsed by Australia's National Health and Medical Research Council (NHMRC).

Jordan Belisle is an associate professor at Missouri State University in the Psychology Department and cofounder of the Institute for Dynamic Behavior Science. He has published over 100 articles and book chapters on topics ranging from supporting language and cognitive development in children, to human altruism, prejudice and discrimination, and the climate change crisis. Dr. Belisle has coauthored two books, including *Acceptance and Commitment Therapy for Behavior Analysts* and *Research Methods for the Practicing Behavior Analyst*, and he has presented this work and research nationally and internationally along with his students and collaborators.

Leandra N. Berry is currently an assistant professor in the section of psychology within the Department of Pediatrics at Baylor College of Medicine (BCM). She is also a licensed psychologist and the associate director of clinical services for the Autism Center at Texas Children's Hospital (TCH). Dr. Berry provides clinical assessments to patients in the Autism Center and conducts evaluations for ASD phenotyping studies. Dr. Berry obtained her bachelor's degree in psychology from Texas Lutheran University in 2000 and her master's degree in clinical psychology from Southern Methodist University in 2003. In 2009, she obtained her doctorate in clinical psychology from the University of Connecticut following completion of her clinical internship at Texas Children's Hospital. During her doctoral training, Dr. Berry served as a research assistant on a project investigating the M-CHAT as a screening measure for ASD in toddlers under the supervision of Deborah Fein, PhD. Dr. Berry completed a 2-year specialized fellowship in autism and neuropsychology at the Center for Autism Research at the Children's Hospital of Philadelphia (CHOP) under the mentorship of Robert Schultz, PhD, and Judith Miller, PhD. Before joining the BCM faculty in April 2012, Dr. Berry worked as a pediatric neuropsychologist and scientist at CHOP's Center for Autism Research, where she was involved in several multisite ASD research projects, including the Infant Brain Imaging Study and the Autism Treatment Network. Dr. Berry's research interests include early identification and diagnosis of ASD, comorbid conditions such as anxiety, evidence-based interventions, and factors associated with positive treatment outcomes.

Camille Blouet is a French child psychiatrist, currently a clinical instructor in the Child and Adolescent Psychiatry Department of the University Hospital Center of Caen Normandy. She obtained a MS in neuroscience from the University of Caen Normandy in 2020.

Edward Bovey is the associate director of the PELE Center at the University of Denver. Ted has been working with young children, children with autism, children with disabilities, and families for over 30 years as an inclusive preschool teacher, early interventionist, researcher, trainer, and consultant. Ted has extensive experience in the use of evidence-based practices for young children with autism and other disabilities, in coaching classrooms to utilize evidence-based instructional strategies, and in supporting classrooms, programs, and districts in the implementation of the LEAP Preschool model.

Matthew E. Brock is an associate professor of special education at Ohio State University and a faculty fellow at the Crane Center for Early Childhood Research and Policy. He has two lines of research that both focus on students with significant disabilities who have diagnoses of autism, intellectual disability, or multiple disabilities. First, he develops and tests peer-mediated interventions that support children with and without disabilities to learn and play together. Second, he studies how best to prepare and support paraeducators to use evidence-based practices that improve outcomes for students with significant disabilities. Dr. Brock currently leads a large federally funded efficacy study of FLIP Recess, an intervention to improve communication and social outcomes at recess for elementary students with significant disabilities. He also leads a training grant focused on preparing future university faculty in the areas of special education for students with significant disabilities and advanced quantitative research methods. Prior to receiving his doctorate, Dr. Brock worked as a preschool teacher, elementary school teacher, and taught through the US Peace Corps in St. Kitts and Nevis. He has published more than 50 peer-reviewed journal articles. He was the recipient of the 2023 Martin J. Kaufman Distinguished Early Career Research Award from the Council for Exceptional Children Division for Research, and he was named in Stanford University's list of Top 2% of Scientists Worldwide.

Natascia Brondino is associate professor of psychiatry, University of Pavia, Italy.

Deborah J. Bubela has been a physical therapist for over 40 years and a board-certified clinical specialist in pediatric physical therapy since 2002. While she has provided therapy for people of all ages, she has specialized in working with children in various settings, including early intervention, schools, and rehabilitation settings. Deborah became a faculty member at the University of Connecticut in 2002 and is now an emeritus associate professor in residence. While at the university she was responsible for the pediatric component of the curriculum along with several other courses. She coauthored *Physical Therapy in Connecticut Schools—Best Practices and Resources*. Her research involved children with and without disabilities. As an educator in a research-based institution, she tried to bridge the research-to-practice gap through empirical study of "real-world issues" and translation of research to serve students' education and clinical practice. She worked with national funding sources (NIH, OSERS, etc.) to perform large-scale studies relating to personnel preparation and development of assessment tools (NIH Motor Toolbox). She also contributed to research relating to community-based wellness program initiatives for school-aged children and adults.

Mary Isaac Cargill is a doctoral student in Montclair State University's PhD program for clinical psychology. Previously, Mary Isaac received dual degrees in psychology and English from the University of Virginia. Her clinical work includes therapy and assessment with autistic people across the lifespan from early childhood into adulthood. Her research interests include identifying phenotypic differences in autism across different genders, sexualities, and cultures, as well as developing assessments that reflect those differences. She is also interested in understanding perceptions of autism in order to reduce stigma surrounding the condition. She plans to utilize these findings to develop specialized, evidence-based interventions to improve the quality of life of autistic people.

Amarie Carnett is the program director and a senior lecturer in educational psychology at Victoria University of Wellington, New Zealand, and a research affiliate at the University of Texas San Antonio in the applied behavior analysis program. She is a doctorate-level Board-Certified Behavior Analyst (BCBA-D). She has over 15 years of experience working in the field of behavior science and autism/developmental disabilities. Her research is focused on developing interventions to help individuals develop autonomy within their environments and increase their overall quality of life. She believes this is best achieved by interventions that target issues associated to generalization of skills, as well as ensuring social significance through stakeholder participation. Her research interest can be classified into two overlapping categories (1) communication interventions and (2) adaptive functioning. Dr. Carnett has 46 peer-reviewed journal articles related to communication interventions and adaptive functioning. Dr. Carnett serves her research community and professional community in several leadership roles (e.g., journal reviewer, special issue editor, international conference convenor, ethics committee member). Since returning to New Zealand, Dr. Carnett has worked in collaboration with colleagues to develop the Society of Behaviour Analysis Aotearo, New Zealand, an organization aimed at establishing professional practice standards for behavior analysis. She currently serves as chair for this organization.

Mark Carter has contributed to the field of special education for over 40 years as an early interventionist, special educator, teacher educator, and researcher. He is currently the dean of the Academy for the Science of Instruction at MultiLit Pty Ltd, an honorary associate professor in the School of Education at the University of Wollongong, and an expert panel member at the Institute of Special Educators in Australia. He has a range of research interests, including educational issues in autism spectrum disorder, evidence-based practice, controversial practices, and educational decision-making. Mark has over 150 refereed publications and book chapters and has contributed to a wide range of conference presentations. He has also contributed extensively to the translation of research into accessible information for practitioners through publications providing summaries and syntheses of research. Mark has served in an editorial capacity on a range of journals and edited special issues. He has also acted as a grant application reviewer for a number of organizations, including the Australian Research Council, has made contributions to government enquiries and reviews, and has been involved in consultancies evaluating government-sponsored programs.

Mirela Cengher, PhD, is an assistant professor in psychology at the University of Maryland, Baltimore County (UMBC). She is a Board-Certified Behavior Analyst–Doctoral Level and a licensed behavior analyst in the state of Maryland. Dr. Cengher first became interested in behavior analysis when she began working with children with developmental disabilities as an undergraduate student in Romania. She then moved to the United States to pursue graduate training in behavior analysis. Dr. Cengher received her doctorate in psychology from The Graduate Center, City University of New York, and completed her postdoctoral fellowship at Kennedy Krieger Institute and Johns Hopkins University School of Medicine. Dr. Cengher has over 15 years of research and clinical experience with individuals with developmental disabilities. Her primary research interest is at the intersection of verbal behavior and stimulus control—specifically, in her research, she evaluates variables that affect the acquisition of verbal behavior and the development of emergent relations. One of the main lines of research in Dr. Cengher's lab is the acquisition of foreign languages in children from bilingual households. Dr. Cengher serves as a guest associate editor and as an editorial board member for several scientific journals (e.g., *Journal of Applied Behavior Analysis, The Analysis of Verbal Behavior,* and *Behavior Analysis in Practice*).

An-An Chang is a distinguished scholar and practitioner in the field of applied behavior analysis (ABA), holding an MS degree from California State University, Northridge (CSUN). She currently practices ABA as an associate clinical supervisor working with Easterseals Southern California. As a research fellow on CSUN ARCS: Autonomy Research Center for STEAHM, An-An co-led student researchers in collaboration with NASA and JPL scientists to study active human-AI team communication dynamics. As a senior researcher at KLab: Behavior Science and Technology Lab CSUN, she made significant contributions to the fields of organizational behavior management, autonomous training technology, and conflict resolution. Currently, she is building Octobit, a virtual simulation training platform that will enable standardized and scalable behavior skills training. An-An is credited as the first author of "The Effectiveness of Virtual Reality Training: A Systematic Review," published in the *Journal of Organizational Behavior Management.* She is also a passionate advocate to uplift disabled gamers and foster inclusivity, leading her to collaborations with Easterseals Gaming Initiative.

Jennifer L. Cook earned a master of science (St Cloud State University) and PhD (University of South Florida), with a major in applied behavior analysis for both degrees. She is certified as a doctoral-level Board-Certified Behavior Analyst (BCBA-D). She has nearly 20 years of clinical experience and is currently an assistant professor at the University of Manitoba in Winnipeg, Canada. Her research primarily involves conjugate schedules of reinforcement, assessment, and interventions to improve performance or exercise adherence in the area of health, sports, and fitness, as well as assessment and treatment for children and youth with autism spectrum disorders or those with other behavioral challenges.

Shoumitro (Shoumi) Deb is a visiting professor of neuropsychiatry at the Imperial College London, UK. His seminal works include (a) the first-ever evidence-based practice guidelines for intellectual disabilities (ID) in the UK NHS, (b) the first-ever comprehensive assessment of psychopathology in adults with ID and epilepsy, (c) a dementia screening questionnaire for adults with ID (DSQIID) translated into more than 24 languages and validated, (d) the first-ever freely available online accessible psychotropic medication information leaflets (http://www.ld-medication.bham.ac.uk), (e) the first-ever European Guideline (and recent update in *European Journal of Psychiatry*, 2022, *36*, 11–25) on the assessment and diagnosis of psychiatric disorders in adults with ID, (f) national and international guidelines on the use of psychotropic medication in adults with ID (*World Psychiatry,* 2009, *8*(3), 181–186), (g) the first-ever online training, SPECTROM for caregivers to help reduce the overmedication of people with ID (https://spectrom.wixsite.com/project), (h) the first-ever comprehensive neuropsychiatric outcome study in adults with traumatic brain injury (TBI), (i) patient and carer-determined outcome measures for patients with TBI, and (j) the only published randomized controlled trial (feasibility) on risperidone versus placebo to treat aggression in adults with traumatic brain injury. He has over 330 publications and has made over 250 presentations at national and international conferences. He ran several MSc programs in three UK universities. He was a member of the first UK NICE GDG on epilepsy and other NICE guidelines, a fellow of the UK National Institute for Health and Care ResearchR, vice-chair of the World Psychiatric Association SPID, and a member of the WHO Working Group on ICD-11.

Janet DeLany is professor emerita from Towson University in Towson, Maryland. At the University, she served as dean of graduate studies from 2012 to 2019, director of the doctoral program in occupational science and director of the postbaccalaureate program in autism studies. She directed the occupational therapy assistant program and the occupational therapy program at Pennsylvania State University. She has practiced as an occupational therapist since 1975, specializing in children, youth, and families. Her research focused on women's leadership, autism, and children and families. She has been the recipient of multiple awards at the state and national level for her leadership in education and practice.

Rhona Dempsey is a research fellow in the School of Psychology, Trinity College, Dublin, who focuses on research that develops novel and innovative assistive technologies spanning education, psychology and disability with a primary aim of improving quality of life and outcomes for people with neurodevelopmental conditions. Her interests include broadening the reach of scientific evidential principles through developing practical applications. One such strand includes innovations in smartphone applications and deliveries in an inclusive accessible format to vested stakeholders spanning people with lived experience, families, and communities as well as professionals in the fields of education, psychology, and disability. Rhona contributes lectures within the Schools of Psychology, Medicine, and Education. Her extensive background in policy and research facilitates her invitation to and active roles across government and nongovernmental organization steering committees charged with influencing change to the benefit of disabled communities and wider society, including for example via legislative instrument.

Mark R. Dixon is a Board-Certified Behavior Analyst and a clinical professor at the Department of Disability and Human Development. Dr. Dixon has published 12 books, over 250 peer-reviewed journal articles, and delivered thousands of presentations around the globe. His research and/or expert opinions have been featured in *Time* Magazine, *Newsweek*, *The New York Times*, National Public Radio, *This American Life*, and Netflix's series *Bill Nye Saves the World*. Dr. Dixon cares for individuals and their families impacted by autism and other developmental disabilities through his innovative research that guides practice. He has generated millions of dollars of funding to infuse behavior analysis within local schools and treatment facilities, and he has created multiple clinics for persons diagnosed with autism and related conditions.

Johann M. D'Souza earned a bachelor's degree from University of Dallas in theology, a master's degree in psychology from Boston University, and a master's degree and PhD in clinical psychology from the University of Houston on a presidential fellowship. He completed his clinical internship at the Obsessive-Compulsive Disorder specialty clinic of Baylor College of Medicine under the direction of Dr. Eric Storch and completed a postdoctoral fellowship at Psychology Houston, PC, where he specialized in obsessive-compulsive and related disorders. His publications focus on the psychological benefits of resilience factors such as hope and optimism as protective against anxiety. Johann is a research affiliate at Harvard's Human Flourishing Program, a coach for OptimalWork, and the founder of Values First Therapy, where he uses cognitive-behavioral therapy (CBT) and acceptance and commitment therapy (ACT) to treat teens with anxiety and obsessive-compulsive disorder.

Sarah R. Edmunds is an assistant professor in the Department of Psychology at the University of South Carolina. Dr. Edmunds received her doctorate in clinical psychology from the University of Washington. She completed her predoctoral internship at Duke University Medical Center and her postdoctoral fellowship at Boston Children's Hospital and Harvard Medical School. Dr. Edmunds received her bachelor's degree in psychology from Cornell University. Dr. Edmunds studies neurodiversity-informed interventions that address the functional impairments that are associated with autism spectrum disorder (e.g., in social communication, social skills, flexibility, emotion regulation, and anxiety). Broadly, her research investigates how we can best implement these interventions within early intervention, school, and mental healthcare systems, in ways that are tailored to each community and support equitable access for all autistic children and teens. Her research explores the balance between fidelity (i.e., staying "true" to an intervention as it was designed) and fit (i.e., adapting aspects of the intervention to better fit the child, family, and organization that provides it). Dr. Edmunds is a licensed psychologist with expertise in a broad range of evidence-based interventions to support social communication, executive functioning, and emotion regulation in children and teens, including several naturalistic developmental behavioral interventions, behavioral parent training, cognitive-behavioral therapy adapted for autistic individuals, exposure and response prevention for obsessive-compulsive disorder and anxiety, and behavioral activation for depression.

Craig A. Erickson is an associate professor at the University of Cincinnati Department of Psychiatry and Behavioral Neuroscience. He specializes in translational treatment development in neurodevelopmental disorders and is considered an international expert in the clinical treatment of fragile X syndrome and fragile X–specific clinical trial development. He and his colleagues have moved forward several repurposed molecules for study in fragile X syndrome and autism spectrum disorder, including work with acamprosate, riluzole, ketamine, D cycloserine, and N acetyl cysteine, among other repurposed molecules. He also is working now to move several novel molecules into autism and fragile X-specific study using proprietary compounds abandoned from initially intended use that may hold promise in the disorders which he and his colleagues study.

Kristen H. Erps earned a BA in psychology from Western Kentucky University and a PhD in school psychology from the University of Houston. She completed an internship at the Nationwide Children's Hospital on the pediatric acute treatment track. She is currently a postdoctoral fellow at Nationwide Children's Hospital as well. Her research interests broadly focus on the identification of at-risk youth and mental health comorbidities for youth with neurodevelopmental disorders.

Terry S. Falcomata received a BS degree in middle school education from the Illinois State University in 1997, a MS degree in behavior analysis and therapy from Southern Illinois University in 2002, and a doctorate in school psychology from the University of Iowa in 2008, under the supervision of David Wacker. He held a postdoctoral research position at the Munroe-Meyer Institute at the University of Nebraska Medical Center with Wayne Fisher and Henry Roane in 2008–2009. He is currently a professor of special education at the University of Texas at Austin, where he has been on faculty since 2009. He serves as the editor-in-chief of the *Journal of Behavioral Education* (JOBE); he has served an as associate editor of *Behavior Analysis in Practice*, JOBE, and the *Journal of Developmental and Physical Disabilities*; and he has served on the board of editors for numerous journals, including the *Journal of Applied Behavior Analysis*, *Behavior Modification*, and the *Review Journal for Autism and Developmental Disabilities*. Dr. Falcomata's research interests include the assessment and treatment of problem behavior displayed by individuals with ASD/DD, methods for increasing behavioral variability in individuals with ASD/DD, and methods for preventing clinical relapse pertaining to challenging behavior.

Julia L. Ferguson is the research and assessment coordinator for Autism Partnership Foundation and the associate director of the Progressive Behavior Analyst Autism Council. Julia received her bachelor's degree in applied behavior analysis and her master's degree in behavior analysis from the University of North Texas. Julia is currently pursuing her PhD in applied behavior analysis at Endicott College under the advisement of Dr. Mary Jane Weiss. Julia has over 10 years of experience working with children diagnosed with autism in home, community, and clinical settings. Her research interests include evaluating social skills interventions, evaluating progressive approaches to behavioral interventions, and comparing different teaching methodologies for individuals diagnosed with autism. Julia has published over 50 peer-reviewed research articles, book chapters, and books and has presented at national and international conferences.

Aaron J. Fischer has been working with individuals with mental health and social, emotional, and behavioral problems, and their families, for over 15 years. Dr. Fischer completed his master's and doctoral degree in school psychology at Louisiana State University, where he provided multitiered school metal and behavior health supports to schools across Louisiana. Before arriving at the University of Utah in 2014, he completed his predoctoral internship in clinical psychology at the May Institute in Massachusetts. His internship and graduate work focused on providing evidence-based practices in schools, hospitals, and mental health clinics to children with disabilities and their families. Specifically, Dr. Fischer's practice and research interests concentrate on culturally responsive assessment and treatment to support children and adolescents with social-emotional and behavioral concerns, as well as providing consultation support and training to caregivers and educators. Dr. Fischer's work specifically focuses on teleconsultation and telehealth for school-based MTSS services. Currently, Dr. Fischer is an associate professor of school psychology and adjunct associate professor of psychiatry. He serves as the director of the University of Utah Technology in Training, Education, and Consultation (U-TTEC) Lab and directs the Utah School Mental Health Collaborative, which partners with numerous school districts across Utah to provide technical assistance, training, and support for education settings. Also, Dr. Fischer directs the Huntsman Mental Health Institute HOME interdisciplinary pediatric feeding disorders clinic. Dr. Fischer is a licensed psychologist and licensed Board-Certified Behavior Analyst who has have extensive experience in research and development, data analysis, and support implementation as evidenced by his almost 20 years working to provide mental and behavior health MTSS supports in schools.

Kyle M. Frost is currently a postdoctoral fellow at the Eunice Kennedy Shriver Center at the University of Massachusetts Chan Medical School. She received her doctorate from the Department of Psychology at Michigan State University in the clinical science program area. She completed her predoctoral internship at the University of Colorado School of Medicine. The overarching goal of Dr. Frost's research is to improve the efficacy and reach of early interventions for supporting social communication development and to increase equitable access to high-quality autism services. Her research examines the core features of effective interventions, the mechanistic processes through which they affect change, and how evidence-based practices can be implemented in community systems of care. Dr. Frost is particularly interested in system- and organization-level factors that might affect receipt of quality services as a target for implementation interventions. Community engagement is a core value in her work, and she frequently applies mixed-methods approaches that incorporate shareholder perspectives. Dr. Frost has extensive clinical training in diagnostic assessment, intervention, and supports for individuals with intellectual and developmental disabilities across the lifespan. Particular areas of expertise include naturalistic developmental behavioral interventions, cognitive-behavioral therapy, and parent coaching or parent-mediated approaches for supporting young autistic children and their families. Dr. Frost also has experience disseminating best practices in early social communication intervention to community providers via professional workshops and consultation.

Laura Fusar-Poli is an associate professor of psychiatry at the University of Pavia, Italy.

Siobhan Gardner is a PhD candidate at Te Herenga Waka Victoria University of Wellington. She completed a master of educational psychology in 2021 at Te Herenga Waka Victoria University of Wellington. Siobhan has practical experience working with children with developmental disabilities across a range of sectors. She has provided support in schools and homes. Siobhan currently works at Victoria University of Wellington's Autism Te Rāngai Takiwātanga clinic providing early intervention support for young autistic children and their families. Siobhan's research interests include communication, naturalistic supports, and supporting parents of children with disabilities. Her PhD research focuses on parents' experiences and perceptions of augmentative and alternative communication for their autistic children.

Jessica E. Graber is a licensed psychologist in the Complex Behavior Program at the Center for Autism Spectrum Disorders at Nationwide Children's Hospital. She directs the Complex Behavior Consultation service, which provides evidence-based interventions for children with neurodevelopmental differences such as autism, who also have an intellectual disability diagnosis and present with complex behavioral needs.

Fabian Guénolé is a French psychiatrist, head of the Department of Child and Adolescent Psychiatry at the Centre Hospitalier Universitaire de Caen Normandie, professor at Caen Normandy University, and a member of the research unit "Neuropsychology and imaging of the human memory" (UMR-1077 INSERM-EPHE-UNICAEN). Dr Guenole received an MS in biology from the Caen Normandy University in 2004, an MD from the Lyon faculty of medicine in 2007, and a PhD from the University of Versailles in 2018. She was certified in child and adolescent psychiatry in 2012. Dr Guenole's fields of interest are child and adolescent psychopathology, affective neuroscience, and the emotional aspects of self and identity. She supports an integrative view of psychopathology, regarding both understanding and treatment, and collaborates with psychiatrists, neurologists, pediatricians, clinical and experimental psychologists, psychoanalysts, methodologists, physiologists, and engineers.

Cecilia Guiot is a psychiatric trainee at the University of Pavia, Italy.

Andrew G. Guzick is a clinical psychologist and assistant professor in the Department of Psychiatry at the University of Pennsylvania. Dr. Guzick completed his bachelor's degree in psychology at Vassar College and his doctoral degree in clinical psychology at the University of Florida. He went on to complete his doctoral internship at Baylor College of Medicine (BCM)/Texas Children's Hospital and his postdoctoral fellowship at BCM, where he was also on the faculty for 2 years. His research has focused on understanding and optimizing exposure therapy for children and adults with anxiety and obsessive-compulsive disorder, low-cost and innovative methods to increase access to cognitive-behavioral therapy (CBT), adaptations to CBT for anxiety among autistic youth, and patient-centered research for youth with misophonia and other problems related to sensory over-responsivity. He has received foundation and state funding to support this work and has published over 60 peer-reviewed publications and 10 chapters on these topics. Dr. Guzick is also a practicing clinical psychologist with a specialization in cognitive-behavioral therapy for youth and adults with anxiety and obsessive-compulsive disorders.

Jennifer Hamrick received her BS degree in interdisciplinary studies from Southwest Texas State University in 2000, an MS degree in criminal justice and applied behavior analysis from Saint Joseph's University in 2012, and a doctorate degree in special education from the University of Texas at Austin in 2016, under the supervision of Terry Falcomata. She is currently an assistant professor of special education at Texas Tech University, where she has been on faculty since 2018. She serves as the director of the Burkhart Center for Autism Education and Research and currently serves on the board for the Autism Society of Texas. Dr. Hamrick's research interests include addressing the needs of individuals with autism spectrum disorders and/or developmental disabilities in rural special education settings while providing parent and educator training via telehealth.

Olive Healy is a behavioral psychologist and Doctoral Board-Certified Behavior Analyst® with 25 years of clinical expertise in neurodevelopmental conditions, including autism. She is director of the MSc program in applied behavior analysis at the School of Psychology, Trinity College Dublin. After serving for 7 years as lecturer in psychology (2006–2013) at the University of Galway, Olive joined the School of Psychology, Trinity College, the University of Dublin and is now an associate professor in psychology. She now acts as principal investigator of numerous clinical evaluations under the project InterAcT (Accomplish & Thrive) within Trinity College Dublin. She is associate editor of four leading international journals contributing to peer review and research dissemination in the field of behavioral psychology. She has authored over 90 academic papers and book chapters published in both behavior-analytic and mainstream psychology journals.

Erin A. Henneberry specializes in child and adolescent psychiatry and is at the Cincinnati Children's Hospital – Department of Child and Adolescent Psychiatry.

Celia Heyman teaches several graduate-level applied behavior analysis (ABA) courses, including behavior analytic assessments and interventions. She has taught various ABA courses at Rider University, Behavioral Momentum India, and the Institute per la Ricerca in Italy. Celia obtained her training in public schools, where she continues to provide consultations, focusing on the dissemination of the practical functional assessment, skill-based treatment, and other assent-based interventions to address interfering behaviors. Her clinical skills include parent and staff training. She is a lead consultant and predoctoral fellow with FTF Behavioral Consulting, under the mentorship of Drs. Greg Hanley and Anthony Cammilleri. Celia has presented in various international conferences. Her research interests include emerging learning instruction, acceptance commitment training, and functional analysis. Celia is on the advisory board of the BF Skinner Foundation and is the Students Committee chairperson with the World Behavior Analysis Day Alliance. She was a guest editor of the *Behavior Analysis in Practice* special issue on compassion. In her spare time, Celia has cultivated an online study group for aspiring behavior analysts, reaching over 54,000 members worldwide.

Ashley E. Hinten is a postdoctoral fellow in the Faculty of Health at the University of Canterbury, New Zealand. She is researching early identification and support for young autistic children in Aotearoa New Zealand under the guidance of Professor Laurie McLay. Dr Hinten completed her doctoral research in the Department of Psychology at the University of Otago under the supervision of Associate Professor Damian Scarf and Professor Elaine Reese. Her thesis examined the short- and long-term effects of screen media pace (frequency of camera cuts and scene changes) and fantasy rates (frequency of unrealistic events) on child viewers' executive functioning (e.g., abilities to problem-solve and follow instructions). In her earlier honors and master's degrees, she studied children's and undergraduates' social evaluations of helping and hindering characters. Through her developmental psychology research experience and teaching roles, she has developed a keen interest in teaching others about science, and she aspires to be a science communicator. In addition to publishing her research in academic journals and presenting at conferences, she is exploring opportunities to develop her science communication skills in multiple mediums for a range of audiences.

Jennifer Holloway is a chartered behavioral psychologist and Board-Certified Behavior Analyst, currently working in Geneva, Switzerland. Jennifer is the CEO of ASK-All Special Kids, which is a nonprofit association focused on the provision of evidence-based interventions to teach and improve socially significant objectives for children and adults with neurodevelopmental diagnoses. She has worked with individuals with special needs for over 25 years as a clinician and researcher. Working across clinical settings, homes, schools, and corporations, Jennifer has dedicated her career to developing and implementing best practices to improve meaningful inclusion for individuals with additional and complex needs. Jennifer continues to contribute to the training and professional development of psychologists, teachers, and other professionals through her work within a number of universities and organizations.

Yoon-Suk Hwang is an adjunct research fellow at the University of Queensland, Australia, and a practitioner in mindfulness, behavioral support, special education needs, and inclusive education. Her research interests include the applications of mindfulness for empowering individuals with social, emotional, behavioral and learning difficulties, student voices and engagement, special needs and family support, bullying and autism spectrum, and arts-based inquiry. She has served a role as an associate editor for international journals.

Britney Jeyanayagam is a first-year student in the clinical psychology PhD program at St. John's University. Britney previously received her bachelor of science in life sciences at Queen's University in 2019. After graduating, she worked as a research assistant at the University of Toronto for two years prior to pursuing her master of arts in clinical psychology, concentrated in child and adolescent psychology, at Montclair State University, where she worked as a research assistant under the supervision of Dr. Erin Kang. Over the past several years, Britney has participated in multiple research projects, conference presentations, and publications largely focusing on correlates of cognitive flexibility and social anxiety, parent psychopathology and child risk, and protective factors against victimization in autistic and non-autistic youth. She has also worked closely with autistic individuals and individuals with developmental disabilities from under-resourced populations in hospital and community settings, providing assistance with daily living, academic support, and assisting with intervention delivery. Through her ongoing research and clinical work, she hopes to help improve the quality of life and long-term mental health outcomes of autistic youth through targeted, evidence-based intervention.

Beth Johnson is a senior research fellow at the School of Psychological Sciences and Department of Pediatrics at Monash University. Dr. Johnson has moved progressively from cellular and molecular understandings of brain function, from "bench to bedside" into their current research linking clinical, neurocognitive, genetic, and psychoeducational models of neurodevelopment and disability. Their primary focus is on improving the diagnosis and care of neurodivergent children and their families, centering on understanding and addressing the limitations of current diagnostic practices and access to care. Collaborating with clinicians, educators, and individuals with lived experiences, Dr. Johnson leads the Monash Autism ADHD Genetics and Neurodevelopment (MAGNET) Project, with an interest in enhancing diagnosis through the discovery of transdiagnostic markers and innovative data-informed perspectives on neurodevelopmental conditions. The goal is to create comprehensive phenotypic profiling for conditions such as autism, attention-deficit/hyperactivity disorder, and intellectual disabilities to develop novel interventions and prognosis tools.

Erin Kang is an assistant professor in the Psychology Department at Montclair State University, where she directs the Autism and Neurodevelopment Lab. Dr. Kang also cofounded and leads the Autism Interdisciplinary Group at Montclair State University. Dr. Kang received her PhD in clinical psychology from Stony Brook University in 2020 with an advanced graduate certificate in quantitative methods. Her research focuses on integrating science and practice by understanding factors that shape clinical presentations in autistic individuals and investigating neural mechanisms of clinical phenotypes and plasticity in this population, and applying these insights to refining evidence-based interventions for social functioning. She has published 25 peer-reviewed publications and book chapters and has more than 100 presentations at conferences and meetings. She also serves on the Editorial Board of the *Journal of Autism and Developmental Disorders*. She has received several awards and grants, including the Slifka/Ritvo Innovation in Autism Research Award from the International Society for Autism Research, Small Grants Program for Early Career Scholars from the Society for Research in Child Development, and Brain & Behavior Research Foundation (NARSAD) Young Investigator Grant, and other awards including the *Journal of Clinical Child and Adolescent Psychology* Future Directions Launch Award and from the Association for Behavioral and Cognitive Therapies Autism Spectrum and Developmental Disorders Special Interest Group, as well as several internal awards and grants from Montclair State University for her research.

Ellie Kazemi, PhD, is the Chief Science Officer at Behavioral Health Center of Excellence (BHCOE), an accrediting organization focused on improving the quality of behavior analytic services. She is also a professor at California State University, Northridge (CSUN), where she founded the M.S. in applied behavior analysis (ABA) program and has been teaching undergraduate and graduate coursework in research methodology, organizational behavior management, and behavior therapy for over 15 years. She has received several mentorship awards, including the ABAI Best Mentor Award, the Outstanding Faculty Award, the Outstanding Teaching Award, and the Outstanding Service Award. Her applied research interests involve the identification of efficient, effective strategies for practical training and supervision of staff, which includes leveraging computer technology and artificial intelligence (e.g., robotics, virtual or augmented reality). She has worked on several nationwide large projects (e.g., with FEMA and NASA) with a focus on effective training and measurement of intervention outcomes. Currently, she leads BHCOE's efforts in quality measure development and conducting reliable, valid evaluations for accreditation.

Sophia Kennedy is a PhD candidate at Te Herenga Waka Victoria University of Wellington, New Zealand, where she received her master's degree in educational psychology in 2021. She has worked in schools, residential settings, and family homes with children and adults with intellectual and developmental disabilities. Sophia's interests include support for challenging behaviors and improving quality of life for adults with intellectual or developmental disabilities, particularly those with high support needs. Her PhD research is centered on training residential support staff to improve the quality of life of the people they support as an antecedent intervention for challenging behaviors.

Lee Kern is a professor of special education and director of the Center for Promoting Research to Practice and Lehigh University Autism Services. She has extensive experience with children and youth with emotional and behavioral disorders, autism, and other disabilities. She has worked in the field of education/special education for over 35 years as a paraprofessional, general and special education teacher, behavior specialist, consultant, and researcher. Dr. Kern has received approximately $25 million in grant support from the Institute of Education Sciences, the National Institutes of Mental Health, and other agencies to conduct research in the area of intervention for child and adolescents with disabilities. Her research primarily focuses on reducing behavioral and mental health problems in children and adolescents using positive behavior support strategies. In addition, her recent research includes developing and evaluating college and career readiness interventions for high school students with and at-risk for emotional and behavioral problems. In 2018 Dr. Kern received the James Kaufman Research Award for excellence in research. She has written numerous articles, book chapters, and four books. Dr. Kern is past Editor of *Journal of Positive Behavior Interventions* and serves on the editorial boards of ten journals in the fields of education and disabilities.

Lynn Kern Koegel is a clinical professor at the Stanford University School of Medicine and the editor in chief of the *Journal of Autism and Developmental Disorders*. She has been active in the development of programs to improve communication in children with autism, including the development of first words, grammatical structures, pragmatics, and social conversation. In addition to her published books and articles in the area of communication and language development, she has developed and published procedures and field manuals in the area of first words, initiations, self-management, and functional analysis that are used in school districts and by parents throughout the United States, as well as translated in other major languages. Dr. Lynn Koegel is the author of *Overcoming Autism and Growing Up on the Spectrum*, published by Viking/Penguin, and most recently *Hidden Brilliance*, published by Harper Wave with parent Claire LaZebnik. Lynn Koegel and her husband, Robert, are the developers of pivotal response treatment, which focuses on motivation. The Koegels have been the recipients of many awards, including the first annual Children's Television Workshop Sesame Street Award for "Brightening the Lives of Children," the first annual Autism Speaks Award for "Science and Research," and the Association for Behavior Analysis International (ABAI) Award for Enduring Programmatic Contributions in Behavior Analysis. Dr. Lynn Koegel appeared on ABC's hit show *Supernanny* working with a child with autism. Their work has also been showcased on ABC, CBS, NBC, PBS, and the Discovery Channel.

Sadaf Khawar is a Board-Certified Behavior Analyst and New York State licensed behavior analyst who has extensive experience in conducting assessments and delivering evidence-based interventions to neurodiverse individuals in a variety of home, school, and mental health settings across the United States. Sadaf is committed to her goal of developing accessible, effective, and culturally sensitive interventions that would improve the quality of life of youth, caregivers, and families, particularly from disadvantaged backgrounds. Notably, Sadaf is a fifth-year doctoral candidate in the clinical psychology PhD program at Montclair State University, New Jersey, and has received clinical training at prestigious sites like the Autism Spectrum Disorder Service at the New York University's Child Study Center and Kennedy Krieger Institute at Johns Hopkins University School of Medicine, with a special focus on psychosocial interventions. Sadaf's exceptional clinical work, social justice initiatives, and commitment to include underrepresented communities in research has garnered her numerous grants and awards from organizations like International Society of Autism Research, Society of Clinical Child and Adolescent Psychology, and Association of Behavior Cognitive Therapies. Further, Sadaf has taught multiple introductory and advanced-level undergraduate psychology courses, engaged in various community service projects, and advocated mobilizing resources at the grassroots level to support families with differently abled youth.

Hunter King is a Board-Certified Behavior Analyst and earned his PhD in school psychology from the University of Utah. He currently works as a research fellow in the Neurobehavioral Unit-Inpatient at the Kennedy Krieger Institute. His research and clinical interests include evaluating antecedent and consequent variables associated with the reemergence of challenging behavior following successful treatment. Within this area, he is also interested in the promotion of treatment outcomes in community settings and how technology can be harnessed to increase access to behavioral supports.

Alan Kinsella is a Board-Certified Behavior Analyst and New York State Licensed Behavior Analyst. He has a BA in psychology from the University of Connecticut, an MS in applied behavior analysis (ABA) from Western New England University, and is currently enrolled in Endicott College's PhD program under the advisement of Dr. Mary Jane Weiss. Alan has worked in the field of autism treatment with a wide age range since 2012 across residential, in-home, and private day school settings. His roles have included direct care staff and classroom teacher, and he is currently employed as the voordinator of BCBA Supervision at The Manhattan Childrens Center in New York City. His research interests include the improvement and evaluation of BCBA supervision, performance management, procedural integrity, leadership, and collaboration. Alan also teaches as an adjunct faculty member for Endicott College's master's program in ABA. He resides in New Jersey.

Ioulia Koniou is a doctoral candidate in the applied human sciences program at the Université de Montréal. Her doctoral thesis is centered on the exploration of virtual reality's potential as a tool for decreasing stigma and fostering positive attitudes toward autism. She is actively engaged in a diverse array of research initiatives, collaborating closely with Saint-Justine Hospital in Montreal and InterActions. Through these collaborations, she is deeply involved in multiple projects that delve into the complexities of stigmatization and exclusion faced by individuals on the autism spectrum. Additionally, she is dedicated to enhancing social inclusion and streamlining access to essential general services for autistic individuals. She has also received training in both cognitive-behavioral therapy and applied behavior analysis. She has worked as clinical consultant in private schools both in France and Montreal, utilizing evidence-based cognitive and behavioral therapeutic strategies.

Elizabeth M. Kryszak is a psychologist at the Nationwide Children's Hospital Child Development Center (CDC) and a clinical associate professor at the Ohio State University. Dr. Kryszak's clinical and research work focuses on the evaluation and assessment of children with developmental disabilities, including autism, with a particular focus on creating system changes to increase access to quality assessment and treatment services for children with developmental disabilities and their families. More recently, Dr. Kryszak led her clinic's transition to assessment through telehealth during the COVID-19 pandemic in order to prevent loss of access to care, developing an observation protocol that allowed clinicians to partner with parents to assess for symptoms of autism in a home environment. She currently leads a national Project ECHO module that has created a learning community of professionals to foster continued use of telehealth assessment tools to increase access to families with barriers to in-clinic care. Through her work promoting access to evidence-based assessment and intervention for children with developmental disabilities, she developed a passion for battling misinformation about autism and exposing pseudoscience interventions. She has coauthored several book chapters focused on teaching professionals and families to understand the differences between evidence-based and unsupported treatments for neurodevelopmental disabilities to avoid the misuse of families' valuable time, energy, and money. She also serves on the executive committee of Division 25 of the American Psychological Association, focused on promoting the science and application of applied behavior analysis across the field of psychology.

Russell Lang, PhD, is a professor of special education and the director of the Clinic for Autism, Research, Evaluation, and Support (CARES) at Texas State University. Dr. Lang received his PhD from the University at Texas at Austin and then completed a postdoctoral researcher position at the University of California, Santa Barbara. He earned his doctoral-level board certification in applied behavior analysis (BCBA-D) in 2009 and has extensive experience in the provision of behavioral services to children and youth with developmental disabilities in schools and clinical settings. Dr. Lang's research has primarily focused on treating challenging behavior, supporting development of play and communication skills, and the systematic identification of evidence-based practices for education and treatment of children with developmental disabilities. He is a former editor-in-chief of *Developmental Neurorehabilitation* and a current editor of *Evidence-Based Communication Assessment and Intervention.* Dr. Lang has served as an associate editor of *Journal of Child and Family Sciences, Journal of Developmental and Physical Disabilities,* and is currently an associate editor of *Advances in Neurodevelopmental Disorders.* He has received the Association of Positive Behavioral Supports' annual Ted Carr Research Award and Texas State University's Presidential Award for Excellence in Scholarly Activity. Dr. Lang's previous books include *Autism: Teaching Makes a Difference, Early Intervention for Young Children With Autism, Play and Social Skills for Children With Autism,* and *Adaptive Behavior Strategies for Individuals With Intellectual and Developmental Disabilities: Evidence-Based Practices Across the Life Span.*

Marc J. Lanovaz is undergraduate program director and professor in the École de psychoéducation at the Université de Montréal and Researcher at the Centre de recherche de l'Institut universitaire en santé mentale de Montréal. He has also served on the steering committee of the National Network of Expertise in Autism for several years. His work has been funded by multiple major grant agencies, including the Canadian Institutes of Health Research, the Social Sciences and Humanities Research Council, the Québec Research Funds, and the Québec Office for People with Disabilities. His research program currently involves (a) developing and testing machine learning models to improve decision-making; (b) producing and assessing mobile and Web apps to support parents, professionals, and managers; (c) automatically detecting motor and vocal behavior using artificial intelligence; and (d) preventing the occurrence of challenging behavior by using smart sensors. His team has developed new Web, mobile, and virtual reality technologies that have benefited thousands of individuals across the world. Dr. Lanovaz has authored more than 80 articles and chapters on a variety of topics, including musical interventions for children with autism, functional behavior assessment and measurement, machine learning to support decision-making, and single-case methodology in research and practice.

Eric Larsson is the executive director of clinical services at the Lovaas Institute Midwest, where he implements the renowned program of intensive early intervention services with families of children with autism. He is a licensed psychologist and Board-Certified Behavior Analyst–Doctoral. He is conducting a systematic research evaluation of the effects of the high intensity EIBI program, with an emphasis on parent training, dynamic program management, language matrix programming, natural language development, schedules of reinforcement, and generalization of complex social behavior. Dr. Larsson is the current president of the Association for Science in Autism Treatment and serves on the board of directors of the Council of Autism Service Providers and the Fundación Lovaas in Barcelona. He is the chair of the Standards Committee of the Autism Commission on Quality. He has served on the Behavior Analyst Certification Board and has served as associate research director of the NIMH Multi-site Replication Study of the UCLA Young Autism Project. He is on the Clinical Faculty in the Psychology Department at the University of Minnesota. Dr. Larsson actively supports advocacy efforts to increase access to ABA services for autism and consults internationally on clinical programming and evaluation. His Language Matrix Curriculum has been translated into five languages. In 2013 he received the Provider of the Year Award from Autism Speaks in Washington, DC, and the Leadership Award from the California Association for Behavior Analysis (CalABA), in Anaheim, California.

Jennifer Croner Lauriello is the clinical director of Autism Services at Lehigh University. She has over 10 years of experience working with children and adults with special needs. Mrs. Lauriello received her bachelor's degree in neuroscience from Colgate University and her master's degree in applied behavior analysis from Temple University. She is currently a doctoral student in special education at Lehigh University. Mrs. Lauriello has been a Board-Certified Behavior Analyst since 2015 and has worked as a direct care staff, behavior analyst, and administrator in home, school, and community settings. Her research focuses on effective supervision practices and evidence-based teaching strategies.

Matthew D. Lerner is an associate professor and Leader of the Life Course Outcomes Research Program at the AJ Drexel Autism Institute, Drexel University, where he directs the Social Competence and Treatment Lab. He is also a research associate professor of psychology, psychiatry, and pediatrics at Stony Brook University. He has presented at over 150 conferences on topics related to social development and developmental disorders. Dr. Lerner's research focuses on understanding emergence and "real-world" implications of social problems in youth adolescents especially related to autism, as well as development, evaluation, and dissemination of novel, evidence-based approaches for ameliorating those problems. He has published 120+ peer-reviewed articles and book chapters; he serves as associate editor of the *Journal of Autism and Developmental Disorders* and on the editorial boards of seven other academic outlets. Dr. Lerner has received grants from organizations, including the National Institutes of Health (NIH), the Health Resources & Services Administration (HRSA), the Brain and Behavior Research Foundation (BBRF), the Simons Foundation, the American Psychological Association (APA), the Society of Clinical Child and Adolescent Psychology, and the American Academy of Arts and Sciences. He has received numerous acknowledgments and awards, including from the National Institute of Mental Health (NIMH), the Society for Research in Child Development (SRCD), the APA Divisions 12, 33, and 53, the Society for a Science of Clinical Psychology, the BBRF (NARSAD), the International Society for Autism Research, the Autism & Developmental Disabilities SIG of the Association for Behavioral and Cognitive Therapies, and the Association for Psychological Science.

Udi Yehuda Levii is a medical student at the University of Pavia, Italy.

Bharati Limbuis is a research assistant at Imperial College London, UK, and was involved in developing the first free online international psychoeducation program for carers to help reduce the overmedication of people with intellectual disabilities (SPECTROM). She has published several papers, including systematic reviews and meta-analyses, in the field of intellectual disabilities and autism.

James K. Luiselli, EdD, ABPP, BCBA-D, is a licensed psychologist and current director of Clinical Development and Research at Melmark New England and adjunct faculty within the School Psychology Program at William James College. Dr. Luiselli has published 22 books, 60 book chapters, and more than 300 journal articles in the areas of neurodevelopmental disabilities, applied behavior analysis, organizational behavior management, performance improvement, and professional training. He is an associate editor for the *Journal of Child and Family Studies*, and he is on the board of editors of *Journal of Developmental and Physical Disabilities*, *Advances in Neurodevelopmental Disorders*, *Mindfulness*, *Child and Family Behavior Therapy*, and *Clinical Case Studies.*

Davide Marisca is a psychiatric trainee at the University of Pavia, Italy.

Meredith Matthews is currently a doctoral student and the research coordinator at the Cognition Behavior and Mindfulness Clinic at the University of Illinois Chicago. Meredith received her master's degree from Missouri State University's applied behavior analysis program and has worked with children, adolescents, and young adults with disabilities for the past 5 years. Her research interests include acceptance and commitment therapy, evidence-based practices for autistic individuals, and broader social issues such as climate change.

Melissa Maye is an assistant scientist at the Center for Health Policy and Health Services within Henry Ford Health and dually appointed as an assistant professor of research of pediatrics within the College of Human Medicine at Michigan State University as part of the HFH and MSU University Health Sciences. She received her doctorate in clinical psychology from the University of Massachusetts, Boston. She completed her predoctoral internship at the Children's Hospital of Philadelphia and her postdoctoral fellowship at the University of Pennsylvania. Dr. Maye received her bachelor's degree in psychology from the University of Michigan. Dr. Maye's program of research aims to increase access and equity of evidence-based interventions by leveraging implementation science methods to incorporate neurodevelopmental interventions into community spaces where infants and young children already spend a substantial period of time (e.g., childcare classrooms, preschools, neonatal intensive care units). Dr. Maye is also a licensed clinical psychologist with specific expertise in diagnosis of autism spectrum disorder, including differential diagnosis of other neurodevelopmental disorders.

Eric McCoy is a research associate at Easterseals Southern California's Research Division. He is passionate about using research to improve the lives of individuals with disabilities and their families. His research interests include the use of technology to support intervention, the development of evidence-based practices, and the evaluation of intervention effectiveness. Eric is currently working on a project that uses a robot named Hans to teach social skills to children with autism spectrum disorder. He is also involved in a study that is evaluating the effectiveness of a new intervention for children with attention-deficit/hyperactivity disorder. Eric is committed to diversity, equity, and inclusion in research. He believes that all individuals should have equal access to high-quality interventions, regardless of their background or circumstances. He is working to ensure that his research is inclusive and representative of the populations it serves.

Rachel McDonald is a fourth-year doctoral candidate in the clinical psychology PhD program at Montclair State University. Her research focuses on underlying mechanisms of co-occurring mental health disorders in autism, specifically transdiagnostic factors such as emotion dysregulation. She plans to utilize these findings to develop specialized interventions targeting transdiagnostic constructs to improve the mental health and quality of life of autistic individuals. Clinically, Rachel has several years of experience working with autistic people across a variety of outpatient and medical settings.

Laurie McLay is a senior research fellow and associate director of the Child Well-Being Research Institute at the University of Canterbury, New Zealand. She has worked with autistic children and their families for over 20 years. Most recently, her research has focused on evaluating the effectiveness and acceptability of digitally delivered supports for autistic children and their caregivers. This includes a particular focus on sleep and other health-promoting behaviors. Dr. McLay has been awarded over 5.2 million NZ dollars in grant funding (1.48 million as principal investigator) to support her research, including Health Research Council NZ, Marsden Royal Society, and Cure Kids grants. Dr McLay has published over 50 journal articles and most recently coedited a book focused on behavioral sleep interventions for autistic children. She is passionate about continuing to conduct research that can enhance the well-being of autistic children and their families.

Aoife McTiernan is a lecturer in psychology at the University of Galway, Ireland. She is a chartered behavioral psychologist with the Psychological Society of Ireland (PSI) and Board-Certified Behavior Analyst–Doctoral. She has worked with educational settings and disability services for over 15 years in both early intervention and positive behavior supports for children and adolescents with autism and intellectual disabilities. She is the current president of the European Association for Behavior Analysis and director of the MSc and PhD in Applied Behavior Analysis at the University of Galway, Ireland.

Britany Melton is the director of research and training at Journeys Autism Center, located in Mishawaka, Indiana. She received her master's degree from Endicott College in special education and applied behavior analysis. She is currently pursuing her PhD in applied behavior analysis at the Institute for Behavioral Science at Endicott College under the advisement of Dr. Mary Jane Weiss. Britany has experience across special education settings, residential placements, and clinic settings. Her research interests include analyzing and teaching compassionate care skills to interventionists and registered behavior technicians (RBTs), effective interventions for the reduction of severe behaviors, and ensuring quality applied behavior analysis practices.

Raymond G. Miltenberger, PhD, BCBA-D, is a professor of child and family studies and the director of the Applied Behavior Analysis program at the University of South Florida. He is a fellow and past president of the Association for Behavior Analysis International (ABAI) and a fellow of the American Association for Advancement of Science. His current research focuses on behavioral approaches for teaching safety skills, increasing physical activity for health promotion, and enhancing sports performance. He has published over 270 journal articles and chapters and has written a behavior modification textbook, now in its seventh edition and published in six languages. Dr. Miltenberger has received numerous teaching, research, and mentoring awards, including the APA Division 25 Award for Distinguished Contributions to Applied Behavioral Research, the ABAI Outstanding Mentorship Award, and the FABA Award for Outstanding Contributions to Behavior Analysis.

David Ray Miranda is a doctoral student at Purdue University majoring in special education. He currently holds a Board-Certified Behavior Analyst credential. David has experience designing and implementing behavioral interventions in residential, clinical, and school settings. David's primary research interests explore (a) the effectiveness of behavioral interventions within natural contexts and (b) how service providers can identify and integrate children's preferences and choices within the services they provide.

Fereshteh Mohammadzaheri is a licensed speech language specialist who earned her PhD from Tehran University of Medical Science. She was ranked first in her undergraduate class at Jundishapur University of Medical Sciences and received the university's Presidential Award for outstanding academic performance as an undergraduate student. She was awarded high honors for her bachelor of science thesis that focused on the treatment of stuttering and high honors for her master of science thesis that focused on the treatment of autism. She was awarded the Excellence in Teaching Award by the president of Hamadan University of Medical Science based on her teaching in the Speech Therapy Department and has been approved as an elite person by Iran's National Elite Foundation. Dr. Mohammadzaheri has numerous publications in the area of autism and has conducted several randomized clinical trials in the Iranian public schools researching the effects of pivotal response treatment on communication and brain changes using electroencephalograms. She has translated and validated tests and questionnaires and published these findings, so that they are available to Farsi-speaking individuals. In addition to her publications, she has translated pivotal response treatment field manuals for use research and to support Iranian children and their families. Dr. Mohammadzaheri lectures throughout Iran on language development, communication, play, and academic challenges in children on the autism spectrum. She has been a faculty member in the speech therapy departments of Iranian universities for several years and organizes an annual autism evaluation and treatment webinar for training Farsi-speaking speech therapists.

Edgar Moussaoui is a child psychiatrist at the Department of Child and Adolescent Psychiatry of the Caen University Hospital Center in France. He earned a doctor of medicine degree in 2000, with a specialization in psychiatry. His professional focus centers on individuals with autism spectrum disorder. He leads a clinical team for diagnosing severe neurodevelopmental disorders in infants aged 0 to 3 years. Additionally, he is the medical coordinator of the local Autism Resource Center. He participates in various research initiatives within the realm of neuropsychology and clinical epidemiology. His approach draws from diverse theoretical frameworks, including neuroscience and systemic human sciences, reflecting a commitment to an open-minded and integrative perspective.

Reem Muharib is an assistant professor of Special Education in the Department of Curriculum and Instruction at Texas State University. She is a Board-Certified Behavior Analyst-Doctoral (BCBA-D). She earned her doctoral degree in Special Education from the University of North Carolina- Charlotte. She has taught classes in undergraduate and graduate special education programs in topics related to classroom management, autism and severe disabilities, applied behavior analysis, and single-case research designs. Muharib has published over 25 peer-reviewed research articles and her research interests include applied behavior analysis, single-case research designs, autism, and functional skills for individuals with Autism and other developmental disabilities.

James A. Mulick is professor emeritus in pediatrics at The Ohio State University. He studied psychology as an undergraduate at Rutgers College (AB, 1970) in New Brunswick, NJ, and general psychology specializing in developmental psychobiology and learning at the University of Vermont (PhD, 1975). He completed a postdoctoral fellowship in clinical child psychology at the University of North Carolina (1977). His professional career has been spent in teaching, research, and clinical service in developmental disabilities.

Matthew J. O'Brien is a licensed psychologist and clinical associate professor of pediatrics in the Carver College of Medicine at The University of Iowa. He directs outpatient and day treatment clinics which focus on the assessment and treatment of challenging behavior displayed by individuals with disabilities. His research focuses on assessment and treatment of severe challenging behavior.

Katherine Pickard is a licensed psychologist and assistant professor in the Department of Pediatrics at the Emory University School of Medicine. She received her doctorate in clinical psychology from Michigan State University and completed a two-year postdoctoral fellowship at JFK Partners at the University of Colorado School of Medicine. Her primary research interest is in the translation of evidence-based practices into community systems that are naturally positioned to serve autistic children and their families. This interest is rooted in a long-standing commitment to supporting more equitable access to autism services. Dr. Pickard's research is grounded in community engagement and is guided by dissemination and implementation science. At the Marcus Autism Center, Dr. Pickard leads and collaborates on research examining mechanisms that foster the adoption, implementation, and sustainment of evidence-based practices within a variety of community systems, including early intervention and public school systems. She is particularly interested in the role of families and community partners in shaping interventions as they are implemented within the community, and in system-level factors that impact the reach and sustainability of translation efforts. Clinically, Dr. Pickard is a licensed psychologist and has a strong background in supporting individuals with ASD across the lifespan. She holds specific expertise in naturalistic, developmental, and behavioral principles (known as NDBIs) and is a certified trainer in Project ImPACT, an evidence-based practice for young autistic children and their families. In addition to working with young children and their families, Dr. Pickard has expertise in cognitive-behavioral therapy (CBT) for autistic youth and co-occurring anxiety.

Katrina Phillips is a registered psychologist and Board-Certified Behavior Analyst (BCBA). For over 15 years, she has worked both as a clinician with people with disability (people with intellectual disabilities, brain injury and dementia, and autistic individuals) and in academia teaching and supervising students to become psychologists and certified behavior analysts. She received her clinical qualification through the University of Auckland in 2007. After working as a clinician, she returned to complete her PhD, which investigated methods for assessing data quality and started her lecture position in 2017. She is currently the director of the Behavioral Psychology Program in the School of Psychology and is actively involved in supporting the vocational training cafes for people with disability through the creation of *Nga Mātauranga ou Mahi*, a manual created alongside people with disability to support their inclusion in the work environment.

Pierluigi Politi is full professor of psychiatry and head of the School of Specialization in Psychiatry, University of Pavia, Italy. He is also the head of the Department of Mental Health and Addictions, ASST Pavia, Italy.

Suzanne C. Purdy (Te Rarawa, NgāiTūhoe) is a professor in the School of Psychology at the University of Auckland. Previously she was head of school (2018–2023) and head of discipline of speech science (2003–2018) in the School of Psychology. She has broad interests in hearing, communication, and neuroscience, including communication difficulties in children and adults, auditory processing, and auditory electrophysiology. She is a principal investigator with the Centre for Brain Research (CBR) at the University of Auckland. Current research projects include investigations of therapies for people with neurological conditions, sensory processing in people with mild cognitive impairment, and auditory processing in adults and children. She has an interest in the evaluation and delivery of ethical evidence-based interventions for children and adults. Her international reputation in the field of hearing science has been recognized through her election as a fellow of the Acoustical Society of America and the New Zealand Psychological Society.

Eve-Marie Quintin is an associate professor and graduate program director in the Department of Educational and Counseling Psychology at McGill University. She leads the McGill Behaviour, Autism, and NeuroDevelopment (BAND) Research Group and primarily teaches and supervises graduate students enrolled in the school/applied child psychology program. Her research aims to investigate the musical profile of neurodiverse youth and to quantify the effects of music programs on their cognitive, social, and brain functioning; with music programs taking place in noninclusive or socially inclusive settings where youth with and without neurodiverse needs complete a music program together. Her work adopts a strength-based approach to support the well-being of neurodiverse persons. Her research has been supported by grant agencies, including the Social Sciences and Humanities Research Council of Canada, the Quebec Research Funds for Health and for Society and Culture, and the Quebec Office for People with Disabilities, and McGill University's William Dawson Scholar Program. Dr. Quintin has authored multiple scientific publications and presented her research in knowledge translation activities covering topics including the musical and language profiles of children and adolescents on the autism spectrum across all levels of support needs; the cognitive, behavioral, and brain functioning of children, adolescents, and young adults with fragile X syndrome; and the cognitive, personality, and neural correlates of creativity within the general population.

John T. Rapp received his doctoral degree in behavior analysis from the University of Florida in 2003. He currently serves as the director of the Applied Behavior Analysis program and a full professor in the Cognitive and Behavior Sciences program in the Department of Psychological Sciences at Auburn University. He is a doctoral-level Board-Certified Behavior Analyst and a licensed behavior analyst in Alabama, and a full professor. He is also the primary investigator and project director for the Alabama Psychiatric Medication Review Team (APMRT) with the Alabama Department of Human Resources and the primary investigator for Accountability Based Sex Offense Prevention Program (ABSOPP) with the Department of Youth Services in Alabama. To date, he has coauthored over 140 peer-reviewed articles. His current research interests include (a) translational study of conjugate schedules, as well as the development of conjugate preparations; (b) assessment of self-control behavior in justice-involved juveniles; and (c) assessment of social perceptions of individuals' eye contact and body movements during social interactions.

Elizabeth Reyes, PhD, is a clinical assistant professor of special education in the Department of Educational and Developmental Science at The University of South Carolina. She has taught classes in undergraduate and graduate special education programs in topics related to classroom management, literacy, and single-case research designs. Reyes was previously involved in grant work for the TIES Center, a national technical assistance center focused on Increasing Time, Instructional Effectiveness, Engagement, and State Support for Inclusive Practices for Students with Significant Cognitive Disabilities (TIES). She earned her PhD in special education from UNC Charlotte. In her time as an educator, Reyes taught students with various high-incidence and low-incidence disabilities in Title I schools in both rural and urban areas in self-contained, resource, and inclusive settings. In her time as an administrator, she was the director of a kindergarten through 12th grade inclusion program for students with a range of disabilities in two different private schools. Her current research interests include training a variety of interventionists in effective implementation of evidence-based practices in inclusive settings for students with disabilities. Reyes is also a wife and mother of three young children.

Mandy J. Rispoli is the Quantitative Foundation Bicentennial Professor of Special Education at the University of Virginia and a Board-Certified Behavior Analyst–Doctoral Level. Operating from a behavior analytic framework, Dr. Rispoli's scholarship is built upon sustained university–community partnerships to improve teacher and caregiver meaningful involvement in functional behavior assessment and intervention and to promote positive outcomes for young children with autism and developmental disabilities. Dr. Rispoli's research explores (a) improving the efficiency, effectiveness, and feasibility of functional behavior assessments and function-based interventions in educational settings, and (b) innovations in professional development for teachers of young children with autism and challenging behavior. Dr. Rispoli has published over 130 peer-reviewed research articles and book chapters concerning behavioral interventions for children with autism and developmental disabilities.

Henry Roane received his PhD in psychology with an emphasis in applied behavior analysis from Louisiana State University. He completed a predoctoral internship at the Kennedy Krieger Institute and the Johns Hopkins University School of Medicine. He has held previous clinical and faculty positions at the Marcus Institute/Emory University School of Medicine and the Munroe-Meyer Institute/University of Nebraska Medical Center. Dr. Roane is the editor-in-chief of *Behavioral Development*, an academic journal published by the American Psychological Association. He is a current associate editor for the *Journal of Developmental and Physical Disabilities*, a former associate editor for the *Journal of Applied Behavior Analysis* and *Behavior Analysis in Practice*, and on the editorial boards of several journals in the field of behavior analysis and pediatrics, including the *Journal of Pediatrics.* He serves on the board of directors for the Society for the Experimental Analysis of Behavior, and he has previously served on the board of directors for the Behavior Analysis Certification Board and the Association of Professional Behavior Analysts. He has been the principal investigator on grants funded by National Institute of Health and the New York State Department of Health, and he serves as a consultant to programs across the United States. He is a fellow of the Association for Behavior Analysis–International and was elected to membership in the Society for Pediatric Research. He is also the 2022 recipient of the Nate Azrin Distinguished Contributions to Applied Behavior Analysis Award given by Division 25 of the American Psychological Association.

Matthew Roberts is in his third year of the University of Utah School psychology program. He is currently working toward his PhD and BCBA certification, with which he hopes to continue supporting children and adolescents on the autism spectrum across a variety of settings. Matthew earned his bachelor's degree in psychology from Gonzaga University in 2019, followed by a master's degree in school psychology from Sam Houston State University in 2021. While he is currently engaged in several research projects, including a systematic PBIS evaluation for his dissertation, he has always toed the line between research and practice, hoping to dedicate his early career to addressing the research-to-practice gap. His current research interests include behavior interventions, technological supports for individuals on the autism spectrum, and strategies for closing the research-to-practice gap. His interest in harnessing technology to support individuals on the autism spectrum was sparked by the COVID-19 pandemic when virtual technology took the field by storm. He feels that if we are to fully embrace technology in our interventions and supports, it is critical to fully understand the contingencies involved when delivering services.

Victor Rodríguez García is a licensed psychologist and a speech and language therapist trained at the Universitat Ramon Llull in Barcelona. He has dedicated his professional career to the delivery of autism services with a focus on early intensive behavioral intervention. He is a behavior analyst trained at LIFE, The Lovaas Institute for Early Intervention Midwest (Minneapolis, Minnesota) under the direct mentorship of its executive director, Dr. Eric V. Larsson. He is clinical director at Lovaas Foundation (Barcelona), and UCLA Young Autism Project Official Replication Site Barcelona. He is also the academic director of the teaching branch of Lovaas Foundation, Young Autism Program. He is an international speaker and consultant working for numerous autism services programs in Europe and Latin America. Víctor is a long-term advocate and a constant presence in the Spanish-speaking media about evidence-based services for autism.

Meera Roy has been a consultant in intellectual disability psychiatry since 1989 and has worked in several NHS trusts in the Midlands in the United Kingdom. She is now an honorary consultant at Worcestershire Health and Care NHS Trust, Worcester, UK. She has published several papers in the field of autism and intellectual disabilities.

Aoife Ryan is a Board-Certified Behavior Analyst® living and working in Galway, Ireland. She has worked with adults and children with autism and intellectual & developmental disabilities across educational and social care settings for seven years. Aoife graduated from the University of Galway with a MSc in applied behavior analysis. She is currently completing a PhD at the University of Galway. Her research examines the provision of behavior analysis services to adults with additional needs via telehealth, and the barriers and facilitators to accessing telehealth-based behavioral supports.

Angela Arnold-Saritepe is a Board-Certified Behavior Analyst (BCBA-D) and New Zealand registered psychologist with over 30 years of experience working with people with neurodiversity, such as autism, intellectual disability, brain injury, and mental unwellness. She has worked across the United States, Canada, and New Zealand supporting individuals, their families, and professionals where behavior has interfered with quality of life. She has experience in severe behavior units, founding autism services, and in providing and establishing community services. She has been a faculty member in the Behavior and Learning Programme, Department of Psychology, University of Auckland, New Zealand, since 2004, where she supervises students completing graduate studies in applied behavior analysis. Her current research interests lie in supporting neurodiverse people to have the information and knowledge they require to pursue relationships, in addition to social validity and ethics in applied behavior analysis.

Kelly M. Schieltz is a licensed psychologist and an assistant professor of pediatrics in the Carver College of Medicine at The University of Iowa. She directs a brief outpatient clinic which focuses on the assessment and treatment of challenging behavior displayed by children with and without developmental differences. Her research focuses on the assessment and treatment of severe challenging behavior displayed by children with developmental disabilities with emphasis on parent training both in vivo and via telehealth, as well as long-term maintenance of treatment effects.

Sophie C. Schneider received her PhD in psychology from Macquarie University in 2016. She began her postdoctoral training at the University of South Florida, before moving to Baylor College of Medicine to complete her training and begin a faculty position. Her research has focused on the early detection and treatment of mental health disorders in young people, particularly anxiety disorders, obsessive-compulsive disorder, and body dysmorphic disorder. Early intervention is crucial as it is a powerful method by which to reduce the negative impacts of mental health disorders over the lifespan. Dr. Schneider has a particular interest in developing and evaluating different models of delivering evidence-based treatment to young people, such as through teletherapy and Internet-delivered treatment adaptations of cognitive-behavioral therapy. Her research has included multiple funded research studies and publications examining mental health among youth with autism spectrum disorder (ASD). Her interest in mental health in youth with ASD led to multiple funded research studies evaluating how best to provide treatment for anxious youth with ASD, and the development of treatment resources specifically designed for youth with ASD. The aim of such research is to ensure that treatment materials are engaging and useful and meet the specific needs of those with ASD.

Elise Settanni is a doctoral candidate at Lehigh University and a Board-Certified Behavior Analyst for Lehigh University Autism Services. Ms. Settanni has over 15 years of experience spanning clinic, school, home, and community-based services and supports for individuals with developmental and intellectual disabilities. She has provided these supports in the role of behavior specialist, special education teacher, and behavior analyst. As a researcher, she is interested in studying how class-wide interventions can reduce autism stigma. As a behavior analyst, she is dedicated to centering her clients' needs by being their chief advocate at home, at school, and out in the world. Ms. Settanni is a member of the Community Against Prejudice Towards Autistic People (CAPTAP), an advocacy group comprised of researchers, autistic individuals, autistic researchers, and practitioners. She is a member of the Association for Positive Behavior Support, the Council for Exceptional Children, and the International Association of Special Education. She has coauthored papers published in the *Journal of Autism and Developmental Disorders, School Mental Health, Review Journal of Autism and Developmental Disorders*, and *Topics in Early Childhood Special Education.* Ms. Settanni received her bachelor of arts in psychology and master of education in special education from the Pennsylvania State University.

Rebecca Sharp is a Board-Certified Behavior Analyst (BCBA-D) and New Zealand registered psychologist who received her training from the University of Auckland. She spent 7 years as a senior lecturer and the director of the Applied Behavior Analysis program at Bangor University in Wales. Rebecca is currently a senior lecturer at the University of Auckland. She is an experienced and innovative teacher for both undergraduate and postgraduate students, with a passion for behavioral pedagogy. Rebecca has served on editorial boards for journals such as the *European Journal of Behavior Analysis.* She served on the UK Society for Behavior Analysis Board of Directors and is a senior fellow of the Higher Education Authority. Rebecca has been an invited speaker in research and clinical settings around the world, and her research interests include expanding the application of behavioral science, stimulus control, behavior-analytic approaches to working with people with dementia and traumatic brain injury, the translation of clinical and laboratory research to applied settings, applied animal behavior, and teaching behavior analysis. Rebecca has been a consultant for the Welsh Government's Behavioral Science unit, and as a clinician, she has worked with recidivist youth offenders, with adults and children with brain injury, adults with dementia, and adults and children with intellectual disabilities.

Daniel J. Sheridan worked with autistic individuals, their families, and many professionals and paraprofessionals across multiple continents, providing behavior-analytic services for nearly a decade. Currently, Dan is a doctoral student and a graduate research assistant in the Department of Psychological Sciences, Auburn University. Dan provides behavior-analytic services and training to justice-involved youth and direct-care staff at a juvenile residential treatment facility while also engaging in and promoting evidence-based assessment and treatment for underserved populations.

Nirbhay N. Singh is clinical professor of psychiatry and health behavior at the Medical College of Georgia, Augusta University, Georgia. His research interests include mindfulness, behavioral treatment of individuals with disabilities, and assistive technology for supporting individuals with severe/profound and multiple disabilities. He has been the founding editor of four international journals and is currently the editor of three Springer book series: *Mindfulness in Behavioral Health, Evidence-Based Practice in Behavioral Health*, and *Children and Families.* He has 790 publications, including 31 books. His most recent books include *Mindfulness in the Classroom: An Evidence-Based Program to Reduce Disruptive Behavior and Increase Academic Engagement* (with Felver) and *Mindfulness-Based Interventions With Children and Adolescents: Research and Practice* (with Singh Joy). He is the editor of *Encyclopedia of Mindfulness, Buddhism, and Other Contemplative Practices.*

Sudha M. Srinivasan is an assistant professor in the physical therapy program within the Department of Kinesiology at the University of Connecticut. She is a physical therapist by training with a specialization in neuroscience and pediatrics. Following her undergraduate and master's-level training in the field of physical therapy in India, she pursued her PhD at the University of Connecticut with a specialization in autism spectrum disorder. She pursued two postdoctoral fellowships, first at the University of Delaware and next, a UNICEF-funded postdoc at the Indian Institute of Technology Bombay. Her doctoral and postdoctoral research has focused on the assessment of the movement system in school-age children with autism, development of embodied, whole-body movement-based interventions for children with autism, early detection of signs of risk of autism, assessment of needs of young adults with autism, and development of novel assistive technologies and communication aids for nonverbal children with autism. She joined the faculty at the University of Connecticut in 2019 and is involved in delivering the pediatric curriculum along with other foundational courses within the physical therapy program. Her current research focuses on developing innovative, playful, creative, and intrinsically motivating movement-based interventions and assistive technologies for young children with disabilities, including children with autism and cerebral palsy. She has worked as part of interdisciplinary teams on projects funded through federal grants, including NIH, Autism Speaks, UNICEF, and the American Academy of Cerebral Palsy & Developmental Medicine.

Lily Stadlober is a New Zealand registered psychologist and Board-Certified Behavior Analyst (BCBA). She graduated from the University of Auckland's Behavior and Learning Program in early 2015. Lily has supported children, youth, and adults across various settings, including early intervention centers, supported living, dementia care, and family homes. She has experience working in both New Zealand and the United Kingdom, where she has overseen service delivery and provided clinical supervision to practitioners. Lily provided home-based early intervention services to neurodiverse children in New Zealand, before moving overseas in 2018. In the United Kingdom, she worked in the National Health System (NHS), providing and overseeing Positive Behavior Support services for adults with intellectual disabilities. Currently, Lily is the clinical manager at Acorn Charitable Trust. Acorn is an interdisciplinary center that provides ABA services, speech and language therapy, and occupational therapy for neurodiverse children and youth in Aotearoa, New Zealand. Lily is passionate about empowering individuals to lead meaningful lives, through the application of behavior science.

Haley M. K. Steinhauser is director of clinical services at Melmark New England. She obtained her PhD in behavior analysis at Western New England University. Her research has been primarily focused on individuals with autism spectrum disorder, working to promote learning and decrease interfering repetitive behavior (i.e., stereotypy). She is an adjunct lecturer at Regis College, developing an online course in verbal behavior and teaching it during summer term. She is also interested in user research and behavior change design focused on health-related behavior.

Jennifer Stephenson has been involved in special education for over 30 years as a special educator, teacher educator, and researcher. She is an honorary associate professor at Macquarie University and a director of the Institute of Special Educators (InSpEd) in Australia. Her research interests include augmentative and alternative communication for students with high support needs, the education of students with autism spectrum disorder, teacher education, the preparation of special educators, the use of evidence-based practices, and the use of controversial practices in special education. She has over 120 refereed publications, as well as book chapters, conference papers, and articles that translate research to practice for practitioners. She has served as a journal editor and as a grant application reviewer. She has been involved in advocacy for quality special education services through the Australian Association of Special Education and InSpEd and has written submissions for or contributed to many government enquiries and reviews relevant to special education and teacher education. She has been a member of advisory groups related to special education, teacher education, and the Australian curriculum. She has partnered with schools in research projects and in providing consultancy and professional learning to teachers.

Eric A. Storch is professor and McIngvale Presidential Endowed Chair in the Department of Psychiatry and Behavioral Sciences at Baylor College of Medicine (BCM). He serves as vice chair and head of psychology and co-directs the Obsessive-Compulsive and Related Disorders program at BCM. Dr. Storch specializes in the nature and treatment of childhood and adult obsessive-compulsive disorder, anxiety disorders, misophonia, posttraumatic stress disorder, and anxiety among youth with autism. In addition to over 850 published articles and chapters and 22 books, he has received multiple federal grants to investigate treatment efficacy, mechanisms of action, genetics, bioethics, innovative approaches to phenotyping, and how to enhance outcomes for those struggling with obsessive-compulsive disorder and related conditions.

Phillip S. Strain is professor of educational psychology and psychiatry at the University of Colorado Denver and director of the Positive Early Learning Experiences Center. He is the author of more than 300 professional papers in the early intervention field, has served on the editorial boards of more than 20 professional journals, has been the principal investigator of grants totaling more than $50 million, and has been recognized with distinguished career awards on three separate occasions. He authored the original grant that funded the development of the LEAP model in 1980 and recently received funding to conduct a long-term follow-up on participants in the randomized trial.

Diondra Straiton is a PhD candidate in the clinical science program in the Psychology Department at Michigan State University. She holds a master's degree in clinical psychology from Michigan State University and a bachelor's degree from Swarthmore College in psychology and educational studies. She is currently completing her clinical psychology predoctoral internship in the Department of Psychiatry at the University of Pennsylvania. Diondra is a certified elementary school teacher and a master trainer for an evidence-based parent-mediated naturalistic developmental behavioral intervention (NDBI) called Project ImPACT. Diondra is passionate about leveraging implementation science to improve autism services for marginalized autistic youth. Her research and clinical work focus on improving health equity for traditionally underserved autistic youth by optimizing training efforts for clinicians working in under-resourced settings. Most of this work focuses on parent coaching interventions and NDBIs. Her recent projects have investigated which training activities in group consultation sessions are most effective at supporting clinicians to implement Project ImPACT via telehealth with low-income families in the Medicaid system. Diondra has clinical expertise in working with neurodivergent and typically developing youth, including parent-mediated NDBIs, cognitive-behavioral therapy, exposure therapy, and evidence-based practices in classroom settings. She has partnered with clinicians in various community settings, including the Medicaid system, the community mental health system, the early intervention system, public elementary schools, and applied behavior analysis clinics.

Peter Sturmey is professor of psychology at the Graduate Center and Queens College, City University of New York. He has published over 30 authored and edited books, is the series editor for Springer's *Advances an Prevention in Violence and Aggression* series, has published over 200 journal articles and 80 chapters, and has given over 300 presentations at national and international conferences. He consults widely with services for children and adults with autism and intellectual disabilities. He is interested in applied behavior analysis, caregiver training, evidence-based practices, and aggression and violence.

Alyssa N. Suess is a licensed psychologist and co-owner of Milestone Health Partners in North Dakota. Her clinical focus includes therapy and psychological testing services for children with emphasis in the areas of autism spectrum disorder, emotion and behavior regulation concerns, anxiety, and attention-deficit/hyperactivity disorder.

Thomas G. Szabo is a peer-reviewed ACT trainer, Board-Certified Behavior Analyst, a behavior analysis professor, and founder of *ACT Now ABA*. Tom received his master's and doctorate degrees at the University of Nevada, Reno, where he studied under W. Larry Williams and Steven C. Hayes. Over the last 15 years, Tom has focused his practice on teaching people ways to ignite psychological flexibility in their personal lives and with others in clinical practice, schools, board rooms, shop floors, and community centers. He has developed iterations of ACTr for autistic people, their parents and caregivers, siblings, and staff members. His research focuses on the development of ACTr functional analysis and treatment that addresses issues related to race, gender, class, ethnicity, neurodiversity, disability, language, and dialect. With the Commit and Act Foundation, Tom has trained therapists in Sierra Leone working with individuals who have committed acts of gender-based violence, and he is currently conducting funded research on ways to reduce intrafamilial violence. He has published empirical and conceptual papers, as well as several book chapters and a new book, *ACT and Applied Behavior Analysis: A Practical Guide to Ensuring Better Outcomes Using Acceptance and Commitment Training*, published by New Harbinger Press.

Aida Tarifa-Rodríguez is a Board-Certified Behavior Analyst and a qualified behavior analyst with over 15 years of experience in the field of applied behavior analysis, working with children, adolescents, and adults with disabilities, autism spectrum disorder (ASD), and brain injuries. Over the past 6 years, she has held the position of student care director at ABA España. She is a member of the Qualified Applied Behavior Analysis Committee and currently serves as the research coordinator at the Mohammed bin Rashid Center for Special Education operated by the New England Center for Children (MRC-NECC). In addition, she collaborates on research projects with the University Hospital La Paz (Madrid) and provides university training at the Valencia International University (VIU) and the Universidad de Cádiz (UCA). Her primary research interest lies in language acquisition and functional communication, encompassing individuals diagnosed with ASD, intellectual disabilities, and aphasia. Her recent research focused on the feasibility, effectiveness, and acceptability of a multicomponent behavioral intervention package that opens new avenues for effective online postgraduate student training capitalizing in the safe use of reinforcement in social media. Dr. Tarifa Rodriguez is the author of *Nala and Her Behavior Analyst: Finding My Voice*.

Allie N. Townsend is a licensed clinical psychologist and assistant professor in the Menninger Department of Psychiatry and Behavioral Sciences at Baylor College of Medicine (BCM). She completed her doctoral degree in clinical psychology from the Chicago School of Professional Psychology in Washington, DC. Her primary research and clinical interests include the nature and treatment of individuals with anxiety, obsessive-compulsive disorder (OCD), and related disorders across the lifespan. She provides evidence-based therapy within the BCM OCD program and provides clinical supervision to trainees. Additionally, she leads BCM's ARPA program through the TCHATT initiative of the Texas Child Mental Health Care Consortium.

Javier Virues-Ortega is associate professor and research fellow at the University of Auckland (New Zealand). Previously, he has been assistant professor of psychology at the University of Manitoba (Canada) and postdoctoral researcher at the Instituto de Salud Carlos III (Spain). His research focuses on the evaluation of interventions based on applied behavior analysis (ABA) for people with and without disabilities. He has an interest in transferring mainstream outcome research methods into ABA, as well as other forms of translational research. He is the author of over 150 specialized publications. His work has been cited over 5,000 times and has been featured in the health coverage policies and authoritative advice of international organizations, including UnitedHealthcare, Blue Cross Blue Shield, ICHOM, CASP, and others. Dr. Virues-Ortega has served as associate editor or member of the editorial board in eight leading behavioral journals and has served as member of the board of directors and executive committees of leading professional organizations, including the Behavior Analyst Certification Board and the European Association for Behavior Analysis.

Lee E. Wachtel received her undergraduate degree in 1993 in Romance languages and literatures from Princeton University, and she received her medical degree from the Johns Hopkins University School of Medicine in Baltimore, Maryland, in 1998. She completed general, and child and adolescent psychiatry training at the University of Maryland psychiatry residency training program in Baltimore. She joined the Kennedy Krieger Institute in 2003, where she serves as medical director of the Neurobehavioral Unit, specializing in the care of children, adolescents, and young adults with autism and intellectual disability who present with concomitant severe psychiatric and behavioral disturbance. Dr. Wachtel is a professor of psychiatry at the Johns Hopkins School of Medicine. Her clinical and research interests focus on pediatric catatonia, particularly in autism spectrum disorders, with emphasis on repetitive self-injurious behaviors and optimal catatonia treatment paradigms, including electroconvulsive therapy. Dr. Wachtel is the author of more than three dozen scientific manuscripts and textbook chapters and has lectured extensively throughout the United States and abroad.

Mary Jane Weiss is the dean of the Institute for Applied Behavioral Science and director of the PhD program in applied behavior analysis (ABA) at Endicott College, where she has been for 12 years. She also does research with the team at Melmark. She has worked in the field of ABA and autism for 38 years. She received her PhD in clinical psychology from Rutgers University in 1990, and she became a Board-Certified Behavior Analyst in 2000. She previously worked for 16 years at the Douglass Developmental Disabilities Center at Rutgers University. Her clinical and research interests center on defining best practice and humane ABA techniques, integrating compassionate care and cultural responsiveness into ABA service delivery, exploring ways to enhance the ethical conduct of practitioners, training staff to be optimally effective at instruction and at collaboration, and maximizing family members' expertise and adaptation. She is also interested in finding interventions that clients and families find to be meaningful, enjoyable, and accessible. She presents regularly at regional and national conferences and is on the editorial board of several journals. She serves on the Scientific Council of the Organization for Autism Research, is on the board of Association for Science in Autism Treatment, is a regular contributor to the ABA Ethics Hotline, is on the editorial board of *Behavior Analysis in Practice*, and is an advisor to the Cambridge Center for Behavioral Studies.

Katrina Williams is a pediatrician and public health physician who has worked and trained in Darwin, Sydney, London, and Melbourne. Katrina is currently the head of the Department of Paediatrics at Monash University and the research director and a developmental pediatrician at Monash Children's Hospital, Australia. In her academic role she oversees the education in child health for medical students and clinically she works as part of a multidisciplinary team. She is a coauthor and editor of methodology and evidence-based textbooks, and coauthor of a book for parents about autism. Her research focuses on children with neurodevelopmental differences and complex needs. She completes clinical and population epidemiology research, making best use of existing data and evidence and establishing new studies. Her research has provided new knowledge about the incidence and prevalence of autism in Australia, and prognosis, diagnosis, and effective interventions, including research with a focus on equity and caregiver needs. She has leadership roles in research and clinical care and works with community advocacy organizations. Her research has been incorporated into international clinical practice directives and guidelines, leading to improved care, and has changed services and influenced policy in Australia. Her vision is to generate evidence that informs delivery of best care for children and their families by embedding research and training in healthcare for children and youth.

Yi Zhihui is a Board-Certified Behavior Analyst and the clinical coordinator of the Cognition Behavior and Mindfulness Clinic at the IDHD Family Clinic at the University of Illinois Chicago (UIC). Zhihui received his master's degree from Arizona State University's applied behavior analysis program and is currently a doctoral candidate in the rehabilitation science program at UIC. Zhihui is dedicated to promoting access and disseminating evidence-based intervention for persons with autism, especially among minority groups. Zhihui's research interests include relational frame theory, early intervention, and the neurological impact of behavior therapy.

1

Lifespan Treatment of Autism Spectrum Disorder

Introduction

Peter Sturmey
The Graduate Center and Queens College, City University of New York

Russell Lang
Texas State University, San Marcos

James K. Luiselli
Melmark New England

Upon receiving an autism spectrum disorder (ASD) diagnosis, many families will begin an extended and emotionally challenging search for effective interventions. The journey can be a rollercoaster ride of undelivered promises, false leads, and frustrations. The first third of Catherine Maurice's classic book, *Let Me Hear Your Voice*, describes a family's search for how to find effective help for their daughter with ASD and the false prophets, professional egos, and ineffective treatments with little reliable guidance for the family or professionals to discriminate the wheat from the chaff. New professional and paraprofessional staff in early intervention, education, and adults services face similar challenges when they enter the field, often with little explicit guidance other than "This is what we do here." State agencies face similar questions when they have to decide which interventions and programs to fund, as do professional organizations that publish guidelines as to which therapies practitioners should and should not use. Ultimately, society invests vast resources in attempting to provide effective service options for people with ASD. Many individuals with ASD receive lifelong services, including early intervention, special education, and adult services (e.g., placement in residential services).

Cakir et al. (2020) used a cost analysis model to compute a baseline and then to estimate future costs associated with ASD in the United States. They reported that the estimated 2 million new cases of ASD identified between 1990 and 2019 have had a cost of over $7 trillion. Further, if current prevalence and service options remain unchanged, the costs could reach $15 trillion by 2029. For an individual family, the lifelong cost associated with care and services for a family member with

Peter Sturmey, Russell Lang, and James K. Luiselli, *Lifespan Treatment of Autism Spectrum Disorder*. In: *Lifespan Treatment for Autistic Individuals*. Edited by: Peter Sturmey, Russell Lang, and James K. Luiselli, Oxford University Press.
© Oxford University Press (2025). DOI: 10.1093/oso/9780197635841.003.0001

ASD can be of the order of several million dollars—reflecting both direct costs, such as the costs of staff, medications, and material resources, and indirect costs, such as loss of family member income, administration, and building maintenance. Also, costs for individuals in special education and residential care can be substantially higher due to the need for specialized resources and staff (Horlin et al., 2014). Indeed, the adoption of some interventions, such as supported employment for adults with ASD, is sometimes justified on economic grounds (Jacob et al., 2015). Finally, some interventions result in physical or psychological harms to individuals with ASD and their caregivers, and hence there is an ethical obligation to identify these harmful treatments to prevent harm to all concerned. In short, there are many good reasons to identify EBPs for individuals with ASD.

1.1 What Is Evidence-Based Practice?

Evidence-based practice (EBP) derives from evidence-based medicine and is often attributed to the work of Archibald Cochrane (1909–1988), who was one of the first researcher-practitioners to organize systematic searches and repositories of evidence. He used the evidence from systematic searches and reviews of randomized controlled trials (RCTs) in medicine to guide clinical practice in adopting the most effective and efficient treatments (Stavrou et al., 2014). These ideas have proliferated within and beyond medicine. Many healthcare organizations now maintain databases of RCTs and use them to identify the most effective treatments available. This process has become more formalized. For example, Sacket et al. (1996) defined evidence-based medicine as "the conscientious explicit and judicious use of current best evidence in making decisions about the care of individual patients" with definitions of the qualifying terms as "Conscientious" (being careful, and thorough, in what you do), "Explicit" (being up-front, open, clear, and transparent), and "Judicious" (using good judgement and common sense) (Cochrane.org, 2023). Originally sprouting from medicine, EBP is now a pervasive social movement, with its defining principle of basing practice on the best available evidence, now firmly rooted across many fields. For example, we now see the application of evidence-based approaches in diverse areas, such as evidence-based policing, evidence-based policymaking, and evidence-based nursing.

EBP uses highly characteristic and formalized methods, typically involving the following procedures and operations:

- Formulation of a clear question to be answered, often using the PICO (Problem/Population, Intervention, Comparison, Outcome) acronym.
- Applying a systematic and fully described search strategy with clear search terms and inclusion criteria often summarized in a flow diagram of the results from each step of the search and with reliability coding data.

- Identification of well-conducted experiments evaluating treatment effectiveness, some of which retain only RCTs and others of which retain both RCTs and experimental single-case research designs.
- Explicit description of the literature retained which may include measures of the experimental rigor (quality) of the retained studies.
- Calculation of magnitude or consistency of effects, usually by means of effect sizes, combination of effect sizes into one overall grand effect size, and often disaggregation of effect sizes by relevant features of the literature such as treatment type and study quality.
- Some evaluation of the risks and benefits of each treatment and the risks and benefits of failure to implement preferred treatments.
- A statement of which treatment(s) are to be preferred for what problems and under what circumstances and perhaps some practice guidelines or algorithm making suggestions as to the order in which treatments are to be implemented, which perhaps includes some evaluation of the likely risks and benefits of the treatment(s) considered.
- Economic analyses of the EBPs that consider the direct financial costs, such as the costs of staffing, treatment materials and medications, and indirect costs of treatment compared to no treatment or other treatments, such as underemployment of family members who provide care.
- Recommendations for how practitioners can effectively apply and widely share EBPs.

The preceding list and aspirations are a tall order, and the outcomes of such attempts to identify EBPs vary considerably from one field to another and from one treatment to another.

1.2 Evidence-Based Practice and Autism Spectrum Disorders

The influence of the EBP movement on the diagnosis and treatment of autism can be considered by noting how much progress has been made. In the 1950s, under the influence of the then dominant model of psychotherapy, autism was considered to be an emotional disorder. Using the emotional disorder paradigm, the now infamous Bruno Bettelheim proposed a milieu treatment approach that was widely adopted. Bettelheim's theory took the view that autism developed as an emotional response when a child's mother was cold and unloving. These mothers were referred to as "Refrigerator Mothers," and the suggested approach to milieu therapy consisted of removing children from said mothers and placing them in separate residential treatment with surrogate parents while persuading mothers to recognize their guilt (Bettelheim, 1967). Bettelheim's scientific publications were very limited, yet his perspectives, to some degree, reflected the prevailing interest in psychoanalysis within the popular culture of that era. Despite the lack of scientific basis for his theory and therapy, he was quite successful in promoting his ideas to the general public through publication in popular magazines and widely watched television shows of the day. Only after his death was it widely publicly acknowledged that he had no appropriate degree (only a degree in art history and no degrees in psychology), that he worked as a lumber dealer rather than as a mental health professional in Vienna, and that he was a bully to his colleagues and possibly abusive to children (Severson, Aune, & Jodlowski, 2008).

In the absence of EBPs in the 1950s, the outlook for affected families was pessimistic. Even into the 1970s, many clinicians were unlikely and unwilling to diagnose autism, in part, due to stigma still associated with Bettelheim's debunked theories and to a lack of effective treatment options. In short, accurate data regarding prevalence and presentation of ASD were scarce because there was little good to be done and some risk of harm in diagnosing a child with ASD.

Bettelheim's debunked theory and unevaluated recommendations provide an early example of how dissemination of a non-evidence-based treatment to the public can be highly influential and harmful to families and children with autism. Although widely repudiated in many circles today, Bettelheim's ideas currently remain alive in France (Briggs, 2020), and they probably have negative influences, such as the exclusion of children with autism from some educational services and settings and until recently the adoption of "packing," another non-evidence-based psychoanalytic treatment (Chamak, 2019). These ideas also spread into the work of the Tinbergens (Tinbergen & Tinbergen, 1983) and other dubious, unevaluated, and apparently stressful treatments, such as holding therapy or "regulatory bonding therapy" (Welch & Mark, 1988), which have been shown to be ineffective (Lilienfeld, 2005) and may have resulted in some child deaths (Mercer, 2014).

At around the same time, concern regarding the effects of psychotherapy was beginning to be voiced in reviews of the research literature elsewhere. The British psychologist Hans Eysenck (1952) reached pessimistic conclusions concerning evidence for adult psychotherapy. At the same time, the development of alternatives to traditional psychotherapy for neuroses which emphasized objectivity and learning as part of therapy challenged the then dominant model empirically (Wolpe, 1952). Thus, the movement away from nonempirical psychotherapies toward empirically based psychotherapies was underway during the 1950s and 1960s.

Therapeutic nihilism in autism was challenged by early behavioral studies. For example, Lovaas et al. (1965) demonstrated that self-injury in three children with autism was responsive to reinforcement and extinction. In the next year, Lovaas et al. (1966) demonstrated that social interaction could be established as a conditioned reinforcer in two autistic children. These studies were revolutionary at that time because they showed that young autistic children could benefit from therapy based on learning theory. Subsequently, Lovaas abandoned this piecemeal approach to treating autism response by response (Lovaas, 1993). He moved out of institutions to work with families in the natural environment with the goal of remediating autism through intensive (40 hours a week) and extensive (50 weeks of the year for 2–4 years) applied behavior analytic therapy. He had trained students to conduct the initial therapy sessions using discrete trial teaching and then, based on child progress, moved to a more naturalistic set of interventions and greater parental involvement as the child progressed. The goal was to place the child in mainstream education by first grade. Lovaas (1987) reported that autistic children who were placed in early intensive behavioral intervention (EIBI) had much better outcomes than autistic children in two control groups. Children in all groups were severely impaired at baseline with average IQs of around 55 at age 33 months. The most important finding was that 47% (9/19) of children "achieved normal intellectual and educational functioning, with normal-range IQ scores and successful first grade performance in public schools," whereas only 2% of children in the control groups achieved this outcome. Further, when McEachin et al. (1993) followed up with the children at age 11.5 years, these robust effects were maintained with evidence of little residual psychopathology. Unsurprisingly, this study has been extensively cited in the literature and received detailed scrutiny and commentary (e.g., Schopler et al., 1989). Lovaas (1987) challenged the prevailing notion of the time where little to no effort was made to educate children with autism, by demonstrating their potential to learn new skills with effective treatment.

As in other fields, EBP has been highly influential in fields related to the education and treatment of ASD. There is a vast array—indeed, hundreds—of ASD treatments! The scientific support for these treatment options varies widely, from rigorously evaluated EBPs, to unevaluated or perpetually experimental approaches, to promising approaches that are still inadequately evaluated, to potentially dangerous pseudoscientific methods. The field is also shifting considerably in response to the increasing number of outcomes studies. For treatment approaches with a robust evidence base, we know what outcomes to expect, what risks need to be considered, and how to deliver procedures with fidelity. Further, although there are relatively few economic analyses of interventions, when there are sufficient economic data available, we can compare costs versus benefits of competing treatment options. Unfortunately, many treatments have not been similarly evaluated, and the potential for wasted resources and direct harm to individuals with ASD remains unknown in too many instances. In other cases, a substantial amount of research has identified notable risk of harm and/or has failed to produce any reliable benefit, yet the treatment approach may still be widely adopted by families, schools, and other service providers.

Interpreting the corpus of ASD treatment research is complicated by differences in research norms across disciplines, competing theoretical underpinnings, and a notable amount of misleading information available from mainstream popular media sources (e.g., Hemsley & Dann, 2015). In addition, the evidence base changes over time. Treatments that previously did not meet the criteria for EBP may subsequently meet criteria for EBP, new treatments may be developed and evaluated, and, as well-conducted research accumulates for established treatments, we may understand the outcomes in greater detail than in the past. For example, over the last 25 years, early intervention for children with ASD has been greatly influenced by developmentally informed naturalistic models of early intervention. These new models have developed curricula that are distinct from that of Lovaas in that they rely less on intensive discrete trial teaching and focus more on lower density and greater variety of trials within a naturalistic environment.

Overall, these issues contribute to a gap between the outcomes demonstrated in tightly controlled scientific studies and what is typically achieved in real-world homes, schools, and other applied settings. Specifically, the enormity and complexity of this field of research complicate the training of future professionals, obscure genuine advances in treatment science, and dissuade individuals without extensive formal scientific training from attempting to address their questions or improve their practice by turning to the literature.

Professional practitioners and family members need to be informed about treatment efficacy in order to select treatments that are procedurally and ethically best suited for their individual clients. Indeed, many professional codes of conduct require ASD practitioners to be knowledgeable and competent in implementing evidence-based treatments. Yet professional training often does not prepare practitioners fully for this expectation. Further, research into treating ASD has been accelerating in both quantity and complexity for several decades, and systematic reviews, authoritative statements, and new practice guidelines continue to emerge but are usually nested within specific disciplines. Accordingly, ASD professionals need resources to meet their ethical obligation to provide EBPs, avoid harm to their clients, and help ensure most efficient use of treatment resources (e.g., therapist and client time and service money).

1.3 Current Status of the Intervention Evidence Base

Over the last 50 years, there has been an accumulation of research and practice statements attempting to identify EBPs for autism. Some of these have a very broad focus, attempting to summarize the entire field of autism and outcome research, and some of these concentrate on the effects of a particular treatment, such as behavioral self-management, or the best treatment options for a specific target area, such as promoting play.

Some examples of professional and state agency statements for EBPs and autism include the following. Several organizations have concluded that EIBI is an EBP (Lang, Hancock, & Singh, 2016). For example, following the publication of Lovaas (1987) and subsequent studies, several professional organizations, including the American Psychological Association, the American Academy of Child and Adolescent Psychiatry, the US Surgeon General, the New York State Department of Health, among others, all concluded that EIBI was an EBP and should be adopted for many children with autism (Larsson, 2013). Additionally, some professional organizations have questioned or even condemned certain forms of therapy. For example, the American Academy of Pediatrics (Section on Complementary and Integrative Medicine, Council on Children with Disabilities, 2012) concluded that sensory integration therapy (SIT) was popular but questioned the existence of the alleged disorder which SIT was supposed to treat and that the evidence to support its use is limited. Similar statements have been issued for facilitated communication and hyperbaric oxygen therapy among others, which are not merely ineffective but in various ways positively harmful to some autistic individuals (see Chapter 38 by Krszak and Mulick for a review of such statements).

There are also at least two groups of researchers and practitioners who have published influential reports on EBP and autism. The National Standards Project is a group of researchers and practitioners who have published two major systematic reviews of EBPs and autism (National Autism Center, 2015). Phase 1, published in 2009, reviewed research with children published from 1957 through 2007, and Phase 2 reviewed research published research published between 2007 and February 2012 and included research with autistic adults. Both projects used explicit methodologies to search the literature and identify experimental studies, used trained experts to extract data, identified treatment targets for both adaptive and maladaptive behavior, rated the quality of the studies and identified EBPs using explicit and reliable public criteria, and rated the strength of the evidence as established, emerging, or unestablished. Phase 2 concluded that there were 14 established, 18 emerging, and 13 unestablished interventions. The established interventions for children were behavioral interventions, cognitive-behavioral intervention package, comprehensive behavioral treatment for young children, language training (production), modeling, natural teaching strategies, parent training, peer training package, pivotal response training, schedules, scripting, self-management, social skills package, and story-based intervention. For adults, there was only one established, four emerging, and four unestablished interventions. The established intervention for adults was behavior interventions package to teach skills and reduce problem behavior. Phase 3, which undertakes to comprehensively review research up to 2018, is currently underway as of 2023.

The second notable group is Odom's group, which has published and updated comprehensive reviews of EBPs to identify which ones should be disseminated (Hume et al., 2021; Odom et al., 2010; Steinbrenner et al., 2020; Wong et al., 2015). The last review (Hume et al., 2021) identified 28 EBPs for children with ASD, specifically antecedent-based interventions; augmentative and alternative communication; behavioral momentum intervention; cognitive-behavioral/instructional strategies; differential reinforcement of alternative, incompatible, or other behavior; direct instruction; discrete trial training; exercise and movement; extinction; functional behavior assessment; functional communication training; modeling; music-mediated intervention; naturalistic intervention; parent-mediated intervention; peer-based instruction and intervention; prompting; reinforcement;

self-management; sensory integration; social narratives; social skills training; task analysis; technology-aided instruction and intervention; time delay; video modeling; and visual supports.

The EBPs that these two groups identified broadly overlap with one another, although details shift between revisions as evidence accumulates. Further, specific intervention procedures (e.g., prompting and reinforcement) are often components of larger multiple-component interventions, and this complicates isolation of the mechanisms of action that underlie the empirically demonstrated benefits of an intervention approach. Ultimately, this overlap necessitates a more nuanced discussion regarding an intervention's empirical support. For example, pivotal response training (PRT) is a naturalistic developmental behavioral intervention that utilizes several well-established EBPs like prompting, modeling, environmental arrangement, reinforcement, and parent involvement. PRT utilizes evidence-based intervention components in a unique way to improve motivation and to target specific pivotal behaviors. The PRT literature accurately cites support for the effectiveness of specific procedures from research not necessarily done in the context of the full PRT intervention (see Chapter 15 by Kern Koegel and Mohammadzaheri). Although incorporating well-established evidence-based procedures into a multicomponent intervention does provide support for some claims regarding efficacy, additional research directly focused on an intervention's overall or unique claims of benefit (e.g., PRT's claims of collateral generalized improvement in wide range of behaviors) is still necessary prior to classification of the practice as an EBP.

1.4 The Challenge of Dissemination of Evidence-Based Practices

Some autism treatments are now well established and with rigorous and replicable research literature supporting their use. We know what the treatments are, as well as the intensity and extensivity of implementation needed to achieve certain known outcomes. We also know the likely outcomes and the social value of these outcomes. To date, these EBPs are predominantly but not exclusively those based on applied behavior analysis (ABA). Indeed, many autistic children now receive some version of these EBPs with varying degrees of treatment integrity and effectiveness. However, most autistic children and adults do not receive any EBPs, and a sizable minority receives ineffective treatments such as SIT and psychopharmacology; a few continue to receive harmful interventions such as chelation and facilitated communication (see Chapter 38 by Kryszak and Mulick). Thus, there is some cause for optimism but also much left to be done in terms of disseminating EBPs.

There are examples of large-scale implementation of EBPs in other literatures which could act as models for how to disseminate EBPs to autistic children and adults. For example, the Improving Access to Psychological Therapies project in the British National Health Service has identified and disseminated EBPs for depression and anxiety. EBPs were identified through systematic reviews and meta-analyses, economic analyses produced evidence in favor of implementation (primarily through savings from returning people to work), and national implementation of evidence-based psychotherapies with large effect sizes during implementation from numerous studies using typical local therapists and psychiatric nurses as the prime agents of change who were trained in a manualized form of cognitive-behavioral therapy (Clark, 2011; Wakefield et al., 2021). Such projects can be models for how to proceed in disseminating EBPs for individuals with ASD.

Some notable progress has been made in disseminating EBPs for autistic children and adults. Odom's group took the results of their multiple systematic review and used them as the basis for dissemination of EBPs in the Autism Focused Intervention Resources Module (AFIRM) project (Sam et al., 2020). Using online training, the AFIRM project (Sam et al., 2020) has successfully disseminated knowledge of EBPs to a large number of practitioners. The AFIRM modules provide information on 27 EBPs for children with ASD. Each module has a standard four-lesson format which covers (1) definition and description of the practice; (2) how to plan use of the practice; (3) how to use the EBP using a step-by-step approach; and (4) steps to monitor practice. Since 2015, there have been over 64,000 registered users mostly from the United States who were most often special education teachers and university students. Users rate the modules to be of very high quality. AFIRM offered over 87,000 certificates and almost 200,000 hours of professional training hours. The most commonly completed modules were antecedent-based intervention, visual supports, reinforcement, prompting, and functional behavior assessment. This widespread dissemination of knowledge is indeed impressive. To date, however, there are no data on changes in practitioner behavior when delivering EBPs and corresponding changes in child behavior.

As well as university-based centers funded with grant money such as the AFIRM project, large-scale dissemination of EBPs can be undertaken using either state-funded services or for-profit businesses funded by private equity. In the first approach, a state passes laws to fund and regulate EBPs, such as EIBI, and a state agency oversees service provision, sometimes with the state agency providing the services and sometimes with contracted private agencies of nonprofits providing services. In the second approach, an existing clinic or other private agency claims to provide services that are based on EBP, often expands to multiple sites, and then seeks out private equity to fund further expansion of services for profit. In both approaches, problems exist. The biggest problem for both approaches is that often pilot work and evaluation are not conducted before large-scale implementation. Thus, the exact procedures to disseminate EBPs are unspecified, resulting in problems with treatment integrity and program drift. In the case of state-funded services, the services may be inefficient, and there may be little incentive to be effective or efficient. In the case of equity-funded services, there may be pressure to maximize profits through rapid expansion, the use of the cheapest labor available, and economies of scale.

These typical approaches to disseminating EBPs are not the only approach. One approach to disseminating EBPs is illustrated by Achievement Place, a program for youth who are at risk for delinquency and criminal behavior. The program adopted EBPs such as token economies, codified these practices, evaluated their effectiveness in pilot studies, and monitored the program integrity and treatment outcomes during the development of the first house. Replication across numerous sites revealed both successes and failures, which allowed program revision such as clustering programs geographically where a group of skilled practitioners could support one another rather than work in isolation. Over time, the number of replication sites has gradually increased using quality assurance mechanisms and certification of programs that met predetermined criteria (Fixsen & Blasé, 2019). Similar approaches have been used to replicate the EBPs used in the Princeton Child Development Institute program (McClannahan & Krantz, 1997). Perhaps this approach to replication of EBPs, although slower and steadier than typical approaches, might be one worth considering when it comes to disseminating EBPs and autism.

A final potential avenue for dissemination of EBPs includes professional and postqualification training of a wide range of mental health professionals who work with individuals with ASD. Although many professional training programs and postgraduate/continuing education training programs recognize the importance of EBPs, the requirements for such training are often quite weak. Thus, accredited programs may be required to provide information or a certain number of practicum hours about EBPs, but there may often be no requirement to train practitioners to master these skills to criterion. Indeed, very often assessment of student performance is often based on verbal behavior such as written responses, term papers, and in-class presentations, rather than direct assessment of clinical skills and outcomes with a variety of clients. Similarly, assessment of practicum training is often based on hours of practiced and participation in supervision rather than observation and mastery of clinical skills. Thus, although professional training has the potential to disseminate EBPs to professionals with ASD, current practices do not make this a likely effective avenue to do so unless training requirements and their accreditation change substantially.

Finally, an aspect of disseminating EBPs which receives little direct acknowledgment is the discouragement and suppression of ineffective and harmful treatments. Lawsuits and research have been quite effective in limiting but not eradicating positively harmful treatments such as holding therapy and facilitative communication. In contrast, SIT, despite being quite well evaluated and found to be ineffective but not positively harmful, remains a common practice for occupational therapists despite the conclusion from many researchers, practitioners, and professional organizations that this is not an EBP.

1.5 Overview of the Present Volume

Lifespan Treatment of Autism Spectrum Disorder: An Evidence-Based Guide to Professionals and Families is intended as an authoritative compendium that appraises this corpus of literature across multiple disciplines (e.g., psychology, education, and medicine) and identifies treatment approaches evaluated against EBP standards by recognized experts. Uniformly organized chapters, each focused on a specific treatment approach, provide a *Consumer Reports*–style reference specifically designed to be useful for a wide range of scholars, practitioners, and other stakeholders interested in ensuring positive and efficient treatment outcomes for individuals with ASD. The book (a) focuses on evidence-based interventions for ASD as well as emerging, ineffective, and harmful interventions across multiple fields of practice, (b) details the application of each included treatment approach by providing a concise description of the EBP, (c) offers practitioners a singular resource capable of quickly addressing essential elements and considerations for each treatment option, (d) gives parents and the general public a plain-language summary of ASD interventions that can be used to inform decisions related to treatment selection for individuals as well as the design of programs serving multiple persons, and (e) recommends directions for future research and practice.

As volume editors, we grouped treatments into learning-based, cognitive/cog nitive-behavioral, sensory-based, psychopharmacology, and other biological categories. With regard to chapter structure, authors followed a standardized format comprised of a technical structured abstract, plain-language summary for nonprofessionals, treatment summary table, treatment overview, research background, and practice implications. A second organizational decision was to exclude treatments and therapies that have been evaluated and found to be ineffective or harmful. SIT, for example, was excluded because a series of systematic reviews concluded that there was insufficient evidence (Barton et al., 2015; Lang et al., 2012; Leong et al., 2015a, 2015b; Wan Yunus et al., 2015), and the American Academy of Pediatrics (Zimmer et al., 2012) policy statement on SIT concluded: "Parents should be informed that the amount of research regarding the effectiveness of sensory integration therapy is limited and inconclusive" (p.1186). We also did not solicit a chapter on facilitated communication (FC) and rapid prompting method (RPM) as recent reviews concluded a lack of evidence in support of either method (Hemsley, 2016; Hemsley et al., 2018; Schlosser et al., 2019). Concerning treatment with hyperbarometric oxygen, three systematic reviews concluded that, although there are trials, the designs are weak, outcomes are mixed, and evidence support is lacking (Ghanizadeh, 2012; Goldfarb et al., 2016; Podgórska-Bednarz & Perenc, 2021). Chelation is another biological treatment with little support, with two systematic reviews determining that it is not effective and may be associated with potentially dangerous side effects (Davis et al., 2013; James et al., 2015). Further, we excluded a chapter on holding therapy, given the lack of empirical evidence (Lilienfeld, 2005) and suggestion of harm to children with autism (Mercer, 2014). Finally, the area of new medications is a very active one which often does not correspond to clinical practice. Although we included chapters on current conventional psychopharmacology and agents, including cannabis, we did not include chapters on other new drugs such as medications typically used for Alzheimer disease (Rossignol & Frye, 2014), and oxytocin, which has been evaluated for its effects on prosocial behavior (Ooi et al., 2017; Preti et al., 2014).

The primary audience for this book includes professional practitioners serving individuals with ASD, as well as researchers, university faculty, graduate students, and postgraduate trainees. With chapters that feature a plain-language summary, the book also is directed at parents of children and adults with ASD, program administrators, community organizers, and other stakeholders in search of cross-discipline treatment approaches for specific needs. Our hope is that the book appeals to the widest readership possible, advances effective ASD treatments across the lifespan, and promotes user-inspired research valued by the autism community.

1.6 References

Barton, E., Reichow, B., Schnitz, A., Smith, I., & Sherlock, D. (2015). A systematic review of sensory-based treatments for children with disabilities. *Research in Developmental Disabilities, 37*, 64–80.

Bettelheim, B. (1967). *Empty fortress*. New York: Simon and Schuster.

Briggs, J. (2020). The enduring fortress: The influence of Bruno Bettelheim in the politics of autism in France. *Modern Intellectual History, 17*(4), 1163–1191.

Cakir, J., Frye, R. E., & Walker, S. J. (2020). The lifetime social cost of autism: 1990–2029. *Research in Autism Spectrum Disorders, 72*, 101502. https://doi.org/10.1016/j.rasd.2019.101502

Chamak, B. (2019). Lobbying by association: The case of autism and the controversy over packing therapy in France. *Social Science & Medicine, 230*, 256–263.

Clark, D. M. (2011). Implementing NICE guidelines for the psychological treatment of depression and anxiety disorders: The IAPT experience. *International Review of Psychiatry, 23*(4), 318–327.

Cochrane.org. (2023). What is evidence-based medicine? https://s4be.cochrane.org/starthere/what-is-evidence-based-medicine/

Davis, T. N., O'Reilly, M., Kang, S., Lang, R., Rispoli, M., Sigafoos, J., Lancioni, G., Copeland, D., Shanna, A. & Mulloy, A. (2013). Chelation treatment for autism spectrum disorders: A systematic review. *Research in Autism Spectrum Disorders, 7*(1), 49–55.

Eysenck, H. J. (1952). The effects of psychotherapy: An evaluation. *Journal of Consulting Psychology, 16*(5), 319.

Fixsen, D. L., & Blase, K. A. (2019). The teaching-family model: The first 50 years. *Perspectives on Behavior Science, 42*(2), 189–211.

Ghanizadeh, A. (2012). Hyperbaric oxygen therapy for treatment of children with autism: a systematic review of randomized trials. *Medical Gas Research, 2*(1), 1–8.

Goldfarb, C., Genore, L., Hunt, C., Flanagan, J., Handley-Derry, M., Jethwa, A.Jones,-Stokreef, N., Kirkpatrick, S.M.L., Rojnica, R.L., Schwartz, C., Shawn, D., Superina-Bell, D., Young, E., & Anagnostou, E. (2016). Hyperbaric oxygen therapy for the treatment of children and youth with Autism Spectrum Disorders: An evidence-based systematic review. *Research in Autism Spectrum Disorders, 29*, 1–7.

Hemsley, B. (2016). Evidence does not support the use of Rapid Prompting Method (RPM) as an intervention for students with autism spectrum disorder and further primary research is not justified. *Evidence-Based Communication Assessment and Intervention, 10*(3–4), 122–130.

Hemsley, B., Bryant, L., Schlosser, R. W., Shane, H. C., Lang, R., Paul, D., Banajee, M., & Ireland, M. (2018). Systematic review of facilitated communication 2014–2018 finds no new evidence that messages delivered using facilitated communication are authored by the person with disability. *Autism & Developmental Language Impairments, 3*, 2396941518821570.

Hemsley, B., & Dann, S. (2015). Social media and social marketing in relation to facilitated communication: Harnessing the affordances of social media for knowledge translation. *Evidence based Communication Assessment and Intervention, 8*(4), 187–206. https://doi.org/10.1080/17489539.2015.1023988

Horlin, C., Falkmer, M., Parsons, R., Albrecht, M. A., & Falkmer, T. (2014). The cost of autism spectrum disorders. *PloS One, 9*(9), e106552.

Hume, K., Steinbrenner, J. R., Odom, S. L., Morin, K. L., Nowell, S. W., Tomaszewski, B., Szendrey, S, McIntyre, N. S., Yücesoy-Özkan, S., Savage, M. N. (2021). Evidence-based practices for children, youth, and young adults with autism: Third generation review. *Journal of Autism and Developmental Disorders, 51*(11), 4013–4032.

Jacob, A., Scott, M., Falkmer, M., & Falkmer, T. (2015). The costs and benefits of employing an adult with autism spectrum disorder: A systematic review. *PloS One, 10*(10), e0139896.

James, S., Stevenson, S. W., Silove, N., & Williams, K. (2015). Chelation for autism spectrum disorder (ASD). *Cochrane Database of Systematic Reviews, 5.*

Kirigin, K. A., Phillips, E. L., Timbers, G. D., Fixsen, D. L., & Wolf, M. M. (2020). Achievement place: The modification of academic behavior problems of delinquent youths in a group home setting. In B. C. Etzel, J. M., LeBlanc, & D. M. Baer (Eds.), *New developments in behavioral research: Theory, method and application: in honor of Sidney W. Bijou* (pp. 473–487). Abingdon, UK: Routledge.

Lang, R., Hancock, T. B., & Singh, N. N. (Eds.). (2016). *Early intervention for young children with autism spectrum disorder.* Cham: Springer.

Lang, R., O'Reilly, M., Healy, O., Rispoli, M., Lydon, H., Streusand, W., Davis, T., Kang, S., Sigafoos, J., Lancioni, G., Didden, R., & Giesbers, S. (2012). Sensory integration therapy for autism spectrum disorders: A systematic review. *Research in Autism Spectrum Disorders, 6*(3), 1004–1018.

Larsson, E. V. (2013). Is applied behavior analysis (ABA) and early intensive behavioral intervention (EIBI) an effective treatment for autism? A cumulative history of impartial independent reviews. *Autism, 27*(1), 168–1792.

Leong, H. M., Carter, M. C., & Stephenson, J. (2015a). Systematic review of sensory integration therapy for individuals with disabilities: Single case design studies. *Research in Developmental Disabilities, 47*, 334–351. http://dx.doi.org.libproxy.txstate.edu/10.1016/j.ridd.2015.09.022

Leong, H. M., Carter, M. C., & Stephenson, J. (2015b). Meta-analysis of research on sensory integration therapy for individuals with developmental and learning disabilities. *Journal of Developmental and Physical Disabilities, 27*(2), 183–206. http://dx.doi.org.libproxy.txstate.edu/10.1007/s10882-014-9408-y

Lilienfeld, S. O. (2005). Scientifically unsupported and supported interventions for childhood psychopathology: A summary. *Pediatrics, 115*(3), 761–764.

Lovaas, O. I. (1987). Behavioral treatment and normal educational and intellectual functioning in young autistic children. *Journal of Consulting and Clinical Psychology, 55*(1), 3–9. https://doi.org/10.1037/0022-006X.55.1.3

Lovaas, O. I. (1993). The development of a treatment-research project for developmentally disabled and autistic children. *Journal of Applied Behavior Analysis, 26*(4), 617–630.

Lovaas, O. I., Freitag, G., Gold, V. J., & Kassorla, I. C. (1965). Experimental studies in childhood schizophrenia: Analysis of self-destructive behavior. *Journal of Experimental Child Psychology, 2*(1), 67–84.

Lovaas, O. I., Freitag, G., Kinder, M. I., Rubenstein, B. D., Schaeffer, B., & Simmons, J. Q. (1966). Establishment of social reinforcers in two schizophrenic children on the basis of food. *Journal of Experimental Child Psychology, 4*(2), 109–125.

McClannahan, L. E., & Krantz, P. J. (1997). Princeton Child Development Institute. *Behavior and Social Issues, 7*, 65–68.

McEachin, J. J., Smith, T., & Lovaas, O. I. (1993). Long-term outcome for children with autism who received early intensive behavioral treatment. *American Journal of Mental Retardation, 97*(4), 359–372.

Mercer, J. (2014). International concerns about holding therapy. *Research on Social Work Practice, 24*(2), 188–191.

National Autism Center. (2015). *Findings and conclusions: National standards project, phase 2.* Randolph, MA: Author.

Odom, S. L., Collet-Klingenberg, L., Rogers, S. J., & Hatton, D. D. (2010). Evidence-based practices in interventions for children and youth with autism spectrum disorders. *Preventing School Failure: Alternative Education for Children and Youth, 54*(4), 275–282.

Ooi, Y. P., Weng, S. J., Kossowsky, J., Gerger, H., & Sung, M. (2017). Oxytocin and autism spectrum disorders: A systematic review and meta-analysis of randomized controlled trials. *Pharmacopsychiatry, 50*(1), 5–13.

Podgórska-Bednarz, J., & Perenc, L. (2021). Hyperbaric oxygen therapy for children and youth with autism spectrum disorder: a review. *Brain Sciences, 11*(7), 916.

Preti, A., Melis, M., Siddi, S., Vellante, M., Doneddu, G., & Fadda, R. (2014). Oxytocin and autism: A systematic review of randomized controlled trials. *Journal of Child and Adolescent Psychopharmacology, 24*(2), 54–68.

Rossignol, D. A., & Frye, R. E. (2014). The use of medications approved for Alzheimer's disease in autism spectrum disorder: A systematic review. *Frontiers in Pediatrics, 2*, 87.

Sackett, D., Rosenberg, W., Gray, M., Haynes, B., & Richardson, S. (1996). Evidence based medicine: What it is and what it isn' t. *British Medical Journal, 312*, 71.

Sam, A. M., Cox, A. W., Savage, M. N., Waters, V., & Odom, S. L. (2020). Disseminating information on evidence-based practices for children and youth with autism spectrum disorder: AFIRM. *Journal of Autism and Developmental Disorders, 50*, 1931–1940.

Sandberg, E. H., & Spritz, B. L. (2012). *A Brief Guide to Autism Treatments*. Philadelphia: Jessica Kingsley Publications.

Schlosser, R. W., Hemsley, B., Shane, H., Todd, J., Lang, R., Lilienfeld, S. O., Trembath, D., Mostert, M., Fong, S., & Odom, S. (2019). Rapid prompting method and autism spectrum disorder: Systematic review exposes lack of evidence. *Review Journal of Autism & Developmental Disorders, 6*, 403–412.

Schopler, E., Short, A., & Mesibov, G. (1989). Relation of behavioral treatment to "normal functioning": Comment on Lovaas. *Journal of Consulting and Clinical Psychology, 57*(1), 162–164.

Severson, K., Aune, J., & Jodlowski, D. (2008). Bruno Bettelheim, autism, and the rhetoric of scientific authority. *Autism and Representation*.

Stavrou, A., Challoumas, D., & Dimitrakakis, G. (2014). Archibald Cochrane (1909–1988): The father of evidence-based medicine. *Interactive Cardiovascular and Thoracic Surgery, 18*(1), 121–124.

Steinbrenner, J. R., Hume, K., Odom, S. L., Morin, K. L., Nowell, S. W., Tomaszewski, B., Szendrey, S., McIntyre, N. S., Yücesoy-Özkan, S., & Savage, M. N. (2020). Evidence-based practices for children, youth, and young adults with Autism. *FPG Child Development Institute*. https://files.eric.ed.gov/fulltext/ED609029.pdf.

Tinbergen, N., & Tinbergen, E. A. (1983). *Autistic children: New hope for a cure*. New South Wales, Australia: Allen & Unwin.

Wakefield, S., Kellett, S., Simmonds-Buckley, M., Stockton, D., Bradbury, A., & Delgadillo, J. (2021). Improving Access to Psychological Therapies (IAPT) in the United Kingdom: A systematic review and meta-analysis of 10-years of practice-based evidence. *British Journal of Clinical Psychology, 60*(1), 1–37.

Wan Yunus, F., Liu, K. P. Y., Bissett, M., & Penkala, S. (2015). Sensory-based intervention for children with behavioral problems: A systematic review. *Journal of Autism and Developmental Disorders, 45*(11), 3565–3579.

Welch, M. G., & Mark, M. E. (1988). *Holding time: How to eliminate conflict, temper tantrums, and sibling rivalry and raise happy, loving, successful children*. New York: Simon & Schuster.

Wolpe, J. (1952). Objective psychotherapy of the neuroses. *South African Medical Journal, 26*(42), 825–829.

Wong, C., Odom, S. L., Hume, K. A., Cox, A. W., Fettig, A., Kucharczyk, S., Brock, M. E., Plavnick, J. B., Fleury, V. P., & Schultz, T. R. (2015). Evidence-based practices for children, youth, and young adults with autism spectrum disorder: A comprehensive review. *Journal of Autism and Developmental Disorders, 45*, 1951–1966. DOI: 10.1007/s10803-014-2351-z

Zimmer, M., Desch, L., Rosen, L.D., Bailey, M. L., Becker, D., Culbert, T. P., McClafferty, H., Sahler, O. J. Z., Vohra, S., Liptak, G. S., Adams, R. C., Burke, R. T., Friedman, S. L., Houtrow, A. J., Kalichman, M. A., Kuo, D. Z., Levy, S. E., Norwood, K. W., Turchi, R. M., & Wiley, S. E. (2012). Sensory integration therapies for children with developmental and behavioral disorders. *Pediatrics, 129*(6). 1186–1189. DOI: 10.1542/peds.2012-0876

2

Antecedent Interventions

Lee Kern, Elise Settanni, and Jennifer Croner Lauriello
Lehigh University

2.1 Technical Abstract

Background: Antecedent interventions alter antecedent or setting events/establishing operations associated with challenging behavior. They are preventive because they are implemented prior to challenging behavior occurring and are designed to preclude the opportunity and/or motivation to engage in challenging behavior. **Method:** To describe research and applications of antecedent interventions, we identified 20 literature reviews or meta-analyses on antecedent-only interventions or multicomponent interventions that included antecedent interventions implemented with individuals with autism spectrum disorder (ASD). **Results:** Hundreds of studies have been conducted evaluating numerous variations of antecedent-only or multicomponent (including antecedent) interventions. As a whole, the literature indicates antecedent interventions are moderately to highly effective across age groups (preschool age to adults) and a large number of target behaviors. However, a limited number of studies reported no or small effects, likely due to behaviors that are resistant to intervention. **Discussion:** Research suggests antecedent interventions offer an excellent option for improving behavior. Additional research is needed to ascertain what antecedent intervention approaches are most likely to occasion desirable change for specific target behaviors and evaluate the additive effects of additional components. **Practitioner recommendations:** Antecedent interventions have been successfully implemented by a variety of practitioners (e.g., caregivers, teachers, paraprofessionals) with limited intervention expertise. Linking antecedent interventions to a challenging behavior's operant function and adding components, such as instruction and consequences, may increase effectiveness.

2.2 Layperson Summary

Antecedent interventions alter events that occur prior to challenging behavior. This may involve events that occur just before challenging behavior, referred to as antecedent events, or those that are not necessarily immediately proximal to

Lee Kern, Elise Settanni, and Jennifer Croner Lauriello, *Antecedent Interventions*. In: *Lifespan Treatment for Autistic Individuals*. Edited by: Peter Sturmey, Russell Lang, and James K. Luiselli, Oxford University Press. © Oxford University Press (2025). DOI: 10.1093/oso/9780197635841.003.0002 challenging behavior, referred to as setting events or establishing operations. In this way, they reduce motivation and/or remove opportunities for challenging behavior and thereby prevent its occurrence.

We conducted a literature search to ascertain how antecedent interventions have been used with individuals with ASD and appraised the rigor of research studies on the topic. Our search identified 20 literature reviews or meta-analyses that assessed antecedent-only interventions or multicomponent interventions that included antecedent interventions. The research literature contains hundreds of studies across a large scope of target behaviors, such as aggression, self-injury, sleep problems, stereotypy, and social behaviors. Antecedent interventions were successfully implemented by a variety of individuals, including peers, paraprofessionals, teachers, and parents/care providers, suggesting ease of implementation in the absence of extensive training. However, it should be noted that these individuals did not necessarily design the intervention, a task that may require additional expertise, such as training in applied behavior analysis (ABA).

Many of the reviews/meta-analyses evaluated the quality of the included research studies using standards established by professional organizations. Some reviews/meta-analyses included only studies that met a threshold of acceptable quality. Overall, the majority of studies evaluated for experimental rigor met standards or did so with only some reservations. Thus, a sufficient number of studies have been conducted to provide strong evidence for the effectiveness of antecedent interventions.

Collectively, the research suggests that practitioners can expect fairly large reductions in challenging behaviors after implementation of antecedent interventions. These foreseeable effects hold true for a large age range, from preschool children to adults. Smaller effects may occur with behaviors targeted for increase, such as social skills. In addition, some behaviors (e.g., restrictive and repetitive behaviors with automatic reinforcement contingencies) may be more resistant to intervention. No reviews/meta-analyses identified any side effects. For additional information, see referenced articles with an asterisk.

2.3 Treatment Summary Table

Treatment summary: Antecedent Interventions

Treatment description: Antecedent interventions alter events that occur prior to challenging behavior. Identified events are then either eliminated or modified such that they no longer occasion challenging behavior. In this way, antecedent interventions prevent challenging behavior.

Expected outcomes: The reviews and meta-analyses that calculated the effectiveness of antecedent interventions indicated moderate to large reductions in challenging behaviors. A caveat, however, is that the wide range of target behaviors and antecedent strategies employed complicates efforts to identify a specific set of antecedent intervention procedures as best practice.

Methods: A literature search yielded 20 literature reviews and meta-analyses summarizing the research on antecedent interventions. The identified reviews/meta-analyses each contained multiple articles (as many as 113). We collated and analyzed information and data across the reviews/meta-analyses to inform this chapter.

Expertise required to implement treatment: Antecedent interventions have been implemented by a variety of individuals, including peers, paraprofessionals, teachers, parents/care providers, and researchers. No implementation difficulties were noted in the reviews/meta-analyses. This suggests that forms of antecedent interventions can be implemented by individuals without training or intervention expertise. However, implementation differs from intervention design, which may require additional skills.

Risks and negative side effects: None of the reviews/meta-analyses noted negative side effects as a result of antecedent interventions. It should be noted, however, that generalization and maintenance may be limited unless antecedent interventions are implemented as part of a multicomponent package, including skill instruction.

Additional considerations and limitations: A large number of antecedent interventions were described in the literature, implemented for a wide range of challenging behaviors, hindering conclusions about the effectiveness of a specific antecedent intervention for a specific targeted behavior. Some reviews/meta-analyses suggested increased effectiveness of antecedent intervention when linked to operant function of challenging behavior and with the inclusion of additional intervention components (e.g., functional communication training).

2.4 Introduction

2.4.1 Intervention Description

Although there are many potential processes that influence behavior (e.g., physiology, systemic practices), the role of environmental events has been well established. A model of environmental determinants that govern challenging (and other) behavior has been described in terms of a four-term contingency. In this equation, setting events or establishing operations (term 1) combine with antecedent events (term 2), which occasion challenging behavior (term 3) that is subject to some type of maintaining consequence, generally reinforcement (term 4). Setting events or establishing operations are events or circumstances that alter the value of reinforcement. These events or circumstances do not directly lead to challenging behavior, but when combined with particular antecedents, increase the likelihood of challenging behavior. Setting events/establishing operations occur either at an earlier time (e.g., lack of sleep) or concurrent with (e.g., noisy environment) the antecedent (expectation to complete a particular task). Antecedent events are stimuli immediately present in the environment that directly occasion challenging behavior. For example, issuing a request to complete a task can promptly result in aggression. The final term of the contingency, maintaining consequences, represents conditions following challenging behavior that reinforce and hence maintain the behavior. Specifically, in the aforementioned example, if the task is withdrawn, aggression will be reinforced, increasing the likelihood it will occur again when the task is requested. Antecedent interventions represent the class of interventions applied to the first two terms of the contingency, setting events/establishing operations and antecedents.

2.4.2 Rationale and Objectives

Historically, interventions to reduce challenging behavior focused on maintaining consequences (term 4), such as exerting punishment to suppress behavior, removing reinforcement for the behavior (extinction), or reinforcing alternative behavior that displaces or supplants challenging behavior. As the field's understanding of the four-term contingency evolved, so did the value of antecedent interventions. That is, the process of functional behavioral assessment (Dunlap et al., 1991; Iwata et al., 1994) heightened our appreciation of the many avenues of intervention that may reduce challenging behavior beyond altering consequences alone. Considering that environmental events can trigger challenging behavior, the use of antecedent interventions has emerged as a powerful approach for resolving behavioral challenges.

The mechanism underlying antecedent and setting event/establishing operation interventions lies in the removal or alteration of the antecedent or setting event/establishing operation that is associated with challenging behavior. For example, the antecedent event of participating in a loud music class might be removed from an individual's schedule. Similarly, the setting event of bright fluorescent lights in the library could be removed by allowing a student to study in a dimly lit classroom. A lengthy task can be altered by chunking, such that portions of the task are completed with embedded breaks.

Kern and Clarke (2021) enumerated four advantages of antecedent interventions. First, they prevent challenging behavior in that they remove or alter the antecedents and/or establishing operations/setting events that occasion that behavior. This obviates the need to encounter challenging behavior in order to apply an aversive consequence. Second, the removal or alteration of antecedents to challenging behavior often results in a rapid reduction of challenging behavior. Third, antecedent interventions can resolve problematic features of the environment, as in the request for work that is beyond an individual's skill set. Finally, the removal or alteration of problematic antecedents and setting events can create a more enjoyable and motivating environment.

2.4.3 Considerations for Implementation

As noted above, antecedent interventions involve removing or altering events that trigger challenging behavior. Sometimes antecedent interventions can be implemented without fully understanding the specific events associated with the challenging behavior, as in the case of behavioral momentum. That is, presenting a series of tasks with high previous compliance increases the likelihood of compliance with a subsequently presented low compliance task, even though little may be known about why the reasons for noncompliance (e.g., task is difficult, lack of clear instruction to complete task, task is repetitive, task is not part of typical schedule). More often, interventions are developed by identifying the events that precede and are associated with challenging behavior. On occasion, these events are evident, as in the situation where an individual reliably engages in self-injury when told to wash dishes. More often, however, events that lead to challenging behavior are far less clear because they may inconsistently occasion challenging behavior, or they entail multiple antecedents and/or establishing operations/setting events. Thus, a functional behavioral assessment is generally required to determine the relative probability that particular events are associated with challenging behavior. As we describe below, research suggests information about behavioral function (i.e., antecedents, maintaining consequences) increases the effectiveness of antecedent interventions.

An additional consideration pertains to setting event/establishing operations. Such events unquestionably play a role in challenging behavior, as we all have familiar experiences of fatigue, hunger, or pain that, when coupled with immediate events (e.g., difficult tasks, failure to reach the doctor by phone), increase the chances of an undesirable reaction. Because internal conditions—like pain and hunger—are not readily observable and their influence on challenging behavior is often less frequent or consistent than antecedents, their influence on challenging behavior is difficult to identify. Further, their role is difficult to determine through experimentation because they are generally more difficult or unethical to manipulate. For instance, pain cannot be programmed in the way that lack of attention or the presentation of a particular task can for the purpose of evaluating its role in challenging behavior. In addition, setting events/establishing operations often need to be self-reported, as in the instance of pain, or presumed, such as the presence of ambient noise. This is particularly challenging for the subset of individuals with ASD who are nonspeaking. Further, setting events/establishing operations are often difficult to precisely identify and characterize. An example is when a certain level of social anxiety makes entering a workplace filled with many employees and customers especially unbearable. These difficulties have resulted in limited research and guidance on the topic.

Another consideration is that best practice suggests that support plans are comprised of multicomponent interventions (Bambara & Kern, 2021). This means that, in addition to antecedent interventions, individuals must learn alternative and appropriate strategies to replace challenging behavior (e.g., politely requesting attention, asking for assistance with a difficult task, presenting a picture card to request a desired item). Response strategies also must be in place to assure challenging behavior is not reinforced. For example, if a child continues to receive attention for screaming, despite an antecedent intervention that provides attention on a predesignated schedule and instruction in how to gain attention using photos of family and staff, then screaming is likely to continue. Below, we describe research to support the value of multicomponent interventions, compared with antecedent only.

A final consideration is whether antecedent interventions should be faded. In some situations, it is appropriate and responsible to maintain the intervention. An example is eliminating work that is too difficult or allowing an individual to use headphones or earplugs in extremely noisy environments. Other times, however, it is important to fade antecedent interventions. Kern and Clarke (2021) posed five considerations for determining whether to fade an antecedent intervention. These include determining whether (a) the altered or eliminated skill is one needed for future success, (b) the intervention will limit participation in inclusive settings, (c) the intervention could be stigmatizing, (d) the individual has a well-established alternative response to replace the challenging behavior, and (e) the individual has learned general skills so that the antecedent event no longer leads to challenging behavior. As we describe below, research provides limited information about maintenance of the effects of antecedent interventions and when and how they should be faded. Nonetheless, fading should be considered in practice.

2.5 Research Background

2.5.1 Search Procedures

To evaluate the state of research on antecedent interventions, we conducted a comprehensive literature search of PsychINFO and ERIC using the search terms (1) "autism" OR "ASD"OR "autism spectrum disorder" OR "PDD-NOS" OR "pervasive developmental disorder" OR "Asperger"; (2) "antecedent based interventions" OR "antecedent-based intervention" OR "antecedent" OR "multicomponent"; and (3) "review" OR "systematic review" OR "Literature review" OR "review of the literature" OR "meta-analysis." This search yielded 206 studies, including 27 literature reviews or meta-analyses. Examination of the reviews/meta-analyses indicated that 20 pertained to both ASD and antecedent interventions. These were used to extract and summarize data and information for the current chapter.

2.5.2 Overview of Studies Identified

The included reviews/meta-analyses indicate an extensive number of research studies have been conducted on antecedent interventions. For example, the reviews included as many as 113 articles containing 263 studies (Ledford et al., 2016). It should be noted, however, that the majority of included studies implemented multicomponent interventions. That is, although all of the studies implemented an antecedent component, other components may have been included, such as an instructional strategy or consequence following challenging behavior. As we will discuss later in this section, this makes it more difficult to parcel out the overall effectiveness of antecedent interventions alone; however, some reviews/meta-analyses evaluate antecedent-only interventions or compared antecedent-only with multicomponent interventions. Publication of the reviews spanned 14 years, with the earliest appearing in 2007 (Machalicek et al.) and the most recent in 2021 (Wei et al.). This suggests enduring interest in antecedent interventions.

Most of the reviews/meta-analyses were focused on the effectiveness of antecedent interventions for a specific target behavior, and a large range was targeted across the reviews/meta-analyses. Behaviors examined in one or more singularly focused review/meta-analysis included aggression, self-injurious behavior, sleep problems, stereotypy, vocal stereotypy, vocal challenging behavior, noncompliance, restricted and repetitive behaviors and interests, social communication skills, transitions, and behavioral variability. Two reviews targeted challenging behavior broadly, one examining challenging behavior in school settings. Other behaviors targeted in studies across the reviews/meta-analyses were a range of social behaviors (e.g., conversation, interactions, initiations and responses, joint attention, social engagement, responses to affective stimuli, answering/asking targeted questions, engaging in trained helping/sympathetic behaviors), on-task behavior, or vocalizations (e.g., mands, intraverbals, phonemes, tacts). Thus, antecedent interventions have been applied for behaviors targeted for both decrease and increase.

Three reviews examined the effectiveness of a particular type of antecedent strategy. These focused on behavioral momentum (Cowan et al., 2017), choice (Howell et al., 2019), and antecedent exercise (Kasner et al., 2012). Numerous other types of antecedent interventions were examined across the reviews. These included, but were not limited to, priming, prompting or cueing, environmental enrichment, interspersal (requests), visual schedule, Social Stories, video-based interventions, advanced warning, response effort manipulation, embedding preferred materials in tasks, scripts, preferred activities or peers during transitions, presession access to reinforcement, noncontingent reinforcement, and modifying events around sleep (e.g., faded bedtime, sleep environment).

2.5.3 Participants

Seventeen of the 20 reviews/meta-analyses described participant age. Participants ranged in age from 2 years old to adulthood (i.e., over age 18). A large majority of studies included younger or school-age children (2–21 years old); however, adults were included in six reviews/meta-analyses. Disability severity also widely ranged, with some described as above average and other as having a severe intellectual disability. These data suggest broad applicability of antecedent interventions, regardless of age and level of functioning.

2.5.4 Design

Almost all of the individual research studies included in the reviews/meta-analyses utilized single-case design methodology. Only four reviews included a limited number of group design studies. Specifically, Ford et al. (2021) included one between-groups design and one pretest/posttest design study, in addition to 10 single-case design studies in their review of antecedent modifications to address sleep problems. Kasner and colleagues (2012) included two group and 10 single-case design studies in their review of antecedent exercise. Among the 60 studies in the Lanovaz et al. (2013) review examining whether interventions that reduced stereotypy also had a collateral effect on other behaviors, three were group designs. Turner and Johnson (2012) reviewed one group and three single-case design studies to examine antecedent interventions for sleep problems. Among the studies employing single-case design methodologies, a variety of designs were used. These included reversal, multielement, multiple baseline, multiple schedule, and a number of variations of these designs.

2.5.5 Interventionist

Approximately half of the reviews/meta-analyses provided information about the interventionist. Three of these examined interventions implemented in school settings. Each of these reviews broadly examined challenging behavior among students with ASD. Specifically, in a meta-analysis conducted by de Bruin et al. (2013) focused on interventions for adolescents and young adults, interventionists were described as school personnel (n = 7) and peers (n = 9 in a single study using trained peers). Machalicek et al. (2007) found that interventionists in studies conducted with students 5–12 years old were both teachers and researchers. Finally, Rivera et al. (2019) examined interventions used with adolescent students. They found that interventionists in most studies were described as teachers (k = 5) and researchers (k = 5), followed by teaching assistants (k = 3) and school personnel (k = 1).

Tullis and colleagues (2015) examined antecedent and other interventions for between-task transitions in both school and community settings. Interventionists were reported as teachers (k = 13), experimenters (k = 6), teaching assistants (k = 2), vocational supervisors (k = 2), caregivers (k = 1), parents (k = 1), and therapists (k = 1). Three additional studies either did not specify the intervention setting or indicated that studies were conducted across settings. Vanderkerken et al. (2013) reported the intervention agent for each participant in their evaluation of strategies to reduce vocal challenging behavior. Interventionists were researchers (n = 32), parents (n = 3), teachers (n = 12), therapists (n = 23), and staff or combination of the aforementioned (n = 4). Wei et al. (2021) evaluated interventions to reduce restricted and repetitive behaviors and interests. Interventionists, summarized by study, were clinicians in 84% of studies ($k = 26$). In the remaining five studies, special education teachers and parents served as interventionists. Wolfe and colleagues (2014) investigated interventions to promote varied social communication. Interventionists were described as researcher or research assistant in 78% ($k = 14$) of studies and as therapist in 22% ($k = 4$) of studies. The broad range of implementors suggests that diverse individuals without extensive intervention expertise can implement antecedent intervention strategies. It should be noted, however, that none of the reviews/meta-analyses described the process of intervention development. Designing or selecting an appropriate antecedent intervention (and multicomponent intervention) unquestionably requires more skill than implementing an intervention, particularly when design includes completing a functional behavioral assessment.

2.5.6 Outcomes

The 20 reviews/meta-analyses summarized the outcomes of the included studies in a variety of ways. Some simply indicated whether studies reported positive outcomes or a functional relationship (Howell et al., 2019). Others calculated the number/percentage of participants or studies that showed improvement (e.g., Brosnan & Healy, 2011). Finally, some reviews calculated effect sizes across the studies (Cowan et al., 2017; Wolfe et al., 2014). About half of the reviews/meta-analyses reported the outcomes of antecedent-based interventions alone, either because only single-component antecedent interventions were included in the review (e.g., review of behavioral momentum) or the authors reported results of the antecedent intervention studies included in their reviews independent of other singular interventions (e.g., consequence-based) or multicomponent interventions. Many studies reported the effects of all interventions, single or multicomponent, collectively. Finally, two studies compared the effect sizes of antecedent interventions with other singular or multicomponent interventions.

Overall, regardless of the strategy used to evaluate outcomes, all of the reviews concluded that antecedent interventions or multicomponent interventions that included antecedent strategies resulted in favorable outcomes. Several reviews (i.e., Machalicek et al., 2007; Martinez et al., 2016; Tullis et al., 2015; Vanderkerken et al., 2013) reported that *all* participants showed favorable outcomes. Among the reviews that reported outcomes across number of participants or number of studies, the authors indicated that the majority of participants or studies resulted in reductions in behaviors targeted for decrease (e.g., aggression, self-injury, sleep problems, stereotypy) as well as improvement in behaviors targeted for increase (e.g., social skills, communication).

Effect sizes were calculated in six reviews, providing more detailed information about the strength of some of the interventions. Four reviews calculated effect sizes for antecedent-only interventions alone. de Bruin et al. (2013) examined school-based interventions for adolescents and young adults (ages 12 to 22 years) that intended to introduce or improve a skill or influence behavior affecting school functioning. Effect sizes of 11 antecedent-only intervention studies that included 23 single-case designs ranged from 0.24 to 0.95, with eight individual effect sizes considered strong, seven moderate, four small, and four negligible. The average weighted effect size was 0.67, which the authors concluded was a "moderately large" overall effect.

In their examination of the effectiveness of behavioral momentum, Cowan et al. (2017) found an overall mean omnibus improvement rate difference (IRD) of 0.8 [CI = 0.74–0.87], indicating a large to very large effect across the studies. Individual studies ranged from 0.45 to 1.0, indicating moderate to very large effect sizes. It should be noted that Cowan et al. did not report behaviors targeted in the studies.

Ledford and colleagues (2016) examined antecedent social skills interventions. Tau-*U* effect sizes were calculated for each of the single-case design studies (over 250) included in 113 articles. Effect sizes ranged from 0 to 1.0. Specifically, 114 studies showed strong effects, 79 showed medium effects, 27 showed weak effects, and 43 demonstrated noneffects. One caveat is that numerous antecedent and combinations of antecedent interventions were included in the analysis, and target behaviors varied widely (i.e., conversation, interactions, initiations, responses, joint attention, social engagement, responses to affective stimuli, answering/asking questions, helping/sympathetic behaviors). Therefore, it is difficult to conclude the specific type of antecedent intervention that is effective and the target behavior for which it is effective. Instead, Ledford et al.'s review should be interpreted as supporting the underlying logic of antecedent intervention (i.e., altering the first two terms in the aforementioned four-term contingency to preclude challenging behavior) as opposed to supporting a specific type set of antecedent intervention procedures.

Finally, Vanderkerken et al. (2013) examined interventions to reduce vocal challenging behavior (e.g., screaming). Among the included studies, 32 participants received an antecedent-only intervention. To ascertain effect size of antecedent interventions, a multilevel analysis was conducted with antecedent interventions used as a moderator. Specifically, antecedent alone interventions were tested against other types of interventions (i.e., consequence and combined). The average effect of antecedent interventions was −1.94, indicating a very large reduction in vocal challenging behavior.

Two reviews/meta-analyses compared the effects of antecedent-only interventions with other interventions. In the aforementioned study, Vanderkerken et al. (2013) compared antecedent-only interventions with consequence-only and combined antecedent and consequence interventions. The effectiveness of antecedent-only interventions was not significantly different from consequence-only interventions; however, combined antecedent and consequence interventions were significantly more effective than either antecedent or consequence alone.

Wei et al. (2021) examined intervention effectiveness for restricted and repetitive patterns of behavior (RRB). Only one difference was identified when comparing antecedent and consequence interventions. The authors concluded that antecedent interventions (e.g., presession access to RRB, noncontingent reinforcement) were not as effective as consequence interventions (e.g., response interruption and redirection, inhibitory stimulus control) for reducing lower order RRB; however, they noted that data analysis methods may play a role in the amount of reduction in stereotypy and that the nature of RRB may also contribute to intervention effectiveness. Specifically, response interruption and redirection appeared to be less effective for individuals with stereotypy that occurred in bouts. Further, rates of RRBs differed at baseline, making comparisons difficult.

2.5.7 Generalization

Data on generalization were mentioned in only eight of the 20 reviews/meta-analyses. In fact, although Brosnan and Healy (2011) did not report data on generalization, they noted that it was rarely included in the studies in their review. This was consistent across the reviews, in that generalization was reported to have been assessed with a small number of participants or in a limited percentage of studies. Specifically, reporting of generalization ranged from 15% of participants in the Erturk et al. (2018) review to 23% of studies in the Martinez et al. (2016) review. Further, none of the reviews included detailed data regarding generalization.

Among the eight studies reporting generalization, only two reviews included antecedent interventions alone or parceled out data for antecedent-only interventions, and specific information was limited. In their review of a variety of antecedent interventions to promote compliance with adult requests, Radley and Dart (2016) noted that one particular procedure, errorless compliance training, resulted in generalization to untrained requests issued by researchers. The authors did not report how many studies described generalization nor did they provide specific data. It also should be noted that generalization of strategy implementation was assessed, not skill generalization among individuals with ASD. Similarly, in an examination of a variety of public school-based interventions implemented with adolescents or young adults, de Bruin et al. (2013) indicated that 13 of the 34 (38%) studies evaluating antecedent interventions included generalization data. They reported only that generalization was "positive" in 11 of the 13 studies.

2.5.8 Maintenance

Twelve reviews/meta-analyses reported information on maintenance. Six indicated only that maintenance data were collected and did not report the results or reported only the duration of time that elapsed between the termination of intervention and assessment of maintenance. Two reviews/meta-analyses assessed maintenance of antecedent-only interventions. Ford et al. (2021) indicated that antecedent modifications to address sleep problems resulted in maintenance of improvements at follow-up for all participants for whom data were collected; however, they did not report the number of participants or articles for which maintenance was assessed. Radley and Dart (2016) reported that 21 of 42 studies examining compliance with adult requests reported maintenance. Four of the 21 studies were conducted with participants with ASD. Intervention effects maintained in all four studies during all follow-up assessments that ranged from 1 week to 6 months post intervention.

The remaining 10 studies using multicomponent interventions resulted in mixed outcomes regarding maintenance. For example, in their review of behavioral interventions designed to reduce aggression among individuals with developmental disabilities, Brosnan and Healy (2011) indicated that four studies provided information on follow-up, and aggression was maintained at low or near zero levels in all. Similarly, Erturk et al. (2018) reviewed interventions to reduce challenging behaviors in school settings. They reported maintenance in two studies. Although not explicitly stated, presumably these were the only two among the included 26 studies that assessed maintenance. They indicated that in one study tantrums among participants either continued to decrease or maintained at 0 levels. In the other study, challenging behaviors continued to decrease, but engagement was similar to intervention. In contrast, de Bruin et al. (2013) reported that among the nine studies assessing maintenance of public school–based interventions for adolescents and young adults, only three reported positive results.

2.5.9 Social Validity

A total of seven of the reviews/meta-analyses reported social validity information. As with generalization and maintenance, limited information was provided. Three of the studies indicated only whether social validity data were collected. One of these (Kasner et al., 2012) reported social validity with respect to Council for Exceptional Children quality indicators (Cook et al., 2014) for each included study. In particular, they coded four dimensions of social validity (i.e., whether the dependent variable was socially important, whether magnitude of change was socially important, whether the independent variable was practical and cost-efficient, and implementation over extended time by typical agents in typical contexts). Among the 10 studies reviewed, all received positive ratings on at least three of the four dimensions. It should be noted, however, that valuative judgments may have been required by the article coders.

Four studies provided some information about social validity outcomes. Three of the four studies evaluated antecedent-only interventions. Ford et al. (2021) indicated that social validity was assessed in six of the 12 studies evaluating antecedent interventions for sleep problems. A variety of assessments were used, and all indicated high levels of satisfaction and acceptability, with the exception of one child who rated the intervention as moderately acceptable. Machalicek et al.

(2007) stated that social validity of interventions to reduce challenging behaviors in school settings, reported in eight studies, was positive. Finally, Turner and Johnson (2012) reported social validity in only one included study, indicating that parents were satisfied with the intervention of scheduled awakenings to address sleep disturbances.

Examining multicomponent school-based interventions to reduce challenging behavior of older students, Rivera et al. (2019) reported that four of their 12 included studies reported social validity. The interventions were rated effective and acceptable by all teachers and school staff.

One caveat in the aforementioned findings is that several authors pointed out that the research largely employed informal assessments. For example, Brosnan and Healy (2011) indicated that only one of 18 studies assessed social validity, and an informal measure was used. This also was the case for Machalicek et al. (2007), who indicated that among the eight studies in their review only one used a formal assessment.

2.5.10 Functional Assessment

Although some antecedent interventions (e.g., behavioral momentum) can be implemented in the absence of a functional behavioral assessment, others (e.g., scheduled attention) require knowledge of the challenging behavior's operant function. Further, it is possible that information about function might facilitate identification of a potentially effective antecedent or multicomponent intervention. Therefore, we were interested in whether information about a functional behavioral assessment was included in the reviews/meta-analyses. Nine studies mentioned function and/or the process to identify function. Erturk et al. (2018) noted that studies were included regardless of whether functional behavioral assessment was conducted, and Lanovaz and Sladeczek (2012) recommended that one be conducted.

The remaining seven reviews/meta-analyses reported the number or percentage of studies and/or participants in which some form of functional behavioral assessment/functional analysis was conducted. They ranged from a low of 9% of studies in the review/meta on interventions for between-task transitions conducted by Tullis et al. (2015) to a high of 92% of participants in the review on behavioral interventions for self-injurious behavior conducted by Erturk et al. (2018).

In their review of interventions for aggression, Brosnan and Healy (2011) reported that 13 of the 18 total studies (2 of 7 studies with antecedent-only strategies) conducted some form of functional assessment. Comparing studies that did to those that did not rely on information about function to select an intervention, the authors noted outcomes were more favorable when function was assessed. Specifically, interventions linked to function resulted in lower rates of challenging behavior, more rapid intervention effects, or more participants who were responsive to intervention. They concluded that variability of intervention effects across studies might be explained, at least in part, by the absence of assessment information.

2.5.11 Discrepant Outcomes

As described above, among the studies that calculated effect sizes of antecedent interventions, most were moderate to strong. However, a relatively small number of studies showed small or no effects. It appears that this might partly be attributable to the topography of targeted behavior (e.g., social skills, lower order restrictive and repetitive patterns of behavior) that may be more challenging to ameliorate. The wide range of intervention procedures also might explain why some studies yielded outcomes that are more favorable. That is, it is unclear whether all antecedent interventions are similarly effective. In addition, as Brosnan and Healy (2011) concluded, perhaps the most important variable explaining discrepancies in outcomes might be the absence of functional assessment information. Finally, although maintenance of intervention effects was seldom assessed, effects maintained in most studies, but not all. Ultimately, these discrepant outcomes suggest the need for more nuanced studies in a number of areas. For example, the circumstances under which a functional behavioral assessment is essential are not yet clear. Also, whether particular antecedent interventions are best matched to specific target behaviors warrants further research.

2.5.12 Quality of Research

Thirteen of the 20 reviews/meta-analyses considered research quality of included studies. One meta-analysis (Vanderkerken et al., 2013), examining psychosocial interventions for reducing vocal challenging behavior, did not report specific findings because they examined study quality as a moderator of intervention effectiveness. Three other reviews/meta-analyses only included studies that met quality indicators. Thus, the 34 multicomponent studies examining public school-based interventions in the de Bruin et al. (2013) meta-analysis (including 11 studies using antecedent-only interventions) met What Works Clearinghouse (WWC; Kratochwill et al., 2010) standards either fully or with reservations. Identical standards were used by Wolfe et al. (2019) in their review of 32 studies of social communication interventions, indicating that 65% met without reservations. Ledford et al. (2016) included antecedent social skills studies that met WWC standards of having at least three data points per phase, a stable or nontherapeutic baseline trend, and evidence of reliability of the depending variable for a minimum of 20% of sessions, resulting in 113 articles containing 263 studies.

Six of the remaining 10 reviews/meta-analyses applied WWC standards while three applied alternative standards. Alternative standards included the Scientific

Merit Rating Scale developed by the National Standards Report (Turner & Johnson, 2012), criteria developed by Reichow et al. (2008) in the study by Ford et al. (2021), and 14 questions for single-case research designed developed by Logan et al. (2008) in Howell et al. (2019).

Among the six studies that applied WWC standards, five reported on antecedent-only interventions. Cowan et al. (2017) reported that four of the 16 (25%) reviews in their meta-analysis on behavioral momentum adequately addressed all 10 of the quality indicators. Martinez et al. (2016) differentiated antecedent intervention quality in their review of school-based interventions. Among the four studies employing antecedent interventions, three met all CEC standards while one did not. Rivera et al. (2019) found that four antecedent school-based intervention studies met WWC standards, four met with reservations, and four did not meet. Reviewing 12 studies on antecedent exercise with self-stimulatory behavior as the dependent variable, Kasner et al. (2012) found that 48% of group experimental design studies and 82% of single-case designs met quality indicators. Finally, Wei et al (2021) reported that all (12 of 12) studies examining interventions for restricted and repetitive patterns of behavior and interests met standards or met standards with reservations. The remaining review examined multicomponent interventions. Erturk et al. (2018) found that among the 46 studies examining interventions to reduce challenging behaviors in school settings, 14 met standards, 19 met standards with reservations, and 12 did not meet standards.

Analyses of quality suggest that a large number of studies employing both antecedent-only interventions and multicomponent interventions were good quality. Still, many did not meet established standards. However, as Kasner et al. (2012) pointed out, several indicators were difficult to interpret and require definitions that are more precise. Further, Cohen et al. (2017) also noted that a large number of studies in their meta-analysis may have failed to meet quality indicators because they were published prior to the recommendations and associated guiding documents (e.g., Cook et al., 2014; Horner et al., 2005; Kratochwill et al., 2013). This was likely the case for all the reviews/meta-analyses and is consistent with findings from other reviews and meta-analyses (Carter & Kern, 2022; Kern et al., in press).

2.6 Practice Implications

2.6.1 Treatment Outcomes

Overall, the research indicates that antecedent interventions are effective for reducing a wide range of challenging behaviors and increasing a small range of desirable behaviors (social skills, engagement). Further, there is research to support the effectiveness of antecedent interventions across all age groups, with studies conducted with preschool age children (i.e., 2 years old) to adults (i.e., over 18). Among the studies that calculated effect sizes, the majority were large, particularly when reduction of challenging behavior was targeted. In contrast, few studies/meta-analyses resulted in small or no effects. Therefore, practitioners can expect a sizeable reduction in challenging behavior following implementation of an antecedent intervention. No reviews/meta-analyses suggested any conditions under which antecedent interventions are contraindicated nor did they mention any side effects.

2.6.2 Practice Implication Guidelines

Several guidelines may assist practitioners when considering implementing antecedent interventions. First, antecedent interventions have been implemented by a variety of individuals, such as paraprofessionals, parents/care providers, and peers. These individuals typically do not have formal intervention training and expertise. This suggests ease of implementation of many antecedent interventions. A consideration, however, is that additional expertise may be required to develop the intervention.

Second, despite their effectiveness, a limited number of research studies showed no or weak effects. The reason for the variability is not clear; however, as suggested by Lanovaz and Sladeczek (2012), antecedent interventions need to be carefully selected. Some studies suggest arbitrary selection, for example to evaluate the effectiveness of a specific antecedent intervention. Intentional effort to identify antecedent interventions matched to contextual variables, such as participant characteristics and preferences, setting parameters, caregiver/interventionist preferences, and behavioral function may render antecedent interventions more effective. It should be noted, however, that research provides little guidance on procedures for designing antecedent interventions. The exception might be matching intervention to behavioral function (e.g., Bambara & Kern, 2021).

Third, as noted above, antecedent interventions are likely to be more effective if intervention is linked to the results of a functional behavioral assessment. Although this recommendation relies on comparative data from a single study (Brosnan & Healy, 2011), it aligns conceptually with the logic of antecedent interventions and is consistent with findings from meta-analyses of consequence-based interventions (e.g., Hurl et al., 2015). That is, prevention of challenging behavior requires alteration of the variables that trigger those behaviors, most readily identified through assessment of function.

Fourth, many studies in our review implemented multicomponent interventions. One study (Vanderkerken et al., 2013) compared antecedent-only interventions with consequence-only interventions as well as combined antecedent and consequence interventions, experimentally revealing the advantage of multicomponent interventions. Again, comparative research is limited, but multicomponent interventions are consistent with best practice, in which antecedent environmental modifications are combined with interventions that teach replacement and adaptive behaviors and also assure that responses do not reinforce challenging behavior (Bambara & Kern, 2021).

Finally, generalization and maintenance data are limited. Almost no studies examined generalization. Most studies assessed continued improvements after intervention ended, but not all. Practitioners should determine whether the interventions should be faded, considering criteria suggested by Kern and Clarke (2021), as noted above. This includes (a) future need for the skill, (b) whether the intervention will limit participation in inclusive settings, (c) potential stigma of the intervention, (d) the participant's alternative responses that replace the challenging behavior, and (e) increases in general skills that have reduced triggers. If fading is needed, data should be collected and closely monitored to assure challenging behaviors continue to decline or maintained at low and acceptable rates.

2.7 References

**Denotes literature reviews and meta-analyses used in review.*

Bambara, L. M., & Kern, L. (Eds.) (2021). *Individualized supports for students with problem behavior.* Baltimore, MD: Paul H. Brookes.

*Brosnan, J., & Healy, O. (2011). A review of behavioral interventions for the treatment of aggression in individuals with developmental disabilities. *Research in Developmental Disabilities, 32*, 437–446. https://doi.org/10.1016/j.ridd.2010.12.023

*de Bruin, C. L., Deppeler, J. M., Moore, D. W., & Diamond, N. T. (2013). Public school-based interventions for adolescents and young adults with an autism spectrum disorder: A meta-analysis. *Review of Educational Research, 83*(4), 521–550. https://doi.org/10.3102/0034654313498621

Carter, D., & Kern, L. (January, 2022). The color of evidence-based practices for students with emotional and behavioral problems: A systematic review. Presented at the Conference for Exceptional Children, Orlando, FL.

Cook, B., Buysse, V., Klingner, J., Landrum, T., McWilliam, R., Tankersley, M., & Test, D. (2014). Council for Exceptional Children: Standards for evidence-based practices in special education. *Teaching Exceptional Children, 46*(6), 206.

*Cowan, R. J., Abel, L., & Candel, L. (2017). A meta-analysis of single-subject research on behavioral momentum to enhance success in students with autism. *Journal of Autism and Developmental Disorders, 47*, 1464–1477. https://doi.org/10.1007/s10803-017-3076-6

Dunlap, G., Kern L., Clarke, S., & Robbins, F. R. (1991). Functional assessment, curricular revision, and severe behavior problems. *Journal of Applied Behavior Analysis, 24*, 387–397.

*Erturk, B., Machalicek, W., & Drew, C. (2018). Self-injurious behavior in children with developmental disabilities: A systematic review of behavioral intervention literature. *Behavior Modification, 42*(4), 498–542. https://doi.org/10.1177/0145445517741474

*Ford, K. A. M., McLay, L. K., France, K. G., Blampied, N. M., & Gibbs, R. M. (2022). Systematic review of the effect of modification of antecedents in the treatment of sleep problems among children on the autism spectrum. *Advances in Neurodevelopmental Disorders.*, 6, 253-269.https://doi.org/10.1007/s41252-021-00224-8

Horner, R. H., Carr, E. G., Halle, J., McGee, G., Odom, S., & Wolery, M. (2005). The use of single-subject research to identify evidence-based practice in special education. *Exceptional Children, 71*(2), 165–179.

*Howell, M., Dounavi, K., & Storey, C. (2019). To choose or not to choose? A systematic literature review considering the effects of antecedent and consequence choice upon on-task and problem behavior. *Review Journal of Autism and Developmental Disorders, 6*, 63–84. https://doi.org/10.1007/s40489-018-00154-7

Hurl, K., Wightman, J., Haynes, S. N., & Virues-Ortega, J. (2015). Does a pre-intervention functional assessment increase intervention effectiveness? A meta-analysis of within-subject interrupted time-series studies. *Clinical Psychology Review*, *47*, 71–84. https://doi.org/10.1016/j.cpr.2016.05.003

Iwata, B. A., Dorsey, M. F., Slifer, K. J., Bauman, K. E., & Richman, G. S. (1994). Toward a functional analysis of self-injury. *Journal of Applied Behavior Analysis*, *27*(2), 197–209.

*Kasner, M., Reid, G., & MacDonald, C. (2012). Evidence-based practice: Quality indicator analysis of antecedent exercise in autism spectrum disorders. *Research in Autism Spectrum Disorders*, *6*, 1418–1425. https://doi.org/10.1016/j.rasd.2012.02.001

Kern, L., & Clarke, S. (2021). Antecedent and setting event interventions. In L. M. Bambara & L. Kern (Eds.), *Individualized supports for students with problem behavior* (pp. 280–320). Baltimore, MD: Paul H. Brookes.

Kern, L., Kelly, S., Rosati, S.A., Shera, S., Fluharty, M., Gabrilowitz, R., Carter, D., Liang, C. T. H., & Freeman, J. (2023). College and career readiness interventions for students with or at-risk for emotional and behavioral disorders. *Career Development and Transition for Exceptional Individuals*, *46*(3), 155–168.

Kratochwill, T. R., Hitchcock, J., Horner, R. H., Levin, J. R., Odom, S. L., Rindskopf, D. M. & Shadish, W. R. (2010). Single-case designs technical documentation. Retrieved from What Works Clearinghouse website: http://ies.ed.gov/ncee/wwc/pdf/wwc_scd.pdf.

Kratochwill, T. R., Hitchcock, J. H., Horner, R. H., Levin, J. R., Odom, S. L., Rindskopf, D. M., & Shadish, W. R. (2013). Single-case intervention research design standards. *Remedial and Special Education*, *34*(1), 26–38. https://doi.org/10.1177/0741932512452794

*Lanovaz, M. J., Robertson, K. M., Soerono, K., & Watkins, N. (2013). Effects of reducing stereotypy on other behaviors: A systematic review. *Research in Autism Spectrum Disorders*, *7*, 1234–1243. http://dx.doi.org/10.1016/j.rasd.2013.07.009

*Lanovaz, M. J., & Sladeczek, I. E. (2012). Vocal stereotypy in individuals with autism spectrum disorders: A review of behavioral interventions. *Behavior Modification*, *36*(2), 146–164. https://doi.org/10.1177/0145445511427192

*Ledford, J. R., King, S., Harbin, E. R., & Zimmerman, K. N. (2016). Antecedent social skills interventions for individuals with ASD: What works, for whom, and under what conditions? *Focus on Autism and Other Developmental Disabilities*, *33*(1), 3–13. https://doi.org/10.1177/1088357616634024

Logan, L. R., Hickman, R. R., Harris, S. R., & Heriza, C. B. (2008). Single-subject research design: Recommendations for levels of evidence and quality rating. *Developmental Medicine & Child Neurology*, *50*(2), 99–103. https://doi.org/10.1111/j.1469-8749.2007.02005.x

*Machalicek, W., O'Reilly, M. F., Beretvas, N., Sigafoos, J., & Lancioni, G. E. (2007). A review of interventions to reduce challenging behavior in school settings for students with autism spectrum disorders. *Research in Autism Spectrum Disorders*, *1*(3), 229–246. https://doi.org/10.1016/j.rasd.2006.10.005

*Martinez, J. R., Werch, B. L., & Conroy, M. A. (2016). School-based interventions targeting challenging behaviors exhibited by young children with autism spectrum disorder: A systematic literature review. *Education and Training in Autism and Developmental Disabilities*, *51*(3), 265–280. http://www.jstor.org/stable/24827523

*Radley, K. C., & Dart, E. H. (2016). Antecedent strategies to promote children's and adolescents' compliance with adult requests: A review of the literature. *Clinical Child and Family Psychology Review*, *19*, 39–54. https://doi.org/10.1007/s10567-015-0197-3

Reichow, B., Volkmar, F. R., & Cicchetti, D. V. (2008). Development of the evaluative method for evaluating and determining evidence-based practices in autism. *Journal of Autism and Developmental Disorders*, *38*(7), 1311–1319. https://doi.org/10.1007/s10803-007-0517-7

*Rivera, G., Gerow, S., & Kirkpatrick, M. (2019). A review of school-based interventions to reduce challenging behavior for adolescents with ASD. *Journal of Developmental and Physical Disabilities*, *31*, 1–21. https://doi.org/10.1007/s10882-018-9626-9

*Tullis, C. A., Cannella-Malone, H. L., & Payne, D. O. (2015). Literature review of interventions for between-task transitioning for individuals with intellectual and developmental disabilities including autism spectrum disorders. *Review Journal of Autism and Developmental Disabilities*, *2*, 91–102. https://doi.org/10.1007/s40489-014-0039-0

*Turner, K. S., & Johnson, C. R. (2012). Behavioral interventions to address sleep disturbances in children with autism spectrum disorders: A review. *Topics in Early Childhood Special Education*, *33*(3), 144–152.

*Vanderkerken, L., Heyvaert, M., Maes, B., & Onghena, P. (2013). Psychosocial interventions for reducing vocal challenging behavior in persons with autistic disorder: A multilevel meta-analysis of single-based experiments. *Research in Developmental Disabilities, 34*(12), 4515–4533. https://doi.org/10.1016/j.ridd.2013.09.030

*Wei, Q., Machalicek, W., Crowe, B., Kunze, M., & Rispoli, M. (2021). Restricted and repetitive patterns of behavior and interests in children with autism spectrum disorder: A systematic review of behavioral interventions. *Education and Training in Autism and Developmental Disabilities, 56*(2), 115–139.

*Wolfe, K., Pound, S., McCammon, M. N., Chezan, L. C., & Drasgow, E. (2019). A systematic review of interventions to promote varied social-communication behavior in individuals with autism spectrum disorder. *Behavior Modification, 43*(6), 790–818. https://doi.org/10.1177/0145445519859803

*Wolfe, K., Slocum, T. A., & Kunnavatana, S. S. (2014). Promoting behavioral variability in individuals with autism spectrum disorders: A literature review. *Focus on Autism and Other Developmental Disabilities, 29*(3), 180–190. https://doi.org/10.1177/1088357614525661

3

Differential Schedules of Reinforcement

Charlene N. Agnew
SUNY Upstate Medical University

Mirela Cengher
University of Maryland, Baltimore County

Henry Roane
SUNY Upstate Medical University

3.1 Technical Abstract

Background: Differential reinforcement refers to a specific approach to intervention based on operant conditioning that involves programming two reinforcement contingencies. When implementing differential reinforcement, clinicians program a better quality, higher magnitude, or denser schedule of reinforcement for behaviors targeted for an increase as compared to behaviors targeted for reduction. **Method:** The National Standards Project (2015) review of empirically supported interventions for individuals with autism as well as systematic reviews and recent single-case design studies focused on differential reinforcement were used to inform this chapter. **Results:** Differential reinforcement has been used to effectively increase and decrease numerous types of target behavior (e.g., language, making choices, sports) and has been found beneficial across populations (e.g., individuals with autism with low to high support needs), ages (e.g., early childhood to adulthood), and settings (e.g., clinics, schools, home or residential centers). **Discussion:** Differential reinforcement is a flexible approach to intervention that should be individualized based on behavioral assessment and implemented by a qualified practitioner or well-trained caregiver.

3.2 Layperson Summary

Differential reinforcement procedures are at the core of most clinical interventions designed to change behavior. Differential reinforcement schedules can increase or decrease behavior in terms dimensions such as frequency, duration, and variability. There are many variations of simple differential reinforcement procedures that allow clinicians to tailor intervention to individual client's needs. Further, there are specialized approaches that allow clinicians to fade reinforcement to

Charlene N. Agnew, Mirela Cengher, and Henry Roane, *Differential Schedules of Reinforcement*. In: *Lifespan Treatment for Autistic Individuals*. Edited by: Peter Sturmey, Russell Lang, and James K. Luiselli, Oxford University Press.
© Oxford University Press (2025). DOI: 10.1093/oso/9780197635841.003.0003

practical levels, which is crucial for the maintenance of desirable outcomes in real-world environments. Expert clinicians design interventions that prevent or mitigate problematic interactive effects. When interventions that entail differential reinforcement schedules are not implemented as prescribed (i.e., poor treatment integrity), there is a high risk that the desired change in behavior will not occur. Some treatment integrity failures result in relapse and resurgence of previously reduced problem behavior. We provide recommendations to maintain high levels of treatment integrity, which in turn should minimize the risk of relapse and resurgence.

3.3 Treatment Summary Table

Treatment summary: Differential Reinforcement

Treatment description: Choice and reinforcement are the key ingredients to differential reinforcement. When implementing differential reinforcement, clinicians arrange reinforcement contingencies that are better quality, higher magnitude, or a denser schedule of reinforcement for behaviors targeted for an increase as compared to behaviors targeted for reduction (Johnson et al., 2017).

Expected outcomes: Differential reinforcement procedures produce better clinical outcomes as compared to interventions that program identical reinforcers for desirable and undesirable behaviors (Hausman et al., 2014; Karsten & Carr, 2009; Olenick & Pear, 1980; Touchette & Howard, 1984). Differential reinforcement has two effects: (1) increasing desirable target behaviors, and (2) reducing behaviors that limit a person's independence or quality of life (i.e., problematic behaviors). Change in frequency or rate of behaviors, duration, latency, topography, interresponse time, or intensity of behaviors can be achieved.

Methods: To appraise the evidence base related to differential reinforcement, we considered the findings of the National Standards Project (National Autism Center, 2015) that identified 13 interventions with empirical support for individuals with autism spectrum disorder (ASD). Results of recent single-case design research as well as systematic reviews of the literature also informed this chapter (e.g., Petscher et al., 2009).

Expertise required to implement treatment: Differential reinforcement interventions should be individualized and designed by a behavior analyst with board certification in behavior analysis (BCBA). Parents, teachers, and other caregivers have been taught to successfully implement differential reinforcement, but they should do so with the support of a qualified professional.

Risks and negative side effects: When differential reinforcement involves extinction, there is a risk of temporary increase in behavior targeted for reduction. However, this risk is substantially mitigated with the inclusion of sufficiently powerful reinforcement contingencies for the behavior targeted for increase. When differential reinforcement schedules are not implemented as prescribed (i.e., poor treatment integrity), there is a high risk that the desired change in behavior will not occur. Treatment integrity failures can result in relapse and resurgence of problem behavior.

Additional considerations and limitations: Ongoing data collection and progress monitoring is essential to ensuring safe, successful, and sustained behavior change.

3.4 Introduction

3.4.1 History and Key Concepts

Nearly 100 years ago, Skinner made the groundbreaking observation that behavior is sensitive to environmental variables (Skinner, 1938). This process, called *operant selection* or *selection by consequences*, was a parallel to natural selection coined by Darwin and Kebler (1859) in that both emphasize that the organism's behaviors and other features change as a function of environmental variables. These changes increase the organism's adaptability to the environment and, implicitly, chances of survival. Operant and natural selection differ in their level of analysis; operant selection describes learning that occurs during an individual's life (i.e., ontogeny), whereas natural selection describes learning that occurs across generations within the same species (i.e., phylogeny). The concept of operant selection is a synonym for behavior change; therefore, from a clinical standpoint, operant selection opened the door for therapeutic intervention.

Consequences are at the forefront of operant selection and, implicitly, therapeutic intervention. Consequences can have one of three effects on behavior: no change, increase in the strength of the behavior, or decrease in the strength of the behavior. The consequences that strengthen behavior are called *reinforcers*. Behaviors can be reinforced by the introduction or removal of stimuli. *Positive reinforcement* occurs when behavior results in access to appetitive, preferred stimuli; as a result, behavior increases in strength. For example, a child may cry and, as a result, receive comfort from the caregiver. In the future, the child may be more likely to cry to access comfort, suggesting that the caregiver's attention functions as a positive reinforcer. *Negative reinforcement* occurs when behavior results in the removal, postponement, or avoidance of an aversive stimulus; as a result, the behavior increases in strength. For example, a child may cry while asked to do homework and, as a result, the caregiver provides a break. In the future, the child may be more likely to cry when asked to do homework, which will result in postponement or removal of the demand. In this scenario, the removal of the demand functions as a negative reinforcer. Most behaviors that one has learned, from the most simple to the most complex, are due to positive and negative reinforcement. Additional detail regarding reinforcement as it relates to prompting strategies (e.g., errorless learning) is provided in Chapter 4 of this text.

Selection by consequences heavily influences the choices we make. Specifically, most individuals have multiple options to choose from at all times; for example, you could choose to continue reading this chapter, watch TV, or text your friends. All other things being equal, the choice you make is a function of what is most reinforcing at the moment. We sometimes choose among different behaviors that result in different reinforcers, as in the example above, and sometimes between different behaviors that result in the same reinforcer. The behaviors that result in the same consequence are called a *response class*. For example, you can turn on a switch, ask your roommate, or ask a voice-activated device (e.g., Alexa©) to turn on the lamp. All other things being equal, the choice you make is a function of which behavior(s) have a longer or more consistent history of reinforcement.

Choice and reinforcement are the key ingredients to differential reinforcement. When implementing differential reinforcement, clinicians program a better quality, higher magnitude, or denser schedule of reinforcement for some behaviors as compared to others (Johnson et al., 2017). For example, assume that a child can ask or can throw a tantrum to get their caregiver to buy preferred snacks from the grocery store. To increase the frequency of desirable behavior and reduce unwanted behavior, the caregiver could implement a differential-reinforcement procedure whereby asking for snacks results in reinforcement and tantrums no longer do (i.e., extinction). When implemented consistently and correctly, this procedure will have two effects: increase the frequency of appropriate requests for snacks, and reduce the frequency of tantrums.

Differential reinforcement procedures are commonly applied to change the frequency or rate of behaviors, such as in the example above; however, all dimensions of behavior are amenable to change. As such, clinicians can implement differential reinforcement procedures to change the duration, latency, topography, interresponse time, or intensity of behaviors. Clinicians should consider the dimension(s) of the behavior that would benefit most from behavior change. For example, it could be that a child responds when asked questions in class, but that their latency to respond is very long. A clinician could differentially reinforce shorter latencies and gradually change the criterion for reinforcement to shorter and shorter latencies until the child responds in time to benefit from natural contingencies of responding to questions.

Generally, differential reinforcement procedures produce better clinical outcomes as compared to nondifferential reinforcement procedures (i.e., those that program identical reinforcers for desirable and undesirable behaviors; Hausman et al., 2014; Kasten & Carr, 2009; Olenick & Pear, 1980; Touchette & Howard, 1984). Because there are at least three variables that can be manipulated when designing differential reinforcement schedules—schedule, magnitude, or quality of reinforcement—it is important to know which one(s) is better, in what context(s), and why. Researchers arrange reinforcers that are more frequent, in larger quantities, or of better quality following desirable behaviors as compared to the reinforcers programmed for the undesirable behaviors. An example of a schedule of reinforcement manipulation is providing snacks every time a child asks for them (i.e., continuous schedule of reinforcement) and withholding snacks when they tantrum (i.e., extinction). An example of quality manipulation is providing the most preferred snack when the child asks for one and providing the least preferred snack when they tantrum. An example of magnitude manipulation is providing an entire pack of chips when the child asks for it and providing only one chip when they tantrum. Researchers compared these different arrangements in several studies and found that all are effective when teaching new skills. However, efficiency outcomes were variable across participants (Boudreau et al.,

2015; Campanaro et al., 2020; Cividini-Motta & Ahearn, 2013; Fiske et al., 2014; Johnson et al., 2017). The variability in outcomes across participants suggests that the most efficient differential reinforcement procedure is learner specific; as such, clinicians should develop individualized assessments to identify the optimal procedure for each learner (for a tutorial on developing individualized assessments of instructional arrangements, see Kodak & Halbur, 2021).

When used as an intervention component, differential reinforcement procedures can be implemented from the onset of intervention or at a later point. Campanaro et al. (2020) compared immediate, early, and late onset of differential reinforcement on skill acquisition in children with ASD. Across conditions, differential reinforcement was introduced from the onset of intervention (immediate), when the participants demonstrated 33% correct responding for two consecutive sessions (early), and when the participants demonstrated 50% correct responding for two consecutive sessions (late). The authors compared these conditions across two different dependent variables for each of the three participants, yielding a total of six comparisons. The immediate onset condition produced the most efficient acquisition of behavior for six of seven comparisons.

Virtually all skill acquisition and behavior reduction goals for individuals with intellectual and developmental disabilities include some form of differential reinforcement procedures. In research targeting skill acquisition, experimenters typically select a clinical goal and outcome, such as teaching a child to label six common objects in the environment. Then, experimenters develop teaching procedures that consist of a combination of differential reinforcement and prompting procedures. For example, Hanney et al. (2019) taught participants to label auditory stimuli. On each trial presentation, the experimenter asked the participant "What do you hear?" and then immediately presented an auditory stimulus (e.g., the sound of a siren). The participant had 3 seconds to respond. If the participant responded correctly and independently, the experimenter provided enthusiastic praise and access to a preferred stimulus for 30 seconds. If the participant did not respond within 3 seconds or responded incorrectly, the experimenter provided a prompt (i.e., also called error correction) and, contingent on a prompted response, provided enthusiastic praise. Therefore, participants were exposed to a differential reinforcement schedule whereby they received praise and access to preferred stimuli for correct independent responses, and praise only for responses following error correction. Under these arrangements, both participants learned how to label auditory stimuli.

In research targeting behavior reduction, experimenters begin by conducting a functional behavior assessment to identify the reason(s) why participants demonstrate problematic behavior. Problematic behavior can take many forms, such as aggression, self-injury, or property destruction. Once function(s) for problematic behavior are identified, experimenters develop function-based, individualized interventions. These interventions typically consist of teaching a functional communication response to replace problematic behavior. This response serves the same function as problematic behavior (i.e., is part of the same response class) and is socially acceptable. For example, Cengher et al. (2022) conducted a functional assessment that confirmed that participants' problematic behavior was maintained by escape from attention (also called social avoidance in the literature). Then, the experimenter implemented functional communication training to teach the participant to ask to be left alone when others were present. Concurrently, the experimenter placed problematic behavior on extinction by no longer leaving the participants alone when it occurred. This differential reinforcement procedure increased the frequency of appropriate communication and decreased problematic behavior.

In many differential reinforcement procedures for behavior reduction, such as the one described above, one of the key components is extinction for problematic behavior. Extinction is highly effective in reducing behavior; however, it can result in temporary unwanted effects when it is first introduced. These effects are called *extinction burst* and consist of a temporary increase in the frequency, magnitude, and duration of problematic behavior. In addition, novel forms of problematic behavior may emerge during the extinction burst; for example, a child who never bit before may demonstrate biting (Lloveras et al., 2022). When extinction is implemented consistently and correctly, the extinction burst is followed by a rapid suppression of problematic behavior; however, extinction cannot be implemented safely with all participants, in all environments, and by all intervention agents (Vollmer et al., 2020). In addition, some question the ethics of implementing extinction (e.g., Rajaraman & Austin, 2022). As such, depending on the individual circumstances surrounding each case, clinicians may choose to design a differential reinforcement procedure that does not entail extinction. For example, Athens and Vollmer (2010) manipulated the duration, magnitude, and quality of reinforcement for functional communication while continuing to reinforce problematic behavior. The authors found that participants were sensitive to manipulation of all of these three variables in isolation, but the greatest magnitude of behavior change was observed when the functional communication response resulted in consequences that encapsulated all of these variables (i.e., greater duration, magnitude, and quality). Another recent approach consists of the enhanced choice model; for example, Rajaraman et al. (2022) allowed participants to choose among (a) treatment that consisted of differential reinforcement, (b) noncontingent access to reinforcers (without adult attention), and (c) leave the therapeutic space. Participants reliably chose treatment, which increased functional communication and a decrease in problematic behavior.

3.5 Research Background

The effectiveness of differential reinforcement procedures has been demonstrated across numerous dependent variables (e.g., language, making choices, playing tennis; Buzas & Ayllon, 1981; Karsina et al., 2011; Johnson et al., 2017), populations (e.g., individuals with autism, college students, adult employees;

Campanaro et al., 2020; Eikenhout & Austin, 2005; Karsina et al., 2011), and settings (e.g., clinics, schools, home or residential centers; Cengher et al., 2022; Meyer, 1999; O'Reilly, 1995). Indeed, of the 13 interventions identified as benefitting from empirical support for individuals with ASD by National Standards Project (2015), almost all of them include a differential reinforcement procedure as part of the treatment package (see also Petscher et al., 2009). In what follows, we will describe variations of these procedures and their clinical benefit.

3.5 Practice Implications

3.5.1 Simple Differential Schedules of Reinforcement

Differential reinforcement schedules entail concurrent arrangements, whereby the learner can choose how to allocate their responses between two or more options, each associated with a different schedule of reinforcement. Most of these schedules of reinforcement are applied to increase the strength of desirable response(s) (e.g., communication) while decreasing the strength of others (e.g., problematic behavior). Typically, clinicians program positive reinforcers when designing these schedules; however, all procedures described in this chapter are amendable to negative reinforcement contingencies as well.

Differential reinforcement procedures begin with the identification of the target behavior to be decreased and an appropriate data collection system for tracking changes. Depending on the type of differential reinforcement procedure selected, choices need to be made regarding variations of treatment. Each of these variations has benefits and costs and will be informed by the individual's characteristics and the context in which they behave.

Defining behavior in a way that facilitates objective and reliable data collection is key to ensuring that we can evaluate the effectiveness of the differential reinforcement treatment. Although differential reinforcement treatments are supported by a large body of research, a poorly designed or implemented treatment may not be effective. Data collection allows us to identify when a differential reinforcement treatment is not working and make modifications to increase effectiveness.

3.5.2 Differential Reinforcement of Alternative Behavior (DRA)

DRA is a behavior reduction procedure involving an alternative behavior that is within the same response class as the challenging behavior (i.e., that serves the same function for the individual). As the goal is to reduce behavior, as described earlier in this chapter, functional behavior assessments are used to identify maintaining reinforcement contingencies. Without knowing the function of behavior, it would be difficult to identify the appropriate alternative behavior to teach. For example, we might deduce that Mari is throwing tantrums because it is the most effective way for her to get adults to rush over and pay attention to her. However, it is possible that tantrums also occur when Mari is asked to complete math worksheets or sit for circle time. Likewise, tantrums may occur to get her access to a "calm down" corner filled with all of her favorite sensory items. After functional behavior assessment has been completed, treatment can begin.

Although it can be tempting for some to prevent Mari from accessing this same reinforcer (after all, it may be desirable for Mari to participate in circle time, be able to work on her own without adult attention, or spend less time in the sensory area), it is important to emphasize at this time that the goal is to help the individual learn how to meet their own needs and ask for what they want in a way that will be less dangerous to themselves and others, and that will be more adaptive. As treatment progresses, the individual can learn other skills such as participating in circle time or working independently.

After an alternative behavior has been identified, it is important to decide how that response will be taught. Considerations include what types of prompts should be used and how your learner's current behavior will align with the teaching procedure. For example, do they easily imitate vocal or verbal words and sounds, or do they follow peer models? You will also want to determine an appropriate reinforcement schedule for contingent delivery of preferred items. When first implementing the schedule, aim for a very rich schedule of reinforcement (Hanley & Tiger, 2011) to make it easier for your learner to get what they want by using the alternative behavior and more difficult to do so using the challenging behavior. Over time, the reinforcement schedule is thinned, or decreased, so that the individual learns to tolerate times when they do not get what they want.

3.5.3 Differential Reinforcement of Other Behavior (DRO)

Another procedural variation is DRO or omission training. DRO is similar to DRA in that both procedures are intended to decrease a target behavior, but DRO does not specify an alternative behavior that is reinforced. Instead, reinforcers are delivered after the passage of a predetermined interval when the target behavior is absent (Reynolds, 1961). Generally, that interval is selected based on the interval of time the child can refrain from engaging in challenging behavior. For example, if a child is currently able to refrain from calling out in class for approximately 5.5 minutes, one may provide tokens every 5 minutes that a child does not call out in class and then increase this duration requirement throughout treatment. Although the full mechanisms that are responsible for behavior reductions seen when DRO procedures are implemented are yet unknown, DRO is useful for behaviors maintained by consequences that are difficult to identify or control, or to weaken excess behavior (Jessel et al., 2015).

Technically, DRO does not require the assessment of the function of the target behavior. For example, let's assume that Errol's problem behavior is maintained by attention from adults. One could implement a DRO procedure where the reinforcer for the absence of problem behavior consists of access to the iPad (i.e., nonfunctional reinforcer) or one where the reinforcer for the absence of problem behavior consists of attention (i.e., functional reinforcer). Austin et al. (2015) found that both variations described above work, but that using the functional reinforcer increases the effectiveness of training. In addition, DRO treatments are aimed to reduce problematic behavior; however, because reinforcers are provided on a time-based schedule, it is plausible to assume that other behaviors are superstitiously reinforced. Indeed, Jessel et al. (2015) found that effect in a basic study. In clinical practice, we recommend measuring other desirable and undesirable behaviors to ensure treatment procedures do not incidentally increase other undesirable behaviors.

Jessel and Ingvarsson (2016) described several other components of DRO treatments that can be varied. A therapist can reset the interval if the target behavior occurs within the time, or not. For example, assume that Amy receives a reinforcer every 10 minutes that she does not swear. If she happened to swear during the 10-minute interval, one could reset the interval and only provide reinforcers if Amy does not swear by the completion of the next interval. In the latter example, if Amy swore during the interval, the therapist would let the time elapse, not provide any reinforcers at the end of it, and then begin a new interval with a new opportunity for reinforcement. Further, the therapist could schedule reinforcers using fixed intervals (e.g., every 10 minutes), or variable intervals (e.g., after 7 minutes, 12 minutes, 15 minutes, and 7 minutes; where the average is 10 minutes). Another component that can be varied is how behavior is tracked; specifically, one could provide reinforcers if the target behavior does not happen only at the end of the interval (i.e., momentary time sampling), or throughout the interval (i.e., whole interval time sampling). For example, say that the therapist set a 10-minute fixed interval DRO. The therapist could reinforce Amy's absence of swearing if she does not swear at the end of 10 minutes or throughout the 10-minute interval. Finally, clinicians could consider providing instructions or signals. Research shows that signals associated with each schedule make them more effective in changing behavior (Becraft et al., 2018). However, while generally instructions increase the effectiveness of a schedule, with a momentary time sampling, a child may learn to omit the undesirable behavior only at the end of the interval.

3.5.4 Differential Reinforcement of Low or High Rates of Behavior (DRL/DRH)

Some behaviors are not problematic in and of themselves, but their frequency can be. For example, teachers typically want their students to participate in class, but only to some degree. When students participate too frequently or too infrequently, there is a need for intervention. This is where DRL or DRH schedules come in place. DRL schedules are meant to reduce behaviors to a practical level, without eliminating them. For example, Austin and Bevan (2011) implemented a DRL schedule to reduce children's rate of requests for attention in a classroom. The DRL schedule consisted of providing a reinforcer if requests for attention occurred less than a predetermined number of times in a given time interval. The intervention was successful at reducing rates of requests for attention in children, and teachers rated the intervention highly as well, suggesting it had good social validity.

There are two variations of DRL schedules: *full session* and *spaced responding*. In full-session DRL, a reinforcer is provided if the target behavior occurs less than a predetermined number of times in a given time interval. For example, the reinforcer is provided if requests for attention occur less than 3 times in 15 minutes. In the spaced-responding DRL, the reinforcer is provided if a predetermined interresponse time occurs in between behaviors. For example, the clinician could provide the reinforcer if a child requests attention every 5 minutes, at a minimum. Jessel and Borrero (2014) compared these two DRL procedures and found that full-session DRL has the potential to eliminate behavior, whereas the spaced-responding DRL procedure does not. As such, if the goal is to reduce but not eliminate behavior, implementation of spaced-responding DRL is desirable as compared to full-session DRL.

DRH is used when the goal is to increase the frequency of behavior. For example, Girolami et al. (2009) noted that a common problem in feeding interventions is that children feed themselves too slowly, which in turn can affect caregivers' adherence to treatment. As such, the authors implemented a DRH schedule, which increased the pace of self-feeding and decreased the overall duration of mealtime.

3.5.5 Differential Reinforcement of Incompatible Behavior (DRI)

DRI can also be used to decrease challenging behaviors (e.g., Young & Wincze, 1974). Incompatible behaviors cannot co-occur; therefore, this procedure can maximize the odds that the challenging behaviors are reduced or eliminated. As such, the use of incompatible behaviors in differential reinforcement treatments can make intuitive sense to practitioners and parents. For example, a teacher may not want their students to wander in the class and would instead prefer that they sit in their seats. As long as sitting is occurring, walking cannot physically occur simultaneously. However, although these behaviors are topographically incompatible, they are not necessarily functionally related. In one early study, Smith (1987) taught an individual with pica to engage in incompatible behaviors such as working with his hands and keeping his mouth clear to access arbitrary reinforcers such as praise, food, drink, or activities. While this successfully reduced consumption of nonfood items for this individual, practitioners considering this approach may also wish to select the incompatible response carefully to ensure that they do not select a behavior that is also incompatible with other functional skills.

3.5.6 Lag Schedules of Reinforcement

Response variability is an important characteristic of behavior that can be supported by schedules of reinforcement (Lee et al., 2007). A lag schedule of reinforcement programs reinforcers for a response, or response chain, if it differs from a predetermined number of responses. Such schedules of reinforcement can be useful for clinical populations, such as individuals with developmental disabilities, who show restrictive patterns of behavior (e.g., restrictive and repetitive play or language; Galizio et al., 2020). For example, Baruni et al. (2014) implemented a lag schedule to promote play variability in children with ASD who, before the intervention, demonstrated restricted play skills. Initially, the authors implemented a lag 1 schedule, whereby each play action was reinforced if it differed from the one before. This intervention resulted in an increase in play variability across participants. Then, the authors implemented a lag 2 schedule, whereby each play action was reinforced if it was different from the two play actions emitted before. This intervention increased variability in play across participants, albeit to a small degree. These outcomes suggest that a lag 1 schedule is sufficient to produce response variability.

3.5.7 Schedule Combinations

So far, we described several variations of simple differential reinforcement schedules. These simple schedules can, and often are, used in combination. In *a multiple schedule of reinforcement*, two or more simple schedules are in effect, one at a time (i.e., nonconcurrently; Bloom & Lambert, 2015). Each of these simple schedules is indicated by a specific stimulus, which helps discriminate between them. The schedules are alternated based on a time schedule; for example, one schedule can be in effect for 5 minutes, and the following one can be in effect for 3 minutes.

Multiple schedules are frequently used to make treatments for problematic behavior practical. For example, recall that the treatment for problematic behavior typically consists of teaching a functional communication response while placing problematic behavior on extinction. When this treatment is successful, it results in high rates of functional communication responses. It is not practical or even possible for caregivers or teachers to reinforce such a high rate of functional communication responses, and research shows that failure to reinforce these requests results in resurgence of problematic behavior (Bloom & Lambert, 2015). As such, it is important to develop procedures that ensure that treatments are practical and feasible for all parties involved. A multiple schedule of reinforcement is often used to fade the schedule of reinforcement for functional communication responses to a practical level. For example, Cengher et al. (2022) reinforced functional communication responses to be left alone, while problematic behavior that served the same function was placed on extinction. Once the authors observed low rates of problematic behavior and high rates of requests, they implemented a multiple schedule of reinforcement which had two components, each signaled by a different color. In the green component, the experimenter reinforced all functional communication responses while continuing to place problematic behavior on extinction. In the red component, both functional communication responses and problematic behavior were extinguished. Initially, the red component was introduced briefly (20 seconds), and then it gradually increased to 80% of the duration of treatment sessions. At the end of treatment, participants demonstrated low rates of problematic behavior and practical rates of functional communication responses; this suggests that they learned to tolerate relatively long intervals of reinforcement unavailability.

A *chained schedule of reinforcement* also consists of two or more simple schedules, each signaled. However, the change from one schedule to another is based on a response requirement rather than time (as is the case with multiple schedules of reinforcement). For example, Slaton and Hanley (2016) compared the effects of chained and multiple schedules on stereotypy and item engagement in children with developmental disabilities. Across these two schedule combinations, the authors alternated between a signaled discriminative stimulus component, wherein participants were allowed to engage in stereotypy, and a delta component, whereby participants were blocked from engaging in stereotypy. In the chained schedule condition, participants had to earn a predetermined number of tokens for not engaging in stereotypy (DRO) during the delta component so that they could access the discriminative stimulus component. In the multiple schedule condition, the discriminative and delta stimulus components were alternated based on units of time that were yoked to the chained schedule. The results showed that the chained schedule of reinforcement was better at establishing discriminative responding, with lower rates of stereotypy in the delta component as compared to the discriminative stimulus component. Further, this condition also resulted in better item engagement. Therefore, both multiple and chained schedules are effective at reducing behaviors to practical levels, with an advantage for the chained schedule of reinforcement.

3.6 Practice Implications

3.6.1 Behavioral Contrast and Reinforcement History Effects

In practice, it is important to be aware that schedules of reinforcement can interact. *Behavioral contrast* occurs during the process of discrimination between two or more, typically concurrently presented, stimuli or schedules of reinforcement. For example, assume that a child begins school and the teacher implements a differential reinforcement procedure, whereby she reinforces appropriate requests for attention and places problematic behavior on extinction. At home, the child may have a long history of receiving attention for both appropriate requests and problematic behavior. Since the child began school, the parents observed an increase in problematic behavior, even though they have not changed their approach to parenting. This change was caused by the introduction of the intervention at school. Both behavioral contrast and reinforcement history effects benefit from extensive basic research, but there are few applied studies investigating their applicability in clinical settings (see call for translational research by Pipkin & Vollmer, 2009). As such, we recommend that clinicians make judgments about their clinical utility cautiously.

Behavioral contrast can limit the generality of treatment effects outside of the therapeutic place. For example, Koegel et al. (1980) hypothesized that failure to generalize treatment effects across settings may be due to behavioral contrast, especially when the reinforcement procedures in one setting are highly discriminable from the ones in another setting. The authors developed an experiment that confirmed this hypothesis. Further, the authors demonstrated that behavioral contrast can be eliminated if the reinforcement procedures are held constant from the onset of treatment across settings. Therefore, treatments must be implemented consistently across settings and intervention agents to prevent behavioral contrast and to demonstrate good generalization.

Reinforcement history effects are similar, in that responding under one schedule of reinforcement is affected by another schedule of reinforcement. However, the two (or more) schedules are programmed consequently, rather than concurrently (Pipkin et al., 2010). For example, assume that a teacher decides to reinforce appropriate requests every 5 minutes while withholding programmed consequences for problematic behavior. The teacher observes that this differential reinforcement procedure does not result in a reduction in problematic behavior or an increase in appropriate requests. As a result, she may change the schedule so that every request is reinforced, while she continues to withhold programmed consequences for problematic behavior. Due to reinforcement history effects, the child persists in engaging in problem behavior while refraining from making appropriate requests, despite the schedule change. Research shows that reinforcement history effects are relatively brief, and with repeated exposure to the new schedule, the participant eventually allocates their behavior according to the schedule. In addition, discriminative stimuli associated with each schedule help reduce reinforcement history effects. In the example above, the teacher could use a green board along with instructions to describe the first differential reinforcement schedule and use a purple board along with corresponding instructions to describe the second differential reinforcement schedule.

3.6.2 Relapse and Resurgence

The durability of treatment effects is one of the primary goals of treatment. A treatment cannot be said to be successful if it does not continue to produce the desirable effects over time, across environments, and with new individuals. However, relapse of challenging behavior often tends to co-occur with disruption of alternative responding (Mitteer et al., 2022). Several models for explaining relapse exist, including resurgence as choice (RaC; Shahan & Craig, 2017), behavioral momentum theory (BMT), or context theory (Bouton et al., 2012). Although full exploration of the models attempting to account for relapse is beyond the scope of this chapter, these models have proven useful for evaluating the variables that contribute to relapse and therefore can be considered when developing treatments.

Relapse mitigation strategies can be categorized as reinforcement contingencies, environmental stimuli, or a combination of the two. While initial differential reinforcement treatments can and should provide rich schedules of reinforcement for the absence of target behavior or engagement in alternative behavior, this rate is likely to be unsustainable over time and in other environments. For example, the reinforcer may not be a desirable long-term choice for the child's well-being, as in the case of unhealthy food items or access to an item that interferes with skill development or escape from a learning context. As mentioned above, thinning the schedule of reinforcement is necessary to maintain treatment effects. However, while thinning increases the likelihood of sustainable effects, it also disrupts the response-reinforcer contingency, which may lead to relapse of challenging behavior. Chained and multiple schedules as described above are two approaches to mitigating the effect of thinning reinforcement schedules on differential reinforcement outcomes.

In an evaluation of how to promote rapid treatment effect transfer to other contexts, Greer et al. (2019) taught caregivers to implement functional communication training, a variation of DRA, and used discriminative stimuli to support the transfer of the treatment into other settings. The authors provided behavioral skills training to caregivers to teach them to assess and treat problem behavior. Throughout treatment, they signaled the availability and nonavailability of reinforcement for an alternative functional communication response with colored shirts, poster boards, and light covers. They found that systematically introducing these schedule-correlated stimuli helped facilitate the transfer of treatment effects.

3.6.3 Treatment Integrity

Treatment integrity is the extent to which the treatment is delivered as intended. Errors in treatment integrity impact the efficacy and effectiveness of differential reinforcement procedures. Often, this influence is due to a disruption between the response and reinforcement contingency. Pipkin et al. (2010) evaluated the effects of errors of commission (delivering reinforcement when it should not be delivered) and errors of omission (failing to deliver reinforcement when it should be delivered) to better understand how errors impacted DRA. The authors looked at various levels of treatment integrity failure by varying the percentage and type of errors made. In both laboratory and clinical settings, they compared errors of commission alone to errors of omission alone to combinations of commission and omission. Overall, the authors found lower alternative behavior and higher problem behavior with an increased number of errors of commission or combined commission and omission in translational and clinical settings. Errors of omission were less detrimental to treatment effects. The authors also found that higher levels of treatment integrity earlier in treatment attenuated the effects of later errors. Ensuring that individuals implementing treatment are prepared and fully trained can increase the likelihood of successful treatment.

3.6.4 Practitioner Summary

In summary, differential reinforcement procedures are at the core of any clinical intervention aimed to change behaviors. Differential reinforcement schedules can increase or decrease several dimensions of behavior, including frequency, duration, and variability. There are many variations of simple differential reinforcement procedures that allow clinicians to tailor their intervention to their clients' needs. Further, there are variations of combinations of schedules that allow clinicians to fade the schedules of reinforcement to practical levels, which is crucial for the maintenance and effectiveness of interventions in clinical settings. Schedules of reinforcement interact when they co-occur, and when they are presented sequentially; clinicians need to design interventions that can prevent or mitigate these interactive effects. Finally, when interventions that entail differential reinforcement schedules are not implemented as prescribed (i.e., poor treatment integrity), there is a high risk that the desired change in behavior will not occur. Oftentimes, these treatment integrity failures result in relapse and resurgence. We provide recommendations to maintain high levels of treatment integrity, which in turn should minimize the risk of relapse and resurgence.

3.7 References

Athens, E. S., & Vollmer, T. R. (2010). An investigation of differential reinforcement of alternative behavior without extinction. *Journal of Applied Behavior Analysis, 43*(4), 569–589.

Austin, J. L., & Bevan, D. (2011). Using differential reinforcement of low rates to reduce children's requests for teacher attention. *Journal of Applied Behavior Analysis, 44*(3), 451–461.

Austin, J. L., Groves, E. A., Reynish, L. C., & Francis, L. L. (2015). Validating trial-based functional analyses in mainstream primary school classrooms. *Journal of Applied Behavior Analysis, 48*(2), 274–288.

Baruni, R. R., Rapp, C., Lipe, S. L., & Novotny, M. (2014). Using lag schedules to increase toy play variability for children with intellectual disabilities. *Behavioral Interventions, 29*(1), 21–35. https://doi.org/10.1002/bin.1377

Becraft, J. L., Borrero, J. C., Davis, B. J., Mendres-Smith, A. E., & Castillo, M. I. (2018). The role of signals in two variations of differential-reinforcement-of-low-rate procedures. *Journal of Applied Behavior Analysis, 51*(1), 3–24.

Bloom, S. E., & Lambert, J. M. (2015). Implications for practice: Resurgence and differential reinforcement of alternative responding. *Journal of Applied Behavior Analysis, 48*(4), 781–784.

Boudreau, B. A., Vladescu, J. C., Kodak, T. M., Argott, P. J., & Kisamore, A. N. (2015). A comparison of differential reinforcement procedures with children with autism. *Journal of Applied Behavior Analysis, 48*(4), 918–923. https://doi.org/10.1002/jaba.232

Bouton, M. E., Winterbauer, N. E., & Todd, T. P. (2012). Relapse processes after the extinction of instrumental learning: renewal, resurgence, and reacquisition. *Behavioural Processes, 90*(1), 130–141.

Buzas, H. P., & Ayllon, T. (1981). Differential reinforcement in coaching tennis skills. *Behavior Modification, 5*(3), 372–385.

Campanaro, A. M., Vladescu, J. C., Kodak, T., DeBar, R. M., & Nippes, K. C. (2020). Comparing skill acquisition under varying onsets of differential reinforcement: A preliminary analysis. *Journal of Applied Behavior Analysis, 53*(2), 690–706.

Cengher, M., O'Connor, J. T., & Strohmeier, C. W. (2022). Assessment and treatment of problem behavior maintained by escape from attention. *Behavioral Interventions, 37*(2), 204–221.

Cividini-Motta, C., & Ahearn, W. H. (2013). Effects of two variations of differential reinforcement on prompt dependency. *Journal of Applied Behavior Analysis, 46*(3), 640–650. https://doi.org/10.1002/jaba.67

Darwin, C., & Kebler, L. (1859) On the origin of species by means of natural selection, or, The preservation of favoured races in the struggle for life. London: J. Murray. https://www.loc.gov/item/06017473/

Eikenhout, N., & Austin, J. (2005). Using goals, feedback, reinforcement, and a performance matrix to improve customer service in a large department store. *Journal of Organizational Behavior Management, 24*(3), 27–62.

Fiske, K. E., Cohen, A. P., Bamond, M. J., Delmolino, L., LaRue, R. H., & Sloman, K. N. (2014). The effects of magnitude-based differential reinforcement on the skill acquisition of children with autism. *Journal of Behavioral Education, 23*(4), 470–487.

Galizio, A., Higbee, T. S., & Odum, A. L. (2020). Choice for reinforced behavioral variability in children with autism spectrum disorder. *Journal of the Experimental Analysis of Behavior, 113*(3), 495–514.

Girolami, K. M., Kahng, S., Hilker, K. A., & Girolami, P. A. (2009). Differential reinforcement of high rate behavior to increase the pace of self-feeding. *Behavioral Interventions: Theory & Practice in Residential & Community-Based Clinical Programs, 24*(1), 17–22.

Greer, B. D., Fisher, W. W., Briggs, A. M., Lichtblau, K. R., Phillips, L. A., & Mitteer, D. R. (2019). Using schedule-correlated stimuli during functional communication training to promote the rapid transfer of treatment effects. *Behavioral Development, 24*(2), 100–119.

Greer, B. D., & Shahan, T. A. (2019). Resurgence as choice: Implications for promoting durable behavior change. *Journal of Applied Behavior Analysis, 52*(3), 816–846.

Hanley, G. P., & Tiger, J. H. (2011). Differential reinforcement procedures. In W. W. Fisher, C. Piazza, & H. S. Roane (Eds.), Handbook of applied behavior analysis (pp. 229–249). New York: Guilford Press.

Hanney, N. M., Carr, J. E., & LeBlanc, L. A. (2019). Teaching children with autism spectrum disorder to tact auditory stimuli. *Journal of Applied Behavior Analysis, 52*(3), 733–738.

Hausman, N. L., Ingvarsson, E. T., & Kahng, S. (2014). A comparison of reinforcement schedules to increase independent responding in individuals with intellectual disabilities. *Journal of Applied Behavior Analysis, 47*(1), 155–159.

Jessel, J., & Borrero, J. C. (2014). A laboratory comparison of response-reducing differential-reinforcement techniques. *Journal of Applied Behavior Analysis, 47*(2), 314–324.

Jessel, J., Borrero, J. C., & Becraft, J. L. (2015). Differential reinforcement of other behavior increases untargeted behavior. *Journal of Applied Behavior Analysis, 48*(2), 402–416.

Jessel J., & Ingvarsson, 2016. Recent advances in applied research on DRO procedures. *Journal of Applied Behavior Analysis, 46*(4), 991–995.

Johnson, K. A., Vladescu, J. C., Kodak, T., & Sidener, T. M. (2017). An assessment of differential reinforcement procedures for learners with autism spectrum disorder. *Journal of Applied Behavior Analysis, 50*(2), 290–303.

Karsina, A., Thompson, R. H., & Rodriguez, N. M. (2011). Effects of a history of differential reinforcement on preference for choice. *Journal of the Experimental Analysis of Behavior, 95*(2), 189–202.

Karsten, A. M., & Carr, J. E. (2009). The effects of differential reinforcement of unprompted responding on the skill acquisition of children with autism. *Journal of Applied Behavior Analysis, 42*(2), 327–334.

Kodak, T., & Halbur, M. (2021). A tutorial for the design and use of assessment-based instruction in practice. *Behavior Analysis in Practice, 14*(1), 166–180.

Koegel, R. L., Egel, A. L., & Williams, J. A. (1980). Behavioral contrast and generalization across settings in the treatment of autistic children. *Journal of Experimental Child Psychology, 30*(3), 422–437.

Lee, R., Sturmey, P., & Fields, L. (2007). Schedule-induced and operant mechanisms that influence response variability: A review and implications for future investigations. *The Psychological Record, 57*(3), 429–455.

Lloveras, L. A., Slanzi, C. M., & Vollmer, T. R. (2022). New (old) perspectives on self-injurious and aggressive biting. *Journal of Applied Behavior Analysis, 55*, 674–687.

Meyer, K. A. (1999). Functional analysis and treatment of problem behavior exhibited by elementary school children. *Journal of Applied Behavior Analysis, 32*(2), 229–232.

Mitteer, D. R., Greer, B. D., Randall, K. R., & Haney, S. D. (2022). On the scope and characteristics of relapse when treating severe destructive behavior. *Journal of Applied Behavior* Analysis, *55*, 688–703.

National Autism Center. (2015). *National standards project findings and conclusions: Phase 2*. Randolph, MA: Author.

O'Reilly, M. F. (1995). Functional analysis and treatment of escape-maintained aggression correlated with sleep deprivation. *Journal of Applied Behavior Analysis, 28*(2), 225–226.

Olenick, D. L., & Pear, J. J. (1980). Differential reinforcement of correct responses to probes and prompts in picture-name training with severely retarded children. *Journal of Applied Behavior Analysis, 13*(1), 77–89.

Petscher, E. S., Rey, C., & Bailey, J. S. (2009). A review of empirical support for differential reinforcement of alternative behavior. *Research in Developmental Disabilities, 30*(3), 409–425.

Pipkin, C. S. P., & Vollmer, T. R. (2009). Applied implications of reinforcement history effects. *Journal of Applied Behavior Analysis, 42*(1), 83–103.

Pipkin, C. S. P., Vollmer, T. R., & Sloman, K. N. (2010). Effects of treatment integrity failures during differential reinforcement of alternative behavior: A translational model. *Journal of Applied Behavior Analysis, 43*(1), 47–70.

Rajaraman, A., Austin, J. L., Gover, H. C., Cammilleri, A. P., Donnelly, D. R., & Hanley, G. P. (2022). Toward trauma-informed applications of behavior analysis. *Journal of Applied Behavior Analysis, 55*(1), 40–61. https://doi.org/10.1002/jaba.881

Rajaraman, A., Hanley, G. P., Gover, H. C., Staubitz, J. L., Staubitz, J. E., Simcoe, K. M., & Metras, R. (2022). Minimizing escalation by treating dangerous problem behavior within an enhanced choice model. *Behavior Analysis in Practice, 15*(1), 219–242.

Reynolds, G. S. (1961). Behavioral contrast. *Journal of the Experimental Analysis of Behavior, 4*(1), 57–71.

Shahan, T. A., & Craig, A. R. (2017). Resurgence as choice. *Behavioural Processes, 141*(1), 100–127.

Skinner, B. F. (1938). *The behavior of organisms: An experimental analysis*. Seventh printing (1966). East Norwalk, CT: Appleton-Century Crofts.

Slaton, J. D., & Hanley, G. P. (2016). Effects of multiple versus chained schedules on stereotypy and item engagement. *Journal of Applied Behavior Analysis, 49*(4), 927–946.

Smith, M. D. (1987). Treatment of pica in an adult disabled by autism by differential reinforcement of incompatible behavior. *Journal of Behavior Therapy and Experimental Psychiatry, 18*, 285–288. https://doi.org/10.1016/0005-7916(87)90012-7

Touchette, P. E., & Howard, J. S. (1984). Errorless learning: Reinforcement contingencies and stimulus control transfer in delayed prompting. *Journal of Applied Behavior Analysis, 17*(2), 175–188.

Vollmer, T. R., Peters, K. P., Kronfli, F. R., Lloveras, L. A., & Ibanez, V. F. (2020). On the definition of differential reinforcement of alternative behavior. *Journal of Applied Behavior Analysis, 53*(3), 1299–1303.

Young, J., & Wincze, J. (1974). The effects of the reinforcement of compatible and incompatible alternative behaviors on the self-injurious and related behaviors of a profoundly retarded female adult. *Behavior Therapy, 5*(5), 614–623.

4

Prompting, Errorless Learning, Time Delay, and Reinforcement

David Ray Miranda
University of Missouri

John Augustine
University of Missouri

Mandy J. Rispoli
The University of Virginia

4.1 Technical Abstract

Background: Prompting and reinforcement are foundational teaching procedures that have been incorporated as components into numerous intervention packages. Prompts include spoken reminders, gestures (e.g., pointing), physical guidance, and other stimuli intended to occasion a target response. Prompts are applied in systematic hierarchies individualized based on the learner's support needs and target behavior. Contingent reinforcement refers to a process in which a particular response or behavior is reinforced or strengthened by the presentation (positive reinforcement) or withdrawal (negative reinforcement) of a stimulus immediately following that behavior. Errorless learning and time delay refer to specific implementations of prompting and reinforcement. **Method:** This chapter utilizes peer-reviewed intervention research and existing evidence-based practice reviews (e.g., Steinbrenner et al., 2020) to synthesize research on prompting and reinforcement in education and treatment for people with autism spectrum disorder (ASD). **Results:** Prompting and reinforcement have been used together in focused behavioral interventions to teach skills related to daily living, academics, communication, and other domains. Further, these two procedures are integral intervention components in most multifaceted comprehensive intervention approaches. **Discussion:** Prompting and reinforcement met criteria to be classified as evidence-based practices in ASD education and treatment. Prompt timing, type or form of prompt, and nature of reinforcement influence outcomes and highlight the need for individualization. **Practitioner recommendations:** Practitioners should determine the most appropriate prompt hierarchy and reinforcement contingencies based on factors such as the learner's repertoire, prior learning history, and the importance of error prevention. Data collection and

David Ray Miranda, John Augustine, and Mandy J. Rispoli, *Prompting, Errorless Learning, Time Delay, and Reinforcement*. In: *Lifespan Treatment for Autistic Individuals*. Edited by: Peter Sturmey, Russell Lang, and James K. Luiselli, Oxford University Press. © Oxford University Press (2025). DOI: 10.1093/oso/9780197635841.003.0004 analysis are necessary to inform adjustments to prompting and reinforcement procedures.

4.2 Layperson Summary

Prompting and reinforcement refer to a set of teaching procedures integrated into many different approaches to education and treatment involving people with autism spectrum disorder (ASD). Prompts include spoken reminders, gestures, physical guidance, and other forms of support that help encourage a selected behavior to occur (response prompt) or to draw the learner's attention to specific things in the environment (stimulus prompt). Prompts are used in a step-by-step manner (prompting hierarchy) and are individualized based on the learner's support needs, environment, and the specific skill or behavior being taught.

Contingent reinforcement refers to a learning process that involves rewarding (reinforcing) occurrences of behaviors and skills selected for instruction (e.g., daily-living skills, academics, spoken language). Reinforcement involves either giving something valuable or desirable (positive reinforcement) or taking away something unwanted (negative reinforcement) to increase behavior. Factors such as when to prompt, the type of prompt to use, and the type of reinforcer (e.g., praise, token, activity access) will affect outcomes, and it is important to individualize procedures. Specifically, clinicians should adjust prompting and reinforcement procedures based on an individual's existing skills, preferences, and previous learning experiences as well as other instructional factors (e.g., whether it is necessary to prevent errors during instruction). Data collection and monitoring are necessary to inform decisions regarding when and what types of prompts and reinforcers to use. Excessive prompting or failure to stop prompting (usually by gradually over time) can result in dependency and prevent independence. Similarly, overuse of reinforcement or failure to reduce reinforcement to natural contingencies can result in instructional and behavioral complications (e.g., reinforcer loses value diminishing outcomes).

4.3 Treatment Summary Table

Treatment summary: Prompting, Errorless Learning, Reinforcement, and Time Delay

Treatment description: Prompts function to occasion correct responses by cueing or signaling the selected behavior to the learner. Least-to-most prompting is a hierarchical strategy that involves incrementally increasing prompting support until effective. Errorless learning involves high support initially and then systematically fades prompting to minimize or eliminate errors during instruction. Time-delay procedures introduce a deliberate pause between the instruction and the prompt to provide an opportunity for independent responses. Contingent reinforcement is a technique where specific behavior is strengthened, either by contingent presentation of a desired stimulus (positive reinforcement) or by withdrawal of an unwanted stimulus (negative reinforcement).

Expected outcomes: Prompting and reinforcement interventions in the education and treatment of people with ASD are expected to facilitate the acquisition of specific skills and behaviors. These can include teaching communication, social interaction, daily-living skills, and self-management to individuals across various age groups and support needs. These procedures can be implemented by educators, therapists, and caregivers across different settings, including schools, therapy centers, and home environments.

Methods: Prompts include spoken reminders, gestures (e.g., pointing), physical guidance, and other stimuli intended to occasion a target response. Prompts are applied in systematic hierarchies individualized based on the learner's support needs, preferences, environment, and target behavior. Least-to-most prompting starts with minimal guidance and increases support incrementally as needed until successful; then it gradually reduces prompting support until the learner can do the skill independently. In time-delay procedures, an initial instruction is given and then a pause is introduced before any additional prompt is provided to allow the learner an opportunity to respond independently. Contingent reinforcement is a technique where specific behavior is either strengthened by immediate presentation of a desired stimulus (positive reinforcement) or withdrawal of an unwanted stimulus (negative reinforcement) contingent on target behavior.

Expertise required to implement treatment: Necessary expertise typically involves education in behavioral principles and training in the application of specific prompting and reinforcement procedures. Board-Certified Behavior Analysts (BCBAs) and special education teachers often receive this training. However, family members, peers, and others have been trained to deliver basic prompting and reinforcement protocols across home, school, and community settings.

Risks and negative side effects: Excessive prompting or failure to withdraw prompting can result in prompt dependency, where the learner becomes reliant on the prompt, hindering the ability to perform the target skill independently. Similarly, misuse of reinforcement can lead to satiation (where the learner becomes less responsive to a reinforcer over time because it's used too often) or to unintended reinforcement of undesired behaviors. Careful planning, data monitoring, and regular procedural adjustments based on the individual's progress mitigate these potential issues.

4.4 Introduction

4.4.1 Treatment Description

Prompting and reinforcement are versatile procedures that can be employed independently or be integrated within complex multicomponent intervention packages (e.g., Pivotal Response Training and Discrete Trial Training). Prompting and reinforcement can be described from a behavioral perspective within the context of the three-term contingency. Specifically, a discriminative stimulus (S^D) is presented, which occasions a specific response (R), and the contingent consequence (C) influences the future probability of that response. Within this model, a prompt is a "functional but irrelevant" stimulus that occasions a target response (Mayer et al., 2022, p. 385).

Prompts function to occasion correct responses by cueing or signaling the selected behavior to the learner. A variety of prompt forms are applied in systematic hierarchies individualized based on the learner's support needs and target behavior. *Least-to-Most Prompting* begins with minimal guidance and increases support until effective, allowing for attempts at independent behavior. *Errorless*

Learning initiates with high support and subsequently fades to minimize or eliminate errors. *Time-Delay* procedures involve a deliberate pause between S^D and prompts, affording an opportunity for independent responses. Reinforcement strategies are employed to both instruct new skills and to enhance existing ones by altering (adding or removing) environmental stimuli contingent on the occurrence of specific behavior. For instance, a teacher might use positive reinforcement by giving praise immediately after a student answers a question correctly. A parent may implement negative reinforcement by removing a disliked chore when a child completes homework on time.

In the context of the three-term contingency, prompting serves to guide the learner in recognizing the correct response to a discriminative stimulus (S^D), while reinforcement ensures the strengthening of this response (R) through contingent consequences (C). For example, a behavior analyst working with an individual with autism might initially use a prompt to elicit the correct response to a given instruction. Upon successful response, a positive reinforcer is provided (e.g., a desired item or praise), making it more likely that the correct response will occur again when S^D is present. Over time, with the strategic integration of these procedures, prompts may be faded to allow the learner to respond independently to the S^D. The careful coordination of prompting and reinforcement forms a flexible approach that tailors the learning experience to the individual needs and progress of the learner.

4.4.2 Rationale and Objectives

We begin this chapter by introducing key terms and vocabulary related to prompting and reinforcement. *Response prompts* are supplemental antecedent stimuli to aid learners in responding to an S^D (Cooper et al., 2020). Commonly used response prompts include *physical prompting* (e.g., teacher physically guides the learner to engage in the response), *modeling* (e.g., teacher demonstrates target response), *gestures* (e.g., teacher points or gestures to help learner engage in the target response), *verbal prompts* (e.g., teacher uses words to help learner engage in target response), and time-delay prompts (e.g., teacher waits expectantly for a specified period of time before providing a prompt). Each of these response prompts varies in terms of intrusiveness and level of support provided. More intrusive prompts provide a high level of support to reduce or preclude errors. Less intrusive prompts provide lower levels of support to allow opportunity for independence in responding (Collins et al., 2018). See Figure 4.1 for a display of prompt hierarchies.

A *prompt hierarchy* allows for the systematic evaluation of performance (e.g., correct responding and errors) and creates an objective guideline to determine the level of prompting to use during the next learning trial (Libby et al., 2008; Wolery & Gast, 1984). Specifically, a prompt hierarchy allows the teacher or interventionist to adjust procedures by identifying the prompts associated with the most errors

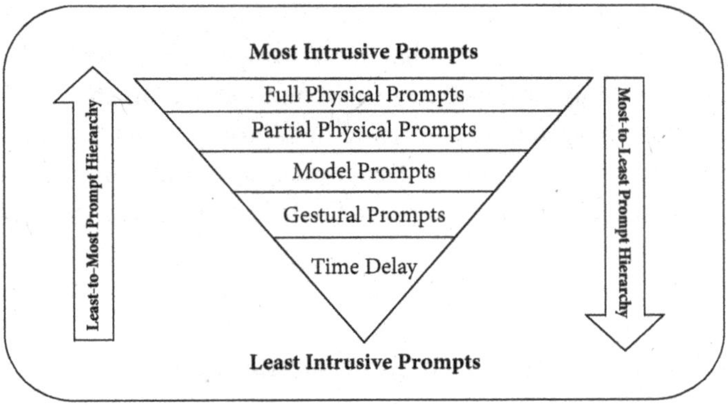

Figure 4.1 Prompt hierarchies

and those more likely to result in correct responses. Furthermore, prompt hierarchies help to increase the likelihood of achieving independence with target skills by reducing probability of becoming prompt dependent (Wolery & Gast, 1984). The four types of prompt hierarchies are most-to-least prompting, least-to-most prompting, graduated guidance, and time delay (Wolery & Gast, 1984).

Most-to-least prompting begins with the most intrusive prompt needed to ensure the correct response, followed by systematic reductions in prompt intensity as the skill is acquired. This approach is used to avoid errors during the early stages of instruction. As the learner practices the correct response with full prompt support rather than making errors, they are more likely to receive reinforcement for accurate responding (Libby et al., 2008).

Graduated guidance refers to another errorless learning procedure in which physical prompts are provided as needed to help the learner complete the target response (Cooper et al., 2020). This prompting hierarchy is typically used with chained skills or behaviors that contain multiple steps. Examples of chained skills may include teeth brushing, making a phone call, or preparing a meal. In the graduated guidance approach, the instructor applies prompts for each task step using a most-to-least sequence and then fades the level of prompt support depending on the learners' immediate response (Morales et al., 2016).

Least-to-most prompting involves beginning with the least intrusive prompt necessary to occasion the target behavior. Prompt support is then systematically adjusted depending on the learner's performance following each attempt. If the learner responds correctly, prompts are reduced. This approach may lead to more errors initially compared to the most-to-least hierarchy (Libby et al., 2008), but the learner's responses are more likely to come under control of the natural S^D rather than the prompt itself (Charlop & Walsh, 1986).

Time delay refers to the systematic application of prompt timing. Rather than changing the type of prompt (e.g., verbal to gestural), time-delay procedures alter the timing of prompt delivery (Snell & Gast, 1981). In time delay, prompts are delivered after a predetermined delay (e.g., immediately, after 5 seconds, or after

10 seconds) following the S^D. In the progressive time delay, the prompt is provided after a delay that is systematically increased. That is, following the first presentation of the S^D, the instructor prompts immediately (0 second delay). On the second presentation of the S^D, they may wait 3 seconds and then prompt, then 5 seconds, and so forth. Alternatively, within the constant time-delay approach, prompts are delivered following the same delay period after each S^D presentation (Cooper et al., 2020).

4.4.3 Considerations for Implementation

There are several factors that practitioners must consider when creating and delivering individualized interventions that involve prompting and reinforcement. First, assessment should precede any intervention to determine the specific needs, preferences, and current abilities of the individual. Intervention procedures must be tailored to the unique needs of each person while accounting for the environment and target behaviors. This includes choosing the appropriate type and level of prompts, considering prompt intrusiveness, and identifying effective and practical reinforcers for the individual.

Determining the most suitable prompting method (e.g., most-to-least or least-to-most) and reinforcement strategy requires careful consideration of the learner's developmental stage, the complexity of the skill being taught, and the context in which the skill is to be applied. Practitioners must be aware of the potential benefits and drawbacks of each prompting and reinforcement approach and how they align with the targeted outcomes (Charlop & Walsh, 1986; Libby et al., 2008). Prompting and reinforcement integration involves selecting prompts that will effectively lead to the desired response and coupling them with reinforcement that will sustain and promote that response (Cooper et al., 2020).

Continuous data collection, monitoring, and analysis are vital to ensure that learning is progressing as intended. Practitioners should be prepared to adapt procedures as needed, whether by fading or increasing prompts, altering reinforcement strategies, or making other adjustments based on ongoing assessment of the learner's performance (Morales et al., 2016). Ultimately, the goal is for the individual to apply the learned skill or behavior across various settings and maintain it over time without prompting or contrived reinforcement contingencies (i.e., independence). Strategies for generalization should be built into the intervention (e.g., varying the instructional stimuli), and reinforcement should be faded until it is aligned with the expectations of the natural environment (Stokes & Baer, 1977).

Effective intervention often involves collaboration among various professionals, including teachers, behavior analysts, speech therapists, and parents. Coordinated efforts and clear communication are essential for consistency in implementation. Additionally, those directly involved with the intervention may require training and ongoing support to ensure that they are competent in the techniques being used. Finally, all interventions must be implemented with adherence to ethical guidelines, respecting the dignity, autonomy, and individual preferences of the person with autism. Any potential risks associated with the chosen prompting and reinforcement strategies must be carefully weighed against the expected benefits, and informed consent must be obtained where appropriate.

4.5 Research Background and Treatment Outcomes

The research on prompting and reinforcement is extensive because prompting and reinforcement strategies are near ubiquitous components across options for teaching and treatment approaches (Steinbrenner, 2020). This section will (a) broadly discuss the evidence base and (b) highlight research on the social validity, service delivery, and dissemination of prompting and reinforcement.

The National Clearinghouse on Autism and Evidence and Practice (NCAEP; Steinbrenner et al., 2020) and the National Standards Program (NSP; National Autism Center, 2015) conducted a comprehensive review of hundreds of research articles. From this review, both organizations identified prompting, time-delay prompts, and reinforcement as evidence-based practices that clearly demonstrated positive benefits and were supported by multiple high-quality studies (Steinbrenner et al., 2020). Prompting, time delay, and reinforcement procedures can be implemented individually, but many studies on response prompting also incorporate reinforcement procedures (see Steinbrenner et al., 2020). Individual studies that have combined prompting procedures with reinforcement have demonstrated positive outcomes for people with ASD.

For prompting hierarchies, positive outcomes were found for most-to-least prompting with reinforcement (e.g., Akmanoglu & Batu, 2004; Jerome et al., 2007), least-to-most prompting with reinforcement (e.g., Barton, 2015; Ford et al., 2021), and graduated guidance with reinforcement (e.g., Boutain et al., 2020; LaLonde et al., 2020). For time-delay procedures, positive outcomes were found for progressive time delay with reinforcement (e.g., Silbaugh & Falcomata, 2019) and constant time delay with reinforcement (e.g., Horn et al., 2020). Collectively, these studies demonstrated positive outcomes across a broad range of outcome domains, including academic skills (e.g., Akmanoglu & Batu, 2004), play skills (Barton, 2015), social skills (e.g., LaLonde et al., 2020; Taylor & Harris, 1995), and daily living or vocational skills (e.g., Ford et al., 2021; Horn et al., 2020).

In addition to positive outcomes, studies have also identified the generalizability and maintenance of results. Some studies have demonstrated that participants were able to apply the learned skills with untaught sets (i.e., generalization) (e.g., Akmanoglu & Batu, 2004; Jerome et al., 2007; Taylor & Harris, 1995). For instance, Jerome et al. (2007) used most-to-least prompting to teach adults with ASD to access an online website, and participants were able to complete this task even with a different computer. Other studies have demonstrated that learners may also maintain these skills after intervention (e.g., Ford et al., 2021; LaLonde et al., 2020). After teaching adults with ASD to complete daily living skills, Ford et al. (2021) found that participants maintained these skills 2 to 11 weeks after the end of the intervention. Finally, recent studies have evaluated whether learners both generalize and maintain these outcomes (e.g., Barton, 2015; Horn et al., 2020). After children with ASD were taught to engage in pretend play skills, Barton (2015) reported that participants continued to engage in the pretend play activity without prompting and engaged in play skills to novel toys and play settings (e.g., classroom).

Literature reviews and meta-analyses that aggregate the results of individual studies also suggest some positive outcomes for some prompting, time delay, and/or reinforcement procedures, specifically for people with ASD. For instance, Watkins et al. (2019) conducted a meta-analysis evaluating interventions for students with ASD who are placed in inclusive classroom settings. Watkins et al. (2019) found that many interventions that incorporated prompting, modeling, and/or reinforcement had positive maintenance and generalization effect and more robust generalization effects in comparison to intervention with fewer instances of prompting and reinforcement. Additionally, Walker (2008) reviewed the constant time-delay and progressive time-delay research literature and found that all learners with ASD who received constant time delay or progressive time delay were able to meet skill mastery, although learners made fewer errors with progressive time-delay procedures.

When considering the social validity and accessibility of prompting, time delay, and reinforcement strategies, results are promising. Multiple studies have evaluated the social acceptability of the procedures and outcomes (e.g., Boutain et al., 2020; Ford et al., 2021; Horn et al., 2020). Across all studies we are aware of that have evaluated social validity of procedures, positive ratings from participants, parents, and other caregivers were reported. For example, a recent survey found that special educators rated prompting, time delay, and reinforcement positively in terms of acceptability, feasibility, and contextual alignment (McNeill, 2019). Furthermore, prompting and reinforcement were rated in the top four of highly rated evidence-based practices for students with ASD (McNeill, 2019).

For service delivery and dissemination, researchers have also utilized advances in technology to further increase the accessibility of interventions using prompting, time delay, and reinforcement. For instance, researchers have used electronic devices (e.g., tablets and phones) as ways to deliver video-based prompts. These video-based prompts have been used to effectively teach functional skills (Weng & Bouck, 2014), vocational skills (Stauch & Plavnick, 2020), play skills (Fragale, 2014), and perspective taking (LeBlanc et al., 2003). Furthermore, researchers have started providing interventions remotely through telecommunication platforms (e.g., Zoom and Skype). Emerging research (e.g., Ferguson et al., 2020; Ford et al., 2021) shows promising effects, but more research is needed to evaluate the effectiveness of interventions provided directly through telehealth.

Research has also examined whether family and community members (e.g., parents, caregivers, and teachers) can be trained to implement prompting and reinforcement strategies with people who have ASD. Researchers have demonstrated that (a) caregivers (e.g., Harriage et al., 2016) and educators (e.g., Horn et al., 2020; Seaman et al., 2017) can be trained to implement behavioral interventions, (b) these non-researcher-implemented interventions have led to positive outcomes for participants with ASD, and (c) the intervention and resulting outcomes were rated positively by the participant, parent, and/or educator. Additionally, to further increase access to these trainings, researchers have also started evaluating the effectiveness of remote parent training and coaching interventions (e.g., Boutain et al., 2020; Gerow et al., 2021; Wainer & Ingersoll, 2015).

4.6 Practice Implications

When teaching a new skill to a learner, one should consider the three-term contingency discussed earlier: (a) the S^D and prompts, (b) the target behavior, and (c) the consequence (i.e., reinforcer). For each learning trial, the S^D is present, the teacher provides an appropriate prompt (if needed), the learner exhibits the target behavior, and receives reinforcement for engaging in the behavior. To set up a learning trial, one must identify the target behavior, determine the most appropriate prompt, and determine the appropriate reinforcement.

To construct a learning trial, one must identify the behavior the learner will engage in during the learning trial and identify situations in which behavior occurs. By identifying relevant situations, one can determine the S^D needed for learning trials. After identifying the behavior and S^D, one should select the most appropriate prompt hierarchy to support learners in acquiring the target skill. When selecting the prompt hierarchy, one should consider factors such as prior learning history, the learner's skill repertoire, and the importance of preventing errors.

Most-to-least prompts may be best for learners who may frequently make errors, learners who may need immediate prompts, or learners acquiring a new skill (Collins et al., 2018). Additionally, the most-to-least prompt hierarchy may be utilized if the learner's prior learning history is not known (Libby et al., 2008). However, because the most intrusive prompts are utilized at the beginning of the learner trial, learners may become prompt dependent because of the reliance of the prompt, rather than the S^D (Oppenhiemer et al., 1993). To reduce the likelihood of prompt dependency, prompts should be systematically faded or reduced so participants are likely to engage in the correct response when the intrusiveness of the prompts is reduced (Libby et al., 2008).

A limitation to the most-to-least prompt procedure is the learner becomes prompt dependent if the prompt is not systematically reduced or removed. Therefore, a criterion should be set to reduce the prompt type or intensity. For instance, the change agent could set the criterion of three correct responses before the prompt is reduced to the partial-physical prompt. Therefore, prompts can be reduced or removed, and the S^D can serve as the opportunity to respond.

Least-to-most prompting may be used for learners who may readily learn skills by imitating others' actions (Wolery & Gast, 1984) and for teaching discrete or multistep responses (Collins et al., 2018). However, one must note that the learner may engage in more error during the least-to-most prompt procedure (Libby et al., 2008). The least-to-most prompt procedure utilizes the least intrusive prompt first and then systematically increases or decreases the intrusiveness of the prompt based on the learner performance.

Within a least-to-most prompt procedure, learners can demonstrate many responses; therefore, it is important to record each response for monitoring progress. An unprompted correct response is a response that is emitted by the learner without a prompt being provided by the change agent. Another response is a prompted correct, which is any correct response after a prompting sequence has been initiated. For example, if a learner does not respond to the initial instructional cue and the teacher must prompt the learner, any correct response would be scored as a prompted correct response. Unprompted errors, prompted errors, and no response by the learner should also be recorded. This will provide information regarding the learner's performance and progress.

Although least-to-most prompt procedures are supplementary stimuli to aid learners, there may be some limitations. Common problems that are faced when implementing a least-to-most procedure include the learner consistently makes errors or waits for a prompt without emitting an independent response. If the learner makes an error at the final level of the prompt hierarchy, the teacher should utilize a more intrusive prompt. If the learner consistently makes errors in the middle of the prompt hierarchy, the change agent can select a new prompt or examine the instructional level of the learner and the difficulty of the task. Finally, if the learner consistently does not emit an independent response, the teacher can eliminate reinforcers for prompted correct responses.

Graduated guidance is commonly used when teaching chained skills (i.e., skills comprised of several behaviors together to form a more complex skill) and can help to quickly reduce prompts. However, this prompting hierarchy does not include a structured outline of when to prompt and which prompt to provide. Additionally, this prompting hierarchy also requires the person providing the prompts to have a competent understanding and momentary awareness of when prompts are necessary (Morales et al., 2016).

A critical step of graduated guidance is to select reinforcers, as it should be as natural as possible. Meaning, it should be related to the activity being implemented.

With chained skills or behaviors and graduated guidance, the completion of the behavior chain is the terminal reinforcer. For example, a learner may be required to tie their shoes before they can go out for recess. Therefore, the chain of tying shoes leads to the natural reinforcer of recess. However, the completion of the chain may not be reinforcing for some learners. As the example used previously, there are multiple steps to transition to a new classroom setting after the bell rang, but the new setting may be less preferred to the learner. Therefore, additional reinforcers may need to be utilized to increase the future likelihood of the behavior occurring. For example, after the student exhibits the transition skills, they may be provided with a reinforcer of a break during class.

The next step to implement graduated guidance is to identify the controlling prompt. This prompt should ensure that the learner provides the correct response during the behavioral chain. Graduated guidance typically involves a physical prompt, but they can also involve less intrusive prompts such as a gesture or model. To reduce the likelihood the learner does not become prompt dependent, practitioners must determine how they will fade the prompts. This can be done by reducing the intensity of the prompt, changing the prompt to a less intrusive prompt, or removing the prompt.

Finally, time delay is a practice that is utilized within prompt hierarchies to systematically fade prompts and includes two types: progressive time delay and constant time delay. Progressive time delay is a procedure for transferring the control from the prompt to the naturally existing S^D (Cooper et al., 2020). Progressive time delay aligns with most-to-least prompting as prompts are initially delivered immediately after the S^D and the delay between the S^D and prompt systematically increases (O'Neill et al., 2020. For example, if a BCBA utilizes a most-to-least prompt procedure to aid a correct response in adding clothes to the wash machine, they may increase the delay of the prompt to provide an opportunity for the learner to engage in the behavior independently.

Like the progressive time delay, a constant time delay transfers the control from the first, or controlling prompt, to the naturally occurring stimulus (Cooper et al., 2020). Constant time delay has two features: Initial learning trials are presented with the naturally occurring stimulus followed by the controlling prompt and, on later trials, the naturally occurring stimulus is presented followed by a fixed time (e.g., after 3 seconds) by the controlling prompt. Constant time delay aligns with least-to-most prompting since prompts are delivered only after a set delay period (e.g., after 5 seconds), which provides an opportunity for the learner to independently respond (Collins et al., 2018). This type of prompt may be effective for learners who can wait for a prompt when they do not know how to respond (Chazin & Ledford, 2021).

A general concern when implementing a prompting procedure is that a learner with ASD may become prompt dependent. This means that the learner may rely on the prompt rather than the S^D to evoke the correct response. Therefore, it is important that practitioners collect data on the learner's performance after each learning trial and systematically fade the prompt, so the learner more independently engages in the correct response.

To increase the likelihood of a behavior occurring in the future, change agents must provide access to a reinforcer and how frequently a correct response should be reinforced (i.e., schedules of reinforcement). When identifying reinforcers, one should consider the natural reinforcers and other stimuli that are more highly preferred by the learner. Change agents must determine when to deliver the reinforcer. If a teacher is teaching a new skill to a learner, it is recommended to reinforce correct responses immediately after the behavior occurs and after each correct response (continuous reinforcement; Cooper et al., 2020; Mayer et al., 2022). For example, after each correct response for a learner to identify a letter in the alphabet, the teacher provides the learner with behavior specific praise and a highly preferred stimulus. Over time, reinforcers can be faded but should still be delivered immediately. Practice implications of prompting procedures and reinforcement are discussed below.

4.6.1 Practice Implication Guidelines

A most-to-least prompt procedure can be utilized if a change agent does not know the learner's learning history or if the learner makes errors. This prompt strategy can be used to reduce the number of learner errors, but it is important to fade prompts over time. Step-by-step procedures to implement the most-to-least prompt procedure are displayed in Figure 4.2.

The least-to-most prompt procedure can be utilized for single behaviors or chained behaviors (i.e., a sequence/series of behaviors). There are three levels of the least-to-most prompt procedure: independent response (i.e., no response), sequence of least amount of help to the most amount of help, and the controlling

Most-to-Least Prompt Procedure

1. Approach the learner and use an attention-getting statement such as "Time to work, Billy."
2. Provide the discriminative stimulus to the learner. For example, "Touch your nose."
3. After immediately providing the discriminative stimulus, provide the prompt. For this example, the teacher would gently grab the learner's hand to touch their nose.
4. Provide praise and reinforcement for the task, e.g., "Good job touching your nose!"
5. Fade the intrusiveness of the prompt.
6. After a certain criterion, e.g., 5 times in a row, reduce the intrusiveness of the prompt.

Figure 4.2 Most-to-least prompt procedure

Least-to-Most Prompt Procedure

1. Establish the learner's attention
   a. Saying the learner's name (e.g., "Look, Bryan")
   b. Delivering the target stimulus
2. Once attention is secured from the learner, present the cue or task to let the learner what they are going to do. For example, a teacher says, "Look, Bryan." Bryan looks at the teacher, as he presents a toy car and toy ball and says, "Touch the car, Bryan."
3. Wait 3–5 seconds for a response.
4. Respond to the learner's attempts in the trials:
   a. If the learner is correct, immediately provide reinforcement (e.g., praise, access to toys, token) and
   b. State what the learner did (e.g., "You touched the car, that's right!")
5. If the learner's response is incorrect:
   a. Interrupt the incorrect response (e.g., block the student from selecting the incorrect response)
   b. Provide a neutral statement (e.g., "That's not the car")
   c. Deliver the next most intrusive prompt in the prompt hierarchy. For example, if the learner incorrectly answered on a gestural prompt, the next prompt would be a model
6. If the learner does not respond, implement the next prompt in the prompt hierarchy
7. Continue through the prompt hierarchy until a correct response is performed.
   a. always reinforce the correct response

Figure 4.3 Least-to-most prompt procedure

prompt, or the prompt that aids the learner in a correct response. The least-to-most prompt procedure is displayed in Figure 4.3.

The graduated guidance prompt procedure is most commonly associated with chained behaviors (see Figure 4.4). This procedure requires change agents to make decisions during learning trials about that prompts that are to be utilized. One must be skillful in the implementation of graduated guidance to implement with high fidelity.

Both time-delay procedures, constant and progressive, include a prompt to get the learner's attention and emit the behavior, the behavior demonstrated by the learner, and feedback (i.e., behavior specific praise and feedback). Steps to implement a time-delay prompt procedure are described in Figure 4.5.

Graduated Guidance

1. Establish the learner's attention
    a. Say the learner's name (e.g., "Jason, time to work")
2. Present the stimulus to the learner, or direct the learner's attention to the stimulus (e.g., "Your shoe is untied, Jason")
3. Deliver the direction of the task
    a. e.g., "Tie your shoes"
    b. e.g., "Wash your hands"
    c. e.g., "Fold your laundry"
4. Provide a wait-time for the learner to independently perform the chained sequence

If the learner does not respond to the task or step in the chained sequence:

7. Provide the type of prompt needed to get the learner to start performing the task
    a. Full-physical
    b. Model
8. Once the learner starts the task, reduce the level or intensity of the prompt
9. Immediately provide the amount and type of prompt if the learner stops responding during the chained sequence
10. Block any incorrect responses by the learner during the chain response
11. Provide behavior specific praise to all unprompted or prompted correct responses
    a. E.g., "Great job tying your shoes!"
    b. E.g., "You did a fantastic job of folding your clothes!"
12. Provide additional reinforcement for the completion of the entire chained sequence

Figure 4.4 Graduated guidance

4.7 Conclusion

Prompting and reinforcement are two behavioral strategies that are anchored within an operant conditioning framework. Through operant conditioning, learning occurs through a three-term contingency consisting of an S^D, a response, and a consequence. Specifically, an S^D signals or evokes a response, the learner engages in a response, and there is a consequence that either reinforces (i.e., increases

Implementing Time Delay

1. Establish the learner's attention
    a. Use attention-getting strategy (e.g., say name and present task)
2. Immediately deliver the controlling prompt
3. Provide reinforcement and behavior specific praise if the learner's response is correct
4. Ignore any incorrect responses or no response by the learner

Increasing the Constant Time Delay

1. Present the task to the learner
    a. E.g., "Touch the green car"
2. Wait 3–5 seconds for the learner to respond
3. If correct, provide behavior specific praise and reinforcement
    a. E.g., "Great job, that is the green car! You have can have your coloring book for 1 minute"
4. Deliver the controlling prompt if the learner does not respond
5. If the learner responds correctly to the prompt, provide reinforcement
6. If the learner responds incorrectly to the prompt, ignore the response and move to the next trial

Progressive Time Delay

1. Present the task to the learner
2. Wait with increased delay time before prompting
3. Provide behavior specific praise and reinforcement for correct responses
4. Ignore and continue to next trial following an incorrect response

Figure 4.5 Time-delay procedures

the future occurrences) or punishes (i.e., decreases the future occurrences) the response. To support the development of new responses, prompts or cues may be delivered after the S^D but before the learner's response to help the learner engage in the correct response. If learners engage in the correct response, reinforcement is the process that makes the behavior more likely to occur in the presence of the S^D.

Within the context of teaching people with ASD skills, change agents can design learning trials that contain the three-term contingency. First, change agents determine the target response and the contexts in which the behavior should occur (i.e., identify the appropriate discriminative stimuli). Next, change agents should determine the appropriate prompts and prompting hierarchy to use to support the learner. In this chapter we describe the general procedures, research, advantages, and disadvantages of four prompting hierarchies: most-to-least prompting, least-to-most prompting, graduated guidance, and time delay. Change agents should determine the appropriate prompt hierarchy based on various factors, including the target response, the learner's learning history, the learner's prerequisite skills, and the advantages and disadvantages of the prompt hierarchy. Finally, change agents should determine how reinforcement is delivered by identifying the reinforcers and the reinforcement schedule (i.e., when reinforcers are delivered). Change agents should consider the natural contingencies for the response (i.e., typical reinforcers when the response occurs and how often these reinforcers are delivered in an environment) and should initially provide multiple opportunities for the learner to contact reinforcement.

When implementing prompting and reinforcement strategies, there are some important considerations. First, reinforcement strategies may be used with prompting to help teach new skills and are commonly considered to be essential components to skill acquisition. Second, prompts should be systematically faded so the learner does not become prompt dependent (i.e., learner engages in the response after prompt is presented) and can engage in the response independently. Practitioners and change agents should collect data on the learner's performance and current prompt level and make data-based decisions on when to increase or decrease prompts. Finally, reinforcement should be faded to match the natural contingencies of the learner's environment. When the learner is first learning a new response, the learner may receive preferred reinforcers in addition to the natural reinforcer and/or may receive reinforcers more frequently than what the environment typically provides. As the learner becomes more independent and masters the response, reinforcement should also be systematically faded to match the natural reinforcement contingencies. This fading process helps ensure that the natural reinforcement contingencies maintain the response over time.

The research literature demonstrates that prompting, time delay, and reinforcement are strategies that may lead to positive outcomes for people with ASD. The National Clearinghouse on Autism and Evidence and Practice (NCAEP; Steinbrenner et al., 2020) and the National Standards Program (NSP; National Autism Center, 2015) have identified prompting, time delay, and reinforcement as evidence-based practices that lead to positive benefits for people with ASD. When examining specific prompting, time-delay, and reinforcement procedures, the literature supports the use of these strategies to support people with ASD develop skills across multiple outcome domains, including academics, play, and daily living or vocational skills. Research studies have demonstrated that participants with ASD may maintain these responses after intervention and may generalize the responses to novel contexts (e.g., Barton, 2015; Ford et al., 2021; Jerome et al., 2007; Taylor & Harris, 1995). When considering social validity, interventions containing prompting, time delay, and/or reinforcement were reported to be socially acceptable (e.g., Boutain et al., 2020), and special educators tended to rate these behavioral strategies favorably to support students with ASD (McNeill, 2019).

Current research has also focused on increasing the accessibility of interventions that use prompting and reinforcement. For instance, researchers have had success integrating technology into how we provide services to people with ASD in ways such as video prompting (e.g., Stauch & Plavnick, 2020; Weng & Bouck, 2014) and providing interventions over telehealth (e.g., Ferguson et al., 2020; Ford et al., 2021). Additionally, researchers have also demonstrated that natural change agents such as families (e.g., Harriage et al., 2016) and educators (e.g., Horn et al., 2020; Seaman et al., 2017) can learn to implement interventions with prompting and reinforcement through remote training and coaching. Future research should continue to investigate and evaluate methods to leverage advances in technology to increase the accessibility of these interventions.

4.8 References

Akmanoglu, N., & Batu, S. (2004). Teaching pointing to numerals to individuals with autism using simultaneous prompting. *Education and Training in Developmental Disabilities, 39*(4), 326–336.

Barton, E. (2015). Teaching generalized pretend play and related behaviors to young children with disabilities. *Exceptional Children*, 81, 489–506. https://doi.org/10.1177/0014402914563694

Boutain, A. R., Sheldon, J. B., & Sherman, J. A. (2020). Evaluation of a telehealth parent training program in teaching self-care skills to children with autism. *Journal of Applied Behavior Analysis, 53*(3), 1259–1275. https://doi.org/10.1002/jaba.743

Charlop, M. H, & Walsh, M. E. (1986). Increasing autistic children's spontaneous verbalizations of affection: An assessment of time delay and peer modeling procedures. *Journal of Applied Behavior Analysis, 19*(3), 307–314. doi: 10.1901/jaba.1986.19-307

Chazin, K. T., & Ledford, J. R. (2021). Constant time delay and system of least prompts: Efficiency and child preference. *Journal of Behavioral Education, 30*(4), 648–707. https://psycnet.apa.org/doi/10.1007/s10864-020-09396-0

Collins, B. C., Lo, Y., Park, G., & Haughney, K. (2018). Response prompting as an ABA-based instructional approach for teaching students with disabilities. *TEACHING Exceptional Children, 50*(6), 343–355. https://doi.org/10.1177%2F0040059918774920

Cooper, J. O., Heron, T. E., & Heward, W. L. (2020). *Applied behavior analysis* (3rd ed.). Hoboken, NJ: Pearson Education.

Ferguson, J. L., Majeski, M. J., McEachin, J., Leaf, R., Cihon, J. H., & Leaf, J. B. (2020). Evaluating discrete trial teaching with instructive feedback delivered in a dyad arrangement via telehealth. *Journal of Applied Behavior Analysis, 53*(4), 1876–1888. https://doi.org/10.1002/jaba.773

Ford, K., Wang, M., Koegel, L. K., Koegel, R. L., & Fedders, A. (2021). Use of a videoconferencing intervention and systematic hierarchy to teach daily living skills to young adults with autism spectrum disorder. *Journal of Positive Behavior Interventions, 23*(2), 81–92. https://doi.org/10.1177%2F1098300720921214

Fragale, C. L. (2014). Video modeling interventions to improve play skills of children with autism spectrum disorders: A systematic literature review. *Review Journal of Autism and Developmental Disorders, 1*, 165–178. https://doi.org/10.1007/s40489-014-0019-4

Gerow, S., Radhakrishnan, S., Akers, J. S., McGinnis, K., & Swensson, R. (2021). Telehealth parent coaching to improve daily living skills for children with ASD. *Journal of Applied Behavior Analysis, 54*(2), 566–581. https://doi.org/10.1002/jaba.813

Harriage, B., Blair, K. C., & Miltenberger, R. (2016). An evaluation of a parent implemented in situ pedestrian safety skills intervention for individuals with autism. *Journal of Autism and Developmental Disorders, 46*, 2017–2027. https://doi.org/10.1007/s10803-016-2730-8

Horn, A. L., Gable, R. A., Bobzien, J. L., Tonelson, S. W., & Rock, M. L. (2020). Teaching young adults job skills using a constant time delay and ecoaching intervention package. *Career Development and Transition for Exceptional Individuals, 43*(1), 29–39. https://doi.org/10.1177%2F2165143419828983

Jerome, J., Frantino, E. P., & Sturmey, P. (2007). The effects of errorless learning and backwards chaining on the acquisition of internet skills in adults with developmental disabilities. *Journal of Applied Behavior Analysis, 40*(1), 185–189. https://doi.org/10.1901/jaba.2007.41-06

LaLonde, K. B., Jones, S., West, L., & Santman, C. (2020). An evaluation of a game-based treatment package on intraverbals in young children with autism. *Behavior Analysis in Practice, 13*(1), 152–157. https://doi.org/10.1007/s40617-019-00397-8

LeBlanc, L. A., Coates, A. M., Daneshvar, S., Charlop-Christy, M. H., Morris, C., & Lancaster, B. M. (2003). Using video modeling and reinforcement to teach perspective-taking skills to children with autism. *Journal of Applied Behavior Analysis, 36*(2), 253–257. https://doi.org/10.1901/jaba.2003.36-253

Libby, M. E., Weiss, J. S., Bancroft, S., & Ahearn, W. H. (2008). A comparison of most-to-least and least-to-most prompting on the acquisition of solitary play skills. *Behavior Analysis in Practice, 1*(1), 37–43. https://doi.org/10.1007/BF03391719

Mayer, R. G., Sulzer-Azaroof, B., & Wallace, M. (2022). *Behavior Analysis for Lasting Change.* Littleton, MA: Cambridge Center for Behavioral Studies.

McNeill, J. (2019). Social validity and teacher's use of evidence-based practices for autism. *Journal of Autism and Developmental Disorders, 49*, 4585–4594. https://doi.org/10.1007/s10803-019-04190-y

Morales, V. A., Ledford, J. R., & Chazi n, K. T. (2016). Graduated guidance. In *Evidence-based instructional practices for young children with autism and other disabilities.* http://ebip.vkcsites.org/graduated-guidance

National Autism Center. (2015). *Findings and conclusions: National standards project, phase 2.* https://www.nationalautismcenter.org/national-standards-project/results-reports/

O'Neill, S. J., McDowell, C., & Leslie, J. C. (2020). A comparison of variations of prompt delay during instruction on an expressive labeling task. *Journal of Behavioral Education, 31*, 404–422. https://doi.org/10.1007/s10864-020-09407-0

Oppenheimer, M., Saunders, R. R., & Spradlin, J. E. (1993). Investigating the generality of the delayed-prompt effect. *Research in Developmental Disabilities, 14*(6), 425–444. https://doi.org/10.1016/0891-4222(93)90036-J

Seaman, R. L., Cannella-Malone, H. I., Brock, M. E., & Dueker, S. A. (2017). Efficacy of paraprofessional-implemented video prompting to teach vocational skills to students with autism spectrum disorders. *Career Development and Transition for Exceptional Individuals, 41*(2), 68–76. https://doi.org/10.1177%2F2165143417708191

Silbaugh, B. C., & Falcomata, T. S. (2019). Effects of a lag schedule with progressive time delay on sign mand variability in a boy with autism. *Behavior Analysis in Practice, 12*, 124–132. https://doi.org/10.1007/s40617-018-00273-x

Snell, M. E., & Gast, D. L. (1981). Applying time delay procedure to the instruction of the severely handicapped. *Research and Practice for Persons with Severe Disabilities, 6*(3), 3–14. https://doi.org/10.1177%2F154079698100600301

Stauch, A., & Plavnick, J. B. (2020). Teaching vocational and social skills to adolescents with autism using video models. *Education and Treatment of Children, 43*, 137–151. https://doi.org/10.1007/s43494-020-00020-4

Steinbrenner, J. R., Hume, K., Odom, S. L., Morin, K. L., Nowell, S. W., Tomaszewski, B., Szendrey, S., McIntyre, N. S., Yücesoy-Özkan, S., & Savage, M. N. (2020). *Evidence-based practices for children, youth, and young adults with autism.* The University of North Carolina, Frank Porter Graham Child Development Institute, National Clearinghouse on Autism Evidence and Practice Review Team. https://ncaep.fpg.unc.edu/sites/ncaep.fpg.unc.edu/files/imce/documents/EBP%20Report%202020.pdf

Stokes, T. F. & Baer, D.M. (1977). An implicit technology of generalization. *Journal of Applied Behavior Analysis, 10*(2), 349–367.

Taylor, B. A., & Harris, S. L. (1995). Teaching children with autism to seek information: Acquisition of novel information and generalization of responding. *Journal of Applied Behavior Analysis, 28*(1), 3–14. https://doi.org/10.1901/jaba.1995.28-3

Wainer, A. L., & Ingersoll, B. R. (2015). Increasing access to an ASD imitation intervention via a telehealth parent training program. *Journal of Autism and Developmental Disorders, 45*, 3877–3890. https://doi.org/10.1007/s10803-014-2186-7

Walker, G. (2008). Constant and progressive time delay procedures for teaching children with autism: A literature review. *Journal of Autism and Developmental Disorders, 38*, 261–275. https://doi.org/10.1007/s10803-007-0390-4

Watkins, L., Ledbetter-Cho, K., O'Reilly, M., Barnard-Brak, L., & Garcia-Grau, P. (2019). Interventions for students with autism in inclusive settings: A best-evidence synthesis and meta-analysis. *Psychological Bulletin, 145*(5), 490–507. https://doi.org/10.1037/bul0000190

Weng, P., & Bouck, E. C. (2014). Using video prompting via iPads to teach price comparison to adolescents with autism. *Research in Autism Spectrum Disorders, 8*(10), 1405–1415. https://doi.org/10.1016/j.rasd.2014.06.014

Wolery, M., & Gast, D. L. (1984). Effective and efficient procedures for the transfer of stimulus control. *Topics in Early Childhood Special Education, 4*(3), 52–77. https://doi.org/10.1177%2F027112148400400305

5

Punishment-Based Behavioral Interventions

Olive Healy
Trinity College Dublin, The University of Dublin

Aoife McTiernan
National University of Ireland Galway

Lorna Barry
ASK, Geneva

Aoife Ryan
National University of Ireland Galway

Jennifer Holloway
ASK, Geneva

Rhona Dempsey
Trinity College Dublin, The University of Dublin

5.1 Technical Abstract

Background: Punishment as defined by Azrin and Holz (1966) may be understood as the contingent application of a specific type of consequence following the occurrence of a response or class of responses that results in a future reduction in the occurrence of such responses. What defines the behavioral process as punishment involves the characteristic effects that subsequently occur to the application of the consequence—that is, an observed reduction or cessation of a specific response or response class. **Method:** The current chapter reviews the general trends in punishment-based behavioral interventions with individuals diagnosed with autism spectrum disorder (ASD). It examines the effectiveness of specific interventions based on the extant literature and provides an updated overview of the use of punishment-based behavioral interventions examining a range of characteristics and outcomes from published studies and reviews. **Results:** A variety of punishment-based interventions are reported to target a spectrum of perceived challenging behavior, including stereotypy, in autistic people. Overall, studies utilizing punishment combined with reinforcement-based procedures show apparent greater effectiveness in target behavior reduction. Infrequent assessment of generalization, maintenance outcomes, and side effects persists. **Discussion:** The outcomes of a range of punishment-based interventions are detailed in the published

Olive Healy et al., *Punishment-Based Behavioral Interventions*. In: *Lifespan Treatment for Autistic Individuals*.
Edited by: Peter Sturmey, Russell Lang, and James K. Luiselli, Oxford University Press. © Oxford University Press (2025).
DOI: 10.1093/oso/9780197635841.003.0005

literature but are not accompanied by guidelines or cautions; therefore, these outcomes must be carefully considered in relation to the protection of human rights of all individuals.

5.2 Layperson Summary

The term *punishment* and its technical description in the field of behavior analysis are controversial. This chapter sets out to describe terminology and how it varies and takes on quite different meanings in everyday language, technical language, and as set out in human rights legislation. The chapter reviews the general trends related to punishment-based behavioral interventions used with people diagnosed with ASD and examines the effectiveness of specific interventions based on the available literature up to 2014. It also provides an updated overview of the more recent use of punishment-based behavioral interventions with autistic people. It subsequently sets out punishment in relation to the United Nations Convention on the Rights of Persons With Disabilities (UNCRPD; United Nations, 2007), an international treaty promoting and protecting the human rights of all persons with disabilities. The chapter indicates professional ethical standards which apply to behavioral interventions and discusses the controversy surrounding the use of programmed punishment interventions to target what is perceived as "challenging behavior" among autistic people. Several limitations are highlighted and noted following review of the included studies. This review establishes that similar to previous reviews and commentaries, only limited conclusions can be drawn about the efficacy of punishment-based procedures due to problematic lack of clarity in the literature regarding how punishment procedures are selected, assessments that identify potential punishment interventions, and factors that influence the effectiveness of those procedures. The chapter ends by attempting to set out recommendations to support professionals in considering the utility of punishment, or other treatments, to selectively reduce particular categories of behavior in autism and related disabilities.

5.3 Treatment Summary Table

Treatment summary: Punishment

Treatment description: The technical description of punishment as a principle of behavior involves the presentation or removal of a stimulus contingent on a specified response. As defined by Azrin and Holz (1966), punishment may be understood as the contingent application of a consequence following a behavior that results in a reduction in the future occurrence of that behavior. What defines the behavioral process as punishment involves the characteristic effects that subsequently occur—that is, an observed reduction or cessation of a specific response or response class following application of the consequence. The stimulus that was presented or removed is therefore often defined as a "punisher" or "aversive stimulus," technical terms that may take on different meanings in everyday parlance.

Expected outcomes: The body of research to date on punishment within the field of behavior analysis demonstrates a wide variety of specific outcomes, usually idiosyncratic. In general, the expected outcome is reduction or suppression of a behavior perceived as "challenging" in some way for the person themselves and/or the context in which they live. The outcomes of a range of punishment-based interventions are detailed in the published literature but are not accompanied by guidelines or cautions; therefore, the outcomes must be carefully considered in relation to the protection of human rights of all individuals.

Methods: A range of punishment-based interventions are reported in the published literature, including, for example, time-out from reinforcement, verbal reprimand, contingent exercise, and response cost. Current approaches to the application of such procedures range widely. Interpreting recommendations from the current body of work gives rise to the following considerations: Punishment-based procedures when implemented should be combined with reinforcement and antecedent-based interventions following completion of an appropriate behavioral assessment to the needs of a person and their individual context; a hierarchy of least restrictive interventions, within a robust framework underpinned by human rights considerations, is a necessity in research and practice.

Expertise required to implement treatment: The credence of the professional code of ethics where punishment-based procedures are implemented involves implementation and oversight from competent and qualified professionals who consider risk-benefit analysis where the intended benefit to the person is considered to outweigh any risks *and* it is a consideration of last resort. The evidence from the literature to date does not seem to align with the guidance outlined in "Minimizing Risk of Behavior Change Interventions" (section 2.15, BACB®, 2020).

Risks and negative side effects: The term "challenging behavior" is a fluid concept in the literature, problematically open to misinterpretation; consequently, the application of punishment procedures currently may be considered to infringe on human rights in some instances. The significant range of effectiveness of such procedures from completely ineffective to total reduction calls to question the sustained gaps in knowledge in the many factors that impact the procedural implementation of these types of approaches to behavior change. The maintenance, generalization, and side effects of these interventions also remain understudied.

Additional considerations and limitations: The protection of the human rights of autistic people is paramount when receiving behavior analytic interventions. "The Right to Effective Behavioral Treatment" originally described by Van Houten et al. (1988) outlines six human rights which are included in the most recent code of ethics for behavior analysts (BACB®, 2020). There is a need for the oversight of fidelity to these standards, especially where behavior reduction or suppression is the goal of intervention.

There are some notable concerns in the body of literature describing the implementation of punishment procedures with autistic people, including their utility without first demonstrating the failure of less restrictive procedures, the young age of participants included in studies, and the disproportionate inclusion of people with moderate to profound disabilities.

It appears that many punishment-based procedures reported in the literature may be considered inappropriate and in breach of both professional and ethical frameworks and standards described above.

Cautions about the application of all punishment-based procedures should be developed and applied to each individual case to ensure a risk-benefit analysis is conducted in an empathetic and insightful way.

5.4 Introduction

In everyday language, the word *punishment* is often used in an equivocal way. The term *punishment* usually denotes the experience of something negative for a person either following their actions (contingent) or in no specific relationship to their actions (noncontingent). There are a few problems encountered when reviewing the literature on punishment. These problems generally arise from the strong feelings and values associated with its use and are often based on many years of traditions and ideas about what punishment as a behavioral process involves. In contrast to everyday language, in behavior analysis, punishment is defined quite precisely. The technical description of punishment as a principle of behavior involves the presentation or removal of a stimulus contingent on a specified response. As defined by Azrin and Holz (1966), punishment may be understood as the contingent application of a consequence to a behavior that results in a reduction in the occurrence of that behavior. What defines the behavioral process as punishment involves the characteristic effects that subsequently occur—that is, an observed reduction or cessation of a specific response or response class (a group of responses sharing the same functional effect). The stimulus that was presented or removed is therefore defined as a "punisher" or "aversive stimulus," again terms that take on different meanings in everyday language.

Importantly, this technical definition of punishment addresses the principle as a process and relies on the behavioral effect observed to determine if punishment has truly occurred. To this end, punishment may be understood either as positive or negative, where the word *positive* is also a scientific term meaning "additive" involving the contingent application of a stimulus, for example, a verbal caution or physical restraint. Alternately, the word *negative* is another scientific term with regard to punishment and involves the contingent "removal" of a reinforcing stimulus, for example, removal of an item the person desires. The words *positive* and *negative* are not synonyms for constructive or helpful; or bad, undesirable, or harmful, respectively but instead are used to designate if something is "added" or "removed," respectively. Furthermore, according to the technical definition, punishment is something that happens to behavior rather than something that is done to a person.

A layperson's traditional view of punishment is whereby someone usually in authority imposes something on someone else as a penalty for a misdeed. It is considered something that is done to people to make them "pay for their misdeed." In such instances, behavior may be somewhat disrupted but not selectively reduced and therefore is not always effective in changing behavior to achieve reduction or suppression. In our everyday lives and throughout our lives, we all will encounter outcomes for our behavior that may reduce our actions in the future or make us less likely to do certain things again (e.g., receiving a speeding fine might cause a person to be more likely to adhere to speed limits in the future). In some instances, our behavior may be punished by its natural consequences; that is, we simply learn from the natural consequences that we encounter (e.g., forgetting a house key could lead to requiring a locksmith to break the lock, so a person is likely to adopt a strategy to mitigate against this reoccurring). The distinction between the procedural experiences of punishment is important, but the differences between naturalistic punishment and programmed punishment have significant implications for how we approach intervention, especially in relation to best practices in raising children, educating across the lifespan, and providing societal motivation for change.

The term *punishment* and its technical description in the field of behavior analysis have caused much controversy among researchers and practitioners both within and outside of the discipline. Indeed, during the last decade a rising number of disability rights and advocacy groups have expressed much concern with applied behavior analysis (ABA) where the utility of negative consequences (including positive and negative punishment interventions) to change human behavior has been observed (see Leaf et al., 2022). In some instances, concerns and distress in relation to these practices are justified. There are many examples in the published literature on ABA that describe behavioral interventions based on the principle of punishment. Much of this research has involved autistic people whereby the goal for the most part has been to reduce or eliminate behaviors that cause harm. In other cases, the focus has been less on high-risk behaviors but on those that are considered to interfere with academic and social learning opportunities (e.g., stereotypies). Both examples have caused much offence to many, particularly among autistic people, and fueled a movement against behavior change, specifically ABA. Nowadays, there is significant and impactful guidance and protection for vulnerable populations from an established human rights framework (e.g., the United Nations Convention on the Rights of Persons With Disabilities; UNCRPD (United Nations, 2007) and ethical guidelines in relation to practices that may seek to change behavior (e.g., Behavior Analyst Certification Board; BACB®). Such frameworks and guidance provide excellent reference points for the use of consequences to improve a person's well-being and ensure the rejection of practices which are not aligned with human rights, and which are against the tenet "Do No Harm." However, such guidance is not always adhered to, and appropriate oversight may be absent. This matters greatly for the field of behavior analysis to responsibly engage in public psychology and to use the fruits of the discipline to address pressing issues related to ensuring excellent support is accessible to autistic people and other populations. Similarly, as will be elaborated on later in this chapter, the term *punishment* has a far broader expanse than what seems to be narrowly implicated in the UNCRPD (2007).

The current chapter will provide a review of the general trends related to punishment-based behavioral interventions with individuals diagnosed with ASD. It will examine the effectiveness of specific interventions based on the extant literature relating to the topic. It will then provide an updated overview of the use of punishment-based behavioral interventions since 2014 examining a range of characteristics and outcomes from studies. It will examine the topic of punishment in relation to UNCRPD, an international treaty promoting and protecting the human rights of all persons with disabilities. The chapter will also discuss the controversy surrounding the use of programmed punishment interventions to target what may be considered problem behavior or behaviors of concern among autistic people. Finally, it will provide a summary of recommendations in relation to the utility of punishment to selectively reduce particular categories of behavior in autism and related disabilities.

5.5 Research Background

5.5.1 General Trends From the 1960s to 2014

An understanding of the research body on punishment is important in order to provide insight into interventions and their outcomes, including identifying variables that impact outcomes, with the aim of informing the role, or otherwise, of punishment in clinical practice and future research priorities in the field. The term *punishment* encompasses both the addition (positive) and removal (negative) of stimuli resulting in a reduction or suppression of a particular response or class of responses in the literature discussed in this section. The most recent review of punishment research was published in 2015 by Lydon and colleagues, who quantitatively examined trends in the evaluation of punishment procedures from the 1960s up to 2014 (Lydon et al., 2015). An earlier literature review in 2002 by Lerman and Vorndran provided a descriptive review of basic and applied research; however, the authors did not assess treatment outcomes or variables that may affect those outcomes (Lerman & Vorndran, 2002). A previous review on the quantitative analysis of punishment effects was also published some 30 years ago (see Matson & Taras, 1989).

Lydon et al. (2015) reviewed the research literature across five decades, starting with the 1960s, evaluating punishment procedures to decrease what was described as challenging behavior for individuals with developmental disabilities. The numbers of studies citing the utility of punishment in this population saw a gradual and consistent decline from a peak in the early 1980s. The authors found since the 1990s on an annual basis that punishment procedures have been reported in fewer than 10 published articles. This finding is consistent with Heyvaert and colleagues (2014), who reported a decrease in the frequency of evaluation of punishment-based interventions over time in their quantitative synthesis of behavioral interventions for the treatment of challenging behaviors in individuals with autism. Similarly, Kahng and colleagues (2002) reported that the use of reinforcement-based interventions had increased during the preceding decade, whereas the use of punishment-based interventions had decreased, albeit slightly; both trends were in line with the corresponding increase in the use of functional behavioral assessments (Kahng et al., 2002).

5.5.2 The Term "Challenging Behavior"

Arising from the review by Lydon et al. (2015), it is clear there is considerable variance in the literature as to what the respective researchers regarded as "challenging behavior" targeted for reduction or elimination; indeed, 16 categorizations were recorded covering a very wide range and diverse topographies such as self-injurious behavior, elopement, noncompliance, or spitting, drooling, or saliva play. A distinction between targeting what were described as more debilitating challenging behaviors compared to those that may be considered less imposing was not clearly evident. The likelihood of treatment was more often cited for challenging behaviors, such as self-injury and aggression, across each decade, except for 2010 onward. However, stereotyped behaviors were also frequently targeted for reduction using punishment-based treatments, particularly after 2010 (up to 2014). As such, there is little evidence of nuance in the examined body of literature as to the selection of least restrictive intervention. This predominance of punishment interventions for self-injury, aggression, and stereotypies concurs with the prior review by Matson and Taras (1989); with Kahng et al. (2002) in their review of behavioral interventions for self-injurious behavior; and with Heyvaert et al.'s (2014) reporting of behavioral interventions for the challenging behavior of persons with autism. In conjunction with other commonalities between Lydon et al. (2015) and Matson and Taras's (1989) respective reviews, this finding possibly points to a mismatch across the decades in terms of punishment interventions keeping pace with knowledge gains and evidence in the field, calling into question practitioner expertise and ethical practices.

Behaviors that are considered relatively harmless, such as stereotypies labeled as "challenging," stand apart from more hazardous behaviors addressed in the literature. This observation aligns with Healy and colleagues (2013) and other researchers, who suggest that the use of punishment interventions may be associated with a failure to accurately identify the source of reinforcement driving these behaviors. Instead, they propose that functional analyses should be employed to correctly identify the underlying causes and develop appropriate interventions based on these analyses (Healy et al., 2013).

To this end, Lydon et al. (2015) examined the consideration of function of behavior by researchers and whether functional assessment methodologies were employed and found mixed results. On the one hand, the authors found that a large proportion of 368 studies reviewed utilized punishment *without* conducting a prior functional assessment or analysis; in the case of 41.5% studies in the 1990s, 24.5% studies in the 2000s and 22.7% studies published between 2010 up to 2014. Lerman and Vorndran (2002) also underscored the importance of functional analysis in order to instruct appropriate interventions. The increased use of functional assessment and functional analysis methodologies across the decades is important because, without determining the function of any targeted behavior, researchers may arrive at selecting interventions in the absence of possible underlying causation.

5.5.3 Intervention Type and Efficacy

Lydon et al. (2015) found that most often and consistently across the decades, except for the 1990s, punishment procedures were used either alone or in combination with other punishment techniques. Multiple punishment-based procedures were selected in close to half of treatment applications (47.8%) in the 2000s. The authors noted their surprise at these findings, particularly in more recent decades, given the known importance of using punishment in combination with reinforcement-based procedures to support beneficial outcomes for the individual (e.g., where the desired source of reinforcement is available to the individual through establishing an alternative behavior). There was also an upward trend toward combining punishment with either antecedent strategies or reinforcement strategies through the decades from 10.3% of treatment applications in the 1970s to 46.0% of treatment applications between 2010 and 2014 in keeping with improved knowledge acquisition in the field.

Lydon et al. (2015) calculated the efficacy of treatments implemented in 78.9% (n = 280) of the 355 studies reviewed employing single-subject research designs by examining mean baseline reduction. They reported a slight decline in treatment efficacy from the 1960s onward and noted that efficacy of punishment-based interventions was variable across the decades with no overt change in trend. This is consistent with Heyvaert et al. (2014), who noted little change in the efficacy of behavioral interventions over time. Lerman and Vorndran (2002) reported that the relative efficacy of treatment with reinforcement versus punishment likely depends on a variety of factors (e.g., history, use of extinction, type, amount, and schedule of the consequence) and noted that there were research gaps to this end.

Lydon et al. (2015) found the use of a punishment procedure alone was least effective, whereas the use of multiple punishment procedures in combination was slightly more effective. Punishment combined with reinforcement-based procedures and/or skills training was the most effective strategy in the literature, followed by punishment combined with antecedent manipulation or changes in instructional context.

In terms of punishment procedures selected by researchers, Lydon et al. (2015) found "time-out" accounted for over one fifth (21%) of all treatment applications (n = 1,768 applications) arising from the studies evaluated; this was followed by "overcorrection" and "verbal reprimand," accounting for 17% and 16%, respectively. Contingent demand, contingent exercise, and guided compliance each accounted for a share of 1% of total applications. Table 5.1 provides a detailed breakdown of the types of punishment procedures employed in previous research studies.

These data further revealed little correlation between a treatment's efficacy and the frequency of its selection. For instance, "time-out" was the most frequently selected punishment intervention yet showed an average decrease in challenging behaviors of only 63.2% when used alone or 82% when used with other strategies. "Contingent demand" was the least frequently selected intervention despite

Table 5.1 Types of punishment procedures identified by Lydon et al. (2015) in the literature from the 1960s to 2014

Punishment Procedure	**Percentage of All Treatment Applications (*n* = 1,768)**
Time-out	21%
Overcorrection	17%
Verbal reprimand	16%
Response cost	13%
Physical restraint	9%
Contingent aversive stimulation	5%
Response blocking	5%
Contingent electric shock	3%
Facial screening	2%
Other restraint	2%
Visual screening	2%
Contingent demand	1%
Contingent exercise	1%
Guided compliance	1%
Other	2%
Total	100%

an average decrease in challenging behavior of 99.1% when used alone and 94.2% when used with other strategies.

A further finding by Lydon et al. (2015) showed all of the interventions evaluated in the reviewed literature were reported to either result in no improvement (mean baseline reduction of 0%) or to entirely remove the target behavior (100% reduction). This finding underscores the *potential* inefficacy of punishment interventions. Both Lydon et al. (2015) and Lerman and Vorndran (2002) underline the vacuum in knowledge of factors influencing the efficacy of punishment procedures. This is far from a cost-neutral position for the individuals concerned and suggests anything other than a person-centered approach that yields positive outcomes for the individual is unsatisfactory.

Where functional assessment was conducted and identified the function, automatically reinforced behaviors were least responsive to punishment interventions (mean baseline reduction of 79.1%) compared to positively (90.6%) and negatively (87.6%) reinforced behaviors.

Across decades, participants were most commonly described as children in studies evaluating punishment-based interventions compared to adolescents and adult age cohorts (Kahng et al., 2002; Lydon et al., 2015; Matson & Taras, 1989). This correlates with research into the use of seclusion and restraint in school settings, where there is an overrepresentation, where data are collected, of children with disabilities and within this cohort of younger children (Bartlett & Ellis, 2020; Verret et al., 2019); and it is contrary to the evidence that challenging behavior typically increase with age in the developmentally disabled population (e.g., Jacobson, 1982; Lydon et al., 2015; Oliver et al., 1987).

In terms of the principle of starting with least restrictive interventions, it is a concern that punishment was seemingly a first approach in approximately half of the 368 studies (Lydon et al., 2015). The authors also flagged that there is a lack of research or guidance on utilizing punishment-based interventions. This recommendation echoes Lerman and Vorndran (2002), who also indicated the need for guidelines and "cautions" about the application of punishment and noted that the potential for undesirable side effects involving caregiver behavior (e.g., overusing punishment, dehumanizing the punished individual) should receive more attention.

Generalization was reported to be understudied and was found by Lydon et al. (2015) in 64 (17.6%) of the studies reviewed, three quarters assessed generalization to other settings. Lerman and Vordran (2002) noted that surprisingly few studies have evaluated strategies to promote generalization since Matson and Taras (1989) lamented this gap in their review. Kahng et al. (2002) also noted the infrequent assessment of generalization and maintenance outcomes.

5.5.4 General Trends From 2014 to 2022

Given the previous findings and recommendations of authors in the field, as well as the growing criticism of the utility of practices based on the behavioral principle of punishment with autistic and other populations, it is pertinent to determine how and in what contexts such interventions are being designed and implemented. The next half of this chapter will examine this issue by providing an overview of related research from 2014 to 2022.

In general, more recent studies report a wide range in what was considered to be "challenging behaviors," ranging from aggression (e.g., Cariveau et al., 2019; Eluri et al., 2016; Quinn et al., 2014), self-injury (e.g., Manente & LaRue, 2017; Saini et al., 2016), bruxism (e.g., Armstrong et al., 2014), pica (e.g., Muething et al., 2020), stereotypies (e.g., Gerow et al., 2019; Laprime & Dittrich, 2014), non-compliance (e.g., Quinn et al., 2014), and sleep disturbance (e.g., Sanberg et al., 2018). This reflects previous findings by Lydon et al. (2015) and proposes that a persistence remains in targeting innocuous behaviors where principles of least restrictive intervention were not applied. The topography of behaviors under each of these categories ranged from what may be considered a dangerous behavior such as pica (e.g., Busch et al., 2018) or bruxism (e.g., Armstrong et al., 2014) to behaviors such as laughing (Shawler et al., 2020), humming, or singing (McNamara & Cividini-Motta, 2019).

Another trend in the more recent published research is that functional analysis is commonly undertaken to determine functional outcomes and inform the design of the punishment-based procedure. Notably, a high proportion identify nonsocial reinforcement as the function of the target behavior (e.g., Hodges et al., 2018; Migan-Gandonou & Leon, 2020; Mitteer et al., 2015); Schmidt et al., 2017).

The trends in the literature also show the use of punishment-based procedures to decrease what was described as challenging behavior, applied in combination with other reinforcement-based procedures rather than in isolation. Table 5.2 provides details of some examples of punishment procedures used in isolation or used as part of a combined treatment package.

Overall, maintenance and generalization remain underreported outcomes in more recent studies from 2014, a similar finding to Lydon et al. (2015), who highlighted this as an important area, which is overlooked in the literature. Where generalization was reported, the authors describe successful outcomes (e.g., Hodges et al., 2018; Muething et al., 2020). Maintenance or follow-up checks for sustained effects of intervention are limited and ranged from 1 month to 5 years (e.g., Migan-Gandonou & Leon, 2020; Schmidt et al., 2017).

Table 5.2 Examples of punishment procedures used in isolation or used as part of a combined treatment package from 2014 to 2022

Punishment in Isolation	
Verbal reprimands	Cook et al.(2014) Dominguez et al. (2014)
Arm-splint belt	Morgan et al. (2017)
Contingent oral hygiene	Migan-Gandonou and Leon (2020)
Response interruption and redirection	Shawler and Miguel (2015)
Treatment Package Including Reinforcement and/or Extinction-Based Procedures	
Response blocking*	Brown (2021) Muething et al. (2020)
Response cost	Cariveau et al. (2019) McNamara and Cividini-Motta (2019)
Verbal reprimand	Hodges et al. (2020) Wilder and Neve (2018)
Response interruption and redirection	Cariveau et al. (2019) McNamara and Cividini-Motta (2019)
Time-out	Dupuis et al. (2015) Hartz et al. (2020)
Facial screening	DeRosa et al. (2019) Mitteer et al. (2015)
Guided compliance	Wilder et al. (2020) Wiskow et al. (2017)
Differential punishment of high rates of challenging behavior	Manente and LaRue (2017)

*There is still debate surrounding the theoretical categorization of response blocking as punishment or extinction.

Social validity (e.g., McNamara & Cividini-Motta, 2019), which is considered an important measure in applied research, also remains an underinvestigated variable in studies examining punishment. The acceptability of procedures used in any intervention is critical to understand, perhaps moreover when considering punishment-based procedures. It is essential that researchers include the voices and perspectives of key stakeholders (e.g., clients and their families) in the acceptability of interventions using such procedures.

The trend in the literature presents a sustained proclivity toward single-case research designs with small numbers of participants included in studies ranging from one participant (e.g., Armstrong et al., 2014; Brown, 2021; DeRosa et al., 2016; Wilder & Neve, 2018) to a few participants (e.g., Saini et al., 2016; Sanberg et al., 2018; Verriden & Roscoe, 2019; Watkins & Rapp, 2014). Although these designs are valuable when describing personalized clinical outcomes, it can be difficult to generalize their findings to wider populations.

While many studies report interobserver agreement on the measurement of frequency of the behavior subject to punishment, few studies report measures of procedural integrity and assessment strategies, making it difficult to interpret how researchers determine type and intensity of "punishers" and whether they are functionally related to the behavior or not.

Similar to the findings of Lydon et al (2015), the rationale for the application of punishment procedures was not always clearly delineated in the majority of recent studies, with poor descriptions of previous treatment, lack of rationale for the selection of specific procedural variations of punishment, and most studies lacking information on the type, intensity, and schedule of the consequence.

Another important trend is the sustained use of punishment on stereotypical patterns of behaviors in autistic people (e.g., Gerow et al., 2019; Laprime & Dittrich, 2014; Watkins & Rapp, 2014). In recent years, the autistic community has voiced concern and objections to the use of interventions on instances of stereotypy in particular (e.g., Cook et al., 2014; Schmidt et al., 2021; Shawler & Miguel, 2015; Watkins & Rapp, 2014). Given the limited rationale for the selection of these behaviors, as described earlier, as well as the limited evaluation of social validity with the autistic participants themselves, this raises yet more concerns.

Key questions remain within the field of ABA, including the acceptability and the necessity for using punishment procedures. Although studies reported during the last decade describe "positive" effects, several key factors remain unclear in many studies that included multicomponent intervention packages, including (a) the mechanism of action responsible for behavior change; (b) the generalization and maintenance of effects; (c) whether side effects and/or adjunctive behaviors were observed or measured; and (d) the parameters for the cessation of the punishment intervention. To overcome these issues, future research should concentrate on elucidating the components of interventions that successfully contribute to behavior change, include stakeholder voices in developing and accessing these procedures, and more clearly outline the decision-making process for considering punishment. There is a need for checks and balances and professional oversight and collaborative decision-making all housed within a human rights framework. Furthermore, as a field, it is crucial to understand the long-term effects of these procedures, and so maintenance and generalization measures are crucial to overcoming this gap in our knowledge.

In line with previous reviews and commentaries, limited conclusions can be drawn about the efficacy of punishment-based procedures due to lack of clarity in the recent literature regarding how punishment procedures are selected, assessments that identify potential punishment interventions, and factors that influence the effectiveness of those procedures (Lerman & Vorndran, 2002; Lydon et al., 2015).

5.6 Practice Implications

5.6.1 Punishment and the Human Rights Framework

The rights of people with disabilities are included in the Universal Declaration of Human Rights (United Nations, 1948); however, the disability community believed a specific convention to protect human rights for persons with disabilities was important, given both the legacy of discrimination and their recurrent higher likelihood of being discriminated against (Lombardi et al., 2019; Sabatello & Schulze, 2014). The UNCRPD is an international treaty to promote, protect, and ensure the full and equal enjoyment of all human rights and fundamental freedoms by all persons with disabilities and to promote respect for their inherent dignity. The Convention and its Optional Protocol were adopted in December 2006. As of January 2022, the UNCRPD has 164 signatories, of which 94 are also signatories to the Optional Protocol (United Nations, 2007).

The UNCRPD is a legally binding policy instrument for both state and private stakeholders, and it is cross-sectoral encompassing all areas of life and living. In theory, it provides a perspective and guiding ethos through which to protect the rights of people with disabilities in providing any therapeutic interventions. This is not a straightforward process. In terms of moving from rhetoric to practice, however, ensuring the implementation of the UNCRPD remains difficult due to societal and systemic issues. Furthermore, from a purely technical viewpoint, as a policy instrument, implementation of the UNCRPD is hindered in part due to abstract concepts and subjective, unclear, or absent definitions (De Maeyer et al., 2017; Lombardi et al., 2019).

Specifically, on the subject of the word *punishment*, it occurs four times in the UNCRPD, three times occurring under Article 15 (United Nations, 2007), which states: "Freedom from torture or cruel, inhuman, or degrading treatment or punishment. 1. No one shall be subjected to torture or to cruel, inhuman or degrading treatment or punishment. In particular, no one shall be subjected without his or her free consent to medical or scientific experimentation. 2. Parties shall take all effective legislative, administrative, judicial or other measures to prevent persons with disabilities, on an equal basis with others, from being subjected to torture or cruel, inhuman or degrading treatment or punishment" (p. 10). Because there is no definition offered for *punishment*, this renders it open to interpretation. The lack of definition or guidance as to what constitutes punishment exposes linguistic issues and aspirations both within the UNCRPD, which is open to different interpretations and hence inevitably open to variances, but also when relating to fields such as behavior analysis. Punishment is clearly defined in the objective scientific field of ABA. Notwithstanding this scientific definition, there remains an element of subjectivity, and this is particularly problematic.

The professional field of behavior analysis is governed by ethics, most notably by the ethical standards of the professional organizations for behavior analysts (i.e., BACB®, 2020). On the subject of the word *punishment*, it occurs three times in the ethical standards, under the heading "Minimizing Risk of Behavior Change Interventions" (section 2.15, BACB®, 2020): "Behavior analysts select, design, and implement behavior-change interventions (including the selection and use of consequences) with a focus on minimizing risk of harm to the client and stakeholders. They recommend and implement restrictive or punishment-based procedures only after demonstrating that desired results have not been obtained using less intrusive means, or when it is determined by an existing intervention team that the risk of harm to the client outweighs the risk associated with the behavior-change intervention. When recommending and implementing restrictive or punishment-based procedures, behavior analysts comply with any required review processes (e.g., a human rights review committee). Behavior analysts must continually evaluate and document the effectiveness of restrictive or punishment-based procedures and modify or discontinue the behavior-change intervention in a timely manner if it is ineffective" (p. 12). It is clear from this code of ethics that punishment-based procedures may be considered permissible if necessary, under *strict* conditions, and by *competent* professionals considering risk-benefit analysis, where the intended benefit to the person is considered to outweigh any risks, and within a framework of review, oversight, and monitoring.

We suggest that there are key considerations in assessing whether the utility of punishment-based procedures is respectful and upholds the human rights of a person in line with the UNCRPD. These include the following:

1. *Linguistic interpretation.* As explained previously, it appears that there are linguistic differences in the concept of punishment as set out in the UNCRPD compared with that expressed in the field of ABA, which is the focus of this chapter;
2. *Ethical standards and rigor.* Ethical standards governing the application of punishment-based procedures by credentialed behavior analysts and punishment procedures, if used at all, should only ever occur as a last resort,

where it is determined it is the right thing to do for the person and to their intended benefit within a framework of scrutiny to ensure the procedure is ethical and effective;

3. *The right to effective treatment.* There are additional resources to support upholding ethical and professional standards, including what we believe to be an excellent "statement of rights" originally outlined by Van Houten et al. (1988, p. 381) encompassing "The Right to Effective Behavioral Treatment."

Van Houten et al. (1988) outlined six human rights for people receiving behavior analytic interventions. Lee et al. (2018) examined the impact of these six rights on practice by comparing the Professional and Ethical Compliance Code for Behavior Analysts at that time (BACB®, 2017) with the six rights described by Van Houten et al. (1988) and concluded that the code clearly includes all six.

These six human rights are described as follows:

1. An individual has a right to a therapeutic environment. Individuals have a right to a safe, supportive physical and social environment.
2. An individual has a right to services whose overriding goal is their personal welfare. The core purpose of any intervention is to support an individual in acquiring functional skills that promote independence for example. Any potential risk to an individual's welfare should be considered and appropriately evaluated before implementing any procedures with review from a suitably qualified group such as a human rights committee or ethics oversight group.
3. An individual has a right to treatment by a competent behavior analyst. Professionals practicing under any BACB® credential (RBT®, BCaBA®, BCBA®, BCBA-D®) are required to conduct and meet the necessary academic and practical training prior to operating at that level. If practicing under any of these credentials and encountering situations outside of one's scope of current knowledge, professionals are obligated to seek assistance from those more experienced.
4. An individual has a right to programs that teach functional skills. Individuals have the right to the selection of goals that target socially significant behaviors that promote the individual's independence.
5. An individual has a right to behavioral assessment and ongoing evaluation. Assessment is a necessary component at the outset of any behavior analytic service. That assessment should include an evaluation of the individual's current skills and needs and the variables underpinning the skill performance.
6. An individual has a right to the most effective treatment procedures available. The field of ABA is considered scientifically validated. The evidence-based treatments associated with behavior analysis should be conducted with the

least restrictiveness possible. Only appropriate evidence-based procedures that will result in the most effective and efficient behavior change should be implemented.

Punishment-based procedures are most often used to reduce "challenging" behavior in populations frequently described as "vulnerable," typically involving autistic people. The body of literature presented herein highlights concerning findings, notably the high propensity to utilize punishment-based procedures without first attempting and demonstrating less restrictive procedures have failed; the young age, often preschool age children, who are more likely to be prone to such a regime (Pokorski & Barton, 2021;Vittrup et al., 2006); and the greater likelihood of individuals who are subjected to punishment-based procedures to have moderate to profound disabilities (Lerman & Vorndran, 2002; Lydon et al., 2015).

In many cited cases, it appears punishment-based procedures are inappropriate and in breach of both professional ethical and "right to effective treatment" standards. In conclusion, where all conditions are satisfied in terms of genuinely meeting all professional ethical standards and codes (e.g., BACB®, 2020) and the "right to effective treatment" standards (Van Houten et al., 1988), then interventions may be considered compatible with the UNCRPD. Compounding assuring ethical practice is the inherent subjectivity involved both to some degree in the behavior analytic field and, to a larger extent, in interpreting the meaning of punishment in the UNCRPD. There is also a paucity of data regarding the prevalence of punishment interventions in the field (Pokorski & Barton, 2021).

5.6.2 Conclusions and Recommendations

Pokorski and Barton (2021) found that researchers demonstrated minimal adherence to ethical standards when implementing punishment-based interventions and noted no improvements over time with the behaviors targeted for change. According to these authors: "all behavioral interventions should be submitted to ethical scrutiny to ensure they are implemented with adherence to ethical guidelines. This is especially important in relation to punishment-based interventions, given: (a) the prevalence of punishment practices, (b) the substantial risk of harm associated with their use, and (c) the vulnerable populations with whom they are regularly implemented" (p. 3).

Punishment procedures are referenced in the literature as being applied by various professionals such as behavior analysts (e.g. Lydon et al., 2015); teachers (Westling et al., 2010); healthcare workers (Pokorski & Barton, 2021); parents (Regalado et al., 2004), and often in settings such as home, school, and care facilities (Pokorski & Barton, 2021; Regalado et al., 2004; Westling et al., 2010). The focus of this chapter is on punishment-based intervention procedures in the behavior analytic field, and there is an urgent need for meeting ethical and right-to-effective-treatment standards in selecting appropriate interventions to best support individuals. Interventions need to be both effective and ethical, and demonstrated as such. Practical guidelines and recommendations such as those proposed by Pokorski and Barton (2021) and Lydon et al. (2015) should be better utilized by researchers and practitioners to support their adhering to BACB® ethical standards and code and the right-to-effective-treatment standards both conceptually and most importantly during and post implementation in order to inform and guide practice.

Practitioners need to demonstrate ethical practice, and the onus is on them to demonstrate that the treatment is appropriate, the least restrictive available, and intended to be to the individual's distinct benefit conducted in an operating framework of continuous and evidenced review and evaluation, including supervision and advice where required. There is an onus in the field to develop toolkits in order for practitioners in the field of behavior analysis to understand the ethics around any intervention, including punishment-based procedures, and the importance of only selecting and qualifying appropriate interventions. Where professional qualifications are regulated outside of a jurisdiction, it is incumbent that there is also a system of national oversight and audit within the profession. As pointed out by Pokorski and Barton (2021), all forms of validity, including ethical validity, are critically important in identifying effective, appropriate interventions. Arguably, the gap between rhetoric and practice of the UNCRPD policy reflects the gap between policy (ethical standards) and practice in cases in the field of behavior analysis. There remains the need for further consideration as to how to ensure alignment between the professional ethical codes and right-to-effective-treatment standards with UNCRPD in implementation and practice.

5.7 References

Armstrong, A., Knapp, V. M., & McAdam, D. B. (2014). Functional analysis and treatment of the diurnal bruxism of a 16-year-old girl with autism. *Journal of Applied Behavior Analysis, 47*(2), 415–419. DOI: 10.1002/jaba.122

Azrin, N. H., & Holz, W. C. (1966). Punishment. In W. K. Honig (Ed.), *Operant behavior: Areas of research and application* (pp. 213–217). New York: Appleton-Century-Crofts.

Bartlett, N., & Ellis, T. F. (2020). Interrogating sanctioned violence: A survey of parents/guardians of children with disabilities about restraint and seclusion in Manitoba's schools. *Canadian Journal of Disability Studies, 9*(5), 121–155. DOI: 10.15353/cjds.v9i5.693

Behavior Analyst Certification Board. (2017). Professional and ethical compliance code for behavior analysts. https://www.bacb.com/wp-content/uploads/BACB-Compliance-Code-english_190318.pdf

Behavior Analyst Certification Board. (2020). *Professional and ethical compliance code for behavior analysts.* https://www.bacb.com/wp-content/uploads/2022/01/Ethics-Code-for-Behavior-Analysts-220316-2.pdf

Brown, K. (2021). The use of isolated and synthesized latency functional analyses in the assessment and treatment of clothing removal exhibited by a child with autism. *Clinical Case Studies, 20*(3), 187–200. DOI: 10.1177/1534650120974448

Busch, L., Saini, V., Zorzos, C., & Duyile, L. (2018). Treatment of life-threatening pica with 5-year follow-up. *Advances in Neurodevelopmental Disorders, 2*(4), 335–343. DOI: 10.1007/s41252-018-0053-9

Cariveau, T., Miller, S. J., Call, N. A., & Alvarez, J. (2019). Assessment and treatment of problem behavior maintained by termination of interruptions. *Developmental Neurorehabilitation, 22*(3), 203–208. DOI: 10.1080/17518423.2019.1566278

Cook, J. L., Rapp, J. T., Gomes, L. A., Frazer, T. J., & Lindblad, T. L. (2014). Effects of verbal reprimands on targeted and untargeted stereotypy. *Behavioral Interventions, 29*(2), 106–124. DOI: 10.1002/bin.1378

DeRosa, N. M., Novak, M. D., Morley, A. J., & Roane, H. S. (2019). Comparing response blocking and response interruption/redirection on levels of motor stereotypy: Effects of data analysis procedures. *Journal of Applied Behavior Analysis, 52*(4), 1021–1033. DOI: 10.1002/jaba.644

DeRosa, N. M., Roane, H. S., Bishop, J. R., & Silkowski, E. L. (2016). The combined effects of noncontingent reinforcement and punishment on the reduction of rumination. *Journal of Applied Behavior Analysis, 49*(3), 680–685. DOI: 10.1002/jaba.304

Dominguez, A., Wilder, D. A., Cheung, K., & Rey, C. (2014). The use of a verbal reprimand to decrease rumination in a child with autism. *Behavioral Interventions, 29*(4), 339–345. DOI: 10.1002/bin.1390

Dupuis, D. L., Lerman, D. C., Tsami, L., & Shireman, M. L. (2015). Reduction of aggression evoked by sounds using noncontingent reinforcement and time-out. *Journal of Applied Behavior Analysis, 48*(3), 669–674. DOI: 10.1002/jaba.220

Eluri, Z., Andrade, I., Trevino, N., & Mahmoud, E. (2016). Assessment and treatment of problem behavior maintained by mand compliance. *Journal of Applied Behavior Analysis, 49*(2), 383–387. DOI: 10.1002/jaba.296

Gerow, S., Rivera, G., Akers, J. S., Kirkpatrick, M., & Radhakrishnan, S. (2019). Parent-implemented treatment for automatically maintained stereotypy. *Behavioral Interventions, 34*(4), 466–474. DOI: 10.1002/bin.1689

Hartz, R. M., Luiselli, J. K., & Harper, J. M. (2020). Behavioral treatment of spitting in a child with autism spectrum disorder: Functional analysis, intervention evaluation, and maintenance assessment. *Behavioral Interventions, 35*(4), 595–603. DOI: 10.1002/bin.1739

Healy, O., Brett, D., & Leader, G. (2013). A comparison of experimental functional analysis and the Questions About Behavioral Function (QABF) in the assessment of challenging behavior of individuals with autism. *Research in Autism Spectrum Disorders, 7*, 66–81. DOI: 10.1016/j.rasd.2012.05.006

Heyvaert, M., Saenen, L., Campbell, J. M., Maes, B., & Onghena, P. (2014). Efficacy of behavioral interventions for reducing problem behavior in persons with autism: An updated quantitative synthesis of single-subject research. *Research in Developmental Disabilities, 35*, 2463–2476. DOI: 10.1016/j.ridd.2014.06.017

Hodges, A., Wilder, D. A., & Ertel, H. (2020). Assessment and treatment of a foot fetish exhibited by an adolescent with autism. *Behavior Analysis in Practice, 13*(4), 961–965. DOI: 10.1007/s40617-020-00468-1

Hodges, A. C., Wilder, D. A., & Ertel, H. (2018). The use of a multiple schedule to decrease toe walking in a child with autism. *Behavioral Interventions, 33*(4), 440–447. DOI: 10.1002/bin.1528

Van Houten, R., Axelrod, S., Bailey, J. S., Favell, J. E., Foxx, R. M., Iwata, B. A., & Lovaas, O. I. (1988). The right to effective behavioral treatment. *The Behavior Analyst, 11*, 111–114. DOI: 10.1901/jaba.1988.21-381

Jacobson, J. W. (1982). Problem behavior and psychiatric impairment within a developmentally disabled population. I: Behavior frequency. *Applied Research in Mental Retardation, 3*, 121–139. DOI: 10.1016/0270-3092(82)90002-9

Kahng, S., Iwata, B. A., & Lewin, A. B. (2002). Behavioral treatment of self-injury, 1964 to 2000. *American Journal on Mental Retardation, 107*, 212–221. DOI: 10.1352/0895-8017(2002)107<0212:BTOSIT>2.0.CO;2

Laprime, A. P., & Dittrich, G. A. (2014). An evaluation of a treatment package consisting of discrimination training and differential reinforcement with response cost and a social story on vocal stereotypy for a preschooler with autism in a preschool classroom. *Education and Treatment of Children*, 37, 407–430. DOI: 10.1353/etc.2014.0028

Leaf, J. B., Cihon, J. H., Leaf, R., McEachin, J., Liu, N., Russell, N., Unumb, L., Shapiro, S., & Khosrowshahi, D. (2022). Concerns about ABA-based intervention: An evaluation and recommendations.

Journal of Autism and Developmental Disorders, 52, 2838–2853. DOI.org/10.1007/s10803-021-05137-y

Lee, G. T., William, D. E., Simmons, J., & Johnson-Patagoc, K. (2018). The right to effective treatment for people with developmental disabilities and severe problem behaviors. *Behavior Analysis: Research and Practice, 18*, 436–447. DOI: 10.1037/bar0000133

Lerman, D. C., & Vorndran, C. M. (2002). On the status of knowledge for using punishment implications for treating behavior disorders. *Journal Applied Behavior Analysis, 35*(4), 431–464. DOI: 10.1901/jaba.2002.35-431

Lombardi, M., Vandenbussche, H., Claes, C., Schalock, R. L., De Maeyer, J., & Vandevelde, S. (2019). The concept of quality of life as framework for implementing the UNCRPD. *Journal of Policy and Practice in Intellectual Disabilities, 16*, 180–190. DOI: 10.1111/jppi.12279

Lydon, S., Healy, O., Moran, L., & Foody, C. (2015). A quantitative examination of punishment research. *Research in Developmental Disabilities, 36*, 470–484. DOI: 10.1016/j.ridd.2014.10.036

De Maeyer, J., Vandenbussche, H., Claes, C., & Reynaert, D. (2017). Human rights, the capability approach and quality of life: An integrated paradigm of support in the quest for social justice. *Therapeutic Communities: The International Journal of Therapeutic Communities, 38*, 1–6. DOI: 10.1108/TC-03-2017-0011

Manente, C. J., & LaRue, R. H. (2017). Treatment of self-injurious behavior using differential punishment of high rates of behavior (DPH). *Behavioral Interventions, 32*(3), 262–271. DOI: 1002/bin.1477

Matson, J. L., & Taras, M. E. (1989). A 20-year review of punishment and alternative methods to treat problem behaviors in developmentally delayed persons. *Research in Developmental Disabilities, 10*(1), 85–104. DOI: 10.1016/0891-4222(89)90031-0

McNamara, K., & Cividini-Motta, C. (2019). Further evaluation of treatments for vocal stereotypy: Response interruption and redirection and response cost. *Behavioral Interventions, 34*(2), 181–197. DOI: 10.1002/bin.1657

Migan-Gandonou, J. A., & Leon, Y. (2020). Empirically derived consequences to treat rumination. *Behavioral Interventions, 35*(1), 166–177. DOI: 10.1002/bin.1698

Mitteer, D. R., Romani, P. W., Greer, B. D., & Fisher, W. W. (2015). Assessment and treatment of pica and destruction of holiday decorations. *Journal of Applied Behavior Analysis, 48*(4), 912–917. DOI: 10.1002/jaba.255

Morgan, A. C., Wilder, D. A., Podlesnik, C. A., & Kelley, M. E. (2017). Evaluation of an arm-splint belt to reduce self-injury. *Behavioral Interventions, 32*(3), 255–261. DOI: 10.1002/bin.1469

Muething, C., Call, N. A., & Clark, S. (2020). An evaluation of differential reinforcement in the treatment of pica. *Developmental Neurorehabilitation, 23*(5), 321–327. DOI: 10.1080/17518423.2019.1689436

Oliver, C., Murphy, G. H., & Corbett, J. A. (1987). Self-injurious behavior in people with mental handicap: a total population study. *Journal of Intellectual Disability Research, 31*, 147–162. DOI: 10.1111/j.1365-2788.1987.tb01351.x

Pokorski, E. A., & Barton, E. E. (2021). A systematic review of the ethics of punishment-based procedures for young children with disabilities. *Remedial and Special Education, 42*(4), 262–275. DOI: 10.1177/0741932520918859

Quinn, C., Nowosielski, A., Kitchen, T., & Belfiore, P. J. (2014). The role of program consistency in a summer therapeutic camp for students with autism spectrum disorder. *Journal of Education and Learning, 3*(3), 95–107. DOI: 10.5539/jel.v3n3p95

Regalado, M., Sareen, H., Inkelas, M., Wissow, L. S., & Halfon, N. (2004). Parents' discipline of young children: Results from the National Survey of Early Childhood Health. *Pediatrics, 113*, 1952–1958. DOI: 10.1542/peds.113.S5.1952

Sabatello, M., & Schulze, M. (2014). *Human rights and disability advocacy*. Philadelphia: University of Pennsylvania Press.

Saini, V., Greer, B. D., Fisher, W. W., Lichtblau, K. R., DeSouza, A. A., & Mitteer, D. R. (2016). Individual and combined effects of noncontingent reinforcement and response blocking on automatically reinforced problem behavior. *Journal of Applied Behavior Analysis, 49*(3), 693–698. DOI: 10.1002/jaba.306

Sanberg, S. A., Kuhn, B. R., & Kennedy, A. E. (2018). Outcomes of a behavioral intervention for sleep disturbances in children with autism spectrum disorder. *Journal of Autism and Developmental Disorders, 48*(12), 4250–4277. DOI: 10.1007/s10803-018-3644-4

Schmidt, J. D., Falligant, J. M., Goetzel, A., Hardisty, S., & Hagopian, L. P. (2021). Decreasing motor stereotypy with competing stimuli and tasks: Analysis of prompted engagement and response blocking. *Behavioral Interventions, 36*(3), 583–594. DOI: 10.1002/bin.1786

Schmidt, J. D., Long, A., Goetzel, A. L., Tung, C., Pizarro, E., Phillips, C., & Hausman, N. (2017). Decreasing pica attempts by manipulating the environment to support prosocial behavior. *Journal of Developmental and Physical Disabilities, 29*(5), 683–697. DOI: 10.1007/s10882-017-9548-y

Shawler, L. A., Dianda, M., & Miguel, C. F. (2020). A comparison of response interruption and redirection and competing items on vocal stereotypy and appropriate vocalizations. *Journal of Applied Behavior Analysis, 53*(1), 355–365. DOI: 10.1002/jaba.596

Shawler, L. A., & Miguel, C. F. (2015). The effects of motor and vocal response interruption and redirection on vocal stereotypy and appropriate vocalizations. *Behavioral Interventions, 30*(2), 112–134. DOI: 10.1002/bin.1407

United Nations General Assembly. (1948). Universal Declaration of Human Rights. December 10, 1948, 217A(III). https://www.refworld.org/docid/3ae6b3712c.html

United Nations General Assembly. (2007). Convention on the Rights of Persons With Disabilities. Resolution adopted by the General Assembly, January 24, 2007, A/RES/61/106. https://www.refworld.org/docid/45f973632.html

Verret, C., Massé, L., Lagacé-Leblanc, J., Delisle, G., & Doyon, J. (2019). The impact of a schoolwide de-escalation intervention plan on the use of seclusion and restraint in a special education school. *Emotional & Behavioral Difficulties, 24*(4), 357–373. DOI: 10.1080/13632752.2019.1628375

Verriden, A. L., & Roscoe, E. M. (2019). An evaluation of a punisher assessment for decreasing automatically reinforced problem behavior. *Journal of Applied Behavior Analysis, 52*(1), 205–226. DOI: 10.1002/jaba.509

Vittrup, B., Holden, G. W., & Buck, J. (2006). Attitudes predict the use of physical punishment: A prospective study of the emergence of disciplinary practices. *Pediatrics, 117*, 2055–2064. DOI: 10.1542/peds.2005-2204

Watkins, N., & Rapp, J. T. (2014). Environmental enrichment and response cost: Immediate and subsequent effects on stereotypy. *Journal of Applied Behavior Analysis, 47*(1), 186–191. DOI: 10.1002/jaba.97

Westling, D. L., Trader, B. R., Smith, C. A., & Marshall, D. S. (2010). Use of restraints, seclusion, and aversive procedures on students with disabilities. *Research and Practice for Persons with Severe Disabilities, 35*, 116–127. DOI: 10.2511/rpsd.35.3-4.116

Wilder, D. A., Ertel, H., & Thomas, R. (2020). Further analysis of modifications to the three-step guided compliance procedure to enhance compliance among children with autism. *Journal of Applied Behavior Analysis, 53*(4), 2339–2348. DOI: 10.1002/jaba.721

Wilder, D. A., & Neve, D. (2018). Assessment and treatment of rumination in a young man with autism. *Behavioral Interventions, 33*(3), 297–305. DOI: 10.1002/bin.1633

Wiskow, K. M., Donaldson, J. M., & Matter, A. L. (2017). An evaluation of generalization of compliance across response types. *Behavior Analysis: Research and Practice, 17*(4), 402. DOI: 10.1037/bar0000087

6

Response Interruption and Redirection

Haley M. K. Steinhauser
Melmark New England; Regis College

William H. Ahearn
The New England Center for Children; Western New England University

6.1 Technical Abstract

Background: Response interruption and redirection (RIRD) is a behavioral intervention designed to interrupt challenging behaviors maintained by automatic reinforcement (e.g., stereotypy) and promote adaptive alternative responses. **Method:** To inform this chapter, 54 peer-reviewed research studies evaluating RIRD alone or as component of a larger intervention were considered along with systematic literature reviews. **Results:** RIRD is an evidence-based practice for treatment of motor and vocal stereotypy. RIRD is most effective when it is paired with a focused effort to increase appropriate behavior. In some cases, targeted stereotypic behavior decreases but other undesirable forms of challenging behavior may emerge during RIRD. Additional research toward elucidating the operant mechanisms responsible for behavior change during RIRD and evaluating the social validity and acceptability of RIRD procedures and treatment goals is warranted. **Discussion:** It is not always necessary or desirable to target stereotypy for reduction. Intervention should be considered when the stereotypy interferes with learning, limits opportunities for inclusion or independence, or negatively affects quality of life. RIRD can be used as a single intervention or as a component of a larger intervention package. RIRD can be resource intensive as it requires ongoing close attention from a caregiver (e.g., parent) or professional (e.g., teacher) to implement as well as oversight from a behavior analyst. **Practitioner recommendations:** Do not assume all forms of stereotypy should be treated and consider using RIRD only when stereotypy is causing problems (e.g., limiting opportunities) for the individual. Redirections should target behaviors that are of value to the individual and are appropriate in the environmental context where stereotypy occurs. Practitioners should consider adding intervention components such as prompting, reinforcement, response blocking, and response cost based on the needs of the individual in the context of specific environments. Ongoing data collection and progress monitoring is necessary to ensure desired behavior change is occurring and to offset risk of unintended increases in other forms of challenging behavior.

Haley M. K. Steinhauser and William H. Ahearn, *Response Interruption and Redirection.* In: *Lifespan Treatment for Autistic Individuals*. Edited by: Peter Sturmey, Russell Lang, and James K. Luiselli, Oxford University Press.
© Oxford University Press (2025). DOI: 10.1093/oso/9780197635841.003.0006

6.2 Layperson Summary

RIRD involves encouraging someone to stop engaging in challenging behavior (stereotypy) and to engage in appropriate alternative behavior instead. RIRD should only be considered when behavior interferes with learning, independence, or quality of life. Research evaluating the outcomes of RIRD has predominantly focused on reduction of repetitive patterns of behavior (stereotypy) and increases in appropriate behavior. In most cases, stereotypy occurs because of the bodily sensations (sensory consequences) it produces (Rapp & Vollmer, 2005). For example, hand flapping and body rocking are examples of stereotypic behaviors frequently observed in individuals with autism spectrum disorder (ASD). These behaviors typically arise due to pleasurable sensations resulting from repetitive body movements or as a means to alleviate discomfort. For example, in terms of more common forms of behavior, swinging on a playground swing produces pleasurable sensations and plugging ears with fingers diminishes volume of unpleasant noises. It is not always necessary to reduce stereotypic behaviors. Caregivers and school staff can be trained to implement RIRD during naturally occurring activities within school, community, or home settings. However, a Board-Certified Behavior Analyst (BCBA) should be involved in designing and tailoring RIRD procedures to best suit the characteristics, preferences, and needs of each individual. A BCBA should also be involved in training others to implement RIRD and in monitoring changes in behavior to ensure RIRD is having the intended effects. For this chapter, we identified and reviewed 54 published peer-reviewed research studies conducted by different groups of researchers that collectively involved more than 100 participants. We also considered conclusions from systematic reviews of the literature focused on the treatment of stereotypy that included RIRD studies. This body of studies and reviews indicates that RIRD can effectively reduce interfering or challenging stereotypic behavior and increase appropriate behavior, such as communication and/or engagement in ongoing activities. However, research has also noted that RIRD may occasion an increase in other interfering or challenging behaviors. To prevent this and to better promote an increase in appropriate behavior, it is crucial to use other individualized teaching strategies, such as prompting and reinforcement, along with RIRD (e.g., Cividini-Motta et al., 2022; Steinhauser & Ahearn, 2021; Tomaszewski et al., 2017).

6.3 Treatment Summary Table

Treatment summary: Response Interruption and Redirection

Treatment description: RIRD is a behavioral intervention that involves interrupting challenging stereotypic behaviors that interfere with an individual's independence, learning, or quality of life while also prompting an increase in appropriate alternative behavior. The appropriate alternative behaviors are individualized and contextualized based on needs and characteristics of the person and their environmental context.

Expected outcomes: The primary goal is to address interfering behavior while simultaneously fostering and reinforcing contextually appropriate alternatives. The RIRD research base indicates a moderate to large reduction in challenging stereotypic behavior and a concurrent increase in appropriate alternative responses (e.g., communication and engagement in ongoing activities).

Methods: A search of the RIRD literature yielded 54 empirical studies that evaluated RIRD procedures as an intervention for stereotypy. The results of those studies informed our summary of considerations for practitioners and classification of RIRD as an evidence-based practice. It is important to note that there are numerous procedural variations and treatment components that affect the efficacy of RIRD.

Expertise required to implement treatment: The implementation of RIRD should be overseen by a BCBA to ensure it is having the intended effects. However, it can be implemented by others with less expertise in behavioral interventions, such as teachers, family members, or other caregivers, so long as they are trained adequately and data are monitored on an ongoing basis by a skilled clinician.

Risks and negative side effects: In some situations, RIRD may evoke aggression and other problem behavior, especially when implemented in the absence of reinforcement for alternative behavior. Lanovaz et al. (2013) suggested that targeting one or a limited set of stereotypic behaviors might result in an increase in other nontargeted stereotypic behaviors.

Additional considerations and limitations: Best practice involves using RIRD within a treatment package that includes teaching procedures that promote engagement in appropriate alternative behavior. Stereotypy that does not interfere with a person's independence, health and safety, quality of life, or other important areas may not require treatment, and close consultation with the individual who would receive treatment and/or their family is necessary. Data collection and monitoring are essential to inform potential intervention changes.

6.4 Introduction

6.4.1 Intervention Description

Behavior maintained by automatic reinforcement persists in the absence of social consequences (Vollmer, 1994). Noncontextual and repetitive body movements and speech maintained by automatic reinforcement are typically referred to as stereotypy (Rapp & Vollmer, 2005). Examples of motor stereotypy include repetitive body rocking, hand flapping, and finger movements as well as restrictive and repetitive patterns of behavior involving items (e.g., lining up or spinning objects). Vocal stereotypy includes repeating nonsensical sounds, words, or noncontextual phrases. Other forms of behavior can also be automatically reinforced, such as pica (i.e., the consumption of inedible items), sexualized behavior, and self-injury. RIRD is a behavioral intervention used to reduce stereotypy and other forms of automatically reinforced behavior while also increasing targeted appropriate behavior (Akers et al., 2020; Steinbrenner, 2020; Tomaszewski et al., 2017; Wang et al., 2020).

The RIRD strategy has primarily been studied in relation to motor and vocal stereotypy. Ahearn et al. (2007) is commonly referenced as the study that introduced the procedures of RIRD. That study focused on interrupting vocal stereotypy and redirecting individuals through prompts to produce sounds, words, or phrases that were more appropriate or functional within a specific context. The outcomes of that first study were a decrease in stereotypy for all participants and a concurrent increase in appropriate vocalizations for three of the four participants. Multiple research groups have conducted evaluations on various iterations of RIRD, encompassing a wide array of factors. These factors include different types and intensities of automatically reinforced target behaviors, varying durations of RIRD procedures, interventions ranging from contrived to naturalistic approaches, and differences in implementer expertise and training, as well as assessing the effectiveness and practicality of RIRD across a range of settings. Although there are many variations, there are several consistent components across RIRD studies. Specifically, RIRD should always involve contingent prompting of alternative responses following the occurrence of the targeted challenging behavior (e.g., stereotypy, pica, self-injury; Steinhauser & Ahearn, 2021). In other words, RIRD involves prompting an individual to do something different when repetitive interfering challenging behavior occurs. RIRD is often implemented in tandem with other treatment procedures, including noncontingent reinforcement, differential reinforcement, response blocking, and response cost. These various components likely affect the efficacy of RIRD and can be used strategically to enhance RIRD efficacy in practice.

6.4.2 Rationale and Objectives

Stereotypic behavior can be challenging to treat, and RIRD is one of several evidence-based treatment options for such behavior. There are individual and contextual considerations to consider when determining if RIRD is the most appropriate treatment option. Behavior and intervention goals vary among individuals and stakeholders. The social validity (acceptability) of different treatment options also varies across individuals and their families. Regardless of the individual or the specific application of RIRD, the ultimate objective should be to improve independence in the community, foster functional engagement in ongoing activities, and reduce interfering behavior to a level that improves access and opportunities for the individual.

The rationale and objectives of RIRD are related to the diagnostic features of ASD, including behavioral deficits in the domains of social communication and behavioral excesses in restrictive and repetitive patterns of behavior and interests (American Psychiatric Association, 2013). While stereotypy is commonly observed in typical development, it becomes more persistent and increases over time in many children with ASD. This may be due to the presence of social deficits and contingent sensory reinforcement produced by stereotypic behaviors (MacDonald et al., 2007). In other words, automatically maintained stereotypic behavior may come to overshadow social behavior in children with ASD due to heightened salience of sensory stimulation (Ahearn et al., 2015). Ostensibly, some individuals with ASD may prioritize sensory stimuli resulting from engagement in stereotypy over socially mediated contingencies. Recognizing that repetitive behavior is a characteristic feature of ASD and is influenced by the salience of stimuli helps us better comprehend automatically reinforced behavior.

Hagopian and colleagues (2015, 2017) developed a model for subtyping self-injurious behavior (SIB) maintained by automatic reinforcement based on clinical and published datasets of functional analysis results and intervention outcomes. The subtyping model categorizes automatically reinforced SIB—and may be applicable to other forms of automatically reinforced behavior—based on the extent other sources of reinforcement or stimulation compete with the automatic reinforcement of that target behavior. In other words, functional analysis results can provide insight on whether an individual will opt to engage in alternative activities rather than the automatically reinforced SIB when other options are available. There are instances where modifying the environment and encouraging alternative responses through reinforcement-based strategies is enough to accomplish treatment objectives related to reducing repetitive or interfering behaviors. These cases are examples of subtype 1 and are likely cases in which RIRD is not warranted. Subtype 2 involves behavior that persists regardless of other sources of stimulation or reinforcement, and RIRD may benefit individuals in those cases. A functional assessment is usually necessary to determine the nature of contingencies maintaining stereotypy.

The operant mechanism(s) that underlie behavior changes resulting from RIRD have been extensively debated in the literature (Ahrens et al., 2011). One possibility is that RIRD reduces stereotypy through punishment. Another possibility is that reinforcement of alternative behavior displaces stereotypy. It is also possible that both punishment and reinforcement contribute to the outcomes to varying degrees. Steinhauser and Ahearn (2021) suggest that the mechanism of behavior change is likely idiosyncratic and is not the same across all individuals who receive RIRD.

6.4.3 Considerations for Implementation

When designing and implementing RIRD, practitioners should take into account interrelated variables associated with the individual, their target behaviors, and the environmental context. These considerations include understanding the functions of the target behaviors, assessing potential risks, and determining the extent to which intervention is required for the proposed target behaviors.

6.4.3.1 Function Considerations

Functional assessment is necessary to determine whether a behavior is maintained by automatic reinforcement. Practitioners in applied settings might consider a variation of the Querim et al. (2013) automatic reinforcement screen to conduct a brief direct assessment to determine whether the target behavior persists in the absence of social consequences. If so, RIRD or some form of redirection may be an appropriate intervention. However, if the target behavior is maintained by a socially mediated function (e.g., to obtain attention or escape from demands), a function-based intervention is likely to be more efficient and effective (see Chapter 11, "Functional Communication Training," by Hamrick and Falcomata). If there is some evidence that socially mediated consequences maintain the behavior, a functional analysis is likely warranted. There are several variations of functional analysis procedures suitable for assessing repetitive patterns of behavior that may be stereotypy, including a brief functional analysis, brief social function test (Cividini-Motta et al., 2020), and a traditional functional analysis (Iwata et al., 1982/1994). Functional analysis procedures should be selected and conducted by a BCBA.

Even when functional assessment reveals an automatic reinforcement function for a behavior, it is possible that socially mediated reinforcement contingencies may still be useful. We suggest clinicians considering RIRD to reduce stereotypy attempt to determine if those reinforcers can be used as competing stimuli—that is, whether other sources of reinforcement compete with the automatic reinforcement produced by the target stereotypic behavior. This is aligned with the automatic reinforcement-subtyping model proposed by Hagopian et al. (2015, 2017). According to that model, automatically reinforced behavior that occurs at lower levels when other sources of reinforcement are available (i.e., subtype 1 of automatic reinforcement) is more likely to respond positively to reinforcement-based procedures. If so, reinforcement procedures that support appropriate alternative behavior might obviate the need to implement RIRD. Conversely, if the frequency of stereotypy is unchanged when reinforcement is available (i.e., subtype 2 of automatic reinforcement), then RIRD may be appropriate or even essential to achieve clinically significant treatment effects.

6.4.3.2 Safety and Risk Assessment Considerations

A risk-benefit analysis that weighs the potential risks and benefits of intervention against the potential risks of not intervening or using a different intervention approach should be conducted. Specifically, if the target behavior itself is harmful (e.g., causes physical injury, destroys property, or restricts opportunity), then RIRD is more likely to be warranted. For behaviors that pose serious risk of harm (e.g., SIB), other intervention components may be needed in tandem with RIRD (e.g., response blocking and response cost). However, if the target behavior can safely occur, such as with most forms of motor and vocal stereotypy, there are more nuanced considerations of whether, when, and how to intervene. It is important to note that, in some cases, the stereotypic behavior itself might not be inherently harmful but may still pose a risk. For instance, an individual engaging in loud vocal stereotypy in the classroom with other students may be at risk of placement in a more restrictive educational setting. Because RIRD may involve physically interrupting or blocking a person's behavior, there may be risk of harm from aggression toward the implementer. In such cases, redirection to an alternative behavior with powerful reinforcement contingency is helpful (Hagopian & Adelinis (2001). A plan for effectively reinforcing appropriate behavior should always be a first consideration before incorporating redirection into the treatment package.

Advocates of the neurodiversity movement have raised ethical concerns regarding the treatment of stereotypy (Leaf et al., 2022). Within this movement, neurodiversity is viewed as a natural and valuable variation of human neurological development. These advocates argue that attempts to suppress or eliminate stereotypic behavior may disregard the individual's unique experiences and preferences, leading to potential harm and a denial of their autonomy. These risks should also be considered in context of the risk of not intervening to reduce behaviors that may cause physical injury, social exclusion, or other adverse outcomes. Relatedly, in some cases, stereotypic behavior is a precursor for other forms of challenging behavior (Richman et al., 2013; Symons et al., 2005), and the potential for escalating risk of untreated stereotypy should also be considered and discussed. There is not a consensus on acceptable levels of risk or regarding the value of certain outcomes typically considered beneficial (e.g., social acceptance). This ethical debate highlights the need for person-centered approaches that prioritize individual autonomy, self-determination, and well-being, while recognizing and respecting the unique experiences and strengths of individuals with neurodevelopmental differences.

6.4.3.3 Context Considerations

When developing an intervention that includes RIRD, it is important to identify the environment and contexts where the automatically maintained challenging behavior interferes with appropriate behavior. Contexts and environments associated with high levels of stereotypy and low levels of functional engagement may be appropriate for RIRD. To help identify appropriate alternative behaviors to reinforce during RIRD, practitioners should determine what constitutes functional engagement in those environments. Further, in those environments, it may be helpful to identify what stimuli or materials are already available. It may be possible to use the available stimuli/materials to compete with the automatic reinforcement of the challenging behavior.

6.4.3.4 Reinforcement Considerations

In the environments and context where automatically maintained challenging behavior is most common, it is important to consider the availability of reinforcement for appropriate behavior and whether the individual regularly accesses it. If reinforcement is available but not accessed by the individual, practitioners should assess to determine if the individual possesses the necessary skills to engage in appropriate behavior. If there are uncertainties about behavioral expectations or deficits impeding the occurrence of those behaviors, the individual may benefit from structured teaching procedures to provide clarity on expectations and to directly teach specific skills.

6.4.3.5 RIRD Procedural Considerations

After addressing these preliminary considerations, further questions arise regarding the components of the RIRD procedure itself. Building upon the earlier inquiries about context, one crucial question to consider is whether the demands of RIRD can be contextually relevant. In other words, can RIRD involve redirecting the individual back to the appropriate activity? This assessment considers both the specific context and the individual's unique attributes and skill levels. Steinhauser et al. (2021) is an example of a study that involved promoting contextually appropriate behavior by redirecting back to the ongoing activity using a contextual redirection (C-RD) procedure that can be conceptualized as a form of RIRD. C-RD is intended to promote response reallocation to appropriate functional engagement and improve the practicality and social acceptability of RIRD. It is also important to know how the individual responds to verbal instruction and physical redirection. RIRD demands can require either motor or vocal responses on the part of the individual experiencing the intervention. Similarly, RIRD demands can involve either physical prompting or verbal directives, allowing individualization of the RIRD procedure suited for individuals with a range of skill levels. If the individual engaging in the automatically reinforced target behavior readily responds to verbal directives, it might be a more socially acceptable and practical approach to present RIRD demands with verbal instructions. However, if an individual has a minimal receptive repertoire and responds well to physical prompts, physical prompts might be best. Finally, it must be determined if it is possible and acceptable to implement RIRD following every instance of the automatically maintained challenging behavior. The findings of some of the RIRD evaluations related to the treatment integrity of RIRD implementation (e.g., Colón & Ahearn, 2019) support the programmed inclusion of high treatment consistency booster sessions to improve and maintain the efficacy of RIRD when diminished treatment integrity is anticipated.

6.4.3.6 Treatment Package Component Considerations

In addition to the RIRD procedure itself, other treatment components are often packaged with RIRD. These components have the potential to improve the efficacy and social acceptability of RIRD. A guiding question that will ensure the inclusion of positive reinforcement in the treatment package is: *How will appropriate alternative behavior be promoted and supported?* This relates to the reinforcement considerations noted above, but this is also a consideration during the design and implementation phases of an RIRD treatment package, and modifications should be made to the reinforcement procedure (e.g., schedule, magnitude) based on individual responding.

Response blocking is an intervention component that may be necessary in some situations. In situations involving notably dangerous behavior with a high risk of harm (e.g., pica and SIB), RIRD might require a response blocking component for safety. Although response blocking may prevent injury, it may also evoke aggressive behavior or emotional responding. It is important to monitor the individual's response to such procedures and make procedural adjustments when there is evidence of aggression or emotional distress following response blocking.

Another treatment component occasionally packaged with RIRD is response cost. Similar to the addition of other contingent interventions like verbal reprimands and response blocking, a response cost component has the potential to enhance the efficacy of an RIRD procedure (e.g., McNamara & Cividini-Motta et al., 2019; Toper-Korkmaz et al., 2018). In practice, this might look like the contingent removal of reinforcers such as preferred leisure items while contingently presenting RIRD demands following the occurrence of automatically reinforced behavior. It is important to note that negative punishment is the mechanism of behavior change in response cost, necessitating additional considerations.

6.4.3.7 RIRD Fading Considerations

It is critical to consider how RIRD will be faded over time as progress toward treatment goals is made. One way to fade RIRD is by reducing the frequency of implementation. In the RIRD literature relating to treatment integrity and consistency, there is evidence that the frequency of contingent RIRD implementation can effectively be faded after initial treatment effects are observed (e.g., Colón & Ahearn, 2019; Gauthier et al., 2020). Similarly, thinning the RIRD demand requirement (e.g., Martinez et al., 2016; Saini et al., 2015), in terms of the number of demands or the length of time-based redirection procedures, can have similar positive effects on the RIRD procedure's practicality and social acceptability.

6.5 Research Background

6.5.1 Search Procedures

To summarize the supporting RIRD literature, 54 empirical studies evaluating RIRD were identified through a systematic search of key term combinations For example, "automatic reinforcement," "pica," and "stereotypy" were combined with "redirection," "response redirection," "response interruption and redirection," "RIRD," and "contingent demands" in the systematic searches of relevant databases and journals (i.e., Academic Search Premier, APA PsycINFO, PubMed, *Journal of Applied Behavior Analysis*, *Behavioral Interventions*, *Behavior Modification*).

6.5.2 Overview of Supporting Literature

Around the year 2000, our research group embarked on a program of research aimed at identifying optimal practices for assessing and treating behavior maintained by automatic reinforcement. This type of behavior, driven by the consequences it produces, poses greater challenges for treatment compared to behavior maintained by social consequences (Vollmer, 1994). We initially chose to concentrate on stereotypic behavior for two reasons. The first was that stereotypy seemed, in our experience, to almost always be automatically maintained. This was later verified by Rapp and Vollmer (2005). The second reason was that automatically reinforced SIB should, in most situations, meet appropriate treatment as soon as it is feasible to do so. We initially started by recruiting participants who were identified by their clinical teams as engaging in stereotypy that interfered with important activities and skill acquisition.

Our first goal was to conduct functional assessments to identify the cause of the individual's behavior. These assessments were then followed up by examining a variety of intervention strategies aimed to find activities the individual would engage in that competed with this repetitive behavior (e.g., Ahearn et al., 2005). These behavioral procedures, however, were not universally effective for finding competing stimuli when targeting automatically reinforced behavior (see, e.g., Jennett et al., 2011). Some previous work had shown that blocking the automatically reinforced response might be a useful alternative when response competition was not enough (e.g., Dorsey et al., 1982; Reid et al., 1993). However, not all topographies of automatically reinforced behavior can be readily blocked (e.g., vocal stereotypy, covert self-injury).

Fellner et al. (1984) attempted to treat four presumably automatically reinforced responses: hand flapping, hyperventilating, slapping hand to mouth, and lip pulling. The authors noted that these responses tended to co-occur, and that other injurious and repetitive responses would often emerge. Ongoing treatment in the clinical setting included differential reinforcement of other behavior (DRO) combined with differential reinforcement of incompatible behavior (DRI). Those procedures were not effective and served as the baseline condition in this study. The authors added what they referred to as a mild interruption procedure in the form of a brief (1 to 2 seconds) redirection during the treatment condition. The results indicated that the inclusion of an interruption procedure led to a decline in challenging behavior, eventually reaching zero occurrences during extended sessions. Furthermore, low levels of responding were maintained during a 4-month follow-up evaluation. Additionally, toy play began to emerge when the DRO + DRI + interruption procedure was added.

Taking the extant literature into consideration, our group then developed a procedure to interrupt and redirect repetitive behavior to other forms of contextually appropriate behavior. Given that interrupting ongoing behavior could be aversive, we individually identified demands that the participant readily complied with independent of prompting and designed our baseline condition to provide naturalistic reinforcement contingencies for acceptable nonrepetitive responses (e.g., answering questions or completing tasks). In Ahearn et al. (2007), this procedure was referred to as RIRD, and the target responses were instances of vocal stereotypy that the clinical teams had referred to as interfering. Similar to Fellner et al. (1984), we saw low levels of vocal stereotypy when RIRD was implemented and, for three of the four participants, nonrepetitive vocalizations occurred more frequently; however, our goal in intervention was never to eliminate stereotypic vocalizations. Staff were trained to implement RIRD, and follow-up evaluations suggested the treatment effects were durable.

Since 2007, there have been numerous variations of the initial RIRD procedures across research studies involving RIRD, including studies that evaluated the extent other intervention components influence outcomes and how RIRD compares to other interventions for challenging automatically reinforced behavior. There have been several literature reviews and book chapters summarizing this line of research and identifying future directions (e.g., Cividini-Motta et al., 2022; Martinez & Betz, 2013; Steinhauser & Ahearn,2021). Steinhauser and Ahearn offer key takeaway points from the RIRD literature. (1) RIRD is an effective intervention, (2) pairing reinforcement procedures with RIRD can make it more effective, and (3) the RIRD variations can inform how to individualize and contextualize it in practice. In terms of RIRD efficacy, the authors outlined that RIRD has been evaluated across many topographies of automatically reinforced behavior (e.g., inappropriate sexualized behavior, pica, stereotypy). Of the 54 studies reviewed, RIRD reduced the target behavior in 91.5% of cases. Although these numbers include procedural variations, the evidence of efficacy is relatively high (Cividini-Motta et al., 2022).

6.5.2.1 Measurement

How behavior is measured directly affects what we can conclude about the effect of an intervention. Likewise, supplemental measures can be insightful in terms of the practicality or social validity of procedures and indirect effects of an intervention. The methods of target behavior measurement and how they relate to interpretations of RIRD efficacy have been an ongoing discussion in the RIRD literature. With RIRD often evaluated with repetitive, or stereotypic, behavior, many responses targeted by RIRD are not discrete; some instances of the target behavior are longer in duration than others. Given this, interval recording methods (e.g., momentary time sampling [MTS], partial interval recording [PIR]) might be used to record the target behavior. Meany-Daboul et al. (2007) compared MTS and PIR to continuous duration recording (CDR) methods, concluding that MTS is the most reflective of CDR. This is informative for practitioners determining practical measurement methods to evaluate interventions, such as RIRD.

One ongoing measurement discussion in the RIRD literature is about whether the target behavior should be measured during redirection. Our research group opted to pause the session timer and not record the targeted vocal stereotypy during redirection in the Ahearn et al. (2007) study. This was based on previous literature in the area of response blocking, with recording the target behavior during a response blocking intervention deflating the measurement of the target behavior. Several research groups have evaluated this practice (i.e., interrupted measurement) within RIRD evaluations to determine if it overestimates the efficacy of RIRD compared to measuring the target behavior during redirection (i.e., uninterrupted measurement). In some studies (e.g., Carroll & Kodak, 2014; Wunderlich & Vollmer, 2015), interrupted measurement was found to overestimate the efficacy of RIRD, but additional evaluations have not consistently supported this finding (e.g., Martinez et al., 2016; McNamara & Cividini-Motta, 2019; Toper-Korkmaz et al., 2018). Nonetheless, it is notable that the manner in which practitioners choose to measure the target behavior in an RIRD evaluation affects the interpretations of its efficacy. For instance, if the uninterrupted measurement method is used, it might be more conservative in terms of the automatically reinforced behavior but also have the possibility of inflating data related to appropriate alternative behavior that is prompted during redirection periods. Another option supported by published studies is to measure the time implementing RIRD (e.g., Steinhauser et al., 2021). This can be an insightful measure on the practicality of the procedure in naturalistic settings.

Published RIRD evaluations have also included supplemental measures of appropriate alternative behavior, with the most common being appropriate vocalizations or verbal responses (e.g., Ahearn et al., 2007; Colón et al., 2012). Other measures of engagement in functional skills in published studies have included leisure and academic engagement (e.g., Gibbs et al., 2018; Steinhauser et al., 2021). Like measuring the effects of RIRD on adaptive alternative responses, several studies have evaluated the effects of RIRD on untargeted forms of automatically reinforced behavior (Cook & Rapp, 2020; Pastrana et al., 2013). This addition of supplemental measures of appropriate alternative responses or other untargeted behavior is supported by the Lanovaz et al. (2013) review's conclusion that the reduction of stereotypy can result in a subsequent increase, or reallocation, of untargeted behavior. Thus, it is good practice to monitor and measure the effects of RIRD on behavior beyond the initial target behavior.

Researchers have utilized dependent measures in RIRD evaluations to assess efficacy and employed measures of untargeted challenging or unsafe behavior as an indicator of social acceptability. Verriden and Roscoe (2019) is an example of a study that enhanced a treatment analysis with a supplemental measure of emotional responding, with the aim of identifying putative punishers that corresponded with minimal challenging behavior. The concept behind this is that an intervention that reduced the targeted automatically reinforced behavior and corresponded with low levels of unsafe or challenging behavior was more acceptable.

6.5.2.2 RIRD Procedural Variations

There are also variations of the RIRD procedure. These procedural variations prompted Steinhauser and Ahearn (2021) to define *redirection* as "prompting of alternative responses contingent on the automatically reinforced response." Some aspects of these key components have been modified within the published RIRD literature, such as the "alternative responses" (i.e., RIRD demands), how they are presented or prompted, and when they are no longer presented.

6.5.2.2.1 RIRD Demands

Ahearn et al. (2007) conducted the initial RIRD evaluation, examining vocal redirection as an alternative to vocal stereotypy. This prompted some research groups to inquire whether the topography of the alternative behavior (i.e., RIRD demands) should match the topography of the targeted automatically reinforced behavior. Several studies have explored the potential impact of this alignment on the efficacy of RIRD (Ahrens et al., 2011; Shawler & Miguel, 2015; Wunderlich & Vollmer, 2015). Across studies, the results suggest that RIRD efficacy is not dependent on the topography of RIRD demands. That is, redirection to any task may be sufficient. This finding empowers flexibility in practitioners' application of RIRD in several ways. First, it supports using an individual's repertoire to inform the alternative responses that you are redirecting them to engage in instead of the interfering or challenging automatically reinforced behavior—for instance, redirecting interfering vocalizations to activities requiring motor movements for a client who emits limited vocal verbal responses. This finding also provides practitioners with the opportunity to redirect back to ongoing activities regardless of what type of responses constitutes contextual engagement (e.g., Cook & Rapp, 2020; Peters & Thompson, 2013; Steinhauser et al., 2021). That is, when redirecting an automatically reinforced motor response during an activity that requires vocal responses (e.g., academic instruction context), the redirection procedure can involve redirecting back to vocal responses dictated by that ongoing activity. Across the RIRD literature, RIRD has also been demonstrated as an effective strategy in studies with RIRD demands involving skills that the individual will readily do (e.g., Ahearn et al., 2007; Cook & Rapp, 2020) and skills that are current teaching targets (e.g., Steinhauser et al., 2021). This also lends to the flexibility of RIRD demand selection in practice.

6.5.2.2.2 RIRD Presentation and Prompting

During the presentation of RIRD demands, some studies have provided an opportunity for independent responding and then moved on to the next demand without prompting (e.g., Ahearn et al., 2007). Other studies have prompted engagement in the RIRD demand (e.g., Ahrens et al., 2011; Cassella et al., 2011; DeRosa et al., 2019; Shawler & Miguel, 2015). Notably, both have been demonstrated to be effective. When implementing RIRD, the best option is likely dictated by individual and contextual factors often determine the most socially valid approach for implementing RIRD. For instance, using physical prompts to redirect interfering motor movements to essential self-care task (e.g., hand washing, feeding oneself) may be socially acceptable in some contexts but not in others, depending on the specific characteristics the individual and environment. Similarly, prompting the completion of the RIRD demand might also be an essential component of RIRD when teaching new skills in the context of RIRD. Prompting the completion of RIRD demands might also be necessary in terms of efficacy, if RIRD without prompting does not shift responding from the automatically reinforced behavior to alternative responses. Conversely, it might be more practical and socially acceptable to move on to the next RIRD task, without prompting compliance, particularly when presenting vocal redirection tasks to an adult engaging in loud interfering vocalizations.

6.5.2.2.3 RIRD Requirement

With the practicality of RIRD procedures directly corresponding to its efficacy in naturalistic settings, the extent to which the approach is practical has been an ongoing topic of discussion and empirical research. There are various aspects of the approach that might make it more or less practical in a given situation; one of these is the criteria to terminate RIRD implementation. In other words, it depends on how long RIRD is presented or what dictates how long it is presented. Variations of the RIRD procedure have involved termination criteria based on the number of RIRD demands (e.g., Ahearn et al., 2007) or duration of redirection (e.g., Cividini-Motta et al., 2020), typically paired with some requirement of the absence of the target behavior. For example, RIRD demands might be implemented for 30 seconds with at least the last 3 seconds of redirection needing to be free of the target behavior, or RIRD demands might be implemented until three demands are completed absent the target behavior.

Several studies have evaluated RIRD requirements and the effects on intervention efficacy. Saini et al. (2015) and Toper-Korkmaz et al. (2018) compared a shorter and longer RIRD requirement, one RIRD demand (RIRD-1) and three RIRD demands (RIRD-3). Both studies found that RIRD-1 was just as effective as RIRD-3, and RIRD-1 corresponded to either less or the same percentage of time redirecting behavior. Other studies have reduced the RIRD requirement after repeated exposure to a more involved RIRD procedure by reducing the number of RIRD demands (e.g., Martinez et al., 2016) or moving to an intermittent RIRD procedure (e.g., Sloman et al., 2017). These results also relate to fading RIRD requirements and to published studies evaluating treatment integrity that lend to social validity considerations (e.g., Ahrens et al., 2011; Colón & Ahearn, 2019; Gauthier et al., 2020).

6.5.2.3 Treatment Packages: RIRD Paired With Other Treatment Components

Treatment components beyond the RIRD procedure itself are often packaged with RIRD. In addition to this being common practice and contributing to improved effects and social acceptability, the empirical body of supporting literature contains numerous evaluations of the additive effects of such components. Although not exhaustive, these treatment package components are often reinforcement-based procedures or other contingent interventions packaged with RIRD.

6.5.2.3.1 RIRD + Reinforcement Procedures

One key takeaway outlined by Steinhauser and Ahearn (2021) is that the addition of reinforcement procedures can enhance the effects of RIRD. This directly relates to the Lanovaz et al. (2013) conclusion that decreasing an automatically reinforced response can result in the response reallocation of untargeted responses; therefore, it is best practice and leads to better clinical outcomes to support appropriate alternative behavior with reinforcement procedures. Another common procedure designed to address behavior maintained by automatic reinforcement involves providing the individual with other items or activities (i.e., competing stimuli, environmental enrichment) with the goal of these stimuli competing with the automatically reinforced target behavior. This approach can be used with or without RIRD. Several studies in the RIRD literature have evaluated the additive effects of combining noncontingent competing stimuli and/or contingent reinforcement for alternative behavior (i.e., DRA) with RIRD. Aside from it being good practice to arrange reinforcement to support appropriate behavior while also aiming to decrease another response, multiple evaluations support the notion that it can enhance the efficacy of RIRD.

Both Love et al. (2012) and Gibbs et al. (2018) evaluated the additive effects of competing stimuli when packaged with RIRD. In the Love et al. evaluation, RIRD with and without competing stimuli effectively decreased stereotypy for both participants. However, the addition of competing stimuli was more effective in one case, corresponding with higher levels of appropriate behavior and requiring less RIRD presentation. Similarly, Gibbs et al. demonstrated that the addition of competing stimuli resulted in lower levels of the targeted automatically reinforced behavior. The arrangement of competing stimuli in an RIRD package can promote response reallocation to responding or engagement with the available putatively competing items or activities. If effective, this can be conceptualized as the reinforcing value of the available stimuli competing with the reinforcement that the individual contacts when engaging in the automatically reinforced target behavior.

Similar to the effects of arranging noncontingent sources of reinforcement (i.e., competing stimuli), delivering reinforcement contingent on appropriate alternative behavior in a DRA arrangement can have similar enhancing effects in an RIRD treatment package. In the published RIRD literature, reinforcement has been arranged for various types of appropriate responses, such as communicative behavior, leisure engagement, academic engagement, and incompatible discard responses in pica interventions. Related to arranging reinforcement in a DRA packaged with RIRD, several studies have included explicit teaching of appropriate responses that are supported and maintained in a DRA (e.g., Colón et al., 2012; Hagopian et al., 2011; Schmidt et al., 2017; Taylor, 2020). Dickman et al. (2012) assessed the additive effects of contingent reinforcement on appropriate alternative behavior within an RIRD treatment package, concluding that additional reinforcement can correspond to higher levels of appropriate behavior and compete with the automatic reinforcement of the targeted behavior. Cividini-Motta et al. (2019) similarly evaluated the effects of DRA on RIRD; however, due to procedural limitations, further evaluations are warranted. Nonetheless, ensuring there is reinforcement available for alternative responses is sound clinical practice.

6.5.2.3.2 RIRD + Contingent Interventions

In the published evaluations of RIRD, it is also often packaged with other contingent interventions such as verbal reprimands, response blocking, and response cost. Like reinforcement-based interventions packaged with RIRD, these additional contingent interventions have the potential to improve treatment effects in terms of further decreases in the automatically reinforced target behavior. In practice, however, it must be considered whether an additional component improves or worsens both the social acceptability and practicality of the treatment package.

In the identified RIRD studies, there were several studies that presented some form of reprimand or directive contingent on the target behavior prior to the presentation of RIRD (e.g., "stop," "don't X"). However, none of the reviewed studies systematically evaluated the additive effect of reprimands on RIRD treatment outcomes. Response blocking has also been combined with RIRD (e.g., Frewing et al., 2015; Gould et al., 2019), especially in cases targeting behavior that cannot safely be allowed to occur such as pica (e.g., Hagopian et al., 2011; Schmidt et al., 2017). Although response blocking is commonly packaged with RIRD, none of the identified studies specifically evaluated the extent it enhances the RIRD procedure. A response cost has also been commonly combined with RIRD. In some studies, the contingent removal of presumably reinforcing stimuli (e.g., leisure items) prior to the presentation of RIRD likely functioned as response cost, or negative punishment, but was not reported as such. Both Toper-Korkmaz et al. (2018) and McNamara and Cividini-Motta (2019) systematically evaluated the effects of adding a response cost component to RIRD. The results were idiosyncratic across participants, but notably, RIRD with response cost was more efficacious than RIRD alone with some individuals. These results suggest that a response cost component can enhance the efficacy of RIRD in some cases.

6.5.2.4 Social Validity: Fading RIRD and Promoting Generalization

Several published studies relate to improved practicality of RIRD by reducing the redirection requirement (i.e., number of demands; e.g., Saini et al., 2015; Toper-Korkmaz et al., 2018) or the frequency of contingent implementation (e.g., Ahrens et al., 2011; Colón & Ahearn, 2019; Gauthier et al., 2020; Sloman et al., 2017). Generally, these studies have demonstrated that the redirection requirement can be reduced, and the procedure remains effective while taking less time to implement in some cases. Both Ahrens et al. and Colón and Ahearn reduced the proportion of stereotypy occurrences followed by contingent RIRD implementation, demonstrating that the target behavior maintained at low levels, supporting the notion that RIRD implementation can be faded while treatment effects remain. This indirectly supports the idea that RIRD might be a feasible option when implemented in naturally occurring activities and across environments when it cannot be practically implemented after every occurrence of the repetitive or challenging target behavior.

In a 2013 review of the early RIRD literature, Martinez and Betz suggested that it needed to be evaluated in naturalistic settings, and this has become more common in the published literature. Similarly, RIRD has been evaluated during other ongoing activities in more recent years. For instance, Steinhauser et al. (2021) evaluated a variation of RIRD during different ongoing activities as an analog to conducting RIRD in a naturalistic school setting. This arrangement of various contexts (e.g., leisure, social, academic) involved arranging the environment with both noncontingent and contingent stimuli, similar to what naturally occurs in a school or other naturalistic setting. Other studies have also progressed to evaluating RIRD in more natural settings (e.g., Hagopian et al., 2011; Martinez et al., 2016), supporting the implementation in naturally occurring settings and activities beyond highly controlled research settings.

6.6 Practice Implications

6.6.1 Treatment Outcomes

Overall, the RIRD research suggests that RIRD is a procedure to consider that can both decrease interfering or dangerous automatically reinforced behavior and promote adaptive behavior. Adaptive alternative behavior that might increase as a result of RIRD implementation can include social interactions or communication, academic responding, or leisure engagement. Response reallocation to these alternative responses can be further improved by packaging RIRD with reinforcement-based procedures that support and maintain appropriate behavior. At times, such as in cases of subtype 1 of automatically reinforced behavior according to Hagopian and colleagues' (2015, 2017) model, reinforcement-based procedures alone might obviate the need to implement RIRD procedures whatsoever. With the possibility of increasing adaptive behavior with RIRD, it might be more socially acceptable than other procedures that emphasize decreasing automatically maintained behavior in some cases (e.g., verbal reprimands, response blocking, response cost). Regardless, the many variations of RIRD procedures in the published literature support the individualization of RIRD in practice for the most efficacious, practical, and socially acceptable implementation of RIRD.

6.6.2 Practice Implication Guidelines

Several broad simple guidelines can assist practitioners when considering an RIRD procedure to address automatically reinforced behavior: (1) assess whether the behavior warrants intervention, (2) ensure reinforcement and teaching procedures are arranged to support alternative behavior, and (3) use the context to inform the procedure (e.g., redirect back to the ongoing activity). Across various published RIRD evaluations, a consistent finding is that the extent to which a particular variation of RIRD is effective is idiosyncratic across participants or individuals. This supports the individualization of the RIRD procedure by a BCBA(R) who designs, oversees, and adjusts the implementation of RIRD based on data and clinical observations. There have been extensive comparative studies evaluating different aspects of the RIRD procedure itself and relative to other interventions altogether. However, clinicians in practice can do this on a case-by-case basis in comparative treatment analyses (e.g., Cividini-Motta et al., 2020; Verriden & Roscoe, 2019) of individually informed and acceptable treatment options to determine which variation of RIRD or intervention is best supported by data on the individual level.

6.7 References

**Denotes empirical studies identified to inform review and considerations for practice.*

Ahearn, W. H., Clark, K. M., DeBar, R., & Florentino, C. (2005). On the role of preference in response competition. *Journal of Applied Behavior Analysis, 38*(2), 247–250.

*Ahearn, W. H., Clark, K. M., MacDonald, R. P. F., & Chung, B. I. (2007). Assessing and treating vocal stereotypy in children with autism. *Journal of Applied Behavior Analysis, 40*(2), 263–275. https://doi.org/10.1901/jaba.2007.30-06

Ahearn, W. H., Parry-Cruwys, D., Toran, T., & MacDonald, J. (2015). Stimulus salience in autism: A social learning disorder. In F. DiGennaro Reed (Ed.), *Autism service delivery: Bridging the gap between science and practice* (pp. 75–111). New York: Springer.

*Ahrens, E. N., Lerman, D. C., Kodak, T., Worsdell, A. S., & Keegan, C. (2011). Further evaluation of response interruption and redirection as treatment for stereotypy. *Journal of Applied Behavior Analysis, 44*(1), 95–108. https://doi.org/10.1901/jaba.2011.44-95

Akers, J. S., Davis, T. N., Gerow, S., & Avery, S. (2020). Decreasing motor stereotypy in individuals with autism spectrum disorder: A systematic review. *Research in Autism Spectrum Disorders, 77*, 101611. https://doi.org/10.1016/j.rasd.2020.101611

American Psychiatric Association. (2013). Diagnostic and statistical manual of mental disorders (DSM-5®). Washington, DC: Author.

*Athens, E. S., Vollmer, T. R., Sloman, K. N., & St. Peter Pipkin, C. (2008). An analysis of vocal stereotypy and therapist fading. *Journal of Applied Behavior Analysis, 41*(2), 291–297. https://doi.org/10.1901/jaba.2008.41-291

*Barszcz, H., Griffith, A. K., Weigand, P., & Garcia, Y. (2021). Generalization of response interruption and redirection procedure with vocal stereotypy. *Behavioral Interventions, 36*(4), 847–866. https://doi.org/10.1002/bin.1814

*Brusa, E., & Richman, D. (2008). Developing stimulus control for occurrences of stereotypy exhibited by a child with autism. *International Journal of Behavioral Consultation and Therapy, 4*(3), 264–269. https://doi/10.1037/h0100855

*Carroll, R. A., & Kodak, T. (2014). An evaluation of interrupted and uninterrupted measurement of vocal stereotypy on perceived treatment outcomes. *Journal of Applied Behavior Analysis, 47*(2), 264–276. https://doi.org/10.1002/jaba.118

*Cassella, M. D., Sidener, T. M., Sidener, D. W., & Progar, P. R. (2011). Response interruption and redirection for vocal stereotypy in children with autism: A systematic replication. *Journal of Applied Behavior Analysis, 44*(1), 169–173. https://doi.org/10.1901/jaba.2011.44-169

*Cividini-Motta, C., Garcia, A. R., Livingston, C., & MacNaul, H. L. (2019). The effect of response interruption and redirection with and without a differential reinforcement of alternative behavior component on stereotypy and appropriate responses. *Behavioral Interventions, 34*(1), 3–18. https://doi.org/10.1002/bin.1654

Cividini-Motta, C., Macnaul, H., Steinhauser, H. M. K., & Ahearn W. H. (2022). Response interruption and redirection. In J. B. Leaf, J. Cihon, J. Ferguson, & M. J. Weiss (Eds.), *Handbook of applied behavior analysis interventions for autism* (pp. 555–575). Cham: Springer. https://doi.org/10.1007/978-3-030-96478-8_29

*Cividini-Motta, C., Moore, K., Fish, L. M., Priehs, J. C., & Ahearn W. H. (2020). Reducing public masturbation in individuals with ASD: An assessment of response interruption procedure. *Behavior Modification, 44*(3), 429–448. https://doi.org/10.1177/0145445518824277

*Colón, C. L., & Ahearn, W. H. (2019). An analysis of treatment integrity of response interruption and redirection. *Journal of Applied Behavior Analysis, 52*(2), 337–354. https://doi.org/10.1002/jaba.537

*Colón, C. L., Ahearn, W. H., Clark, K. M., & Masalasky, J. (2012). The effects of verbal operant training and response interruption and redirection on appropriate and inappropriate vocalizations. *Journal of Applied Behavior Analysis, 45*(1), 107–120. https://doi.org/10.1901/jaba.2012.45-107

*Cook, J. L., & Rapp, J. T. (2020). To what extent do practitioners need to treat stereotypy during academic tasks? *Behavior Modification, 44*(2), 228–264. https://doi.org/10.1177/0145445518808226

*DeRosa, N. M., Novak, M. D., Morley, A. J., & Roane, H. S. (2019). Comparing response blocking and response interruption/redirection on levels of motor stereotypy: Effects of data analysis procedures. *Journal of Applied Behavior Analysis, 52*(4), 1021–1033. https://doi.org/10.1002/jaba.644

*Dickman, S. E., Bright, C. N., Montgomery, D. H., & Miguel, C. F. (2012). The effects of response interruption and redirection (RIRD) and differential reinforcement on vocal stereotypy and appropriate vocalizations. *Behavioral Interventions, 27*(4), 185–192. https://doi.org/10.1002/bin.1348

Dorsey, M. F., Iwata, B. A., Reid, D. H., & Davis, P. A. (1982). Protective equipment: Continuous and contingent application in the treatment of self-injurious behavior. *Journal of Applied Behavior Analysis, 15*(2), 217–230. https://doi.org/10.1901/jaba.1982.15-217

*Esposito, M., Pignotti, L., Mondani, F., D'errico, M., Ricciardi, O., Mirizzi, P., Mazza, M., & Valenti, M. (2021). Stimulus control procedure for reducing vocal stereotypies in an autistic child. *Children, 8*(12), 1–12. https://doi.org/10.3390/children8121107

*Falligant, J. M., & Dommestrup, A. K. (2020). Decreasing motor stereotypy in leisure contexts: Analysis of stimulus control with response interruption and redirection. *Behavioral Interventions, 35*(2), 306–314. https://doi.org/10.1002/bin.1703

Fellner, D. J., Laroche, M., & Sulzer-Azaroff, B. (1984). The effects of adding interruption to differential reinforcement on targeted and novel self-stimulatory behaviors. *Journal of Behavior Therapy and Experimental Psychiatry, 15*(4), 315–321.

*Frewing, T. M., Tanner, A., Bonner, A. C., Baxter, S., & Pastrana, S. J. (2015). The immediate and subsequent effects of response interruption and redirection on vocal stereotypy, motor stereotypy and heart rate. *European Journal of Behavior Analysis, 16*(2), 351–361. https://doi.org/10.1080/15021149.2015.1110407

*Friedman, A., & Luiselli, J. K. (2008). Excessive daytime sleep: Behavioral assessment and intervention in a child with autism. *Behavior Modification, 32*(4), 548–555. https://doi.org/10.1177/0145445507312187

*Gauthier, K. A., Ahearn, W. H., & Colón, C. L. (2020). Further evaluation of treatment integrity of response interruption and redirection. *Behavioral Interventions, 35*(4), 571–580. https://doi.org/10.1002/bin.1738

*Gibbs, A. R., Tullis, C. A., Thomas, R., & Elkins, B. (2018). The effects of noncontingent music and response interruption and redirection on vocal stereotypy. *Journal of Applied Behavior Analysis, 51*(4), 899–914. https://doi.org/10.1002/jaba.485

*Gibney, C., Phillips, K. J., Arnold-Saritepe, A., & Taylor, S. A. (2020). An evaluation of the effects of response interruption redirection and matched stimulation on vocal stereotypy. *Behavioral Interventions, 35*(1), 114–130. https://doi.org/10.1002/bin.1700

*Giles, A., St. Peter, C., Pence, S. T., & Gibson, A. B. (2012). Preference for blocking or response redirection during stereotypy treatment. *Research in Developmental Disabilities, 33*(6), 1691–1700. https://doi.org/10.1016/j.ridd.2012.05.008

*Giles, A., Swain, S., Quinn, L., & Weifenbach, B. (2018). Teacher-implemented response interruption and redirection: Training, evaluation, and descriptive analysis of treatment integrity. *Behavior Modification, 42*(1), 148–169. https://doi.org/10.1177/0145445517731061

*Gould, K. M., Harper, J. M., Gillich, E., & Luiselli, J. K. (2019). Intervention, stimulus control, and generalization effects of response interruption and redirection on motor stereotypy. *Behavioral Interventions, 34*(1), 118–126. https://doi.org/10.1002/bin.1652

*Guzinski, E. M., Cihon, T. M., & Eshleman, J. (2012). The effects of tact training on stereotypic vocalizations in children with autism. *The Analysis of Verbal Behavior, 28*, 101–110. https://doi.org/10.1007/bf03393110

Hagopian, L. P., & Adelinis, J. D. (2001). Response blocking with and without redirection for the treatment of pica. *Journal of Applied Behavior Analysis, 34*(4), 527–530. https://doi.org/10.1901/jaba.2001.34-527

*Hagopian, L. P., González, M. L., Rivet, T. T., Triggs, M., & Clark, S. B. (2011). Response interruption and differential reinforcement of alternative behavior for the treatment of pica. *Behavioral Interventions, 26*(4), 309–325. https://doi.org/10.1002/bin.339

Hagopian, L. P., Rooker, G. W., & Zarcone, J. R. (2015). Delineating subtypes of self-injurious behavior maintained by automatic reinforcement. *Journal of Applied Behavior Analysis, 48*(3), 523–543. https://doi.org/10.1002/jaba.236

Hagopian, L. P., Rooker, G. W., Zarcone, J. R., Bonner, A. C., & Arevalo, A. R. (2017). Further analysis of subtypes of automatically reinforced SIB: A replication and quantitative analysis of published datasets, *Journal of Applied Behavior Analysis, 50*(1), 48–66. https://doi.org/10.1002/jaba.368

*Hagopian, L. P., & Toole, L. M. (2009). Effects of response blocking and competing stimuli on stereotypic behavior. *Behavioral Interventions, 24*(2), 117–125. https://doi.org/10.1002/bin.278

Iwata, B., Dorsey, M., Slifer, K., Bauman, K., & Richman, G. (1982/1994). Toward a functional analysis of self-injury. *Analysis and Intervention in Developmental Disabilities, 2*(1), 3–20. https://doi.org/10.1901/jaba.1994.27-197

*Jeglum, S. R., Luehring, M. C., & Kurtz, P. F. (2022). Using competing stimuli with an adult with stereotypic skin picking: A case study of assessment, treatment, and generalization. *Behavioral Interventions, 37*(3), 898–908. https://doi.org/10.1002/bin.1870

Jennett, H., Jann, K., & Hagopian, L. P. (2013). Evaluation of response blocking and re-presentation in a competing stimulus assessment. *Journal of Applied Behavior Analysis, 44*, 925–929. https://doi.org/10.1901/jaba.2011.44-925

*Lang, R., O'Reilly, M., Sigafoos, J., Lancioni, G. E., Machalicek, W., Rispoli, M., White, P., & Zarcone, J. (2009). Enhancing the effectiveness of a play intervention by abolishing the reinforcing value of stereotypy: A pilot study. *Journal of Applied Behavior Analysis, 42*(4), 889–894. https://doi.org/10.1901/jaba.2009.42-889

*Lang, R., O'Reilly, M., Sigafoos, J., Machalicek, W., Rispoli, M., Lancioni, G. E., Aguilar, J., & Fragale, C. (2010). The effects of an abolishing operation intervention component on play skills, challenging behavior, and stereotypy. *Behavior Modification, 34*(4), 267–289. https://doi.org/10.1177/0145445510370713

Lanovaz, M. J., Robertson, K. M., Soerono, K., & Watkins, N. (2013). Effects of reducing stereotypy on other behaviors: A systematic review. *Research in Autism Spectrum Disorders, 7*(10), 1234–1243. https://doi.org/10.1016/j.rasd.2013.07.009

Leaf, J. B., Cihon, J. H., Leaf, R., McEachin, J., Liu, N., Russell, N., Unumb, L., Shapiro, S., & Khosrowshahi, D. (2022). Concerns about ABA-based intervention: An evaluation and recommendations. *Journal of Autism and Developmental Disorders, 52*(6), 2838–2853. https://doi.org/10.1007/s10803-021-05200-8

*Liu-Gitz, L., & Banda, D. R. (2010). A replication of the RIRD strategy to decrease vocal stereotypy in a student with autism. *Behavioral Intervention, 25*(1), 77–87. https://doi.org/10.1002/bin.297

*Love, J. J., Miguel, C. F., Fernand, J. K., & LaBrie, J. K. (2012). The effects of matched stimulation and response interruption and redirection on vocal stereotypy. *Journal of Applied Behavior of Analysis, 45*(3), 549–564. https://doi.org/10.1901/jaba.2012.45-549

MacDonald, R., Green, G., Mansfield, R., Geckeler, A., Gardenier, N., Anderson, J., Holcomb, W., & Sanchez, J. (2007). Stereotypy in young children with autism and typically developing children. *Research in Developmental Disabilities, 28*(3), 266–277. https://doi.org/10.1016/j.ridd.2006.01.004

Martinez, C. K., & Betz, A. M. (2013). Response interruption and redirection: Current research trends and clinical application. *Journal of Applied Behavior Analysis, 46*(2), 549–554. https://doi.org/10.1002/jaba.38

*Martinez, C. K., Betz, A. M., Liddon, C. J., & Werle, R. L. (2016). A progression to transfer RIRD to the natural environment. *Behavioral Interventions, 31*(2), 144–162. https://doi.org/10.1002/bin.1444

*McNamara, K., & Cividini-Motta, C. (2019). Further evaluation of treatments for vocal stereotypy: Response interruption and redirection and response cost. *Behavioral Interventions, 34*(2), 181–197. https://doi.org/10.1002/bin.1657

*Meany-Daboul, M. G., Roscoe, E. M., Bourret, J. C., & Ahearn, W. H. (2007). A comparison of momentary time sampling and partial-interval recording for evaluating functional relations. *Journal of Applied Behavior Analysis, 40*(3), 501–514. https://doi.org/10.1901/jaba.2007.40-501

*Miguel, C. F., Clark, K., Tereshko, L., & Ahearn, W. H. (2009). The effects of response interruption and redirection and sertraline on vocal stereotypy. *Journal of Applied Behavior Analysis, 42*(4), 883–888. https://doi.org/10.1901/jaba.2009.42-883

*Pastrana, S. J., Rapp, J. T., & Frewing, T. M. (2013). Immediate and subsequent effects of response interruption and redirection on targeted and untargeted forms of stereotypy. *Behavior Modification, 37*(4), 591–610. https://doi.org/10.1177/0145445513485751

*Peters, L. C., & Thompson, R. H. (2013). Some indirect effects of positive practice overcorrection. *Journal of Applied Behavior Analysis, 46*(3), 613–625. https://doi.org/10.1002/jaba.63

Querim, A. C., Iwata, B. A., Roscoe, E. M., Schlichenmeyer, K. J., Ortega, J. V., & Hurl, K. E. (2013). Functional analysis screening for problem behavior maintained by automatic reinforcement. *Journal of Applied Behavior Analysis, 46*(1), 47–60. https://doi.org/10.1002/jaba.26

Rapp, J. T., & Vollmer, T. R. (2005). Stereotypy I: A review of behavioral assessment and treatment. *Research in Developmental Disabilities, 26*(6), 527–547. https://doi.org/10.1016/j.ridd.2004.11.005

Reid, D. H., Parsons, M. B., Phillips, J. F., & Green, C. W. (1993). Reduction of self-injurious hand mouthing using response blocking. *Journal of Applied Behavior Analysis, 26*(1), 139–140. https://doi.org/10.1901/jaba.1993.26-139

Richman, D. M., Barnard-Brak, L., Bosch, A., Thompson, S., Grubb, L., & Abby, L. (2013). Predictors of self-injurious behaviour exhibited by individuals with autism spectrum disorder. *Journal of Intellectual Disability Research, 57*(5), 429–439. https://doi.org/10.1111/j.1365-2788.2012.01628.x

*Saini, V., Gregory, M. K., Uran, K. J., & Fantetti, M. A. (2015). Parametric analysis of response interruption and redirection as treatment for stereotypy. *Journal of Applied Behavior Analysis, 48*(1), 96–106. https://doi.org/10.1002/jaba.186

*Schmidt, J. D., Long, A., Goetzel, A. L., Tung, C., Pizarro, E., Phillips, C., & Hausman, N. (2017). Decreasing pica attempts by manipulating the environment to support prosocial behavior. *Journal of Developmental and Physical Disabilities, 29*, 683–697. https://doi.org/10.1007/s10882-017-9548-y

*Schumacher, B. I., & Rapp, J. T. (2011). Evaluation of the immediate and subsequent effects of response interruption and redirection on vocal stereotypy. *Journal of Applied Behavior Analysis, 44*(3), 681–685. https://doi.org/10.1901/jaba.2011.44-681

*Shawler, L. A., Dianda, M., & Miguel, C. F. (2020). A comparison of response interruption and redirection and competing items on vocal stereotypy and appropriate vocalizations. *Journal of Applied Behavior Analysis, 53*(1), 355–365. https://doi.org/10.1002/jaba.596

*Shawler, L. A., & Miguel, C. G. (2015). The effects of motor and vocal response interruption and redirection on vocal stereotypy and appropriate vocalizations. *Behavioral Interventions, 30*(2), 112–134. https://doi.org/10.1002/bin.1407

*Sivaraman, M., & Rapp, J. T. (2020). Further analysis of immediate and subsequent effect of RIRD on vocal stereotypy. *Behavior Modification, 44*(5), 646–669. https://doi.org/10.1177/0145445519838826

*Sloman, K. N., McGarry, K. M., Kishel, C., & Hawkins, A. (2022). A comparison of RIRD within chained and multiple schedules in the treatment of vocal stereotypy. *Journal of Applied Behavior Analysis, 55*(2), 584–602. https://doi.org/10.1002/jaba.906

*Sloman, K. N., Schulman, R. K., Torres-Viso, M., & Edelstein, M. L. (2017). Evaluation of response interruption and redirection during school and community activities. *Behavior Analysis: Research and Practice, 17*(3), 266–273. https://doi.org/10.1037/bar0000061

Steinbrenner, J. R., Hume, K., Odom, S. L., Morin, K. L., Nowell, S. W., Tomaszewski, B., Szendrey, S., McIntyre, N. S., Yücesoy-Özkan, S., & Savage, M. N. (2020). Evidence-based practices for children, youth, and young adults with Autism. The University of North Carolina at Chapel Hill, Frank Porter Graham Child Development Institute, National Clearinghouse on Autism Evidence and Practice Review Team.

Steinhauser, H. M. K., & Ahearn W. H. (2021). Response interruption and redirection. In J. L. Matson (Ed.), *Handbook of Applied Behavior Analysis. Autism and Child Psychopathology Series* (pp. 269–288). Cham: Springer.

*Steinhauser, H. M. K., Ahearn, W. H., Foster, R. A., Jacobs, M., Doggett, C. G., & Goad, M. S. (2021). Examining stereotypy in naturalistic contexts: Differential reinforcement and context-specific redirection. *Journal of Applied Behavior Analysis, 54*(4), 1420–1436. https://doi.org/10.1002/jaba.847

Symons, F. J., Sperry, L. A., Dropik, P. L., & Bodfish, J. (2005). The early development of stereotypy and self-injury: A review of research methods. *Journal of Intellectual Disability Research*, *49*(2), 144–158. https://doi.org/10.1111/j.1365-2788.2004.00632.x

*Taylor, T. (2020). Assessment and treatment of pica within the home setting in Australia. *Behavioral Development*, *25*(1), 40–51. https://doi.org/10.1037/bdb0000094

Tomaszewski, B., Regan, T., & AFIRM Team. (2017). Response interruption and redirection. Chapel Hill: National Professional Development Center on Autism Spectrum Disorder, FPG Child Development Center, University of North Carolina. http://afirm.fpg.unc.edu/response-interruption-and-redirectio

*Toper-Korkmaz, O., Lerman, D. C., & Tsami, L. (2018). Effects of toy removal and number of demands on vocal stereotypy during response interruption and redirection. *Journal of Applied Behavior Analysis*, *51*, 757–768. https://doi.org/10.1002/jaba.497

*Verriden, A., & Roscoe, E. (2019). An evaluation of a punisher assessment for decreasing automatically reinforced problem behavior. *Journal of Applied Behavior Analysis*, *52*(1), 205–226. https://doi.org/10.1002/jaba.509

Vollmer, T. R. (1994). The concept of automatic reinforcement: Implications for behavioral research in developmental disabilities. *Research in Developmental Disabilities*, *15*(3), 187–207.

Wang, D., Mason, R. A., Lory, C., Kim, S. Y., David, M., & Guo, X. (2020). Vocal stereotypy and autism spectrum disorder: A systematic review of interventions. *Research in Autism Spectrum Disorders*, *78*, 101647. https://doi.org/10.1016/j.rasd.2020.101647

*Wells, J., Collier, L., & Sheehey, P. H. (2016). Decreasing vocal stereotypy of youth with autism in a classroom setting. *Child & Family Behavior Therapy*, *38*(2), 164–174. https://doi.org/10.1080/07317107.2016.1172887

*Wunderlich, K. L., & Vollmer, T. R. (2015). Data analysis of response interruption and redirection as a treatment for vocal stereotypy. *Journal of Applied Behavior Analysis*, *48*(4), 749–764. https://doi.org/10.1002/jaba.227

7

Matched Stimulation

John T. Rapp, Daniel J. Sheridan, and Ashley N. Anderson
Auburn University

7.1 Technical Abstract

Background: In this chapter, authors describe how practitioners and caregivers may use matched stimulation (MS) to decrease noninjurious repetitive behavior for individuals with autism spectrum disorder (ASD) and related neurodevelopmental disabilities. **Method**: To identify interventions for reducing repetitive behavior with MS, authors systematically reviewed electronic databases (e.g., PsycINFO), conducted hand and ancestral searches, and employed expert consultation. Searches involved analysis of peer-reviewed studies with sufficient single-case or group designs. Where applicable, authors also applied the 5-3-30 criteria for determining whether the literature contained sufficient empirical support for a given intervention. **Results**: Researchers have demonstrated that MS can be an effective treatment for reducing stereotypies exhibited by individuals diagnosed with a variety of disorders, including ASD. **Discussion**: Although behavioral interventions with MS can decrease some forms of stereotypy, future research should focus on how MS may be used to establish and develop new behavioral repertoires (e.g., vocal verbal behavior). We conclude the chapter with recommendations for extending the literature for MS. **Practitioner recommendations**: Practitioners should use preference and competing stimulus assessment to identify preferred stimuli that match the product of their clients' repetitive behavior. Thereafter, practitioners should employ antecedent- and consequent-based interventions that provide matched stimuli noncontingently to compete with repetitive behavior, contingently to increase alternative behavior to displace repetitive behavior, or both.

7.2 Layperson Summary

In this chapter, authors describe how practitioners and caregivers may use preferred items and activities that produce stimulation that matches sensory products generated by performing repetitive behavior to decrease noninjurious repetitive behavior for individuals with ASD and related disabilities. The authors identified sources of information that evaluated the use of MS to reduce various noninjurious repetitive behaviors (e.g., hand flapping). Results of this review show that

John T. Rapp, Daniel J. Sheridan, and Ashley N. Anderson, *Matched Stimulation*. In: *Lifespan Treatment for Autistic Individuals*. Edited by: Peter Sturmey, Russell Lang, and James K. Luiselli, Oxford University Press. © Oxford University Press (2025). DOI: 10.1093/oso/9780197635841.003.0007

MS can be an effective way to reduce repetitive behavior displayed by individuals diagnosed with a variety of disorders, including ASD. Although research on MS is promising, there are still areas that require further exploration. For instance, researchers should consider using MS to establish or increase new skills. Collaborate with a licensed behavior analyst to identify preferred items that can be used in various behavioral interventions to decrease repetitive behavior.

7.3 Treatment Summary Table

Treatment summary: Matched Stimulation

Treatment description: MS is a stimulus event that functionally matches the sensory product maintaining a repetitive behavior. Stimulus preference assessments are always indicated as the first step toward identifying matched stimuli. Thereafter, antecedent- and consequent-based interventions that utilize matched stimuli have been shown to reduce stereotypy.

Expected outcomes: A review of the literature indicates that MS tends to produce immediate reductions across a variety of stereotypic behavior. However, it can be difficult to identify items or objects that provide MS for specific forms of stereotypy.

Methods: Authors systematically reviewed electronic databases (e.g., PsycINFO), conducted hand and ancestral searches, and employed expert consultation. Searches involved analysis of peer-reviewed studies with sufficient single-case or group designs.

Expertise required to implement treatment: Research on MS tends to indicate that behaviorally trained individuals implement these procedures, especially depending on the topography of stereotypy. Nonetheless, MS delivered noncontingently can be implemented by many, including paraprofessionals, teachers, and parents/caregivers.

Risks and negative side effects: The primary risk of decreasing forms of motor or vocal stereotypy with MS is that previously less frequent or less probable behavior may increase. This increased behavior, which can be viewed as a side effect, may give rise to the same challenges as the behavior that was initially targeted for intervention.

Additional considerations and limitations: Treatment of repetitive behavior may require long-term intervention with MS. In addition, the intervention may require routine updates to maintain behavior changes.

7.4 Introduction

7.4.1 Intervention Description

Individuals with intellectual disabilities, ASD, or other neurodevelopmental disorders may engage in problem behavior that generates its own stimulus products that, in turn, support that behavior (Rapp et al., 2008). Piazza et al. (1998, 2000) and Patel et al. (2000) introduced procedures for identifying objects that were structurally similar to the putative, overt stimulus products generated by individuals' automatically reinforced problem behavior. In what follows, we describe steps for identifying objects that generate stimulation that functionally matches the stimulus products of automatically reinforced problem behavior (hereafter described generally as target behavior, motor stereotypy [various forms], or vocal stereotypy). Specifically, we outline how to determine the need to intervene, collect data for duration-based target behavior, identify and categorize preferred stimuli, conduct a three-component multiple schedule, and select intervention with either noncontingent or contingent MS for noninjurious target behavior. Ultimately, the goal of such interventions is to produce an abolishing operation for the target behavior of concern (Laraway et al., 2003). We conclude the chapter by outlining caregivers' roles in the assessment and intervention process. We begin this process by providing some guidance about when practitioners should consider intervention for repetitive behavior.

7.4.2 Rationale and Objectives

In general, there is not a consensus position in applied behavior analysis (ABA) about when noninjurious repetitive behavior (e.g., motor stereotypy) warrants intervention (e.g., Rapp & Vollmer, 2005; Raulston & Machalicek, 2018). Broadly, practitioners should consider intervening when engagement in the target behavior (a) interferes with behavior acquisition, (b) diminishes social opportunities, or (c) both (e.g., Cook & Rapp, 2020; Cunningham & Schreibman, 2008; Enloe & Rapp, 2014; Lanovaz et al., 2013; Leaf et al., 2022). Specifically, the individual's target behavior may require intervention when either it disrupts the learning environment for others (Cook & Rapp, 2020) or could be viewed unfavorably by peers (Coon & Rapp, 2020). To this end, Coon and Rapp found that even low levels of motor stereotypy by a child with ASD produced negative ratings of the child's behavior by adults; as the level of stereotypy increased, so did the negativity of the ratings. Other researchers reported similar findings for repetitive behavior displayed by children with ASD and adults with intellectual disabilities (e.g., Grossman, 2015; Jones et al., 1990; Long et al., 1998, 1999). Nevertheless, it may be acceptable for some individuals to engage in noninjurious repetitive behavior during leisure or unstructured time intervals in the absence of peer evaluation. We recommend consulting with stakeholders about the issues noted above.

7.5 Research Background and Clinical Considerations

7.5.1 Data Collection

Given that time allocation to noninjurious repetitive behavior is a determining factor in the need to intervene, we will assume (a) the target behavior in question is a duration-based event and (b) practitioners have developed a clear response definition for that target behavior (see Table 7.1 for a definition bank). Several studies have shown 10-second momentary time sampling (MTS) correctly

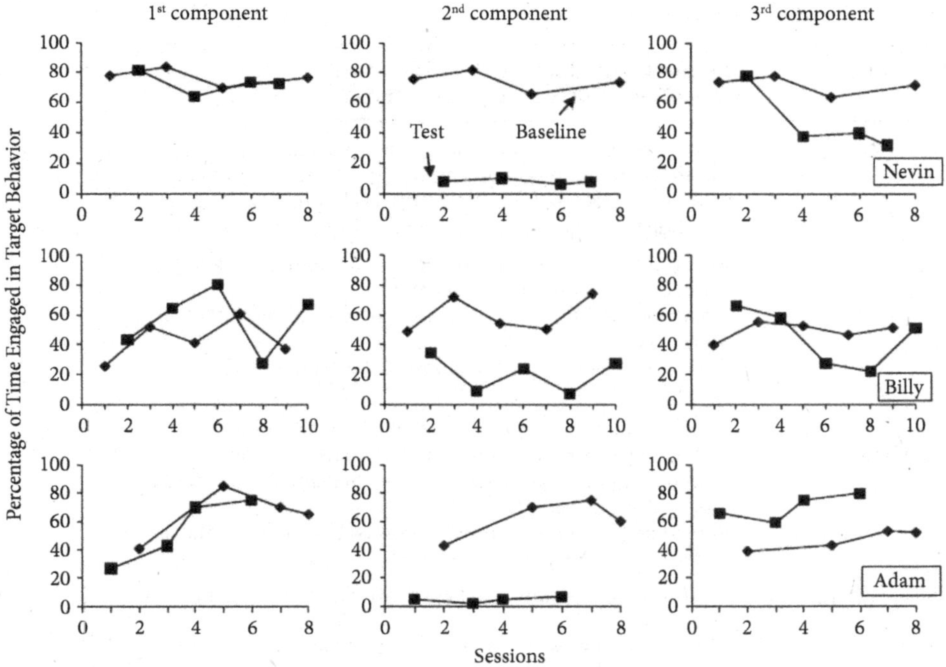

Figure 7.1 Examples of the between-sequence analysis

Note. Between-sequence analysis showing the percentage of time Nevin (three upper [from left to right] panels), Billy (three center panels), and Adam (three lower panels) engaged in the target behavior across the first (left [from top to bottom] panels), second (middle panels), and third (right panels) components of no-interaction (denote Baseline) and intervention-test (denoted Test) sequences. Reprinted with permission from Lanovaz, M. J., Rapp, J. T., & Fletcher, S. M. (2010). Expanding functional analysis of automatically reinforced behavior using a three-component multiple schedule. *European Journal of Behavior Analysis, 11*, 17–27. https://doi.org/10.1080/15021149.2010.11434331

detects various changes in duration events during observations of 10 minutes or longer (e.g., Devine et al., 2011; Rapp et al., 2008). To collect data with MTS, divide the total observation session (e.g., 10 minutes) by small intervals (e.g., 10 seconds) and score a designated second of each interval for the presence of the target behavior (see Figure 7.1). To calculate the percentage of intervals with the target behavior, sum the scored intervals, divide the sum by the total number of intervals (e.g., 60 for a 10-minute session), and multiply that quotient by 100%. Plot this data point in a linear graph and repeat the process for assessment sessions, as well as baseline and intervention sessions.

7.5.2 Categorizing Stimuli

By definition, functionally MS involves sensory stimulation that has been empirically determined to match the sensory product maintaining a target behavior (Lanovaz et al., 2009). The distinctions among nonstructurally, structurally, and functionally matched preferred stimulation can be important because preferred stimuli (nonstructurally or structurally matched) may compete with a target

Table 7.1 Response definition bank

Code	Response Form	Response Definitions for STEREOTYPY (2-s offset for all stereotypy definitions)
vs.	Vocal Stereotypy	Noncontextual vocal utterances or whispering, including unintelligible sounds (e.g., mumbling, humming, growling, yelling), words, phrases, or singing (excluding coughing and sneezing), lasting 2 seconds or more
os.	Object Stereotypy	Repetitive (2 or more within 2 seconds) tapping or hitting a surface with an object held in hand(s); OR Noncontextual spinning or rotating of objects for 2 seconds or more; OR Rotating, posturing, or waving with objects in hand(s) for 2 seconds or more
sc.	Surface Contact (with body)	Licking, mouthing, or sniffing the surface of an object (e.g., toy, table) or structure (e.g., wall) for 2 seconds or more; OR Rubbing or pressing a body part (e.g., fingers) into surfaces for 2 seconds or more; OR Repetitive (2 or more within 2 seconds) tapping or hitting a surface with body part (e.g., palms)
og.	Object Gazing	Holding object within 6 inches of own face for 2 seconds or more; OR Placing own face within 1 foot of a stationary object or surface (e.g., walls, tables, floors) for 2 seconds or more; OR Noncontextual staring at an inactive object (e.g., wall decal) for 2 seconds or more
fl.	Hand/Arm Flapping	Repetitive (2 or more within 2 seconds) waving of both arms/hand, including flapping while bent at the elbows or flapping with straightened arms down at the sides
wf.	Wrist/Finger Movements	Rotating hand (loose or clenched) at the wrist for 2 seconds or more; OR Clenching fingers or hands for 2 seconds or more; OR Wiggling or tensing fingers for 2 seconds or more; OR Repetitive (2 or more within 2 seconds) flicking of thumb and fingers
hp.	Hand Posturing	Straightening or flexing the palm, wrist, or fingers in various positions of tension, including holding the tensed position, for 2 seconds or more (i.e., invariant positioning)
ea.	Ear Covering	Contact of hand(s), or shoulder, with one or both ears for 2 seconds or more
he.	Head Movements	Holding head in a turned position 2 seconds or more; OR Rotating head in partial or full head rolls for 2 seconds or more; OR Repetitive (2 or more within 2 seconds) head nodding (up and down), head shaking (side to side), or head tilting (shoulder to shoulder)
hs.	Hair/Scalp Manipulation	Twirling, rubbing, grasping or gliding fingers on hair or scalp for 2 seconds or more
fo.	Facial/Oral Movements	Blinking, squinting eyes, or furrowing brow for 2 seconds or more; OR Lip positioning including smacking, puckering, or blowing/sucking air for 2 seconds or more; OR Audibly clicking tongue, grinding teeth, or swishing saliva for 2 seconds or more

Code	Response Form	Response Definitions for STEREOTYPY (2-s offset for all stereotypy definitions)
ss.	Spitting/Saliva Play	Expelling (or sucking back expelled) saliva past the plane of the lips for 2 seconds or more; OR Making body contact with saliva once expelled past the plane of the lips for 2 seconds or more
tw.	Twirling Body	Full rotation (360 degrees) of own body while standing, sitting, or kneeling on the floor
ps.	Pacing/Sprinting	Two or more walking or running steps (second step within 2 seconds of first step) in a forward motion
st.	Stomping	One or more instances of impactful foot contact with floor or wall producing a sound
bo.	Body Rocking/Tilting	Repetitive (two or more within 2 seconds) forward and backward or side-to-side full torso or full body movements (bending at waist or stiff body); may be sitting or standing
bp.	Body Posturing	Stiffening or holding partial or full body poses for 2 seconds or more
ju.	Jumping/Bouncing	Repetitive (two or more within 2 seconds) movements in an up and down motion with bent knees (feet may or may not leave on the floor)

behavior but may not produce the same sensory product as that target stereotypy (Lanovaz et al., 2009, 2010).

Practitioners can identify structurally matched stimuli via empirical preference assessments that match the overt product of the target behavior (Lanovaz et al., 2009; Piazza et al., 2000). That is, researchers have demonstrated a reduction in both immediate (while the change agent implements the intervention) and subsequent (after the change agent discontinues the intervention) engagement in the target behavior (e.g., Lanovaz et al., 2009; Rapp, 2007; Rapp et al., 2013, 2017). By definition, functionally matched stimuli compete with stereotypy when available and may continue to exert a decreasing effect after a change agent removes those stimuli. Ideally, practitioners should seek to identify and utilize functionally matched stimuli.

A stimulus preference assessment is a necessary first step toward identifying matched stimuli; however, a preferred stimulus may *increase* target behavior for some individuals. To complicate this issue, such increases can occur while the stimulus is available, after the stimulus is removed, or both (Brogan et al., 2018; Rapp et al., 2013). A preferred stimulus that increases target behavior is, by definition, not functionally matched to that target behavior. Results from free operant competing stimulus assessments (FOCSA) can identify stimuli that reduce the likelihood of inadvertently increasing stereotypy (Brogan et al., 2018; Frewing et al., 2015; Rapp et al., 2013); however, a functionally matched stimulus that reduces immediate and subsequent stereotypy is best identified through a three-component multiple schedule (TCMS) assessment (Lanovaz et al., 2010; Rapp, 2007).

7.5.3 Free Operant Preference Assessment

As previously noted, conducting a preference assessment is the first step in the process of identifying matched stimuli. In general, preference assessments identify stimuli that are likely to function as reinforcers. Potentially matched stimuli should generate overt stimulation resembling the product of the target behavior. For example, if an individual engages in vocal stereotypy, a matched stimulus might produce auditory stimulation, whereas a nonmatched stimulus (e.g., building blocks) might produce tactile stimulation (e.g., Rapp et al., 2013). Practitioners can identify stimuli to include in a preference assessment through the clients' teachers and caregivers using indirect assessments such as the reinforcer assessment for individuals with severe disabilities (RAISD; Fisher et al., 1996). Importantly, practitioners should conduct a free operant preference assessment (FOPA) after identifying items with the RAISD.

The FOPA consists of 10-minute sessions where the client receives access to six or more stimuli concurrently (Roane et al., 1998). Practitioners should collect data on both object engagement and stereotypy using 10-second MTS during the 10-minute sessions (see Figure 7.S2). To avoid scoring incidental engagement with items, we recommend practitioners define engagement as active manipulation of an item (e.g., the client holding an item as opposed to resting their hand on it) or clear consumption of an ambient stimulus (e.g., the client approaching and standing close to a music source). When oriented to the datasheet, the observer should score the column indicating no engagement if the client does not engage with any item. At the end of the session, practitioners should add up all the intervals with engagement for each item separately. Thereafter, divide that value by the total number of intervals (i.e., 60 intervals for a 10-minute session). This calculation gives the percentage of intervals of engagement for each item. Subsequently, the practitioner should rank the stimuli according to the number of intervals engaged for each item. For example, rank the stimulus with the most intervals with engagement as the most preferred stimulus. Practitioners should then rank the stimulus with the second-highest level of engagement as the second preferred stimulus. Practitioners should continue in this fashion until they have ranked all stimuli. Theoretically, the most preferred stimulus is the one with the highest level of engagement; however, the client may not exhibit the strongest preference for structurally matched stimuli (Ahearn et al., 2005; Gibney et al., 2020; Rapp et al., 2013). Practitioners can use the potentially reinforcing stimuli identified through the FOPA in the interventions discussed later in the chapter (see Cook et al. [2019] and Weldy et al. [2014][1] for additional details on conducting FOPAs).

7.5.4 Free Operant Competing Stimulus Assessments

This assessment involves measuring an individual's engagement in noninjurious repetitive behavior while alternative stimuli are available (Brogan et al., 2018;

[1] A demonstration is available from http://repository.stcloudstate.edu/cpcf_gradresearch/1

Frewing et al., 2015). Notably, several studies have found some individuals engage in higher levels of stereotypy in the presence of specific stimuli (Brogan et al., 2018; Cook et al., 2014; Frewing et al., 2015; Lanovaz et al., 2013; Rapp, 2004, 2005; Rapp et al., 2013; Van Camp et al., 2000). If an individual prefers an item that increases their target behavior, it would not be an appropriate stimulus to include in an intervention.

The FOCSA is a multistep assessment for identifying competing stimuli. As with a FOPA, practitioners should establish the operational definition for stereotypy and appropriate item engagement. As the first step, practitioners should conduct three or more sessions without alternative stimuli (Haddock & Hagopian, 2020). Data from these sessions will serve as a baseline to determine the extent to which the target behavior changes in the presence of structurally matched stimuli. The second step is determining which stimuli to include in the FOCSA. Practitioners can identify stimuli through preference assessments, interviews, or both. The stimuli should be safe for the client, controllable by a change agent, matched to the putative overt product of the target behavior, and appropriate for the setting (e.g., home, clinic). The third step consists of conducting three to five, 10-minute FOSCA sessions with at least 6 to 10 items. Certain circumstances may require more sessions (e.g., low engagement with the items). Practitioners should make the same stimuli available simultaneously during all sessions. Additionally, practitioners should record the client's engagement with each individual item and target behavior for the duration of each session using 10-second MTS (see Figure 7.S2).

After completing the series of FOCSA sessions, practitioners should categorize stimuli based on the client's engagement with each stimulus *and* the client's engagement in stereotypy while engaging with each stimulus. To categorize a stimulus as high preference, low stereotypy (HP-LS), use conditional and unconditional percentages (Brogan et al., 2018; Frewing et al., 2015). Practitioners should combine all the FOCSA sessions and calculate the unconditional percentage of stereotypy by dividing the number of intervals engaged in stereotypy by the total number of intervals and then multiplying the quotient by 100% (Brogan et al., 2018). Calculating the unconditional percentage of stereotypy will indicate the approximate amount of time the client engaged in stereotypy regardless of item engagement. Next, practitioners should calculate the conditional percentage for each item by dividing the number of intervals the client engaged in stereotypy while simultaneously engaging with each item (separately) by the total number of intervals the client engaged with the item and multiplying the quotient by 100% (Brogan et al., 2018; Frewing et al., 2015). Thereafter, practitioners should compare the conditional percentages to the unconditional percentage of stereotypy and the baseline levels shown in the control sessions to determine if specific items increase or decrease levels of the target behavior (Brogan et al., 2018; Frewing et al., 2015; Lanovaz et al., 2013). If the conditional percentage of stereotypy for a stimulus is lower than both the unconditional percentage and control sessions, the stimulus will likely decrease the target behavior when presented alone (Brogan et al., 2018).

Date: __________

Start and End Time: _______

DC Initials: _____________

Circle one: Primary/Secondary

Session: _______________

Condition: _______________

Stimuli:	
1	
2	
3	
4	
5	
6	

Interval	1	2	3	4	5	6	NE		VS	MS
Minute 0–1										
10										
20										
30										
40										
50										
60										
Minute 1–2										
10										
20										
30										

Figure 7.S2 Datasheet for FOPA and FOCSA preference assessments

40										
50										
60										
Minute 2–3										
10										
20										
30										
40										
50										
60										
Minute 3–4										
10										
20										
30										
40										
50										
60										
Minute 4–5										
10										
20										

Figure 7.S2 *Continued*

30										
40										
50										
60										

Figure 7.S2 *Continued*

Note. 10-second momentary time sampling datasheet across a 5-minute session. This datasheet can be used for FOPA and FOCSA. NE = no engagement; VS = vocal stereotypy; MS = motor stereotypy. Adapted from Cook, J. L., Rapp, J. T., & Brogan, K. M. (2018). Assessment and treatment of stereotypical behavior displayed by children with autism spectrum disorders. In C. McNeil, L. Quetsch, & C. Anderson (Eds.), *Handbook of parent-child interaction therapy for children on the autism spectrum* (pp. 147-168). Cham: Springer.

7.5.5 Three-Component Multiple Schedule Analysis

As previously noted, target behavior may decrease while an intervention is in place but may return to or surpass baseline levels when intervention is removed (e.g., Enloe & Rapp, 2014; Lanovaz et al., 2009, 2010; Rapp, 2006, 2007). Specifically, providing access to a structurally matched stimulus could decrease an individual's engagement in repetitive behavior; however, after removal of the intervention, the individual may be deprived of stimulation generated by that behavior (e.g., Klatt & Morris, 2001; Rapp, 2007; Rapp et al., 2004). Thus, they may be more likely to emit that target behavior and less likely to engage in appropriate behavior (e.g., academic tasks). To prevent this problem, practitioners can use the TCMS analysis to determine the immediate *and* subsequent effects of stimuli on levels of target behavior (e.g., Lanovaz et al., 2009; Rapp, 2006, 2007; Rapp et al., 2013, 2017; Simmons et al., 2003).

Although a FOCSA can determine immediate effects of an intervention on one or more target behaviors, only a TCMS analysis can assess the subsequent effects of an intervention on those behaviors (Lanovaz et al., 2009, 2010; Rapp, 2007). Like a FOCSA, a TCMS analysis begins with a preference assessment. Thereafter, practitioners should use the items they plan to use as interventions for the target behavior in the TCMS assessment. Practitioners could begin this process with either a brief functional analysis (Iwata & Dozier, 2008) or a series of no-interactions sessions (Querim et al., 2013) to determine if the target behavior persists in the absence of social consequences. Alternatively, the TCMS analysis contains multiple no-interaction components, which are comparable to a no-interaction screening series. Specifically, the TCMS analysis consists of a No-Interaction (NI) sequence and an Intervention-Test sequence (IT), each with three components. The purpose of the NI sequence is to (a) measure the target behavior in the absence of social consequences, (b) evaluate the naturally occurring pattern of the target behavior across the three components, and (c) serve as a baseline against which to evaluate the effects of an intervention. The purpose of the IT sequence is to determine if

Table 7.2 Quick reference guide for practitioners: Three-component multiple schedule analysis

Sequence	Component		
	First	Second	Three
NI (3 or more)	• NI • 5 or 10 minutes • 10-second MTS	• NI • 5 or 10 minutes • 10-second MTS	• NI • 5 or 10 minutes • 10-second MTS
IT (3 or more)	• NI • 10 minutes each • 10-second MTS	• *Intervention* • 10 minutes each • 10-second MTS	• NI • 10 minutes each • 10-second MTS

Note. These guidelines apply to all age groups. Alternate between the sequences over several days. IT = Intervention-Test. MTS = momentary time sampling. NI = no interaction.

the target behavior (a) decreases when the intervention is in effect in the second component and (b) remains low in the third component (after removal of the intervention). Practitioners should conduct only one sequence per day, consistently use either 5- or 10-minute components (see Table 7.2), and alternate sequences across days (Brogan et al., 2018; Rapp et al., 2013, 2017).

In the NI sequence, each component consists of only a no-interaction condition. During the no-interaction components, practitioners should have the client in a room without alternative stimuli or social consequences for engagement in stereotypy. Practitioners should measure the behavior using 10-second MTS (see again Figure 7.S1), then determine the percentage of intervals with the target behavior by dividing the number of scored intervals by the total number of intervals in the session and multiply the quotient by 100% (Rapp et al., 2017). The only difference between the NI and IT sequences is the second component. For the second

Date: ________ Circle one: Primary/Secondary
Start and End Time: ______ Session: ____________
DC Initials: ____________ Sequence: ____________

Seconds	VS	MS	Seconds	VS	MS
10–11	Y N	Y N	310–311	Y N	Y N
20–21	Y N	Y N	320–321	Y N	Y N
30–31	Y N	Y N	330–331	Y N	Y N
40–41	Y N	Y N	340–341	Y N	Y N
50–51	Y N	Y N	350–351	Y N	Y N
60–61	Y N	Y N	360–361	Y N	Y N

Figure 7.S1 *Datasheet for scoring target behaviors*

Seconds	VS	MS	Seconds	VS	MS
70–71	Y N	Y N	370–371	Y N	Y N
80–81	Y N	Y N	380–381	Y N	Y N
90–91	Y N	Y N	390–391	Y N	Y N
100–101	Y N	Y N	400–401	Y N	Y N
110–111	Y N	Y N	410–411	Y N	Y N
120–121	Y N	Y N	420–421	Y N	Y N
Seconds	**VS**	**MS**	**Seconds**	**VS**	**MS**
130–131	Y N	Y N	430–431	Y N	Y N
140–141	Y N	Y N	440–441	Y N	Y N
150–151	Y N	Y N	450–451	Y N	Y N
160–161	Y N	Y N	460–461	Y N	Y N
170–171	Y N	Y N	470–471	Y N	Y N
180–181	Y N	Y N	480–481	Y N	Y N
Seconds	**VS**	**MS**	**Seconds**	**VS**	**MS**
190–191	Y N	Y N	490–491	Y N	Y N
200–201	Y N	Y N	500–501	Y N	Y N
210–211	Y N	Y N	510–511	Y N	Y N
220–221	Y N	Y N	520–521	Y N	Y N
230–231	Y N	Y N	530–531	Y N	Y N
240–241	Y N	Y N	540–541	Y N	Y N
Seconds	**VS**	**MS**	**Seconds**	**VS**	**MS**
250–251	Y N	Y N	550–551	Y N	Y N
260–261	Y N	Y N	560–561	Y N	Y N
270–271	Y N	Y N	570–571	Y N	Y N
280–281	Y N	Y N	580–581	Y N	Y N
290–291	Y N	Y N	590–591	Y N	Y N
300–301	Y N	Y N	600	Y N	Y N

Figure 7.S1 *Continued*

Note. Datasheet for scoring with 10-second momentary time sampling during a 5-minute or 10-minute component or session.

component of the IT sequence, practitioners should implement the intervention with putative MS (e.g., NCR).

7.5.6 Between-Sequence Analysis

Whenever possible, practitioners should use a between-sequence analysis to evaluate the immediate and subsequent effects of putative MS. This process compares patterns from the two sequences within separate multielement line graphs for each component (Lanovaz et al., 2009, 2010; Rapp et al., 2013, 2017). In the absence of a confounding event, the first component should be undifferentiated based on visual inspection. If the NI and IT data paths for the first components appear differentiated, the practitioner should repeat the assessment. If the paths are undifferentiated, practitioners should compare the second components of the two sequences. If the IT data path is lower than the NI data path for the second components, the intervention produced an abolishing operation (AO) for immediate engagement in the target behavior. To determine whether the intervention is a functional match to the target behavior, compare the third components of the two sequences. If the third component of the IT sequence is lower than the third component of the NI sequence, the intervention produced an AO for subsequent engagement in the target behavior. This is the most desirable outcome and indicates that the intervention is likely appropriate. If the third components of the two sequences are undifferentiated, the intervention did *not* produce a subsequent motivating operation (MO) for the targeted behavior. This pattern also indicates that the intervention may be appropriate. By contrast, if the third component of the IT sequence is higher and differentiated from the third component of the NI sequence, the intervention produced as subsequent establishing operation (EO) for the target behavior. This pattern indicates the intervention does not match the product of the target behavior. See Figure 7.1 for examples of immediate decreases in the second components with each of the three subsequent patterns in the third components.

7.5.7 Within-Sequence Analysis

Under time constraints, practitioners can simply conduct three to five IT sequences and then depict the level of behavior in each component for each IT sequence in a bar graph. If data show the target behavior is lower in the second component than in the first component of most sequences, the intervention produced an immediate AO for the target behavior. Thereafter, the practitioner should compare the data for the first and third components (Lanovaz et al., 2010; Morrison et al., 2011; Rapp, 2006, 2007). If the third component is lower than the first component for most IT sequences, the intervention is a functional match to the target behavior. By contrast, if the third component is typically higher than the first component, the

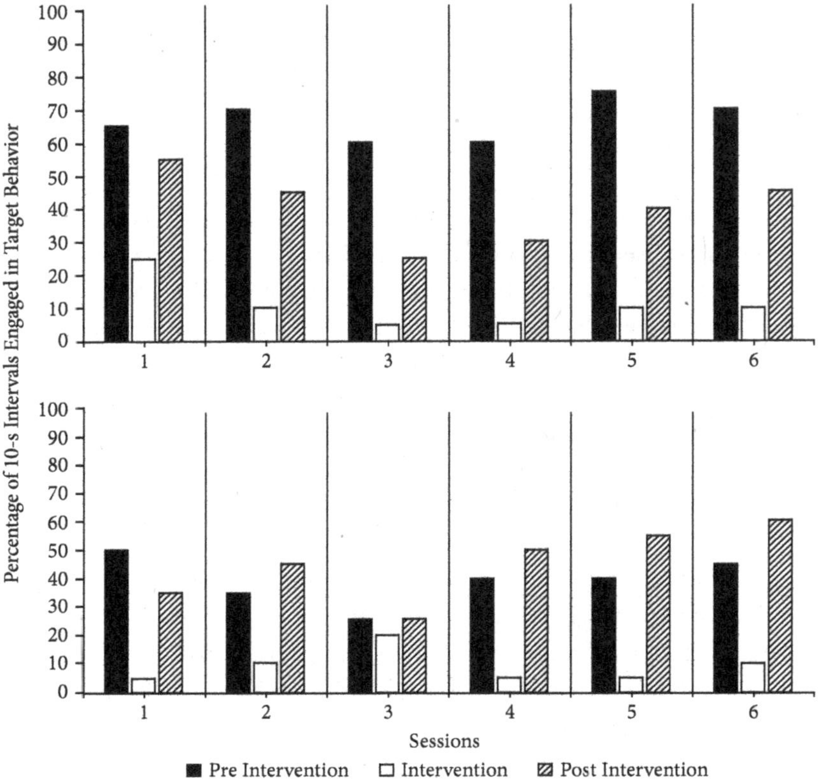

Figure 7.2 Examples of the within-sequence analysis with intervention-test sequences

Note. First and third components are always no-interaction conditions. Second components contain an intervention with a putative matched stimulus. Top panel demonstrates the identification of a matched stimulus in second component because the third component is always lower than the first component. Lower panel demonstrates the identification of a nonmatched stimulus as the third component is higher than the first component. Data in this figure are based on results depicted in Morrison, H., Roscoe, E. M., & Atwell, A. (2011). An evaluation of antecedent exercise on behavior maintained by automatic reinforcement using a three-component multiple schedule. *Journal of Applied Behavior Analysis, 44*, 523–541. https://doi.org/10.1901/jaba.2011.44-523

intervention is not a functional match. See Figure 7.2 for examples of subsequent decreases (upper panel) and subsequent increases (lower panel), which indicate matched and unmatched stimuli, respectively, within IT sequences.

7.5.8 Matched Stimulation for Noninjurious Repetitive Behavior

The literature contains moderate-to-strong empirical support for decreasing automatically reinforced behavior with MS provided either noncontingently (NCR-M) (e.g., Ahearn et al., 2005; Lanovaz & Argumedes, 2010; Llinas et al., 2022; Piazza et al., 2000; Rapp, 2006; Rapp et al., 2017; Slocum et al., 2020) or contingently (e.g., Brogan et al., 2018; Lanovaz & Argumedes, 2010; Rapp et al., 2017). Practitioners should consider treatment context when choosing an intervention (Cook et al.,

2019; Rapp & Lanovaz, 2016). For example, individuals may receive NCR-M as intervention during leisure times. By contrast, they may receive MS contingent on either omitting the target behavior or completing academic or other work-related segments during instructional segments. As a whole, children were the most frequent participants in assessment and treatment studies of MS.

Generally, practitioners should follow the same order of events outlined above regardless of the intervention. That is, practitioners should conduct a preference assessment and competing stimulus assessment. If time is a constraining factor, Rapp et al. (2017) suggests forgoing the FOCSA and using only the TCMS analysis to determine which stimuli functionally match a target behavior. On balance, Brogan et al. (2018) suggested the pre-TCMS FOCSA might be justified to avoid inadvertently using a high preference, high stereotypy (HP-HS) stimulus. Ultimately, practitioners should proceed with the chosen intervention after the identification of a matched stimulus.

Most research has focused on the use of MS as a single-component intervention (e.g., Gibney et al., 2020; Rapp et al., 2013). Although MS is often effective, studies have shown NCR-M may decrease a *targeted* behavior but simultaneously increase previously lower probability behaviors (e.g., Enloe & Rapp, 2014; Lanovaz et al., 2013; Rapp et al., 2013). In anticipation of this problem, practitioners should prepare to observe and measure additional, nontargeted, repetitive response forms (see Table 7.1) during the TCMS analysis (e.g., Rapp et al., 2017).

7.5.9 Noncontingent Reinforcement (NCR)

We recommend conducting a preliminary TCMS analysis to identify the stimulus in the NCR-Matched (NCR-M) intervention. If the TCMS results indicate the stimulus is a functional match to the target behavior, the practitioner can use NCR-M as a broader intervention in a leisure context. Procedurally, NCR-M involves a change agent delivering the empirically identified item independent of the occurrence of the target behavior. Conceptually, the schedule of access to the matched stimulus should be dense enough to reduce the MO for engaging in the target behavior. NCR-M procedures are straightforward to implement and relatively easy to teach to caregivers (Llinas et al., 2022). For optimal effects, practitioners can provide continuous access to the matched stimulus.

An individual's repetitive vocalizing may be either socially or nonsocially maintained. Here, we limit our focus to vocalizing that persists without social consequences and thus meets the definition of vocal stereotypy (Lanovaz & Sladeczek, 2012). Research generally shows NCR-M decreases vocal stereotypy in children (e.g., Lanovaz et al., 2009; Rapp et al., 2017). After practitioners identify a matched stimulus, change agents can provide that stimulus during brief periods either before an activity wherein vocal stereotypy is undesirable or throughout the entire day.

For example, Gibney et al. (2020) identified structurally matched stimuli by using the RAISD with parents and teachers of four adolescents with ASD. Functional analyses confirmed all four participants engaged in automatically maintained vocalizing. Thereafter, Gibney et al. utilized sound effects, music, scripted dialogues, theme songs from television, and movies for their assessment. The researchers then included the stimuli in a 10-minute FOPA on a visual choice board. To identify matched stimuli, the authors rotated target and control conditions: low preference, high preference, along with recorded samples from their own stereotypic behavior. Each phase consisted of three 5-minute control sessions (i.e., no access to auditory stimuli) alternated with three 5-minute auditory access conditions. The authors compared the auditory access conditions to the control sessions and found idiosyncratic results across participants. Interestingly, for two of the participants, the lowest preferred stimuli resulted in the greatest reduction in targeted stereotypy. Subsequently, the authors used the stimulus shown to compete with stereotypy most effectively in NCR-M. The intervention reduced vocal stereotypies for all four participants; however, one participant experienced only a slight reduction. Importantly, the Gibney et al. study illustrates why preference assessments, alone, are not sufficient. One variation of NCR practitioners should strongly consider using to decrease noninjurious repetitive behavior is antecedent exercise. Morrison et al. (2011) outlined a methodology for identifying matched activities that involve the same essential steps described above (see also Neely et al., 2015).

Studies also show that NCR-M decreases in stereotypy for some adolescents. The process for developing the intervention is the same as for children; however, practitioners should use relevant stimuli for the client's age and skill. Most researchers provided the auditory stimulus through earphones and an MP3 player (with only one earphone) during academic periods to minimize interference with learning opportunities and instruction. Additionally, Thomas et al. (2020) used singing to simulate both vocal-auditory and vocal-physical consequences. The individuals participated in singing their choice of song before an event during which vocal stereotypy was undesirable. Thomas et al. found singing decreased vocal stereotypy while simultaneously provided an appropriate replacement behavior.

Chan (2020) noted NCR-M is often socially acceptable intervention in community settings; however, NCR-M is not without potential limitations. For instance, matched stimuli may become less effective with repeated, long-term usage. In addition, as with the initial target behavior, an individual's engagement with matched stimuli could interfere with either academic instruction or social engagement (Rapp et al., 2017). If this is a concern, the practitioner may need to consider an alternative treatment such as differential reinforcement with matched stimuli. To our knowledge, only Lanovaz et al. (2014) used adult participants: Results supported the use of NCR-M with differential reinforcement of other behavior (DRO, described below) as an alternative. Given the limited number of empirical demonstrations with adults, practitioners should proceed with caution. Specifically, practitioners should proceed as though they are conducting an application extension with adult clients.

7.5.10 Differential Reinforcement

Within the context of DRO and differential reinforcement of alternative behavior (DRA) procedures, practitioners should use access to matched stimuli as a contingent event (e.g., Brogan et al., 2018; Lanovaz & Argumedes, 2009; Rapp et al., 2017). Procedurally, DRO involves delivering an item contingent on the omission of a target behavior for a predetermined time interval. Typically, the initial DRO interval is determined by measuring the interresponse time (IRT) of the target behavior in the absence of intervention (Hangen et al., 2020; Rapp et al., 2017). The practitioner should then (a) decide to use either a resetting or nonresetting interval (see Jessel & Ingvarasson, 2016 for a review), (b) establish rules to systematically increase the DRO interval, and (c) determine a practical terminal interval for change agents. For example, practitioners can increase the interval duration by 10% after (a) three to five consecutive successful omission trials or (b) three consecutive 10-minute sessions with target behavior at or below a specific level. Rapp et al. (2017) investigated the effects of a trial-based DRO consisting of functionally matched stimuli. The trial-based DRO with functionally matched stimuli decreased vocal stereotypy, motor stereotypy, or both for three children. That is, DRO may inadvertently *decrease* nontargeted repetitive behavior. Rapp et al. reached a terminal DRO interval of 600 seconds, 300 seconds, and 120 seconds for their three participants. To this end, Rapp and Lanovaz (2016) argued that DRO procedures with terminal intervals shorter than 300 seconds have limited practical utility for change agents. Thus, if practitioners cannot achieve the 300-second criterion, they should consider other intervention options with MS.

Alternatively, practitioners can employ DRA wherein they provide access to MS contingent on the participant's completion of a specified amount work (e.g., five math problems). Likewise, practitioners should establish criteria for increasing the participant's response requirement to access MS while also keeping the schedule sufficiently dense to abate the target behavior. Notably, the literature does not contain clear guidelines for terminal schedules for DRA with MS. Nevertheless, if the context wherein the participant emits the target behavior allows for the development of appropriate behavior, we advise practitioners to opt for DRA over DRO (e.g., see Brogan et al., 2018).

7.5.11 Response Interruption and Redirection

When NCR and differential reinforcement procedures fail to produce meaningful reductions in vocal or motor stereotypy, practitioners can include response interruption and redirection (RIRD). Since its introduction by Ahearn et al. (2007), RIRD has become the most researched intervention for vocal and motor stereotypy. Researchers have determined that RIRD facilitates response reallocation to more socially appropriate behavior with comparable sensory stimulation. Procedurally, RIRD involves (a) interrupting engagement in stereotypy and (b) redirecting the individual to engage in either another activity (e.g., imitating motor responses) or task that matches the sensory consequence of the target behavior. RIRD implementation can involve either prompted (by the change agent) or independent responses by the individual. Studies by Gibbs et al. (2018) and Love et al. (2012) found the combined implementation of MS and RIRD was more effective for decreasing noninjurious repetitive behavior than was either component alone.

From the outset, practitioners should plan to fade one or more dimensions of their intervention with MS. For example, successful implementation of a DRO 5-minute schedule can be readily modified to become a 5-minute momentary DRO schedule wherein the change agent provides the matched stimulus if the respective individual does not emit the target behavior during the last 30 seconds of the 5-minute period. Likewise, studies show that after change agents have provided five repetitions of RIRD, they can maintain low levels of the target behavior with single repetitions of RIRD for several sessions. Additionally, practitioners should include generalization training and recruit social validity data (e.g., ratings of intervention acceptability) from relevant stakeholders (Park & Blair, 2019).

7.5.11 Pivotal Role of Caregivers

Although we acknowledge that only Board-Certified Behavior Analysts (BCBAs) should conduct the aforementioned procedures, caregivers' active engagement in the process is imperative for successful intervention. As with all interventions, caregivers should work with their BCBA to ensure correct implementation. Some interventions such as NCR-M simply require caregivers to make matched stimuli available, whereas differential reinforcement procedures can be more complicated. The following are suggestions on how caregivers can prepare for working with a BCBA.

7.5.12 Identify Alternative Stimuli

To help your BCBA identify items for behavioral interventions, caregivers should expose their children to numerous items with varying sounds to compete with vocal stereotypy and various tactile and motor functions to compete with motor stereotypy. For example, when an individual engages in vocal stereotypy, caregivers can offer toys that vary in sound or different songs and styles of music. Likewise, when an individual engages in motor stereotypy, caregivers can offer alternatives such as items, objects, or instructions that require manipulation or interfere with the stereotypic movement. Caregivers should notate which items the child plays with, seems to enjoy, or asks for the most. Additionally, caregivers should make note if stereotypy decreases when they are playing with particular items or listening to certain songs. This information can be extremely useful in the success of preintervention assessment.

7.5.13 Ongoing Assessment

Under the direction of their consulting BCBA, caregivers can routinely collect data on the target behavior in naturalistic settings using the procedures described above in the "Data Collection" section and in Figure 7.S1. Thereafter, caregivers can share this information with their practitioner to facilitate ongoing discussion about intervention effects. In particular, items used in NCR-M interventions will likely require regular replacement as a form of intervention maintenance. Data collected by caregivers will determine when the BCBA should initiate the change.

7.6 Research Background

7.6.1 Review Procedures

Authors systematically reviewed electronic databases (e.g., PsycINFO) using the following search terms: "matched stimulation, "stereotypy," "repetitive movements," "autism spectrum disorder," "behavioral intervention AND stereotypy," and "behavioral intervention AND noninjurious AND repetitive behavior"; conducted hand and ancestral searches of articles involving MS; and employed expert consultation.

7.6.2 Participants

The preponderance of research on assessment and intervention with MS has focused on children and young adolescents with ASD. The aforementioned research on MS was conducted mainly with autistic individuals. Thus, it is most likely that individuals with ASD will benefit from treatments that utilized MS.

7.6.3 Research Design and Quality

Searches involved peer-reviewed studies with sufficient single-case (predominantly) or group designs containing direct measurement of repetitive behavior with empirically supported data collection systems and secondary observations for baseline and intervention phases or conditions. Authors applied the 5-3-30 criteria (Kratochwill et al., 2010, 2013, 2021) for determining whether the literature contained sufficient empirical support for contingent or noncontingent use of MS for reducing vocal stereotypy or one or more forms of motor stereotypy.

7.6.4 Outcomes

The majority of studies evaluating MS do not include measures of generalization, maintenance, or social validity. The few studies that did assess generalization, treatment effects generalized across locations (e.g., school, home, etc.) and people (e.g., parents, teachers, etc.; Chan, 2020; Gibbs et al., 2018; Gibney et al., 2020; Slocum et al., 2020). Even fewer studies evaluated maintenance over time, but treatment effects remained evident up to 3 months post intervention (Chan, 2020; Slocum et al., 2020). A number of researchers assessed social validity for MS and RIRD and found high ratings from both parents and teachers (Gibbs et al., 2018; Gibney et al., 2020; Love et al., 2012). Additionally, Love et al. (2012) found that parents preferred the combination of these two interventions.

7.6.5 Future Research

Future research should evaluate the effects of procedures with MS for individuals in various stages of adulthood. Similarly, future research should continue to examine conditions under which behavior warrants intervention (e.g., Leaf et al, 2022). More broadly, future research should determine whether active or passive consumption of preferred stimulation is more likely to match the product of target behavior. We speculate that conjugate schedules, which are variations of continuous schedules of reinforcement wherein the behavior proportionally modulates the stimulus products (e.g., Davis et al., 2021; MacAleese et al., 2015), generated by active engagement with preferred stimuli enhance the effectiveness of MS.

7.7 Practice Implications

To summarize, for more accurate identification of matched stimuli, pretreatment preference and competing item assessments are conducted prior to treatment. The context in which stereotypy occurs should be considered as this may influence treatment selection (Rapp & Lanovaz, 2016). It may be more practical to use an NCR procedure during leisure periods, given the dense schedule of reinforcement associated with this arrangement. However, if stereotypy occurs during instructional periods (e.g., academics), then using either a DRO or RIRD procedure may be considered. From the outset, practitioners should plan to systematically fade the intervention. For instance, systematic fading can involve gradual reduction along some dimension(s) of the intervention (e.g., the amount of reinforcement the individual receives). For example, if a DRO procedure is utilized as a treatment option for stereotypy and the initial criterion is set at 60 seconds, once the individual has met the criterion for three consecutive days the practitioner could thin the schedule of reinforcement by 10 seconds. Additionally, practitioners should include generalization training and recruit social validity data from relevant stakeholders (Park & Blair, 2019).

7.8 References

Ahearn, W. H., Clark, K. M., DeBar, R., & Florentino, C. (2005). On the role of preference in response competition. *Journal of Applied Behavior Analysis, 38*(2), 247–250. https://doi.org/10.1901/jaba.2005.36-04

Ahearn, W. H., Clark, K. M., MacDonald, R. P., & Chung, B. I. (2007). Assessing and treating vocal stereotypy in children with autism. *Journal of Applied Behavior Analysis, 40*(2), 263–275. https://doi.org/10.1901/jaba.2007.30-06

Brogan, K. M., Rapp, J. T., Sennott, L. A., Cook, J. L., & Swinkels, E. (2018). Further analysis of the predictive effects of a free-operant competing stimulus assessment on stereotypy. *Behavior Modification, 42*(4), 543–583. https://doi.org/10.1177/0145445517741476

Van Camp, C. M., Lerman, D. C., Kelley, M. E., Roane, H. S., Contrucci, S. A., & Vorndran, C. M. (2000). Further analysis of idiosyncratic antecedent influences during the assessment and treatment of problem behavior. *Journal of Applied Behavior Analysis, 33*(2), 207–221. https://doi.org/10.1901/jaba.2000.33-207

Chan, J. M. (2020). Practical considerations for using noncontingent reinforcement with matched stimulation or response interruption and redirection in school. *Evidence-Based Communication Assessment and Intervention, 14*(4), 218–222. https://doi.org/10.1080/17489539.2020.1834687

Cook, J. L., & Rapp, J. T. (2020). To what extent do practitioners need to treat stereotypy during academic tasks? *Behavior Modification, 44*(2), 228–264. https://doi.org/10.1177/0145445518808226

Cook, J. L., Rapp, J. T., & Brogan, K. M. (2019). Assessment and treatment of stereotypical behavior displayed by children with autism spectrum disorders. In C.B. McNeil, L.B. Quetsch, & C.M. Anderson (Eds.) *Handbook of parent-child interaction therapy for children on the autism spectrum* (pp. 147–168). Cham: Springer. https://doi.org/10.1177/0145445518808226

Cook, J. L., Rapp, J. T., Gomes, L. A., Frazer, T. J., & Lindblad, T. L. (2014). Effects of verbal reprimands on targeted and untargeted stereotypy. *Behavioral Interventions, 29*(2), 106–124. https://doi.org/10.1002/bin.1378

Coon, J. C., & Rapp, J. T. (2020). Brief report: evaluating college students' perceptions of a child displaying stereotypic behaviors: Do changes in stereotypy levels affect ratings? *Journal of Autism and Developmental Disorders, 50*(5), 1827–1833. https://doi.org/10.1007/s10803-019-03916-2

Cunningham, A. B., & Schreibman, L. (2008). Stereotypy in autism: The importance of function. *Research in Autism Spectrum Disorders, 2*(3), 469–479. https://doi.org/10.1016/j.rasd.2007.09.006

Davis, W. T., Rapp, J. T., Brogan, K. M., Pinkston, J. W., & Chinnappan, B. (2021). Comparing stimulus preference and response force in a conjugate preparation. *Journal of the Experimental Analysis of Behavior, 116*(1), 96–113. https://doi.org/10.1002/jeab.705

Devine, S. L., Rapp, J. T., Testa, J. R., Henrickson, M. L., & Schnerch, G. (2011). Detecting changes in simulated events using partial interval recording and momentary time sampling. *Behavioral Interventions, 24*(4), 103–124. https://doi.org/10.1002/bin.328

Enloe, K., & Rapp, J. T. (2014). Effects of noncontingent social interaction on immediate and subsequent engagement in vocal and motor stereotypy in children with autism. *Behavior Modification, 38*(3), 374–391. https://doi.org/10.1177/0145445513514081

Fisher, W. W., Piazza, C. C., Bowman, L. G., & Amari, A. (1996). Integrating caregiver report with a systematic choice assessment to enhance reinforcer identification. *American Journal on Mental Retardation, 101*(1), 15–25.

Frewing, T., Rapp, J. T., & Pastrana, S. J. (2015). Using conditional percentages during free operant stimulus preference assessments to predict the effects of preferred items on stereotypy: Preliminary findings. *Behavior Modification, 39*(1), 740–765. https://doi.org/10.1177/0145445515593511

Gibbs, A. R., Tullis, C. A., Thomas, R., & Elkins, B. (2018). The effects of noncontingent music and response interruption and redirection on vocal stereotypy. *Journal of Applied Behavior Analysis, 51*(4), 899–914. https://doi.org/10.1002/jaba.485

Gibney, C., Phillips, K. J., Arnold-Saritepe, A., & Taylor, S. A. (2020). An evaluation of the effects of response interruption redirection and matched stimulation on vocal stereotypy. *Behavioral Interventions, 35*(1), 114–130. https://doi.org/10.1002/bin.1700

Grossman, R. B. (2015). Judgments of social awkwardness from brief exposure to children with and without high functioning autism. *Autism, 19*(5), 580–587. https://doi.org/10.1177/132361314536937

Haddock, J. N., & Hagopian, L. P. (2020). Competing stimulus assessments: A systematic review. *Journal of Applied Behavior Analysis, 53*(4), 1982–2001. https://doi.org/10.1002/jaba.754

Hangen, M. M., Romero, A. N., Neidert, P. L., & Borrero, J. C. (2020). "Other" behaviorand the DRO: The roles of extinction and reinforcement. *Journal of Applied Behavior Analysis, 53*(4), 2385–2404. https://doi.org/10.1002/jaba.736

Iwata, B. A., & Dozier, C. L. (2008). Clinical application of functional analysis methodology. *Behavior Analysis in Practice, 1*(1), 3–9. https://doi.org/10.1007/BF03391714

Jessel, J., & Ingvarsson, E. T. (2016). Recent advances in applied research on DRO procedures. *Journal of Applied Behavior Analysis, 49*(4), 991–995. https://doi.org/10.1002/jaba.323

Jones, R. S. P., Wint, D., & Ellis, N. C. (1990). The social effects of stereotyped behavior. *Journal of Mental Deficiency Research, 34*, 261–268. https://doi.org/10.1111/j.1365-2788.1990.tb01537.x.

Klatt, K. P., & Morris, E. K. (2001). The Premack principle, response deprivation, and establishing operations. *The Behavior Analyst, 24*(2), 173–180. https://doi.org/10.1007/BF03392028

Kratochwill, T. R., Hitchcock, J., Horner, R. H., Levin, J. R., Odom, S. L., Rindskopf, D. M., & Shadish, W. R. (2010). Single-case designs technical documentation. http://ies.ed.gov/ncee/wwc/pdf/wwc_scd.pdf

Kratochwill, T. R., Hitchcock, J., Horner, R. H., Levin, J. R., Odom, S. L., Rindskopf, D. M., & Shadish, W. R. (2013). Single-case intervention research design standards. *Remedial and Special Education, 34*, 26–38. http://doi.org/10.1177/0741932512452794

Kratochwill, T. R., Horner, R. H., Levin, J. R., Machalicek, W., Ferron, J., & Johnson, A. (2021). Single-case design standards: An update and proposed upgrades. *Journal of School Psychology, 89*, 91–105. https://doi.org/10.1016/j.jsp.2021.10.006

Lanovaz, M. J., & Argumedes, M. (2009). Using the three-component multiple-schedule to examine the effects of treatments on stereotypy. *Journal on Developmental Disabilities, 15*(3), 64–68.

Lanovaz, M. J., & Argumedes, M. (2010). Immediate and subsequent effects of differential reinforcement of other behavior and noncontingent matched stimulation on stereotypy. *Behavioral Interventions, 25*, 229–238. https://doi.org/10.1002/bin.308

Lanovaz, M. J., Fletcher, S. E., & Rapp, J. T. (2009). Identifying stimuli that alter immediate and subsequent levels of vocal stereotypy: A further analysis of functionally matched stimulation. *Behavior Modification, 33*(5), 682–704. https://doi.org/10.1177/0145445509344972

Lanovaz, M. J., Rapp, J. T., & Ferguson, S. (2013). Assessment and treatment of vocal stereotypy evoked by television: A pilot study. *Journal of Applied Behavior Analysis, 46*(2), 544–548. https://doi.org/10.1002/jaba.35

Lanovaz, M. J., Rapp, J. T., & Fletcher, S. E. (2010). Expanding functional analysis of automatically reinforced behavior using a three-component multiple-schedule. *European Journal of Behavior Analysis, 11*(1), 17–27. https://doi.org/10.1080/15021149.2010.11434331

Lanovaz, M. J., Rapp, J. T., Long, E. S., Richling, S. M., & Carroll, R. A. (2014). Preliminary effects of conditioned motivating operations on stereotypy. *The Psychological Record, 64*(2), 209–216. https://doi.org/10.1007/s40732-014-0027-x

Lanovaz, M. J., Sladeczek, I. E., & Rapp, J. T. (2012). Effects of noncontingent music on vocal stereotypy and toy manipulation in children with autism spectrum disorders. *Behavioral Interventions, 27*(4), 207–223. https://doi.org/10.1002/bin.1345

Laraway, S., Snycerski, S., Michael, J., & Poling, A. (2003). Motivating operations and terms to describe them: Some further refinements. *Journal of Applied Behavior Analysis, 36*(3), 407–414. https://doi.org/10.1901/jaba.2003.36-407

Leaf, J. B., Cihon, J. H., Javed, A., Klick, S., Ferguson, J. L., Milne, C., Creem, A. Arthur, S., Saunders, M. S., Olive, M. L., Ross, R., K., Leaf, R., & McEachin, J. (2022) A call for discussion on stereotypic behavior. *European Journal of Behavior Analysis*, 23(2), 156–180. https://doi.org/10.1080/15021149.2022.2112810

Llinas, M., Wilder, D. A., & Walz, R. (2022). A comparison of continuous, dense, and lean schedules of noncontingent access to matched competing stimuli to reduce stereotypy. *Behavioral Interventions*, 37, 1–13. https://doi.org/10.1002/bin.1867

Long, E. S., Miltenberger, R. G., & Rapp, J. T. (1998). A survey of habit behaviors exhibited by individuals with mental retardation. *Behavioral Interventions, 13*, 79–89. https://doi.org/10.1002/(SICI)1099.078x

Long, E. S., Woods, D. W., Miltenberger, R. G., Fuqua, R. W., & Boudjouk, P. J. (1999). Examining the social effects of habit behaviors exhibited by individuals with mental retardation. *Journal of Developmental and Physical Disabilities, 11*, 295–312. https://doi.org/10.1023/A:10218 62723409

Love, J. J., Miguel, C. F., Fernand, J. K., & LaBrie, J. K. (2012). The effects of matched stimulation and response interruption and redirection on vocal stereotypy. *Journal of Applied Behavior Analysis, 45*(3), 549–564. https://doi.org/10.1901/jaba.2012.45-549

MacAleese, K. R., Ghezzi, P. M., & Rapp, J. T. (2015). Revisiting conjugate schedules. *Journal of the Experimental Analysis of Behavior, 104*, 63–73. https://doi.org/10.1002/jeab.160

Morrison, H., Roscoe, E. M., & Atwell, A. (2011). An evaluation of antecedent exercise on behavior maintained by automatic reinforcement using a three component multiple schedule. *Journal of Applied Behavior Analysis, 44*, 523–541. https://doi.org/10.1901/jaba.2011.44-523

Neely, L., Rispoli, M., Gerow, S., & Ninci, J. (2015). Effects of antecedent exercise on academic engagement and stereotypy during instruction. *Behavior Modification, 39*(1), 98–116. https://doi.org/10.1177/0145445514552891

Park, E. Y., & Blair, K. S. C. (2019). Social validity assessment in behavior interventions for young children: A systematic review. *Topics in Early Childhood Special Education, 39*(3), 156–169. https://doi.org/10.1177/0271121419860195

Patel, M. R., Carr, J. E., Kim, C., Robles, A., & Eastridge, D. (2000). Functional analysis of aberrant behavior maintained by automatic reinforcement: Assessments of specific sensory reinforcers. *Research in Developmental Disabilities, 21*(5), 393–407. https://doi.org/10.1016/s0891-4222(00)00051-2

Piazza, C. C., Adelinis, J. D., Hanley, G. P., Goh, H. L., & Delia, M. D. (2000). An evaluation of the effects of matched stimuli on behaviors maintained by automatic reinforcement. *Journal of Applied Behavior Analysis, 33*(1), 13–27. https://doi.org/10.1901/jaba.2000.33-13

Piazza, C. C., Fisher, W. W., Hanley, G. P., LeBlanc, L. A., Worsdell, A. S., Lindauer, S. E., & Keeney, K. M. (1998). Treatment of pica through multiple analyses of its reinforcing functions. *Journal of Applied Behavior Analysis, 31*(2), 165–189. https://doi.org/10.1901/jaba.1998.31-165

Querim, A. C., Iwata, B. A., Roscoe, E. M., Schlichenmeyer, K. J., Ortega, J. V., & Hurl, K. E. (2013). Functional analysis screening for problem behavior maintained by automatic reinforcement. *Journal of Applied Behavior Analysis, 46*(1), 47–60. https://doi.org/10.1002/jaba.26

Rapp, J. T. (2004). Effects of prior access and environmental enrichment on stereotypy. *Behavioral Interventions, 19*, 287–295. https://doi.org/10.1002/bin.166

Rapp, J. T. (2005). Some effects of audio and visual stimulation on multiple forms of stereotypy. *Behavioral Interventions, 20*(4), 255–272. https://doi.org/10.1002/bin.196

Rapp, J. T. (2006). Toward an empirical method for identifying matched stimulation for automatically reinforced behavior: A preliminary investigation. *Journal of Applied Behavior Analysis, 39*(1), 137–140. https://doi.org/10.1901/jaba.2006.37-05

Rapp, J. T. (2007). Further evaluation of methods to identify matched stimulation. *Journal of Applied Behavior Analysis, 40*(1), 73–88. https://doi.org/10.1901/jaba.2007.142-05

Rapp, J. T., Colby-Dirksen, A. M., Michalski, D. N., Carroll, R. A., & Lindenberg, A. M. (2008). Detecting changes in simulated events using partial interval recording and momentary time sampling. *Behavioral Interventions, 23*(4), 237–269. https://doi.org/10.1002/bin269

Rapp, J. T., Cook, J. L., McHugh, M., & Mann, K. (2017). Decreasing stereotypy using NCR and DRO with functionally matched stimulation: Effects on targeted and nontargeted stereotypy. *Behavior Modification, 41*(1), 45–83. https://doi.org/10.1177/0145445516652370

Rapp, J. T., & Lanovaz, M. J. (2016). Evidence-based practices in behavioral health: Stereotypy. In N. Singh (Ed.), *Clinical handbook of evidence-based practices for individuals with intellectual disabilities* (pp. 751–780). Cham: Springer.

Rapp, J. T., Swanson, G., Sheridan, S. M., Enloe, K. A., Maltese, D., Sennott, L. A., Shrader, L., Carroll, R. A., Richling, S. M., Long, E. S., & Lanovaz, M. J. (2013). Immediate and subsequent effects of matched and unmatched stimuli on targeted vocal stereotypy and untargeted motor stereotypy. *Behavior Modification, 37*(4), 543–567. https://doi.org/10.1177/0145445512461650

Rapp, J. T., & Vollmer, T. R. (2005). Stereotypy I: A review of behavioral assessment and treatment. *Research in Developmental Disabilities*, *26*(6), 527–547. https://doi.org/10.1016/j.ridd.2004.11.005

Rapp, J. T., Vollmer, T. R., St Peter, C., Dozier, C. L., & Cotnoir, N. M. (2004). Analysis of response allocation in individuals with multiple forms of stereotyped behavior. *Journal of Applied Behavior Analysis*, *37*(4), 481–501. https://doi.org/10.1901/jaba.2004.37-481

Raulston, T. J., & Machlalicek, W. (2018). Early intervention for repetitive behavior in autism spectrum disorder: A conceptual model. *Journal of Developmental and Physical Disabilities*, *30*(1), 89–109. https://doi.org/10.1007/s10882-017-9566-9

Roane, H. S., Vollmer, T. R., Ringdahl, J. E., & Marcus, B. A. (1998). Evaluation of a brief stimulus preference assessment. *Journal of Applied Behavior Analysis*, *31*(4), 605–620. https://doi.org/10.1901/jaba.1998.31-605

Simmons, J. N., Smith, R. G., & Kliethermes, L. (2003). A multiple-schedule evaluation of immediate and subsequent effects of fixed-time food presentation on automatically maintained mouthing. *Journal of Applied Behavior Analysis*, *36*, 541–544. https://doi.org/10.1901/jaba.2003.36-541

Slocum, S., Yatros, N., & Scheithauer, Mindy. (2020). Developing a treatment for hand-clapping maintained by automatic reinforcement using sensory analysis, noncontingent reinforcement, and thinning. *Behavioral Interventions*, *36*(1), 228–241. https://doi.org/10.1002/bin.1749

Thomas, B. R., Charlop, M. H., Lim, N., & Gumaer, C. (2020). Effects of socially appropriate singing on the vocal stereotypy of children with autism spectrum disorder. *Behavioral Interventions*, *35*(2), 249–262. https://doi.org/10.1002/bin.1709

Weldy, C. R., Rapp, J. T., & Capocasa, K. C. (2014). Training staff to implement brief stimulus preference assessments. *Journal of Applied Behavior Analysis*, *47*(1), 214–218. https://doi.org/10.1002/jaba.98

8

Imitation-Based Interventions

Modeling, Video Modeling, and Self-Modeling

Reem Muharib
Texas State University

Elizabeth Reyes
University of South Carolina

8.1 Technical Abstract

Background: Video modeling can be used to teach a range of skills across domains (e.g., play, social skills, and vocational skills) and involves showing a video of a person performing a target behavior while a learner observes and imitates. Variations involve different models (e.g., peers, teachers, and self-modeling) and vantage points (e.g., point of view and third-person view). **Method**: Combinations of keywords related to video modeling (e.g., model*) and ASD (e.g., autis*) were searched in eight databases to identify studies where participants with ASD received video modeling. Studies were evaluated using the What Works Clearinghouse (WWC) standards. **Results**: Across 50 studies, video modeling was used to successfully teach social communication, vocational skills, adaptive behavior, safety skills, play, and mathematics to people with autism spectrum disorder (ASD). Social validity, generalization, and maintenance data are limited. **Discussion**: This review supports previous reviews identifying video modeling as an evidence-based practice. Portable tablets and smartphones have made video modeling more practical in applied settings and more cost-efficient. **Practitioner recommendations**: The model (e.g., peer or self) and perspective (e.g., point of view or third person) should be considered in context of the target skill (e.g., first-person perspective for tying shoes and third-person perspective for social interactions). Video self-modeling requires more time and expertise to produce. Prompting and reinforcing imitation of the model are not always necessary but may improve outcomes.

Reem Muharib, and Elizabeth Reyes, *Imitation-Based Interventions*. In: *Lifespan Treatment for Autistic Individuals*.
Edited by: Peter Sturmey, Russell Lang, and James K. Luiselli, Oxford University Press. © Oxford University Press (2025).
DOI: 10.1093/oso/9780197635841.003.0008

8.2 Layperson Summary

8.2.1 General Description of Treatment

Imitation is an important learning mechanism involved in the acquisition of many skills across a person's lifetime. Video modeling is a teaching strategy that utilizes imitation by showing a video of a person performing a target skill to a learner who observes and imitates that skill. Video modeling can be used for priming in the natural environment and is often supported by prompting and/or reinforcement contingent on imitation. Expertise required to implement video modeling includes (a) the technological knowledge to record, edit, and play videos; (b) ability to deliver prompts and reinforcers with fidelity; and (c) familiarity with variations of video modeling in order to tailor treatment to individual needs of the learner. Video modeling procedures and variations are described in more detail below.

8.2.2 Video Priming

Video priming involves showing a video model immediately before an opportunity for the target skill/tasks occurs in the natural environment. Priming can be used to increase or decrease a target behavior. For example, in a study by Schreibman and colleagues (2000), three children with ASD who engaged in challenging behavior (i.e., disruptive tantrums) when transitioning to different settings or activities watched videos of successful transitions immediately before they were expected to transition to a new setting (e.g., leave their home to go to a public place). Participants learned to transition without challenging behavior following video priming.

8.2.3 Prompting in Video Modeling Interventions

Prompting can be added to a video modeling intervention to facilitate observation and imitation. Prompts are designed to cue learners' behaviors. Prompts may be in the form of gestures (e.g., pointing to the video to redirect the learners' attention), verbal (i.e., spoken instructions), physical (e.g., guiding hands while tying shoes), or other more subtle supports (e.g., eye gaze). Prompts can be used to direct a learner's attention to the video; for example, verbally prompting the learner to "do what the person in the video did." Prompts may also be used to redirect off task behavior or to give more support in completing multistep tasks. For example, if the learner makes an error when imitating the video model, the interventionist may provide a vocal prompt (e.g., saying "turn off the faucet" after the individual finishes washing his/her hands). For the learner to be able to perform the skill independently, prompts must be gradually reduced until the learner is able to perform the target behavior without support.

Another form of prompting associated with video modeling involves breaking down the full video into smaller clips displaying one step in a sequence of steps at a time and then pausing to allow imitation. Video priming may include voice or text narrative instructions for each step (Le Grice & Blampied, 1994). When teaching complex multistep tasks, teaching one step at a time may be more effective than expecting the learner to imitate the entire behavior chain involved in the task. Video prompting clips can also be used for error correction. For example, after an individual with ASD makes an error while working through steps to tie shoes, a practitioner may show the individual a clip wherein the model performs the step causing difficulty correctly. However, for less complex skills, the additional effort to break videos into clips may not be necessary and playing the whole video at once may be more efficient as less support from the interventionist is needed (Bellini & Akullian, 2007). Further, because there are fewer prompts in video modeling than in video prompting, it may be easier to fade intervention as the learner's skill improves.

8.2.4 Reinforcement Contingent on Imitation

In many cases, the interventionist provides reinforcement-contingent accurate imitation of the target skill. Reinforcement is usually a small reward that increases probability of a target behavior occurring again. For example, an interventionist might use praise (e.g., "Great job cooking your food!") or give the learner access to a preferred item or activity. When possible, the specific reinforcer used should be related to the natural occurring outcome of the skill. For example, the natural reinforcer for properly cooking a meal could be eating the food that was prepared, and the natural reinforcer for cleaning a room could be the opportunity to play with a preferred toy in the new clean space. However, in many cases, the natural consequence is not sufficient to reinforce the behavior. This occurs when the learner does not value the outcome of the behavior enough for it to function as a reinforcer and increase the behavior. For example, access to a preferred food is only reinforcing when someone is hungry, and some children are just as happy playing in messy rooms as clean rooms. In those cases, arbitrary reinforcers unrelated to the target skill may be necessary, for example, giving a gold star sticker for brushing teeth. When possible, it is helpful to pair the arbitrary reinforcer with the natural reinforcer, for example reinforcing with a gold star while also delivering praise that highlights the natural contingency (e.g., "Wow, your breath smells so fresh and clean!"). Reinforcement should be gradually faded to ensure maintenance of the target skills in the absence of arbitrary reinforcers. More detail on prompting and reinforcement can be found in Chapter 4 of this text.

8.2.5 Implementer Training and Credentials

Most of the studies were implemented by a research team member with a doctoral or a master's degree in special education or applied behavior analysis (ABA).

In studies wherein a parent or practitioner implemented the intervention, they were provided with training by a researcher which typically involved a behavioral skills training (BST; instruction, modeling, role-play, feedback). The required skills include those related to recording, editing, and playing videos as well as sufficient understanding of strengths and weakness of variations of video modeling. There are no particular certifications or licensures required, but a background in special education, ABA, and/or social learning theory is likely helpful.

8.2.6 Research Quantity and Quality

Search procedures yielded 60 single-case design studies. Those 60 studies were screened using the WWC standards (Kratochwill et al., 2013) to ensure only sufficiently rigorous research was considered in this review. Ten of the 60 studies did not meet the WWC standards and were excluded due to limitations in research design (e.g., less than three attempts to demonstrate intervention effects or fewer than three data points per phase). Of the 50 studies that were included, 18 met WWC standards with reservations (36%) and 32 met standards without reservations (64%). In addition to the 50 single-case studies included, 11 literature reviews and meta-analyses met inclusion criteria.

8.2.7 Likely Outcomes and Potential Risks

Video modeling has been effective at improving social-communication skills, job-related skills, daily living skills, safety skills, play skills and some academic skills for individuals with ASD. Due to limitations in the research base, the social acceptability of video modeling, generalization, and maintenance of skills may require additional consideration. Concerns about screen time of children in general and for children with ASD in particular have been raised, but there appears to be no evidence of negative side effects related to video modeling interventions documented in the literature.

8.3 Treatment Summary Table

Treatment summary: Video Modeling

Treatment description: In video modeling, the learner watches a video demonstration (model) of someone (i.e., adult, peer, or self-model) performing a target skill. Videos are typically displayed on portable tablet computers or smartphones. After observing the video, the learner with ASD is prompted to perform the skill/task by imitating the model. Video prompting is a variation in which the learner observes and imitates the first step of the target skill/task before moving on to the next step in the task sequence. Video priming is a variation that involves showing the video immediately prior to the opportunity to engage in the target skill/task in the natural environment. The person modeling in the video can be an adult, child, or the learner themselves (self-modeling). Self-modeling usually involves editing a recording of the learner to remove errors and provide a correct video demonstration. The vantage of the recording can be first-person point of view (i.e., seen from the perspective of the model) or third-person point of view (i.e., the model can be seen). Prompting to observe the model and stay on task, as well as reinforcement contingent on imitation, is likely to improve efficiency of skill acquisition in video modeling.

Expected outcomes: Video modeling has been effective at improving social communication skills, job-related skills, daily living skills, safety skills, play skills, and some academic skills for individuals with ASD. Due to limitations in the research base, the social acceptability of video modeling, generalization, and maintenance of skills may require additional consideration.

Methods: Boolean combinations of keywords related to video modeling (e.g., model*) and ASD (e.g., autis*) were searched in eight databases (i.e., Academic Search Complete, APA PsycInfo, Complementary Index, Education Source, Scopus®, ERIC, MEDLINE Complete, and Springer Nature Journals). Studies meeting the inclusion criteria (i.e., involved video modeling and participants with ASD) were coded for (a) participant characteristics (e.g., age and severity of ASD); (b) target skills, behaviors, or tasks; (c) type of video modeling (e.g., video modeling, priming, or prompting), (d) perspective (i.e., first- or third-person vantage); (e) model type (adult, child, or self-modeling); (f) technology used (e.g., portable tablet); (g) context (i.e., setting and interventionist characteristics); (h) any augmentative intervention components (e.g., reinforcement, least-to-most prompting hierarchy); and (i) data related to social validity, generalization, maintenance, and treatment fidelity.

Expertise required to implement treatment: Majority of research in video modeling has been implemented by teams of researchers with considerable training and expertise. In some studies, a parent or a practitioner (e.g., teacher or paraprofessional) implemented the treatment after receiving training from a research team. Training often involved BST (i.e., instruction, modeling, role-play, and feedback). The ability to record and edit videos and sufficient familiarity with various forms of video modeling to empower individualization of treatment are usually necessary. There are no certifications or licensure requirements to implement video modeling, but the majority of the research was done from a behavior analytic perspective and a Board-Certified Behavior Analyst (BCBA) may help to optimize intervention.

Risks and negative side effects: Concerns about the screen time of children in general and for children with ASD in particular have been raised, but there appears to be no evidence of negative side effects documented in the literature related to video modeling.

Additional considerations and limitations: Video modeling is often more effective when accompanied by reinforcement contingencies for imitation and/or when the model in the video is reinforced (e.g., vicarious reinforcement). In most cases, videos have ranged from 30 seconds to 3 minutes, and it is unclear if duration of video affects outcomes.

8.4 Introduction

8.4.1 Treatment Description

Imitation is a type of social learning which requires a "frame of reference" or the ability to understand the context and viewpoint to guide the viewer to completing a task as the model shows (McCoy & Hermansen, 2007). Video modeling is rooted in Bandura and Walter's (1977) social learning theory, which suggested humans learn by observing others model behaviors and observing consequences that follow. Video modeling involves showing a video of the performance of a targeted skill to a student. Videos can be created on several technology platforms, including personal cell phones and iPads. After watching the video, the student has the opportunity to perform the task. At this point, the practitioner can use response-prompting procedures to support the student through performing the skill. Video modeling has important applications in educational settings because students with disabilities have been shown to initiate, maintain, and generalize skills across learning environments from a single video model made for a specific setting (Carnahan et al., 2012). Video modeling is appealing to practitioners and parents because it is convenient and noninvasive; videos can be recorded and edited with relative ease and then shown to the student quickly with little disruption to routine (Banda et al., 2007). Additional benefits of video modeling include the ability to obtain students' attention and control over the initial stimuli (Dorwrick, 1991).

8.4.2 Rationale and Objectives

The ability to observe and imitate behaviors of others either is acquired during infancy or innate at birth (Slaughter, 2021). Children with ASD may prefer imitating behavior observed in a video more than from a live model (McDowell et al., 2015). Therefore, the objective of video modeling is to teach new skills using imitation as a learning mechanism. Video models can be presented in several formats, including video modeling of others (VMO), point of view video modeling (POV-VM), and video self-modeling (VSM).

8.4.3 Video Modeling of Others

Among the different types of video modeling, VMO is the easiest to create, as it does not require video editing or configuring a way to record from a first-person point-of-view perspective. VMO involves video recording another person, adult or peer, performing the targeted task and then playing this video model for the student with a disability receiving the intervention (McCoy & Hermansen, 2007). One advantage to using this type of video modeling is that it does not require the student to perform any parts of the targeted task at intervention onset, but rather relies on another student or adult to model the targeted task to create the initial video model. It may be beneficial to use a peer with similar characteristics to the student or possibly a favorite peer/adult (e.g., matched to culture, race, age, and/or gender) as the model.

8.4.4 Point-of-View Modeling

POV modeling or first-person perspective modeling is a variation of video modeling wherein, rather than having the student observe a scene with an individual modeling the targeted task, the modeled actions are seen from the student's point of view. POV modeling includes visual images seen from the perspective of the student (e.g., images of hands demonstrating a specific task; McCoy & Hermansen, 2007). POV modeling is likely to be more effective when paired with explicit instruction and immediate feedback.

8.4.5 Video Self-Modeling

VSM refers to "the observation of images of oneself engaged in adaptive behavior" (Hitchcock et al., 2003, p. 37). VSM requires the individual to perform the targeted skill in some way in order to be recorded. This might involve prompting each individual step in a task analysis of the target skill and then editing out prompts, so the video shows the student performing the whole task without prompts. The majority of VSM interventions have been conducted with individuals with ASD focusing on self-help and daily-living skills (McCoy & Hermansen, 2007; Park et al., 2019); however, it has also been used to support academic skills. Of the different types of video models, VSM seems to be the most successful across behaviors and allows for more applications of generalization to other settings and situations. However, conclusions regarding the best approach to video modeling are limited by a paucity of studies directly comparing variations of video modeling, and it is possible that individual characteristics of the learner (e.g., preferences and attention span) more directly affect relative efficacy between options.

8.4.6 Considerations for Implementation

Regardless of what form of video modeling a practitioner chooses, the steps to creating a video model are similar. Hall et al. (2019) defined the following stages required to implement a video modeling intervention:

- Identification of needed skill that needs to be taught (i.e., unpacking bookbag)
- Preparing the video by setting up a good view of the model and editing videos as needed
- Implementation in an environment without distractions
- Ongoing data collection from baseline through cessation of intervention and maintenance
- Fading of the intervention supports as the target skill improves

For practitioners, this means making time to prepare for this type of intervention, as well as having access to adequate technology and the ability to use it. Luckily, creating and editing videos is easier now due to advancements of applications on hand-held devices. After a video model is created, it is usually used for the duration of an intervention and can be implemented with the help of various adults in school or clinical settings.

8.5 Research Background

8.5.1 Search Procedures and Inclusion Criteria

A systematic search was conducted to identify rigorous peer-reviewed research evaluating the effects of video modeling for people with ASD. The search was restricted to the last 10 years (2012–2022) to focus on the most recent technology. Search procedures yielded 60 single-case design studies. Those 60 studies were screened using the WWC standards to ensure only sufficiently rigorous research was considered in this review. Ten of the 60 studies did not meet the WWC standards and were excluded due to limitations in research design (e.g., less than three attempts to demonstrate intervention effects or fewer than three data points per phase). Of the 50 studies that were included, 18 met WWC standards with reservations (36%) and 32 met standards without reservations (64%; see Table 8.1). In addition to the 50 single-case studies included, 11 literature reviews and meta-analyses met the inclusion criteria. Studies were categorized based on the domain of the target skill; (a) social communication, (b) play, (c) adaptive, (e) job-related, (f) academic, (g) safety, and (h) other functional skills.

8.5.2 Effects on Social Communication Skills

Eight single-case design intervention studies and one meta-analysis were included in this review. Across the eight intervention studies, 31 individuals with ASD (ages 3 to 19 years) received video modeling that targeted social communication skills, including social initiations, eye contact, vocalizations, manding, and texting. Models included self-modeling, peers, and adults, and videos were filmed from the point of view of the model or from a third-person perspective. Videos were recorded and played on smartphones, laptops, and tablets. In the majority of studies (75%), video modeling was implemented by researchers in a clinic or school setting. In all eight studies, video modeling was effective at increasing social communication skills of individuals with ASD; however, generalization

Table 8.1 Number of video modeling experimental studies

Target Skill	N of Studies	N of Studies Meeting WWC Standards
Social communication skills	11	8
Play skills	9	8
Adaptive skills	14	13
Job-related skills	10	9
Academic skills	7	7
Safety skills	4	3
Other functional skills	5	2

WWC = What Works Clearinghouse.

and maintenance data varied across studies and target behaviors within studies. Additionally, because video modeling was only implemented by practitioners in one study (Wilson et al., 2013), further research is warranted to determine whether video modeling can be effective when implemented by practitioners or parents to teach social communication skills to individuals with ASD. Qi and colleagues (2018) conducted a meta-analysis of 18 studies involving 52 school-aged individuals with ASD by calculating Tau-U to estimate effect sizes (Parker et al., 2011). Video modeling was found to be moderately effective at improving social communication skills in school-age individuals with ASD (*Tau-U* = 0.63).

8.5.3 Effects on Play Skills

Eight single-case design intervention studies involving 27 participants with ASD (ages 5 to 11 years) evaluated the effects of video modeling on play skills. Targeted play skills included functional play, pretend play, and video gaming, as well as collateral engagement and vocalizations during play. In all eight studies, video modeling was used as a form of priming wherein participants observed videos before being presented with opportunities to play. Regardless of technology (e.g., phone, tablet) or type of model (i.e., self, peer, or adult), targeted play skills improved and maintained. All eight studies were carried out by researchers, and therefore, further research evaluating effects when implemented by a parent or a practitioner in applied settings is warranted.

8.5.4 Effects on Adaptive Skills

Thirteen studies including 30 participants with ASD (ages 5 to 21 years old) evaluated the effects of video modeling on adaptive skills. Targeted adaptive skills included cleaning, cooking, shopping, doing laundry, and tying shoes. For the majority of participants (83%), supplemental procedures were implemented such as least-to-most prompts, graduated guidance, and reinforcement. For all but one participant, the video model was a familiar (e.g., parent) or unfamiliar adult. Self-modeling was only used for one participant. Video modeling was effective at increasing adaptive skills for individuals with ASD regardless of the technology used (e.g., tablet, desktop) or the implementer of the intervention (e.g., parent, researcher). The literature also suggests that adaptive skills generalize across novel contexts and maintain after the withdrawal of video modeling. Several meta-analyses were conducted in the area of adaptive skills. For example, Aljehany et al. (2019) reported strong effects for video modeling to teach adaptive skills (*Tau-U* = 0.92) and found no statistical differences whether it was combined with error correction procedures (e.g., prompts). Hong et al. (2016) found video modeling using a third-person perspective (*Tau-U* = 0.89) to outperform point of view video modeling (*Tau-U* = 0.77) to teach adaptive skills.

8.5.5 Effects on Vocational Skills

Effects of video modeling were evaluated on vocational (job-related) skills for 29 individuals with ASD ages 13 to 26 years in nine studies. Examples of job-related skills included sorting mail, taking phone calls, sending email, greeting customers, and gardening. Intervention was conducted by a researcher and took place at school or job site. With the exception of two participants who did not show behavior change, job-related skills increased for all participants using video modeling regardless of the technology used to view the videos (e.g., tablet, phone). Job-related skills maintained for all participants, but generalization data varied across participants. More research is needed to evaluate outcomes when implemented by an employer, parent, or teacher.

8.5.6 Effects on Academic Skills

Seven studies evaluated video modeling on academic skills with 16 individuals with ASD ages 5 to 16 years. Academic skills included mathematics (e.g., addition, fractions), reading, science, and writing. Models were either an adult or self-modeling. Intervention was carried out at school by either a researcher or practitioner (i.e., teacher, paraprofessional). Video modeling was effective in teaching mathematics skills, and Wright et al. (2020) concluded that video modeling could be classified as an evidence-based practice to teach mathematics skills. However, more research is needed to assess utility with more advanced mathematics and for learners across a wide range of support needs. From the available research, video modeling appears to be ineffective at increasing other academic skills (e.g., was ineffective at improving reading fluency), and more research is warranted in this area.

8.5.7 Effects on Safety Skills

Recent studies evaluated the effects of video modeling on safety skills such as responding appropriately to stranger lures and seeking help when lost. Sixteen participants with ASD ages 3 to 14 years were included in three studies. Models were adults and peers, and videos were shown on an iPad or desktop from a third-person or first-person perspective. Across all three studies and all 16 participants, video modeling was effective at increasing safety skills, and maintenance and generalization data across untrained locations and people were evident. It is worth noting that intervention was implemented by a researcher for all participants, and the addition of supplemental procedures (e.g., prompts) was necessary for some participants.

8.5.8 Effects on Other Functional Skills

Video modeling has also been used to teach other functional skills such as entering data, writing a check (Spriggs et al., 2016), and changing computer memory (Smith et al., 2015). Overall, video modeling was effective but required the use of prompts and reinforcement.

8.5.9 Fidelity and Social Validity

Video modeling was delivered in-person in all the reviewed single-case design studies, and most studies (84%, $n = 42$) reported data on treatment fidelity. Averages of treatment fidelity were high between 92% and 100% across studies. It is worth noting that studies were often implemented by a research team member with a doctoral or master's degree in a related field (e.g., ABA). When video modeling was implemented by practitioners or parents, they were provided with training by a researcher which often involved some or all steps of BST (i.e., instruction, modeling, role-play, and feedback) in a simulated context. That is, training was conducted in a one-on-one format (i.e., researcher and parent or practitioner) until the practitioner/parent reached a certain mastery criterion before they would implement the intervention with the participants.

Studies (70%, $n = 35$) often reported data on social validity in regard to the importance of the targeted skills, acceptance of the procedures, effectiveness, and cost-effectiveness. Data were collected using interviews or questionnaires and completed by parents, practitioners, or the participants with ASD. Overall, video modeling was found to be socially valid. Parents and practitioners often reported video modeling to be cost-effective (e.g., Abadir et al., 2021; Carlile et al., 2018; Knight et al., 2018). In only one study (Kouo, 2019), parents and practitioners reported variable social validity responses in regard to effectiveness of video modeling on child outcomes in the area of social communication skills.

8.5.10 Effect Moderators

Regardless of the skill targeted, video modeling with reinforcement was found to produce greater effects than when used alone (Mason et al., 2012; Mason, Ganz et al., 2013). Researchers also found that video modeling with an adult as the model to be more effective than self-video modeling (Mason, Ganz et al., 2013). As noted earlier, video modeling can be implemented using priming (watching the entire video before practicing the skill) or prompting (watching one segment and practicing one step of a task). A meta-analysis found a statistically significant difference between priming and prompting, with prompting yielding a greater magnitude of change (Mason, Davis, et al., 2013). Based on results of meta-analyses, video modeling appears to be most effective at increasing adaptive skills and least effective at increasing academic skills. For example, Mason, Davis et al. (2013) found a statistically significant difference between video modeling for adaptive skills and social communication skills, with adaptive skills having a larger effect size. Statistically significant difference was also found among adaptive, social communication, and academic skills, with academic skills yielding the least magnitude of change (Mason et al., 2016).

8.6 Practice Implications

8.6.1 Treatment Outcomes

Video modeling has been used across a wide range of ages and support needs. Overall, video modeling appears to be most effective at increasing adaptive skills (Maston, Davis, et al., 2013). Video modeling was also found to be effective for social communication, play, safety, job-related skills, and mathematics. Caution should be exercised when using video modeling for academic skills as research in this area lacks sufficient replications. There are no known side effects of video modeling. However, video modeling may require substantial time in creating video models, especially in self-modeling. Because in self-modeling, the model is the individual with ASD who needs to acquire the target skill, more time and effort are needed to prompt the individual to perform the skill while videotaping and then to edit the video so that prompts are not shown in the video. Although video modeling alone can be effective, it may be more effective to include reinforcement, and it may be necessary to include prompts for some individuals with ASD. If included, reinforcement and prompts must be faded gradually so that the individual does not become prompt-dependent and to ensure the maintenance of skills without the need for contrived reinforcement or prompts. In addition, practitioners should ensure that the individual has the prerequisite skills that are necessary for video modeling, as video modeling may fail when (a) the individual does not have generalized imitation skills, (b) there are contingencies of punishment or extinction for modeling, and (c) the individual has not acquired relevant higher order stimulus control of modeling (e.g., don't say "no" to parents, but say "no" to strangers; do your own laundry, don't do your roommate's laundry).

8.6.2 Practice Implication Guidelines

Video modeling can be classified as an evidence-based practice for individuals with ASD in the areas of social communication skills, job-related skills, adaptive skills, safety skills, play skills, and simple mathematics. Practitioners may use video modeling from the first-person or third-person perspective based on the target skill. For example, it may be more appropriate to use a first-person perspective to show a video model tying his/her shoes as this can provide a closer look at the steps of tying shoes. Conversely, it may be more appropriate to use a third-person perspective to show a video model engaging in a social interaction with another individual. Practitioners can select between a number of inexpensive and accessible technologies to create and show videos (e.g., tablet devices, smartphones, or desktop computers). Selection is based on consideration of learner's characteristics, the target skill, and criterion environment. For example, a practitioner that wants to teach an individual with ASD how to perform a job-related skill (e.g., cleaning tables, greeting customers) at the worksite may select a smartphone to show the videos because it is portable and less intrusive than other options (e.g., laptop). A practitioner may use self-modeling or select an adult or peer who is proficient in the target skill to be the video model. The latter may be more time efficient as the practitioner does not need to provide prompts to the model and spend less time editing compared to self-modeling. Videos should be short (usually between 30 seconds and 3 minutes) and can be shown using priming or prompting methods. Research does suggest that prompting may be more effective than the priming, especially for longer videos and tasks with complex steps. In such cases, the prompting method allows the learner to perform one step at a time after watching each segment. Regardless of the skill targeted, a practitioner must ensure that the individual with ASD has the prerequisite skills before using video modeling. These are (a) the ability to imitate, (b) the ability to pay attention long enough to watch the video, and (c) the ability to discriminate between contexts to engage in the target behavior (i.e., stimulus control). In addition, a practitioner should create a task analysis consisting of all steps of the target skill prior to using video modeling. This serves two purposes: (a) It ensures that all steps of the skill are included in the video, and (b) it serves as a data collection sheet to collect data on the individual's skill level in baseline, during the implementation of video modeling, and after the withdrawal of video modeling.

Data collection is key to determining the effectives of video modeling and making data-informed decisions. Using data, practitioners can make modifications to video modeling such as combining it with prompts and/or reinforcement. Similarly, a practitioner should create a treatment fidelity sheet that lists all the steps of how to implement video modeling. This can be used as a cue sheet to help the practitioner remember all the steps to be implemented and to collect data on steps implemented correctly by the practitioner.

8.7 References

Abadir, C. M., DeBar, R. M., Vladescu, J. C., Reeve, S. A., & Kupferman, D. M. (2021). Effects of video modeling on abduction-prevention skills by individuals with autism spectrum disorder. *Journal of Applied Behavior Analysis*, *54*(3), 1139–1156. https://doi.org/10.1002/jaba.822

Aljehany, M. S., & Bennett, K. D. (2019). Meta-Analysis of Video Prompting to Teach Daily Living Skills to Individuals With Autism Spectrum Disorder. *Journal of Special Education Technology*, *34*(1), 17–26. https://doi.org/10.1177/0162643418780495

Banda, D. R., Matuszny, R. M., & Turkan, S. (2007). Video modeling strategies to enhance appropriate behaviors in children with autism spectrum disorders. *Teaching Exceptional Children*, *39*(6), 47–52. https://doi.org/10.1177/004005990703900607

Bandura, A., & Walters, R. H. (1977). *Social learning theory*. Englewood Cliffs, NJ: Prentice Hall.

Bellini, S., & Akullian, J. (2007). A meta-analysis of video modeling and video self-modeling interventions for children and adolescents with autism spectrum disorders. *Exceptional Children*, *73*(3), 264–287. https://doi.org/10.1177/001440290707300301

Carlile, K. A., DeBar, R. M., Reeve, S. A., Reeve, K. F., & Meyer, L. S. (2018). Teaching help-seeking when lost to individuals with autism spectrum disorder. *Journal of Applied Behavior Analysis*, *51*(2), 191–206. https://doi.org/10.1002/jaba.447

Carnahan, C. R., Basham, J. D., Christman, J., & Hollingshead, A. (2012). Overcoming challenges: Going mobile with your own video models. *Teaching Exceptional Children*, *45*(2), 50–59. https://doi.org/10.1177/004005991204500207

Dorwick, P. W. (1991). *Practical guide to using video in the behavioral sciences*. New York: John Wiley & Sons.

Hall, C., Hollingshead, A., & Christman, J. (2019). Implementing video modeling to improve transitions within activities in inclusive classrooms. *Intervention in School and Clinic, 54*(4), 235–240. https://doi.org/10.1177/1053451217736870

Hitchcock, C. H., Dowrick, P. W., & Prater, M. A. (2003). Video self-modeling intervention in school-based settings: A review. *Remedial and Special Education, 24*(1), 36–46. https://doi.org/10.1177/074193250302400104

Hong, E. A., Ganz, J. B., Mason, R., Morin, K., Davis, J. L., Ninci, J., Neely, L. C., Boles, M. B., & Gilliland, W. D. (2016). The effects of video modeling in teaching functional living skills to persons with ASD: A meta-analysis of single-case studies. *Research in Developmental Disabilities, 57*, 158–169.

Knight, V. F., Kuntz, E. M., & Brown, M. (2018). Paraprofessional-delivered video prompting to teach academics to students with severe disabilities in inclusive settings. *Journal of Autism and Developmental Disorders, 48*, 2203–2216. https://doi.org/10.1007/s10803-018-3476-2

Kouo, J. L. (2019). The effectiveness of a packaged intervention including point-of-view video modeling in teaching social initiation skills to children with autism spectrum disorders. *Focus on Autism and Other Developmental Disabilities, 34*(3), 141–152. https://doi.org/10.1177/1088357618815887

Kratochwill, T. R., Hitchcock, J. H., Horner, R. H., Levin, J. R., Odom, S. L., Rindskoff, D. M., & Shadish, W. R. (2013). Single-case intervention research design standards. *Remedial and Special Education, 34*, 26–38. doi:10.1177/0741932512452794

Le Grice, B., & Blampied, N. M. (1994). Training pupils with intellectual disability to operate educational technology using video prompting. *Education and Training in Mental Retardation and Developmental Disabilities, 29*(4), 321–330.

Mason, R. A., Davis, H. S., Boles, M. B., & Goodwyn, F. (2013). Efficacy of point-of-view video modeling: A meta-analysis. *Remedial and Special Education, 34*(6), 333–345. https://doi.org/10.1177/0741932513486298

Mason, R.A., Rispoli, M., Ganz, J.B., Boles, M.B., & Orr, K. (2012). Effects of video modeling on communicative social skills of college students with Asperger syndrome. *Developmental Neurorehabilitation, 15*(6):425–434. https://doi.org/10.3109/17518423.2012.704530

McCoy, K., & Hermansen, E. (2007). Video modeling for individuals with autism: A review of model types and effects. *Education & Treatment of Children, 30*(4), 183–213. https://doi.org/10.1353/etc.2007.0029

McDowell, L. S., Gutierrez, A., & Bennett, K. D. (2015). Analysis of live modeling plus prompting and video modeling for teaching imitation to children with autism. *Behavioral Interventions, 30*, 333–351. http://dx.doi.org/10.1002/bin.1419

Park, J., Bouck, E., & Duenas, A. (2019). The effect of video modeling and video prompting interventions on individuals with intellectual disability: A systematic literature review. *Journal of Special Education Technology, 34*(1), 3–16. https://doi.org/10.1177/0162643418780464

Parker, R., Vannest, K., Davis, J., & Sauber, S. B. (2011). Combining nonoverlap and trend for single-case research: Tau-U. *Behavior Therapy, 42*(2), 284–299.

Qi, C. H., Barton, E. E., Collier, M. A., & Yi-Ling, L. (2018). A Systematic Review of Single-Case Research Studies on Using Video Modeling Interventions to Improve Social Communication Skills for Individuals with Autism Spectrum Disorder. *Focus on Autism and Other Developmental Disabilities, 33*(4), 249–257. https://doi.org/10.1177/1088357617741282

Schreibman, L., Whalen, C., & Stahmer, A. C. (2000). The use of video priming to reduce disruptive transition behavior in children with autism. *Journal of Positive Behavior Supports, 2*, 3–11. https://doi.org/10.1177/109830070000200102

Slaughter, V. (2021). Do newborns have the ability to imitate? *Trends in Cognitive Sciences, 25*, 377–387. https://doi.org/10.1016/j.tics.2021.02.006

Smith, K. A., Shepley, S. B., Alexander, J. L., Davis, A. D., & Ayers, K. M. (2015). Self-instruction using mobile technology to learn functional skills. *Research in Autism Spectrum Disorders, 11*, 93–100.

Spriggs, A. D., Gast, D. L., & Knight, V. F. (2016). Video modeling and observational learning to teach gaming access to students with ASD. *Journal of Autism and Developmental Disorders, 46*(9), 2845–2858. https://doi.org/10.1007/s10803-016-2824-3

Wilson, K. P., (2013). Incorporating video modeling into a school-based intervention for students with autism spectrum disorders. *Language speech Hearing Services in School, 44*(1), 105–117. https://doi.org/10.1044/0161-1461(2012/11-0098

Wright, J., Knight, V. F., & Barton, E. E. (2020). A review of video modeling to teach STEM to students with autism and intellectual disability. *Research in Autism Spectrum Disordes, 70*, 101476.

9

Behavioral Skills Training

Raymond G. Miltenberger, Jennifer L. Cook, and Rasha R. Baruni
University of South Florida

9.1 Technical Abstract

Background: Behavioral skills training (BST) is a teaching procedure that has been used to teach a wide range of skills to individuals with and without developmental and intellectual disabilities, including individuals with autism spectrum disorders (ASD). **Method**: We searched the literature using combinations of terms related to BST and ASD. An ancestry search was then conducted to identify relevant studies cited by those articles. Particular attention was given to peer-reviewed literature reviews focused on BST. **Results**: BST is a robust procedure with established effectiveness for teaching skills to individuals with ASD and for teaching skills to staff and teachers who work with individuals with ASD. **Discussion**: The effectiveness of BST procedures varies across studies and can be enhanced with in-situ training, tangible reinforcers, prompting, and fading procedures to improve generalization. **Practitioner recommendations**: BST is appropriate for any client able to attend to instructions, imitate a model, and participate in role-play. Reinforcement is provided contingent on correct responses and corrective feedback is used following errors during training. Practitioners are advised to measure generalization of target skills during and after training and to incorporate additional strategies into BST as needed to promote generalization to natural environments.

9.2 Layperson Summary

BST consists of four primary components: written or vocal instructions, modeling, rehearsal and role-play, and feedback. BST has been used to teach a range of skills to individuals with ASD and to train staff who work with individuals with ASD. BST is typically implemented by behavior analysts or by caregivers trained by behavior analysts. Substantial research supports the efficacy of BST and variations of BST (e.g., in-situ training) for teaching skills and promoting generalization, and it has no identified side effects.

Raymond G. Miltenberger, Jennifer L. Cook, and Rasha R. Baruni, *Behavioral Skills Training*. In: *Lifespan Treatment for Autistic Individuals*. Edited by: Peter Sturmey, Russell Lang, and James K. Luiselli, Oxford University Press.
© Oxford University Press (2025). DOI: 10.1093/oso/9780197635841.003.0009

9.3 Treatment Summary Table

Treatment summary: Behavioral Skills Training

Treatment description: BST consisting of instructions, modeling, rehearsal, and feedback is used to teach skills to individuals with autism spectrum disorder and individuals who work with individuals with ASD. Instructions and modeling evoke the correct response in a role-play context and praise is used to strengthen the behavior. Corrective feedback (i.e., further instruction) is delivered to correct errors.

Expected outcomes: BST is effective for teaching a wide variety of behaviors and promoting generalization. However, additional intervention components are sometimes necessary to support generalization to the natural environment.

Methods: BST is implemented in the context of a role-play that simulates the discriminative stimuli (S^Ds) that should evoke the behavior in the natural environment. Instructions and modeling facilitate correct rehearsals in the presence of the simulated S^Ds. Immediate feedback involves reinforcement to strengthen target skills or error correction to facilitate correct performance in the subsequent rehearsals. In-situ training, consisting of BST conducted in the natural environment, facilitates generalization of the target skills.

Expertise required to implement treatment: BST should be implemented by a Board-Certified Behavior Analyst (BCBA) or other professional with specific training in implementing BST.

Risks and negative side effects: None identified.

Additional considerations and limitations: Modifications to BST may include additional prompting strategies, addition of tangible reinforcers, and fading during training to promote generalization.

9.4 Introduction

9.4.1 Treatment Description

BST is an instructional method used to teach a range of skills (Miltenberger, 2016). BST consists of instructions, modeling, rehearsal, and feedback. In the role-play context, the learner performs the skills in the presence of a discriminative stimulus (S^D; environmental cues that signal when a target behavior should occur). The opportunity to engage in target skills in the presence of the S^D and receive reinforcement (e.g., praise) when performed correctly, or receive corrective feedback when errors occur, underlies the effectiveness of BST (Miltenberger, 2016). For the first component (i.e., instructions), the trainer provides vocal and/or written details about the target behavior (i.e., skills to be learned) and the context in which it should be performed. The instructions describe the behaviors in sufficient detail so that the learner understands what they are expected to do. For example, when teaching a child firearm safety skills, the trainer would instruct the child to not touch the firearm, move safely away, and tell an adult. Modeling involves the trainer demonstrating the skill in a role-play context while the learner observes and then imitates. Modeling can be delivered live in-person or via video modeling. For example, following the information provided about behaving safely when encountering a firearm, the trainer would demonstrate walking up to a firearm and not touching it, moving away, and reporting to a trusted adult.

Following instructions and modeling, the learner is provided with multiple opportunities to practice the skill in role-play with the relevant S^D and receive feedback (Baruni & Miltenberger, 2022; Miltenberger et al., 2020). This part of training allows the trainer to observe the learner engaging in the skills and assess if additional practice is needed. The trainer provides praise for correct behaviors and corrective feedback for errors. Praise and other reinforcers are delivered immediately following correct performance of the skill to increase the likelihood of occurrence in the presence of the S^D in the future. Corrective feedback involves identification of what was done incorrectly as well as what to do differently and functions as instructions for correct behavior in subsequent rehearsals.

One complementary intervention often used with BST is in-situ training (IST). IST occurs when a learner does not perform the skill correctly during an assessment in the natural environment and involves a previously unseen trainer that enters the situation and turns the assessment into a training opportunity. The learner practices the skill again in the natural environment in the presence of the S^D and receives reinforcement or corrective feedback. During IST, the trainer should have the learner practice until meeting mastery criteria (e.g., three to five consecutive rehearsals with correct responses). IST has been utilized primarily to teach safety skills (e.g., Beck & Miltenberger, 2009; Gatheridge et al., 2004; Gunby & Rapp, 2014; Himle et al., 2004; Miltenberger et al., 2004, 2005, 2009), but it has also been used to improve social and vocational skills (e.g., Lerman et al., 2013; Ryan et al., 2019).

9.4.2 Rationale and Objectives

Although BST occurs in a training environment using a role-play context, ultimately, the goal of BST is for the learner to demonstrate skills in the natural environment (e.g., community and home). Thus, before completing BST, the trainer should ensure that the learner has exhibited the skills with reinforcement across multiple rehearsals with different variations of the S^D (multiple exemplars) that sample the range of stimuli in the natural environment to promote generalization. When the mastery criterion has been achieved and correct performance occurs in the presence of multiple relevant S^Ds, the effects of training are more likely to generalize to the natural environment. Because BST usually occurs first in situations contrived to resemble the natural environment, it is necessary to assess target skills in the actual natural environment using in-situ assessment before considering the skill mastered. For example, after training a child to engage in abduction prevention skills in a contrived clinical setting, the child would need to perform the skill in a real-world setting before considering it mastered. Specifically, the child should be able to demonstrate the skill when they are lured by a confederate stranger (i.e., a person unknown to the child assisting with the assessment) in the community (e.g., local park or a grocery store). Because an in-situ assessment occurs without the original trainer present and without the individual aware that an assessment is occurring (Baruni & Miltenberger, 2022), reactivity is not a problem (e.g., Bracket et al., 2007; Miltenberger, 2016). Thus, in-situ assessments are more likely to predict whether an individual will engage in the target skill in the event of an actual safety threat. When an individual fails to demonstrate the skill during an in-situ assessment, IST should be conducted.

9.4.3 Considerations for Implementation.

BST should be implemented in the context of data-based decision-making in which ongoing assessment informs the progression from BST to IST or other complementary interventions (Baruni & Miltenberger, 2022). For example, research indicates BST alone is not always effective and IST may be needed to produce the generalized use of the skills during in-situ assessments (Miltenberger, 2008). Furthermore, in some cases, IST is not effective until tangible reinforcers are added (e.g., Miltenberger et al., 2004). Therefore, a critical consideration for implementation is using ongoing data collection to guide intervention in an iterative process.

Research indicates enhancements to BST may be needed with individuals with ASD in some cases, particularly when targeting safety skills (Bergstrom et al., 2014; Ledbetter-Cho et al., 2016; Miltenberger et al., 1999; Summers et al., 2011), social skills (Kassardjian et al., 2014; Leaf et al., 2009, 2010; Ryan et al., 2019), sports skills (Thomas et al., 2016), and vocational skills (Lerman et al., 2015). Due to limited repertoires exhibited by some individuals with ASD, generalizing skills to the natural environment may be challenging (Gunning et al., 2019). In a recent review of training safety skills to children with disabilities, Baruni and Miltenberger (2022) defined enhancements to BST as procedures that are embedded within training rather than those that are added after a training failure. Some examples of enhancements to BST that have been cited in the literature are prompting and prompt fading procedures (e.g., Grob et al., 2019; Ledbetter-Cho et al., 2021), tangible reinforcers (e.g., Dotson et al., 2013; Miltenberger et al., 1999; Morosohk & Miltenberger, 2021), video feedback (e.g., Thomas et al., 2016), and video modeling (e.g., Ledbetter-Cho et al., 2016). Researchers have reported success with these procedures to teach individuals with disabilities poison prevention (e.g., Petit-Frere & Miltenberger, 2021), social skills (Ryan et al., 2019), vocational skills (Lerman et al., 2015), and athletic skills (Thomas et al., 2016).

Research has also demonstrated that complementary interventions, those that are added after a BST failure, have positive outcomes for individuals with disabilities (Baruni & Miltenberger, 2022). One example of a complementary intervention to BST that has been effective is IST (Dancho et al., 2008; Gunby & Rapp, 2014).

As described previously, IST has been used to promote generalization of skills when the individual does not perform the skills in the natural environment following BST (Gatheridge et al., 2004; Miltenberger et al., 2020). For example, Gunby and Rapp (2014) used BST to train three children with ASD to respond safely to abduction lures and found that BST alone was not effective for producing correct responses to the lures. Following the addition of IST sessions, all three participants' safety scores increased across four different types of lures. When researchers combine BST and IST to teach safety skills, the outcomes are more likely to be positive (Baruni & Miltenberger, 2022; Giannakakos et al., 2020). In response to errors during assessment, other modifications include adding prompts and tangible reinforcers (e.g., Roberts et al., 2021). Modifications to BST should be considered when designing interventions to teach skills to individuals with ASD.

9.5 Research Background

9.5.1 Social Skills

Deficits in social communication and interaction are included in the diagnostic criteria for ASD (American Psychological Association [APA], 2013). Such impairments can adversely affect an individual's ability to develop and maintain relationships with others, which may limit contact with social sources of reinforcement and impede a higher quality life (Kornacki et al., 2013; Ryan et al., 2019). Along with other interventions such as video modeling (Apple et al., 2005), social stories (Barry & Burlew, 2004), and discrete trial teaching (Lovaas, 1987), the use of BST has been shown to be effective for teaching social skills to children and adults with ASD (Hassan et al., 2018; Peters & Thompson, 2015; Ryan et al., 2019). Research has targeted a variety of social skills such as initiating and maintaining conversations (Nuernberger et al., 2013; Ryan et al., 2019), eye contact (Ryan et al., 2019), play skills (Kassardjian et al., 2014; Leaf et al., 2009), responding to conversation partners (Peters & Thompson, 2015), and asking questions during conversation (Palmen et al., 2008). Furthermore, BST has been implemented successfully with children, adolescents, and adults with ASD (Hassan et al., 2018; Kasssardjian et al., 2014; Nuernberger et al., 2013; Palmen et al., 2008; Peters & Thompson, 2015; Ryan et al., 2019).

Ryan et al. (2019) evaluated the effects of a BST package on teaching conversation skills to six adults with ASD. The conversation skills included approaching a peer, making eye contact, greeting the peer, posing a question or making a statement, waiting for a response, and ending conversation when appropriate. The intervention consisted of dyadic BST, IST, and reinforcement. During BST, the participants rehearsed the conversation steps by taking turns with a researcher. While one participant was performing the conversations steps, the other observed the conversation exchange. If the participant performed the steps correctly, the researcher delivered praise. If the participant did not perform the steps correctly, the researcher provided verbal and gestural prompts directed at correcting the specific error. After participants engaged in 80% of the conversation task analysis steps across three consecutive sessions or 100% in one session, IST was initiated. Specifically, IST was implemented by carrying out identical procedures to the BST phase but was provided in the natural environment. Participants completed IST when they performed the skills to mastery criteria. Thereafter, follow-up probes were conducted with a peer once a week for 4 weeks, and results indicated BST was effective for increasing and maintaining conversation skills. Specifically, five participants performed all the steps correctly during follow-up probes, and one participant required booster sessions.

Another variation of BST aimed at teaching social skills to children and adults is called the teaching interaction (TI) procedure (Kassardjian et al., 2014; Leaf et al., 2009, 2010). Similar to BST, TI consists of instructions, modeling, rehearsal, and feedback. In the TI procedure, the trainer describes the target skill, provides a rationale, models the skill for the participant, instructs the participant to rehearse the skill, and provides feedback (Leaf et al., 2012). For example, Kassardjian et al. (2014) taught participants to engage in social skills that included inviting a peer to play a structured game and changing the game when the peer appeared bored. The authors compared the TI procedure to a social stories intervention and found the TI procedure to be more effective. Furthermore, participants maintained the skills during probes for up to 4 months. Similarly, Leaf et al. (2012) compared the TI procedure to social stories for teaching 18 social skills to six boys with ASD. Their results also indicated TI was more effective than social stories procedure for teaching social skills. The authors noted that the success of the TI procedure for increasing and maintaining social skills may be attributed to the rehearsal and feedback components.

In summary, researchers have established the effectiveness of BST and similar procedures for teaching a number of social skills to individuals with ASD. Component analyses of BST have found that some participants experience outcomes that are more positive when fewer BST components are implemented (e.g., (Kornacki et al., 2013). Thus, further component analyses of BST may provide insight on increasing efficiency when teaching social skills to individuals with ASD.

9.5.2 Safety Skills

Unintentional injuries resulting from safety threats in the environment are the leading cause of death among children (World Health Organization, 2008), and individuals with ASD are at even greater risk (Lee et al., 2008; Tekin-Iftar et al.,

2020). Some safety threats are low incidence but highly dangerous such as encountering a dangerous item (e.g., a firearm or poisonous household chemical) or an abduction lure (Miltenberger, 2008; Miltenberger et al., 2020). Although parents and caregivers should strive to keep environments safe, children can learn skills to respond safely to such threats (Gatheridge et al., 2004; Himle et al., 2004).

To improve safety, individuals can learn to (a) identify and avoid a safety threat, (b) safely move away from the threat, and (c) report the threat to a trusted adult (Baruni & Miltenberger, 2022; Miltenberger, 2008). Research has shown that BST and IST are effective for teaching individuals with ASD safety skills across a number of safety threats such as abduction lures (e.g., Gunby & Rapp, 2014; Sanchez & Miltenberger, 2015), sexual abuse lures (e.g., Egemo-Helm et al., 2007; Miltenberger et al., 1999), poisonous substances (e.g., Petit-Frere & Miltenberger, 2021; Summers et al., 2011), and firearms (e.g., Rossi et al., 2017). However, much of the research has focused on teaching abduction prevention skills (Giannakakos et al., 2020).

Haseltine and Miltenberger (1990) evaluated BST to teach abduction prevention skills to eight adults with disabilities. The training program consisted of BST with the addition of an informational video from which participants were instructed to identify the safety skills exhibited in the video. In the presence of abduction lures, participants were taught to refuse the lure, move away from the abductor, and inform a staff member. BST was successful for five of the eight participants, and BST combined with IST was effective with two more participants. In another example, Sanchez and Miltenberger (2015) taught four young adults with disabilities to engage in the same abduction prevention skill and found that BST with IST was more effective than BST alone. Their finding is consistent across other studies evaluating BST and IST for abduction prevention (Baruni & Miltenberger, 2022). In a similar fashion, a few studies evaluated BST and IST for teaching sexual abuse prevention skills to women with disabilities (Egemo-Helm et al., 2007; Kim, 2016; Miltenberger et al., 1999). The women were taught to say "no," get away quickly, and tell a trusted staff member. Egemo-Helm et al. (2007) and Miltenberger et al. (1999) showed that, even though the women performed the skills successfully during role-plays in the presence of the researcher, they did not exhibit the skills during in-situ assessments until IST was implemented. Conversely, Kim (2016) showed that BST was effective in promoting the safety skill during role-plays and that it generalized to in-situ assessments. These differing results underscore the importance of ongoing data collection and data-based decision-making to determine what level of training is necessary.

Researchers have also evaluated BST and IST for teaching poison prevention and firearm safety skills and incorporated other behavioral procedures such as prompting, prompt fading, and use of tangible reinforcers (Morosohk & Miltenbeger, 2021; Petit-Frere & Miltenberger, 2020; Summers et al., 2011). For example, Morosohk and Miltenberger (2021) evaluated generalization enhanced BST to teach poison safety skills to three children with ASD. The researchers enhanced BST by adding a tangible reinforcer for performing the safety responses during training and in-situ assessments. Additionally, the researchers incorporated a fading procedure wherein the trainer faded their presence by moving further away from the participant during the reporting component of the safety response chain. These procedures were effective for teaching children with ASD to respond correctly when encountering poisonous substances.

In a study that used prompts and prompt fading procedures, Summers et al. (2011) evaluated a training to teach three children with ASD to respond safely when encountering common poisonous household cleaning chemicals. The authors utilized BST with a least-to-most prompting procedure to teach children to refrain from touching the chemical, leave the area, and tell a parent. Following BST with prompts, two of the three children responded safely to the poisonous chemicals. In a similar evaluation of BST with least-to-most prompting and fading, Petit-Frere and Miltenberger (2021) showed that this procedure was effective in teaching poison prevention skills to three children with ASD. We identified one study that evaluated BST to teach firearm safety skills to children with ASD. Rossi et al. (2017) evaluated BST for teaching skills to respond safely to firearm and other safety threats, such as lighters and poison, to three children with ASD. The authors incorporated multiple exemplars of firearms (e.g., handguns and rifles) during training and evaluated effects with in-situ assessments. All participants performed the safety skills in the presence of multiple exemplars of firearms and successfully completed 2- and 4-week follow-up probes.

These studies demonstrate the effectiveness of using BST and IST to teach safety responses for several safety threats (e.g., sexual abuse, abduction, poison, and firearm). Additionally, researchers have reported positive outcomes for teaching safety skills when BST is combined with other teaching procedures such as prompting and prompt fading, adding tangible reinforcers, and video modeling. Furthermore, much of the research has focused on teaching individuals with ASD and related disabilities abduction prevention. Considering the dangerous consequences of physical safety threats (i.e., encountering a poisonous substances or unattended loaded firearm) and sexual abuse, future research should continue to evaluate BST, enhancements to BST, and IST to teach these skills to individuals with ASD.

9.5.3 Vocational Skills

There are numerous programs for individuals with ASD that are designed to teach vocational skills and prevocational skills (i.e., how to obtain and maintain employment). These programs include, HeroX, Workplace Inclusion Now™ (Autism Speaks, 2022), and Project SEARCH (2018), as well as government initiatives, including the Vocational Rehabilitation Agency for each state (Council of State Administrators of Vocational Rehabilitation, 2022) and the Individuals with Disabilities Education Act transition guide (IDEA; US Department of Education, 2020). Despite these and other resources, adults with ASD have the highest rate of unemployment when compared to same-aged peers with other disabilities (Office for National Statistics, 2021; Roux et al., 2015). In response to this crisis, as well as citing concerns for quality vocational programs for people with ASD, Campanaro et al. (2021) reviewed the literature to identify interventions in this area and found that BST was among the interventions identified as effective for teaching vocational skills. Across 50 articles encompassing 53 experiments, they identified 10 articles containing 12 experiments, which used BST alone or in combination with other intervention components. As a whole, those 10 articles demonstrated improvements in a range of vocational skills for 35 adults ranging in age from 17 to 30 years old with ASD or another similar neurodevelopmental disabilities.

Prevocational skills are abilities that are expected to be in a person's repertoire prior to learning any specific job tasks. Campanaro et al. (2021) classified three BST articles as targeting prevocational skills, including job interview skills (Roberts et al., 2021; Rosales & Whitlow, 2019) and basic computer skills (Sump et al., 2019). For example, Rosales and Whitlow (2019) initially evaluated a commercially available software program designed to teach job interview skills with a video self-evaluation approach. Results suggested that this technology was ineffective across all six adult participants with ASD. The experimenters then supplemented the software with a live feedback component, which produced improvements, but, ultimately, the complete BST package (i.e., instructions, modeling, role-play, and feedback) was required for all participants to meet mastery criterion.

In addition to the three BST articles identified as prevocational by Campanaro et al. (2021), we suggest recategorizing two other articles as prevocational (rather than vocational). The first of these, Grob et al. (2019), sought to increase responses of adults with ASD such as asking for help or confirming they understood a directive, targets which were identified in an assessment designed for job-related social skills (Lerman et al., 2017). These responses were taught to three adults with ASD, using BST and stimulus prompts in simulated workspaces within a clinic. Second, Shireman et al. (2016) evaluated BST to teach adults how to build rapport by playfully engaging with children with ASD. Results showed BST increased these prevocational skills for the adults with ASD to the point that they could be successfully interact with children. Further, the children showed an increase in play skills.

Our search procedures identified five articles that evaluated BST to teach adults with ASD skills required for specific job tasks. This research shows BST to be an effective intervention to train several vocation skills for adults with ASD, including custodial, clerical, and supervisory work (Dotson et al., 2013), restaurant service tasks (Morgan & Wine, 2018), and evidenced-based teaching techniques for teaching children with ASD language and academic skills (Lerman et al., 2013, 2015).

Burke et al. (2010) evaluated BST to teach six adults with ASD to perform as a FirePal Mascott for fire prevention educational presentations. Although BST improved performance for all three adults, a Performance Cue System (PCS) was a more effective intervention for two of the three participants. The PCS intervention involved an app on a smartphone placed inside the mascot costume that provided cues on what to do throughout their performance. For Study 2, the PCS was presented as the first intervention for the remaining three adults, prior to implementing BST. Use of the PCS device was immediately effective for two participants, precluding the need for BST. For the final participant, a combined PCS plus BST intervention was required to improve performance. After BST, the PCT device remained to mediate the performance cues. Indeed, ongoing use of a PCS device continued for all but the one participant who was successful with BST alone.

Although the PCS device was generally a more effective and efficient intervention than BST in these studies, it is possible that the performer who learned from BST alone may have developed a performing repertoire that was more independent and spontaneous than the other performers, given that no additional prompts were required to maintain the skill. Although BST is an effective approach to training vocational skills, the results of Burke et al. (2010) and Rosales and Whitlow (2019) suggest that researchers should evaluate the relative effectiveness of potentially efficient technologies versus BST for teaching prevocational and vocational skills. Such research could evaluate technology applications alone and in conjunction with BST to determine their effects on acquisition, maintenance, and generalization of the skills.

9.5.4 Athletic Skills

According to the Centers for Disease Control and Prevention (2022), participating in sports and physical activity provides numerous health, mental health, and cognitive benefits throughout a person's lifetime. However, Stanish et al. (2017) found that adolescents with ASD engaged in recommended levels of activity for significantly less time than neurotypical peers. They subsequently called for research to establish evidenced-based interventions designed to foster sustained physical activity for individuals with ASD. Fortunately, several studies have demonstrated success in teaching individuals with ASD the athletic skills necessary to participate in physical activities (Birkan et al., 2010; Lambert et al., 2016; MacDonald et al., 2012; Matshushita & Sonoyama, 2010; Miltenberger & Charlop, 2014; Thomas et al., 2022).

Two studies have evaluated BST to teach athletic skills to individuals with ASD (i.e., Chambers & Radley, 2020; Thomas et al., 2016). Thomas et al. (2016) used BST to teach five skateboarding skills to an 11-year-old boy with ASD. Baseline assessments consisted of written and spoken instructions and praise for performing steps correctly. The BST intervention was comprised of the same procedures from baseline but was followed by a review of the descriptive feedback data (praise and corrections) from the previous session. The experimenter then modeled the skill three times. Subsequently, the participant tried the skill three times with immediate descriptive feedback from the trainer. This process (model, attempt, feedback) continued for a 10-minute period. Each BST session was followed with three assessments, which also included praise from the trainer for correct performances (as in baseline). The participant improved from low or zero levels to at least 70% across all five skills and demonstrated at least one performance at 100% for each of the skills. The addition of modeling and repeated attempts at the skill with descriptive feedback was a salient component distinguishing the BST intervention from baseline. This supports the literature that instructions alone are typically insufficient for training new skills (Baruni & Miltenberger, 2022; Miltenberger, 2016).

Chambers and Radley (2020) used a two-tiered BST approach. First, BST was used to teach a neurotypical female youth how to perform three target soccer skills (i.e., throwing the ball from the sideline, kicking the ball in an intended direction, and defending a shot on goal). Next, BST was used to teach her how to implement BST with others as a peer-trainer. Finally, she used BST to teach the same three soccer skills to three male youth with ASD. BST was successful at every phase of training, and all three individuals with ASD demonstrated substantial improvements in the targeted soccer skills.

In summary, when using BST for teaching athletic skills to individuals with ASD, intervention should incorporate the four BST components in an intensive teaching session, allowing for plenty of opportunities to practice the skill with additional instructions, modeling, and feedback, as needed. Furthermore, post-BST assessments should not include any BST components or include only the components that were available in baseline and/or those that could be expected in the natural environment (e.g., praise; Thomas et al., 2016). Finally, the addition of other efficacious strategies such as utilization of a peer mediator (Chambers & Radley, 2020) or video feedback (Thomas et al., 2016) may enhance the utility of BST for training athletic skills to individuals with ASD.

9.5.5 Caregiver and Staff Training

BST is also an approach that can be used to train staff to deliver services and/or provide care to individuals with ASD. Multiple exemplars of such target skills can be presented in role-play for promoting generalization. BST can train staff to engage in the wide range of skills they will need on the job. Substantial research has established the effectiveness of BST for training staff (Shaefer & Andzik, 2021) and teachers (Kirkpatrick et al., 2019).

Many practitioners are familiar with BST as a training model for training others to implement evidenced-based procedures for clients, both with and without disabilities. Two recent literature reviews on the efficacy of BST as a training tool showed strong support for the use of BST for training teachers (Kirkpatrick et al., 2019) and caregivers (Schaefer & Andzik, 2021). Furthermore, BST has been shown to be effective as a train-the-trainer model, referred to as pyramidal BST, which can greatly benefit training staff in human service settings (e.g., Erath et al., 2020). Similarly, pyramidal BST has been used to extend training to additional family members (e.g., Conklin & Wallace, 2019) and for teachers and paraprofessionals (e.g., Lerman et al., 2020).

Recent research has considered methods and technology for advancing the use of BST for training others to be more efficient and practical. For example, Erath et al. (2020) demonstrated an improved method using a limited one-time group training to make pyramidal BST more accessible to human service facilities. And the integration of telehealth technology with BST for training others to implement interventions (e.g., Lloveras et al., 2022) has been instrumental in satisfying the urgent need to train practitioners and staff during the COVID-19 pandemic. Before the pandemic made telehealth an essential means of service delivery, there was already a growing body of literature evaluating telehealth as a means to make behavior analytic services accessible to populations in urban areas (e.g., Barretto et al., 2006) and worldwide where in-person services are difficult to access (Tsami et al., 2019).

Telehealth has varied definitions within the broader healthcare industry (Rispoli & Machalicek, 2020). In behavior analysis, telehealth is described as "real-time sharing of video and audio information to deliver services" (Rios et al., 2020, p. 450). Telehealth has primarily been used for training caregivers or staff in providing interventions (Rispoli & Machalicek, 2020), but since the onset of the COVID-19 pandemic, telehealth has expanded to service models for delivering behavior analytic interventions directly to the client, while interacting with them in the connected monitor (Bergmann et al., 2021). Concurrently, multiple resource options have been emerging to improve telehealth services, such as tutorials to deliver direct services remotely (Bergmann et al., 2021; Mattson et al., 2020; Neely et al., 2022; Rodriguez, 2020) and novel technology adaptations such a telepresence robots (Zoder-Martell et al., 2020). Behavioral services provided over telehealth have been shown to be effective, rated with high acceptability, and accessible regionally and internationally (e.g., Akemoglu et al., 2020; Alnemary et al., 2015; Neely et al., 2021; Sivaraman et al., 2021; Sump et al., 2018; Tsami et al., 2019).

Training via telehealth for caregivers and practitioners has often been delivered using variations or select aspects of BST, but only a few studies have evaluated a fully remote systematic iteration of BST (e.g., Alnemary et al., 2015; Boutain et al., 2020; Lloveras et al., 2022; Rios et al., 2020; Sump et al., 2018). Earlier versions of fully remote BST contained adaptations or less than ideal versions of the components. For example, Alnemary et al. (2015) used video models and a large group format for all aspects of the initial training, including role-play. These adaptations may have compromised individual active responding opportunities, which are likely important to skill acquisition. Moreover, post-BST assessments occurred after only the initial three of the four components were delivered. Contingent on failing to meet the mastery criterion during assessments, the final feedback component was implemented, resulting in at least a 2-day delay after the training. However, advancements in technology have made possible the implementation of remote BST with a fully interactive experience just short of onsite live versions. In a recent example, Lloveras et al. (2022) provided models that can be demonstrated live by the experimenter with opportunity for discussion as needed. They also provided a comprehensive model for conducting individualized rehearsal and feedback components by using virtual "break-out" rooms. In summary, the COVID-19 pandemic has facilitated a rapid evolution of telehealth research, giving practitioners, caregivers, and clients an effective and efficient mode to provide services. Evidenced-based practitioner and caregiver training models, such as a BST, are critical to the ongoing success telehealth. Likewise, current telehealth technology has become a vital platform for remotely delivering effective BST interventions, as evidenced by the outcomes and acceptability measures reported in the research.

9.6 Practice Implications

9.6.1 Treatment Outcomes

BST is appropriate for individuals capable of attending to instructions and imitating models, and it can be used to target behaviors that can be rehearsed in a role-play. BST alone is an appropriate intervention when generalization is likely to occur from the training context to the natural environment once the behavior occurs fluently in the training context. BST is not the appropriate training approach for individuals with more severe disabilities who require intensive approaches for skill acquisition and for skills unlikely to generalize to natural environments.

9.6.2 Practice Guidelines

Following are guidelines for implementing BST. Specifically, these guidelines include (a) identifying the target skill and its antecedents; (b) assessing the learner's present level of skill performance; (c) conducting BST; and (d) conducting follow-up assessment.

Identify Target Skill. Identify the specific skills for the learner to acquire, including all variations of the skills that might be needed in different contexts.

Identify Antecedents (Relevant Contexts and S^Ds). Identify the relevant contexts in which the skills are needed. The goal of BST is to teach the skills and promote generalization to all relevant contexts. Identify the S^Ds to which the learner will be required to respond in each context. Once identified, train in scenarios involving the full range of S^Ds.

Assess Skills. Assess the level of the target skill in the relevant contexts before training. When possible, assess the skills when the trainees do not know they are being assessed. As knowledge of the assessment and the presence of an assessor may influence the emission of skills through reactivity, the use of in-situ assessments is usually desirable. Research in safety skills and in staff training and management suggests that participants often perform better when they know they are being watched (Brackett et al., 2007). Depending on the learner's ability and the difficulty of the skill, consider if enhancements to BST should be incorporated in the training. Prompts, tangible reinforcers, or video modeling and video feedback are all possible enhancements that may facilitate the acquisition of a skill. However, a learner may also respond only with this additional support and steps may be required to fade enhancements before an in-situ assessment.

Conduct BST Session. Utilize the four components of BST to train the target skills. For each component, engage the learning by requiring an active response. First, describe to the learner how the skill should be performed and in what circumstances. Ask the learner to repeat the instructions back to you, if possible. Second, provide a live or video model of the behavior in the relevant context showing positive consequences (i.e., reinforcement) for the modeled behavior and ask the learner to describe the critical aspects of the model's behavior. Third, have the learner practice the skill in the presence of the S^D in role-play. Fourth, provide feedback after each rehearsal consisting of behavior-specific praise for correct performance and corrective feedback (further instruction) for incorrect performance. Rehearsal and feedback should continue until the skill is performed independently and accurately in response to relevant S^Ds. Utilize tangible reinforcers when needed. The termination of training occurs when appropriately set mastery criterion are met. Typically, a mastery criterion includes a competency measure consisting of a number of correct performances across a range of relevant S^Ds and is based on consideration of the specific target skill and contingencies in the natural environment. For example, skills necessary to safely cross a busy street (e.g., finding a crosswalk, waiting on light, and looking both ways) should not be considered mastered until they reach 100% accuracy.

9.6.3 Post-BST Assessment and Follow-Up

Post-BST assessments are critical to evaluate the effects of the training and should consist of in-situ assessments that sample the range of contexts in which the behavior should occur. Finally, the effects of BST should be periodically assessed to determine if the behavior maintains over time. Assessments that yield lower levels of performance indicate the need for BST booster sessions.

9.7 References

Akemoglu, Y., Muharib, R., & Meadan, H. (2020). A systematic and quality review of parent-implemented language and communication interventions conducted via telepractice. *Journal of Behavioral Education, 29*(2), 282–316. https://doi.org/10.1007/s10864-019-09356-3

Alnemary, F. M., Wallace, M., Symon, J. B. G., & Barry, L. M. (2015). Using international videoconferencing to provide staff training on functional behavioral assessment. *Behavioral Interventions, 30*(1), 73–86. https://doi.org/10.1002/bin.1403

American Psychiatric Association. (2013). *Diagnostic and statistical manual of mental disorders* (5th ed.). Washington, DC: Author. https://doi.org/10.1176/appi.books.9780890425596

Apple, A. L., Billingsley, F., Schwartz, I. S., & Carr, E. G. (2005). Effects of video modeling alone and with self-management on compliment-giving behaviors of children with high functioning ASD. *Journal of Positive Behavior Interventions, 7*(1), 33–46. https://doi.org/10.1177/10983007050070010401

Autism Speaks. (2022.) Job seekers, students & employees. https://www.autismspeaks.org/job-seekers-students-employees

Barretto, A., Wacker, D. P., Harding, J., Lee, J., & Berg, W. K. (2006). Using telemedicine to conduct behavioral assessments. *Journal of Applied Behavior Analysis, 39*(3), 333–340. https://doi.org/10.1901/jaba.2006.173-04

Barry, L. M., & Burlew, S. B. (2004). Using social stories to teach choice and play skills to children with autism. *Focus on Autism and Other Developmental Disabilities, 19*(1), 45–51. https://doi.org/10.1177/10883576040190010601

Baruni, R. R., & Miltenberger, R. G. (2022). Teaching safety skills to children: A discussion of critical features and practice recommendations. *Behavior Analysis in Practice.* https://doi.org/10.1007/s40617-021-00667-4

Beck, K., & Miltenberger, R. (2009). Evaluation of a commercially available program and in situ training by parents to teach abduction prevention skills to children. *Journal of Applied Behavior Analysis, 42*(4), 761–772. https://doi.org/10.1901/jaba.2009.42-761

Bergmann, S., Toussaint, K. A., Niland, H., Sansing, E. M., Armshaw, G., & Baltazar, M. (2021). Adapting direct services for telehealth: A practical tutorial. *Behavior Analysis in Practice, 14*(4), 1010–1046. https://doi.org/10.1007/s40617-020-00529-5

Bergstrom, R., Nardjowski, A. C., & Tarbox, J. (2014). A systematic replication of teaching children with autism to respond appropriately to lures from strangers. *Journal of Applied Behavior Analysis, 47*(4), 861–865. https://doi.org/10.1002/jaba.175

Birkan, B., Yılmaz, İ, Konukman, F., Birkan, B., Özen, A., Yanardağ, M., & Çamursoy, İ. (2010). Effects of constant time delay procedure on the halliwick's method of swimming rotation skills for children with autism. *Education and Training in Autism and Developmental Disabilities, 45*(1), 124–135. http://www.jstor.org/stable/23880156

Boutain, A. R., Sheldon, J. B., & Sherman, J. A. (2020). Evaluation of a telehealth parent training program in teaching self-care skills to children with autism. *Journal of Applied Behavior Analysis, 53*, 1259–1275.

Brackett, L., Reid, D. H., & Green, C. W. (2007). Effects of reactivity to observations on staff performance. *Journal of Applied Behavior Analysis, 40*(1), 191–195. https://doi.org/10.1901/jaba.2007.112-05

Burke, R. V., Andersen, M. N., Bowen, S. L., Howard, M. R., & Allen, K. D. (2010). Evaluation of two instruction methods to increase employment options for young adults with autism spectrum disorders. *Research in Developmental Disabilities, 31*(6), 1223–1233. https://doi.org/10.1016/j.ridd.2010.07.023

Campanaro, A. M., Vladescu, J. C., Manente, C. J., Deshais, M. A., & DeBar, R. M. (2021). A review of the literature on vocational training interventions with individuals with autism spectrum disorder. *Behavioral Interventions, 36*(3), 675–696. https://doi.org/10.1002/bin.1795

Center of Disease Control and Prevention. (2022). Benefits of physical activity. https://www.cdc.gov/physicalactivity/basics/pa-health/index.htm

Chambers, C., & Radley, K. C. (2020). Training soccer skills to adolescents with autism spectrum disorder via peer-mediated behavioral skills training. *Behavior Analysis in Practice, 13*(2), 454–461. https://doi.org/10.1007/s40617-019-00381-2

Conklin, S. M., & Wallace, M. D. (2019). Pyramidal parent training using behavioral skills training: Training caregivers in the use of a differential reinforcement procedure. *Behavioral Interventions, 34*(3), 377–387. https://doi.org/10.1002/bin.1668

Council of State Administrators of Vocational Rehabilitation. (2022). Resources. https://www.csavr.org/resources

Dancho, K., Thompson, R., & Rhoades, M. (2008). Teaching preschool children to avoid poison hazards. *Journal of Applied Behavior Analysis, 41*(2), 267–271. https://doi.org/10.1901/jaba.2008.41-267

Dotson, W. H., Richman, D. M., Abby, L., Thompson, S., & Plotner, A. (2013). Teaching skills related to self-employment to adults with developmental disabilities: An analog analysis. *Research in Developmental Disabilities, 34*(8), 2336–2350. https://doi.org/10.1016/j.ridd.2013.04.009

Egemo-Helm, K. R., Miltenberger R. G., Knudson, P., Finstrom N., Jostad, C., & Johnson, B. (2007). An evaluation of in situ training to teach sexual abuse prevention skills to women with mental retardation. *Behavioral Interventions, 22*(2), 99–119. https://doi.org/10.1002/bin.234

Erath, T. G., DiGennaro Reed, F. D., Sundermeyer, H. W., Brand, D., Novak, M. D., Harbison, M. J., & Shears, R. (2020). Enhancing the training integrity of human service staff using pyramidal behavioral skills training. *Journal of Applied Behavior Analysis, 53*(1), 449–464. https://doi.org/10.1002/jaba.608

Gatheridge, B. J., Miltenberger, R. G., Huneke, D. F., Satterlund, M. J., Mattern, A. R., Johnson, B. M., & Flessner, C. A. (2004). Comparison of two programs to teach firearm injury prevention skills to 6-and 7-year old children. *Pediatrics, 114*(3), 294–299. https://doi.org/10.1542/peds.2003-0635-L

Giannakakos, A. R., Vladescu, J. C., Kisamore, A. N., Reeve, K. F., & Fienup, D. M. (2020). A review of the literature on safety response training. *Journal of Behavioral Education, 29*(1), 64–121. https://doi.org/10.1007/s10864-019-09347-4

Grob, C. M., Lerman, D. C., Langlinais, C. A., & Villante, N. K. (2019). Assessing and teaching job-related social skills to adults with autism spectrum disorder. *Journal of Applied Behavior Analysis, 52*(1), 150–172. https://doi.org/10.1002/jaba.503

Gunby, K. V., & Rapp, J. T. (2014). The use of behavioral skills training and in situ feedback to protect children with autism from abduction lures. *Journal of Applied Behavior Analysis, 47*(4), 856–860. https://doi.org/10.1002/jaba.173

Gunning, C., Holloway, J., Fee, B., Breathnach, O., Bergin, C. M., Greene, I., & Ní Bheoláin, R. N. (2019). A systematic review of generalization and maintenance outcomes of social skills interventions for preschool children with autism spectrum disorder. *Review Journal of Autism and Developmental Disorders, 6*(2), 172–199. https://doi.org/10.1007/s40489-019-00162-1

Haseltine, B., & Miltenberger, R. G. (1990). Teaching self- protection skills to persons with mental retardation. *Journal of Mental Retardation, 95*(2), 188–197. https://doi.org/10.1007/BF02234094

Hassan, M., Simpson, A., Danaher, K., Haesen, J., Makela, T., & Thomson, K. (2018). An evaluation of behavioral skills training for teaching caregivers how to support social skill development in their child with autism spectrum disorder. *Journal of Autism and Developmental Disorders, 48*(6), 1957–1970. https://doi.org/10.1007/s10803-017-3455

Himle, M., Miltenberger, R., Flessner, C., & Gatheridge, B. (2004). Teaching safety skills to children to prevent gun play. *Journal of Applied Behavior Analysis, 37*(1), 1–9.https://doi.org/10.1901/jaba.2004.37-1

Himle, M., Miltenberger, R., Gatheridge, B., & Flessner, C. (2004). An evaluation of two procedures for training skills to prevent gun play in children. *Pediatrics, 113*(1), 70–77. https://doi.org/10.1542/peds.113.1.70

Kassardjian, A., Leaf, J. B., Ravid, D., Leaf, J. A., Alcalay, A., Dale, S., Tsuji, K., Taubman, M., Leaf, R., McEachin, J., & Oppenheim-Leaf, M. L. (2014). Comparing the teaching interaction procedure to social stories: A replication study. *Journal of Autism and Developmental Disorders, 44*(9), 2329–2340. https://doi.org/10.1007/s10803-014-2103-0

Kim, Y. (2016). Evaluation of a sexual abuse prevention program for children with intellectual disabilities. *Behavioral Interventions, 31*(2), 195–209. https://doi.org/10.1002/bin.1439

Kirkpatrick, M., Akers, J., & Rivera, G. (2019). Use of behavioral skills training with teachers: A systematic review. *Journal of Behavioral Education, 28*(3), 344–361. https://doi.org/10.1007/s10864-019-09322-z

Kornacki, L. T., Ringdahl, J. E., Sjostrom, A., & Nuernberger, J. E. (2013). A component analysis of a behavioral skills training package used to teach conversation skills to young adults with autism spectrum and other developmental disorders. *Research in Autism Spectrum Disorders, 7*(11), 1370–1376. https://doi.org/10.1016/j.rasd.2013.07.012

Lambert, J. M., Copeland, B. A., Karp, E. L., Finley, C. I., Houchins-Juarez, N. J., & Ledford, J. R. (2016). Chaining functional basketball sequences (with embedded conditional discriminations) in an adolescent with autism. *Behavior Analysis in Practice, 9*(3), 199–210. https://doi.org/10.1007/s40617-016-0125-0.

Leaf, J. B., Dotson, W. H., Oppeneheim, M. L., Sheldon, J. B., & Sherman, J. A. (2010). The effectiveness of a group teaching interaction procedure for teaching social skills to young children with a pervasive developmental disorder. *Research in Autism Spectrum Disorders, 4*(2), 186–198. https://doi.org/10.1016/j.rasd.2009.09.003

Leaf, J. B., Oppenheim-Leaf, M. L., Call, N. A., Sheldon, J. B., Sherman, J. A., Taubman, M., McEachin, J., Dayharsh, J., & Leaf, R. (2012). Comparing the teaching interaction procedure to social stories for people with autism. *Journal of Applied Behavior Analysis, 45*(2), 281–298. https://doi.org/10.1901/jaba.2012.45-281

Leaf, J. B., Taubman, M., Bloomfield, S., Palos-Rafuse, L., Leaf, R., McEachin, J., & Oppenheim, M. L. (2009). Increasing social skills and pro-social behavior for three children diagnosed with autism through the use of a teaching package. *Research in Autism Spectrum Disorders, 3*(1), 275–289. https://doi.org/10.1016/j.rasd.2008.07.003

Ledbetter-Cho, K., Lang, K., Davenport, K., Moore, M., Lee, A., O-Reilly, M., Watkins, L., & Falcomata, T. (2016). Behavior skills training to improve the abduction-prevention skills of children with autism. *Behavior Analysis in Practice, 9*(3), 266–270. https://doi.org/10.1007/s40617-016-0128-x

Ledbetter-Cho, K., Lang, R., Lee, A., Murphy, C., Davenport, K., Kirkpatrick, M., Schollian, M., Moore, M., Billingsley, G., & O'Reilly, M. (2021). Teaching children with autism abduction-prevention skills may result in overgeneralization of the target response. *Behavior Modification, 45*(3), 438–461. https://doi.org.10.1177/0145445519865165

Lee, L., Harrington, R. A., Chang, J. J., & Connors, S. L. (2008) Increased risk of injury in children with developmental disabilities. *Research in Developmental Disabilities, 29*(3), 247–255. https://doi.org/10.1016/j.ridd.2007.05.002

Lerman, D. C., Hawkins, L., Hillman, C., Shireman, M., & Nissen, M. A. (2015). Adults with autism spectrum disorder as behavior technicians for young children with autism: Outcomes of a behavioral skills training program. *Journal of Applied Behavior Analysis, 48*(2), 233–256. https://doi.org/10.1002/jaba.196

Lerman, D. C., Hawkins, L., Hoffman, R., & Caccavale, M. (2013). Training adults with an autism spectrum disorder to conduct discrete-trial training for young children with autism: A pilot study. *Journal of Applied Behavior Analysis, 46*(2), 465–478. https://doi.org/10.1002/jaba.50

Lerman, D. C., O'Brien, M. J., Neely, L., Call, N. A., Tsami, L., Schieltz, K.M., Berg, W. K., Graber, J., Huang, P., Kopelman, T., & Cooper-Brown, L. J. (2020). Remote coaching of caregivers via telehealth: Challenges and potential solutions. *Journal of Behavioral Education, 29*(2), 195–221. https://doi.org/10.1007/s10864-020-09378-2.

Lerman, D. C., White, B., Grob, C., & Laudont, C. (2017). A clinic-based assessment for evaluating job-related social skills in adolescents and adults with autism. *Behavior Analysis in Practice, 10*(4), 323–336. https://doi.org/10.1007/s40617-017-0177-9

Lloveras, L. A., Tate, S. A., Vollmer, T. R., King, M., Jones, H., & Peters, K. P. (2022). Training behavior analysts to conduct functional analyses using a remote group behavioral skills training package. *Journal of Applied Behavior Analysis, 55*(1), 290–304. https://doi.org/10.1002/jaba.893

Lovaas, O. I. (1987). Behavioral treatment and normal educational and intellectual functioning in young autistic children. *Journal of Consulting and Clinical Psychology, 55*(1), 3–9. https://doi.org/10.1037/0022-006X.55.1.3

MacDonald, M., Esposito, P., Hauck, J., Jeong, I., Hornyak, J., Argento, A., & Ulrich, D. A. (2012). Bicycle training for youth with Down syndrome and autism spectrum disorders. *Focus on Autism and Other Developmental Disabilities, 27*(1), 12–21. https://doi.org/10.1177/1088357611428333

Matshushita, H., & Sonoyama, S. (2010). Teaching ball-throwing skills to a boy with asperger's disorder: A case study. *Japanese Journal of Special Education, 47*(6), 495–508. https://doi.org/10.6033/tokkyou.47.495

Mattson, S. L., Higbee, T. S., Aguilar, J., Nichols, B., Campbell, V. E., Nix, L. D., Reinert, K. S., Peck, S., & Lewis, K. (2020). Creating and sharing digital ABA instructional activities: A practical tutorial. *Behavior Analysis in Practice, 13*(4), 1–27. https://doi.org/10.1007/s40617-020-00440-z

Miltenberger, C. A., & Charlop, M. H. (2014). Increasing the athletic group play of children with autism. *Journal of Autism and Developmental Disorders, 44*(1), 41–54. https://doi.org/10.1007/s10803-013-1850-7.

Miltenberger, R., Roberts, J., Ellingson, S., Galensky, T., Rapp, J., Long, E., & Lumley, V. (1999). Training and generalization of sexual abuse prevention skills for women with mental retardation. *Journal of Applied Behavior Analysis, 32*(3), 385–388. https://doi.org/10.1901/jaba.1999.32-385

Miltenberger, R., Sanchez, S., & Valbuena, D. (2020). Pediatric prevention: Teaching safety skills. *Pediatric Clinics of North America, 67*(3), 573–584. https://doi.org/10.1016/j.pcl.2020.02.011

Miltenberger, R. G. (2008). Teaching safety skills to children: Prevention of firearm injury as an exemplar of best practice in assessment, training, and generalization of safety skills. *Behavior Analysis in Practice, 1*(1), 30–36. https://doi.org/10.1007/BF03391718

Miltenberger, R. G. (2016). *Behavior modification: Principles and procedures* (6th ed.). Boston: Cengage Learning.

Miltenberger, R. G., Flessner, C., Gatheridge, B., Johnson, B., Satterlund, M., & Egemo, K. (2004). Evaluation of behavioral skills training to prevent gun play in children. *Journal of Applied Behavior Analysis, 37*(4), 513–516. https://doi.org/10.1901/jaba.2004.37-513

Miltenberger, R. G., Gatheridge, B. J., Satterlund, M, Egemo-Helm, K. R., Johnson, B. M., Jostad, C., Kelso, P., & Flessner, C. A. (2005). Teaching safety skills to children to prevent gun play: An evaluation of in situ training. *Journal of Applied Behavior Analysis, 38*(3), 395–398. https://doi.org/10.1901/jaba.2005.130-04

Miltenberger, R. G., Gross, A., Knudson, P., Bosch, A., Jostad, C., & Breitwieser C. B. (2009). Evaluating behavioral skills training with and without simulated in situ training for teaching safety skills to children. *Education and Treatment of Children, 32*(1), 63–75. https://doi.org/10.1353/etc.0.0049

Morgan, C. A., & Wine, B. (2018). Evaluation of behavior skills training for teaching work skills to a student with autism spectrum disorder. *Education and Treatment of Children, 41*(2), 223–232. https://doi.org/10.1353/etc.2018.0009

Morosohk, E., & Miltenberger, R. G. (2021). Using generalization-enhanced behavioral skills training to teach poison safety skills to children with autism. *Journal of Autism and Developmental Disorders, 52*(1), 283–290. https://doi.org/10.1007/s10803-021-04938-5

Neely, L., MacNaul, H., Gregori, E., & Cantrell, K. (2021). Effects of telehealth mediated behavior analytic interventions and assessments on subject outcomes. *Journal of Applied Behavior Analysis, 54*(2), 484–510. https://doi.org/10.1002/jaba.818

Neely, L., Tsami, L., Graber, J., & Lerman, D. C. (2022). Towards the development of a curriculum to train behavior analysts to provide services via telehealth. *Journal of Applied Behavior Analysis, 55*(2), 395–411. https://doi.org/10.1002/jaba.904

Nuernberger, J. E., Ringdahl, J. E., Vargo, K. K., Crumpecker, A. C., & Gunnarsson, K. F. (2013). Using a behavioral skills training package to teach conversation skills to young adults with autism spectrum disorders. *Research in Autism Spectrum Disorders, 7*(2), 411–417. https://doi.org/10.1016/j.rasd.2012.09.004

Office for National Statistics. (2021). *Outcomes for disabled people in the UK: 2020.* https://www.ons.gov.uk/peoplepopulationandcommunity/healthandsocialcare/disability/rticles/outcomesfordisabledpeopleintheuk/2020#employment

Palmen, A., Didden, R., & Arts, M. (2008). Improving question asking in high-functioning adolescents with autism spectrum disorders: Effectiveness of small-group training. *Autism, 12*(1), 83–98. https://doi.org/10.1177/1362361307085265

Peters, L. C., & Thompson, R. H. (2015). Teaching children with autism to respond to conversation partners' interest. *Journal of Applied Behavior Analysis, 48*(3), 544–562. https://doi.org/10.1002/jaba.235

Petit-Frere, P., & Miltenberger, R. G. (2021). Evaluating a modified behavioral skills training procedure for teaching poison prevention skills to children with autism. *Journal of Applied Behavior Analysis, 54*(2), 783–792. https://doi.org/10.1002/jaba.799

Project SEARCH. (2018). Preparing young people with significant disabilities for success in competitive integrated employment. https://projectsearch.us/

Rios, D., Schenk, Y. A., Eldridge, R. R., & Peterson, S. M. (2020). The effects of remote behavioral skills training on conducting functional analyses. *Journal of Behavioral Education, 29*(1), 449–468. https://doi.org/10.1007/s10864-020-09385-3

Rispoli, M., & Machalicek, W. (2020). Advances in telehealth and behavioral assessment and intervention in education: Introduction to the special issue. *Journal of Behavioral Education, 29*(2), 189–194. https://doi.org/10.1007/s10864-020-09383-5

Roberts, K., DeQuinzio, J. A., Taylor, B. A., & Petroski, J. (2021). Using behavioral skills training to teach interview skills to young adults with autism. *Journal of Behavioral Education, 30*(4), 664–683. https://doi.org/10.1007/s10864-020-09389-z

Rodriguez, K. A. (2020). Maintaining treatment integrity in the face of crisis: A treatment selection model for transitioning direct ABA services to telehealth. *Behavior Analysis in Practice, 13*(2), 291–298. https://doi.org/10.1007/s40617-020-00429-8

Rosales, R., & Whitlow, H. (2019). A component analysis of job interview training for young adults with autism spectrum disorder. *Behavioral Interventions, 34*(2), 147–162. https://doi.org/10.1002/bin.1658

Rossi, M. R., Vladescu, J. C., Reeve, K. F., & Gross, A. C. (2017). Teaching safety responding to children with autism spectrum disorder. *Education & Treatment of Children, 40*(2), 187–208. https://doi.org/10.1353/etc.2017.0009.

Roux, A. M., Shattuck, P. T., Rast, J. E., Rava, J. A., & Anderson, K. A. (2015). *National autism indicators report: Transition into young adulthood.* https://drexel.edu/~/media/Files/autismoutcomes/publications/LCO%20Fact%20Sheet%0Employment.ashx

Ryan, G., Brady, S., Holloway, J., & Lydon, H. (2019). Increasing appropriate conversation skills using a behavioral skills training package for adults with intellectual disability and autism spectrum disorder. *Journal of Intellectual Disabilities, 23*(4), 567–580. https://doi.org/10.1177/1744629517750744

Sanchez, S., & Miltenberger, R. G. (2015). Evaluating the effectiveness of an abduction prevention program for young adults with intellectual disabilities. *Child & Family Behavior Therapy, 37*(3), 197–207. https://doi.org/10.1080/07317107.2015.1071178

Schaefer, J. M., & Andzik, N. R. (2021). Evaluating behavioral skills training as an evidence-based practice when training parents to intervene with their children. *Behavior Modification, 45*(6), 887–910. https://doi.org/10.1177/0145445520923996

Shireman, M. L., Lerman, D. C., & Hillman, C. B. (2016). Teaching social play skills to adults and children with autism as an approach to building rapport. *Journal of Applied Behavior Analysis, 49*(3), 512–531. https://doi.org/10.1002/jaba.299

Sivaraman, M., Virues-Ortega, J., & Roeyers, H. (2021). Telehealth mask wearing training for children with autism during the COVID-19 pandemic. *Journal of Applied Behavior Analysis, 54*(1), 70–86. https://doi.org/10.1002/jaba.802

Stanish, H. I., Curtin, C., Must, A., Phillips, S., Maslin, M., & Bandini, L. G. (2017). Physical activity levels, frequency, and type among adolescents with and without autism spectrum disorder. *Journal of Autism and Developmental Disorders, 47*(3), 785–794. https://doi.org/10.1007/s10803-016-3001-4

Summers, J., Tarbox, J., Findel-Pyles, R. S., Wilke, A. E., Bergstrom, R., & Williams, W. L. (2011). Teaching two household safety skills to children with autism. *Research in Autism Spectrum Disorders, 5*(1), 629–632. https://doi.org/10.1016/j.rasd.2010.07.008

Sump, L. A., Richman, D. M., Schaefer, A. M., Grubb, L. M., & Brewer, A. T. (2018). Telehealth and in-person training outcomes for novice discrete trial training therapists. *Journal of Applied Behavior Analysis, 51*(3), 466–481. https://doi.org/10.1002/jaba.461

Sump, L. S., Mottau, B. C., & LeBlanc, L. A. (2019). Evaluating behavioral skills training to teach basic computer skills to a young adult with autism. *Behavior Analysis in Practice, 12*(2), 331–334. https://doi.org/10.1007/s40617-018-00295-5

Tekin-Iftar, E., Olcay, S., Sirin, N., Bilmez, H., Degirmenci, D., & Collins, B.C. (2020). Systematic review of safety skill interventions for individuals with autism spectrum disorder. *The Journal of Special Education, 54*(4), 239–250. https://doi.org/10.1177/0022466920918247

Thomas, B. R., Gumaer, C., & Charlop, M. H. (2022). Teaching basketball shooting skills to children with autism spectrum disorder. *Journal of Developmental and Physical Disabilities, 34*(1), 113–125. https://doi.org/10.1007/s10882-021-09792-y

Thomas, B. R., Lafasakis, M., & Spector, V. (2016). Brief report: Using behavioral skills training to teach skateboarding skills to a child with autism spectrum disorder. *Journal of Autism and Developmental Disorders, 46*(12), 3824–3829. https://doi.org/10.1007/s10803-016-2900-8

Tsami, L., Lerman, D., & Toper-Korkmaz, O. (2019). Effectiveness and acceptability of a parent training via telehealth among families around the world. *Journal of Applied Behavior Analysis, 52*(4), 1113–1129. https://doi.org/10.1002/jaba.645

U.S. Department of Education, Office of Special Education and Rehabilitative Services. (2020). *A Transition Guide to Postsecondary Education and Employment for Students and Youth with Disabilities.* https://sites.ed.gov/idea/files/postsecondary-transition-guide-august-2020.pdf

World Health Organization. (2008). *World report on child injury prevention.* https://www.who.int/violence_injury_prevention/child/injury/world_report/en/

Zoder-Martell, K. A., Markelz, A. M., Floress, M. T., Skriba, H. A., & Sayyah, L. E. (2020). Technology to facilitate telehealth in applied behavior analysis. *Behavior Analysis in Practice, 13*(3), 596–603. https://doi.org/10.1007/s40617-020-00449-4

10

Self-Management Interventions

Amarie Carnett, Sophia Kennedy, and Siobhan Gardner
Faculty of Education, Educational Psychology, Victoria University of Wellington

10.1 Technical Abstract

Background: Self-management interventions are used to promote an individual's ability to manage their own behavior through self-monitoring, self-evaluation, and self-reinforcement. **Method:** Peer-reviewed studies investigating self-management interventions by people with autism were analyzed for this chapter. To identify studies, electronic databases (e.g., Psych Info, ERIC, Google Scholar) were searched using relevant keywords (e.g., autism, self-management, self-monitoring, self-control, self-evaluation, and self-reinforcement). **Results:** Research literature indicates that self-management intervention for individuals with autism meets the National Professional Development Center's criteria to be classified as an evidence-based practice. **Discussion:** Self-management interventions have been used by individuals with autism to improve adaptive behavior, increase task completion and productivity, reduce challenging behavior, and improve social interactions, particularly for children and adolescents between 4 and 18 years of age without severe intellectual disability. These interventions have been successful when applied in homes, schools, and other community settings. Additional research is needed to address issues related to social validity, generalization, and maintenance of self-management skills. **Practitioner recommendations:** When designing and implementing interventions, practitioners should take into account the following factors: (a) individualizing intervention contexts and components, (b) enabling learners to select self-management goals, and (c) employing teaching procedures that facilitate the acquisition of self-monitoring and self-evaluation skills.

10.2 Layperson Summary

Self-management interventions involve strategies designed to help individuals with autism improve their ability to control, change, and reinforce their own behavior. Self-management interventions involve several general procedures. First, individuals are taught specific skills like self-monitoring, where they learn to monitor and record their own behavior. They also learn self-evaluation, which involves

Amarie Carnett, Sophia Kennedy, and Siobhan Gardner, *Self-Management Interventions*. In: *Lifespan Treatment for Autistic Individuals*. Edited by: Peter Sturmey, Russell Lang, and James K. Luiselli, Oxford University Press.
© Oxford University Press (2025). DOI: 10.1093/oso/9780197635841.003.0010

assessing their behavior against predetermined goals or criteria. Additionally, individuals are trained in self-administered consequences, such as rewarding themselves for desired behavior or applying appropriate consequences for undesirable behavior. Teaching procedures for self-management have involved some combination of regular feedback, reward (reinforcement), visual aids, prompts, and gradual fading of support. Overall, self-management interventions are designed to empower individuals to actively participate in changing their own behavior, and they have been used to improve academics, communication, daily living skills, and social skills, as well as to reduce challenging behavior. Various individuals, including teachers, therapists, and parents, have been trained to provide guidance and assistance during the self-management process. Self-management interventions should be personalized by considering the individual's characteristics, preferences, and goals through individualization of self-management procedures, contingencies, and other contextual details. Self-management interventions are recognized as evidence-based practices by the National Professional Development Center (Steinbrenner et al., 2020; Wong et al., 2015) and the National Autism Center (2015). Although effective in most cases, there is limited evidence regarding the extent to which outcomes of self-management interventions maintain over time and generalize. Specifically, individuals may struggle to apply self-management strategies consistently and effectively in different contexts or when faced with unexpected challenges. Further, there is less evidence to support the use of self-management interventions by individuals with severe intellectual and developmental disabilities.

10.3 Treatment Summary Table

Treatment summary: Self-Management

Treatment description: Self-management interventions involve the systematic teaching of skills related to self-monitoring, self-evaluation, and self-administration of contingent consequences (e.g., self-reinforcement) that an individual then applies to produce a meaningful change in their own behavior.

Expected outcomes: Research has demonstrated that self-management interventions can be used to improve adaptive behavior, increase task completion and productivity, reduce challenging behavior, and improve social interactions. The strongest evidence is available for children ages 4 to 18 years. Evidence of social validity, maintenance, and generalization of acquired self-management strategies to new goals and novel contexts is limited, particularly for individuals with higher support needs.

Methods: Self-management interventions involve a systematic approach to teaching individuals with autism how to regulate their own behavior. This includes teaching skills such as self-monitoring (awareness of one's own behavior), self-evaluation (assessing performance or progress), and self-administered consequences (applying rewards or reinforcements). The teaching procedures typically include providing clear instructions, setting specific goals, using visual supports, implementing reinforcement strategies, and providing feedback and support.

Expertise required to implement treatment: Implementing a self-management intervention with a person with autism spectrum disorder (ASD) requires expertise from professionals who have a strong understanding of ASD, evidence-based teaching procedures, and the specific self-management techniques being employed. This expertise, combined with a collaborative and individualized approach, contributes to the successful implementation of self-management interventions for individuals with ASD.

Risks and negative side effects: Although no specific negative side effects have been noted in the literature, there may be difficulties in generalizing self-management skills from structured settings (e.g., therapy sessions) to real-life situations and to new target behaviors without additional targeted support.

Additional considerations and limitations: Considerations and limitations for self-management interventions in individuals with ASD include the need to assess and teach prerequisite skills required for successful self-management. Individualization of teaching procedures is crucial, as strategies must be tailored to the unique needs and abilities of the individual. Visual aids and other environmental supports should be in place to facilitate the acquisition and application of self-management skills, ensuring the intervention is feasible and achievable. Additionally, careful planning for generalization and maintenance of acquired skills is essential to promote long-term independence and effectiveness.

10.4 Introduction

10.4.1 Treatment Description

Self-management is commonly defined as the self-application of behavior change tactics to produce a desired change (Briesch & Briesch, 2016; Epstein, 1997; Harchik et al., 1992; Lee et al., 2007). Simply stated, *self-management* allows an individual to manage their own behaviors (Aljadeff-Abergel et al., 2015). *Self-control* is sometimes used synonymously with the term *self-management*; however, distinction of these terms has been highlighted in the literature (e.g., Brigham, 1982; Esptein, 1997). The term *self-control* implies that a person has full control of their own behavior, reducing emphasis on environmental variables (e.g., availability of choices and learning history). Additionally, self-control is often used to refer to a person's ability to delay gratification (e.g., having enough self-control to limit how much dessert you eat) or as the ability to restrain from engaging in a behavior (i.e., impulse control). Thus, within the context of self-management, it is possible that a person might achieve self-control (Baer, 1984). Self-management interventions can incorporate a range of self-administered supports ranging from simple strategies (e.g., making a to-do list) to complex multicomponent supports to address planning, implementation, and monitoring of a desired behavior change.

The literature highlights various components within the realm of self-management interventions (Baer, 1984; Fantuzzo et al., 1987). Specifically, three major components are *self-monitoring, self-evaluation*, and *self-administered consequences* (Cooper et al., 2020; Lee et al., 2007; Southall & Gast, 2011). Self-monitoring involves the individual's awareness of their behavior and subsequent recording of its occurrences or nonoccurrences (Cooper et al., 2020; Maag, 2016). This tactic can be used alone or in conjunction with other techniques so an individual can collect data on their performance. Similarly, an individual might also engage in self-evaluation (e.g., self-assessment) to determine the degree to which their target behavior has reached a predetermined level, rate, or standard of performance (Cooper et al., 2020; Southall & Gast, 2011). Finally, *self-administered consequences* are a critical component of a self-management program. When using this tactic, an individual arranges a specific consequence to follow the occurrence or nonoccurrence of the targeted behavior (Cooper et al., 2020; Jones et al., 1977; Maag, 2016). For example, if an individual is working to increase the amount of time they engage in study behavior, they might use *self-monitoring* to record the amount of time spent studying each day, *self-evaluation* to determine if study time is consistent with their goal, and then *self-reinforcement* to support the future occurrence of studying. Alternatively, a person might also use *self-reinforcement* to decrease the occurrence of an undesirable behavior, such as spending too much time on social media. This can be done by delivering reinforcement for reducing or refraining from a target behavior. For example, having a special dessert on days when social media use is less than a targeted amount of time. In some cases, individuals might also choose to utilize a mild form of self-punishment. For example, if an individual is trying to decrease their use of swear words, they might use a response cost procedure, where they put money in a jar contingent on saying a swear word. Regardless of the consequence the individual selects, considerations should be given in terms of the type, quality, quantity, and delivery methods employed.

Self-management interventions may encompass antecedent-based tactics, such as environmental planning, as an additional component (Baer, 1984). This involves arranging the environment in a way that supports and promotes the desired behavior. For example, if a self-management plan was created to increase the frequency of exercising at the gym, environmental arrangement could involve packing a gym bag the night before and setting it by the door. Doing so reduces the effort necessary to go to the gym that day and functions as a prompt (reminder) as the individual leaves their home. Additionally, self-management interventions may incorporate motivational strategies that influence the probability of their engagement in desired behavior. For example, if a person's self-management goal is related to eating healthy foods, they might schedule grocery shopping for times when they do not expect to be hungry (e.g., after lunch) so that they are less motivated to buy unhealthy snack foods due to hunger. Lastly, as part of a self-management program, individuals may incorporate specific prompting tactics to cue their target behavior. Self-arranged prompts, such as visual, auditory, textual, or symbolic cues, can support self-management (Cooper et al., 2020; Maag, 2016). For example, if an individual's self-management plan involves increasing their water consumption throughout the day, they might set an alarm on their phone or watch to provide alerts to remind them to drink a glass of water at predetermined times.

10.4.2 Rationale and Objectives

Two competing theories have been posited to account for behavior change resulting from self-management, broadly operant models (Skinner, 1953), and cognitive models (Hughes & Lloyd, 1993). The operant (behavioral) conceptualization of self-management involves arranging consequences to reinforce desired behavior and arranging antecedent variables (environments) to signal when a target behavior should or should not occur (Cooper et al., 2020). In contrast, the cognitive perspective emphasizes the internal thought processes involved when a person is engaged in self-monitoring, self-reinforcement, and self-evaluation (Maag, 2016). Regardless of the theoretical underpinnings, it is widely accepted that including self-management interventions within educational programs for individuals with autism is important to self-determination, independence, and other factors that influence the quality of life (Lee et al., 2007; Turnbull & Turnbull, 2001).

In practice, most self-management intervention components and procedures used with individuals with ASD in the research literature are similar, regardless of which theoretical perspective (operant or cognitive) underlies the approach. The components and procedures described in this chapter were identified through analysis of the research literature, with particular emphasis given to meta-analyses and systematic reviews (e.g., Lee et al., 2007; Southall & Gast, 2011).

Self-management interventions for individuals with ASD typically involve some form and combination of the following components.

1. *Goal Setting*: Setting clear and achievable goals is important. The individual (*self-determination*) or their family identifies specific behavioral targets they believe will make a meaningful difference in the person's life. For example, these goals may be related to academics, social skills, or daily routines.
2. *Self-Monitoring*: The individual learns to observe and track their own behavior or progress. This involves the use of checklists, timers, or other tools to record and monitor their actions.
3. *Self-Prompting*: Using self-generated cues or prompts helps individuals initiate or maintain target behaviors. Visual supports, reminders, and self-instructions aid in prompting desired actions.
4. *Self-Evaluation*: Individuals engage in self-reflection to assess their own performance or progress toward their goals. They evaluate their own behavior to identify progress and areas for improvement.
5. *Self-Reinforcement*: Implementing self-administered reinforcement is a key component. Individuals select meaningful rewards for themselves and allocate them upon achieving their predetermined goals.
6. *Self-Correction*: Individuals learn to identify and correct errors or deviations from desired behaviors. They develop strategies to adjust their actions when necessary.

These components are typically used together in some combination, but the specific emphasis and implementation of these components vary based on the individual's goals, characteristics (e.g., developmental level, age, and preferences), and context (e.g., home, school, or work).

10.5 Research Background

Self-management is classified as an evidence-based practice by both the National Professional Development Center on Autism Spectrum Disorder (Steinbrenner et al., 2020; Wong et al., 2015) and the National Autism Center (National Autism Center, 2015). The following section provides examples of peer-reviewed self-management intervention research across a variety of contexts and skill domains (e.g., communication, play, problem behavior) and self-management skills (e.g., self-monitoring, self-reinforcement, self-evaluation). Intervention findings are summarized, and implications are discussed.

10.5.1 Social Communication and Engagement Skills

Self-management intervention approaches have been used to help improve social communication and engagement behaviors in children with autism. For example, Liu et al. (2015) evaluated a self-management intervention for improving social skills with a 9-year-old girl with ASD. The intervention involved video modeling and was partially implemented by the girl's parents. Liu and colleagues utilized a multiple baseline across behaviors research design to assess the targeted social behaviors, including interruptions, asking for opinions, and greeting unfamiliar adults. The participant was taught to self-reinforce contingent on the desired behavior. Results indicated the intervention was associated with improvements in all target behaviors with a strong overall treatment effect. Moreover, behavior gains were generalized to a nontraining setting and maintained during the fading and follow-up phases.

Likewise, Koegel et al. (1992) used self-management to improve social skills and, in turn, reduce disruptive behavior for four children with ASD. Specifically, the study evaluated a self-management intervention's effects on responsiveness to verbal initiations from others in the community, home, and school settings. After an assessment to identify reinforcers, the children were taught to discriminate between correct and incorrect social responses. Then they were taught to self-monitor their own behavior with a wrister counter to record instances of appropriate behavior. The total occurrence of the target behavior, as recorded on the wrist counter, was then converted to tokens/points to be used in the token exchange reinforcement system. The schedule of reinforcement was thinned as the target skill developed, and prompts were eventually faded out entirely. The results show that the children were able to learn to self-manage responsivity across multiple settings without a treatment provider present, and improvements were associated with reductions in disruptive behavior.

Koegel et al. (2014) conducted a study to examine the effectiveness of self-management in enhancing reciprocal social conversations. The researchers focused on improving on-topic responsiveness to conversation partners, expanding conversational topics, and asking on-topic questions. The study employed a multiple-baseline design involving two children and one adolescent with ASD who had previously struggled to exhibit appropriate reciprocal social conversational skills. Self-management was taught using a procedure similar to Koegel et al. (1992). Participants were asked to identify a highly preferred item or activity that could be earned through the exchange of conversation points that were awarded when the participant demonstrated appropriate conversation. The participants followed a self-management schematic with child-friendly definitions. The findings revealed enhancements in reciprocal social conversation, characterized by improved elaborated responses and on-topic question asking. The acquired skills generalized across multiple community settings and maintained over time. Additionally, social validity data were collected from naïve observers using a rating scale. Their ratings indicated the intervention led to meaningful improvements for the participants.

A hallmark characteristic of ASD is a preference for sameness and routine, leading to limited variability in social communication and engagement. Newman et al. (2000) employed self-management techniques to promote increased variability in responding, targeting play and language skills in children with ASD. Within a multiple-baseline design, the authors taught three children between 6 and 8 years old to self-monitor and self-manage skills related to play and language. Reinforcement consisting of verbal praise and a token system was used. During baseline, tokens were available regardless of behavior. When the self-management intervention was initiated, tokens were made contingent on variations in the topography of the target behavior. During baseline and self-management conditions, students were asked to vary their responding (e.g., tell me something different). For the first 6 days, students were verbally prompted to take a token when demonstrating variability in target behavior. Attempts to take a token when variability was not demonstrated were blocked. All students experienced an increase in variability during the self-management phases. The improved variability was maintained at 1-month follow-up, but data on generalizability and social validity were not reported.

10.5.2 Play Skills

Self-management interventions have been used in the context of play to help improve social behaviors toward peers, including turn taking, sharing, and appropriate play. For example, Stahmer and Schreibman (1992) evaluated the effects of a treatment package targeting self-management to improve play skills for three children (ages 7 to 13 years) with autism. Discrimination training was first implemented to ensure each child could discriminate between targeted forms of play (e.g., feeding the baby pretend food) and inappropriate challenging behaviors (e.g., throwing the doll) using a variety of different toys (e.g., baby doll, toy spaceship, games, and puzzles). Following this training phase, self-management skills were targeted. During this phase, each child was given a wristwatch with an interval timer, which sounded an alarm to signal the beginning and end of a time interval. During the interval, reinforcement was provided if the child engaged in the targeted form of play behavior. After the children consistently engaged in high levels of appropriate play, the interval duration was gradually increased, and children were given control over obtaining reinforcement independently. Specifically, a tray of preferred foods and stickers was placed in the room with the children, and the children retrieved their own reinforcer at the end of each successful interval. After the children demonstrated self-monitoring during 85% of intervals, the reinforcement schedule was thinned by increasing the criteria for reinforcement to consecutive intervals. Further, the experimenter's presence in the room was faded after 20 minutes of appropriate play. Initially, the experimenter left for 30 seconds (while the child was being observed via a one-way mirror or video monitor) and, upon returning, would ask the child if they played appropriately while they were gone. In the last phase, the self-management materials (e.g., watch, monitoring sheet) were removed, and reinforcement was provided if the child engaged in two consecutive intervals (20 minutes) of appropriate play. Follow-up data and generalization measures across settings and new toys were evaluated a month after intervention cessation. Results indicated each child learned to engage in appropriate play behaviors, and these behaviors generalized to new settings and toys, and for two of the children, their behavior maintained after 1 month.

Similarly, Reinecke and colleagues (1999) evaluated the effects of self-management to teach sharing to three preschool-aged children with ASD. During the intervention, a token economy was incorporated into a play activity where the children were able to reinforce themselves with a token each time they shared with a peer or sibling. All children increased the frequency of independent sharing behaviors during the self-management phase.

Newman et al. (2020) taught self-monitoring and self-management to three children with ASD to increase variability in play and social language. Specifically, one participant was taught to use self-management to increase the variety of imaginative play scenarios when playing with a toy robot. During the intervention, he was taught to self-reinforce using a token economy system to increase play variation. The result showed increased rates of play variability. However, the accuracy of the child's self-management did not exceed 60% because the child sometimes forgot to take a token for engaging in the target behavior. All the same, there is a clear indication that the use of self-monitoring did result in increases of varied responding.

Although each of these single case studies exemplifies the utility of teaching self-management to increase play behaviors for children with autism, only one of these examples (i.e., Stahmer & Schreibaman, 1992) assessed generalization and the effects of the intervention over time via follow-up data collection. Further, measurement of social validity was not included in any of these examples. Thus, although the findings are positive in that teaching self-monitoring can be used to improve play, there is still a need for more rigorous research to further evaluate the effects of teaching self-management in the context of play skills.

10.5.3 Problem Behavior

Self-management techniques have also been used to reduce a range of problem behaviors. For example, Lin and Koegel (2018) used a self-management procedure to address higher-order restrictive and repetitive behavior (H-RRB) with associated challenging behavior. Three children diagnosed with ASD between 4 and 6 years of age received treatment to increase behavioral flexibility. Before treatment, children were demonstrating H-RRB in the form of restricted preferences and insistence on repetitive routines with their toys. Around 90% of the time, these restrictive and repetitive behaviors were interrupted, the children engaged in problem behaviors (i.e., crying, yelling, aggression, and avoidance). During the intervention, children were given a tracking sheet and taught to record their engagement in flexible behavior (i.e., "trying something new while keeping your cool"). While children engaged with their toys, parents provided opportunities to be flexible in play (e.g., "Here's your chance to get your point, I'm going to add a different train to the railroad track"). If the child appropriately engaged in their parents' bid to vary their routine (e.g., accepted the different train) within 10 seconds and did not display challenging behavior, the child was praised and encouraged to mark a point on their sheet. After earning a certain number of points, the child could choose a reward such as snacks or stickers. Throughout the intervention, behavioral flexibility increased from baseline (10–13% of opportunities) to an average of 77–92% of opportunities during the intervention. Two weeks after the intervention, the self-management tool was no longer used, and the children continued to demonstrate behavioral flexibility in 80–96% of opportunities. This study also reported an improvement in both child and parent affect. The findings of this study are promising, but replication with larger and varied (e.g., different age groups and characteristics) sample sizes is needed.

Several studies have used self-management techniques to reduce stereotypic or self-stimulatory behaviors (e.g., rocking, hand flapping, and inappropriate vocalizations) that impeded access to inclusive settings and opportunities for social engagement. For example, Koegel and Koegel (1990) found an intervention using a paper self-monitoring tool and contingent reinforcement to be effective in reducing stereotypic behavior in children 9 to 14 years old with ASD and intellectual disability. Shabani et al. (2001) replicated this procedure and found it effective in reducing instances of body rocking in a 12-year-old boy with ASD in multiple settings. Mancina et al. (2000) also adapted Koegel and Koegel's (1990) intervention, effectively reducing high rates of inappropriate vocalizations in a 12-year-old girl with ASD.

It should be noted that there has been discussion concerning whether the self-monitoring component of the intervention is responsible for the reduction of stereotypic behavior or, more so, the reinforcement component of the intervention. The functional relationship between the self-monitoring system and reduction in stereotypy alone was investigated by Fritz et al. (2012). Findings from their study supported their hypothesis that the reduction in stereotypic behavior was attributable to reinforcement of other behaviors but not the self-monitoring tool itself. However, a more recent study by Crutchfield et al. (2014) has reported contradicting results. The study used a self-monitoring tool called "i-connect" to effectively reduce stereotypic behavior that was interfering with the independent work of two 14-year-old boys with autism. No programmed reinforcement was used in the intervention, yet the implementation of the self-monitoring system had an immediate reduction on the boy's stereotypic behavior. Importantly, the intervention was also reported to be acceptable (socially valid) by both the participants themselves and their teachers.

Mindfulness-based interventions have also been used within the context of self-management. For example, Singh et al. (2011) and Singh et al. (2019) used a mindfulness-focused self-management intervention to reduce verbal and physical aggression in adolescent males 14 to 17 years of age with ASD. Specifically, these interventions were based on teaching informal mindfulness practices called *meditation on the soles of the feet (Sof)* (Singh et al., 2003) and *Surfing the Urge* (Singh et al., 2019). With some individual differences, these interventions involved teaching mindfulness practices based on focusing on the body in times of anger, observing the emotion, and waiting for it to dissipate. Both studies involved intensive training in the mindfulness method, which was delivered by the mother. After training, the adolescents practiced the mindfulness techniques when they experienced the onset of anger and aggression. Prior to the interventions, participants in the *SoF* study were engaged in 14 to 20 acts of aggression per week. These acts reduced to 4 to 6 per week during the training period and, beginning at 30 weeks, no instances occurred for over a month. In terms of maintenance, an average of one act of aggression per year was recorded for each participant over a 3-year period. In the *Surfing the Urge* study, baseline rates of aggression ranged from an average of 2.8 to 6.7 instances per week. During the intervention, these instances reduced to an average of between 1.1 and 3.2 per week. By the 25th week of practicing *Surfing the Urge*. all three participants of the study had discontinued psychotropic medication due to reduction in aggression. The above studies show promise for the feasibility of mindfulness practices as part of a self-management approach to reducing aggressive behavior in adolescents with ASD. Replications of these findings in more varied populations and larger samples are needed to demonstrate efficacy.

Research syntheses and reviews have compiled and analyzed studies that investigate the use of self-monitoring strategies for reducing problem behavior. For example, Carr (2016) conducted a meta-analysis that examined 12 studies reporting positive effects, particularly in the reduction of stereotypy. The review provided substantial evidence to support the classification of self-management techniques as an evidence-based practice for reducing challenging behavior in children and adolescents within the age range of 4 to 18 years. However, assessment of social validity from the perspective of participants and their family has been understudied.

10.5.4 Functional Skills

Self-management interventions have also been used to support functional daily living skills of children with ASD. A study by Pierce and Schreibman (1994) used a self-management system to teach three boys with ASD and intellectual disability (6 to 9 years old) a range of daily living skills. Three target skills were chosen for each child, including some combination of getting dressed, setting the table, making lunch, making the bed, and doing laundry. In a baseline condition, children were told to complete the task (e.g., "Go get dressed"), and the therapist directed their attention to the self-management materials by pointing. On-task behavior was reported at an average of 0% of occasions in this condition. The training phase taught children to use a task analysis book containing pictures related to each step of the target skill, as well as engage in self-reinforcement. First, children were taught to discriminate between the pictures related to their future tasks (e.g., "Point to the plates") and were reinforced after every three correct responses. This phase continued until children reached 100% of the time engaged in on-task behavior. Next, children were empowered to choose their own reinforcer (e.g., snacks and toys), independently turn book pages, perform actions depicted in the book, and self-reinforce upon completion. A chaining procedure with least-to-most prompting was used where children were first reinforced for opening the book, then for opening the book and pointing to the action inside the book, and then for imitating a single action in the book. After completing the task, they were taught to turn to the final page of the booklet, which depicted a smiley face that indicated that they could access reinforcement. This procedure was repeated until the child could repeat the process, including self-reinforcement independently, then an additional picture/task was added to the book. The final phase of training faded the presence of the therapist, initially leaving the room for 20-second periods and then gradually increasing time away until they were absent for the duration of the task time. After acquiring the first of the three skills, the following two skills were acquired in fewer sessions than the first. The time taken to reach criterion on the different training steps ranged from a single session to 16 sessions. Posttreatment probes found that children completed their target tasks between 60% and 100% of the time. Generalization probes collected in the home and clinic indicated that skills generalized between environments with little to no additional training. Follow-up at 2 months revealed that children had maintained the skills. This study provides promising evidence for the use of self-monitoring interventions for teaching daily living skills and suggests that the intervention can be generalized to a range of different skills. It should be noted that in follow-up sessions, children's accuracy dropped significantly upon removal of the booklet, indicating the need for further studies.

More recently, a similar self-monitoring intervention was used in China to teach eight children with autism, ages 6 to 8 years old, to wash dishes (Lee et al., 2018). For this intervention, a task analysis sheet showing eight steps of a dishwashing task in picture form with descriptive text appropriate to the child's reading level was used. In a preintervention baseline assessment, children successfully completed between 0 and 2 (25% of the steps). The intervention phase involved teaching all steps involved in dishwashing and how to self-monitor progress in learning the skill. Each of the steps in the task analysis was initially modeled for the child, and physical prompting was used when needed. Teaching self-monitoring involved the child watching a video of themselves completing the task alongside the instructor. They evaluated each step individually and, if correct, assigned the step a smiley face on their recording sheet. If both the instructor and child agreed on successful completion of a step, the child was given a reward. Agreement between child and observer was initially variable but consistently less than 50% agreement. However, after 14 to 16 sessions, agreement increased to 75%, and children began independently self-monitoring without video self-feedback. After agreement reached 75%, the density of reinforcement was gradually reduced to one reward after at least seven of eight steps were completed and recorded accurately. Follow-up trials were conducted after accuracy reached 100% for three consecutive days, and all children maintained their performance in self-monitoring with 100% accuracy. Dishwashing itself was completed with 87–100% accuracy. Further, parents indicated that skills were maintained for at least 1 month. A range of social validity variables were measured with the parents indicating that they were highly satisfied with both the procedure and results of the intervention. Parents also reported using the same technique to teach their children different daily living skills, including morning and bedtime routines.

The above studies provide promising evidence for the use of self-monitoring to improve daily living skills. Pierce and Schreibman (1994) provide evidence to suggest that self-monitoring can be applied to a wide range of daily living skills and generalized to different environments. Lee et al. (2018) provide findings that support application of this intervention outside of a Western context and provide evidence of social validity.

10.5.5 Academic Skills

The ability to self-manage is an essential component of academic success in schools. As such, research has investigated the use of interventions that target self-management in the context of academic skills. For example, Hampshire et al. (2016) assessed the effectiveness of an intervention package including both parent training and self-management strategies. The participants were five middle schoolers and their parents. The intervention aimed to increase students' ability to independently complete homework. The self-management strategy entailed the students monitoring, evaluating, and rewarding their own behavior. The parent monitored the child's use of the self-management strategy following training. Students received access to a preselected reinforcer following completion of the homework task or earned a point on their tally sheet. The results evidenced an increase in task independence following the implementation of the self-management intervention. Prior to the implementation of the study, parents reported students seldom completed their homework without extensive parental support. Social validity was measured by both parents and teachers. Results indicated that stakeholders felt the intervention was helpful and effective, and they would continue to use the strategy learned.

Simmons et al. (2022) also investigated a parent-supported self-management intervention for on-task behavior that targeted independent schoolwork in the home. The intervention consisted of self-monitoring, self-evaluation, and contingent reinforcement. The parent had a portable smart device (e.g., phone, tablet) that displayed live video of the child in their workroom and used variable momentary-time sampling with intervals of 3 minutes. At the end of 15-minute periods, both the parent and child completed self-monitoring datasheets. For the self-evaluation training, the researchers provided descriptive examples and nonexamples of on-task behavior and explained the difference to the child. The researchers also used video examples and asked the child to self-evaluate if they were on task or not and used verbal praise to reinforce correct answers. The results showed that the intervention successfully increased on-task behavior for each participant, and the improvement was maintained post intervention. Furthermore, parents were able to implement the intervention with high fidelity, and the video observations resulted in high degree of correspondence between parent and child ratings. Social validity was reported as "highly acceptable" by both the children and their parents.

Finally, Holifield et al. (2010) used a self-monitoring procedure to increase attendance to task and academic accuracy for children with ASD. The participant was given a self-monitoring sheet before the teacher verbally prompted them to start the independent work. The teacher also provided a gestural prompt by pointing to the assignment sheet. The participant was expected to circle "yes" or "no" regarding the occurrence of the target behavior. Verbal praise was provided when the participant accurately circled "yes." Results indicated that self-monitoring increased attendance to tasks and task accuracy for both students.

The studies provided above offer promising evidence for the use of self-management in the context of academic skills. However, future replications and extensions should evaluate maintenance and generalization in this area also.

10.5.6 Technology

A variety of technology can be used to support self-management across a range of environments (e.g., home, school, community). Given the rise in touchscreen devices and apps to support productivity and organization, it is not surprising to see the use of these tools embedded within the context of self-management interventions. Research has evaluated the use of smartphone apps and digital activity schedules to support self-management skills for individuals with ASD across a range of contexts. For example, Cheung et al. (2016) evaluated the use of a digital self-management activity schedule to improve community skills for two children with ASD. Specifically, the children were taught how to effectively order food items at a local bakery using an iPhone loaded with a six-page activity schedule. Each page of the activity schedule also included written instructions for the steps of the task. Teaching sessions were conducted in a classroom that simulated the activity. A combination of least-to-most prompting procedures and total task presentation was employed for each step of the activity schedule. Additionally, self-management procedures were utilized to focus on reading the instructions on the activity schedule, performing the corresponding step, and self-monitoring the completion of each step by progressing to the next page on the activity schedule until the activity was finished. Reinforcement was provided for completing all the steps of the activity. Following mastery of purchasing skills, community training at a bakery was conducted. Generalization was assessed at a different community bakery, and maintenance checks were conducted 2 weeks after the intervention phase. Probes where the iPhone activity schedule was not provided were conducted between 2 and 5 weeks later. Both participants learned to independently order items, and generalization to a novel bakery was reported. Additionally, both participants were able to continue to complete each step of the activity independently in the follow-up sessions without the iPhone activity schedule. This study highlights the use of touchscreen technology to teach self-management and generalization of these skills across environments, as well as how to fade out the use of technology when independence has been achieved.

More recently, Chia et al. (2018) reviewed the literature on technology used to support self-management for individuals with autism. In that review, 12 studies were evaluated using the What Works Clearinghouse (WWC) standards for single-case methodology rigor. The evaluated studies utilized a variety of technology: however, most studies used touchscreen devices with self-management applications, such as I-Connect, Upad, and Wunderlist (e.g., Bouck et al., 2014; Clemons et al., 2015; Hampshire & Allred, 2018). The second most common technology reported was the use of wristwatches with alarms or counters (e.g., Finn et al., 2015; Koegel et al., 1992; Stahmer & Schreibman, 1992). General findings showed that the use of technology to support self-management for individuals with ASD is effective. However, of note, only three of the studies evaluated generalization, and only six of the studies evaluated maintenance of the skill post intervention, which is an important aspect of self-management. Further, when evaluated for quality standards using the WWC framework, only eight of the 12 studies met standards without reservations, suggesting a need for more rigorous research in this area.

Although the use of technology to support self-management skills is promising, more research is needed for replication and extensions to this area of self-management. In particular, data on long-term maintenance and generalization to other environments and across other behaviors are needed.

10.6 Practice Implications

10.6.1 Treatment Outcomes

As outlined in the previous section, self-management interventions can be used in the home, community, and school to address a range of behaviors (e.g., communication, academic skills, and functional skills). Self-management interventions include a variety of teaching components. As indicated by reviews of the literature (i.e., Lee et al., 2007; Southall & Gast, 2011) and studies highlighted in this chapter, self-management interventions are an effective treatment to increase appropriate behaviors. However, there remains a need for longitudinal research on maintenance of positive outcomes over time (Baer, 1984; Lee et al., 2018; Vargas, 2020).

10.6.2 Practice Implication Guidelines

Practitioners should consider a few important factors during the design and implementation of self-management interventions. First, individualization is crucial when selecting intervention contexts and components. For instance, when incorporating self-monitoring, it is important to assess and teach any necessary prerequisites to ensure individuals can accurately and independently record their own behavior (Lee et al., 2007). Second, careful consideration should be given to selecting realistic and specific self-management goals, including the timeframe for achieving them (Cooper et al., 2020). Teaching goal selection and prioritization can be an integral part of self-management interventions. Third, alongside the long-term benefits of self-management, the inclusion of supports, such as coaching or peer assistance, should be considered. For example, some individuals may require support with progress monitoring, accountability, or plan adjustments to ensure sustained effectiveness (Vargas, 2020). Lastly, the implementation of self-management may incorporate many teaching elements to help learners with ASD acquire the skills needed to manage their own behavior. For example, teaching procedures, such as arranging antecedent variables, using systematic instruction, prompting, modeling, reinforcement, and incorporating technology, have been described in the literature.

10.7 Conclusion

Self-management plays a crucial role in promoting autonomy and self-determination, which are essential aspects of functional living. Interventions aimed at fostering self-management skills in individuals with autism have demonstrated effectiveness and are recognized as evidence-based practices. Although a substantial body of literature exists on this topic, further research is needed to comprehensively explore the impacts and benefits of self-management interventions for individuals with ASD across a range of abilities.

10.8 References

Aljadeff-Abergel, E., Schenk, Y., Walmsley, C., Peterson, S. M., Frieder, J. E., & Acker, N. (2015). The effectiveness of self-management interventions for children with autism—A literature review. *Research in Autism Spectrum Disorders, 18*, 34–50. https://doi.org/10.1016/j.rasd.2015.07.001

Baer, D. M. (1984). Does research on self-control need more control? *Analysis and Intervention in Developmental Disabilities, 4*(2), 211–218. https://doi.org/10.1016/0270-4684(84)90042-9

Bouck, E. C., Savage, M., Meyer, N. K., Taber-Doughty, T., & Hunley, M. (2014). High-tech or low-tech? Comparing self-monitoring systems to increase task independence for students with autism. *Focus on Autism and Other Developmental Disabilities, 29*(3), 156–167. https://doi.org/10.1177/1088357614528797

Briesch, A. M., & Briesch, J. M. (2016). Meta-analysis of behavioral self-management interventions in single-case research. *School Psychology Review, 45*(1), 3–18. https://doi.org/10.17105/spr45-1.3-18

Brigham, T. (1982). Self-management: A radical behavioral perspective. In P. Karoly & F. H. Kanfer (Eds.), *Self-management and behavior change: From theory to practice* (pp. 32–59). New York: Pergamon.

Carr, M. E. (2016). Self-management of challenging behaviours associated with autism spectrum disorder: A meta-analysis. *Australian Psychologist, 51*(4), 316–333. https://doi.org/10.1111/ap.12227

Cheung, Y., Schulze, K. A., Leaf, J. B., & Rudrud, E. (2016). Teaching community skills to two young children with autism using a digital self-managed activity schedule. *Exceptionality, 24*(4), 241–250. https://doi.org/10.1080/09362835.2016.1215654

Chia, G. L. C., Anderson, A., & McLean, L. A. (2018). Use of technology to support self-management in individuals with autism: Systematic review. *Review Journal of Autism and Developmental Disorders, 5*, 142–155. https://doi.org/10.1007/s40489-018-0129-5

Clemons, L. L., Mason, B. A., Garrison-Kane, L., & Wills, H. P. (2015). Self-monitoring for high school students with disabilities. *Journal of Positive Behavior Interventions, 18*(3), 145–155. https://doi.org/10.1177/1098300715596134

Cooper, J. O., Heron, T. E., & Heward, W. L. (2020). *Applied behavior analysis* (3rd ed.). Hoboken, NJ: Pearson Education.

Crutchfield, S. A., Mason, R. A., Chambers, A., Wills, H. P., & Mason, B. A. (2014). Use of a self-monitoring application to reduce stereotypic behavior in adolescents with autism: A preliminary investigation of I-connect. *Journal of Autism and Developmental Disorders, 45*(5), 1146–1155. https://doi.org/10.1007/s10803-014-2272-x

Epstein, R. (1997). Skinner as self-manager. *Journal of Applied Behavior Analysis, 30*(3), 545–568. https://doi.org/10.1901/jaba.1997.30-545

Fantuzzo, J. W., Rohrbeck, C. A., & Azar, S. T. (1987). A component analysis of behavioral self-management interventions with elementary school students. *Child & Family Behavior Therapy, 9*, 33–43. https://doi.org/10.1300/j019v09n01_03

Finn, L., Ramasamy, R., Dukes, C., & Scott, J. (2015). Using WatchMinder to increase the on-task behavior of students with autism spectrum disorder. *Journal of Autism and Developmental Disorders, 45*(5), 1408–1418. https://doi.org/10.1007/s10803-014-2300–x

Fritz, J. N., Iwata, B. A., Rolider, N. U., Camp, E. M., & Neidert, P. L. (2012). Analysis of self-recording in self-management interventions for stereotypy. *Journal of Applied Behavior Analysis, 45*(1), 55–68. https://doi.org/10.1901/jaba.2012.45-55

Hampshire, P. K., & Allred, K. W. (2018). A parent-implemented, technology-mediated approach to increasing self-management homework skills in middle school students with autism. *Exceptionality, 26*(2), 119–136. https://doi.org/10.1080/09362835.2016.1216848

Hampshire, P. K., Butera, G. D., & Bellini, S. (2016). Self-management and parents as interventionists to improve homework independence in students with autism spectrum disorders. *Preventing School Failure, 60*(1), 22–34. https://doi.org/10.1080/1045988X.2014.954515

Harchik, A. E., Sherman, J. A., & Sheldon, J. B. (1992). The use of self-management procedures by people with developmental disabilities: A brief review. *Research in Developmental Disabilities, 13*(3), 211–227. https://doi.org/10.1016/0891-4222(92)90026-3

Holifield, C., Goodman, J., Hazelkorn, M., & Heflin, L. J. (2010). Using self-monitoring to increase attending to task and academic accuracy in children with autism. *Focus on Autism and Other Developmental Disabilities, 25*(4), 230–238. https://doi.org/10.1177/1088357610380137

Hughes, C., & Lloyd, J. W. (1993). An analysis of self-management. *Journal of Behavioral Education, 3*(4), 405–425.

Jones, R. T., Nelson, R. E., & Kazdin, A. E. (1977). The role of external variables in self-reinforcement: A review. *Behavior Modification, 1*(2), 147–178. https://doi.org/10.1177/014544557712001

Koegel, L., Koegel, R., Hurley, C., & Frea William. (1992). Improving social skills and disruptive behavior in children with autism through self-management. *Journal of Applied Behavior Analysis, 25*(2), 341–353.

Koegel, L. K., Park, M. N., & Koegel, R. L. (2014). Using self-management to improve the reciprocal social conversation of children with autism spectrum disorder. *Journal of Autism and Developmental Disorders, 44*(5), 1055–1063. https://doi.org/10.1007/s10803-013-1956-y

Koegel, R. L., & Koegel, L. K. (1990). Extended reductions in stereotypic behavior of students with autism through a self-management treatment package. *Journal of Applied Behavior Analysis, 23*(1), 119–127. https://doi.org/10.1901/jaba.1990.23-119

Lee, G. T., Chen, J., Xu, S., Feng, H., & Guo, Z. (2018). Effects of self-monitoring intervention on independent completion of a daily living skill for children with autism spectrum disorders in China. *Child and Family Behavior Therapy, 40*(2), 148–165. https://doi.org/10.1080/07317107.2018.1477352

Lee, S. H., Simpson, R. L., & Shogren, K. A. (2007). Effects and implications of self-management for students with autism: A meta-analysis. *Focus on Autism and Other Developmental Disabilities, 22*(1), 2–13. https://doi.org/10.1177/10883576070220010101

Lin, C. E., & Koegel, R. (2018). Treatment for higher-order restricted repetitive behaviors (H-RRB) in children with autism spectrum disorder. *Journal of Autism and Developmental Disorders, 48*(11), 3831–3845. https://doi.org/10.1007/s10803-018-3637-3

Liu, Y., Moore, D. W., & Anderson, A. (2015). Improving social skills in a child with autism spectrum disorder through self-management training. *Behaviour Change, 32*(4), 273–284. https://doi.org/10.1017/bec.2015.14

Maag, J. W. (2016). *Behavior management: From theoretical implications to practical applications* (3rd ed.). Boston: Cengage Learning.

Mancina, C., Tankersley, M., Kamps, D., Kravits, T., & Parrett, J. (2000). Brief report: Reduction of inappropriate vocalizations for a child with autism using a self-management treatment program. *Journal of Autism and Developmental Disorders, 30*(6), 599–606.

Moore, D. W., Anderson, A., Glassenbury, M., Lang, R., & Didden, R. (2013). Increasing on-task behavior in students in a regular classroom: effectiveness of a self-management procedure using a tactile prompt. *Journal of Behavioral Education, 22*(4), 302–311. https://doi.org/10.1007/s10864-013-9180-6

National Autism Center. (2015). *Findings and conclusions: National standards project, phase 2*. Randolph, MA: Author.

Newman, B., Reinecke, D. R., & Meinberg, D. L. (2000). Self-management of varied responding in three students with autism. *Behavioral Interventions, 15*(2), 145–151. https://doi.org/10.1002/(SICI)1099-078X(200004/06)15:2<145:AID-BIN50>3.0.CO;2-3

Pierce, K. L., & Schreibman, L. (1994). Teaching daily living skills to children with autism in unsupervised settings through pictorial self-management. *Journal of Applied Behavior Analysis, 27*(3), 471–481. https://doi.org/10.1901/jaba.1994.27-471

Reinecke, D. R., Newman, B., & Meinberg, D. L. (1999). Self-management of sharing in three preschoolers with autism. *Education and Training in Mental Retardation and Developmental Disabilities, 34*(3), 312–317.

Shabani, D. B., Wilder, D. A., & Flood, W. A. (2001). Reducing stereotypic behavior through discrimination training, differential reinforcement of other behavior, and self-monitoring. *Behavioral Interventions, 16*(4), 279–286. https://doi.org/10.1002/bin.96

Simmons, C. A., Ardoin, S. P., Ayres, K. M., & Powell, L. E. (2022). Parent-implemented self- management intervention on the on-task behavior of students with autism. *School Psychology, 37*(3), 273–284. https://doi.org/10.1037/spq0000501

Singh, N. N., Lancioni, G. E., Karazsia, B. T., Myers, R. E., Kim, E., Chan, J., Jackman, M. M., McPherson, C. L., & Janson, M. (2019). Surfing the urge: An informal mindfulness practice for the self-management of aggression by adolescents with autism spectrum disorder. *Journal of Contextual Behavioral Science, 12*, 170–177. https://doi.org/10.1016/j.jcbs.2018.10.003

Singh, N. N., Lancioni, G. E., Manikam, R., Winton, A. S. W., Singh, A. N. A., Singh, J., & Singh, A. D. A. (2011). A mindfulness-based strategy for self-management of aggressive behavior in adolescents with autism. *Research in Autism Spectrum Disorders, 5*(3), 1153–1158. https://doi.org/10.1016/j.rasd.2010.12.012

Singh, N. N., Wahler, R. G., Adkins, A. D., & Myers, R. E. (2003). Soles of the feet: A mindfulness-based self-control intervention for aggression by an individual with mild mental retardation and mental illness. *Research in Developmental Disabilities, 24*(3), 158–169. https://doi.org/10.1016/S0891-4222(03)00026-X

Skinner, B. F. (1953). *Science and human behavior.* New York: Macmillan.

Southall, C. M., & Gast, D. L. (2011). Self-management procedures: A comparison across the autism spectrum. *Education and Training in Autism and Developmental Disabilities, 46*(2), 155–171.

Stahmer, A. C., & Schreibman, L. (1992). Teaching children with autism appropriate play in unsupervised environments using a self-management treatment package. *Journal of Applied Behavior Analysis, 25*(2), 447–459. https://doi.org/10.1901/jaba.1992.25-447

Steinbrenner, J. R., Hume, K., Odom, S. L., Morin, K. L., Nowell, S. W., Tomaszewski, B., Szendrey, S., McIntyre, N.S., Yücesoy-Özkan, S., & Savage, M. N. (2020). *Evidence-based practices for children, youth, and young adults with autism.* The University of North Carolina at Chapel Hill, Frank Porter Graham Child Development Institute, National Clearinghouse on Autism Evidence and Practice Review Team.

Turnbull, H. R., & Turnbull, A. P. (2001). Self-determination for individuals with significant cognitive disabilities and their families. *Journal of the Association for Persons With Severe Handicaps, 26*(1), 56–62. https://doi.org/10.2511/rpsd.26.1.56

Vargas, J. S. (2020). *Behavior analysis for effective teaching* (3rd ed.). New York: Routledge.

Wong, C., Odom, S. L., Hume, K. A., Cox, A. W., Fettig, A., Kucharczyk, S., Brock, M., Plavnik, J. B., Fleury, V. P., & Schultz, T. R. (2015). Evidence-based practices for children, youth, and young adults with autism spectrum disorder: A comprehensive review. *Journal of Autism and Developmental Disorders, 45*(7), 1951–1966. https://doi.org/10.1007/s10803-014-2351-z

11

Functional Communication Training

Jennifer Hamrick
Texas Tech University

Terry S. Falcomata
University of Texas at Austin

11.1 Technical Abstract

Background: Functional communication training (FCT) is a reinforcement-based treatment for problem behavior. The purpose of FCT is to teach individuals appropriate communicative responses to replace problem behavior in their behavioral repertoires. **Method:** We conducted a search of the literature pertaining to FCT via Google Scholar, literature reviews, meta-analyses, and forward citation searches with seminal studies. We considered literature reviews, meta-analyses, clinical case review-based methods, and studies that utilized experimental methodologies, including single-subject designs and randomized clinical trials. **Results:** FCT has been shown to be an effective intervention for a variety of problem behaviors exhibited by individuals with autism spectrum disorder (ASD) across a variety of settings, with the treatment implemented by a variety of individuals. **Discussion:** Strengths of FCT include its conceptual basis in operant mechanisms/principles as well as its focus on communication skills aligning it with diagnostic characteristics of ASD. A weakness includes its susceptibility to treatment relapse in the form of resurgence and renewal. Although studies focusing on mitigating treatment relapse pertaining to FCT are growing, continued future work is needed. **Practitioner recommendations:** Included in the findings below, studies have shown that parents, special educators, and paraprofessionals are able to learn the steps and processes for implementation of FCT in home and school settings. High treatment fidelity is key to the effectiveness of FCT. Findings indicate the use of behavioral skills training (BST) can improve and maintain treatment fidelity across a variety of care providers trained to use FCT with individuals of varied ages and disabilities. By following practice guidelines for FCT, multiple levels of practitioners can implement FCT to decrease problem behaviors for individuals with disabilities.

Jennifer Hamrick, and Terry S. Falcomata, *Functional Communication Training*. In: *Lifespan Treatment for Autistic Individuals*. Edited by: Peter Sturmey, Russell Lang, and James K. Luiselli, Oxford University Press. © Oxford University Press (2025). DOI: 10.1093/oso/9780197635841.003.0011

11.2 Layperson Summary

One of the diagnostic characteristics of ASD includes deficits in social communication skills, and some individuals with ASD can have difficulties communicating their wants and needs. At times, individuals with ASD engage in problem behavior that is reinforced, often inadvertently, by care providers. For example, individuals might engage in problem behavior that results in attention, access to preferred activities, or escape from nonpreferred activities. As a result, the problem behavior is reinforced, maintains, and becomes "communicative" for the individual. The purpose of FCT is to teach individuals appropriate communication skills that allow them to access preferred outcomes. In essence, appropriate communication replaces problem behavior for the individual. Before FCT is conducted, the function(s) of problem behavior (e.g., attention, access to preferred activities; escape) are identified. Next, the individual is taught to use an appropriate communicative response which can consist of a variety of modalities (e.g., sign language; device-based [e.g., iPad] communication applications; communication card exchange system; voice output device; vocal/verbal). Care providers consistently reinforce appropriate communication to strengthen the individual's ability to use the skill to produce preferred outcomes. Alternatively, to the extent possible, the same preferred outcomes are withheld from the individual when problem behavior occurs so as to break the relations between problem behavior and preferred outcomes. Although the formal identification of functions of problem behavior typically requires trained clinicians or educational personnel, FCT can be implemented by a variety of individuals, including parents, other family members, teachers, paraprofessionals, and other relevant care providers. The likely outcome of FCT is a decrease in problem behavior and acquisition of appropriate communication which replaces the problem behavior. Negative side effects can include (a) high rates of communication that can be difficult to honor and (b) unforeseen challenges (e.g., drained iPad battery; misplaced communication materials) that can result in relapse of problem behavior.

11.3 Treatment Summary Table

Treatment summary: Functional Communication Training

Treatment description: FCT teaches communicative responses as an alternative to problem behavior in order for individuals to advocate for their basic needs.

Expected outcomes: Functional and appropriate communication is reinforced while problem behaviors no longer contact reinforcement; therefore, making problem behavior less efficient and, over time, eliminated while communicative attempts increase to access reinforcement.

Methods: While various practice guidelines and recommendations have been published, the primary criteria and recommendations remain consistent:

1. Conduct functional analysis to identify function of problem behavior.
2. Identify the most efficient mode of communication via modality assessment.
3. Teach FCT across multiple opportunities in order to promote rapid acquisition of the identified communicative response.

Expertise required to implement treatment: Additional training in identifying function of the problem behavior prior to intervention is crucial, but actual implementation of FCT is possible from a variety of individuals to include parents, other caretakers, and all levels of educators, including teachers and paraprofessionals.

Risks and negative side effects: While rates or problem behavior typically decreases significantly with continued use of FCT, resurgence of problem behavior does sometimes occur.

Additional considerations and limitations: Generalization of the communicative response across settings and caregivers is crucial for continued reduction of problem behavior. FCT alone may not be effective for everyone, and considerations for including punishing procedures along with FCT may be necessary for some.

11.4 Introduction

11.4.1 Treatment Description

FCT (Carr & Durand, 1985) is an evidence-based treatment approach for problem behavior (Durand, 2012; Durand & Moskowitz, 2015; Gerow et al., 2018a; Hutchins & Prelock, 2014) and among the most common reinforcement-based treatments for problem behavior in the behavioral literature (Tiger et al., 2008). FCT typically consists of a two-step process of (a) identifying the functional reinforcer(s) responsible for the maintenance of problem behavior and then (b) delivering the same class of reinforcement contingent on an appropriate communicative response (Carr & Durand, 1985). The first step involves the assessment of problem behavior to identify why the individual is engaging in problem behavior (i.e., what positive outcomes are produced as a result of engagement in problem behavior?). Said another way, the goal of assessment is to identify the function of problem behavior. Assessments methods can include direct experimental procedures such as functional analysis (FA; e.g., analogue FA, Iwata et al., 1994; brief FA, Northup et al., 1991; trial-based FA, LaRue et al., 2010) and antecedent analysis (e.g., Carr & Durand, 1985); and indirect methods such as interviews (e.g., O'Neill et al., 1997) and rating scales (e.g., Matson & Vollmer, 1995). Problem behavior can function to produce a variety of preferred outcomes (i.e., reinforcement) for individuals who engage in the behavior, including attention, access to preferred items, escape from nonpreferred items, and access to stereotypy.

The second step, following the identification of the function(s) of problem behavior, involves training the individual to utilize an appropriate communication response (e.g., manual sign; card exchange; device-based communication application; vocal/verbal; voice-output device) to access the same positive outcomes (i.e., reinforcers) that were previously produced by problem behavior. Thus, FCT is implemented with the purpose of replacing problem behavior with appropriate communication within the individual's behavioral repertoire. In addition to training and reinforcing appropriate communicative responses, FCT typically also involves the withholding of the identified functional reinforcers when problem behavior occurs (i.e., extinction). Subsequently, as appropriate communication is reinforced and problem behaviors no longer produce reinforcement, (a) appropriate communication is strengthened, (b) the relation between problem behavior and reinforcement is weakened, and (c) over time, problem behavior is eliminated.

11.4.2 Rationale and Objectives

Although it is not one of the core diagnostic features of ASD according to the *Diagnostic and Statistical Manual of Mental Disorders*, 5th ed. (*DSM-5*; American Psychiatric Association, 2013), many individuals with ASD exhibit problem behavior. In general, individuals with disabilities are significantly more likely to exhibit problem behavior than their neurotypical peers (e.g., Alimovic, 2013; Lowe et al., 2007; Matson et al., 2009) with rates among individuals with intellectual disability reported to be as high as 52% of individuals demonstrating some form of problem behavior (Dworschak et al., 2016). With regard to ASD specifically, research has shown prevalence rates of problem behavior among individuals with ASD as high as 94% of individuals demonstrating some form of problem behavior (Matson et al., 2009). Problem behaviors exhibited by individuals with ASD can include a range of behaviors on a continuum of severity, including self-injurious behavior (SIB), aggression, pica (i.e., the ingestion of inedible objects), coprophagia (ingestion of feces), elopement, property destruction at the more severe end of the continuum; and tantrums, noncompliance, off-task behavior, and inappropriate vocalizations at the relatively less severe end of the continuum. Engagement in problem behavior can produce a variety of negative side effects for the individuals who display the behaviors as well as their families and other care providers (e.g., educational personnel), including health risks to the individual (in the case of SIB, pica, coprophagia), family members, and peers (in the case of aggression); social isolation for the individual and the individual's family; restriction from educational, social, and vocational skills programming, which can result in further enhancement of skills deficits across domains; and social stigmatism of the individual and family. Thus, there is often a significant need for effective treatments for problem behavior.

The core features of ASD and the functional approach to problem behavior. FCT is based on several conceptualizations, including an assumption regarding the *functional* nature of problem behavior. As mentioned above, problem behavior is not a core feature of ASD. However, it may be considered a secondary feature of the disorder because of the relation between problem behavior and the core features of ASD. Specifically, one of the core features of ASD is communication deficits. Despite experiencing communication skill deficits, individuals with ASD have wants and needs just as their neurotypical peers do. Unfortunately, however, individuals with ASD often struggle to express their wants and needs due to deficits in communication skills. As a result, individuals with ASD learn, via interactions with individuals in their environment, alternative means of communication to obtain wants and needs. To illustrate, consider a 4-year-old child with ASD and limited communicative skills who is motivated to obtain attention from her mother or father. However, the child does not have the skills to request attention from a parent. Over time, however, the child learns that if she engages in problem behavior (e.g., SIB; tantrum behavior), it reliably produces attention from her parents. This can happen naturally as her parents may intervene upon problem behavior in ways that are "natural" to them (e.g., comforting a child that is demonstrating distress in the form of SIB or tantrum behavior to alleviate the distress). Unfortunately, a direct effect of the parents' response is that problem behavior is reinforced with attention, strengthened over time, and comes to serve the function of producing attention for the child. Said another way, the problem behavior is now *communicative* in that the child, who is experiencing communication skills deficits (a core feature of ASD), has learned to use problem behavior as an alternative means of communication. Thus, although not a core feature of ASD, problem behavior emerges and maintains as a direct result of one of the core features of ASD. In addition to attention, other functions of problem behavior can include access to preferred items (i.e., tangible function), escape from non-preferred activities, and access to stereotypy. The functional conceptualization of problem behavior rejects the notion that the behavior occurs as a result of a particular disorder in favor of one characterized by a "purposeful" nature of problem behavior (Carr, 1994). As Wacker et al. (1996) stated, "rather than attributing the behavior to the child's mental retardation, diagnostic group, or home life, we define behavior as occurring in response to specific events in the child's environment; that is, the behavior serves a purpose or has a function for the child" (p. 328).

Operant learning theory, problem behavior, and ASD. The function-based approach to problem behavior exhibited by individuals with ASD is grounded in operant learning theory. Operant conditioning is the process through which behavior and the environment interact to shape the behavior and behavioral repertoire of an individual or other organism (Skinner, 1953). Applied behavior analysis (ABA), one of the three branches of the discipline of behavior analysis (with the other two being behaviorism [i.e., the philosophical focus behavior analysis; e.g., radical behaviorism, Chiesa, 1994]) and basic experimental analysis of behavior [EAB]), focuses on functional relations between environment-based variables and socially relevant behaviors (Roane & Betz, 2012). More specifically, ABA involves the application of behavioral principles and mechanisms (e.g., positive reinforcement; negative reinforcement; stimulus control) to social relevant issues.

Reinforcement is a basic component of operant conditioning (Skinner, 1953) and has been characterized as the most vital principle of behavior in terms of applied behavioral programming (Cooper et al., 2007; Roane & Betz, 2012). The two types of reinforcement, positive and negative, are distinct in terms of their inherent mechanisms of action.

Positive reinforcement can be determined to have occurred if the presentation of a stimulus following a behavior increases the likelihood that the behavior will occur in the future (Skinner, 1953). For example, if an individual requests access to a leisure item and a care provider immediately provides the individual with the item following the request, the future probability that the individual will request access to the item in the future increases; therefore, positive reinforcement has occurred. For individuals with ASD, positive reinforcers can include attention, access to preferred items, and access to preferred edibles. Negative reinforcement can be determined to have occurred if the removal of a stimulus following a behavior increases the likelihood that the behavior will occur in the future (Skinner, 1953). For example, if an individual asks for a break from a task and the individual's care provider immediately honors the request and provides a break, the future probability that the individual will request a break in the future increases; therefore, negative reinforcement has occurred. For individuals with ASD, negative reinforcers can include escape from nonpreferred activities such as self-care tasks (e.g., tooth brushing); academic, social, or vocational skill acquisition programming; and other aversive events.

Problem behavior exhibited by individuals with ASD is often occasioned by deprivation from a preferred outcome (i.e., establishing operations; e.g., diverted attention; restricted access to preferred items; presentations of nonpreferred activities) and subsequently maintained by access to those same preferred outcomes (i.e., reinforcement). In this way, the occurrence of problem behavior is a byproduct of a combination of (a) communication deficits implicit to ASD (i.e., as a core diagnostic feature of the disorder) and (b) interaction between problem behavior and environmental variables (i.e., deprivation from preferred outcomes; access to preferred outcomes contingent on problem behavior). In other words, the core features of ASD and naturally occurring behavioral phenomena (i.e., deprivation; reinforcement) interact to produce and maintain problem behavior exhibited by individuals with ASD. It should be noted that in addition to positive and negative reinforcement, there are numerous other behavioral mechanisms (e.g., stimulus control; punishment; schedules of reinforcement) that play a role in the occurrence of problem behavior and FCT; however, a full discussion of these mechanisms is beyond the scope of the current chapter.

11.4.3 Considerations for Implementation

In their seminal study on FCT, Carr and Durand (1985) treated the severe problem behavior exhibited by four children with developmental disabilities. An antecedent assessment was conducted with each child to identify conditions that were associated with the occurrence of problem behavior. The results of the assessment suggested that for one child, restricted teacher attention was associated with the occurrence of problem behavior. For two children, the results suggested that work situations were associated with the occurrence of severe problem behavior. For the fourth child, the results suggested that problem behavior was associated with both restricted teacher attention and work. For the children whose behavior was associated with restricted teacher attention, a communicative response was taught (i.e., "Am I doing good work?") that resulted in teacher attention. For the children whose behavior was correlated with work situations, a communicative response was taught ("I don't understand") that resulted in teacher assistance. Each of the children successfully acquired and exhibited the communicative responses, and each displayed substantially reduced problem behavior.

Typically, when FCT is utilized, an antecedent (e.g., Carr & Durand, 1985) or functional (e.g., Iwata et al., 1994; Northup et al., 1991) analysis is first conducted to identify the variable(s) that are occasioning and maintaining problem behavior. An appropriate communicative response (e.g., signs, card exchange, voice output device activation), or function-based communicative response (FCR), is then taught, permitting the individual to access the functional reinforcer via communication; and problem behavior is placed on extinction (e.g., Fisher et al., 1993; Hagopian et al., 1998); punished (e.g., Wacker et al., 1990); or reinforced but in ways that are distinct from how FCRs are reinforced (e.g., schedule of reinforcement, quality of reinforcement, delay to reinforcement, magnitude of reinforcement; e.g., Athens & Vollmer, 2010; Davis et al., 2012; Worsdell et al., 2000).

The initial studies of FCT (e.g., Carr & Durand, 1985; Durand & Carr, 1991, 1992; Wacker et al., 1990), or first-generation FCT studies, demonstrated that the procedures would effectively reduce problem behavior by replacing it with FCRs. Studies published during the subsequent three decades have demonstrated the effectiveness of FCT across subgroups (e.g., Hagopian et al. 1998; Kurtz et al. 2003), topographies of behavior (e.g., Derby et al., 1997; Hagopian et al. 1998; Kurtz et al., 2003), and settings (e.g., Wacker et al., 2005). Second-generation FCT studies, also published during the subsequent three decades, have evaluated different components and parameters associated with FCT to determine their influence on the effects of the treatment. For example, studies have evaluated aspects of the FCR itself (e.g., Bailey et al., 2002; Buckley & Newchok, 2005; Falcomata et al., 2018; Horner & Day, 1991; Horner et al., 1990; Ringdahl et al., 2009; Winborn et al., 2002) and specific consequences (e.g., Athens & Vollmer, 2010; Davis et al., 2012; Fisher et al., 1993; Hagopian et al., 1998; Wacker et al., 1990; Worsdell et al., 2000) incorporated into the treatment package. Other second-generation FCT studies have investigated generalization and maintenance of FCT treatment effects (e.g., Berg et al., 2007; Falcomata & Wacker, 2013; Lambert et al., 2015; Neely et al., 2018; Wacker et al., 2005), clinical relapse pertaining to problem behavior during FCT and potential methods for preventing relapse (e.g., Berg et al., 2015; Hoffman & Falcomata, 2014; Radhakrishnan et al., 2020; Ringdahl et al., 2018; Wacker et al., 2011), and telehealth-based delivery formats for aspects of the treatment (e.g., Gerow et al., 2021; Lindgren et al., 2016; Lindgren et al., 2020; Machalicek et al., 2016; Unholz et al., 2020).

FCR-based variables. Relative to the FCR component, several variables have been shown to impact FCT. These include response effort (e.g., Bailey et al., 2002; Buckley & Newchok, 2005; Horner & Day, 1991; Horner et al., 1990), novelty of FCRs (Winborn et al., 2002), and the proficiency with which individuals can utilize respective FCR modalities (e.g., Falcomata et al., 2018; Ringdahl et al., 2009). Other FCR-related variables that have been shown to impact FCT include preference for FCRs (e.g., Kunnavatana et al., 2018; Ringdahl et al., 2016; Torelli et al., 2016), variability across FCRs (e.g., Adami et al., 2017; Falcomata et al., 2018; Muething et al., 2018), and the complexity of the FCR (e.g., Ghaemmaghami et al., 2018; Randall et al., 2021). Overall, studies focusing on FCR-based variables have shown that practitioners should consider a variety of factors when selecting FCRs to target during FCT both in terms of modality and number for inclusion.

Consequence-based variables. With regard to consequence-based variables, the presence of reductive components such as extinction (Day et al., 1994; Durand, 1999; Hagopian et al., 1998; Wacker et al., 1990) and punishment (Fisher et al., 1993; Hagopian et al., 1998; Wacker et al., 1990) have been shown, at times, to be necessary to the effectiveness of FCT. Other studies have shown that extinction and/or punishment may not be necessary, at times, when reinforcement-based variables associated with FCRs and problem behavior are modified to favor FCRs. Such modifications have included schedules of reinforcement (e.g., Rooker et al., 2013; Worsdell et al., 2000); magnitude of reinforcement (e.g., Davis et al., 2012); and quality, delay, duration, or a combination of other reinforcement-based variables (Athens & Vollmer, 2010). Taken together, previous studies focusing on consequence-based variables suggest that decisions regarding the application of consequences should be determined on an individual basis based on assessment and ongoing evaluation of response to treatment.

Generalization and maintenance. Studies have shown that FCT can produce stimulus generalization across different stimulus conditions, including settings, tasks, and people (Falcomata & Wacker, 2013; Neely et al., 2018). Although generalization of FCT effects can occur without additional programming (e.g., Moes & Frea, 2002), studies have shown that generalization should not be assumed following FCT (e.g., Schindler & Horner, 2005). Thus, researchers have evaluated the use of specific tactics to program specifically for generalization (Stokes & Baer, 1977; Stokes & Osnes, 1989) of FCT treatment effects (in addition to the tactic of recruiting natural consequences inherent to FCT; Falcomata & Wacker, 2013). Stokes and Osnes (1989) described three general principles of generalization with related tactics that have been applied effectively to FCT. *Exploitation of current functional contingencies* includes tactics that have been effectively applied to FCT, including (a) recruiting natural consequences (Moes & Frea, 2002); (b) modifying maladaptive consequences (e.g., Wacker et al., 2005); and (c) contact natural consequences and reinforcement of occurrences of generalization (e.g., Schindler & Horner, 2005). *Training diversely* includes tactics that have been effectively applied to FCT, including (a) use of sufficient stimulus exemplars (e.g., Wacker et al., 2005) and (b) the use of sufficient response exemplars (e.g., Dyches et al., 2002). Last, *incorporating functional mediators* includes tactics that been effectively applied to FCT, including the (a) incorporation of comment salient physical stimuli (e.g., Durand, 1999; Falcomata et al., 2010) and (b) incorporation of common salient social stimuli (Durand & Carr, 1991). Overall, studies focusing on generalization and maintenance of FCT treatment effects have shown that although the treatment can result in generalized effects, additional programmed tactics may be necessary to produce positive outcomes across stimuli and time. A variety of tactics have been shown to be effective in producing generalization and maintenance.

Relapse/resurgence. Studies have shown that relapse of problem behavior can occur during and subsequent to FCT (e.g., Radhakrishnan et al., 2020; Volkert et al., 2009) in the form of resurgence (i.e., the recovery of a previously reinforced and extinguished response during extinction of a second previously reinforced response [Epstein, 1983]). For example, Volkert et al. (2009) demonstrated resurgence of problem behavior when trained FCRs were placed on extinction following FCT showing how clinical relapse in the form of problem behavior can occur as a result of a challenge to treatment (e.g., extinction of FCRs during FCT; Wacker et al., 2011). Thus, researchers have evaluated potential methods for preventing or delaying resurgence of problem behavior. Procedures aimed at preventing or delaying resurgence during and following FCT have included training multiple modalities of FCRs (e.g., Berg et al., 2015; Falcomata et al., 2018; Hoffman & Falcomata, 2014; Lambert et al., 2015), FCR fading (e.g., Wacker et al., 2011, 2013b), programming for the presence of FCRs (e.g., Wacker et al., 2013b), modifying baseline schedules of reinforcement (e.g., Fisher et al., 2019), language-based factors (e.g., Neely et al., 2020; Padilla Dalmau et al., 2011), and prior contact with extinction (e.g., Wacker et al., 2011). Taken together, the still-emerging literature pertaining to FCT and clinical relapse has shown that (a) the treatment can be susceptible to resurgence and (b) modifications to the basic FCT arrangement can be made that can mitigate resurgence.

Telehealth. The last 10 years have seen significant growth in the area of telehealth (i.e., telepractice; telemedicine) as a delivery model for FCT. Wacker and colleagues first showed that parents, while being coached via telehealth by ABA consultants, could successfully implement assessment and treatment procedures in their home including (a) FA of problem behavior (Wacker et al., 2013a) and

(b) FCT based on the results of the FA (Wacker et al., 2013b). Subsequent to their seminal papers, Wacker and colleagues, as well as researchers from other sites, have conducted studies of different aspects of telehealth-based FCT, including additional demonstration studies (e.g., Lindgren et al., 2016, 2020; Machalicek et al., 2016), evaluations of treatment fidelity of care provider-implemented FCT (e.g., Suess et al., 2014), and comparative evaluations focusing on cost per model (e.g., Lindgren et al., 2016). Taken together, studies of telehealth-based FCT have shown that (a) care providers can successfully implement the treatment when coached via telehealth by behavioral consultants resulting in reductions of problem behavior exhibited by individuals with ASD, (b) care providers can implement the treatment with high fidelity via this model, and (c) telehealth-based models (i.e., in-home telehealth; clinic-based telehealth) can be cost-effective relative to alternative models (e.g., in-home therapy).

11.5 Research Background

Numerous systematic reviews and meta-analyses have focused on different aspects of FCT, including (a) general treatment effects pertaining to different populations (e.g., Gerow et al., 2018a; Gregori et al., 2020; Heath et al., 2015; Luo et al., 2019; Mancil, 2006); (b) generalization and maintenance of treatment effects (e.g., Falcomata & Wacker, 2013; Neely et al., 2018); (c) evaluations of resurgence following FCT (Radhakrishnan et al., 2020); (d) the effects of parent-implemented FCT (Gerow et al., 2018b); (e) telehealth-based delivery of the treatment (Schieltz & Wacker, 2020; Simacek et al., 2021; Sutherland et al., 2018); and (f) procedures for training tolerance of delay-to-reinforcement and reinforcement schedule thinning (Hagopian et al., 2011). Below, we describe and summarize treatment outcomes, quality of research, and evidence pertaining to the effects of FCT across specific areas and aspects of the treatment as indicated by topic-specific reviews of the literature and meta-analyses.

11.5.1 FCT Treatment Effects and Population-Specific Findings

Several literature reviews and meta-analyses have been conducted that have examined the overall effects of FCT as well as the treatment's effects pertaining to specific populations. These include evaluations of the overall effects of FCT (Gerow et al., 2018b; Heath et al., 2015; Kurtz et al., 2011; Mancil, 2006) as well as evaluations with specific foci on adult populations (Gregori et al., 2020), early childhood (Luo et al., 2019), and children with ASD diagnoses (Mancil, 2006).

Overall effects of FCT: Existing evidence. Several reviews of the literature have determined that the evidence supporting FCT as an evidence-based practice is clear and exceeds criteria for categorization as an evidence-based treatment (e.g.,

Gerow et al., 2018; Kurtz et al., 2011; Steinbrenner et al., 2020). Gerow et al. (2018) conducted a systematic review of the literature pertaining to the overall effects of FCT on problem behavior exhibited by individuals diagnosed with disabilities and including an evaluation of strength of the evidence based on the What Works Clearinghouse (WWC; 2017) design and evidence standards. Gerow et al. identified 215 studies that contained 482 individual experiments. The authors rated 78 experiments as *meets standards*, 135 as *meets standards with reservations*, and 269 as *does not meet standards*. The authors reviewed and rated, using visual analysis, the results of the 212 experiments that they rated as *meets standards* or *meets standards with reservations*. Gerow et al. rated 64% (*n* =135) of the 212 experiments as providing *strong* or *moderate evidence* (i.e., 62% [*n* =132] were rated as having *strong evidence*; 1% [*n* = 3] were rated as having *moderate evidence*). The authors rated the remaining 36% (*n* = 77) as having *no evidence*. With regard to their evaluation of the extent to which FCT meets the definition for an evidence-based practice (20 or more participants across five or more articles and across three or more research teams) across disability categories, Gerow et al. determined that "FCT was considered an evidence-based practice for individuals with ASD, intellectual disability (ID), other health impairments, and multiple disabilities" (p. 96). Specifically, all four disability categories included 20 or more participants (i.e., ASD = 77 participants; intellectual disability = 55 participants; other health impairments = 20 participants; multiple disabilities = 56 participants; Gerow et al., 2018).

The results of Gerow et al. were consistent with other findings determining FCT to be an evidence-based practice (e.g., Kurtz et al., 2011; Steinbrenner et al., 2020). For example, Steinbrenner et al. (2020) and the Frank Porter Graham Institute at the University of North Carolina identified evidence-based practices to address problem behavior exhibited by individuals with ASD. Based on their review of the published literature, Steinbrenner et al. (2020) identified FCT as an evidence-based practice. Additionally, Kurtz et al. (2011) conducted a review of the literature to determine the extent to which evidence supporting FCT met criteria for *empirically supported treatments* (Kratochwill & Stoiber, 2002; Task Force, 1995) with individuals with ID and ASD. Similar to Gerow et al., Kurtz et al. revealed evidence that showed "that there is sufficient empirical support to characterize FCT as a well-established treatment for a range of problem behavior exhibited by persons with ID" (p. 2940), and "in fact, 28 studies of sufficient quality were identified, far exceeding the criteria needed to characterize an intervention as well established. In particular, it is a *well-established* treatment for children and adolescents with ID, and individuals with ASD. FCT with adults (over 18) can be categorized as *probably efficacious*" (p. 2940).

Extending Kurtz et al.'s (2011) findings specific to adult populations, Gregori et al. (2020) conducted a systematic review and quality appraisal of the evidence pertaining to FCT as a treatment for problem behavior exhibited by adults with ASD. Gregori et al. identified and synthesized 20 studies and evaluated them using the WWC design and evidence standards. Based on the WWC standards, the results showed that eight experiments were found to entail *moderate* or *strong* evidence of effectiveness. Thus, the authors asserted that their results suggested that the literature "provided some evidence for the efficacy of FCT in reducing challenging behavior for adults with ASD, but additional research in this area is warranted" (p. 1). Of note, Gregori et al. reported that the most common issue that resulted in the failure of studies to meet standards was the number of data points included across phases (i.e., WWC DS 3; "a minimum of three attempts were made to demonstrate an intervention effect between baseline and intervention at three different points in time"). It should be noted that WWC DS 3 ("a minimum of three attempts were made to demonstrate an intervention effect between baseline and intervention at three different points in time") does not indicate whether experimental control has been established via the control of threats to internal validity and demonstration of functional relations. Specifically, the presence of a "minimum of three attempts to demonstrate an intervention effect" is not pertinent to the demonstration of prediction, verification, and replication, which are the actual standards in terms of logic and rationale for demonstrating effects using single-subject design methodologies rather than the arbitrarily determined "three effects" standard. Specifically, experimental control, the control for threats to internal validity, and the demonstration of functional relations can be demonstrated without "a minimum of three attempts to demonstrate an intervention effect." For example, three studies (i.e., Ghaemmaghami et al., 2016; Langdon et al., 2008; Petursson & Eldevik, 2018) that appeared in Gregori et al. demonstrated prediction, verification, and replication (i.e., experimental control) using designs that did not entail "three demonstrations of effects." Ghaemmaghami et al. (2016) and Petursson and Eldevik (2018) utilized a BAB design; or BAB design logic (i.e., the last three phases of Petursson & Eldevik, 2018). Langdon et al. (2008) utilized a two-tier multiple-baseline design. Both the BAB and two-tier multiple baseline design allow for the demonstration of prediction, verification, and replication elements; and, subsequently, the demonstration of functional relations and experimental control. Thus, the lower rating of certain studies in Gregori et al. that demonstrated functional relations between FCT and positive outcomes pertaining to problem behavior should be interpreted with caution.

In another population-specific study, Luo et al. (2019) conducted a systematic review and quality appraisal of the evidence pertaining to FCT as a treatment for problem behavior exhibited by children in early care and educational settings. Luo et al. identified 20 studies and, similar to Gregori et al. (2020), evaluated the studies using the WWC standards. In addition, the authors calculated effect sizes using nonoverlapping data and Tau-U statistical analysis procedures. Although Luo et al. found strong effects via statistical analysis, their evaluation via the WWC standards suggested that the strength of evidence based on the 20 studies was not strong. Specifically, the authors found that none of the 20 studies were rated as *Meets Design Standards without Reservations* while eight and 12 studies were rated as *Meets Design Standards with Reservations* and *Does Not Meet Design Standards*, respectively. Luo et al. used visual analysis to evaluate the effects demonstrated in the 8 studies rated as *Meets Design Standards with Reservations. Strong evidence* was determined with 3 studies and *moderate evidence* with 1. The 6 studies were rated as having *no evidence*. It should be noted that several studies were rated twice because they included multiple applications or experiments (i.e., Radstaake et al., 2013; Volkert et al., 2009). It should also be noted that functional relations were demonstrated between the independent and dependent variables via prediction, verification, and replication with several of the studies that were rated as having *no evidence* (e.g., Durand, 1993; Lambert et al., 2012); and these studies had sufficient interobserver agreement (IOA) to demonstrate reliability of measurement. In addition, several studies that were not included in the final analysis because of low WWC-based ratings also demonstrated experimental control/functional relations via prediction, verification, and replication with viable designs and sufficient steady-state within-phase data with sufficient IOA (e.g., Langdon et al., 2008; O'Neill & Sweetland-Baker, 2001). Thus, similar to Gregori et al., the restriction of some studies from full analysis because of WWC standards and lower rating of certain studies that demonstrated experimental control and sufficient IOA should be interpreted with caution.

Other general findings and evidence. Heath et al. (2015) conducted a meta-analysis of FCT with a focus on effects pertaining to age, disability, and modality of communication. Heath et al. identified 36 studies that evaluated the effects of FCT on problem behavior exhibited by individuals with disabilities and determined effects via robust improvement rate difference (IRD) effect size. The meta-analysis findings indicated (a) strong overall effects, (b) stronger effects with primary-aged versus elementary-aged individuals, (c) stronger effects with elementary-aged as well as secondary-aged individuals versus adult-aged individuals, (d) no differences between treatment effects with secondary-aged individuals versus primary- and elementary-aged individuals, and (e) better results with individuals with ASD versus intellectual disabilities. Heath et al. also found that stronger effects were found with vocal versus aided augmentative and alternative communication (AAC) and unaided AAC modalities of communication; and stronger effects with aided AAC versus unaided AAC modalities.

11.5.2 Generalization and Maintenance of FCT Treatment Effects

Several previous reviews of the literature have evaluated FCT and tactics for programming maintenance and generalization effects (i.e., Falcomata & Wacker, 2013; Heath et al., 2015; Neely et al., 2018). Falcomata and Wacker (2013) conducted a review of the FCT literature with a specific focus on the principles and tactics for programming for generalization. Using the framework provided by Stokes and Osnes (1989), the authors identified, analyzed, and summarized 10 studies that utilized and specifically evaluated the effects of tactics for programming for generalization during FCT. Falcomata and Wacker found that in addition to the inherent tactic of recruiting natural contingencies, tactics described by Stokes and Osnes that have been evaluated with FCT included training sufficient *stimulus exemplars, modification of maladaptive consequences*, reinforcement of occurrences of generalization, *programming common physical stimuli*, and *programming common social stimuli*. Overall, the results of the studies showed that generalization of FCT treatment effects can be facilitated by specific tactics for programming for generalization. Falcomata and Wacker also found that the tactic of recruiting natural consequences can be sufficient absent other specific tactics; but in some cases, additional tactics are needed. Neely et al. (2018) extended Falcomata and Wacker by conducting a systematic review and synthesis of 37 studies and (a) categorizing and summarizing the tactics for programming for generalization used in the identified studies based on categories described by Stokes and Baer (1977) and Stokes and Osnes (1989) and (b) evaluating the studies using the WWC standards (Kratochwill et al., 2013) with adaptions described by Maggin et al. (2013). Neely et al. found that 30 of the 37 identified studies "met standards or met standards with reservations" (p. 1116). In addition, using standards they developed for use in their review based on existing WWC standards, the authors found that (a) 20 studies met generalization standards, (b) 16 studies met maintenance standards, and (c) only six studies met all maintenance *and* generalization standards (with only four of those demonstrating positive effects). Similar to Falcomata and Wacker, Neely et al. found that of the nine possible tactics and strategies described by Stokes and Baer and Stokes and Osnes, only four were evaluated across the 37 identified studies. including train and hope, sequential modification, programming common stimuli, and training sufficient exemplars. Overall, Neely et al. concluded that limitations of the literature pertaining to FCT and maintenance and generalization included (a) "the rigor of the maintenance and generalization data collected" (p. 127); and (b) the relatively small number of studies that met design standards and the limited number of tactics that have been evaluated. The findings of Neely et al. as well as Falcomata and Wacker suggest that additional research is needed in the area(s) of maintenance and generalization with FCT.

11.5.3 FCT and Resurgence

Resurgence is the recurrence of a previously reinforced behavior during the application of extinction to a second, subsequently reinforced behavior (Epstein, 1983), or the "transient recurrence, with consideration of the stimulus context, of some dimension of previously established but not currently occurring activity when reinforcement conditions of current behavior are worsened" (Lattal et al., 2017, p. 90). Resurgence has been demonstrated across a variety of behaviors, including problem behavior (e.g., Hoffman & Falcomata, 2014; Lieving et al., 2004; Ringdahl et al., 2018; Volkert et al., 2009; Wacker et al., 2011). With regard to FCT, certain challenges to treatment can result in the resurgence of problem behavior (e.g., Volkert et al., 2009; Wacker et al., 2011). Challenges to treatment can occur during FCT when changes in the environment disrupt relations between FCRs and functional reinforcers (e.g., lapses in treatment integrity). Such challenges can include unplanned periods of extinction of FCRs (e.g., augmentative alternative communication [AAC] device malfunction or loss; loss of communication card; unintentional implementation of extinction by caregivers) or delays to reinforcement. When FCRs trained via FCT contact extinction, increases and/or the reemergence (i.e., resurgence) of problem behavior can occur (e.g., Volkert et al., 2009; Wacker et al., 2011). Given the potential susceptibility of FCT to treatment relapse in the form of resurgence, a relatively recent and growing number of studies have sought to evaluate procedures aimed at preventing or mitigating resurgence during FCT. Tactics that have been evaluated have included the use of multiple modalities of communication (e.g., Fuhrman et al., 2022; Hoffman & Falcomata, 2014; Lambert et al., 2015, 2017), stimulus control-based procedures via multiple schedules (e.g., Fisher et al., 2020), modification of reinforcement rates during baseline (e.g., Fisher et al., 2019; Lambert et al., 2020), duration of treatment (e.g., Greer et al., 2020), and the combination of multiple adaptions of FCT (e.g., schedule of reinforcement during baseline and treatment; length of treatment; Fisher et al., 2018).

Several previous reviews of the literature have focused on resurgence of problem behavior during or following FCT (e.g., Kestner & Peterson, 2017; Radhakrishnan et al., 2020). For example, Radhakrishnan et al. (2020) conducted a review of the literature in which they examined studies that evaluated resurgence following FCT. The authors identified 14 studies that met inclusion criteria. Radhakrishnan et al.'s review identified six variables and/or procedures that have been evaluated for their impact on resurgence, including (a) demand fading, (b) language of instruction, (c) the presence stimuli previously paired with treatment, (d) prior exposure to extinction, (e) baseline schedules of reinforcement, and (f) the inclusion of multiple FCRs during treatment. The 14 studies identified by Radhakrishnan et al. included a total of 42 participants. Overall, Radhakrishnan et al. found reliable effects with (a) language of instruction (i.e., participant's first language; Padilla Dalmau et al., 2011) and (b) the presence of stimuli previously paired with treatment (Wacker et al., 2013). The authors found mixed results with regard to other variables/procedures (i.e., prior exposures to extinction; demand fading; baseline schedules of reinforcement). Thus, despite a growing number of studies that have evaluated the effects of a variety of procedures aimed at preventing and/or mitigating resurgence during FCT, Radhakrishnan et al.'s findings suggested that more research is needed in this area.

11.5.4 Parent-Implemented FCT

Given that parents play a prominent role in the lives of many individuals who engage in problem behavior and are tasked with implementing FCT, an emphasis on parent implementation is vital. Several previous literature reviews and syntheses have examined research pertaining to parent-implemented FCT (i.e., Fettig & Barton, 2014; Gerow et al., 2018b). Gerow et al. (2018b) synthesized and evaluated 26 studies that focused on parent-implemented FCT. The 26 studies included a total of 78 parents who implemented FCT with 69 participants. Overall, Gerow et al. found that the results of the 26 studies they reviewed indicated (a) parent-implemented FCT was effective at decreasing problem behavior and (b) maintenance and generalization to novel settings and implementers occurred in some instances. The authors also found that the results of the synthesis indicated that the inclusion of treatment integrity data was limited across the reviewed studies. Further, Gerow et al. found that although FCT was often implemented by "natural change agents in typical settings, parent training is often provided by professionals not typically accessible to parents" (p. 336). Last, they found that parents indicated that FCT was effective, practical, and they were likely to continue using the treatment. Gerow et al. identified several areas pertaining to parent-implemented FCT in need of additional research, including (a) the inclusion of fathers as implementers, (b) evaluations of methods for including parents in the development of FCT procedures, (c) a specific focus on ways to enhance treatment integrity demonstrated by parents, and (d) more research focusing on the inclusion of parent training during clinical services that include FCT.

11.5.5 Telehealth-Based FCT

No previous reviews of the literature have examined telehealth formats with an exclusive focus on FCT. However, several reviews of the literature have evaluated telehealth-based approaches to ABA and/or communication training-based service delivery, including assessment and treatment of problem behavior with subfoci on the effectiveness of FCT (e.g., Schieltz & Wacker, 2020; Simacek et al., 2021; Sutherland et al., 2018). For example, Schieltz and Wacker (2020) conducted a review of the literature pertaining to function-based approaches to assessment and treatment of problem behavior delivered via telehealth formats. The authors reviewed 18 studies that involved telehealth-delivered assessment and treatment procedures. Thirteen of the 18 reviewed studies evaluated a function-based treatment; 12 of those 13 studies utilized FCT as a treatment with a total of approximately 96 participants across a variety of functions. Schieltz and Wacker reported percentage reductions of problem behavior from six of the 12 studies that utilized FCT. The overall mean reduction across the six studies, which included 83 total participants, was 87.2% (range = 65–100%). For the other six studies that utilized FCT, percentage reductions were not reported. However, four of the six reported decreases in problem behavior; one reported treatment failure; and one focused exclusively on parent training with results showing high levels of treatment fidelity demonstrated by the parents. Thus, Schieltz and Wacker found that of 96 participants who were provided with FCT via telehealth format, 98.9% experienced reductions in problem behavior. Overall, Schieltz and Wacker asserted, "the historically positive results reported across research projects at the University of Iowa and across other research groups consistently show that practitioners can provide FA plus FCT via telehealth for most young children with ASD displaying problem behavior. These data suggest that behavior analysts can shift their clinical services that target challenging behavior to a telehealth modality, as is needed and/or desired" (p. 1251). The authors also suggested several factors should be taken into account when practitioners consider transitioning to telehealth-based formats, including technology, ethical considerations, and best-fit service model. Schieltz and Wacker also provided several areas in need of future research, including "caregiver stress, caregiver preference for types of services, stimulus generalization for both caregiver and child behavior, and procedures that best promote generalization" (p. 1253). Last, their review showed that several different models have been used for telehealth-based training which included a variety of components and combinations of components. Thus, Schieltz and Wacker suggested additional research is needed focusing on various training models.

11.5.6 Delay-to-Reinforcement Training and Reinforcement Schedule Thinning

Delay training and/or reinforcement schedule thinning procedures are important to consider when implementing FCT to enhance the likelihood of generalization and maintenance of treatment effects. Specifically, delay training and schedule thinning procedures are intended to (a) prepare individuals for success in the natural environment by promoting their ability to tolerate delays to reinforcement, (b) decrease rates of responding to manageable levels while maintaining reductions in problem behavior, and (c) enhance the "user-friendliness" of the procedures for caregivers in the individual's environment, thereby enhancing treatment fidelity. Several reviews of the literature have examined studies focusing on delay training and/or schedule thinning during/following FCT (e.g., Hagopian et al., 2011). Hagopian et al. (2011) conducted a review of the literature pertaining to reinforcement schedule thinning and discussed commonly used schedule thinning arrangements. The authors identified 76 studies that focused on FCT and were published between 1985 and 2009; 19 of the identified 76 studies included schedule thinning procedures. Hagopian et al. found that across the 19 studies, four arrangements were typically utilized, including (a) delay-to-reinforcement procedures (i.e., delays to reinforcement are implemented following FCRs), (b) chain schedules of reinforcement (i.e., requirements for compliance prior to reinforcement of FCRs are systematically increased), (c) multiple schedules of reinforcement (i.e., periods of reinforcement of FCRs and extinction are signaled and systematic increases in extinction components are implemented), and (d) the restriction of FCR materials for increasing periods of time. Overall, Hagopian et al. found that practical reductions in rates of FCRs can be maintained via schedule thinning procedures while decreased levels of problem behavior are concurrently maintained. The authors also found that (a) in some cases, systematic reductions in reinforcer density for FCRs can result in the recurrence of problem behavior and (b) schedule thinning methods procedures can sometimes benefit from supplemental procedures (e.g., the provision of alternative reinforcers during thinning).

11.6 Practice Implications

11.6.1 Treatment Outcomes

Successful treatment outcomes of FCT are characterized by demonstrations of consistent increases in functional communication and decreases in problem behavior exhibited by the individual (e.g., Carr & Durand, 1985), with outcomes resulting from the proper use of FCT that include long-term maintenance and generalization of treatment effects (Wacker et al., 2011). Numerous studies have demonstrated positive FCT outcomes across a large range of age, demographics, and populations, including multiple disabilities such as (but not limited to) ASD, intellectual disabilities, other health impairments, and individuals with multiple disabilities (e.g., Heath et al., 2015; Luo et al., 2019). FCT has been demonstrated to be effective (a) in combination with extinction as well as punishment procedures (when the results demonstrate the need for a punishment-based component), (b) without the use punishment-based procedures for many individuals, and (c) without, at times, extinction (e.g., Fisher et al., 1993; Gerow et al., 2018b).

There may be times when FCT is contraindicated and the procedures could be ineffective depending on the function(s) of the problem behavior. For example, if an individual exhibits problem behavior that serves more than one function, it may be challenging for care providers to identify the possible function(s) at play during particular instances of problem behavior that occur in naturalistic settings; with subsequent implications for FCT-based teaching procedures during those instances. FCT also requires the individual with problem behavior to learn new FCRs that may, at times, be less efficient and more effortful than engaging in problem behavior. An additional potential limitation pertaining to FCT is clinical relapse in the form of resurgence of problem behavior (i.e., problem behavior may reappear quickly during some treatment conditions when challenges to treatment occur). If and when resurgence does occur, it may indicate low levels of treatment fidelity (e.g., intermittent reinforcement of problem behavior; failure to reinforce FCRs; technical failures) requiring care providers to explore possible sources for the resurgence.

11.6.2 Practice Implication Guidelines

Multiple publications have identified practice guidelines to assist practitioners when implementing FCT with individuals with disabilities (e.g., Dunlap & Duda, 2004; Durand, 1990; Franzone, 2009; Mancil & Boman, 2010; Reichle & Wacker, 2017; Tiger et al., 2008). Each describes processes and considerations for use of FCT to reduce problem behavior. Taken together, along with the wider findings of studies that comprise the FCT literature, they indicate that the basic implementation procedures consist of the following steps:

Step 1: Functional Behavioral Assessment

The defining characteristic of FCT that distinguishes it from typical language- and communication-based skill acquisition programming is that a communicative response is specifically taught to serve as an alternative to or replace a functionally equivalent problem behavior. In other words, when (a) the function of the problem behavior has been identified, (b) an alternative functionally equivalent FCR is designated, and (c) the FCR is taught using practice guidelines for FCT, substantial reductions of the problem behavior should occur. Therefore, the procedures for FCT should be individualized to clients based on the results of their functional behavioral assessments (FBA). Thus, prior to development of an individualized plan for FCT, an FBA of problem behavior must be completed to determine its function. FBAs are typically completed via direct (e.g., functional analysis; naturalistic observations; assessment of antecedents, behaviors, and consequences) and indirect (e.g., interviews; rating scales) assessment of environmental contingencies that occasion and maintain problem behavior. Individual training for the implementation of FBA procedures is crucial for correctly identifying the function(s) of problem behavior. That said, research has shown that a variety of individuals ranging from parents to all levels of educators can be trained to conduct such assessments (e.g., Bloom et al., 2013; Wacker et al., 2011).

Step 2: Identifying FCRs

When the function of the problem behavior has been identified, determining the most appropriate FCR is critical. There are several considerations when determining the modality of communication to target during FCT to replace problem behavior. When determining which modality of communication will be utilized during FCT, considerations should include the individual's current communication abilities, or skill levels. If they have no or limited vocal communication skills, alternative modalities of communication should be considered (e.g., picture exchange, manual sign, device-based communication system, voice output device). Pre-FCT assessment of proficiency with which individuals can utilize different modalities of communication may be beneficial (see Ringdahl et al., 2009; Falcomata et al., 2017; and Reichle & Wacker, 2017 for additional information for conducting modality proficiency assessment). FCT has been shown to be effective across a variety of FCRs, including vocal responses, sign language, picture exchange, and alternative communication devices (Durand & Moskowitz, 2015). Not only will identifying and using the most proficient communicative response increase the probability of communication by the individual, it should also increase the likelihood that others in the individual's natural settings will understand the response, and thereby facilitate generalization. At a minimum, the extent to which FCRs are more or less effortful to exhibit than problem behavior should be considered (see Horner & Day, 1991 for further discussion).

Step 3: Teaching the FCR and Implementing FCT

Crucial considerations regarding the teaching of FCRs include (a) the development of a detailed plan and protocol for implementation, (b) identification of care providers who will be responsible for implementing teaching/practice trials (i.e., designated time blocks during the individual's day in which FCT is conducted), (c) determination of settings in which FCT will be initially introduced (i.e., controlled/analogue vs. natural setting), (d) the protocol for responding if the individual demonstrates problem behavior during FCT (e.g., extinction, blocking), (e) an emphasis on seeking opportunities to implement training trials during naturally occurring situations and reinforcement of FCRs outside of the teaching/practice trials (i.e., to actively program for generalization via promotion and reinforcement of FCRs throughout the day), (f) determination of data collection procedures for both problem behavior and FCRs that inform intervention decisions (e.g., treatment modification; reinforcement schedule thinning; delay fading), and (g) actively planning for generalization across people and settings.

The programming of multiple opportunities for the individual to utilize the FCR throughout the day is an important consideration. Arranging and facilitating situations that would typically evoke problem behavior to provide learning opportunities to prompt use of the FCRs (and subsequent reinforcement of the FCR) will strengthen the FCR response in the individual's repertoire. For example, if it has been determined that the function of the student's problem behavior is escape from nonpreferred academic tasks (e.g., math), the educator may start by presenting math activities more often to prompt the individual to request breaks via the FCR.

11.6.3 Other Considerations

What if the communicative response does not align with speech pathology recommendations and/or preferred communication caretakers? The ultimate goal of FCT is the reduction of problem behavior. Often times, when working with an individual with limited vocal communication, the most efficient and effective FCR for implementation during FCT will align with current communication goals. However, there may be times when the most efficient means to reduce problem behavior will take a different form or response than what has been utilized for typical communication. Collaboration with speech pathologists when assessing and determining the most efficient means of communication to reduce problem behavior is crucial (LaRue et al., 2009).

Are there any negative side effects to FCT? Depending on an individual's history of reinforcement, "extinction bursts" may occur during FCT. Specifically, when reinforcement is withheld following instances of reinforcement, escalation in rate and severity of behavior can occur. It is important that care providers be aware, prior to the implementation of FCT, that such bursts are possible. Being aware that bursts may occur will, ideally, prevent care providers from abandoning the treatment because of perceptions that it is failing. The possibility that extinction bursts might occur should not hinder the use of FCT; rather, it should emphasize considerations on how to properly respond to bursts of problem behavior when they occur, including the identification of safety measures and training of care providers on those measures.

What if it does not appear to be working? As with all evidence-based interventions, program decisions and planning should be based assessment of ongoing data. If the data indicate that the intervention is not effective, it may be necessary to reevaluate the FBA (to ensure the correct function has been identified), training procedures, and/or treatment protocol. It is also vital that treatment integrity/fidelity be assessed on an ongoing basis to ensure that those responsible for the intervention are implementing it as intended (see also Durand, 1990).

11.7 References

Adami, S., Falcomata, T. S., Muething, C. S., & Hoffman, K. (2017). An evaluation of lag schedules of reinforcement during functional communication training: Effects on varied mand responding and challenging behavior. *Behavior Analysis in Practice, 10*(3), 209–213. https://doi.org/10.1007/s40617-017-0179-7

Alimovic, S. (2013). Emotional and behavioural problems in children with visual impairment, intellectual and multiple disabilities. *Journal of Intellectual Disability Research, 57*(2), 153–160. https://doi.org/10.1111/j.1365-2788.2012.01562.x

American Psychiatric Association. (2013). *Diagnostic and statistical manual of mental disorders* (5th ed.). Washington, DC: Author. https://doi.org/10.1176/appi.books.9780890425596

Athens, E. S., & Vollmer, T. R. (2010). An investigation of differential reinforcement of alternative behavior without extinction. *Journal of Applied Behavior Analysis, 43*(4), 569–589. https://doi.org/10.1901/jaba.2010.43-569

Bailey, J., McComas, J. J., Benavides, C., & Lovascz, C. (2002). Functional assessment in a residential setting: Identifying an effective communicative replacement response for aggressive behavior. *Journal of Developmental and Physical Disabilities, 14*(4), 353–369. https://doi.org/10.1023/A:1020382819146

Berg, W. K., Ringdahl, J. E., Ryan, S. E., Ing, A. D., Lustig, N., Romani, P., Wacker, D. P., Andersen, J. K., & Durako, E. (2015). Resurgence of mands following functional communication training. *Mexican Journal of Behavior Analysis, 41*(2), 166.

Berg, W. K., Wacker, D. P., Harding, J. W., Ganzer, J., & Barretto, A. (2007). An evaluation of multiple dependent variables across distinct classes of antecedent stimuli pre and post functional communication training. *Journal of Early and Intensive Behavior Intervention, 3*, 305–333. https://doi.org/10.1037/h0100346

Bloom, S. E., Lambert, J. M., Dayton, E., & Samaha, A. L. (2013). Teacher-conducted trial-based functional analyses as the basis for intervention. *Journal of Applied Behavior Analysis, 46*(1), 208–218. https://doi.org/10.1002/jaba.21

Buckley, S. D., & Newchok, D. K. (2005). Differential impact of response effort within a response chain on use of mands in a student with autism. *Research in Developmental Disabilities, 26*(1), 77–85. https://doi.org/10.1016/j.ridd.2004.07.004

Carr, E. G. (1994). The purposeful nature of problem behavior: Conceptual and empirical background. In E. G. Carr, L. Levin, G. McConnachie, J. I. Carlson, D. C. Kemp, & C. E. Smith (Eds.), *Communication-based interventions for problem behavior: A user's guide for producing positive change* (pp. 17–29). Baltimore: Paul H. Brookes.

Carr, E. G., & Durand, V. M. (1985). Reducing behavior problems through functional communication training. *Journal of Applied Behavior Analysis, 18*(2), 111–126. https://doi.org/10.1901/jaba.1985.18-111

Chiesa, M. (1994). *Radical behaviorism: The philosophy and the science.* Southborough, MA: Authors Cooperative.

Cooper, J. O., Heron, T. E., & Heward, W. L. (2007). *Applied behavior analysis* (2nd ed.). Upper Saddle River, NJ: Prentice-Hall.

Davis, D. H., Fredrick, L. D., Alberto, P. A., & Gama, R. (2012). Functional communication training without extinction using concurrent schedules of differing magnitudes of reinforcement in classrooms. *Journal of Positive Behavior Interventions, 14*(3), 162–172. https://doi.org/10.1177/1098300711429597

Day, H. M., Horner, R. H., & O'Neill, R. E. (1994). Multiple functions of problem behaviors: Assessment and intervention. *Journal of Applied Behavior Analysis, 27*(2), 279–289. https://doi.org/10.1901/jaba.1994.27-279

Derby, K. M., Wacker, D. P., Berg, W., Deraad, A., Ulrich, S., Asmus, J., Harding, J., Prouty, A., Laffey, P., & Stoner, E. A. (1997). The long-term effects of functional communication training in home settings. *Journal of Applied Behavior Analysis, 30*(3), 507–531. https://doi.org/10.1901/jaba.1997.30-507

Dunlap, G., & Duda, M. (2004). Using functional communication training to replace Challenging behavior. [Conference Paper]. WHAT WORKS BRIEF #11.

Durand, V. M. (1990). *Severe behavior problems: A functional communication training approach.* New York: Guilford Press.

Durand, V. M. (1993). Functional communication training using assistive devices: Effects on challenging behavior and affect. *AAC: Augmentative and Alternative Communication, 9*, 168–176. https://doi.org10.1080/07434619312331276571

Durand, V. M. (1999). Functional communication training using assistive devices: recruiting natural communities of reinforcement. *Journal of Applied Behavior Analysis, 32*, 247–267. https://doi.org/10.1901/jaba.1999.32-247

Durand V. M. (2012). Functional communication training: treating challenging behavior. In P. A. Prelock & R. J. McCauley (Eds.), *Treatment of autism spectrum disorders: evidence-based intervention strategies for communication and social interaction* (pp. 107–138). Baltimore: Paul H. Brookes.

Durand, V. M., & Carr, E. G. (1991). Functional communication training to reduce challenging behavior: Maintenance and application in new settings. *Journal of Applied Behavior Analysis, 24*(2), 251–264. https://doi.org/10.1901/jaba.1991.24-251

Durand, V. M., & Carr, E. G. (1992). An analysis of maintenance following functional communication training. *Journal of Applied Behavior Analysis, 25*(4), 777–794. https://doi.org/10.1901/jaba.1992.25-777

Durand, V. M., & Moskowitz, L. (2015). Functional communication training: Thirty years of treating challenging behavior. *Topics in Early Childhood Special Education*, *35*(2), 116–126. https://doi.org/10.1177/0271121415569509

Dworschak, W., Ratz, C., & Wagner, M. (2016). Prevalence and putative risk markers of challenging behavior in students with intellectual disabilities. *Research in Developmental Disabilities, 58*, 94–103. https://doi:10.1016/j.ridd.2016.08.006

Dyches, T. T., Davis, A., Lucido, B., & Young, J. R. (2002). Generalization of skills using pictographic and voice output communication devices. *Augmentative and Alternative Communication, 18*, 124–131. https://doi.org/10.1080/07434610212331281211

Epstein, R. (1983). Resurgence of previously reinforced behavior during extinction. *Behaviour Analysis Letters, 3*(6), 391–397.

Falcomata, T. S., Muething, C. S., Silbaugh, B. C., Adami, S., Hoffman, K., Shpall, C., & Ringdahl, J. E. (2018). Lag schedules and functional communication training: Persistence of mands and relapse of problem behavior. *Behavior Modification, 42*(3), 314–334. https://doi.org/10.1177/0145445517741475

Falcomata, T. S., Roane, H. S., Feeney, B. J., & Stephenson, K. M. (2010). Assessment and treatment of elopement maintained by access to stereotypy. *Journal of Applied Behavior Analysis, 43*(3), 513–517. https://doi.org/10.1901/jaba.2010.43-513

Falcomata, T. S., Shpall, C. S., Ringdahl, J. E., Ferguson, R. H., Wingate, H. V., & Swinnea, S. B. (2017). A comparison of high and low-proficiency mands during functional communication training across multiple functions of problem behavior. *Journal of Developmental and Physical Disabilities, 29*(6), 983–1002. https://doi.org/10.1007/s10882-017-9571-z

Falcomata, T. S., & Wacker, D. P. (2013). On the use of strategies for programming generalization during functional communication training: A review of the literature. *Journal of Developmental and Physical Disabilities, 25*(1), 5–15. https://doi.org/10.1007/s10882-012-9311-3

Fettig, A., & Barton, E. E. (2014). Parent implementation of function-based intervention to reduce children's challenging behavior: A literature review. *Topics in Early Childhood Special Education, 34*(1), 49–61. https://doi.org/10.1177/0271121413513037

Fisher, W., Piazza, C., Cataldo, M., Harrell, R., Jefferson, G., & Conner, R. (1993). Functional communication training with and without extinction and punishment. *Journal of Applied Behavior Analysis, 26*(1), 23–36. https://doi.org/10.1901/jaba.1993.26-23

Fisher, W. W., Fuhrman, A. M., Greer, B. D., Mitteer, D. R., & Piazza, C. C. (2020). Mitigating resurgence of destructive behavior using the discriminative stimuli of a multiple schedule. *Journal of the Experimental Analysis of Behavior, 113*(1), 263–277. https://doi.org/10.1002/jeab.552

Fisher, W. W., Greer, B. D., Fuhrman, A. M., Saini, V., & Simmons, C. A. (2018). Minimizing resurgence of destructive behavior using behavioral momentum theory. *Journal of Applied Behavior Analysis, 51*(4), 831–853. https://doi.org/10.1002/jaba.499

Fisher, W. W., Saini, V., Greer, B. D., Sullivan, W. E., Roane, H. S., Fuhrman, A. M., Criag, A. R., & Kimball, R. T. (2019). Baseline reinforcement rate and resurgence of destructive behavior. *Journal of the Experimental Analysis of Behavior, 111*(1), 75–93. https://doi.org/10.1002/jeab.488

Franzone, E. (2009). *Steps for implementation: Functional communication training*. Madison: The National Professional Development Center on Autism Spectrum Disorders, Waisman Center, University of Wisconsin.

Fuhrman, A. M., Lambert, J. M., & Greer, B. D. (2022). A brief review of expanded-operant Treatments for mitigating resurgence. *The Psychological Record, 72* (1), 319–323. https://doi.org/10.1007/s40732-021-00456-z

Gerow, S., Davis, T., Radhakrishnan, S., Gregori, E., & Rivera, G. (2018a). Functional communication training: The strength of evidence across disabilities. *Exceptional Children, 85*(1), 86–103. https://doi.org/10.1177/0014402918793399

Gerow, S., Hagan-Burke, S., Rispoli, M., Gregori, E., Mason, R., & Ninci, J. (2018b). A systematic review of parent-implemented functional communication training for children with ASD. *Behavior Modification, 42*(3), 335–363. https://doi.org/10.1177/0145445517740872

Gerow, S., Radhakrishnan, S., Akers, J., McGinnis, K., & Swensson, R. (2021). Telehealth parent coaching to improve daily living skills for children with ASD. *Journal of Applied Behavior Analysis, 54*(2), 566–581. https://doi.org/10.1002/jaba.813

Ghaemmaghami, M., Hanley, G. P., & Jessel, J. (2016). Contingencies promote delay tolerance. *Journal of Applied Behavior Analysis, 49*(3), 548–575. https://doi.org/10.1002/jaba.333

Ghaemmaghami, M., Hanley, G. P., Jessel, J., & Landa, R. (2018). Shaping complex functional communication responses. *Journal of Applied Behavior Analysis, 51*(3), 502–520. https://doi.org/10.1002/jaba.468

Greer, B. D., Fisher, W. W., Retzlaff, B. J., & Fuhrman, A. M. (2020). A preliminary evaluation of treatment duration on the resurgence of destructive behavior. *Journal of the Experimental Analysis of Behavior, 113*(1), 251–262. https://doi.org/10.1002/jeab.567

Gregori, E., Wendt, O., Gerow, S., Peltier, C., Genc-Tosun, D., Lory, C., & Gold, Z. S. (2020). Functional communication training for adults with autism spectrum disorder: A systematic review and quality appraisal. *Journal of Behavioral Education, 29*(1), 42–63. https://doi.org/10.1007/s10864-019-09339-4

Hagopian, L. P., Boelter, E. W., & Jarmolowicz, D. P. (2011). Reinforcement schedule thinning following functional communication training: Review and recommendations. *Behavior Analysis in Practice, 4*(1), 4–16. https://doi.org/10.1007/BF03391770

Hagopian, L. P., Fisher, W. W., Sullivan, M. T., Acquisto, J., & LeBlanc, L. A. (1998). Effectiveness of functional communication training with and without extinction and punishment: A summary of 21 inpatient cases. *Journal of Applied Behavior Analysis, 31*, 211–235. https://doi.org/10.1901/jaba.1998.31-211

Heath, A. K., Ganz, J. B., Parker, R., Burke, M., & Ninci, J. (2015). A meta-analytic review of functional communication training across mode of communication, age, and disability. *Review Journal of Autism and Developmental Disorders, 2*(2), 155–166. https://doi.org/10.1007/s40489-014-0044-3

Hoffman, K., & Falcomata, T. S. (2014). An evaluation of resurgence of appropriate communication in individuals with autism who exhibit severe problem behavior. *Journal of Applied Behavior Analysis, 47*, 651–656. https://doi.org10.1002/jaba.144

Horner, R. H., & Day, H. M. (1991). The effects of response efficiency on functionally equivalent competing behaviors. *Journal of Applied Behavior Analysis, 24*(4), 719–732. https://doi.org/10.1901/jaba.1991.24-719

Horner, R. H., Sprague, J. R., O'Brien, M., & Heathfield, L. T. (1990). The role of response efficiency in the reduction of problem behaviors through functional equivalence training: A case study. *Journal of the Association for Persons with Severe Handicaps, 15*(2), 91–97. https://doi.org/10.1177/154079699001500205

Hutchins, T. L., & Prelock, P. A. (2014). Using communication to reduce challenging behaviors in individuals with autism spectrum disorders and intellectual disability. *Child and Adolescent Psychiatric Clinics, 23*(1), 41–55. https://doi.org/10.1016/j.chc.2013.07.003

Iwata, B. A., Dorsey, M. F., Slifer, K. J., Bauman, K. E., & Richman, G. S. (1994). Toward a functional analysis of self-injury. *Journal of Applied Behavior Analysis, 27*(2), 197–209. https://doi.org/10.1901/jaba.1994.27-197

Kestner, K. M., & Peterson, S. M. (2017). A review of resurgence literature with human participants. *Behavior Analysis: Research and Practice, 17*(1), 1–17. https://doi.org/10.1037/bar0000039

Kratochwill, T. R., Hitchcock, J. H., Horner, R. H., Levin, J. R., Odom, S. L., Rindskopf, D. M., & Shadish, W. R. (2013). Single-case intervention research design standards. *Remedial and Special Education, 34*(1), 26–38. https://doi.org/10.1177/0741932512452794

Kratochwill, T. R., & Stoiber, K. C. (2002). Evidence-based interventions in school psychology: Conceptual foundations of the procedural and coding manual of division 16 and the society for the study of school psychology task force. *School Psychology Quarterly, 17*(4), 341. https://doi.org/10.1521/scpq.17.4.341.20872

Kunnavatana, S. S., Wolfe, K., & Aguilar, A. N. (2018). Assessing mand topography preference when developing a functional communication training intervention. *Behavior Modification, 42*(3), 364–381. https://doi.org/10.1177/0145445517751437

Kurtz, P. F., Boelter, E. W., Jarmolowicz, D. P., Chin, M. D., & Hagopian, L. P. (2011). An analysis of functional communication training as an empirically supported treatment for problem behavior displayed by individuals with intellectual disabilities. *Research in Developmental Disabilities, 32*(6), 2935–2942. https://doi.org/10.1016/j.ridd.2011.05.009

Kurtz, P. F., Chin, M. D., Huete, J. M., Tarbox, R. S. F., O'Connor, J. T., Paclawskyj, T. R., & Rush, K. S. (2003). Functional analysis and treatment of self-injurious behavior in young children: A summary of 30 cases. *Journal of Applied Behavior Analysis, 36*, 205–219. https://doi.org/10.1901/jaba.2003.36-205

Lambert, J. M., Bloom, S. E., & Irvin, J. (2012). Trial-based functional analysis and functional communication training in an early childhood setting. *Journal of Applied Behavior Analysis, 45*, 579–584. https://doi.org/10.1901/jaba.2012.45-579

Lambert, J. M., Bloom, S. E., Samaha, A. L., & Dayton, E. (2017). Serial functional communication training: Extending serial DRA to mands and problem behavior. *Behavioral Interventions, 32*(4), 311–325. https://doi.org/10.1002/bin.1493

Lambert, J. M., Bloom, S. E., Samaha, A. L., Dayton, E., & Rodewald, A. M. (2015). Serial alternative response training as intervention for target response resurgence. *Journal of Applied Behavior Analysis, 48*, 765–780. https://doi.org/10.1002/jaba.253

Lambert, J. M., Pericozzi, H. G., Bailey, K. M., Standish, C. M., & Perry, E. C. (2020). Evaluating duration of baseline as a moderator of resurgence following serial training. *Behavioral Development, 25*(2), 52. https://doi.org/10.1037/bdb0000096

Langdon, N. A., Carr, E. G., & Owen-Deschryver, J. S. (2008). Functional analysis of precursors for serious problem behavior and related intervention. *Behavior Modifcation, 32*(6), 804–827. https://doi.org/10.1177/0145445508317943

LaRue, R., Weiss, M. J., & Cable, M. K. (2009). Functional communication training: The role of speech pathologists and behavior analysts in serving students with autism. *Journal of Speech and Language Pathology—Applied Behavior Analysis, 3*(2–3), 164–172. https://doi.org/10.1037/h0100244

LaRue, R. H., Lenard, K., Weiss, M. J., Bamond, M., Palmieri, M., & Kelley, M. E. (2010). Comparison of traditional and trial-based methodologies for conducting functional analyses. *Research in Developmental Disabilities, 31*, 480–487. https://doi.org/10.1016/j.ridd.2009.10.020

Lattal, K. A., Cançado, C. R., Cook, J. E., Kincaid, S. L., Nighbor, T. D., & Oliver, A. C. (2017). On defining resurgence. *Behavioural Processes, 141*, 85–91. https://doi.org/10.1016/j.beproc.2017.04.018

Lieving, G. A., Hagopian, L. P., Long, E. S., & O'Connor, J. (2004). Response-class hierarchies and resurgence of severe problem behavior. *The Psychological Record, 54*(4), 621–634. https://doi.org/10.1007/BF03395495

Lindgren, S., Wacker, D., Schieltz, K., Suess, A., Pelzel, K., Kopelman, T., Lee, J., Romani, P., & O'Brien, M. (2020). A randomized controlled trial of functional communication training via telehealth for young children with autism spectrum disorder. *Journal of Autism and Developmental Disorders, 50*(12), 4449–4462. https://doi.org/10.1007/s10803-020-04451-1

Lindgren, S., Wacker, D., Suess, A., Schieltz, K., Pelzel, K., Kopelman, T., Lee, J., Romani, P., & Waldron, D. (2016). Telehealth and autism: Treating challenging behavior at lower cost. *Pediatrics, 137*, S167–S175. https://doi.org/10.1542/peds.2015-28510

Lowe, K., Allen, D., Jones, E., Brophy, S., Moore, K., & James, W. (2007). Challenging behaviours: Prevalence and topographies. *Journal of Intellectual Disability Research, 51*(8), 625–636. https://doi.org/10.1111/j.1365-2788.2006.00948.x

Luo, L., Gage, N. A., & Prykanowski, D. A. (2019). Systematic review of functional communication training in early care and education settings. *Education and Training in Autism and Developmental Disabilities, 54*(4), 358–376. https://www.jstor.org/stable/26822514

Machalicek, W., Lequia, J., Pinkelman, S., Knowles, C., Raulston, T., Davis, T., & Alresheed, F. (2016). Behavioral telehealth consultation with families of children with autism spectrum disorder. *Behavioral Interventions, 31*(3), 223–250. https://doi.org/10.1002/bin.1450

Maggin, D. M., Briesch, A. M., & Chafouleas, S. M. (2013). An application of the What Works Clearinghouse standards for evaluating single-subject research: Synthesis of the self-management literature base. *Remedial and Special Education, 34*(1), 44–58. https://doi.org/10.1177/0741932511435176

Mancil, G. R. (2006). Functional communication training: A review of the literature related to children with autism. *Education and Training in Developmental Disabilities, 41*(3), 213–224. http://www.jstor.org/stable/23880196

Mancil, G. R., & Boman, M. (2010). Functional communication training in the classroom: A guide for success. Preventing School Failure: Alternative Education for Children and *Youth, 54*(4), 238–246. https://doi.org/10.1080/10459881003745195

Matson, J. L., & Vollmer, T. R. (1995). Questions About Behavioral Function (QABF). *APA PsycTests*. https://doi.org/10.1037/t64275-000

Matson, J. L., Wilkins, J., & Macken, J. (2009). The relationship of challenging behaviors to severity and symptoms of autism spectrum disorders. *Journal of Mental Health Research in Intellectual Disabilities, 2*, 29–44. https://doi.org/10.1080/19315860802611415

Moes, D. R., & Frea, W. D. (2002). Contextualized behavioral support in early intervention for children with autism and their families. *Journal of Autism and Developmental Disorders, 32*, 519–533. https://doi.org/10.1023/A:1021298729297

Muething, C. S., Falcomata, T. S., Ferguson, R., Swinnea, S., & Shpall, C. (2018). An evaluation of delay to reinforcement and mand variability during functional communication training. *Journal of Applied Behavior Analysis, 51*(2), 263–275. https://doi.org/10.1002/jaba.441

Neely, L., Garcia, E., Bankston, B., & Green, A. (2018). Generalization and maintenance of functional communication training for individuals with developmental disabilities: A systematic and quality review. *Research in Developmental Disabilities, 79*, 116–129. https://doi.org/10.1016/j.ridd.2018.02.002

Neely, L., Graber, J., Kunnavatana, S., & Cantrell, K. (2020). Impact of language on behavior treatment outcomes. *Journal of Applied Behavior Analysis, 53*(2), 796–810. https://doi.org/10.1002/jaba.626

Northup, J., Wacker, D., Sasso, G., Steege, M., Cigrand, K., Cook, J., & DeRaad, A. (1991). A brief functional analysis of aggressive and alternative behavior in an outclinic setting. *Journal of Applied Behavior Analysis, 24*(3), 509–522. https://doi.org/10.1901/jaba.1991.24-509

O'Neill, R. E., Horner, R. H., Albin, R. W., Sprague, J. R., Storey, K., & Newton, J. S. (1997). *Functional assessment and program development for problem behavior: A practical handbook.* Pacific Grove, CA: Brooks/Cole.

O'Neill, R. E., & Sweetland-Baker, M. (2001). Brief report: An assessment of stimulus generalization and contingency effects in functional communication training with two students with autism. *Journal of Autism and Developmental Disorders, 31*(2), 235–240. https://doi.org/10.1023/A:1010711518182

Padilla Dalmau, Y. C., Wacker, D. P., Harding, J. W., Berg, W. K., Schieltz, K. M., Lee, J. F., Breznican, G. P., & Kramer, A. R. (2011). A preliminary evaluation of functional communication training effectiveness and language preference when Spanish and English are manipulated. *Journal of Behavioral Education, 20*(4), 233–251. https://doi.org/10.1007/s10864-011-9131-z

Petursson, P. I., & Eldevik, S. (2018). Functional analysis and communication training to reduce problem behavior and time in restraint: A case study. *Behavior Analysis: Research and Practice*, 19(1), 114–122. https://doi.org/10.1037/bar0000139

Radhakrishnan, S., Gerow, S., & Weston, R. (2020). Resurgence of challenging behavior following functional communication training for children with disabilities: A literature review. *Journal of Developmental and Physical Disabilities, 32*(2), 213–239. https://doi.org/10.1007/s10882-019-09685-1

Radstaake, M., Didden, R., Lang, R., O'Reilly, M., Sigafoos, J., Lancioni, G. E., Appels, N., & Curfs, L. M. (2013). Functional analysis and functional communication training in the classroom for three children with Angelman syndrome. *Journal of Developmental and Physical Disabilities, 25*(1), 49–63. https://doi.org/10.1007/s10882-012-9302-4

Randall, K. R., Greer, B. D., Smith, S. W., & Kimball, R. T. (2021). Sustaining behavior reduction by transitioning the topography of the functional communication response. *Journal of Applied Behavior Analysis, 54*(3), 1013–1031. https://doi.org/10.1002/jaba.824

Reichle, J., & Wacker, D. P. (2017). *Functional communication training for problem behavior.* New York: Guilford Press.

Ringdahl, J. E., Berg, W. K., Wacker, D. P., Crook, K., Molony, M. A., Vargo, K. K., Neurnberger, J. E., Zabala, K., & Taylor, C. J. (2018). Effects of response preference on resistance to change. *Journal of the Experimental Analysis of Behavior, 109*(1), 265–280. https://doi.org/10.1002/jeab.308

Ringdahl, J. E., Berg, W. K., Wacker, D. P., Ryan, S., Ryan, A., Crook, K., & Molony, M. (2016). Further demonstrations of individual preference among mand modalities during functional communication training. *Journal of Developmental and Physical Disabilities, 28*(6), 905–917. https://doi.org/10.1007/s10882-016-9518-9

Ringdahl, J. E., Falcomata, T. S., Christensen, T. J., Bass-Ringdahl, S. M., Lentz, A., Dutt, A., & Schuh-Claus, J. (2009). Evaluation of a pre-treatment assessment to select mand topographies for functional communication training. *Research in Developmental Disabilities, 30*(2), 330–341. https://doi.org/10.1016/j.ridd.2008.06.002

Roane, H. S., & Betz, A. M. (2012). Behavior analysis. In V. S. Ramachandran (Ed.), *Encyclopedia of human behavior* (2nd ed.) (pp. 267–273). Kidlington, UK: Elsevier Press.

Rooker, G. W., Jessel, J., Kurtz, P. F., & Hagopian, L. P. (2013). Functional communication training with and without alternative reinforcement and punishment: An analysis of 58 applications. *Journal of Applied Behavior Analysis, 46*, 708–722. https://doi.org/10.1002/jaba.76

Schieltz, K. M., & Wacker, D. P. (2020). Functional assessment and function-based treatment delivered via telehealth: A brief summary. *Journal of Applied Behavior Analysis, 53*(3), 1242–1258. https://doi.org/10.1002/jaba.742

Schindler, H. S., & Horner, R. H. (2005). Generalized reduction of challenging behavior of young children with autism: Building transituational interventions. *American Journal on Mental Retardation, 110*, 36–47. https://doi.org/10.1352/0895-8017(2005)110<36:GROPBO>2.0.CO;2

Simacek, J., Elmquist, M., Dimian, A. F., & Reichle, J. (2021). Current trends in telehealth applications to deliver social communication interventions for young children with or at risk for autism spectrum disorder. *Current Developmental Disorders Reports, 8*(1), 15–23. https://doi.org/10.1007/s40474-020-00214-w

Skinner, B. F. (1953). *Science and human behavior*. New York: Simon and Schuster.

Steinbrenner, J. R., Hume, K., Odom, S. L., Morin, K. L., Nowell, S. W., Tomaszewski, B., Szendrey, S., McIntyre, N. S., Yücesoy-Özkan, S., & Savage, M. N. (2020). *Evidence-based practices for children, youth, and young adults with autism*. Chapel Hill: The University of North Carolina, Frank Porter Graham Child Development Institute, National Clearinghouse on Autism Evidence and Practice Review Team.

Stokes, T. F., & Baer, D. M. (1977). An implicit technology of generalization. *Journal of Applied Behavior Analysis, 10*, 349–367. https://doi.org/10.1901/jaba.1977.10-349

Stokes, T. F., & Osnes, P. G. (1989). An operant pursuit of generalization. *Behavior Therapy, 20*(3), 337–355. https://doi.org/10.1016/S0005-7894(89)80054-1

Suess, A. N., Romani, P. W., Wacker, D. P., Dyson, S. M., Kuhle, J. L., Lee, J. F., Lindgren, S. D., Kopelman, T. G., Pelzel, K. E., & Waldron, D. B. (2014). Evaluating the treatment fidelity of parents who conduct in-home functional communication training with coaching via telehealth. *Journal of Behavioral Education, 23*(1), 34–59. https://doi.org/10.1007/s10864-013-9183-3

Sutherland, R., Trembath, D., & Roberts, J. (2018). Telehealth and autism: A systematic search and review of the literature. *International Journal of Speech-Language Pathology, 20*(3), 324–336. https://doi.org/10.1080/17549507.2018.1465123

Task Force on Promotion and Dissemination of Psychological Procedures. (1995). Training in and dissemination of empirically-validated psychological treatments. *The Clinical Psychologist, 48*, 3–23.

Tiger, J. H., Hanley, G. P., & Bruzek, J. (2008). Functional communication training: A review and practical guide. *Behavior Analysis in Practice, 1*(1), 16–23. https://doi.org/10.1007/BF03391716

Torelli, J. N., Lambert, J. M., Da Fonte, M. A., Denham, K. N., Jedrzynski, T. M., & Houchins-Juarez, N. J. (2016). Assessing acquisition of and preference for mand topographies during functional communication training. *Behavior Analysis in Practice, 9*(2), 165–168. https://doi.org/10.1007/s40617-015-0083-y

Unholz-Bowden, E., McComas, J. J., McMaster, K. L., Girtler, S. N., Kolb, R. L., & Shipchandler, A. (2020). Caregiver training via telehealth on behavioral procedures: A systematic review. *Journal of Behavioral Education, 29*(2), 246–281. https://doi.org/10.1007/s10864-020-09381-7

Volkert, V. M., Lerman, D. C., Call, N. A., & Trosclair-Lasserre, N. (2009). An evaluation of resurgence during treatment with functional communication training. *Journal of Applied Behavior Analysis, 42*, 145–160. https://doi.org/10.1901/jaba.2009.42-145

Wacker, D., McMahon, C., Steege, M., Berg, W., Sasso, G., & Melloy, K. (1990). Applications of a sequential alternating treatments design. *Journal of Applied Behavior Analysis, 23*(3), 333–339. https://doi.org/10.1901/jaba.1990.23-333

Wacker, D. P., Berg, W. K., Harding, J., & Asmus, J. (1996). A functional approach to dealing with severe challenging behavior. In S. Stainback & W. Stainback (Eds.), *Inclusion: A guide for educators* (pp. 327–342). Baltimore: Paul H. Brookes.

Wacker, D. P., Berg, W. K., Harding, J. W., Barretto, A., Rankin, B., & Ganzer, J. (2005). Treatment effectiveness, stimulus generalization, and acceptability to parents of functional communication training. *Educational Psychology, 25*(2-3), 233–256. https://doi.org/10.1080/0144341042000301184

Wacker, D. P., Harding, J. W., Berg, W. K., Lee, J. F., Schieltz, K. M., Padilla, Y. C., Nevin, J. A., & Shahan, T. A. (2011). An evaluation of persistence of treatment effects during long-term treatment of destructive behavior. *Journal of the Experimental Analysis of Behavior, 96*, 261–282. https://doi.org/10.1901/jeab.2011.96-261

Wacker, D. P., Lee, J. F., Dalmau, Y. C. P., Kopelman, T. G., Lindgren, S. D., Kuhle, J., Pelzel, K. E., & Waldron, D. B. (2013a). Conducting functional analyses of problem behavior via telehealth. *Journal of Applied Behavior Analysis, 46*(1), 31–46. https://doi.org/10.1002/jaba.29

Wacker, D. P., Lee, J. F., Padilla Dalmau, Y. C., Kopelman, T. G., Lindgren, S. D., Kuhle, J., Pelzel, K. E., Dyson, S., Schieltz, K. M., & Waldron, D. B. (2013b). Conducting functional communication training via telehealth to reduce the problem behavior of young children with autism. *Journal of Developmental and Physical Disabilities, 25*(1), 35–48. https://doi.org/10.1007/s10882-012-9314-0

What Works Clearinghouse. (2017). *What Works Clearinghouse™ standards handbook (Version 4.0)*. https://ies.ed.gov/ncee/wwc/docs/referenceresources/wwc_procedures_handbook_v4.pdf

Winborn, L., Wacker, D. P., Richman, D. M., Asmus, J., & Geier, D. (2002). Assessment of mand selection for functional communication training packages. *Journal of Applied Behavior Analysis, 35*(3), 295–298. https://doi.org/10.1901/jaba.2002.35-295

Worsdell, A. S., Iwata, B. A., Hanley, G. P., Thompson, R. H., & Kahng, S. (2000). Effects of continuous and intermittent reinforcement for problem behavior during functional communication training. *Journal of Applied Behavior Analysis, 33*(2), 167–179. https://doi.org/10.1901/jaba.2000.33-167

12
Discrete Trial Teaching

Mary Jane Weiss, Julia L. Ferguson, Alan Kinsella, Eilis O'Connell-Sussman, and Britany Melton
Endicott College, Institute of Behavioral Studies

12.1 Technical Abstract

Background: Discrete trial teaching (DTT) is a systematic form of instruction in which an interventionist provides an instruction, provides an opportunity for the learner to respond, and then provides a corresponding consequence based on the learner's response. This form of instruction has been used to teach children with autism spectrum disorder (ASD) a variety of skills. **Method:** To identify sources of information, "discrete trial teaching," "discrete trial training," and "discrete trial instruction" were searched in a variety of databases to identify articles, best practice guidelines, literature reviews, and previous commentaries and chapters written on the topic. **Results:** DTT is an evidence-based and effective instructional procedure that can be used to teach a variety of skills across a variety of contexts to children with ASD. **Discussion:** Strengths of the research on DTT are the variety of skills it has been used to teach and the level of evidence that supports its effectiveness over 50 years. In addition, the procedure allows for many learning opportunities. Current weaknesses and limitations on the use of DTT include limited generalization data, the fact that it is often implemented in more structured (and less natural) settings, and limited application toward more complex skills such as teaching executive functioning. **Practitioner recommendations:** DTT is an effective procedure for teaching a wide variety of skills to individuals with autism. It is especially well suited to this population of learners, who often need many instructional opportunities to learn new material and who may have difficulty learning when they are not intrinsically interested in the content. DTT has been applied to a wide variety of skills, and it is effective in teaching a broad array of instructional targets. It is also highly efficient. While there have been limitations noted, these can be addressed with additional instructional strategies.

12.2 Layperson Summary

DTT is an evidence-based applied behavior analytic (ABA) approach to teaching skills frequently used with individuals with ASD. DTT is an interventionist-led

Mary Jane Weiss et al., *Discrete Trial Teaching*. In: *Lifespan Treatment for Autistic Individuals*. Edited by: Peter Sturmey, Russell Lang, and James K. Luiselli, Oxford University Press. © Oxford University Press (2025).
DOI: 10.1093/oso/9780197635841.003.0012

systematic form of instruction that breaks complex skills down into small components that are presented repeatedly in order to build fluency and mastery. DTT is commonly implemented by paraprofessionals who may be credentialed by the Behavior Analyst Certification Board (BACB) as registered behavior technicians (RBTs). There are hundreds of published peer-reviewed studies demonstrating the effectiveness of DTT to teach a broad array of skills, including learning-how-to-learn skills, language and communication skills, play and social skills, academic skills, and self-help skills. DTT has been identified under the umbrella of behavioral interventions as an effective and evidence-based intervention for children with ASD (National Autism Council, 2009, 2015; Steinbrenner et al., 2020). Limitations associated with the use of DTT include the lack of generalized outcomes, overuse of the procedure by some interventionists, and reliance on interventionist-led instructions instead of child-initiated behaviors. DTT has evolved immensely over the past decades since it was first introduced, and many misconceptions exist and persist that reflect its historical origins. State-of-the-art DTT is implemented in a flexible and naturalistic manner that does not lead to robotic outcomes and can be engaging and motivating for the child. The Association for Science in Autism Treatment (ASAT), Autism New Jersey, evidence-based practice reports for the treatment of ASD (e.g., National Standards Project, National Clearinghouse on Autism Evidence and Practice Review Team), and the Association of Behavior Analysis International Autism Special Interest Group Parent Guidelines all provide resources and additional information for parents and other providers regarding the evidence and use of DTT.

12.3 Treatment Summary Table

Treatment summary: Discrete Trial Teaching

Treatment description: DTT is an intervention strategy in the field of ABA that consists of three main components: (a) an instruction provided by an interventionist, (b) the learner's response, and (c) an interventionist-provided consequence that is contingent on the learner's response (Smith, 2001). In addition to the three main components of a discrete trial, optional components include the provision of a prompt after the instruction is provided and the use of error correction procedures (Leaf et al., 2016). Each trial is discrete in that it begins with the interventionist providing an instruction and ends with an interventionist-provided consequence. This discrete format allows the interventionist to provide many opportunities for a learner to practice and acquire new skills and focuses on establishing early learning repertories and learning-how-to-learn skills for autistic children (Leaf & McEachin, 1999; Lerman et al., 2016). This foundational early-learning repertoire established through DTT helps to facilitate higher rates of skill acquisition in the future and allows opportunities to demonstrate fluency for the targeted skills (Lerman et al., 2016).

Expected outcomes: Overall DTT has been demonstrated to be a highly effective procedure at teaching new communication skills (e.g., Bak et al., 2021), teaching relevant discriminations (e.g., Grow et al., 2011), social skills (Shillingsburg et al., 2014), play skills (Weiss et al., 2017), and daily living skills (e.g., Magiati et al., 2007) to children diagnosed with ASD. Past and current research implementing DTT to teach new skills to autistic children indicates that this intervention is likely to be successful for learners to acquire new skills (National Autism Center, 2015). Skill acquisition should be monitored with data collection, child assent measures (e.g., approach, affect, choice), and the interventionist should use a program for generalization and maintenance of the learned skills.

Methods: The core components of DTT remain the same (i.e., instruction, response, consequence), but there are vast differences in the way DTT is implemented across programs, organizations, and learners. Some learners may receive only several minutes of DTT per day, while others may receive longer sessions of DTT up to several hours per day (Smith, 2001). Additionally, DTT can be implemented in very systematic and inflexible methods (e.g., only 10 trials at a time, repeated target, only at table) or in flexible and responsive ways (e.g., flexible prompt fading, targets selected based on learner's responding, conducted on floor). Additional components of a discrete trial include an intertrial interval and often the provision of a prompt to increase the likelihood the learner will respond correctly. An intertrial interval is the amount of time that separates each discrete trial. Intertrial intervals can range from just 1 second up to 30 seconds or longer depending on the interventionist's behavior. During the intertrial interval, the interventionist can provide reinforcement for the learner's previous response, collect data on learner responding, change or alter the stimulus array (if applicable), decide on the next target, and determine if a prompt will be needed for the next trial (Leaf & McEachin, 1999). Prompts are often provided during DTT after the instruction is provided to increase the likelihood of correct responding. A prompt is defined as anything the interventionist does to promote correct responding from the learner (Leaf & McEachin, 1999). Prompts can be visual, positional, gestures, verbal, models, within-stimulus, physical, and more. Typically, prompts are used within a prompting system which outlines a hierarchy of prompt types and guidelines for when to provide or fade prompts. These prompting systems include constant time delay (Wolery et al., 1992), progressive time delay (Walker, 2008), most-to-least prompting (e.g., Foran-Conn et al., 2021), least-to-most prompting (Shepley et al., 2019), no-no prompt (e.g., Leaf et al.,2011), simultaneous prompting (Morse & Schuster, 2004), and flexible prompt fading (Soluaga et al., 2008).

Expertise required to implement treatment: The expertise required to implement DTT has varied across the available literature (Leaf et al., 2019). Populations that have commonly been trained to implement DTT include parents (e.g., Ward-Horner & Sturmey, 2008), students (e.g., Downs et al., 2008), paraprofessionals (e.g., Thomas, 2013), therapists/technicians (Severtson & Carr, 2012), and teachers (e.g., Ryan & Hemmes, 2005). The education level of individuals who have been trained to implement DTT has also varied. The education level of individuals who have successfully learned to implement DTT has included a high school level of education (Nosik & Williams, 2011), some college (Crockett et al., 2007), bachelor's degree (Catania et al., 2009), master's degree (Eldevik et al., 2013), and doctoral-level education (Subramaniam et al., 2017). Currently, the Registered Behavior Technician (RBT) certification created by the BACB has DTT on the task list (Behavior Analyst Certification Board, 2018) and is present on the RBT Initial Competency Assessment as a component to be assessed with a client or via role-play (Behavior Analyst Certification Board, 2019). Currently the initial qualifications to apply to become an RBT only require an individual to be 18 years of age, have a high-school diploma, pass a background check, and complete the relevant training and assessment components (Behavior Analyst Certification Board, 2021). Training is required in order to be able to implement DTT with fidelity and proficiency (Smith, 2001). In a review of the DTT training literature, Leaf and colleagues (2019) found that in research reporting training times it took anywhere from 30 minutes to 25 hours for participants to meet the mastery criteria when implementing DTT. Others have noted that it may take 25 to 60 hours of supervised experience for technicians to be able to implement DTT proficiently (Koegel et al., 1977; Smith, 2001). Additionally, more education and training is likely needed when implementing DTT without a protocol and having an interventionist use clinical judgement and in-the-moment assessment to determine the target, trial order, prompt level, reinforcement provided, and so on (Leaf et al., 2016).

Risks and negative side effects: DTT is a procedure that is interventionist initiated, not child initiated. This could lead to a child with ASD being dependent on instructions from the interventionist to engage in targeted behaviors (Smith, 2001). Since DTT is interventionist initiated, other behavior analytic procedures would need to be used alongside DTT (e.g., natural environment training, incidental teaching) to teach skills such as initiation, independence, and engagement in the targeted skills in the absence of instruction from the interventionist. Generalization of targeted behaviors taught through DTT to other environments, instructors, and contexts has also been found lacking (Koegel & Rincover, 1977). When implementing DTT, generalization will need to be specifically programmed in order for the targeted skills to generalize to additional contexts (Stokes & Baer, 1977). Another common critique of DTT is the rigidity of the procedure. Critics of DTT discuss the procedure as leading to robotic behavior, being monotonous (e.g., always same instruction, mass trials, same target), and having a historic absence of assent from the child leading to overcompliance (e.g., Sandoval-Norton et al.,2019). Although these are misconceptions about DTT, it is important for behavior analysts to be aware of the commonly purported misconceptions and work to improve our reputation and address the misconceptions with compassion.

Additional considerations and limitations: Although DTT is an evidence-based and effective procedure to teach children with ASD new skills, it should not be the only ABA procedure implemented to teach autistic children new skills. DTT can and should be implemented alongside other evidence-based ABA procedures such as incidental teaching, social skills groups, behavioral skills training, and pivotal response training. Maintenance and generalization of the targeted skills should also be considered and programmed. This can be accomplished through interspersed maintenance trials once skills have been learned and through moving programming to contexts that are more naturalistic. Generalization should also be planned for in terms of the stimuli used (e.g., various pictures, 2D, 3D), the instructors teaching the targets, and the setting in which the child is learning. Using a flexible and progressive approach to DTT (Leaf et al., 2016) can help to facilitate generalization of learned skills through the use of naturalistic language provided during instructions, varying the instructions, and teaching toward a busy environment.

12.4 Introduction

12.4.1 Treatment Description

DTT is a systematic way of teaching a variety of skills that consists of three distinct components: (a) instruction (or discriminative stimulus), (b) a response from the learner, and (c) a consequence immediately following the learner's response (Leaf & McEachin, 1999). In correlation with the science of ABA, the type of consequence provided to the learner contingent on their response will make the behavior more likely to occur in the future (i.e., positive reinforcement for correct responding) or less likely to occur in the future (i.e., punishment and absence of positive reinforcement for incorrect responding). Additionally, instructors of DTT can utilize different prompting strategies that are embedded after instruction is provided and before the learner's response (Leaf & McEachin, 1999). There are a variety of prompting strategies that can be utilized, including no-no prompting, simultaneous prompting, least-to-most prompting, time delay, and most-to-least prompting. If incorrect responding occurs, error correction may be provided, which results in corrective feedback to the learner and the reintroduction of the instruction with a prompt for the learner to respond correctly. There are a variety of error correction procedures that may be utilized within DTT, including vocal feedback (e.g., "no" after an incorrect response), brief time-out from instruction (e.g., the instructor turns away from student for number of seconds), modeling the correct response, and remedial trials (e.g., after instructors model, the learner is required to respond for a number of times) (Carroll et al., 2015). The purpose of the error correction is to ensure that incorrect responding no longer persists in the future and the learner learns the correct response for future trials.

DTT methods fall into the category of structured, adult-led approaches that incorporate breaking down complex tasks and utilizing repeated learning trials (Ryan & Hemmes, 2005) versus naturalistic approaches, such as incidental teaching (Weiss, 2005). As research advances, it is important to incorporate the feedback of participants and stakeholders about the variety of methods we utilize within ABA, including DTT. We will discuss the following considerations for DTT in relation to early intensive behavioral intervention (EIBI): incorporating a progressive ABA approach to DTT, types of skills targeted within DTT for young learners, and cultural considerations.

A variety of criticisms exist about DTT, some of which are related to early applications of the procedure. However, many center on the focus that DTT has on building responsiveness to teacher direction, rather than on the establishment of reciprocal interactions. DTT teaches responsivity to instructions very well, but it does not target initiation as effectively. Toward that end, DTT and naturalistic instructional approaches can both be used, resulting in strengthening of both the responsivity and initiation response classes.

DTT has been criticized as leading to robotic answers, and as being characterized by an odd tone on the instructor's part. As with most myths, there is an element of truth in this, based on the earliest historical attempts at DTT. In the early days of instruction, it was thought that using a special tone of voice might make it more salient to the learner that a response was expected. Additionally, instructions were often kept as brief as possible to assist the learner in comprehending the instruction. For the same reason, instructions were not altered over trials. Ultimately, this proved ineffective, as learners then failed to respond to more naturalistically delivered instructions and did not learn a generalized understanding of the instructions. Today, instructions are delivered in a naturalistic manner, with a wide variety of language and variable wording whenever possible. In this way, instructors program for generalization from the onset of instruction.

DTT has been criticized as leading to automatic responding. For example, a learner may anticipate that a particular question will be asked repeatedly. They may then simply answer the question that has recently been presented, instead of listening well for the specific question. (Historically, clinicians did sometimes present blocks of unchanging trials, inadvertently leading to this issue.) This can be prevented with the use of trial interspersal. In this procedure, new targets of instruction are interspersed with known material. This procedure can be individualized for learners who struggle with new content, so that the ratio of new material to well-known material can be adjusted over time as tolerance builds. For learners who can easily manage new material, interspersal can also extend to multiple new targets of instruction.

In today's application, DTT is used in a maximally naturalistic manner that facilitates generalization. Some of the concerns about DTT remain, namely that generalization must be assessed and initiation skills must be emphasized through other instructional approaches. Nevertheless, DTT remains a backbone instructional approach in teaching learners with autism, and it is highly effective, efficient, and important.

12.4.2 Rationale and Objectives

The first case report of the use of DTT to teach a child with autism was conducted by Wolf et al. (1963). Wolf and colleagues described a case report of a child, Dicky, who engaged in high rates of problem behavior (i.e., tantrums, self-destructive episodes, bedtime problems), would not wear his glasses which he needed to see, and did not engage in consistent or socially appropriate verbal behavior when they first began working with him. Among a variety of other ABA-based interventions (e.g., shaping, time-out, positive reinforcement, extinction), Wolf and his colleagues described the first use of discrete trial teaching to increase Dickey's socially appropriate verbal behavior. The authors described the instructor presenting pictures one at a time, providing an instruction, a prompt, and waiting until Dicky imitated the correct verbal response. The instructor would then provide praise and give him a contingent bite of his meal. The authors also describe the instructor fading their verbal prompt, increasing the number of pictures Dicky was learning, and progressing the targets to objects/items in books, things around the house, and then more abstract concepts (Wolf et al., 1963). This approach was developed due to the lack of communication opportunities available when Dicky initiated on his own. This form of instruction allowed the interventionists to provide repeated, structured opportunities for Dicky to communicate, and the interventionists to reinforce his verbal behavior. This case study and approach to breaking down a skill and repeatedly practicing set the foundation for hundreds of future studies demonstrating the effectiveness of DTT.

The term *DTT* was first introduced by Lovaas (1981) when working with children with developmental disabilities. Lovaas found that providing structured, systematic instruction based on the principles of ABA to young learners with developmental disabilities taught them a variety of skills (Lovaas, 1987). Longitudinal data were reported in 1993 that demonstrated the experimental group receiving intensive intervention, including DTT, preserving their gains time (McEachin et al., 1993). These seminal articles informed the future trajectory of autism intervention, specifically for young children newly diagnosed with autism. Today, treatment models suggested to parents of newly diagnosed children are based on EIBI and deemed evidenced-based (Hyman et al., 2020). Based on the longitudinal studies of Lovaas and colleagues (1981, 1987, 1993), EIBI would incorporate intensive intervention hours (i.e., the more hours of intervention, the greater the gains demonstrated). It is important to note the heterogeneity of the ASD phenotype and how treatment intensity may vary based on the individual learners' needs and their clinical data (Hyman et al., 2020).

12.4.3 Considerations for Implementation

DTT has been demonstrated to effectively teach a variety of skills, including play (Leaf et al., 2016; Nuzzolo-Gomez et al., 2002), joint attention (Milne et al., 2017), communication (Cihon et al., 2020), labeling (Leaf et al., 2018), and discrimination (Kodak et al., 2011). DTT individualizes and simplifies instruction to ensure skill acquisition for complex skills (Carroll et al., 2015), and, at times, it has been criticized for its fixed and rigid manner (e.g., Wilkenfeld & McCarthy, 2020). DTT's repetition and simplification of instruction is beneficial for learners, but multiple steps can be taken by practitioners to ensure that instruction is not provided in a "fixed" manner that is outlined by Leaf and colleagues (2016). First, ensure the trial targets and placement of stimuli is based upon your individual learner's needs. Practitioners should consult the learner's data on previous trials and allow this to guide decision-making on how to set up future trials (Leaf et al., 2016). Practitioners should ensure stimuli are arranged in a manner that does not leave to response bias, which should also be done in an evolving manner based on learner responding.

Another helpful step in a progressive DTT approach is utilizing natural language whenever possible (Leaf et al., 2016). The first component of DTT is the practitioner providing an instruction to the learner. Some research (Green, 2001) has suggested limiting the auditory stimulus utilized within instruction as it may be difficult for the learner to discriminate complex instructions. Again, this highlights the importance of individualizing your learner's needs and current levels within DTT programs rather than following strict protocols. For example, you may have a young learner newly diagnosed with autism with extremely limited skills that requires succinct instructions but, as they progress in their programming, can respond to instructions that are more complex. In fact, incorporating more complex language may lead to greater generalization of skills and prepare students for incidental learning situations (Leaf & McEachin, 1999). Practitioners should regularly assess what forms of instruction will lead to the most efficient and effective learning outcomes for their learners across all their programs, which may incorporate multiple variables like attending, verbal repertoires, and promoting generalization (Leaf et al., 2016). Practitioners should also be ensuring that their instructions are varied for learners as soon as possible (Leaf et al., 2016). This can lead to generalization to incidental learning and greater maintenance of skill acquisition. Practitioners should take into account if acquisition is slowed by more varied instruction, and they may begin to systematically embed the variety of instructions over time (Leaf et al., 2016).

Optional procedures embedded into DTT, such as prompting and error correction, should also be incorporated within a flexible and individualized manner. Prompting procedures can include within-stimulus prompts and extra-stimulus prompts. Within-stimulus prompts will alter some dimensions of the stimuli's critical features (e.g., making one target larger than the other) and extra-stimulus prompts add dimensions to the stimuli (e.g., putting a square around the correct target) and can include vocally stating or pointing to the correct response (Leaf et al., 2016; Touchette & Howard, 1984). Practitioners should be assessing what types of prompts work best for their learners and when to fade prompts determined on learner responding versus prescribed protocols to follow. Leaf and colleagues (2016) describe flexible prompt fading (FPF) as a prompting system that provides therapists with general guidelines as follows: freedom to use any and all prompt styles that are effective for the learner related to a given skill, ensuring the learner responds correctly on 80% of trials utilizing prompts as needed for accuracy; utilizing the least assistive prompts possible for correct responding, therapists utilize prompts when they are unsure if the learner will respond correctly without prompting; and, lastly, fade prompts quickly while ensuring learner success.

While DTT offers a robust potential to teach a variety of skills across domains with students of all skill levels, it demands particular curation toward ensuring that acquired targets can generalize to practical environments. Such acquisition without programming for generalization may be a futile endeavor otherwise. Fienup and Carr (2021) point to the inclusion of *supplementary variables* in programming—additional stimuli in the presence of which the initial components of a target must be met (e.g., other therapists, multiple days, settings). These variables may vary across several nuanced characteristics (e.g., magnitude, rate of delivery), thus requiring specification of their value and defining features. Programming for such may help preserve a technological procedure that can be replicated by other professionals (Baer et al., 1968). When examining the effects of supplementary variables on a target behavior, for instance during DTT programming, Fienup and Carr (2021) suggest including baseline and posttreatment assessments of stimulus generalization to determine the full extent of the effect.

The aforementioned procedure demonstrates a systematic approach toward training for generalization. Firat and Ergenekon (2021) support the use of naturalistic instructional approaches that incorporate all facets of the learner's environment: practicing acquisition programs at home, at school, and the community. The authors suggest adopting embedded instruction in which the skills are directly incorporated "into daily routines, planned activities, play activities, and/or transitions" (p. 2). This provides opportunities to emit the target behavior in "meaningful contexts" (p. 2). This may involve teaching functional entry-level learning skills in the classroom, self-care tasks in a home bathroom, and purchasing skills in a local store. Firat and Egenekon (2021) highlight the importance of practicing an activity "in the natural setting where the activity is being realized" (p. 2). This provides further evaluation of maintenance and efficacy of training under relevant circumstances.

Ward and Mehta (2019) demonstrated the importance of using multiple exemplars from the beginning to strengthen targets such as communication (e.g., manding). They also utilized strong motivating operations by restricting access to highly reinforcing items to during intervention periods only. Other methods included contriving stronger motivating operations by using visible or out-of-view items, and fading the physical proximity of the item.

In short, generalization is an essential component of an overall acquisition program (Stokes & Baer, 1977), and it should be highly considered when developing a DTT curriculum. Supplemental variables should be identified ahead of time in order to test quickly and recognize necessary circumstances where the target behavior may be evaluated. An appropriate designed curriculum sequence will allow for systematic generalization of one's program. As stated above, a practitioner should collect baseline data under all planned data collection environments, if possible, to determine the full effect of the intervention.

12.5 Research Background

DTT has been commonly evaluated using single-subject designs. For example, Hume and colleagues (2021) reported on 36 single-subject design studies evaluating DTT with individuals with ASD between the years of 1990 to 2017. In a synthesis of this single-case research, Steinbrenner et al. (2020) found that DTT has demonstrated positive outcomes for autistic individuals in the skills of communication across ages 3 to 22, social skills across the ages of 0 to 22, joint attention skills for individuals between the ages of 0 to 11, and play skills for children ages 3 to 11. Additional skills taught through the use of DTT for children with ASD between the ages of 3 to 11 include cognitive skills, school readiness, academic skills, self-help skills, decreasing challenging behavior, and vocational skills (Steinbrenner et al., 2020). In general, the single-subject research is often focused on its treatment effectiveness through targeting specific outcome areas.

Although DTT has been found to be a successful method to teach a vast number of skills, the single-case research still has gaps when it comes to DTT for young adults and high school aged autistic individuals (Steinbrenner et al., 2020). Although the research on DTT with adults and adolescents is limited, research examples have been published. For example, Lambert and colleagues (2016) creatively taught a young male adolescent with ASD to play basketball using a chaining procedure with embedded conditional discriminations. Given that basketball requires the mastery of many skills with complex discriminations, the authors mapped out the required prerequisites for offense and defense and taught those skills to fluency prior to chaining. Phase one of this study taught skills like "pass" and "get open" and shoot with clear operational definitions. Details such as jersey color were presented in counterbalancing fashion so that the participant cued to the most relevant stimuli rather than the person. Using a least-to-most prompting strategy, the participant was taught the component skills (prerequisites) that comprised the larger response chains required. For example, the participant was taught to pass, dribble, and shoot all independently prior to chaining those skills together. Once those skills were mastered in discrete trial formats, longer response chains were taught to comprise both offense and defensive plays. This study demonstrates that DTT can be used to teach adolescents complex leisure/recreational skills and provide a nice outline of how prerequisite skills of a chain are necessary for completion of the entire task. However, given this thorough and effective teaching procedure, DTT as a teaching methodology for adolescents and adults is not well described in the research or perhaps. In fact, a review conducted by Matson and colleagues (2012) does not mention the use of DTT in teaching leisure, self-help, work, or hygiene in adolescents and adults with ASD. This could be accounted for by practitioners choosing chaining methods over discrete trial methods to teach skills that are more complex. Like the study by Lambert and colleagues (2016), it may behoove clinicians to teach component skills to mastery in efficient learning environments like DTT and then move to chaining those mastered skills into more complex and generalizable skills.

The common narrative behind the removal of DTT as a teaching procedure for adolescents is that it does not typically emulate real-life situations. However, with creative and applied teaching procedures, this teaching strategy can be effective in teaching safety skills. Taylor and colleagues (2004) taught three participants (ages 17, 13, and 14 years old) to respond to a vibrating pager to seek assistance from another person when separated from their parent or caregiver. When the participants were paged, they were taught to hand over a communication card to an unknown person or community member indicating that they were lost. In doing this, the authors used a form of discrete trials in the teaching phase. The skill was first taught in a structured school setting with more formal DTT procedures and then generalized to the community setting using novel adults. This study demonstrates that even complex skills, like safety, can be taught using discrete trial formats.

Gerhardt and Lanier (2011) cited a possible reason for the lack of use of DTT in adolescents and adults. For early learners, DTT is efficient and effective in providing multiple and repeated interactions with a learning contingency. For adolescents and adults, the skills being taught often require community settings as the teaching environment, which may increase cost and decrease efficiency. This should be taken into consideration for future research conducted using DTT to teach skills to children and adolescents diagnosed with ASD.

Several group studies evaluating DTT have also been conducted. For example, DTT has been compared to other behavior analytic procedures such as direct instruction (Flores & Ganz, 2014). Flores and Ganz (2014) compared direct instruction to DTT for 13 children diagnosed with ASD. Seven children participated in the DTT group, and six students participated in the direct instruction group. The researchers found no statistical differences between the groups prior to intervention. Intervention for the direct instruction condition consisted of teachers using the direct instruction script to present instructions, ask the participants to respond to questions, engage in tasks, and use signals to prompt group responses. If any errors occurred during direct instruction, error correction procedures were used which included modeling of the correct responses. Intervention for the DTT condition consisted of one-on-one instruction of DTT, most-to-least prompting, reinforcement (i.e., praise and tangible items), and error correction for incorrect responses. Each teaching session (i.e., DTT or direct instruction) lasted 15 minutes and language targets were taught to the participants in both conditions. Results of this study showed that the participants in the DTT condition improved 15% from pretest to posttest and students in the direct instruction group improved 34% from pretest to posttest. The authors found statistical differences between the groups on posttest responding. Delprato (2001) reviewed studies that compared DTT to normalized behavioral language interventions for young children on the autism spectrum (Delprato, 2001). In this review, DTT consisted of structured direct teaching using discrete trials, teacher led instruction, response shaping, and contrived reinforcers. The normalized interventions consisted of loosely structured teaching sessions, child initiated communication, and the use of natural reinforcers. Delprato (2001) found that across eight studies the normalized language training interventions were overall more effective than DTT when it came to language responses. It may be the case that for developing spontaneous, child-initiated language, DTT may not be the most efficient teaching strategy due to the procedure being instructor led and the reinforcers used often being contrived. In addition to comparison group studies between DTT and other behavior analytic procedures, other group studies have been conducted comparing DTT components. For example, group studies have been conducted between various prompting procedures used in DTT (e.g., Cihon et al., 2020) and between errorless learning and error correction procedures used in DTT (e.g., Leaf et al., 2020). When components of DTT have been compared to one another (e.g., prompting systems), the research has found idiosyncratic effects across groups and participants with no statistically significant differences between groups (Cihon et al., 2020; Leaf et al., 2020). This research highlights (a) the positive effects of DTT in that participants acquire the targeted skills when they are targeted systematically through DTT, and (b) the components of DTT should be altered and adjusted based on the specific client you are working with. Since various prompting systems (e.g., most-to-least, time delay, flexible prompt fading) and teaching strategies (e.g., errorless learning, error correction) have been demonstrated to be effective, when it comes to clinical application, the prompting or teaching strategy used during DTT should be adapted to what is most effective and efficient for that particular learner while also taking into account client preference for the teaching strategies.

DTT has been found to be an effective teaching method in-person in one-to-one settings (e.g., Spooner et al., 2012) and in group settings (e.g., Leaf et al., 2017); recently, it has been demonstrated to be effective when delivered via telehealth (Ferguson et al., 2020). This demonstrates the flexibility of DTT when it comes to its implementation across in-person and telehealth modalities as well as individual and group settings. Additionally, when DTT has been implemented in group settings, opportunities for observational learning occurs which has been shown to be effective for children with ASD not only to learn their directly taught targets but also learn the targets of their peers in the group (e.g., Albarran & Sandbank, 2019; Leaf et al., 2017). School and social skill group settings are environments where group DTT could be especially beneficial for children with ASD to learn several targets at once without any additional teaching.

Currently the DTT research lacks an evaluation of social validity of the acceptability of the goals, procedures, and effects from clients and caregivers. Future researchers should focus on incorporating measures of social validity in order to assess how clients and caregivers feel about the acceptability of the procedures. It will be especially important to collect social validity data on the variety of ways DTT has been implemented clinically and in the research. It may be the case that when DTT is implemented in naturalistic and flexible ways (e.g., Leaf et al., 2016), it is more socially valid than when DTT is implemented in a more structured and less flexible manner (e.g., mass trials, always at table). Generalization of skills taught via DTT is also an area that continues to need more research. While maintenance is often assessed within the research, generalization is less often measured. Future researchers should also evaluate and measure if skills learned using DTT generalize to new contexts, with new people, and different stimuli and the conditions under which generalization occurs or does not occur.

When it comes to training others to implement DTT, several formats have emerged as effective methods for teaching professionals and caregivers to implement DTT procedures. These tactics have ranged from traditional group instruction and lecture to self-instruction and multimedia formats. While the efficacy of each tactic depends on the context in which it is practiced and the goals of the community impacted, some options have proven to be more time-efficient and result in quicker acquisition. Further, higher levels of fidelity "should result in greater educational success for the students served" (Catania et al., 2009, p. 387). Research on improving procedural integrity and training staff and caregivers to implement behavior analytic procedures has been extensive. Miller et al. (2014) used incentives (entering a drawing for gift certificates) to improve implantation of skill acquisition procedures (e.g., prompt hierarchy, accuracy of data collection, correct delivery of prompts, prescribing next session). Other tactics demonstrated to teach implementation of discrete-trial instruction have included behavior skills training (Sarokoff & Sturmey, 2004; Subramaniam et al., 2017) and self-instruction manuals (Thiessen et al., 2009). Video instruction and modeling has also been demonstrated to be an effective tactic to teach procedures such as preference assessments (Hansard & Kazemi, 2018; Lavie & Sturmey, 2002; Rosales et al., 2015), behavioral intervention (DiGennaro-Reed et al., 2010) and discrete trial instruction (Vladescu et al., 2012). However, the format of such methods varies considerably, and it may be limited by the cost and time associated with developing videos or the time-consuming implementation demanding a live trainer.

12.6 Practice Implications

12.6.1 Treatment Outcomes

DTT is an effective and efficient procedure that teaches a wide variety of skills to learners with autism. It is especially good for teaching foundational skills, for teaching necessary content when there are limited natural opportunities for instruction, and for providing many practice opportunities to build fluency with material.

The main limitation to DTT is that it primarily targets responsivity. The methodology does not permit much focus on building initiation skills. Hence, an overemphasis on DTT can limit the development of learner-initiated interactions. This limitation, however, should not be interpreted as a fatal flaw. Instead, one needs to view each instructional procedure as having unique applications and associated strengths and limitations. DTT simply needs to be paired with other instructional procedures that focus on initiation building, such as natural environment training, mand training, and pivotal response training. A combination of all of these procedures (DTT and the naturalistic models of instruction) ensures that both responsivity and initiation repertoires are solidly established and continue to flourish in the learner.

Another potential limitation of DTT is limited generalization. In other words, some attention to instructional detail must be given, so that generalization can be fostered. It is important to teach within DTT as naturalistically as possible, including using natural tones and varied instructions. In addition, it is important to present instructions in an interspersed format, so that the learner remains engaged and attentive. Indeed, much of DTT is now done in a thematic or modular manner, with many different types of instruction across the content. In this way, the advantages of the approach for efficiency and effectiveness are preserved, while potential limitations are minimized.

It is also important that assessment be continuous, so that the application of DTT for each individual is altered to ensure success, comfort, and happiness of the learner. Occasionally, a learner may respond poorly to the structure of DTT.

When this is the case, it may be possible to rely more heavily on the naturalistic procedures initially and to build tolerance for structured teaching over time. It may also be possible to ensure that the instructional content selected is high interest and motivating for the learner.

There are several other issues relevant to treatment outcomes. First, there is the issue of qualifications. DTT can be implemented by caregivers and by behavior technicians. Training is needed to understand the rationale, procedures, and state-of-the-art implementation. The most effective and efficient methods for teaching require modeling and rehearsal, and evaluation should include measures of performance-based mastery. In addition, supervision is needed to assess the individual application of the DTI procedures and to provide feedback to enhance instruction. Quality of instruction is a complex and essential element of intervention. Oversight by an experienced supervisor can ensure that DTI's potential is fully realized, that the learner is maximally engaged, and that the learning context is exciting, engaging, positive, and pleasant.

12.6.2 Practice Implication Guidelines

The list below contains the top 10 clinical best practice guidelines:

1. *Continue to use DTT.* DTT is effective and efficient, and it is a necessary instructional procedure in the education of individuals with autism. State-of-the-art implementation has reduced the limitations of the procedure. It remains an integral part of the array of instructional procedures within ABA, and it should be used especially for foundational skills, skills requiring repetition, and skills where the naturally occurring opportunities are insufficient for mastery.
2. *Use state-of-the-art instructional strategies within DTT.* DTT should be done with naturalistic, embedded procedures such as natural tone of voice, varied language, and trial interspersal. It should also incorporate learner preferences, use intrinsically motivating materials, and utilize natural reinforcers whenever possible.
3. *Balance DTT with naturalistic strategies.* As DTT builds responsivity, it is important to balance instruction with procedures that build initiation skills. Both instructional procedures build essential skills, and both are needed for comprehensive intervention.
4. *Program for generalization within DTT.* DTT does have some inherent limitations regarding generalization. Hence, it is important to program for generalization in every possible way. Using a variety of instructions, materials, instructors, settings, and response modalities can address this limitation. It is important to assess for generality, so that additional procedures can be added when necessary.

5. *Ensure learner engagement and assent.* The repetition of DTT may make it less appealing at times. For this reason, continual attention to learner engagement is essential. In addition, there should be continuous efforts at rapport building and assessment of learner happiness. Assent should be routinely assessed, and withdrawals of assent should be monitored, honored, and used to revamp procedures.
6. *Incorporate naturalistic reinforcers into all instructional modalities, including DTT.* Many of the procedures used in naturalistic instruction can also be used in DTT. Whenever possible, naturalistic reinforcers should be embedded into instructional sequences.
7. *Incorporate preference of the learner into all instructional modalities, including DTT.* Learner preferences should influence every aspect of teaching within DTT. Content, materials, and reinforcers should all reflect the learner's preferences and interests.
8. *Do not confuse instructional procedure with the application setting/context.* DTT simply refers to an instructional sequence. It is not determined by setting or context. DTT can be done on the floor, in the backyard, in the cafeteria, at the park, or on a walk. The defining feature is the instructional sequence. It can be applied in any situation, and in any context or environment.
9. *Always monitor the quality of the instructional context.* DTT should be regularly observed, evaluated, and adjusted.
10. *Ensure that every teaching context is dynamic and responsive.* Good instruction is dynamic and responsive to the learner's needs. It is important that the implementation is regularly observed and adjusted.

12.7 References

Albarran, S. A., & Sandbank, M. P. (2019). Teaching non-target information to children with disabilities: An examination of instructive feedback. *Journal of Behavior Education, 28*, 107–140. https://doi.org/10.1007/s10864-018-9301-3

Baer, D. M., Wolf, M. M., & Risley, T. R. (1968). Some current dimensions of applied behavior analysis. *Journal of Applied Behavior Analysis, 1*(1), 91–97. https://doi.org/10.1901/jaba.1968.1-91

Bak, M. Y. S., Dueñas, A. D., Avendaño, S. M., Graham, A. C., & Stanley, T. (2021). Tact instruction for children with autism spectrum disorder: A review. *Autism and Developmental Language Impairments, 6.* https://doi.org/10.1177/2396941521999010

Behavior Analyst Certification Board. (2018). *RBT™ task list* (2nd ed.). Randolph, MA: Author.

Behavior Analyst Certification Board. (2019). *RBT™ initial competency assessment packet.* Randolph, MA: Author.

Behavior Analyst Certification Board. (2021). *RBT: Registered behavior technician™ handbook.* Randolph, MA: Author.

Carroll, R. A., Joachim, B. T., St. Peter, C., C., & Robinson, N. (2015). A comparison of error-correction procedures on skill acquisition during discrete-trial instruction. *Journal of Applied Behavior Analysis, 48*(2), 257–273. https://doi.org/10.1002/jaba.205

Catania, C. N., Almeida, D., Liu-Constant, B., & DiGennaro Reed, F. D. (2009). Video modeling to train staff to implement discrete-trial instruction. *Journal of Applied Behavior Analysis, 42*(2), 387–392. https://doi.org/10.1901/jaba.2009.42-387

Cihon, J. H., Ferguson, J. L., Leaf, J. B., Milne, C. M., Leaf, R., & McEachin, J. (2020). A randomized clinical trial of three prompting systems to teach tact relations. *Journal of Applied Behavior Analysis, 53*(2), 727–743. https://doi.org/10.1002/jaba.617

Crockett, J. L., Fleming, R. K., Doepke, K. J., & Stevens, J. S. (2007). Parent training: Acquisition and generalization of discrete trials teaching skills with parents of children with autism. *Research in Developmental Disabilities, 28*(1), 23–26. https://doi.org/10.1016/j.ridd.2005.10.003

Delprato, D. J. (2001). Comparisons of discrete-trial and normalized behavioral language intervention for young children with autism. *Journal of Autism and Developmental Disorders, 31*(3), 315–325.

DiGennaro-Reed, F. D., Codding, R., Catania, C. N., & Maguire, H. (2010). Effects of video modeling on treatment integrity of behavioral interventions. *Journal of Applied Behavior Analysis, 43*(2), 291–295. https://doi.org/10.1901/jaba.2010.43-291

Downs, A., Downs, R. C., & Rau, K. (2008). Effects of training and feedback on discrete trial teaching skills and student performance. *Research in Developmental Disabilities, 29*(3), 235–246. https://doi.org/10.1016/j.ridd.2007.05.001

Eldevik, S., Ondire, I., Hughes, J. C., Grindle, C. F., Randell, T., & Remington, B. (2013). Effects of computer simulation training on in vivo discrete trial teaching. *Journal of Autism and Developmental Disorders, 43*(3), 569–578. https://doi.org/10.1007/s10803-012-1593-x

Ferguson, J. L., Majeski, M. J., McEachin, J., Leaf, R., Cihon, J. H., & Leaf, J. B. (2020). Evaluating discrete trial teaching with instructive feedback delivered in a dyad arrangement via telehealth. *Journal of Applied Behavior Analysis, 53*(4), 1876–1888. https://doi.org/10.1002/jaba.773

Fienup, D. M., & Carr, J. E. (2021). The use of performance criteria for determining "mastery" in discrete-trial instruction: A call for research. *Behavioral Interventions, 36*(4), 756–763. https://doi.org/10.1002/bin.1827

Firat, Ö. A., & Ergenekon, Y. (2021). Effectiveness of the embedded instructions provided by preschool teachers on the acquisition of target behaviors by inclusion students. *Education and Science, 46*(207), 1–20.

Flores, M. M., & Ganz, J. B. (2014). Comparison of direct instruction and discrete trial teaching on the curriculum-based assessment of language performance of students with autism. *Exceptionality: A Special Education Journal, 22*(4), 191–204. https://doi.org/10.1080/09362835.2013.865533

Foran-Conn, D., Hoerger, M., Kelly, E., Cross, R. R., Jones, S., Walley, H., & Firth, L. (2021). A comparison of most to least prompting, no-no prompting and responsive prompt delay procedures. *Behavioral Interventions, 36*(4), 1024–1041. https://doi.org/10.1002/bin.1808

Gerhardt, P. F., & Lanier, I. (2011). Addressing the needs of adolescents and adults with autism: A crisis on the horizon. *Journal of Contemporary Psychotherapy, 41*, 37–45. https://doi.org/10.1007/s10879-010-9160-2

Green, G. (2001). Behavior analytic instruction for learners with autism: Advances in stimulus control technology. *Focus on Autism and Other Developmental Disabilities, 16*(2), 72–85. https://doi.org/10.1177/108835760101600203

Grow, L. L., Carr, J. E., Kodak, T. B., Jostad, C. M., & Kisamore, A. N. (2011). A comparison of methods for teaching receptive labeling to children with autism spectrum disorder. *Journal of Applied Behavior Analysis, 44*(3), 475–498. https://doi.org/10.1901/jaba.2011.44-475

Hansard, C., & Kazemi, E. (2018). Evaluation of video self-instruction for implementing paired-stimulus preference assessments. *Journal of Applied Behavior Analysis, 51*(3), 675–680. https://doi.org/10.1002/jaba.476

Hume, K., Steinbrenner, J. R., Odom, S., Morin, K. L., Nowell, S. W., Tomaszewski, B., Szendrey, S., McIntyre, N., Yücesoy-Özkan, S., & Savage, M. N. (2021). Evidence-based practices for children, youth, and young adults with autism: third generation review. *Journal of Autism & Developmental Disorders, 51*(11), 4013–4032. https://doi.org/10.1007/s10803-020-04844-2

Hyman, S. L., Levy, S. E., & Myers, S. M. (2020). Identification, evaluation, and management of children with autism spectrum disorder. *Pediatrics, 145*(1), 1–4. https://doi.org/10.1542/peds.2019-3447

Kodak, T., Fisher, W.W., Clements, A., Paden, A., & Dickes, N. R. (2011). Functional assessment of instructional variables: Linking assessment and treatment. *Research in Autism Spectrum Disorders, 5*(3), 1059–1077. http://dx.doi.org/10.1016/j.rasd.2010.11.012

Koegel, R. L., & Rincover, A. (1977). Research on the difference between generalization and maintenance in extra-therapy responding. *Journal of Applied Behavior Analysis, 10*(1), 1–12. https://doi.org/10.1901/jaba.1977.10-1

Koegel, R. L., Russo, D. C., & Rincover, A. (1977). Assessing and training teachers in the generalized use of behavior modification with autistic children. *Journal of Applied Behavior Analysis, 10*(2), 197–205. https://doi.org/10.1901/jaba.1977.10-197

Lambert, J. M., Copeland, B. A., Karp, E. L., Finley, C. I., Houchins-Juarez, N. J., & Ledford, J. R. (2016). Chaining functional basketball sequences (with embedded conditional discriminations) in an adolescent with autism. *Behavior Analysis in Practice, 9*(3), 199–210. https://doi.org/10.1007/s40617-016-0125-0

Lavie, T., & Sturmey, P. (2002). Training staff to conduct a paired-stimulus preference assessment. *Journal of Applied Behavior Analysis, 35*(2), 209–211. https://doi.org/10.1901/jaba.2002.35-209

Leaf, J. B., Aljohani, W. A., Milne, C. M., Ferguson, J. L., Cihon, J. H., Oppenheim-Leaf, M. L., McEachin, J., & Leaf, R. (2019). Training behavior change agents and parents to implement discrete trial teaching: A literature review. *Review Journal of Autism and Developmental Disorders, 6*, 26–39. https://doi.org/10.1007/s40489-018-0152-6

Leaf, J. B., Cihon, J. H., Alcalay, A., Mitchell, E., Townley-Cochran, D., Miller, K., Leaf, R., Taubman, M., & McEachin, J. (2017). Instructive feedback embedded within group instruction for children diagnosed with autism spectrum disorder. *Journal of Applied Behavior Analysis, 50*(2), 304–316. https://doi.org/10.1002/jaba.375

Leaf, J. B., Cihon, J. H., Ferguson, J. L., McEachin, J. M., & Leaf, R., & Taubman, M. (2018). Evaluating three methods of stimulus rotation when teaching receptive labels. *Behavior Analysis in Practice, 11*(4), 334–349. https://doi.org/10.1007/s40617-018-0249-5

Leaf, J. B., Cihon, J. H., Ferguson, J. L., Milne, C. M., Leaf, R., & McEachin, J. (2020). Comparing error correction to errorless learning: A randomized clinical trial. *The Analysis of Verbal Behavior, 36*(1), 1–20. https://doi.org/10.1007/s40616-019-00124-y

Leaf, J. B., Cihon, J. H., Leaf, R., McEachin, J., & Taubman, M. (2016). A progressive approach to discrete trial teaching: Some current guidelines. *International Electronic Journal of Elementary Education, 9*(2), 361–372.

Leaf, J. B., Oppenheim-Leaf, M. L., Dotson, W. H., Johnson, V. A., Courtemanche, A. B., Sheldon, J. B., & Sherman, J. A. (2011). Effects of no-no prompting on teaching expressive labeling of facial expressions to children with and without a pervasive developmental disorder. *Education and Training in Autism and Developmental Disabilities, 46*(2), 186–203.

Leaf, R., & McEachin, J. (1999). *A work in progress: Behavior management strategies and a curriculum for intensive behavioral treatment of autism*. New York: Different Roads to Learning.

Lerman, D. C., Valentino, A. L., & LeBlanc, L. A. (2016). Discrete trial training. In R. Lang, T. B. Hancock, & N. N. Singh (Eds.), *Early intervention for young children with autism spectrum disorder* (pp. 47–83). Cham: Springer. https://doi.org/10.1007/978-3-319-30925-5_3

Lovaas, O. I. (1981). *Teaching developmentally disabled children: The ME book*. Dallas: Pro-ED.

Lovaas, O. I. (1987). Behavioral treatment and normal educational and intellectual functioning in young autistic children. *Journal of Consulting and Clinical Psychology, 55*(1), 3–9. https://doi.org/10.1037/0022-006X.55.1.3

Lovaas, O. I. (1993). The development of a treatment-research project for developmentally disabled and autistic children. *Journal of Applied Behavior Analysis, 26*(4), 617–630. https://doi.org/10.1901/jaba.1993.26-617

Magiati, I., Charman, T., & Howlin, P. (2007). A two-year prospective follow-up study of community-based early intensive behavioural intervention and specialist nursery provision for children with autism spectrum disorders. *Journal of Child Psychology and Psychiatry, 48*(8), 803–812. https://doi.org/10.1111/j.1469-7610.2007.01756.x

Matson, J. L., Hattier, M. A., & Belva, B. (2012). Treating adaptive living skills of persons with autism using applied behavior analysis: a review. *Research in Autism Spectrum Disorders, 6*(1), 271–276. https://doi.org/10.1016/j.rasd.2011.05.008

McEachin, J. J., Smith, T., & Lovaas, O. I. (1993). Long-term outcome for children with autism who received early intensive behavioral treatment. *American Journal on Mental Retardation, 97*(4), 359–372.

Miller, M. V., Carlson, J., & Sigurdsson, S. O. (2014). Improving treatment integrity in a human service setting using lottery-based incentives. *Journal of Organizational Behavior Management, 34*(1), 29–38. https://doi.org/10.1080/01608061.2013.873381

Milne, C., Leaf, J. A., Leaf, J. B., Torres, N., Townley-Cochran, D., Taubman, M., Leaf, R., McEachin, J., & Oppeheim-Leaf, M. (2017). Teaching joint attention and peer to peer communication using the cool versus not cool procedure in a large group setting. *Journal Developmental Physical Disabilities, 29*, 777–796. https://doi.org/10.1007/s10882-017-9556-y

Morse, T. E., & Schuster, J. W. (2004). Simultaneous prompting: A review of the literature. *Education and Training in Developmental Disabilities, 39*(2), 153–168.

National Autism Center. (2009). *Findings and conclusions: National standards project, phase 1.* Randolph, MA: Author.

National Autism Center. (2015). *Findings and conclusions: National standards project, phase 2.* Randolph, MA: Author.

Nosik, M. R., & Williams, W. L. (2011). Component evaluation of a computer based format for teaching discrete trial and backward chaining. *Research in Developmental Disabilities, 32*(5), 1694–1702. https://doi.org/10.1016/j.ridd.2011.02.022

Nuzzolo-Gomez, R., Leonard, M. A., Ortiz, E., Rivera, C. M., & Greer, R. D. (2002). Teaching children with autism to prefer books over stereotypy or passivity. *Journal of Positive Behavior Interventions, 4*(2), 80–87. https://doi.org/10.1177/109830070200400203

Rosales, R., Gongola, L., & Homlitas, G. (2015). An evaluation of video modeling with embedded instructions to teach implementation of stimulus preference assessments. *Journal of Applied Behavior Analysis, 48*(1), 209–214. https://doi.org/10.1002/jaba.174

Ryan, C. S., & Hemmes, N. S. (2005). Post-training discrete-trial teaching performance by instructors with young children with autism in early intensive behavioral intervention. *The Behavior Analyst Today, 6*(1), 1–12. https://doi.org/10.1037/h0100052

Sandoval-Norton, A. H., Shkedy, G., & Shkedy, D. (2019). How much compliance is too much compliance: Is long-term ABA therapy abuse? *Cogent Psychology, 6*(1). https://doi.org/10.1080/23311908.2019.1641258

Sarokoff, R. A., & Sturmey, P. (2004). The effects of behavioral skills training on staff implementation of discrete-trial teaching. *Journal of Applied Behavior Analysis, 37*(4), 535–538. https://doi.org/10.1901/jaba.2004.37-535

Severtson, J. M., & Carr, J. E. (2012). Training novice instructors to implement errorless discrete-trial teaching: A sequential analysis. *Behavior Analysis in Practice, 5*(2), 13–23. https://doi.org/10.1007/BF03391820

Shepley, C., Lane, J. D., & Ault, M. J. (2019). A review and critical examination of the system of least prompts. *Remedial and Special Education, 40*(5), 313–327. https://doi.org/10.1177/0741932517751213

Shillingsburg, M. A., Bowen, C. N., & Shapiro, S. K. (2014). Increasing social approach and decreasing social avoidance in children with autism spectrum disorder during discrete trial teaching. *Research in Autism Spectrum Disorders, 8*(11), 1443–1453. https://doi.org/10.1016/j.rasd.2014.07.013

Smith, T. (2001). Discrete trial training in the treatment of autism. *Focus on Autism and Other Developmental Disabilities, 16*(2), 86–92. https://doi.org/10.1177/108835760101600204

Soluaga, D., Leaf, J. B., Taubman, M., McEachin, J., & Leaf, R. (2008). A comparison of flexible prompt fading and constant time delay for five children with autism. *Research in Autism Spectrum Disorders, 2*(4), 753–765. https://doi.org/10.1016/j.rasd.2008.03.005

Spooner, F., Knight, V. F., Browder, D. M., & Smith, B. R. (2012). Evidence-based practice for teaching academics to students with severe developmental disabilities. *Remedial and Special Education, 33*(6), 374–387. https://doi.org/10.1177/0741932511421634

Steinbrenner, J. R., Hume, K., Odom, S. L., Morin, K. L., Nowell, S. W., Tomaszewski, B., Szendrey, S., McIntyre, N. S., Yücesoy-Özakan, S., & Savage, M. N. (2020). *Evidence-based practices for children, youth, and young adults with autism.* Chapel Hill: The University of North Carolina at Chapel Hill, Frank Porter Graham Child Development Institute, National Clearinghouse on Autism Evidence and Practice Review Team.

Stokes, T. F., & Baer, D. M. (1977). An implicit technology of generalization. *Journal of Applied Behavior Analysis, 10*(2), 349–367. https://doi.org/10.1901/jaba.1977.10-349

Subramaniam, S., Brunson, L. Y., Cook, J. E., Larson, N. A., Poe, S. G., & St. Peter, C. C. (2017). Maintenance of parent-implemented discrete-trial instruction during videoconferencing. *Journal of Behavioral Education, 26*, 1–16. https://doi.org/10.1007/s10864-016-9258-z

Taylor, B. A., Hughes, C. E., Richard, E., Hoch, H. (2004). Teaching teenagers with autism to seek assistance when lost. *Journal of Applied Behavior Analysis, 31*, 79–82.

Thiessen, C., Fazzio, D., Arnal, L., Martin, G. L., Yu, C. T., & Keilback, L. (2009). Evaluation of a self-instructional manual for conducting discrete-trials teaching with children with autism. *Behavior Modification, 33*(3), https://doi.org/10.1177/0145445508327443

Thomas, B. R. (2013). Effects of conducting peer behavioral observations on the observer's correct use of discrete trial teaching procedures. *Research in Developmental Disabilities, 34*(7), 2143–2148. https://doi.org/10.1016/j.ridd.2013.03.033

Touchette, P. E., & Howard, J. S. (1984). Errorless learning: Reinforcement contingencies and stimulus control transfer in delayed prompting. *Journal of Applied Behavior Analysis, 17*(2), 175–188. https://doi.org/10.1901/jaba.1984.17-175

Vladescu, J. C., Carroll, R., Paden, A., & Kodak, T. M. (2012). The effects of video modeling with voiceover instruction on accurate implementation of discrete-trial instruction. *Journal of Applied Behavior Analysis, 45*(2), 419–423. https://doi.org/10.1901/jaba.2012.45-419

Walker, G. (2008). Constant and progressive time delay procedures for teaching children with autism: A literature review. *Journal of Autism and Developmental Disorders, 38*, 261–275. https://doi.org/10.1007/s10803-007-0390-4

Ward, K. D., & Mehta, S. S. (2019). The use of a stimulus control transfer procedure to teach motivation controlled mands to children with autism. *Focus on Autism and Other Developmental Disabilities, 34*(4), 215–225. https://doi.org/10.1177/1088357619838273

Ward-Horner, J., & Sturmey, P. (2008). The effects of general-case training and behavioral skills training on the generalization of parents' use of discrete-trial teaching, child correct responses, and child maladaptive behavior. *Behavioral Interventions, 23*(4), 271–284. https://doi.org/10.1002/bin.268

Weiss, M. J. (2005). Comprehensive ABA programs: Integrating and evaluating the implementation of varied instructional approaches. *The Behavior Analyst Today, 6*(4), 249–256. https://doi.org/10.1037/h0100077

Weiss, M. J., Hilton, J., & Russo, S. (2017). Discrete trial teaching and social skill training: Don't throw the baby out with the bathwater. In J. B. Leaf (Ed.), *Handbook of social skills and autism spectrum disorder* (pp. 155–169). Cham: Springer. https://doi.org/10.1007/978-3-319-62995-7_10

Wilkenfeld, D. A., & McCarthy, A. M. (2020). Ethical concerns with applied behavior analysis for autism spectrum "disorder". *Kennedy Institute of Ethics Journal*, 30, 31–69. https://doi.org/10.1353/ken.2020.0000

Wolery, M., Holcombe, A., Cybriwsky, C., Doyle, P. M., Schuster, J. W., Ault, M. J., & Gast, D. L. (1992). Constant time delay with discrete responses: A review of effectiveness and demographic, procedural, and methodological parameters. *Research in Developmental Disabilities, 13*(3), 239–266. https://doi.org/10.1016/0891-4222(92)90028-5

Wolf, M., Risley, T., & Mees, H. (1963). Application of operant conditioning procedures to the behaviour problems of an autistic child. *Behaviour Research and Therapy, 1*(2–4), 305–312. https://doi.org/10.1016/0005-7967(63)90045-7

13

Enhanced Milieu Teaching

Ashley E. Hinten
Te Kaupeka Oranga—The Faculty of Health, University of Canterbury

Cara E. Petrofes
Texas State University

Laurie McLay
Te Kaupeka Oranga—The Faculty of Health, University of Canterbury

13.1 Technical Abstract

Background: Milieu teaching (MT) and its variants are based on the principles of naturalistic developmental behavioral interventions (NDBIs) and are designed to support development of children's language and communication. **Method:** A review of the literature was conducted to examine levels of empirical support for enhanced milieu teaching (EMT) and prelinguistic milieu teaching (PMT) for autistic children. A search of electronic databases and ancestry searching was undertaken using search terms related to MT, EMT, PMT, autism, and developmental disabilities generally. Approximately 60 articles were identified. This included systematic reviews and meta-analyses that included children with developmental disabilities (e.g., autism) as well as relevant individual studies. The key outcomes of these studies are described in this chapter. **Results:** EMT and PMT can enhance autistic children's preverbal and verbal communication. However, effects may vary across children and contexts. **Discussion:** MT strategies confer the advantage of being implemented in natural environments, with natural change agents, resulting in numerous daily learning opportunities. While there is preliminary evidence supporting MT, there is a need for further methodologically rigorous research that includes autistic children. Further research is also needed to explore the intervention components associated with greatest gains. **Practitioner recommendations:** It is important that the intervention targets and the strategies implemented are informed by a comprehensive assessment of each child's language and communication. Moreover, ongoing assessment should be undertaken to monitor therapeutic response.

Ashley E. Hinten, Cara E. Petrofes, and Laurie McLay, *Enhanced Milieu Teaching*. In: *Lifespan Treatment for Autistic Individuals*. Edited by: Peter Sturmey, Russell Lang, and James K. Luiselli, Oxford University Press. © Oxford University Press (2025). DOI: 10.1093/oso/9780197635841.003.0013

13.2 Layperson Summary

EMT and PMT are intervention approaches that use effective instructional procedures in everyday contexts to teach and support developmentally appropriate skills. EMT and PMT are designed to enhance young children's language and communication. Both EMT and PMT draw upon children's interests, attention, initiations, and motivation to facilitate learning. This includes techniques such as environmental arrangement (i.e., management of the environment to create learning opportunities), responsive interaction (i.e., modeling use of language), and incidental teaching (i.e., use of naturally occurring opportunities to support communication). These techniques are embedded within the context of naturally occurring daily routines and social interactions to create language learning opportunities. EMT is designed to be applied with children who have some spoken vocabulary, whereas PMT is designed for children who do not communicate verbally and who communicate nonverbally (e.g., using gestures). EMT and PMT are implemented by therapists from a variety of professional backgrounds (e.g., education, psychology, health) as well as natural change agents (e.g., parents and other family members). People implementing these strategies should be trained in the use of techniques to ensure safe and appropriate implementation. EMT and PMT have been shown to result in improvements in autistic children's preverbal and verbal communication skills. However, the What Works Clearinghouse's (WWC) review noted that the evidence base in support of MT for communication and language of preschool-aged children with disabilities is limited. No risks or negative side effects have been associated with implementation of EMT or PMT, though it is important to ensure that use of these strategies is informed by comprehensive assessment that identifies appropriate goals and strategies for each child.

13.3 Treatment Summary Table

Treatment summary: Enhanced Milieu Teaching

Treatment description: EMT and PMT are naturalistic developmental behavioral interventions designed to improve young children's communication. Both EMT and PMT draw upon children's motivation and interests to create language learning opportunities within the context of everyday routines and social interactions. Prompting, responsive feedback, and modeling are key mechanisms.

Expected outcomes: EMT and PMT have been shown to result in improvements in autistic children's preverbal and verbal communication skills, including when implemented by natural change agents such as caregivers and educators.

Methods: When implementing EMT and PMT, intervention agents use environmental arrangement, responsive interaction, and MT techniques, to support language learning. Four critical prompting strategies are embedded within MT: modeling, mand-modeling, time delay, and incidental teaching. These strategies are embedded in the context of naturally occurring routines. EMT is distinct from PMT in that it is designed for children who have acquired some verbal language and are making attempts at verbal communication. Conversely, PMT is designed for children who do not communicate verbally and who have limited nonverbal communication (e.g., use of gestures).

Expertise required to implement treatment: Those implementing EMT and PMT should be trained to ensure safe, appropriate, and effective use of these therapeutic techniques. Frameworks have been developed to support this training.

Risks and negative side effects: No significant risks or negative side effects were identified.

Additional considerations and limitations: Comprehensive assessment of each child's current language and communication abilities is necessary to determine the type of MT that is most appropriate and to individualize language goals. Likewise, ongoing assessment and monitoring should be used to determine therapeutic response and to ensure that intervention agents are implementing strategies appropriately.

13.4 Introduction

13.4.1 Treatment Description

EMT (Hemmeter & Kaiser, 1994) and PMT (Warren et al., 2006; Yoder & Warren, 1998) are a type of NDBI (Schreibman et al., 2015). They are designed to support language learning by drawing upon children's interests and initiations that occur in the natural environment, during daily social interactions and routines. Both treatments use modeling and prompting strategies, natural reinforcement contingencies for language attempts, and environmental management to support communication. These strategies are embedded within social games and daily activities that occur in the child's natural environment. The selection of language goals and implementation of MT strategies can be modified to accommodate each individual child, meaning it is appropriate for children with a range of neurodiversity (Kaiser et al., 2021).

EMT and PMT are hybrid treatments that have traditionally incorporated three distinct components: environmental arrangement (Ostrosky & Kaiser, 1991), responsive interaction (Kaiser et al., 1996; Weiss, 1981; Wilcox & Shannon, 1998), and MT (Alpert & Kaiser, 1992; Hart & Risley, 1968, 1975; Hart & Rogers-Warren, 1978; Warren, 1991). However, more recently, these core components have been expanded to include greater emphasis on language modeling, language expansion, prompting functional communication, and time delays. Of note, responsive interaction is a core component of EMT, but it is not always used within PMT (Warren et al., 2006). As such, the literature makes a clear distinction between PMT and responsive education and PMT (RPMT).

The following descriptions of core components of EMT and PMT draw substantially upon the formative and subsequent literature published by the creators of these therapies (e.g., EMT: Hancock & Kaiser, 2006; Kaiser et al., 2021; PMT: Warren et al., 2006).

Environmental arrangement describes the processes of selecting, arranging, managing, and positioning of items within the learning environment (Hancock & Kaiser, 2006; Warren et al., 2006). The purpose of environmental arrangement is to create a need for the child to communicate to obtain the items that appeal to them. This is to motivate children's communicative acts and increase opportunities for communication partners to engage in responsive interaction and additional MT strategies (Hancock & Kaiser, 2006). Environmental arrangement can include multiple components.

Item selection involves choosing objects that interest the child (e.g., something they want or need) and could motivate them to communicate (Hancock & Kaiser, 2006; Hart & Risley, 1968; for example, a train set would appeal to a child who likes locomotives). Intricate items like train sets have the added benefit of having many pieces (e.g., trains, track segments, road signs, people, etc.), necessitating multiple communication requests for assistance. When arranging the environment for autistic children, it is important to include a range of items and provide regular choices to maintain motivation and engagement and to ensure multiple opportunities for language modeling (Kaiser et al., 2021). It is also important to attempt to expand their play by modeling different play actions and integrating new and novel activities or items (Kaiser et al., 2021).

Item arrangement is a process in which a physical hurdle is placed between the child and the item so the child cannot access it without communicating with the adult (Hancock & Kaiser, 2006). This could include placing the item on a shelf the child cannot reach or keeping the item in a container that the child cannot open. In these scenarios, the child must communicate their desire to access the item with a communication partner.

Item management is designed to support sustained communication by continuing to control the child's access to the item or its components, so the child is required to persist in expressing their needs (Hancock & Kaiser, 2006). For example, the intervention agent may open the container containing the train set and give the child just two pieces of the track and then close it again. They then wait for the child to request more pieces until the track is complete. Alternatively, the intervention agent can contradict the child's expectations. For example, they might "misplace" the last track pieces making it veer off-course or complete the track but "forget" the trains.

Positioning involves situating the items between the intervention agent and child to encourage the initiation of an interaction (Warren et al., 2006). For example, to instigate joint attention with the child, the intervention agent could face the child, lower their head to the child's eye level, and hold the item between their faces.

The intervention agent can use these environmental arrangement processes during social games and daily routines with the child to create frequent opportunities for communication (Conti-Ramsden & Friel-Patti, 1986; Warren et al., 2006). The child can be taught new gestures, vocalizations (as in PMT), and/or language models (as in EMT) during a routine that the child recognizes and engages in naturally and frequently (Warren et al., 2006). These routines lend themselves to EMT and PMT because the child will be cognizant of modifications to their usual routine (Piaget & Inhelder, 1969). Additionally, the intervention agent and child engage in defined roles and turn taking, these routines occur frequently (e.g., daily basis), and they are predictable for the child, providing a stable context for the intervention (Warren et al., 2006).

Alongside the environmental arrangement processes, the intervention agent is trained in *responsive interaction* (Hancock & Kaiser, 2006; Warren et al., 2006). Responsive interaction is intended to enhance social exchanges between the intervention agent and the child (Hemmeter & Kaiser, 1994; Kaiser et al., 1996; Tannock et al., 1992; Warren et al., 2006; Weiss, 1981). Specifically, it is designed to coach the intervention agent to be highly responsive to the child, rather than directive (Hemmeter & Kaiser, 1994), accurately interpreting what the child is communicating and responding appropriately (Hancock & Kaiser, 2006; Warren et al., 2006). For example, a child sits in the dog's bed, looking around the room and at the intervention agent. A responsive intervention agent might deduce that the child is wondering where the dog is and explain "Rex is sick. He's with the vet." By being highly responsive, accurately interpreting children's verbal and nonverbal communication, and responding in kind to children's communicative efforts, the intervention agent can support children's understanding of the important functions of language (Warren et al., 2006) and encourage them to continue with their communicative efforts (Hancock & Kaiser, 2006).

Responsive interaction techniques can include verbal turn taking, following the child's lead, expansions, mirroring children's actions and linguistic mapping. When *following the child's lead*, communication partners are taught to involve themselves in an activity that the child is already engaged in. In such cases, the focus is on establishing engagement and extending the exchange to provide further opportunities for learning. Within these exchanges, communication partners may *mirror* the child's actions or vocalizations. For example, when the child makes a gesture (e.g., picks up a toy block), the intervention agent can mimic them or modify the movement (e.g., reach for a block but not pick it up, or pick up two blocks and stack them). Likewise, when the child makes a vocalization (e.g., "Tah, tah"), the intervention agent can copy this exactly or modify the vocalization (e.g., walk around and say "Tah" with each step, change their tone of voice or say "Tah toh" instead). This type of modeling may support children to learn new gestures and vocalizations (Warren et al., 2006).

Other responsive interaction techniques, including expansions (i.e., the intervention agent adds to what the child said; Hemmeter & Kaiser, 1994; Kaiser et al., 2021; Tannock et al., 1992) and linguistic mapping (i.e., the intervention agent provides language models for what the child is doing or communicating; Hemmeter & Kaiser, 1994; Kaiser et al., 2021; Warren et al., 2006; Weiss, 1981), overlap with MT strategies and are described below.

13.4.2 Milieu Teaching

There are four MT strategies: modeling, mand-modeling, time delay, and incidental teaching (Hancock & Kaiser, 2006). *Modeling* involves the intervention agent demonstrating an example of a gesture or other form of nonverbal communication (as in PMT) or language (as in EMT) that could be used in the given context

(Hancock & Kaiser, 2006; Warren et al., 2006). Modeling demonstrates for the child exactly what they need to say and when (Hancock & Kaiser, 2006). In EMT, for example, if the child is gesturing toward a toy block that is out of their reach, the intervention agent might say "Want block" to demonstrate the appropriate request. If the child correctly repeats the phrase, the intervention agent expands on the verbal model (e.g., "Want yellow block") and rewards the child by giving them the item they requested (Hancock & Kaiser, 2006). If the child incorrectly imitates the verbal model, the intervention agent presents a *corrective model* by initiating joint attention with the child and repeating the model (e.g., "Say 'want block'"; Hancock & Kaiser, 2006). If the child correctly imitates on this second attempt, the intervention agent can expand on the verbal model by one or two words (e.g., "Want big block") and give them the item (Hancock & Kaiser, 2006; Kaiser et al., 2021). If the child imitates incorrectly on both attempts, the intervention agent provides the child with *corrective feedback* by repeating the verbal model (e.g., "Want block") and then giving the item to the child (Hancock & Kaiser, 2006). The verbal model should be tailored to the child's language level and target goals (Hancock & Kaiser, 2006).

When using *mand-modeling*, the intervention agent provides a mand (request) or asks a question (mand for information) instead of a verbal model (Hancock & Kaiser, 2006). Mand-modeling provides less support than the modeling procedure previously described as the child is not provided with a model of what language could be used (i.e., they are not imitating; Hancock & Kaiser, 2006). Instead, the intervention agent may give the child a choice (e.g., "Do you want the blue car or the red car?"), ask them an open-ended question (e.g., "What do you want to play?"), give them a mand (e.g., "Tell me what is wrong"; Hancock & Kaiser, 2006), or make an incomplete statement (e.g., "I am waving my . . . ; Alpert & Kaiser, 1992).

Time delay and incidental teaching strategies help teach children the function of initiating communication and provide less support than the modeling and mand-modeling strategies (Hancock & Kaiser, 2006). In this way, the intervention agent transitions from most to least supportive prompting as therapy progresses to support the child to become more independent in their language use (Kaiser et al., 2021).

When using *time delay*, the intervention agent joins in on the child's activity but remains silent until the child initiates communication by asking the intervention agent for something or making a comment (Hancock & Kaiser, 2006). If this initiation is at the target level for the child, the intervention agent expands on their request/comment and gives them the item (e.g., "Want fast car"; Hancock & Kaiser, 2006). If the child does not initiate at the expected level, the intervention agent provides the child with a verbal model to be repeated back or gives them a mand (e.g., choice: "Do you want the big car or the little car?," question: "Which car do you want?," or "Tell me what you want") depending on how much support the child needs (Hancock & Kaiser, 2006). Consistent with modeling and mand-modeling procedures, the intervention agent expands on the child's response and gives them the item if they are correct or states the expected response and give them the item if they are incorrect (i.e., corrective model or corrective feedback; Hancock & Kaiser, 2006). More detail on time-delay procedures is available in Chapter 4 of this text.

Once a child is making requests, it is possible for the intervention agent to use *incidental teaching* strategies in combination with the modeling, mand-modeling, and time-delay strategies (Hancock & Kaiser, 2006). When using incidental teaching, the intervention agent is responsive to requests that the child makes during daily routines (Hancock & Kaiser, 2006). When the child makes a request, the intervention agent chooses whether to respond with a high (i.e., modeling), moderate (i.e., mand-modeling), or low level of support (i.e., time-delay procedure) based on the child's language level and target goals (Hancock & Kaiser, 2006).

In recent years, EMT has been further developed to include new strategies that support autistic children's social communication (Fuller & Kaiser, 2020). When implementing EMT with autistic children, the intervention agent will need to be cognizant of the child's current language level and adapt strategies accordingly. These considerations are described further in section 13.4.3 of this chapter.

13.4.3 Prelinguistic Milieu Teaching

PMT is designed to support children to initiate and respond to communication more frequently, to use these modes more clearly, and to learn additional and more complex modes of communication (Warren et al., 2006). For example, increasing the frequency of requests (i.e., indicating they want an item; nonsocial) and comments (i.e., sharing an experience; social; Warren et al., 2006). Sequentially, the child is taught to (1) gesture and vocalize more, (2) make eye contact and engage in joint attention, (3) use conventional (e.g., waving and pointing) and unconventional gestures (e.g., handing items to the intervention agent or miming an action), and finally, to combine all of these components (i.e., to communicate while vocalizing, making eye contact, and gesturing; Warren et al., 2006).

PMT involves modifications to techniques that are used during EMT. For example, verbal models may be replaced or accompanied by gestural or nonverbal prompts (Warren et al., 2006). Similarly, when using *modeling* and *mand-modeling* procedures, the intervention agent could provide a vocalization prompt in place of complete words or sentences (i.e., if the spontaneously says "LAH" and likes to dance, the intervention agent could repeat the syllable within a tune while dancing). When using the *time-delay* technique, if the intervention agent were to intentionally refrain from immediately engaging in play, the child may request the intervention agent to join them by pulling their arm toward the toy or vocalizing as opposed to use of complete words or sentences (Warren et al., 2006). Likewise, intervention agents may provide the child with a gestural model or nonverbal prompt to increase the child's use of communication-adjacent skills such as eye contact, gesturing, and vocalizing or may engage in linguistic mapping rather than expecting the child to reply verbally (Warren et al., 2006).

Finally, when using *incidental teaching* during PMT, and after a routine has been established, the intervention agent may use proto-imperatives and proto-declaratives (Warren et al., 2006). When using proto-imperatives during an established routine, the adult may interrupt the routine and introduce a prompt (i.e., verbal, nonverbal, or time-delay prompt). Once the child starts attempting independent communication, the adult reduces their use of the prompts and responds to the child-initiated communication attempts (Warren et al., 2006). Proto-declaratives can assist children in sharing an affective state with their communication partner (Warren et al., 2006). To do this, the clinician collects items they think the child will find interesting and positions them around the room (Warren et al., 2006). While interacting with the child, the clinician can point to or comment on the items to model communication (Warren et al., 2006). Again, the techniques the adult uses should be selected and individualized based on the child's goals and support needs (Warren et al., 2006).

The intervention agent should follow the same fundamental steps regardless of which MT strategy they are applying (Hancock & Kaiser, 2006). First, the intervention agent needs to engage the child in joint attention (Hancock & Kaiser, 2006). For example, if the child is playing with a toy, the intervention agent can join in the activity. Second, the intervention agent waits for the child to initiate communication verbally or nonverbally (Hancock & Kaiser, 2006) and depending on the level of support the child needs and what is natural for the situation, the intervention agent will try to elicit verbal or nonverbal communication using one of the four prompting strategies (Hancock & Kaiser, 2006; Warren et al., 2006).

13.5 Rationale and Objectives

EMT is designed for children who are acquiring vocabulary and attempting to communicate (Hancock & Kaiser, 2006). By contrast, PMT is designed for children who do not communicate verbally and have limited or inconsistent nonverbal communication (e.g., gestures and nonspeech vocalizations; Warren et al., 2006). Whether children take part in EMT or PMT is dependent on their language development level. The goal of EMT is to increase the duration, rate, independence, diversity, and complexity of communication. This can include expanding their vocabulary, teaching them the function of language in social interactions, increasing initiated social communication and generalization of this communication, and increasing the complexity of language use (i.e., single words to complex sentences; Hancock & Kaiser, 2006), as well as to increase their spontaneous use of language (Kaiser et al., 2021). The goal of PMT is to build on children's prelinguistic communication skills (e.g., gestures and nonspeech vocalizations) and help them to begin acquiring linguistic skills (e.g., vocabulary, communication attempts frequency) and social communication skills (Warren et al., 2006).

EMT is believed to have advantages over other less naturalistic therapies as it facilitates generalization. This is achieved by the use of natural change agents, embedding of strategies within the natural environment (e.g., home or preschool), use of familiar stimulus items, targeting functional responses, and the use of natural and immediately occurring consequences (Hancock & Kaiser, 2006). As such, specific teaching to facilitate generalization across settings, materials, social scenarios, and communication partners is minimized. This is particularly important for autistic children when they are struggling with skill generalization (Hancock & Kaiser, 2006; Kaiser et al., 2021).

EMT is informed by social interactionist, developmental, and behavioral theory, as outlined below. Responsive interaction is rooted in social interactionist theory (Bruner, 1975, 1978; Vygotsky, 1978) and the transactional model of social communication development (McLean & Snyder-McLean, 1978; Sameroff & Chandler, 1975). At the heart of both theories, children develop language skills through communicating and interacting with others in their natural environments. The intervention agent has an important role as the child's communication partner as they can scaffold and adjust procedures as they progress (Kaiser et al., 2021). The intervention agent needs to talk to the child using language at their target level 50% of the time (i.e., the level they are expected to use at their age and development level) and at their *proximal* target half of the time (i.e., just above their current level; Kaiser et al., 2021; Vygotsky, 1978).

Neurotypical children often demonstrate "a smooth bidirectional or transactional flow" when they speak with their caregivers, where the parent can adapt their language to harmonize with their child's language level (Kaiser et al., 2021, p. 258). However, compared to their neurotypical peers, autistic children are less likely to initiate conversation with others, likely to speak at a lower rate, and may struggle with receptive language (Landa, 2007). These differences may complicate the ability of caregivers to determine their autistic child's language level. As a result, these interactions can become less instructive and may occur less frequently, reducing opportunities for learning and development (Kaiser et al., 2021). Caregivers may develop a pattern of low responsiveness (Warren et al., 2006) and high directiveness (Tannock et al., 1992) to their child's communication when they view their attempts to communicate with their child as unsuccessful. Responsiveness training may be particularly beneficial for autistic children's caregivers (Kaiser et al., 2021).

During responsive interaction training, the intervention agent (often the child's parent or teacher) is taught to be attentive and responsive to their child's communication attempts (Warren et al., 2006). If the adult responds quickly and appropriately to the child's attempt (e.g., gives them the item they requested, expands on what they said, listens attentively), the child is more likely to attempt to communicate again (Warren et al., 2006). In turn, this provides the intervention agent with more opportunities to use MT strategies to increase the complexity of their verbal, nonverbal, and gestural models (Warren et al., 2006). The child is reinforced by adults responding to their attempt and learns that language has a purpose (Warren et al., 2006). The caregiver is more likely to try to engage the child in communication because there is evidence that the child is listening and has a desire to talk to them (Warren et al., 2006).

In terms of *behavioral theory of language development*, Skinner (1957) proposed that children's language skills develop when they are reinforced for correct use of language. The MT strategies of EMT are rooted in behavioral principles (Hancock & Kaiser, 2006; Kaiser et al., 2021), specifically the antecedent behavior consequence (ABC) model. This model posits that the child's behavior is related to events that precede a behavior or set the occasion for a behavior to occur (i.e., the antecedent) and changes in the environment as a result of the behavior (e.g., access to social attention, toys, or activities) that function to reinforce (strengthen) or punish (weaken) a behavior (Cooper et al., 2020).

In EMT and PMT, the behavior of interest is the child's communication attempts. The intervention agent provides antecedent stimuli through environmental arrangement (e.g., the child's preferred toys are stored out of their reach, so they need to ask for access to them) and MT (e.g., the intervention agent provides a prompt for the child; Hancock & Kaiser, 2006). These techniques are designed to increase the likelihood that the child will attempt to communicate with the intervention agent. The child may verbally or nonverbally respond to the antecedent stimuli.

The intervention agent also provides the consequence for the child's behavior (Hancock & Kaiser, 2006; Warren et al., 2006). If the child correctly repeats the model or responds to a mand, the intervention agent reinforces their communication attempt by providing them with the item they requested. In EMT, even if the child is initially incorrect, the intervention agent provides a corrective model (e.g., repeats the model to the child and provides them another chance to copy it) or gives corrective feedback (e.g., reiterates the model once more before giving the child the item) and then reinforces their attempt (Hancock & Kaiser, 2006).

Other natural consequences for the child's communication attempts include the adults responsiveness to the child's communication attempt (e.g., listening and watching them) and the adults subsequent efforts to prolong the interaction (e.g., continue talking, expand on what the child said, etc.; Warren et al., 2006). These are natural consequences because they reflect real-life, natural conversation (Warren et al., 2006). It is also possible to "supplement" these natural consequences by giving a specific acknowledgment or engaging in linguistic mapping (Warren et al., 2006). Specific acknowledgments are particularly reinforcing when the child is first learning to use one of the communication components (Warren et al., 2006). When using a specific acknowledgment, the adult reacts to the child's correct use of a component by smiling and verbally reacting to their attempt (Warren et al., 2006). Linguistic mapping involves providing the child with the language to describe what they are trying to communicate immediately after their attempt (Warren et al., 2006). As the training occurs during natural, everyday activities, the child can receive frequent learning opportunities throughout their day (Warren et al., 2006).

In accordance with the principles of responsive interaction, the intervention agent supports the child to respond correctly by prompting them (e.g., giving them the exact language model in the modeling strategy) and the child is rewarded (e.g., given the item they are trying to request) regardless of whether they correctly used the target language (Hancock & Kaiser, 2006). Moreover, the intervention agent should acknowledge all communication attempts and try to prolong the conversation.

Finally, there is *developmental theory*. Before the child begins EMT treatment, it is essential that the child's language skills are assessed (Kaiser et al., 2021). This is because the order children progress through language development is reasonably predictable. To select the appropriate intervention goals and strategies, it is important to have a clear understanding of each child's current communication level and the prerequisite skills for further advancing social communication. Likewise, as children progress, future targets can be informed by our understanding of developmentally appropriate sequences of acquiring language and communication skills.

13.5.1 Considerations for Implementation

One of the first considerations, prior to the child beginning EMT or PMT, is to deduce which approach is best suited to each child and their family. While children who may benefit from PMT will mainly communicate using gestures and nonspeech vocalizations (Warren et al., 2006), children who receive EMT should typically already have some expressive language (Hancock & Kaiser, 2006). For example, they should be able to imitate others' language (i.e., so the child can repeat the intervention agent's phrases during modeling), have some vocabulary (i.e., so the intervention agent can expand on the child's language during training), and already be attempting to communication using an average of 1 to 3.5 word utterances (Hancock & Kaiser, 2006). To determine which approach is most suitable, Kaiser et al. (2021) recommend a comprehensive assessment that includes child observations and transcribing of utterances, standardized measures, parent- or teacher-report measures, measures of global language skills, and measures of specific skills (e.g., vocabulary, mean length of utterances, receptive vs. productive language, etc.; Kaiser et al., 2021). Moreover, assessments should be made during the child's time in the treatment to ensure that the child's language skills are developing, and the adult is still implementing the strategies correctly (Kaiser et al., 2021).

Once the clinician decides which treatment best suits the child, they need to consider the child's current level of language development and what language they need to be able to use to functionally communicate in their natural environment (Hancock & Kaiser, 2006; Warren et al., 2006). These considerations will help to set target goals that are specific to the needs of each child (Hancock & Kaiser, 2006). Making allowances for the child's age or development level is important because early language acquisition occurs in a well-documented order (e.g., vocabulary, then semantics, and then syntax; Hancock & Kaiser, 2006).

Considerations also need to be made for implementation of PMT or EMT with autistic children and those with complex communication needs. This includes consideration of the characteristics of the learner (e.g., current social and communication skills, motivation, and interests); current levels of engagement with objects, activities, and people; and their responsiveness to different teaching strategies (e.g., modeling, prompting, and reinforcement). This may affect strategies that are used to engage the learner, the integration on additional language or communication supports (e.g., speech generating devices), teaching strategies that are used; and the foundational skills that are targeted (i.e., social and communication or language skills) for both children and their communication partners.

Communication partners play a fundamental role in EMT and PMT. Thus far, caregivers, teachers, and therapists have been trained as intervention agents in EMT and PMT (Hancock & Kaiser, 2006). Caregivers are particularly well-placed to implement EMT and PMT because their child spends a large proportion of their time with their caregivers. They already have a relationship for the foundation of the training and can take advantage of the learning opportunities that arise in everyday life (Alpert & Kaiser, 1992; Hancock & Kaiser, 2006; Warren et al., 2006). Moreover, increasing caregiver responsiveness is likely to increase the frequency of the child's communication attempts and create more opportunities for teaching language. To support training in EMT, Kaiser et al. (2021) developed the teach-model-coach-review (TMCR) approach that has been paired with EMT (Kaiser et al., 2021). TMCR (Roberts et al., 2014; Trivette et al., 2009) outlines how each intervention agent can be trained to use EMT by a trained clinician. First, the clinician *teaches* the caregiver by recapping the EMT strategies they will focus on in that session. Second, the clinician *models* the strategies for the caregiver by implementing them with the child. Third, the caregiver is *coached* through using the strategies with their child. Fourth, the clinician and caregiver review how the caregiver's attempt went and plan for when the caregiver could implement the techniques in their daily routines. While there is no requirement for formal training in EMT, such training is likely to be fundamental to its success (Kaiser et al., 2021).

Finally, it is important to consider the cultural context in which EMT is being implemented and the degree of alignment between the program objectives and strategies as well as the cultural norms, values, and linguistic environment of the family. MT approaches are based on a set of Western assumptions about social communication, and the effectiveness and acceptability of EMT may vary across cultures, particularly given the fundamental role of parents in the delivery of EMT or PMT (Johnston & Wong, 2002; van Kleeck, 1994). At a minimum, it is important for families to be asked about their beliefs, values, and preferences, prior to commencing EMT.

13.6 Research Background

To understand the application of MT programs, and associated levels of empirical support, a search of peer-reviewed literature was undertaken. Articles were considered relevant if they empirically analyzed or reviewed the effectiveness of MT programs. Our search included APA PsycINFO, ERIC, MEDLINE Complete, and Psychology and Behavioral Sciences Collection databases. The following search terms were applied in various combinations to identify articles for this chapter: enhanced milieu*, autis*, prelinguistic milieu*, communication dis*, incidental teaching, and milieu training. The focus was on extracting articles that included autistic children as participants. Approximately 60 articles were ultimately reviewed to evaluate the levels of empirical support for MT approaches, but not all included participants with ASD. These studies included children with cleft palate, Down syndrome, hearing and vision impairments, and adults with learning and language delays. The following sections provided an overview of the literature evaluating the effectiveness of PMT or EMT for autistic children, with additional evidence for use with other developmental disabilities described to provide additional context.

13.6.1 Milieu Therapy

Numerous studies have evaluated the effect of MT procedures on the social communication of children with language delays. Generally speaking, this research suggests that MT is effective in supporting children's language developmental and social communication (Fey et al., 2006; Yoder & Stone, 2006).

Two literature reviews were identified that have evaluated the use of MT for autistic children (Goldstein, 2002; Mancil et al., 2009). The first of these reviews evaluated the effectiveness of interventions designed to enhance the speech and language of autistic children (Goldstein2002; e.g., discrete trial training, sign language and MT). The findings of this review suggest that MT was used to teach various preverbal and verbal communicative functions and acts to autistic children, including preverbal skills such as joint attention and eye contact; peer interactions; responses to questions; social graces (e.g., please and thank you); and increased number and repertoire of words, and they have resulted in increased communication repertoires of autistic children. The authors noted that mand-model and time-delay procedures were the strategies most frequently applied with autistic children. Although MT was effective, the review concluded there was no evidence to suggest that MT procedures are superior to other ABA-based procedures designed to support language and highlighted the overlap in procedures with other intervention approaches.

In a second review, Mancil et al., (2009) investigated the effectiveness of MT for autistic children, the characteristics of interventionists and trainers, and the environments in which MT has been implemented. Although only eight studies met inclusion criteria, findings suggest that most studies evaluated interventions that were delivered by natural change agents (i.e., parents or teachers) and implemented in naturalistic settings (i.e., the home and community). Regardless of specific MT strategies used, MT was found to result in improvement in the communication skills of autistic children and, when measured, generalization across people and settings.

13.6.2 Prelinguistic Milieu Teaching

Several studies were identified that have investigated the effectiveness of PMT for children with developmental disabilities and language delay (Fey et al., 2006, 2013; McCathren, 2000; Warren et al., 2008; Yoder & Warren, 2002). Overall, that research has found that PMT is effective in increasing use of intentional communication among children with developmental delays, including minimally verbal children with Down syndrome (Fey et al., 2006), intellectual disabilities (Fey et al., 2013; McCathren, 2000; Warren et al., 2008; Yoder & Warren, 2002), language delays (Kaiser, Ostrosky & Alpert, 1993), and concurrent vision and hearing impairment (Brady & Bashinski, 2008).

Several studies have also investigated the effectiveness of parent- and teacher-implemented PMT for autistic children. These studies have included preschool- and school-aged children and have predominantly evaluated treatment effects using single-case research design studies (e.g., McCathren 2010; Ogletree, Davis et al., 2012). Typically, parent-implemented MT has focused on teaching nonverbal or minimally verbal autistic children to communicate within the context of salient play routines in the home environment (Franco et al., 2013; McDuffie & Yoder, 2010; Yoder & Warren, 1998; Yoder & Warren, 2002). Parents in the majority of studies were taught techniques by the primary researcher or other therapists (McCathren, 2010; Yoder & Stone, 2006a; 2006b; Yoder & Warren, 1998). Study outcomes demonstrated increases in language acquisition and use, sustained attention, joint attention, and parental responsiveness toward communication attempts (McCathren, 2010; Yoder & Stone, 2006; Yoder & Warren, 1998).

A small number of studies have compared PMT with other techniques. For example, Yoder and Stone (2006) compared PECS with RPMT on initiating joint attention, requests, and turn taking for 36 preschool-aged autistic children within a randomized group experiment. Interventions were delivered during 20-minute sessions 3 times per week over the course of 6 months. Although RPMT and PECS were both effective, RPMT resulted in superior outcomes in regard to initiating joint attention, facilitating requesting, and turn taking. However, initiated joint attention was only superior to PECS for children who already demonstrated some existing ability to initiate joint attention.

13.6.3 Enhanced Milieu Teaching

Research into the effectiveness of EMT has included children with Down syndrome (Wright et al., 2013), language delays (Hancock & Kaiser, 2002; Peterson et al., 2005), and autism (Hancock et al., 2002; Kaiser et al., 2000; Kasari et al., 2014), and it has used a variety of intervention agents, including teachers (Olive et al., 2007), therapists (Hancock & Kaiser, 2002; Kasari et al., 2014; Kim et al., 2020), siblings (Hancock & Kaiser, 1996), and parents (Peterson et al., 2005). Moreover, there is evidence to support the use of EMT with children from diverse cultural and linguistic backgrounds (Hampton et al., 2019, 2021; Olive et al., 2010) and among children who are learning multiple languages simultaneously (e.g., Peredo et al., 2018). In many of these studies, EMT is used in conjunction with other interventions such as joint attention, structured play, and emotion regulation (JASPER; Hampton et al., 2021; Kasari et la., 2014); alongside use of additional communication aids (Olive et al., 2007); or embedded within the context of play activities such as reading (Sunyoun et al., 2020).

The majority of research into the effectiveness of EMT has focused on therapist-implemented approaches in the home environment, and they have examined the effect of EMT on language and communication (Hampton et al., 2019; Kasari et al., 2014; Sunyoung et al., 2020). Outcomes of this research suggest that EMT is effective in enhancing the number and variety of words used, including spontaneous utterances in autistic children (Hampton et al., 2019; Kasari et al., 2014; Sunyoung et al., 2020) and children with language delays (Robertson & Weismer, 1999). For example, Hampton et al. (2019) used a single-case, multiple-baseline, across-participants design to evaluate the effectiveness of therapist-implemented EMT on the frequency and variety of spoken words used among three 5–7-year-old autistic children. EMT resulted in an increase in the number of different words and spontaneous utterances across all children, with findings generalized to novel materials and communication partners.

In a significant study, Kasari et al. (2014) compared the effectiveness of JASPER+EMT against JASPER+EMT with a speech-generating device (SGD) for 61 minimally verbal autistic children aged 5–8. The intervention was clinic-based, delivered by therapists, with parents also receiving in-clinic coaching. The study featured a distinctive experimental design, with participants undergoing 12 weeks of their assigned treatment, each stage lasting the same duration. After this period, early responders continued in their group, while slow responders in the JASPER+EMT+SGD group received intensified treatment, and those in the JASPER+EMT alone group were rerandomized to intensified or augmented JASPER+EMT+SGD. The authors found that SGD inclusion led to more spontaneous utterances than the alternative and noted that adding SGD later did not offer the same benefits as implementing it from the beginning.

In a study by Quinn et al. (2021), the effects of caregiver implementation of EMT were examined after a therapist delivered a hybrid training program that combined telepractice and face-to-face sessions. Caregiver outcomes were measured in terms of fidelity, accuracy, and frequency of EMT strategy use, while child outcomes were assessed through communicative acts and the number of different words used. The findings revealed an increase in the use and accuracy of EMT strategies for most caregiver participants and improvements in the measured child outcomes for three of the four autistic children involved in the study.

13.6.4 Milieu Teaching in Educational Contexts

A small number of studies have investigated the effectiveness of MT when delivered by teachers and support staff, within educational settings (McCathren, 2000; Olive et al., 2007). Although the research is relatively limited, preliminary findings suggest that teacher- or teacher assistant–implemented MT can result in positive effects for autistic children. For example, McCathren (2000) investigated the effectiveness of teacher-implemented PMT for a child with language delay. As a result of PMT, this child demonstrated an increase in the rate of intentional communication, as well as collateral improvement in play skills. In a second study, teachers and teacher assistants implemented EMT, combined with an SGD, to teach requesting skills for three autistic children in the classroom setting during 5-minute play sessions. This resulted in increased requests during play sessions for all three children (Olive et al., 2007).

A small number of additional studies have investigated the effect of therapist-implemented MT in educational contexts for children with developmental disabilities. These studies have reported improvement in communication and social interaction (Dubin & Lieberman-Betz, 2020). For example, Lieberman-Betz et al. (2020) investigated the effectiveness of therapist-delivered PMT, implemented in the preschool classroom environment, on early intentional communication among three preschool-aged children who were autistic or had a high likelihood of being autistic. Each of these children increased rates of intentional communication (e.g., purposeful use of vocalizations and gestures), with gains maintained at follow-up for the two participants for whom this was assessed. Importantly, however, generalization to teachers did not occur consistently across participants.

13.6.5 Collateral Effects of Milieu Teaching

So far, in accordance with the goals of EMT and PMT, most research has focused on the immediate impact of these methods on children's social communication and language skills. However, recognizing the interconnected relationship between communication and behavior, MT approaches might also provide collateral benefits. These benefits extend beyond the behaviors explicitly targeted by PMT/EMT and could include improvements in children's internalizing and externalizing behavior as well as their adaptive functioning.

A small number of studies were identified that have investigated the collateral effects of parent-implemented language intervention on children's daytime behavior (Curtis et al., 2019; Mancil et al., 2009), as well as the number of different toys children played with (Dubin et al., 2020). In such studies, improved communication was associated with a reduction in challenging behavior (Mancil & Conroy, 2009), though it was not associated with an increase in the number of toys children played with (Dubin et al., 2020). The collateral effect of PMT on parenting stress has also been investigated, but no collateral benefits were observed (Fey et al., 2006). To date, research is limited in terms of the number of studies but also the potential range of collateral benefits that have been assessed. This is an area worthy of further investigation.

13.6.6 Practice Implications

Based on existing research, there are a number of important considerations for implementation of EMT and PMT. First, there is evidence to suggest that not only is MT able to be effectively embedded in daily activities (e.g., reading books; McLeod et al., 2017; Sunyoung et al., 2020), it may in fact enhance therapeutic outcomes when used in conjunction with other strategies such as SGD (Kasari et al., 2014; Olive et al., 2007) and JASPER (Hampton et al., 2021; Kasari et al., 2014; Wright et al., 2013). As such, it is important to consider the additional benefits of strategies to augment EMT to further enhance outcomes.

Secondly, there is evidence to suggest that the effectiveness of MT may vary according to participant characteristics such as levels of communication (Fey et al., 2013) and that some children may benefit from the addition of strategies such as augmentative and alternative communication (AAC) systems, particularly among those with minimal expressive language (Kasari et al., 2014; Olive et al., 2007).

There are also unanswered questions regarding appropriate intervention dosage/intensity and whether this may vary according to participant characteristics (Fey et al., 2013). There is also evidence that brief interventions, both in terms of session times and period of delivery, can have positive effects for children. For example, in Olive et al. (2007), MT combined with SGD interventions was delivered for approximately 5 minutes per day and over 19 sessions, resulting in improvement in children's use of the SGD to request items within the context of play. In a systematic review of the literature, Parker-McGowan et al. (2014) sought to investigate intervention dosage (i.e., frequency and form of dosage, total duration and cumulative intensive of intervention) within MT interventions for children with developmental disabilities, based on the dosage framework suggested by Warren et al. (2007). However, the authors found that very few studies provide information about dosage parameters; thus, little can be concluded about the role of treatment dosage in outcomes of MT.

13.6.7 Limitations

Although there is preliminary evidence to support the use of MT, this evidence is insufficient to suggest that PMT and EMT are evidence based, and according to WWC, MT has no discernable effects on the communication and language of preschool-aged children with disabilities (retrieved from: https://ies.ed.gov/ncee/wwc/Intervention/764). This conclusion may, in part, reflect the fact that few studies met the necessary research standards of research rigor. Research into the effectiveness of MT approaches, including research with autistic children, is generally marred by small sample sizes which make it difficult to discern the clinical significance and generalizability of the findings. Moreover, while single-case research designs are certainly appropriate for heterogeneous groups, larger-scale, robust group designs such as randomized controlled trial (RCT) studies are conventionally considered the gold standard for determining the effectiveness of a therapeutic approach and there are very few RCT evaluations of MT for autistic children. In addition to issues with sample size and experimental design, there are additional methodological issues. For example, Parker-McGowan et al. (2014) reported that only 35% of single-case research design studies and 75% of group design studies reported treatment fidelity. Moreover, few studies have reported intervention dosage and intensity and, as such, it is difficult to determine the appropriate intervention intensity duration needed to result in therapeutic benefit and to attribute outcomes as being a direct result of therapeutic process. Finally, while there is some evidence that children with language delays may generalize gains in language use across parents, peers, and teachers when participating in EMT (Kaiser & Roberts, 2013; Wright et al., 2013), this has seldom been investigated in autistic children, and there is some evidence to suggest that there is limited generalization across communication partners (Dubin et al., 2020; Hampton et al., 2021).

13.6.8 Areas in Need of Further Research

Building upon extant research, there are a number of areas that require further investigation. First, there is a need for further evaluations of MT within the natural environment (e.g., home or school) as opposed to clinical settings. Likewise, there is a need for further research evaluating the effectiveness of MT when implemented by those that children may typically encounter, such as parents and teachers, or at minimum, further research assessing generalization to these and other communication partners (e.g., peers). Research is also typically limited to preschool-aged children, and there is a need for further research among those who are school-aged who may also logically benefit from MT. Finally, further research is needed to guide implementation, such as the relationship among treatment dosage, participant characteristics, and therapeutic outcome as well as further research into the effectiveness and acceptability of EMT across families from diverse cultural and linguistic backgrounds.

13.7 References

Alpert, C. L., & Kaiser, A. (1992). Training parents as milieu language teachers. *Journal of Early Intervention, 16*(1), 31–52. https://doi.org/10.1177/105381519201600104

American Psychiatric Association. (2013). Autism spectrum disorder. *In Diagnostic and statistical manual of mental disorders* (5th ed.). Washington, DC: Author.

Brady, N. C., & Bashinski, S. M. (2008). Increasing communication in children with concurrent vision and hearing loss. *Research and Practice for Persons with Severe Disabilities, 33*(1–2), 59–70. https://doi.org/10.2511/rpsd.33.1-2.59

Bruner, J. S. (1975). From communication to language: A psychological perspective. *Cognition, 3*(3), 255–387. https://doi.org/10.1016/0010-0277(74)90012-2

Bruner, J. S. (1978). The role of dialogue in language acquisition. In A. Sinclair, R. J. Jarvelle, & W. J. M. Levelt (Eds.), *The child's concept of language.* New York: Springer-Verlag.

Conti-Ramsden, G., & Friel-Patti, S. (1986). Mother-child dialogues: Consideration of cognitive complexity for young language learning children. *British Journal of Disorders of Communication, 21*(2), 245–255. https://doi.org/10.3109/13682828609012281

Cooper, J. O., Heron, T. E., & Heward, W. L. (2020). *Applied Behavior Analysis* (3rd ed.). London: Pearson.

Curtis, P. R., Kaiser, A. P., Estabrook, R., & Roberts, M. Y. (2019). The longitudinal effects of early language intervention on children's problem behaviors. *Child Development, 90*(2), 576–592. https://doi.org/10.1111/cdev.12942

Dubin, A. H., & Lieberman-Betz, R. G. (2020). Naturalistic interventions to improve prelinguistic communication for children with autism spectrum disorder: a systematic review. *Review Journal of Autism and Developmental Disorders, 7,* 151–167. https://doi.org/10.1007/s40489-019-00184-9

Dubin, A. H., Lieberman-Betz, R. G., Ayres, K. M., & Zawoyski, A. (2020). The effects of prelinguistic milieu teaching implemented in classrooms for preschoolers with or at risk for autism spectrum disorder. *Focus on Autism and Other Developmental Disabilities, 35*(2), 79–89. https://doi.org/10.1177/1088357619888917

Fey, M. E., Warren, S. F., Brady, N., Finestack, L. H., Bredin-Oja, S. L., Fairchild, M., Sokol, S., & Yoder, P. J. (2006). Early effects of responsivity education/prelinguistic milieu teaching for children with developmental delays and their parents. *Journal of Speech, Language, and Hearing Research, 49*(3), 526–547. https://doi.org/10.1044/1092-4388(2006/039)

Fey, M. E., Yoder, P. J., Warren, S. F., & Bredin-Oja, S. L. (2013). Is more better? Milieu communication teaching in toddlers with intellectual disabilities. *Journal of Speech, Language, and Hearing Research, 56*(2), 679–693. https://doi.org/10.1044/1092-4388(2012/12-0061)

Franco, J. H., Davis, B. L., & Davis, J. L. (2013). Increasing social interaction using Prelinguistic Milieu Teaching with nonverbal school-age children with autism. *American Journal of Speech-Language Pathology, 22*(3), 489–502. https://doi.org/10.1044/1058-0360(2012/10-0103)

Fuller, E. A., & Kaiser, A. P. (2020). The effects of early intervention on social-communication outcomes for children with autism spectrum disorder: A meta-analysis. *Journal of Autism and Developmental Disabilities, 50*(5), 1683–1700. https://doi.org/10.1007/s10803-019-03927-z

Goldstein, H. (2002). Communication intervention for children with autism: A review of treatment efficacy. *Journal of Autism and Developmental Disorders, 32*(5), 373–396. https://doi.org/10.1023/A:1020589821992

Hampton, L. H., Harty, M., Fuller, E. A., & Kaiser, A. P. (2019). Enhanced milieu teaching for children with autism spectrum disorder in South Africa. *International Journal of Speech Language Pathology, 21*(6), 635–645. https://doi.org/10.1080/17549507.2018.1559357

Hampton, L. H., Kaiser, A. P., Nietfeld, J. P., & Khachoyan, A. (2021). Generalized effects of naturalistic social communication intervention for minimally verbal children with autism. *Journal of Autism and Developmental Disorders, 51*(1), 75–87. https://doi.org/10.1007/s10803-020-04521-4

Hancock, T. B., & Kaiser, A. P. (1996). Siblings' use of milieu teaching at home. *Topics in Early Childhood Special Education, 16*(2), 168–190. https://doi.org/10.1177/027112149601600204

Hancock, T. B., & Kaiser, A. P. (2002). The effects of trainer-implemented enhanced milieu teaching on the social communication of children with autism. *Topics in Early Childhood Special Education, 22*(1), 39–54. https://doi.org/10.1177/027112140202200104

Hancock, T. B., & Kaiser, A. P. (2006). Enhanced milieu teaching. In R.J. McCauley & M.E. Fey (Eds.), *Treatment of language disorders in children* (pp. 203–236). Baltimore: Paul H. Brooks.

Hart, B. M., & Risley, T. R. (1968). Establishing the use of descriptive adjectives in the spontaneous speech of disadvantaged preschool children. *Journal of Applied Behavior Analysis, 1*, 109–120. https://doi.org/10.1901/jaba.1968.1-109

Hart, B. M., & Risley, T. R. (1975). Incidental teaching of language in the preschool. *Journal of Applied Behavior Analysis, 8*, 411–420. https://doi.org/10.1901/jaba.1975.8-411

Hart, B. M., & Rogers-Warren, A. K. (1978). Milieu teaching approaches. In R. L. Schiefelbusch (Ed.), *Bases of language intervention* (Vol. 2, pp. 193–235). Baltimore: University Park Press.

Hemmeter, M. L., & Kaiser, A. P. (1994). Enhanced milieu teaching: Effects of parent-implemented language intervention. *Journal of Early Intervention, 18*, 269–289. https://doi.org/10.1177/105381519401800303

Johnston, J. R., & Wong, M. Y. (2002). Cultural differences in beliefs and practices concerning talk to children. *Journal of Speech Language and Hearing Research, 45*(5), 916–926. https://doi.org/10.1044/1092-4388(2002/074)

Kaiser, A. P. (1993). Functional language. In M. E. Snell (Ed.), *Enhancing children's communication: Research foundations for intervention* (pp. 347–379). Baltimore: Paul H. Brookes.

Kaiser, A. P., Fuller, E. A., & Heidlage, J. K. (2021). Enhanced milieu teaching. In P. A. Prelock & R. J. McCauley (Eds.), *Treatment of autism spectrum disorder: Evidence-based intervention strategies for communication & social interactions* (2nd ed., pp. 255–286). Baltimore: Paul H. Brooks.

Kaiser, A. P., & Hampton, L. H. (2016). Enhanced milieu teaching. In R. McCauley, M. Fey, & R. Gilliam (Eds.), *Treatment of language disorders in children* (2nd ed., pp. 87–120). Baltimore: Paul H. Brookes.

Kaiser, A. P., Hancock, T. B., & Nietfeld, J. P. (2000). The effects of parent-implemented enhanced milieu teaching on the social communication of children who have autism. *Journal of Early Education and Development [Special Issue], 4*, 423–446. https://doi.org/10.1207/s15566935eed1104_4

Kaiser, A. P., Hemmeter, M. L., Ostrosky, M., Fischer, R., Yoder, P. J., & Keefer, M. (1996). The effects of teaching parents to use responsive interaction strategies. *Topics in Early Childhood Special Education, 16*(3), 375–406. https://doi.org/10.1177/027112149601600307

Kaiser, A. P., Ostrosky, M. M., & Alpert, C. L. (1993). Training teachers to use environmental arrangement and milieu teaching with nonvocal preschool children. *Journal of the Association for Persons with Severe Handicaps, 18*(3), 188–199. https://doi.org/10.1177/154079699301800305

Kaiser, A. P., & Roberts, M. Y. (2013). Parent-implemented enhanced milieu teaching with preschool children who have intellectual disabilities. *Journal of Speech, Language, and Hearing Research, 56*(1), 295–309. https://doi.org/10.1044/1092-4388(2012/11-0231)

Kaiser, A. P., & Warren, S. F. (1987). Pragmatics and generalization. In R. L. Schiefelbusch & L. L. Lloyd (Eds.), *Language perspectives: Acquisition, retardation, and intervention* (2nd ed.) (pp. 118–132). Austin, TX: PRO-ED.

Kasari, C., Kaiser, A., Goods, K., Nietfeld, J., Mathy, P., Landa, R., Murphy, S., & Almirall, D. (2014). Communication interventions for minimally verbal children with autism: A sequential multiple assignment randomized trial. *Journal of the American Academy of Child and Adolescent Psychiatry, 53*(6), 635–646. https://doi.org/10.1016/j.jaac.2014.01.019

Kim, S., Kang, V. Y., & McLeod, R. H. (2020). Effects of enhanced milieu teaching with book reading for children with autism spectrum disorder. *Education and Training in Autism and Developmental Disabilities, 55*(4), 451–465. https://doi.org/10.1177/00224669209734

Landa, R. (2007). Early communication developmental and intervention for children with autism. *Mental Retardation and Developmental Disabilities Research Reviews, 13*(1), 16–25. https://doi.org/10.1002/mrdd.20134

Mancil, G. R., Conroy, M. A., & Haydon, T. F. (2009). Effects of a modified milieu therapy intervention on the social communicative behaviors of young children with autism spectrum disorders. *Journal of Autism and Developmental Disorders, 39*(1), 149–163. https://doi.org/10.1007/s10803-008-0613-3

McCathren, R. B. (2000). Teacher-implemented prelinguistic communication intervention. *Focus on Autism and Other Developmental Disabilities, 15*(1), 21–29. https://doi.org/10.1177/108835760001500103

McCathren, R. B. (2010). Case study: Parent-implemented prelinguistic milieu teaching with a high risk dyad. *Communication Disorders Quarterly, 31*(4), 243–252. https://doi.org/10.1177/1525740109337733

McDuffie, A., & Yoder, P. (2010). Types of parent verbal responsiveness that predict language in young children with autism spectrum disorder. *Journal of Speech, Language, and Hearing Research, 53*(4), 1026–1039. https://doi.org/10.1044/1092-4388(2009/09-0023)

McLean, J. E., & Snyder-McLean, L. (1978). *A transactional approach to early language training.* Columbus, OH: Charles E. Merill.

McLeod, R. H., Hardy, J. K., & Kaiser, A. P. (2017). The effects of play-based intervention on vocabulary acquisition by preschoolers at risk for reading and language delays. *Journal of Early Intervention, 39*(2), 147–160. https://doi.org/10.1177/1053815117702927

Ogletree, B. T., Davis, P., Hambrecht, G., & Phillips, E. W. (2012). Using milieu training to promote photograph exchange for a young child with autism. *Focus on Autism and Other Developmental Disabilities, 27*(2), 93–101. https://doi.org/10.1177/1088357612441968

Olive, M. L., de la Cruz, B., Davis, T. N., Chan, J. M., Lang, R. B., O'Reilly, M. F., & Dickson, S. M. (2007). The effects of enhanced milieu teaching and a voice output communication aid on the requesting of three children with autism. *Journal of Autism and Developmental Disorders, 37*(8), 1505–1513. https://doi.org/10.1007/s10803-006-0243-6

Olive, M. L., Lang, R., & Davis, T. (2010). An analysis of the effects of functional communication and a voice output communication aid for a child with autism spectrum disorder. *Research in Autism Spectrum Disorders, 2*(2), 223–236. https://doi.org/10.1016/j.rasd.2007.06.002

Ostrosky, M. M., & Kaiser, A. P. (1991). Preschool classroom environments that promote communication. *Teaching Exceptional Children, 23*(4), 6–10.

Parker-McGowan, Q., Chen, M., Reichle, J., Pandit, S., Johnson, L., & Kreibich, S. (2014). Describing treatment intensity in milieu teaching interventions for children with developmental disabilities: A review. *Language, Speech & Hearing Services in Schools, 45*(4), 351–364. https://doi.org/10.1044/2014_LSHSS-13-0087

Peredo, T. N., Zelaya, M. I., & Kaiser, A. P. (2018). Teaching low-income Spanish-speaking caregivers to implement EMT en español with their young children with language impairment: a pilot study. *American Journal of Speech Language Pathology, 27*(1), 136–153. doi: 10.1044/2017_AJSLP-16-0228.

Peterson, P., Carta, J. J., & Greenwood, C. (2005). Teaching enhanced milieu language teaching skills to parents in multiple risk families. *Journal of Early Intervention, 27*(2), 94–109. https://doi.org/10.1177/105381510502700205

Piaget, J., & Inhelder, B. (1969). *The psychology of the child.* New York: Basic Books.

Quinn, E. D., Kaiser, A. P., & Ledford, J. (2021). Hybrid telepractice delivery of enhanced milieu teaching: Effects on caregiver implementation and child communication. *Journal of Speech, Language, and Hearing Research, 64*(8), 3074–3099. https://doi.org/10.1044/2021_JSLHR-20-00430

Roberts, M. Y., Kaiser, A. P., Wolfe, C., Bryant, J., & Spidalieri, A. (2014). The effects of the Teach-Model-Coach-Review instructional approach on caregiver use of language support strategies and children's expressive language skills. *Journal of Speech, Language, and Hearing Research, 57*(5), 1851–1869. https://doi.org/10.1044/2014_JSLHR-L-13-0113

Robertson, S. B., & Weismer, S. E. (1999). Effects of treatment on linguistic and social skills in toddlers with delayed language development. *Journal of Speech, Language, and Hearing Research, 42*(5), 1234–1248. https://doi.org/10.1044/jslhr.4205.1234

Sameroff, A. J., & Chandler, M. J. (1975). Reproductive risk and the continuum of caretaking casualty. In F.D. Horowitz, E. Hetherington, S. Scarr-Salapatek, & G. Siegel (Eds.), *Review of child development research* (Vol. 4, pp. 187–244). Chicago: University of Chicago Press.

Schreibman, L., Dawson, G., Stahmer, A. C., Landa, R., Rogers, S. J., McGee, G.G., Kasari, C., Ingersoll, B., Kaiser, A. P., Bruinsma, Y., McNerney, E., Wetherby, A., & Halladay, A. (2015). Naturalistic developmental behavioral interventions: Empirically validated treatments for autism spectrum disorder. *Journal of Autism and Developmental Disorders, 45*, 2411–2428. doi: 10.1007/s10803-015-2407-8

Skinner, B. E. (1957). *Verbal behavior*. New York: Appleton-Century-Crofts.

Snow, C. E. (1989). Imitativeness: A trait or a skill? In G.E. Speidel & K.E. Nelson (Eds.), *The many faces of imitation in language learning* (pp. 73–90). New York: Springer-Verlag.

Tannock, R., Girolametto, L., & Siegel, L. S. (1992). Language intervention with children who have developmental delays: Effects of an interactive approach. *American Journal on Mental Retardation, 97*, 145–160.

Trivette, C. M., Dunst, C. J., Hamby, D. W., & O'Herin, C. E. (2009). Characteristics and consequences of adult learning methods and strategies. *Practical Evaluation Reports, 2*(1), 1–32.

van Kleeck, A. (1994). Potential cultural bias in training parents as conversational partners with their children who have delays in language development. *American Journal of Speech-Language Pathology, 3*(1), 67–78. https://doi.org/10.1044/1058-0360.0301.67

Vygotsky, L. S. (1978). *Mind in society: The development of higher psychological processes*. Cambridge, MA: Harvard University Press.

Warren, S. F. (1991). Enhancing communication and language development with milieu teaching procedures. In E. Cipani (Ed.), *A guide for developing language competence in preschool children with severe and moderate handicaps* (pp. 68–98). Springfield, IL: Charles C. Thomas.

Warren, S. F., Bredin-Oja, S. L., Fairchild, M., Finestack, L. H., Fey, M. E., & Brady, N. C. (2006). Responsivity education/prelinguistic milieu teaching. In R. J. McCauley & M. E. Fey (Eds.), *Treatment of language disorders in children* (pp. 47–75). Baltimore: Paul H. Brooks.

Warren, S. F., Fey, M. E., Finestack, L. H., Brady, N. C., Bredin-Oja, S. L., & Fleming, K. K. (2008). A randomized trial of longitudinal effects of low-intensity responsivity education/prelinguistic milieu teaching. *Journal of Speech, Language, and Hearing Research, 51*(2), 451–470. https://doi.org/10.1044/1092-4388(2008/033)

Warren, S. F., Fey, M. E., & Yoder, P. J. (2007). Differential treatment intensity research: A missing link to creating optimally effective communication interventions. *Mental Retardation and Developmental Disabilities Research Reviews, 13*(1), 70–77. https://doi.org/10.1002/mrdd.20139

Weiss, R. S. (1981). INREAL intervention for language handicapped and bilingual children. *Journal of the Division for Early Childhood, 4*(1), 40–51. https://doi.org/10.1177/105381518100400106

Wilcox, M., & Shannon, M. (1998). Facilitating the transition from prelinguistic to linguistic communication. In S. F. Warren & J. Reichle (Series Eds.) & A. M. Wetherby, S. F. Warren, & J. Reichle (Vol. Eds.), *Communication and language intervention series: Vol. 7. Transitions in prelinguistic communication* (pp. 385–416). Baltimore: Paul H. Brooks.

Wright, C. A., Kaiser, A. P., Reikowsky, D. I., & Roberts, M. Y. (2013). Effects of a naturalistic sign intervention on expressive language of toddlers with Down syndrome. *Journal of Speech, Language, and Hearing Research, 56*(3), 994–1008. https://doi.org/10.1044/1092-4388(2012/12-0060)

Yoder, P., & Stone, W. L. (2006a). A randomized comparison of the effect of two prelinguistic communication interventions on the acquisition of spoken communication in preschoolers with ASD. *Journal of Speech, Language, and Hearing Research, 49*(4), 698–711. https://doi.org/10.1044/1092-4388(2006/051)

Yoder, P., & Stone, W. L. (2006b). Randomized comparison of two communication interventions for preschoolers with autism spectrum disorders. *Journal of Consulting and Clinical Psychology, 74*(3), 426–435. https://doi.org/10.1037/0022-006X.74.3.426

Yoder, P. J., & Warren, S. F. (1998). Maternal responsivity predicts the prelinguistic communication intervention that facilitates generalized intentional communication. *Journal of Speech, Language, and Hearing Research, 41*(5), 1207–1219. https://doi.org/10.1044/jslhr.4105.1207

Yoder, P.J., & Warren, S.F. (2002). Effects of prelinguistic milieu teaching and parent responsivity education on dyads involving children with intellectual disabilities. *Journal of Speech Language and Hearing Research, 45*(6), 1158–1174. https://doi.org/10.1044/1092-4388(2002/094)

14

Early Intensive Behavioral Intervention for Autism

Lily Stadlober
Acorn Autism Charitable Trust, Auckland, New Zealand

Angela Arnold-Saritepe, Katrina Phillips, and Rebecca Sharp
The University of Auckland

Victor Rodríguez García
Fundación Lovaas, Barcelona, Spain

Eric Larsson
Lovaas Institute Midwest, Minneapolis, Minnesota

Aida Tarifa-Rodriguez
Universidad Autónoma de Madrid

Suzanne C. Purdy and Javier Virues-Ortega
The University of Auckland

14.1 Technical Abstract

Background: Early intensive behavioral intervention (EIBI) denotes 20 or more weekly hours of educational and therapeutic programming for autistic children, incorporating the principles of applied behavior analysis (ABA). EIBI uses a low child-therapist ratio to teach an individualized therapy program based on the needs of the child. **Method:** We reviewed EIBI evidence across four categories: small-*n* experimental studies, randomized controlled trials (RCTs) focusing on specific elements or facets of EIBI, comprehensive longitudinal RCTs, and comprehensive longitudinal nonrandomized group studies. **Results:** Results from hundreds of small-*n* research studies and tens of group-based studies suggest that EIBI is an effective therapy for autistic individuals, specifically in the areas of language and communication, daily living skills, and social behavior. **Discussion:** More research is needed to identify the long-term outcomes of EIBI for the autistic population in adulthood. Further research is also needed to explore client perspectives and the social validity of EIBI. A shift from manualized curricula towards a less prescriptive and more person-centered approach may be necessary to ensure best practice. **Practitioner recommendations:** EIBI is an effective approach for

Lily Stadlober et al., *Early Intensive Behavioral Intervention for Autism*. In: *Lifespan Treatment for Autistic Individuals*.
Edited by: Peter Sturmey, Russell Lang, and James K. Luiselli, Oxford University Press. © Oxford University Press (2025).
DOI: 10.1093/oso/9780197635841.003.0014

increasing skills across a range of developmental domains, both as a comprehensive or focused therapeutic approach. Involving autistic children and their families in all aspects of assessment and intervention planning is paramount to ensuring that treatment outcomes are person-centered and socially valid.

14.2 Layperson Summary

EIBI is a type of therapeutic intervention for autistic children. EIBI is typically delivered to children as young as 18 months of age over a period of several years for 20 to 40 hours per week. EIBI is based on a science of human learning and behavior known as ABA. A trained therapist will support the child one-to-one or in a small group, working on individualized therapy goals across a range of developmental skill areas. Skills are often broken down into small, teachable steps.

We reviewed the evidence base for EIBI and evaluated the quality of evidence across a range of research designs. Additionally, we explored some of the criticisms and claims against EIBI, including the lack of client involvement in the assessment and intervention process and concerns regarding some treatment goals (e.g., reducing stereotypy or "stimming").

Hundreds of studies have demonstrated the effectiveness of EIBI for autistic individuals. However, a substantial portion of this literature has examined specific elements of the intervention, with only a few participants in each study. These small-*n* studies are often omitted from the EIBI evidence base by researchers who favor evidence from larger studies, resulting in debate as to the current level of evidence that supports EIBI. Several ethical and practical constraints have limited the number of RCTs available for this treatment model.

Despite this debate, research suggests that EIBI results in positive improvements for autistic individuals across a range of areas, including language and communication, daily living skills, and social behavior. Some studies suggest that preintervention functioning and age have a negative correlation with treatment outcomes. Person-centered EIBI should involve autistic children and their families in the assessment and intervention process to ensure intervention goals and approaches are based on client values and preferences.

14.3 Treatment Summary Table

Treatment summary: Early Intensive Behavioral Intervention

Treatment description: EIBI refers to therapeutic services for autistic children based on the principles of applied behavior analysis. Services start as early as possible (typically no earlier than 18 months of age) and consists of 20 to 40 hours per week of intervention. Therapy programs are based on developmental progression and involve breaking skills down into small, teachable steps.

Expected outcomes: Results from hundreds of small-*n* research studies and tens of group-based studies suggest that EIBI is an effective therapy for autistic individuals, specifically in the areas of language and communication, daily living skills, and social behavior. Although research with respect to intervention intensity is mixed, at least 15 hours of intervention has been shown to lead to clinically important changes.

Methods: A review of the existing EIBI literature examined research across four categories: small-*n* experimental studies, RCTs focusing on specific elements or facets of EIBI, comprehensive longitudinal RCTs, and comprehensive longitudinal nonrandomized group studies. Several myths and criticisms pertaining to EIBI were also explored.

Expertise required to implement treatment: EIBI is typically delivered via a tiered service model. EIBI assessment, program development, and case supervision is undertaken by a certified master-level professional. Due to recent changes in the professional certification landscape (i.e., the Behavior Analyst Certification Board is only available in the United States, Canada, United Kingdom, and Australia), some countries are in the process of developing their own national credentials or adopting existing international certification schemes.

Risks and negative side effects: None of the studies reviewed noted negative side effects associated with EIBI. Further research is still needed to understand the long-term outcomes of EIBI. Focused interventions have evaluated restrictive procedures including extinction, which could cause extinction-induced aggression and emotional distress in the absence of appropriate mitigating strategies.

Additional considerations and limitations: In countries where EIBI is not publicly or insurance funded, the cost of EIBI can be prohibitive. Receiving fewer therapy hours or parent training may result in a more focused intervention and can produce slower progress. Clients and their families should be involved in all aspects of the intervention. EIBI based on manualized or prescriptive curricula can limit the individualized nature of the intervention. Parental involvement and stress levels should be assessed as it may have a significant impact on treatment success. Research remains limited on the long-term outcomes of EIBI.

14.4 Introduction

14.4.1 Intervention Description

EIBI refers to educational and therapeutic programming for autistic children first developed as a comprehensive intervention by O. Ivar Lovaas at the University of California (Lovaas, 1987).[1] This approach is based on ABA, a scientific field that uses experimental methodology to facilitate meaningful changes in socially important behaviors. Behavior-analytic interventions have been used in a range of practice areas, including autism, intellectual disability, dementia, brain injury, addiction, fitness training, and organizational behavior management, among others (Roane et al., 2015).

Most EIBI programs are delivered with 1:1 or a low child-therapist ratio for 20 to 40 hours per week over several years (Eldevik et al., 2010; Linstead et al., 2017).

[1] This chapter will use identity-first language based on the recommendations of Autism Terminology Guidance from Aotearoa New Zealand's Autistic community. Preferences in language and terminology differ within the autistic community, and it is respectful to ask an autistic person about their terminology preferences.

Typically, EIBI programs are developed and overseen by a master-level certified behavior analyst and implemented by one or more registered technicians (Council of Autism Service Providers [CASP], 2020). The curriculum of EIBI programs varies based on each child's individual needs. However, most bona fide programs incorporate a set of core elements (Peters-Scheffer et al., 2012), including the ones indicated below:

1. *EIBI programs should be based on behavior-analytic principles*, meaning that interventions are guided by well-established research-based principles within the empirical (mostly experimental) behavioral literature.
2. *EIBI programs are comprehensive*, addressing a wide range of skill domains, including language and communication, play, social relationships, cognitive and academic skills, and activities of daily living. Comprehensive EIBI programs also look to reduce behavioral challenges (i.e., problem behaviors). Focused ABA-based services that address a specific repertoire or need are generally not referred to as EIBI (see CASP, 2020, for a brief distinction between comprehensive and focused programs).
3. *EIBI programs teach skills systematically.* Skills are broken down into small, teachable steps. This scaffolding approach supports the development of simple and subsequently more complex skills. Interventions can be delivered in the home environment or in a dedicated clinic or classroom, with a plan to ensure that skills are transferred to the child's everyday life.
4. *All EIBI goals and teaching procedures are individualized* to the strengths and needs of the individual child and are typically based upon manualized curricula (e.g., Verbal Behavior Milestones Assessment and Placement Program, VB-MAPP; Assessment of Basic Language and Learning Skills, Revised, ABLLS-R) and functional behavioral assessments.
5. *Progress is monitored through data collection and analysis.* Data-based decision-making is critical to evaluate the effectiveness of interventions and ensure timely changes in the behavior plan.
6. *EIBI should start as early as possible.* Research indicates that starting as early as 2 years of age or earlier can lead to the best outcomes (Zwaigenbaum et al., 2015).
7. *A 1:1 child-therapist ratio or small group is common.* Therapy often starts with 1:1 and transitions to small groups when the child has acquired critical prerequisite academic, communication, and play skills.

14.4.2 Rationale and Objectives

EIBI should be construed as a comprehensive, multicomponent, data-based, and individualized approach to behavioral autism services. The practitioner, drawing from an extensive empirical body of literature, uses a plethora of procedures intended to establish or modify developmentally important behaviors. These procedures can be grouped into reinforcement-based and antecedent-based programs. Reinforcement-based programs teach skills by following functional skills or behaviors with a positive outcome. Antecedent-based programs make environmental changes to reduce the likelihood of challenging behaviors occurring and increase the likelihood of positive interactions. Table 14.1 presents a brief overview of this simplified classification of the intervention procedures that make up an EIBI curriculum. A more complete listing of these procedures can be obtained in the professional task list for behavior analysts published by the Behavior Analyst Certification Board (Behavior Analyst Certification Board [BACB], 2023a).

Extensive research dating back to 1987 has demonstrated the effectiveness of EIBI as a comprehensive (or semicomprehensive) approach to working with autistic individuals on skill areas, including expressive and receptive language, intellectual functioning, and other adaptive skills (Virues-Ortega et al., 2022). It is critical to note that the long-term, between-group studies of comprehensive ABA that found the largest effects incorporated extensive weekly hours of direct observation, programing adjustments, therapist training, and parent training by the behavior analysts. These studies also specified extensive ongoing clinical review to ensure treatment fidelity and parent satisfaction.

The overwhelming majority of focused ABA studies (in contrast with group-based EIBI studies) have used small-*n* research designs whereby one or a small number of research participants serve as their own control and are exposed to all conditions of the study. Small-*n* designs are often challenged by mainstream clinical sciences as providing a lesser form of scientific evidence than more established group-based designs used in the medical sciences (e.g., RCTs) (see, for example, Virues-Ortega & Sivaraman, in press). However, due to the high heterogeneity of autism, both research designs have their own value (Zwaigenbaum et al., 2015), with small-*n* studies better suited for treatment component development and evaluation and group-based studies providing an overview of the compounded long-term effect of complex multicomponent interventions.

Historically, EIBI has heavily relied on discrete-trial instruction (DTI), which refers to an approach to teaching whereby the instructor presents a clear instruction, the learner responds, and the response may be followed by a rewarding consequence (see Chapter 12). If the learner provides the desired response, the instructor may grant access to a preferred item or activity for a brief period with the aim of producing a reinforcement effect, meaning that the target skill would become more firmly established in the individual's repertoire. The trials may be repeated at a high rate to maintain the learner's engagement. It may be necessary to introduce a new target skill in "massed trials" (without intervening alternative discrimination trials) without errors, while systematically fading the instructor prompts. As soon as possible, the discrimination is then introduced, expanded, and generalized in order to establish and maintain natural responding (Larsson &

Table 14.1 Simplified classification of intervention procedures composing EIBI curricula

Category	Application	Example Procedure	Example Application
Reinforcement-based program	Establish developmentally appropriate novel behavior.	Shaping	Establish the vowel sound "a" as part of a generalized mand.
	Reduce challenging behavior by introducing an alternative behavior that is equally or more reinforcing than the challenging behavior.	Differential reinforcement	Reduce attention-maintained class disruption by making attention contingent on the student raising their hand.
	Reduce challenging behavior by eliminating subsequent reinforcing events.	Extinction	Adult refrains from providing attention (e.g., eye contact, physical proximity, verbal interaction) upon the occurrence of attention-maintained destructive behavior (e.g., destroying a toy).
Antecedent-based program	Induce developmentally appropriate behavior in relevant contexts.	Mand training	With water present, offering water only when the learner says "water."
	Establish complex stimulus-stimulus relations.	Equivalence-based instruction	Student says the word "car" in the presence of a toy car after having learned to select a toy car in the presence of the word "car."
	Reduce challenging behavior by preventing the behavior from occurring.	Stimulus fading	Reduce task difficulty to reduce disruptive behavior maintained by escape from instructional demands.
	Establish imitation as a generalized class of behavior to teach and maintain complex language and social skills.	Modeling	Provide a model of an offer to share during cooperative play with a natural peer.
Extinction-based program	Reduce challenging behavior by eliminating subsequent reinforcing events.	Planned to ignore	Adult refrains from providing attention (e.g., eye contact, physical proximity, verbal interaction) upon the occurrence of attention-maintained destructive behavior (e.g., destroying a toy).

EIBI = early intensive behavioral intervention.

Wright, 2024). DTI has been criticized for its focus on "rote learning" and lack of generalization of acquired skills beyond the teaching environment when compared to more naturalistic methods (see, for example, Jennett et al., 2008). However, it is a standard of practice that DTI procedures should include built-in generalization strategies such as varying the instructions and contextual cues in which a response is required across learning trials, thereby helping to emulate the diversity of the natural environment. The use of DTI relative to instructional methods that more closely track the natural environment (e.g., natural environment teaching [NET]) should not be thought of as conflicting ABA-based approaches, but as complementary tools at the disposal of the professional. Specifically, DTI can provide the learning opportunities needed for acquiring repertoires that would be lengthy to teach by other means (e.g., acquisition of an age-appropriate vocabulary), while naturalistic strategies can enhance the generalization and ecological validity of the behavioral gains (e.g., naming everyday objects in appropriate social contexts). Like most areas of clinical practice, EIBI has evolved over time, and many practitioners now employ more individualized, naturalistic, and play-based teaching methods, now referred to as naturalistic developmental behavioral interventions (NDBIs) (Schreibman et al., 2015). See Chapter 16 for detailed consideration of NDBI.

With the substantial evidence base that exists for EIBI and the increase in the prevalence of autism diagnoses, it is unsurprising that all 50 states across the United States now require that insurance companies fund EIBI (National Conference of State Legislatures, 2021). Additionally, most states have developed policies for professional licensure and certification (BACB, 2023b). The recent increase in demand for behavioral supports for people with autism and their families has seen a dramatic rise in ABA-based services in North America and elsewhere. This growth has been funded by venture capitalists in some contexts, raising concerns about how the cost-cutting and fast-profit incentives that often underlie private equity firms measure up with the commitment to high-quality ethical services (e.g., Fry, 2022). Further, starting in 2020, the US-based Behavior Analyst Certification Board (BACB) ceased to provide credentialing services to professionals outside the United States and a handful of other countries. These recent changes to credentialing outside North America have raised concerns around ensuring practitioners are appropriately trained, follow best practice, and are accountable to consumers and other stakeholders.

14.4.3 Considerations for Implementation

Although the goal of EIBI is to improve socially valid outcomes for autistic people, EIBI has been the subject of increasing scrutiny from the community. For example, EIBI has been criticized for its focus on the reduction of autistic characteristics such as non-self-injurious stereotypy ("stimming"). More recently, it has been compared to "conversion therapy," and some autism advocates have taken a clear stance against any ABA-based interventions (Conine et al., 2022).

In this chapter, we will present a brief overview of the empirical evidence in support of EIBI services, while highlighting the areas that still require much research, acknowledging the merits (or lack thereof) of common criticisms that have become more apparent in the wake of the unprecedented growth of the professional field in recent decades. We will discuss the importance of social validity and involvement of the clients and their families in the assessment process and during service delivery.

14.5 Research Background

14.5.1 Overview of EIBI Research

The evidence supporting EIBI can be grouped in four major categories: small-*n* experimental studies, RCTs focusing on specific elements or facets of EIBI, comprehensive longitudinal RCTs, and comprehensive longitudinal nonrandomized group studies. A major challenge for the first two categories is that they are seldom recognized by non-behavior analysts as pertaining to EIBI at all and, as a result, this literature, including several hundreds of small-*n* experimental studies, is often dismissed. For example, RCTs evaluating ABA-based interventions for establishing joint attention would rarely be appreciated as relevant to the EIBI outcome literature, even though engaging in joint attention is a common target of EIBI curricula (see a summary of this literature in Murza et al., 2016).

The assessment of evidence in favor of an intervention model is often evaluated through RCTs whereby participants are assigned at random to an intervention or control group. Those in the intervention group would receive the bona fide intervention, whereas those in the control group would receive *treatment as usual*, meaning no new interventions, or a placebo (something that looks like an intervention, but it is not). While RCTs have become the currency of intervention evaluation in the health sciences, they have proved to be incredibly challenging to conduct in the ABA-services context. Specifically, most families and ethics committees find it unacceptable that a child would be deprived of a potentially useful intervention early in the individual's development due to the methodological requirements of the RCT's randomization schedule. Further, where the typical RCT of a medical intervention may only last for a period of weeks or months, comprehensive EIBI typically lasts for 2 to 3 years. This long treatment duration compounds the ethical challenges of an RCT. This and other similar challenges have produced a mixed-outcome research landscape in the field of ABA where most of the evidence comes from small-*n* studies that are generally not recognized by the mainstream clinical sciences, as well as a myriad of nonrandomized group-based studies that provide various degrees of evidence that invariably fall short of the

RCT standard. If we are to attend only to comprehensive and longitudinal RCT studies, this literature is currently limited to Smith et al. (2000).

Meta-analyses, studies that compile the evidence of several individual studies, still describe EIBI simply as a *promising* intervention (Reichow et al., 2018; Shi et al., 2021; Virues-Ortega, 2010) or an intervention that requires further research (Sandback et al., 2020, 2021). These studies regularly call for additional RCTs in what has become a decades-long litany demanding that the meager pool of randomized studies be expanded. In the last few years, a modest but healthy trend of RCTs that focus on specific aspects of EIBI, or on relatively short follow-up periods of wider interventions, is becoming evident. For example, Dixon et al. (2021) reported a multiarm RCT of two approaches to comprehensive ABA-based services (i.e., comprehensive ABA services based on Skinner's (1957) analysis of verbal operants, and comprehensive ABA services that incorporate instruction based on derived stimulus–stimulus relations) over a short 18-week follow-up period. The authors were able to demonstrate clinically significant effects of various ABA-based curricula while circumventing the ethical implications of longer-term RCTs.

In another recent example, Rogers et al. (2021) minimized the ethical concerns regarding randomization by conducting a randomized *clinical* trial (they still use the term *RCT* in their manuscript), meaning that the random assignment was limited to various levels of treatment intensities (15 vs. 25 weekly hours) and styles (EIBI vs Early Start Denver Model), and did not involve a no-intervention control group. In this comparison of two low-intensity treatments, no statistical differences by treatment intensity or treatment style were found (although the higher intensity did improve outcomes for participants at one of the participating sites). While the study ticked several methodological boxes (treatment fidelity checks, blind assessors and coders, multisite recruitment, intention-to-treat analysis), their results were limited by the constrained age range, short follow-up period, absence of a bona fide control group, small number of assessment tools, and borderline statistical power.[2]

Most group-based treatment evaluations are found in the last of the four categories of research proposed at the beginning of this section, nonrandomized studies. Most of this literature (see reviews in Sandbank et al., 2020; Shi et al., 2021; Virues-Ortega, 2010) has focused on standardized scores, such as IQ, receptive and expressive language, and adaptive behavior, including communication, daily living skills, and social repertoires. Fewer studies have used standardized scores of social affect, hyperactivity, and challenging behaviors. There is no consensus in the literature on the standardized outcomes that should be used in comprehensive psychosocial interventions for autistic people. However, cognitive, language, and social/adaptive domains are consistently reported (see Virues-Ortega et al., 2022).

[2] Although not discussed by the authors, an a posteriori power analysis suggests that at least 116 individuals (as opposed to the 87 participants reported) would have been needed for a four-arm RCT where effect differences across groups are expected to be minimal (assumed power: 0.9; expected eta squared effect: 0.15; alpha: 0.05).

The effect sizes among these various domains fall within the moderate to large (0.50 to 0.80) and large (above 0.80) effect size ranges. Sensitivity analyses have shown that these results are robust to study design (nonrandomized controlled trial versus single-arm trial or retrospective observational study) and to the specific standardized outcomes utilized within a particular outcome domain (Virues-Ortega, 2010). One further problem is that the assessment instruments are standardized for the nonautistic population, with the impact that they are not sensitive to the improvements made by many autistic individuals whose baseline measures were more than two standard deviations from the mean.

Two interesting themes are gradually being established within this literature: community-based evaluations and treatment effect moderators. Several nonrandomized large-*n* studies have focused on community-level evaluations of EIBI (Dimian et al., 2021; Plavnick et al., 2020; Yingling et al., 2019). These studies generally validate the preexisting literature with a very diverse set of methodologies (usually observational studies) and outcomes. For example, Dimian et al. (2021) reported a retrospective cohort study ($n = 667$) focusing on the educational outcomes of individuals that had received Medicaid-waved EIBI services. The study showed that individuals who started receiving services sooner had better educational outcomes 4 to 6 years after the onset of services. Other community-based studies generally support the delivery of ABA services at a population scale as indicated by the percentage of use of services (Plavnick et al., 2020) and the demographics of the individuals using subsidized services (arguably an indication of treatment acceptability at the population level when these demographics are found to be comparable to those in the general population) (Yingling et al., 2019).

Studies have also focused on a small range of treatment effect moderators. These include treatment intensity, age at intervention onset, preintervention functioning, and intervention quality, among others. Overall, the evidence available pertaining to intervention intensity has been mixed. Several studies and meta-regression analyses report positive (Shi et al., 2021; Virues-Ortega, 2010; Virues-Ortega et al., 2013a) or mixed results (Rogers et al., 2021; Sandbank et al., 2020, 2021). Here absence of evidence should not be confused with evidence of absence. Specifically, the heterogeneity of the available studies (see a discussion in Virues-Ortega, 2010) cannot be overlooked. Moreover, intensity, usually measured in weekly intervention hours, cannot be dissociated from the personal and clinical contexts of the individuals and families receiving the service. For example, treatment intensity is often dictated by family preference, availability of services, or client characteristics, which are probably co-dependent on the preintervention functioning, intervention quality, and other relevant moderators. The potential for collinearity of these moderator candidates calls into question much of the literature focused narrowly on treatment effect moderators using group-based studies (see, for example, Rogers et al., 2021). An alternative approach might be to focus on intervention duration (e.g., total intervention hours), which has shown dose-dependent characteristics in at least one meta-analysis (see Virues-Ortega, 2010, fig. 3). The effects of age and preintervention functioning are generally less contested as predictors of medium- and long-term intervention effects (Dimian et al., 2021; Tiura et al., 2017; Virues-Ortega et al., 2013a; see Rogers et al., 2021 for a negative result).

An interesting exception in the treatment moderator literature is the study on treatment quality by Långh et al. (2021). They used the York Measure of Quality of Intensive Behavioral Intervention (Penn et al., 2007) to evaluate how the standard of ABA-based intervention impacted treatment outcomes after 4 to 6 months of services. The authors concluded that treatment organization (ability to adapt intervention based on the progress of the child), teaching level (the extent to which the trainer teaches the child skills that are neither too difficult nor too easy for the child), and the use of differential reinforcement were discrete factors correlated with better outcomes, particularly in the areas of *language* and *learning skills* (the RCT by Dixon et al. [2021] could also fall within this category).

Although research syntheses abound, policy decision makers and consumers should sharpen their critical judgment when consuming this literature. Arbitrary methodological decisions can have a huge impact in the evaluation of scientific evidence. For example, Tachibana et al. (2017) restricted their selection of the literature to RCTs and included only two studies within the "behavioral" category in their meta-analysis; one was a long-term comprehensive evaluation study of EIBI (Smith et al., 2000), while the second involved a short-term functional communication treatment evaluation (Reitzel et al., 2013). Furthermore, Sandbank et al. (2020) pooled a variety of comprehensive and focused intervention studies in their meta-analysis of behavior-oriented interventions, ranging from a focused intervention on sleep disturbances in young children with ASD (Johnson et al., 2013) to a longitudinal analysis focusing on postintervention effect maintenance (Kovshoff et al., 2011). This confusion may be attributed to the fact that behavior analysts are leaving it to others (non-behavior analysts) to evaluate EIBI in randomized, non-randomized studies, and meta-analysis (e.g., Rogers et al., 2021; Sandbank et al., 2020). While this provides a veneer of independence, it often results in conceptual misunderstandings in key aspects of the studies, including inclusion criteria, treatment characterization, and treatment fidelity.

14.5.2 Summary and Recommendations

As the subfield of outcome research in ABA-based services slowly matures, a few recommendations and corollaries are emerging that have the potential to orient professionals and consumers. These are briefly summarized below.

1. *Assess the existing evidence in context.* All the designs used in research point to the emerging effectiveness of EIBI for autism, whether they are RCTs (focused or comprehensive-longitudinal), randomized clinical trials, within-subject studies (i.e., small-*n*), or observational community-based studies. A final cautionary note relevant here pertains to the evolving nature of the ABA-based curriculum, a field that is under a constant feedback loop

from the basic and applied sectors of behavior analysis. This is often not fully appreciated in studies characterizing EIBI as a component-based intervention (see, for example, the conceptualization of EIBI treatment fidelity by Rogers et al., 2021).

2. *Consider both focused and comprehensive ABA services when evaluating evidence.* The mainstream outcome literature has systematically missed (or dismissed) focused treatment evaluations, both based in small-*n* experimental designs and group-based studies (randomized and nonrandomized). This body of evidence is rich and relevant to evaluating elements of the EIBI curriculum. It may also be more sensitive to the authentic, person-centered goals of the participants.
3. *We need a greater understanding of when and for whom the intervention is effective.* The EIBI outcome literature falls short in its relevance to service planning for the individual client. Still, it is not too early to indicate that programs of at least 15 hours per week have consistently shown clinically important gains and that individuals with any preintervention functioning can benefit from EIBI. There is also some evidence to suggest that the earlier the intervention starts and the longer it runs, the more positive its impact seems to be.
4. *Standardized outcomes are limited but not flawed.* The heterogeneity of outcomes in the existing EIBI outcome literature is challenged by the omission of all-important domains of functioning that have remained unreported. These include areas such as anxiety and socioemotional development, parental acceptability and stress, and school adaptation and graduation requirements, to mention a few. A valuable attempt to develop a core set of standardized outcomes with some interdisciplinary acceptability and cross-cultural validity has been proposed by International Consortium of Health Outcomes Measurement (2021). It is desirable that comprehensive assessment batteries are implemented in the future.

14.5.3 Research on Social Validity

The field of outcome research of autism services may be at a transition point as person-centered outcomes take priority over the (still-informative) standardized outcomes discussed in the previous section. A standard deviation above the expected postintervention performance in receptive language or general IQ has face value, but what do these outcomes look like for the learner, their family, and those closest to them? Scores on a test or data points on a graph do not generally hold the same value to parents and caregivers as tying shoelaces and asking for a glass of juice.

Research pertaining to parental satisfaction with EIBI is limited. Grey et al. (2019) developed an EIBI parental satisfaction scale (PSS-EIBI) that looked at child outcomes, family outcomes, quality of the intervention model, and relationship with the team. The scale was given to parents during the first and second year of their child's EIBI program, and results indicated parental satisfaction was high across all domains. Similarly, Rogers et al. (2021) reported caregiver satisfaction was high regardless of intervention type or intensity.

Even less research has paid attention to long-term outcomes for autistic people who received EIBI as children. Koudys et al. (2021) looked at the mental health profiles of 12 youth who had previously received EIBI. Overall group means for the autistic youth were not significantly different from the normative sample. On the internalizing index, autistic youth scored significantly worse than the normative group, suggesting that autistic youth may be experiencing more anxiety and depression than their nonautistic peers. Similarly, on follow-up, Smith et al. (2021) found their sample of 19 youth who had received 2 years of EIBI as preschoolers had received no additional psychiatric diagnoses or had been prescribed psychotropic medications. They also found the 19 youth to have maintained the gains they made in EIBI. Both findings contrast with reports of high comorbid psychiatric diagnoses among autistic people (see, for example, Virues-Ortega et al., 2018).

14.5.4 Utility of Manualized Curricula

Numerous resources have been published since Lovaas's (1981) text, *The Me Book*. Examples include *Behavioral Interventions for Children with Autism* (Maurice et al., 1996), *A Work in Progress* (Leaf et al., 1999), and *Teaching Individuals With Developmental Delays* (Lovaas, 2003). These curricula are all based primarily on DTI and fall broadly into the category of EIBI. Further manuals for supporting autistic children have been published that use a naturalistic developmental approach. Examples include the Early Start Denver model (Dawson et al., 2010); Social Communication, Emotional Regulation, and Transactional Support® (SCERTS; Prizant et al. 2003); or ACE® ABA Software System (New England Center for Children, 2023).

Manuals are intended to guide clinicians and parents on how to support young autistic children to acquire skills. They also help to support the integrity of the delivery of interventions. While aspirational, these are not necessarily their only effects, because those following the manual may or may not be skilled practitioners, and the intervention goals and strategies may or may not fit with those of the family. It is therefore important to consider whether manuals can be a barrier to individualized intervention. Each individual lives and behaves in a different context which will impact their learning. A challenge for families and practitioners is that the field of early intervention for autistic children has been divided into various subgroups or micro paradigms, for example, NDBI, verbal behavior, Early

Start Denver model, relational frame theory, CABAS®, and the list goes on. A potential adverse effect of splitting into subapproaches is that following one might also involve rejecting previous approaches, leading to missed opportunities to learn from these previous approaches. A fragmented professional field is particularly disadvantageous for an emerging applied science, such as ABA, in that those self-ascribed to a particular subgroup or niche may not read publications or attend to events from the subgroup or niche "next door" (see Virues-Ortega et al., 2014, for some evidence on closed scientific interaction among ABA subgroups).

14.6 Myths versus Legitimate Criticisms

The field of ABA-based autism services has been heavily criticized over the years. A summary of these criticisms is presented on Table 14.2 along with an appraisal on the merits of these "attacks" (myth vs. fact) and a commentary on the legitimate criticisms and constructive lessons that can be derived from them. Below, we take a more in-depth approach to a selection of these considerations.

Table 14.2 Myths around ABA-based autism services

Myth	Fact	Legitimate Criticism
ABA-based services for autism have not been demonstrated to be effective.	EIBI and other ABA-based services are supported by a large corpus of scientific evidence, including laboratory studies, translational studies, small-*n* experimental studies, within-subject studies, case-control studies, between-group studies without randomization, and, to a lesser extent, focused and comprehensive randomized controlled trials.	There are few longitudinal and randomized controlled trials in the EIBI outcome literature. The field should invest in these kinds of studies in the coming years, owing to their high acceptability for policy decision makers and other stakeholders.
ABA is a therapy for autism that was invented by O. I. Lovaas.	ABA is an applied science and not a therapy directed to a specific clinical population. While O. I. Lovaas did pioneering work in the applications of ABA for autism, there have been other ABA-based interventions studied before Lovaas's work, including studies conducted with autistic children.	Misnomers such as "Lovaas therapy" or "UCLA model" have become mainstream, thereby perpetuating this confusion.
ABA uses punishment and bribes to trick children into engaging in desirable behaviors.	ABA-based services make extensive use of contingent reinforcement and massed trials to modify socially important behaviors. Reinforcement is a	The use of the term *punishment* to denote a technical meaning (reduce a behavior by means of stimulus presentation or reward

Myth	Fact	Legitimate Criticism
	natural process that is part of our daily lives and cannot be misrepresented as bribing. Behavior analysts abide by ethical codes that severely restrict the use of punishment-based procedures.	withdrawal) has been the cause of much confusion. The use of punishment-based procedures, particularly in the early ABA literature, overshadows the understanding of current ABA services. The field should acknowledge and learn from its legacy. Interestingly, other fields of psychology seem to be proud of their unethical legacy, which does not appear to have fueled criticism (e.g., Zimbardo prison's study, Milner's study on compliance to authority).
ABA-based therapy can cure autism.	Autism is a complex multigenic disorder that has no known cure in the traditional medical sense. A fraction of children with a diagnosis of autism may no longer meet the diagnostic criteria for autism after receiving EIBI or may be able to function in mainstream classrooms without additional supports. However, this kind of progress cannot be equated to a "cure."	The traditional emphasis on standardized assessments (i.e., indices of deviation from the statistical norm), as the sole indicators of treatment success, has contributed to a perception that the intervention's primary focus is to "normalize" the learner. More emphasis in patient-centered outcomes in future studies could help to balance this trend.
ABA-based intervention cares only about the "behavior."	ABA focuses on all observable behavior. Nonobservables with face validity (e.g., self-esteem, empathy, abstract thinking) are constructs that may be broken down in specific behavioral indicators. Behavior analysis regards emotions, thoughts, and other nonobservables as behavior, although for practical reasons professionals emphasize the observable by-products of private behavior.	More behavior-analytic research is needed in areas such as indices of happiness (particularly while receiving EIBI), metacognitive skills, creativity, and other areas commonly considered "not behavior" outside the field of ABA. It should be noted that these domains are already part of most ABA-based curricula.
ABA-based services only work with young children and with certain kinds of autism. ABA-based services are not for every child or every family.	As an applied science, ABA is not limited to a specific population. Numerous applications of ABA have been demonstrated with a huge variety of populations and in very diverse contexts. Also, the effects of EIBI have been documented with individuals with diverse preintervention functioning, ages, and cultural backgrounds.	Curriculum design should be tailored to the needs of the individual and family. Most ABA-based research and services for autism has focused on young children. Further research and practice guidelines should be developed to address client diversity due to age, culture, and other factors.

continued

Table 14.2 *continued*

Myth	Fact	Legitimate Criticism
ABA for autism has become a multi-million-dollar industry, putting it at risk of sacrificing standards for profit.	There are legitimate concerns about the scaling up of services through venture-capitalist investments. This is developing trend; the consequences are yet to be evaluated.	Major service providers should play an important role in the assessment of service quality and treatment effects—so far this has not been the case. The scaling up of an economic sector does raise concerns about ethical and quality standards. This is true for other areas, including medical services. Checks and balances should be in place to prevent service delivery standards from being compromised.
ABA causes trauma. ABA is a form of conversion therapy in disguise.	There is no evidence that ABA-based services can cause trauma. However, some autism advocates have informally described ABA services as alienating and traumatic. It is unclear how prevalent these perceptions might be or whether they are the result of direct experience with ABA services.	The field should investigate these reports and allegations and make a sincere effort to understand the relevant contexts. Professionals should embrace trauma-informed approaches to service delivery (see, for example, Rajaraman et al., 2022). The field should readily acknowledge unethical cases from its history whenever it is appropriate to do so and learn valuable lessons from this legacy.
ABA-based services emphasize compliance, rote memory, and robot-like behaviors, and ignore decision-making, emotions, spontaneity, and language generativity.	EIBI curricula typically place a strong emphasis on language, generativity, spontaneity, and generalization (ecological validity).	Not all ABA curricula place the same emphasis on these factors. A greater consensus and greater integration of most recent research would be a positive move. In addition, published ABA curricula should be updated periodically. The authors of these curricula should proactively incorporate all relevant research.
ABA-based services only work if they are delivered intensively (20 hours per week or more).	ABA-based interventions may be focused or comprehensive.	Professionals should be clear about what realistic expectations come with various levels of service.
ABA-based services rely on a bogus and outdated pseudoscience that was refuted back in the 1950s.	The science of behavior analysis has been a part of psychology, although in constant evolution, for many decades. Noam Chomsky published a famous critique to B. F. Skinner book on verbal behavior (language). However, this was a conceptual criticism, not an empirical one.	Behavior analysis is a minority subfield within psychology. While its philosophical basis is comprehensive, its development has been limited to specific areas. The field is divided into numerous groups and micro-paradigms (UCLA model, CABAS, Verbal

Myth	Fact	Legitimate Criticism
	Subsequent studies have demonstrated that Skinner's approach to language can lead to numerous evidence-based procedures for the acquisition of verbal repertoires.	behavior approach, Contextualism, Interbehaviorism, etc.), which may be confusing to the public.

ABA = applied behavior analysis; EIBI = early intensive behavioral intervention.

14.6.1 Lack of Evidence as a Criticism to EIBI

"ABA is abusive and unethical because it aims to 'extinguish' autistic traits and 'normalize' children, otherizes benign behavior, *lacks evidence of effectiveness* [italics added], works against the development of key life skills and independence, and leads to serious, trauma-based mental health phenomena" (Cernius, 2022).

The field of behavior analysis has never been short of critics. As suggested by the *Fortune* magazine excerpt above, the lack-of-evidence argument is often brought to the table. Although much remains to be done, there are numerous studies supporting EIBI effectiveness, and there is no other treatment model with a comparable body of evidence (see, for example, Virues-Ortega et al., 2013b). The authors of the Early Start Denver model and Pre-school Autism Communication Trial (PACT), to mention two evidence-based alternatives, have made definite efforts to evaluate their programs. However, by comparison, their respective bodies of empirical studies are modest (albeit their number of RCTs is comparable to those available for EIBI) (see, for example, Dawson et al., 2010; Green et al., 2010).

There are, however, several lessons to be learned from the lack-of-evidence criticisms received by EIBI (warranted or unwarranted) that should inform scientific decision-making in the future. Some of these are summarized below:

1. *Need for ethically informed methodological standards.* We have briefly reviewed ethical concerns in the use of RCTs. Yet emerging approaches such as focused RCTs and community-based studies are bound to bridge the evidence gap over the next few years. There is also room for improvement in making this new research more relatable to clinical decision-making for the individual client. Are there specific criteria that would make a student ineligible for ABA services? Are EIBI curricula free of potentially restrictive procedures (e.g., extinction, use of intensive establishing operations)? These, and many other questions, could inform the design of future evaluations of effectiveness.
2. *Actively include research standards that inform treatment acceptability.* Future studies should actively evaluate short- and long-term side effects; assess parental involvement, stress, and perceived acceptability; and enforce

consecutive admission or other forms of unbiased participant admission. A more holistic approach to the evaluation of evidence would offset some of the current criticisms and engage in the wider conversation of treatment ethics in autism.

3. *Become mainstream.* Behavior analysts often publish in niche journals and present their work in behavioral conferences rather than speaking to broader audiences. A transition to a more multidisciplinary approach to treatment evaluation would have a favorable impact on dissemination of findings and treatment acceptability. Some steps in this direction may include incorporating multidisciplinary teams in treatment planning and evaluation (see, for example, Taylor et al., 2019), identifying focused intervention evaluations as part of the typical EIBI curriculum, educating stakeholders on the value of single-subject studies, and reaching methodological compromises, for example, by synthesizing small-*n* and group-based studies recognizing the distinct merits of both methodological traditions.

14.6.2 Autism Cure Criticism

A common criticism of EIBI is that it attempts to "cure" autism or teach autistic people how to be neurotypical or indistinguishable from others. Some have compared EIBI to "conversion therapy." Lovaas (1987) did report on the number of individuals who achieved "normal intellectual and educational functioning." With EIBI manualized assessments and curricula focusing on neurotypical development milestones, one could easily imply some of the basis for this misconception. A standard of evidence-based practice in psychology (including ABA) is that practice should integrate "the best available research with clinical expertise in the context of patient characteristics, culture, and preferences" (APA Presidential Task Force on Evidence Based Practice, 2006, p. 273).

An illustration of ecological validity in services to people with intellectual and developmental disability may be provided by Essential for Living (2012). This assessment tool and curriculum focuses on prioritizing and teaching skills based on what matters to the individual. The curriculum breaks skills down into must-haves, should-haves, good-to-haves, and nice-to-haves. It highlights eight essential skills that increase independence and quality of life for both children and adults. The essential eight skills focus on communication, health and safety, and dignity (McGreevey et al., 2012). It differs from developmental assessments such as the The Verbal Behavior Milestones Assessment and Placement Program: The VB-MAPP, which focuses on skills based on developmental milestones (Sundberg, 2008).

14.6.3 Views on "Stimming"

Most autistic individuals engage in self-stimulatory behaviors (often called stereotypy or "stimming"), including but not limited to hand flapping, vocalizations, mouthing inedible items, and body movements such as rocking, among many others (Melo et al., 2020). ABA-based services have been criticized for attempting to suppress self-stimulatory behavior. Self-reports from the autistic community, when they are available, tell us that these behaviors provide comfort and a means for coping with an overwhelming sensory environment (Kapp et al., 2019).

The selection of stereotypy as an intervention target should be supported by an assessment of the behavior's impact on the person's learning and ability to participate in their community (Koegel & Covert, 1972). For example, loud vocalizations are likely to be disruptive in a classroom setting or when watching a movie. In circumstances where the self-stimulatory behaviors are negatively impacting a child, an intervention plan will typically focus on supporting the child to get the same stimulation in a safer or more appropriate way, rather than stopping the self-stimulatory behavior altogether. For example, EIBI curricula may include specific programs to reduce stereotypy by rewarding the omission of stereotypy during periods of instruction (e.g., Butler et al., 2021). Unless self-stimulatory behaviors are negatively impacting a child, skill-building programs should probably take precedence within the EIBI curriculum.

More research is required to understand the nature of self-stimulatory behaviors in the context of social anxiety and language. Preliminary evidence suggests that even short-term reductions in stereotypy can produce increments in social interaction initiations (Tereshko et al., 2021). Also, the presence of stereotypy seems to be negatively correlated with the overall level of functioning of the individual (Melo et al., 2020). Moreover, limited social communication is distinctively linked to higher levels of stereotypy (Martínez-González et al., 2022). These findings are compatible with the view that building skills that produce positive outcomes (whether sensory input, control of the social environment, emotional regulation, or access to preferred items) effectively competes with the self-stimulatory behavior over time. If the function of stereotypy is indeed "self-regulatory," it is possible that these behaviors would abate naturally with the gradual acquisition of verbal and social repertoires.

14.6.4 Unethical Legacy

Another criticism of EIBI is that it is harsh and abusive. This criticism is frequently discussed with reference to the use of punishment. Technically, behavior analysts use the label *punishment* to describe a reduction in behavior occasioned by either presenting a stimulus or withdrawing a reward following the behavior of interest (Cooper et al., 2019). An example may include a parent placing their child away from leisure items for a brief period after having thrown a toy, resulting in the child being less likely to throw the toy again in the future. This definition differs from the more colloquially accepted definition, whereby a penalty or sanction is inflicted for an offense (physical aggressions included). Punishment does not necessarily pertain to something aversive, though it can. For example, if a child hits another child, a parent may say, "We don't hit!" If the child then hits less in the future, saying "We don't hit!" can be classed as punishment (i.e., stimulus presentation resulting in less behavior). Several studies have addressed the fact that the field of ABA often uses terminology and jargon that is abrasive or unpleasant (Becirevic et al., 2016; Doughty et al., 2012), and the term *punishment* is perhaps a prime example where confusion between the ABA definition and colloquial use of the word has been problematic.

Historically, aversive punishment procedures have been used as part of EIBI programs, and there are autistic individuals that have endured or witnessed aversive procedures. The ethics and practice of EIBI have evolved, and aversive procedures are no longer utilized in current EIBI programs. Behavioral practitioners will prioritize reinforcement-based interventions and may resort to including a nonaversive punishment procedure in the context of a schedule of reinforcement. In this context the term *punishment* refers narrowly to strategies that require the presentation or removal of a stimulus resulting in a lower level of a target problem behavior. These may include procedures such as response cost (e.g., losing tokens for engaging in problem behavior) and overcorrection (e.g., correcting the damage caused by destructive behavior), among others. In some cases of dangerous self-injurious behaviors, more intrusive antecedents and punishment procedures may be resorted to, while following strict due process guidelines (see, for example, Malott & Kohler, 2020, p. 139).

14.7 EIBI on the International Stage

Autistic children can access ABA-based interventions across the United States, Canada, and Australia. As discussed, all 50 states in the United States now require insurance cover for ABA therapy services for autism. While the extent of coverage varies across provinces, autism services are also available across Canada. The National Disability Insurance Scheme, which started in 2013 in Australia, provides autistic individuals with needs-based funding that can be used toward ABA-based interventions. Access to this funding has resulted in an exponential increase in the number of ABA service providers across these countries and has allowed autistic children to access EIBI. Canada and the United States have well-established certification programs and licensure schemes in addition to widely used professional and ethical standards (see, for example, Council of Autism Services Providers, 2020, or Behavior Analyst Certification Board, 2020) and public professional registries (see, for example, the professional registries of the BACB or the province-level registries of autism service providers in Canada). These resources provide families with guidance and reassurance when navigating the wide range of therapies and supports that exist for autism, all with varying degrees of evidence.

In countries where EIBI is not currently funded, families are required to privately fund therapy services. For example, EIBI is not currently funded in New Zealand through the public health system or via private health insurance. Due to the intensity of EIBI, privately funding therapy is near impossible for most families as it can cost up to $100,000 a year. This has resulted in families privately funding a lesser number of therapy hours, usually directed toward more focused intervention goals. Families are forced to prioritize goals and progress may be slower. The lack of funding also makes in-center EIBI a challenging and often unsustainable business model due to the high cost of properly trained staff. As a result, very few EIBI service providers currently exist across New Zealand, and many service providers do not have appropriately trained or qualified clinicians. Access to culturally specific training and professional development for qualified clinicians is also limited. Focused parent-training intervention models, sometimes capitalizing on the cost savings of telehealth, can be workable alternatives in some cases (Lindgren et al., 2016; Taylor et al., 2019).

14.8 Practice Implications and Conclusions

14.8.1 Treatment Outcomes

Overall, research indicates that EIBI is an effective intervention for improving language and communication, daily living skills, and social repertoires for autistic preschool and school-age children. Research suggests that 20+ hours per week of intervention results in clinically significant outcomes, and limited research suggests that commencing intervention earlier results in larger improvements. No negative side effects have been reported because of EIBI. However, the long-term outcomes for autistic children that receive EIBI require further research.

14.8.2 Cost-Benefit Analysis

Jacobson and Mulick (2000) discussed the need for comprehensive research to evaluate the effectiveness and cost-efficiency of treatments for individuals with autism. They emphasized the importance of considering the long-term outcomes and societal benefits of interventions. The authors highlighted the significance of developing systematic approaches and cost analysis models to guide decision-making regarding autism treatments.

A few studies have conducted actual cost analyses of EIBI over the last 25 years. Jacobson et al. (1998) evaluated a model estimating the potential financial benefits associated with EIBI implementation, considering factors such as reduced special education costs and long-term benefits. The study concluded that EIBI can lead to substantial savings for society in the long run. Marcus et al. (2000) responded to this analysis by presenting an alternative perspective on cost-benefit analysis in autism services. The authors discussed methodological issues and challenges related to measuring costs and outcomes in the context of autism treatment, highlighting the need for nuanced analysis to understand the economic implications of different interventions. Additionally, Chasson et al. (2007) compared the costs associated with EIBI and special education for children with autism. The study suggests that although EIBI is initially more expensive, it may lead to significant cost savings in the long term due to reduced special education and the cost of other services. Research conducted in the Netherlands by Peters-Scheffer et al. (2012) reported that investing in EIBI for autistic children can save an estimated €1,103,067 throughout the person's lifetime (see also Hodgson et al., 2022, for a less optimistic cost analysis).

Despite the potential for cost benefits across the lifespan, the immediate cost of ABA-based intervention seems to be by far the primary factor preventing a wider dissemination of services. Overall, these studies contribute to the understanding of the economic aspects and cost-effectiveness of treatments for individuals with autism. They emphasize the need for comprehensive research, cost analysis models, and careful consideration of long-term benefits when evaluating interventions for individuals with ASD.

14.8.3 Shifting Focus

Social validity is an essential component of ABA. While research consistently presents positive outcomes following EIBI for autistic children, few have asked the recipients for their perspectives on the intervention. We may have asked parents if they are satisfied, but have they been involved in all aspects of their child's intervention? Have questions been asked about preferred goals and interventions? Have the children been asked? Quality of life (QoL) is at the core of person-centered outcomes, but it can be hard to measure, particularly for people who cannot self-report. One aspect of QoL is happiness, for which there are several measurement approaches (some of which do not require a person to communicate verbally). Parsons et al. (2012) defined indices of happiness (objective indicators of happiness such as smiling) and demonstrated the validity of measuring them in autistic people. Indices of happiness can be used to determine what goals, interventions, and teaching stimuli are most preferred, therefore ensuring social validity of the support provided. Additionally, happiness-informed interventions have been demonstrated to be as effective as those based on the assessment of challenging behavior. Thomas et al. (2021) measured indices of happiness during functional analyses of challenging behavior, which allowed them to identify a possible intervention. Although the challenging behaviors were found to be mostly maintained by access to tangible items, the autistic children in the study showed indices of happiness when provided with attention in the conditions in which this was available. Access to attention was then used successfully to minimize challenging behavior when a preferred tangible was not available. Their study showed that capturing indices of happiness during assessments might be useful to inform socially valid interventions. Carnett et al. (2022) completed a retrospective analysis of happiness in parents and children when parents were taught to implement a skill-building intervention for their children. Parents' indices of happiness increased as fidelity of the implementation of the skill-building intervention grew; however, the child's overall indices of happiness decreased. Their results were consistent with previous findings of lower indices of happiness during work tasks (e.g., Dillon & Carr, 2007). Overall, these studies suggest that objectively measuring indices of happiness can capture happiness as both an indicator of social validity and QoL. EIBI has had a remarkable impact on the lives of autistic children and their families in terms of concrete measures of standardized assessment. It is now time for the use of other measurements such as satisfaction and indices of happiness to be extended so that EIBI can be informed by QoL indicators.

There is a need to establish when, if at all, manualized approaches and prescriptive curricula should be used in EIBI. Perhaps they are best considered as just one tool in the EIBI arsenal, and we caution that a purely manualized approach might result in a loss of individualization. One way to ameliorate the loss of individualization is to ensure the inclusion of autistic children and their families in all aspects of therapy. We add to previous calls for this (e.g., Leaf et al., 2022), because ultimately, it is the person and their family's QoL that we are attempting to enhance. This trend may require acknowledging parental stress and anxiety from a more traditional psychotherapeutic standpoint as a form of support complementary or parallel to EIBI (see, for example, Corti et al., 2018; Yi & Dixon, 2021).

Many of the criticisms can be mitigated by adopting a more collaborative and context-sensitive approach to the procedures and goals that are part of an EIBI program. Two of the defining features of ABA (and therefore EIBI) are that interventions should focus on socially important behavior change and that the intervention outcomes (behaviors that are the focus of the intervention) should be meaningful (Baer et al., 1968). Due to the varied ways in which autism can present, the skills will increase independence and QoL will vary, as will the level of support needed. For example, some autistic individuals can communicate vocally or through augmentative and alternative communication, while others may require additional support to learn how to express their wants, needs, and emotions. Some individuals may need additional support with learning daily living skills such as toilet training. EIBI should therefore be seen as an effective tool for teaching autistic individuals skills important to them that will improve QoL, rather than a predetermined set of skills that "should" be taught. When clients are preverbal or experience difficulties in communicating their wants, needs, and emotions, we can then look to parents/caregivers and to factors such as safety and dignity to guide skills to be targeted.

The professional field of ABA-based services for autism seems to be at a crossroads. Some may find it disorienting that a time when the development and dissemination of services has been the greatest (particularly in the North American context) is also a time when the field has come under fire from fierce critics.

Maybe these two processes are related. As ABA services become mainstream, their weaknesses are more apparent, and the risks of growing too fast are ever so real. While science often stays away from folklore, criticisms about the "lack of evidence" have brought academic behavior analysts closer to the center of this turmoil. Critics are often unmerciful. They do not focus on specific aspects that require improvement, like adding more RCTs to the scientific corpus of EIBI or incorporating patient-centered outcomes, and culturally sensitive curricula as research and practice standards. On the contrary, critics may say that "there is no true evidence," and that the selection of instructional targets is based on "an authoritarian philosophy." Such uncompromising criticism can be very destructive in that it prevents an actual conversation. It is very hard to respond to total criticism, with the resulting silence perhaps taken as "evidence" that the critics are correct. Evidence should be countered with evidence, and researchers and clinicians need to develop their science communication skills so that families can better understand how EIBI could support their autistic child's learning and development. This is challenging as the field of autism services increasingly becomes an industry, and the discussion becomes more political and off centered from the scientific dialectics.

In this chapter we have tried to provide the background, the characters, and some of the themes of the unfolding drama. Hopefully, the language and the information provided can inspire a more critical appreciation of the existing evidence supporting EIBI and, at the same time, a realistic appreciation of the many challenges that lie ahead. The current scenario is complex, and every decision maker, whether a professional or an individual family seeking a better future for their loved one, needs to understand this complexity and act accordingly.

14.9 References

APA Presidential Task Force on Evidence Based Practice. (2006). Evidence-based practice in psychology. *American Psychologist, 61*(4), 271–285. https://doi.org/10.1037/0003-066X.61.4.271

Baer, D. M., Wolf, M. M., & Risley, T. R. (1968). Some current dimensions of applied behavior analysis. *Journal of Applied Behavior Analysis, 1*(1), 91–97. https://doi.org/10.1901/jaba.1968.1-91

Becirevic, A., Critchfield, T. S., & Reed, D. D. (2016). On the social acceptability of behavior-analytic terms: Crowdsourced comparisons of lay and technical language. *The Behavior Analyst, 39*(2), 305–317. https://doi.org/10.1007/s40614-016-0067-4

Behavior Analyst Certification Board. (2020). *Ethics code for behavior analysts*. https://bacb.com/wp-content/ethics-code-for-behavior-analysts/

Behavior Analyst Certification Board. (2023a). *Task list for BACB certifications*. https://www.bacb.com/task-lists/

Behavior Analyst Certification Board. (2023b). *US licensure of behavior analyst*. https://www.bacb.com/u-s-licensure-of-behavior-analysts/

Butler, C., Kobylarz, A., Zaki-Scarpa, C., LaRue, R.H., Manente, C., & Kahng, S. (2021), Differential reinforcement to decrease stereotypy exhibited by an adult with autism spectrum disorder. *Behavioral Interventions, 36*, 261–270. https://doi.org/10.1002/bin.1760

Carnett, A., Neely, L., Chen, M. T., Cantrell, K., Santos, E., & Rosales, S. A. (2022). How might indices of happiness inform early intervention research and decision making? *Advances in Neurodevelopmental Disorders, 6*, 567–576. https://doi.org/10.1007/s41252-022-00288-0

Cernius, A. (2022, May 13). The autistic community is having a reckoning with ABA therapy. We should listen. *Fortune.* https://fortune.com/2022/05/13/autistic-community-reckoning-aba-therapy-rights-autism-insurance-private-equity-ariana-cernius/

Chasson, G. S., Harris, G. E., & Neely, W. J. (2007). Cost comparison of early intensive behavioral intervention and special education for children with autism. *Journal of Child and Family Studies, 16,* 401–413. https://doi.org/10.1007/s10826-006-9094-1

Conine, D. E., Campau, S. C., & Petronelli, A. K. (2022). LGBTQ+ conversion therapy and applied behavior analysis: A call to action. *Journal of Applied Behavior Analysis, 55*(1), 6–18. https://doi.org/10.1002/jaba.876

Cooper, J. O., Heron, T. E., & Heward, W. L. (2019). *Applied behavior analysis* (3rd ed.) London: Pearson.

Corti, C., Pergolizzi, F., Vanzin, L., Cargasacchi, G., Villa, L., Pozzi, M., & Molteni, M. (2018). Acceptance and commitment therapy-oriented parent-training for parents of children with autism. *Journal of Child & Family Studies, 27*(9), 2887–2900. https://doi.org/10.1007/s10826-018-1123-3

Council of Autism Service Providers. (2020). *Applied behavior analysis treatment of autism spectrum disorder: Practice guidelines for healthcare funders and managers* (2nd ed.). https://www.casproviders.org/asd-guidelines

Dawson, G., Rogers, S., Munson, J., Smith, M., Winter, J., Greenson, J., Donaldson, A., & Varley, J. (2010). Randomized, controlled trial of an intervention for toddlers with autism: The Early Start Denver model. *Pediatrics, 125*(1), e17–e23. https://doi.org/10.1542/peds.2009-0958

Dillon C. M, & Carr, J. E. (2007). Assessing indices of happiness and unhappiness in individuals with developmental disabilities: A review. *Behavioral Interventions, 22*(3), 229–244. https://doi.org/10.1002/bin.240

Dimian, A. F., Symons, F. J., & Wolff, J. J. (2021). Delay to early intensive behavioral intervention and educational outcomes for a Medicaid-enrolled cohort of children with Autism. *Journal of Autism and Developmental Disorders, 51*(4), 1054–1066. https://doi.org/10.1007/s10803-020-04586-1

Dixon, M. R., Paliliunas, D., & Barron, B. F. (2021). Randomized controlled trial evaluation of ABA content on IQ gains in children with autism. *Journal of Behavioral Education, 30,* 455–477. https://doi.org/10.1007/s10864-019-09344-7

Doughty, A.H., Holloway, C., Shields, M.C., & Kennedy, L. E. (2012). Marketing behavior analysis requires (really) different talk: A critique of Kohn (2005) and a(nother) call to arms. *Behavior Analysis and Social Issues, 21,* 115–135. https://doi.org/10.5210/bsi.v21i0.3914

Eldevik, S., Jahr, E., Eikeseth, S., Hastings, R. P., & Hughes, C. J. (2010). Cognitive and adaptive behavior outcomes of behavioral intervention for young children with intellectual disability. *Behavior Modification, 34*(1), 16–34. https://doi.org/10.1177/0145445509351961

Fry. E. (2022, July 29). Private equity is the biggest player in a booming autism-therapy industry. Some therapists say the "money grab" is hurting the quality of care. *Fortune.* https://fortune.com/2022/07/29/autism-therapy-care-centers-private-equity-hopebridge

Green, J., Charman, T., McConachie, H., Aldred, C., Slonims, V., Howlin, P., Le Couteur, A., Leadbitter, K., Hudry, K., Byford, S., Barrett, B., Temple, K., Macdonald, W., Pickles, A., & PACT Consortium. (2010). Parent-mediated communication-focused treatment in children with autism (PACT): a randomised controlled trial. *Lancet, 375*(9732), 2152–2160. https://doi.org/10.1016/S0140-6736(10)60587-9

Grey, I., Coughlan, B., Lydon, H., Healy, O., & Thomas, J. (2019). Parental satisfaction with early intensive behavioral intervention. *Journal of Intellectual Disabilities, 23*(3), 373–384. https://doi.org/10.1177/1744629517742813

Hodgson, R., Biswas, M., Palmer, S., Marshall, D., Rodgers, M., Stewart, L., Simmonds, M., Rai, D., & Le Couteur, A. (2022). Intensive behavioral interventions based on applied behavior analysis (ABA) for young children with autism: A cost-effectiveness analysis. *PloS One, 17*(8), e0270833. https://doi.org/10.1371/journal.pone.0270833

International Consortium of Health Outcomes Measurement. (2021). *Autism standard set.* https://connect.ichom.org/standard-sets/autism-spectrum-disorder/

Jacobson, J. W., & Mulick, J. A. (2000). System and cost research issues in treatments for people with autistic disorders. *Journal of Autism and Developmental Disorders, 30*(6), 585. https://doi.org/10.1023/a:1005691411255

Jacobson, J. W., Mulick, J. A., & Green, G. (1998). Cost–benefit estimates for early intensive behavioral intervention for young children with autism—general model and single state case. *Behavioral Interventions, 13*(4), 201–226. https://doi.org/10.1002/(SICI)1099-078X(199811)13:4<201:AID-BIN17>3.0.CO;2-R

Jennett, H. K., Harris, S. L., & Delmolino, L. (2008). Discrete trial instruction vs. mand training for teaching children with autism to make requests. *The Analysis of Verbal Behavior, 24*(1), 69–85. https://doi.org/10.1007/BF03393058

Johnson, C.R., Turner, K.S., Foldes, E., Brooks, M.M., Kronk, R., & Wiggs, L. (2013). Behavioral parent training to address sleep disturbances in young children with autism spectrum disorder: a pilot trial. *Sleep Medicine*, 14, 995–1004. https://doi.org/10.1016/j.sleep.2013.05.013.

Kapp, S. K., Steward, R., Crane, L., Elliott, D., Elphick, C., Pellicano, E., & Russell, G. (2019). "People should be allowed to do what they like": Autistic adults' views and experiences of stimming. *Autism, 23*(7), 1782–1792. https://doi.org/10.1177/1362361319829628

Koegel, R. L., & Covert, A. (1972). The relationship of self-stimulation to learning in autistic children. *Journal of Applied Behavior Analysis, 5*(4), 381–387. https://doi.org/10.1901/jaba.1972.5-381

Koudys, J., Perry, A., Ho, H. S. W., & Charles, M. (2021). Mental health status of youth diagnosed with ASD who received early intensive behavioral intervention as young children. *Child & Family Behavior Therapy, 43*(2), 103–113. https://doi.org/10.1080/07317107.2021.1895

Kovshoff, H., Hastings, R. P., & Remington, B. (2011). Two-year outcomes for children with autism after the cessation of early intensive behavioral intervention. *Behavior Modification, 35*(5), 427-450. https://doi.org/10.1177/0145445511405513

Långh, U., Perry, A., Eikeseth, S., & Bölte, S. (2021). Quality of early intensive behavioral intervention as a predictor of children's outcome. *Behavior Modification, 45*(6), 911–928. https://doi.org/10.1177/0145445520923998

Larsson, E. V. & Wright, L. B. (2024). Early intensive behavioral intervention—The Lovaas Institute. In S. M. Peterson & R. R. Eldridge (Eds.), *Effective programs for treating autism spectrum disorder: Applied behavior analysis models* (2nd ed.) (pp. 230–270). New York: Routledge.

Leaf, J. B., Cihon, J. H., Leaf, R., McEachin, J., Liu, N., Russell, N., Unumb, L., Shapiro, S., & Khosrowshahi, D. (2022). Concerns about ABA-based intervention: An evaluation and recommendations. *Journal of Autism and Developmental Disorders, 52*(6), 2838–2853. https://doi.org/10.1007/s10803-021-05137-y

Leaf, R., McEachin, J., & Harsh, J. D. (1999). *A work in progress: Behavior management strategies and a curriculum for intensive behavioral treatment of autism*. New York: DRL Books.

Lindgren, S., Wacker, D., Suess, A., Schieltz, K., Pelzel, K., Kopelman, T., Lee, J., Romani, P., & Waldron, D. (2016). Telehealth and autism: treating challenging behavior at lower cost. *Pediatrics, 137* (Suppl 2), S167–S175. https://doi.org/10.1542/peds.2015-2851O

Linstead, E., Dixon, D. R., French, R., Granpeesheh, D., Adams, H., German, R., Powell, A., Stevens, E., Tarbox, J., & Kornack, J. (2017). Intensity and learning outcomes in the treatment of children with autism spectrum disorder. *Behavior Modification, 41*(2), 229–252. https://doi.org/10.1177/0145445516667059

Lovaas, O. I. (1981). *Teaching developmentally disabled children: The me book*. University Park, PA: University Park.

Lovaas, O. I. (1987). Behavioral treatment and normal educational and intellectual functioning in young autistic children. *Journal of Consulting and Clinical Psychology, 55*(1), 3–9. https://doi.org/10.1037/0022-006X.55.1.3

Lovaas, O. I. (2003). *Teaching individuals with developmental delays*. Austin, TX: Pro-Ed.

Malott, R. W., & Kohler, K. T. (2020). *Principles of behavior* (8th ed.). London: Routledge.

Marcus, L. M., Rubin, J. S., & Rubin, M. A. (2000). Benefit-cost analysis and autism services: A response to Jacobson and Mulick. *Journal of Autism and Developmental Disorders, 30*(6), 595. https://doi.org/10.1023/a:1005643528093

Martínez-González, A. E., Cervin, M., & Piqueras, J. A. (2022). Relationships between emotion regulation, social communication and repetitive behaviors in autism spectrum disorder. *Journal of Autism and Developmental Disorders, 52*(10), 4519–4527. https://doi.org/10.1007/s10803-021-05340-x

Maurice, C., Green, G., & Luce, S. C. (Eds.). (1996). *Behavioral interventions for children with autism*. Austin, TX: Pro-Ed.

McGreevy, P., Fry, T., & Cornwall, C. (2012). *Essential for living*. Orlando, FL: Patrick McGreevy

Melo, C., Ruano, L., Jorge, J., Pinto Ribeiro, T., Oliveira, G., Azevedo, L., & Temudo, T. (2020). Prevalence and determinants of motor stereotypies in autism spectrum disorder: A systematic review and meta-analysis. *Autism, 24*(3), 569–590. https://doi.org/10.1177/1362361319869118

Murza, K. A., Schwartz, J. B., Hahs-Vaughn, D. L., & Nye, C. (2016). Joint attention interventions for children with autism spectrum disorder: A systematic review and meta-analysis. *International Journal of Language & Communication Disorders, 51*(3), 236–251. https://doi.org/10.1111/1460-6984.12212

National Conference of State Legislatures. (2021). *Autism and insurance coverage state laws*. https://www.ncsl.org/health/autism-and-insurance-coverage-state-laws

New England Center for Children. (2023). *ACE® ABA software system*. https://www.acenecc.org/

Parsons, M. B., Reid, D. H., Bentley, E., Inman, A., & Lattimore, L. P. (2012). Identifying indices of happiness and unhappiness among adults with autism: Potential targets for behavioral assessment and intervention. *Behavior Analysis in Practice*, *5*(1), 15–25. https://doi.org/10.1007/BF03391814

Penn H. E., Prichard E. A., & Perry A. (2007). The reliability and validity of a pilot version of the York Measure of Quality of Intensive Behavioral Intervention. *Journal on Developmental Disabilities*, *13*(3), 149–166.

Peters-Scheffer, N., Didden, R., Korzilius, H., & Matson, J. (2012). Cost comparison of early intensive behavioral intervention and treatment as usual for children with autism spectrum disorder in The Netherlands. *Research in Developmental Disabilities*, *33*(6), 1763–1772. https://doi.org/10.1016/j.ridd.2012.04.006

Plavnick, J. B., Bak, M. Y. S., Avendaño, S. M., Dueñas, A. D., Brodhead, M. T., & Sipila, E. S. (2020). Implementing early intensive behavioral intervention in community settings. *Autism: International Journal of Research and Practice*, *24*(7), 1913–1916. https://doi.org/10.1177/1362361320919243

Prizant, B. M., Wetherby, A. M., Rubin, E., & Laurent, A. C. (2003) The SCERTS model: A transactional, family-centered approach to enhancing communication and socioemotional abilities of children with autism spectrum disorder. *Infants & Young Children*, *16*(4), 296–316.

Rajaraman, A., Austin, J. L., Gover, H. C., Cammilleri, A. P., Donnelly, D. R., & Hanley, G. P. (2022). Toward trauma-informed applications of behavior analysis. *Journal of Applied Behavior Analysis*, *55*(1), 40–61. https://doi.org/10.1002/jaba.881

Reichow, B., Hume, K., Barton, E. E., & Boyd, B. A. (2018). Early intensive behavioral intervention (EIBI) for young children with autism spectrum disorders (ASD). *The Cochrane Database of Systematic Reviews*, *5*(5), CD009260. https://doi.org/10.1002/14651858.CD009260.pub3

Reitzel, J., Summers, J., Lorv, B., Szatmari, P., Zwaigenbaum, L., Georgiades, S., & Duku, E. (2013). Pilot randomized controlled trial of a Functional Behavior Skills Training program for young children with autism spectrum disorder who have significant early learning skill impairments and their families. *Research in Autism Spectrum Disorders*, *7*(11), 1418–1432. https://doi.org/10.1016/j.rasd.2013.07.025

Roane, H. S., Ringdahl, J. L., & Falcomata, T.S. (2015). *Clinical and organizational applications of applied behavior analysis*. New York: Academic Press. https://doi.org/10.1016/C2013-0-09993-8

Rogers, S. J., Yoder, P., Estes, A., Warren, Z., McEachin, J., Munson, J., Rocha, M., Greenson, J., Wallace, L., Gardner, E., Dawson, G., Sugar, C. A., Hellemann, G., & Whelan, F. (2021). A multisite randomized controlled trial comparing the effects of intervention intensity and intervention style on outcomes for young children with autism. *Journal of the American Academy of Child and Adolescent Psychiatry*, *60*(6), 710–722. https://doi.org/10.1016/j.jaac.2020.06.013

Sandbank, M., Bottema-Beutel, K., Crowley, S., Cassidy, M., Dunham, K., Feldman, J. I., Crank, J., Albarran, S. A., Raj, S., Mahbub, P., & Woynaroski, T. G. (2020). Project AIM: Autism intervention meta-analysis for studies of young children. *Psychological Bulletin*, *146*(1), 1–29. https://doi.org/10.1037/bul0000215

Sandbank, M., Bottema-Beutel, K., & Woynaroski, T. (2021). Intervention recommendations for children with autism in light of a changing evidence base. *JAMA Pediatrics*, *175*(4), 341–342. https://doi.org/10.1001/jamapediatrics.2020.4730

Schreibman, L., Dawson, G., Stahmer, A. C., Landa, R., Rogers, S. J., McGee, G. G., Kasari, C., Ingersoll, B., Kaiser, A. P., Bruinsma, Y., McNerney, E., Wetherby, A., & Halladay, A. (2015). Naturalistic developmental behavioral interventions: empirically validated treatments for autism spectrum disorder. *Journal of Autism and Developmental Disorders*, *45*(8), 2411–2428. https://doi.org/10.1007/s10803-015-2407-8

Shi, B., Wu, W., Dai, M., Zeng, J., Luo, J., Cai, L., Wan, B., & Jing, J. (2021). Cognitive, language, and behavioral outcomes in children with autism spectrum disorders exposed to early comprehensive treatment models: A meta-analysis and meta-regression. *Frontiers in Psychiatry*, *12*, 691148. https://doi.org/10.3389/fpsyt.2021.691148

Skinner, B. F. (1957). *Verbal behavior*. Crows Nest, NSW: Appleton-Century-Crofts.

Smith, D. P., Hayward, D. W., Gale, C. M., Eikeseth, S., & Klintwall, L. (2021). Treatment gains from early and intensive behavioral intervention (EIBI) are maintained 10 years later. *Behavior Modification*, *45*(4), 581–601. https://doi.org/10.1177/0145445519882895

Smith, T., Groen, A. D., & Wynn, J. W. (2000). Randomized trial of intensive early intervention for children with pervasive developmental disorder. *American Journal of Mental Retardation, 105*, 269–285. https://doi.org/10.1352/0895-8017(2000)105<0269:RTOIEI>2.0.CO;2

Sundberg, M. L. (2008). *VB-MAPP: Verbal behavior milestones assessment and placement program.* Concord: AVB Press.

Tachibana, Y., Miyazaki, C., Ota, E., Mori, R., Hwang, Y., Kobayashi, E., Terasaka, A., Tang, J., & Kamio, Y. A. (2017). Systematic review and meta-analysis of comprehensive interventions for preschool children with autism spectrum disorder. *PLoS One, 6*(12), e0186502. https://doi.org/10.1371/journal.pone.0186502

Taylor, S. L., Purdy, S., Jackson, B., Phillips, K., & Virues-Ortega, J. (2019). Evaluation of a home-based Behavioral treatment model for children with tube dependency. *Journal of Pediatric Psychology, 44*, 656–668. https://doi.org/10.1093/jpepsy/jsz014

Tereshko, L., Ross, R. K., & Frazee, L. (2021). The effects of a procedure to decrease motor stereotypy on social interactions in a child with autism spectrum disorder. *Behavior analysis in practice, 14*(2), 367–377. https://doi.org/10.1007/s40617-020-00516-w

Thomas, B. R., Charlop, M. H., Lim, N., & Gumaer, C. (2021). Measuring happiness behavior in functional analyses of challenging behavior for children with autism spectrum disorder. *Behavior Modification, 45*(3), 502–530. https://doi.org/10.1177/0145445519878673

Tiura, M., Kim, J., Detmers, D., & Baldi, H. (2017). Predictors of longitudinal ABA treatment outcomes for children with autism: A growth curve analysis. *Research in Developmental Disabilities, 70*, 185–197. https://doi.org/10.1016/j.ridd.2017.09.008

Virues-Ortega, J. (2010). Applied behavior analytic intervention for autism in early childhood: Meta-analysis, meta-regression and dose–response meta-analysis of multiple outcomes. *Clinical Psychology Review, 30*(4), 387–399. http://doi.org/10.1016/j.cpr.2010.01.008

Virues-Ortega, J., Hurtado-Parrado, J., Cox, A. D., & Pear, J. J. (2014). A systematic analysis of the interaction between experimental and applied behavior analysis. *Journal of Applied Behavior Analysis, 47*, 1–24. https://doi.org/10.1002/jaba.124

Virues-Ortega, J., Julio, F., & Pastor, R. (2013b). The TEACCH program for children and adults with autism: A meta-analysis of intervention studies. *Clinical Psychology Review, 33*, 940–953. https://doi.org/10.1016/j.cpr.2013.07.005

Virues-Ortega, J., Lehnert, K., Swan, B., Taylor, M.W., Southee, A., Dougan, D., Taylor, J., Hille, R., Snell, R. G., & Jacobsen, J. J. (2018). The New Zealand Minds for Minds autism spectrum disorder self-reported cohort. *Research in Autism Spectrum Disorder, 36*, 1–7. https://doi.org/10.1016/j.rasd.2016.12.003

Virues-Ortega, J., Moeyaert, M., Sivaraman, M., Tarifa-Rodriguez, & Fernandez Castilla, B. (2023). Quantifying outcomes in applied behavior analysis through visual and statistical analyses: a synthesis. In J. L. Matson (Ed.), *Handbook of applied behavior analysis* (pp. 515–537). New York: SpringerNature. https://doi.org/10.1007/978-3-031-19964-6_28

Virues-Ortega, J., Perez-Bustamante, A., & Tarifa Rodriguez, A. (2022). Evidence-based applied behavior analysis (ABA) autism treatments: An overview of comprehensive and focused meta-analyses. In J. L. Matson & P. Sturmey (Eds.), *Handbook of autism and pervasive developmental* disorders (pp. 631–659). Cham: Springer. https://doi.org/10.1007/978-3-030-88538-0_27

Virues-Ortega, J., Rodríguez, V., & Yu, C. T. (2013a). Prediction of treatment outcomes and longitudinal analysis in children with autism undergoing intensive behavioral intervention. *International Journal of Clinical and Health Psychology, 13*(2), 91–100. https://doi.org/10.1016/s1697-2600(13)70012-7

Virues-Ortega, J., & Sivaraman, M. (in press). The emerging science of outcome research in applied behavior analysis. *Perspective on Behavior Science.*

Yi, Z., & Dixon, M.R., (2021). Developing and enhancing adherence to a telehealth ABA parent training curriculum for caregivers of children with autism. Behavior Analysis in Practice 14, 58–74. https://doi.org/10.1007/s40617-020-00464-5

Yingling, M. E., Bell, B. A., & Hock, R. M. (2019). Comparing neighborhoods of children with autism spectrum disorder in a Medicaid waiver program and a state population, 2007–2015. *Psychiatric Services, 70*(11), 1034–1039. https://doi.org/10.1176/appi.ps.201800479

Zwaigenbaum, L., Bauman, M. L., Stone, W. L., Yirmiya, N., Estes, A., Hansen, R. L., McPartland, J. C., Natowicz, M. R., Choueiri, R., Fein, D., Kasari, C., Pierce, K., Buie, T., Carter, A., Davis, P. A., Granpeesheh, D., Mailloux, Z., Newschaffer, C., Robins, D., Roley, S. S., . . . Wetherby, A. (2015). Early identification of autism spectrum disorder: Recommendations for practice and research. *Pediatrics, 136* (Suppl 1), S10–S40. https://doi.org/10.1542/peds.2014-3667C

15

Pivotal Response Treatment

Lynn Kern Koegel
Department of Psychiatry and Behavioral Sciences, Stanford University School of Medicine

Fereshteh Mohammadzaheri
Department of Speech Therapy, School of Rehabilitation, Tehran University of Medical Sciences

15.1 Technical Abstract

Background: Pivotal response treatment (PRT) was first developed to teach young children with autism spectrum disorder (ASD) to produce first words and initiate verbal communication at an earlier age. PRT is designed to improve motivation for social communication by targeting pivotal areas that, when acquired, occasion collateral gains in other behaviors not directly targeted during intervention. **Method:** To identify PRT studies involving individuals with ASD, we searched relevant terms (e.g., autism and pivotal response) in electronic databases (e.g., PsychInfo). We also considered potentially relevant studies cited by the studies returned from database searches (i.e., ancestry search). Particular attention was given to literature reviews, original laboratory research, and replication and expansion studies of PRT procedures. Peer-reviewed articles using a variety of methodologies, including single-subject, qualitative, and group designs where included. **Results:** The motivational components of PRT have been effective in improving first words, social communication, language, play, initiations, self-help, academics, and other areas. PRT has been effective with individuals with ASD from infancy to adulthood. In addition to improvements in targeted goals, concomitant changes in other nontargeted areas have been shown when PRT motivational components are incorporated. **Discussion:** PRT has been classified as an evidence-based practice for improving communication skills in children with ASD. No side effects have been reported in the literature, but PRT does require specialized training to implement accurately. Challenges related to specific behavioral characteristics and pivotal areas, limitations in research, and directions for future research are discussed. **Practitioner recommendations:** Responsiveness, positive affect, and correct responding improve while interfering and disruptive behaviors decrease during PRT. Thus, incorporating PRT's motivational strategies into intervention is helpful for improved engagement and learning.

Lynn Kern Koegel, and Fereshteh Mohammadzaheri, *Pivotal Response Treatment*. In: *Lifespan Treatment for Autistic Individuals*. Edited by: Peter Sturmey, Russell Lang, and James K. Luiselli, Oxford University Press. © Oxford University Press (2025). DOI: 10.1093/oso/9780197635841.003.0015

15.2 Layperson Summary

PRT is an effective intervention supported by many types of studies. PRT focuses on supporting and teaching behaviors that, once learned, positively influence other behaviors that contribute to learning new skills. Initially, motivation was the main area studied, and research revealed that children with ASD responded better and showed improved affect, engagement, and interest in tasks when specific intervention procedures were applied to improve motivation. These procedures included child choice, task variation, interspersal of easy and difficult tasks, rewarding (reinforcing) attempts, and using natural rewards (reinforcers). Originally, PRT was implemented by graduate-level practitioners, speech and language specialists, and psychologists. However, subsequent research demonstrated that parents, teachers, school aides, siblings, peers, and others could be taught to implement PRT effectively. Many studies have demonstrated positive outcomes for children with ASD during PRT. Those studies have employed a variety of research designs capable of providing different types of evidence, including single-case research and randomized controlled trials. Further, in research that compares outcomes of PRT to those of other intervention options, PRT groups consistently outperform interventions that do not include the motivational intervention procedures (Mohammadzaheri et al., 2014, 2015). In addition to a focus on motivation, PRT targets initiations, self-management, responding to multiple cues, and empathy. These specific areas are the focus of instruction because they have been shown to produce positive changes in other areas not directly targeted (Ledbetter-Cho et al., 2017). For this reason, those targeted areas are also considered "pivotal."

15.3 Treatment Summary Table

Treatment summary: Pivotal Response Treatment

Treatment description: PRT focuses on improving motivation, initiations, self-management, responding to multiple cues, and empathy. These specific areas are the focus of instruction because they have been shown to produce positive changes in other important behaviors and skills.

Expected outcomes: PRT has been used to effectively improve a variety of areas, such as first words, language, mean length of utterance (MLU), play, articulation, academics, socialization, verb use and verb diversity, academics, initiations, and conversation.

Methods: To identify PRT studies involving individuals with ASD, we searched relevant terms (e.g., autism and pivotal response) in electronic databases (e.g., PsychInfo). We also considered potentially relevant studies cited by the studies returned from database searches (i.e., ancestry search). Particular attention was given to literature reviews, original laboratory research, and replication and expansion studies of PRT procedures. Peer-reviewed articles using a variety of methodologies, including single-subject, qualitative, and group designs were included.

Expertise required to implement treatment: Individuals from various backgrounds can learn to motivational procedures implement PRT's fundamental with approximately 25 hours of instruction. However, to ensure successful outcomes, ongoing consultation with a PRT professional may be needed to establish treatment goals and receive feedback on treatment fidelity. Parents, teachers, school aides, siblings, peers, and other individuals can all be effectively taught to implement PRT.

Risks and negative side effects: To date, no reported risks or negative side effects have been associated with PRT. However, it is worth noting that around 10–15% of young children under 5 years old may not acquire verbal spoken words or communication through PRT and may remain nonverbal. Nonetheless, the likelihood of nonverbal outcomes appears to be higher with interventions that lack motivational components.

Additional considerations and limitations: Additional research is necessary to identify behavioral phenotypes that can predict who will likely respond the most rapidly to PRT. Discussions have arisen regarding the potential limitations concerning generalization to other areas. For instance, while PRT may effectively teach a targeted skill (e.g., social initiations), gains in another skill area (e.g., academics) may not occur without direct instruction. However, it is vital to highlight that when motivational components are integrated, individuals often become more motivated to learn overall. Active engagement, responsiveness, and increased positive affect frequently extend to other activities as well.

15.4 Introduction

15.4.1 Treatment Description

PRT strategically identifies and prioritizes pivotal areas in a learner's repertoire to target for instruction. These pivotal areas, once acquired, demonstrate a cascading effect, leading to positive improvements in other nontargeted behaviors. This approach expedites the learning process by focusing on pivotal skills. Central to PRT is the emphasis on enhancing motivation for learning and social interactions by creating an optimal environment for active and engaged participation in learning activities.

PRT incorporates five essential motivational procedures, offering choices, task variation, interspersal of acquisition and maintenance tasks, reinforcement of attempts, and use of naturalistic reinforcers. First, *offering choices* empowers learners to take an active role in their learning experiences and establishes a history of reinforcement for responding to the interventionist. Second, *task variation* in PRT refers to the intentional use of diverse learning activities and instructional exercises within the intervention sessions. By incorporating different tasks, PRT aims to maintain learner engagement and prevent monotony, promoting continuous interest and exploration in the learning process. Third, PRT involves interspersing practice of already mastered skills while addressing new skills that the learner has not yet acquired. This strengthens skill generalization and interrelatedness between different behaviors. Fourth, reinforcing attempts (even when not completely successful) encourages learners to persist in their efforts, even in the face of challenges or errors. This promotes adaptive learning strategies.

Finally, PRT incorporates natural reinforcement contingencies, leveraging naturally occurring reinforcing consequences in the learning process. This promotes motivation and facilitates the transfer of acquired skills to real-life situations. Table 15.1 provides examples of these strategies for infants, children, and adolescents to adults.

In PRT, specific pivotal areas and behaviors are identified and targeted to enhance learning outcomes. One crucial pivotal area involves *responsiveness to multiple cues*, where some individuals with autism may struggle to attend to relevant cues within complex stimuli. PRT aims to expand their responsiveness to these cues, resulting in improved learning outcomes and more efficient progress. Another crucial pivotal area in PRT is *self-management*. Teaching individuals to modify and monitor their own behavior empowers them to take an active role in their learning process. This increased autonomy may result in more meaningful and widespread progress in various domains. *Initiations*, including asking questions, represent another important focal point in PRT interventions. Individuals with autism sometimes struggle to initiate social interactions and engage in conversation. By targeting question asking, language complexity can be increased, pragmatics can be improved, and overall long-term outcomes may be facilitated. Finally, *responding empathetically* is emphasized in PRT to improve social conversation and relationships. Encouraging individuals to express empathy and understanding toward others fosters more meaningful and successful social interactions. By targeting these pivotal areas, PRT aims to holistically enhance social and communication skills, thereby promoting overall developmental progress in individuals with autism and other developmental disabilities. The adaptability of PRT across diverse age groups and settings further underscores its value as a valuable intervention in fostering lasting positive changes in behavioral repertoires.

15.4.2 Rationale and Objectives

PRT was first conceptualized to focus on improving the core diagnostic characteristic of challenges in social communication (Koegel et al., 1987). At that time, PRT was described as the "natural language paradigm" as the intervention targeted verbal communication and appeared similar to natural language interactions. The objective of that research was to evaluate a novel theoretical foundation that considered children with ASD to be more capable than typically assumed at the time. According to the theory being assessed, deficits were predominately attributed to an apparent lack of motivation, referred to as "learned helplessness" (Maier & Seligman, 1976). For example, caregivers often excessively help individuals with autism who exhibit challenges, thereby creating a pattern of avoidance in attempting difficult tasks and a lack of opportunity for problem solving. To counteract this cycle, specific teaching procedures were developed to improve motivation. Specifically, to create a greater connection between the behavior and

Table 15.1 Shows the PRT motivational components with examples for various age groups

PRT Motivational Components	Implementation With an Infant	Implementation With a Child	Implementation With an Adolescent or Adult
Choice	Provide experiences with a variety of toys (e.g., rattles, stuffed animals). Observe which item(s) the infant reaches for or looks at when both are freely available.	Choices for activities, items, and other instructional variables are possible.	Assess preferred interests and activities to design and/or secure social opportunities, language goals, self-help, or other area. Example: the adolescent enjoys anime, so a school club is created around that interest.
Task Variation	Engage in short intervals of various preferred activities. Preferred activities are rotated during sessions or as child chooses.	Vary the learning opportunities so that target goals are not presented repeatedly (e.g., expressive language target can rotate across colors, numbers, and shapes).	Vary social activities where social goals are addressed based on person's interests to address a range of goals.
Interspersal of Acquisition and Maintenance	As the infant displays high affect with parent–child activities, gradually introduce neutral activities (e.g., pairing a less preferred activity with enjoyable ones aims to increase its appeal over time).	Vary challenging tasks with mastered skills. For instance, mixing known object labels with teaching counting, colors, or shapes related to those objects.	Vary more difficult targets already acquired skills (e.g., alternating question-asking with easier tasks like discussing favorite anime characters).
Reinforce Correct Responses and Attempts	Appropriate affect (smiles, giggles, laughing) is reinforced (e.g., a parent's funny face elicits infant laughter).	Immediate rewards follow correct responses or clear attempts (e.g., when a child says "ba" for "ball," they receive a ball promptly).	Still, reinforcement follows any correct response or attempt (e.g., peer mentors support and verbally praise individuals for practicing challenging areas outside the club).
Natural Rewards	Social reinforcers pair with other activities (e.g., walk with parent paired with positive social interactions).	Reinforcement is directly tied to tasks (e.g., when the child says "up," the adult lifts them up in the air).	Reinforcement is directly tied to tasks (e.g., goals related to social relationships addressed in context of interest-based activities with peers).

PRT = pivotal response treatment.

the inherent consequences of that behavior, natural rewards (reinforcement) were provided immediately following occurrences—even attempts—at target behaviors. For example, when teaching initial expressive verbal communication, a child's preferred items and activities are utilized to gain interest, verbal requests for those motivating stimuli are modeled, and then they are provided in a playful and engaging manner. After a verbal attempt or clear word is emitted, access to the item or activity is immediately provided (i.e., contingent positive reinforcement), while early or inappropriate forms of communication (e.g., whining, crying, grabbing, no response) are not reinforced. Measuring improvement involves assessing areas such as decreased response latency, decreases in avoidance/escape behaviors, improved affect, and correct responding.

In addition to improvements in targeted areas, when motivational components are incorporated into teaching, improvements in untargeted areas have also been shown, thereby accelerating the learning process. Some examples of areas that have shown collateral improvement following PRT intervention include increases in joint attention and socialization (Bruinsma, 2004; Ebrahim, 2019; Vismara & Lyons, 2007), improvements in pragmatics (Mohammadzaheri et al., 2014), decreases in off-task and disruptive behavior (Coolican et al., 2010; Koegel et al., 1992; Mohammadzaheri et al., 2015), and improvements in global functioning, attention, and socialization (de Korte et al., 2021). As well, the in-session improvements in engagement, affect, and responsiveness have been correlated with increased generalization of both learned and new behaviors outside of the teaching setting (Ashbaugh et al., 2017; de Korte et al., 2022; Gengoux et al., 2019; Koegel et al., 1998).

The first published PRT study targeted initial verbal communication in minimally and nonverbal children (Koegel et al., 1987). Since that initial study, the general motivational procedures have been applied to many target areas, including improving language and linguistic structures (Hardan et al., 2015; Koegel et al., 1998), receptive and expressive communication (Coolican et al., 2010), play (Pierce & Schreibman, 1997), peer social play interactions in integrated recess settings (Harper et al., 2008), socialization (Ashbaugh et al., 2017), self-initiations (de Korte, 2022), question asking (Koegel et al., 2010; Mohammadzaheri et al., 2022), academics (Koegel et al., 2010), and responsiveness (Kuhn et al., 2008).

Following the initial findings demonstrating improved intervention outcomes by incorporating PRT's motivational components into teaching procedures, studies began searching for other pivotal behaviors that, after being acquired, would result in widespread improvements in untargeted areas. Although the motivational components are considered essential during intervention, other areas have appeared to add value when targeted. These include responsiveness to multiple cues, self-management, initiations, and responding empathetically. For example, difficulty responding to simultaneous multiple cues has long been discussed in the literature, and research has shown that children can be taught to respond to multiple stimuli both within and across modalities (auditory, visual, and tactile)

(Koegel & Wilhelm, 1973; Lovaas et al., 1971). To tackle overselective attention, PRT motivational components are incorporated. For example, if a child enjoys drawing, a variety of long and short markers and pencils of various colors can be provided. The child may be instructed to take the long red pencil. As such, the child must attend and respond to all the multiple relevant cues (color, length, and type of drawing implement) to engage in the preferred activity.

Self-management is another pivotal area that can be used to increase or decrease specific behaviors, and it leads to additional gains in untargeted areas. Self-management assists independence, as the individual can take responsibility for identifying the occurrence or nonoccurrence of a behavior in the absence of a service provider. Some individuals can administer their own reinforcers after self-managing their behavior, making the program completely self-reliant. For individuals with autism, the procedures have been shown to be effective across a wide age range (childhood through adulthood) and with a wide variety of behaviors, including communication, social skills, vocational skills, and for decreasing interfering behaviors (Carr et al., 2014; Koegel et al., 1999, 2024; Southall & Gast, 2011). Although most self-management programs have been implemented with verbal individuals, pictorial self-management can be used for minimally verbal autistic children (Pierce & Schreibman, 1994). For example, pictures depicting various steps of an activity (e.g., table setting, packing lunch) are provided in a book, on a ring, or other format. After each step is completed, the individual can self-manage by moving the picture, indicating the step has been completed. The order of the pictures is changed, and if the individual continues to follow the steps in the new order, it assures self-management is occurring (rather than simply completing the steps). Again, self-management systems can be used to increase or decrease behaviors, and once taught, these can be programed into natural environments in the absence of a service provider.

Self-initiations are also considered a pivotal area. The communication of individuals on the autism spectrum often consists primarily of responses and requests. To expand the linguistic functions of communication, reciprocal interactions, and social initiations, question asking and other initiations have been shown to have widespread positive effects and are thus considered pivotal (Mohammadzaheri et al., 2021). Questions are taught in a developmental order, beginning with the first question produced by typical language learners, "What's that?" with the result of expanding expressive vocabulary (Koegel et al., 1998). Children who are taught a series of questions and initiations appear to have improved long-term outcomes (Koegel et al., 1999) as they can create their own learning opportunities and engage in a greater variety of reciprocal verbal interactions as their language functions are expanded.

Finally, the pivotal area of responding empathetically appears to be helpful for producing gains in social interaction and reported confidence. Specifically, individuals who have challenges verbally responding with empathetic statements can be taught to respond with an empathetic statement and question in response to the emotional state of the speaker (Cohen et al., 2022; Koegel et al., 2016). For example, if a speaker indicates discomfort, such as "I'm feeling kind of sick today," an empathetic response that acknowledges the feeling (e.g., "I'm sorry you're feeling sick") and then adds a question (e.g., "Have you seen a doctor?").

Again, the overall objective of PRT has been to determine specific variables that, when incorporated into the intervention, will result in faster learning in targeted areas as well as collateral gains in untargeted areas.

15.4.3 Considerations for Implementation

PRT involves implementing the various procedures simultaneously with fidelity across settings. For each pivotal area, fidelity of implementation (FoI) has been developed and is scored in 1-minute intervals for 10 uninterrupted minutes. Although a few studies have scored fidelity for only 5 minutes, the longer (10-minute) time periods are recommended so that PRT can be evaluated over a longer, uninterrupted period. For all pivotal areas, individuals must meet at least 80% correct implementation of the procedures in all areas to meet FoI criteria. Studies show that PRT can be implemented with fidelity by graduate students (Koegel et al., 1987), speech therapists (Mohammadzaheri et al., 2014, 2021), peers (Kuhn et al., 2008), paraprofessionals (Murphy et al., 2016; Robinson, 2011), and teachers (Stahmer et al., 2012). However, particular attention is paid to assuring that parents can implement PRT with fidelity, because parents are with their children most often and they can implement the procedures within the context of their everyday activities (Coolican et al., 2010; Hardan et al., 2015; Koegel et al., 1996; Minjarez et al., 2011; Nefdt et al., 2010).

15.5 Research Background

The groundwork for PRT was developed in response to the learners' apparent low interest when trials were presented in a structured, drill-type manner (Lovaas et al., 1966, 1974). These early methods were effective, shifted away from parental causation, and showed that children with autism could learn. However, they were labor intensive, and the children exhibited varying levels of escape and avoidance behavior. To counteract this, a variety studies were conducted targeting responsiveness, engagement, correct responding, and improved affect. This ongoing research and subsequent publications created a foundation for the PRT package.

For example, Dyer et al. (1987) used a repeated reversal design with 11 participants and showed that when preferred topics and activities were included into the intervention, social avoidance was greatly reduced, and social engagement increased. Koegel and Williams (1980) used a variety of tasks in a multiple-baseline design across three children to demonstrate that when the child's response was part of the chain leading to the reinforcer, they consistently demonstrated rapid acquisition of the target behavior when compared to trials when the response was unrelated to the reinforcer. In a follow-up study, Williams et al. (1981) used a multiple-baseline design with a reversal condition across three children and multiple behaviors. This study showed that when the reward was directly related to the child's response (as opposed to indirectly related, such as providing edibles or tokens) the children showed immediate improvements in their correct responding and rate of responding. These early studies began to show that specific attention to arranging direct and functional response–reinforcer relationships created high levels of responding (Koegel & Mentis, 1985).

Other research addressed the drill-type practice of repeated trials, which also seemed to cause avoidance and escape motivated behavior. For example, Dunlap and Koegel (1980) implemented a multiple-baseline design with reversals targeting a variety of behaviors across two children with autism. Specifically, repeatedly presenting the same task was compared to varying the task with different activities from the child's curriculum. This study showed that interspersing maintenance trials (targets that the individual had mastered) with acquisition (new target behaviors) resulted in more efficient learning and improved child affect on objectively scored Likert scales of behavior, interest, and happiness. Similarly, Dunlap (1984) used a simultaneous treatments design with four children involving (1) one new task that was repeatedly drilled; (2) a varied condition with 10 new tasks that were systematically alternated; and (3) a varied condition with five new (acquisition) tasks and five previously learned (maintenance) tasks that were systematically alternated. The results of this study showed that, regardless of task, the varied condition with the new and previously learned behaviors always resulted in learning that is more efficient. Furthermore, the Likert rating scales of enthusiasm, interest, and happiness demonstrated consistently higher affect during the condition with varied acquisition and maintenance tasks. Other research showed that reinforcing all communicative attempts, rather than using a strict shaping paradigm, was greatly more effective for teaching first words (Koegel et al., 1988).

This ongoing research in the 1980s created a foundation for the Koegel et al. (1987) study that first combined these individually researched variables into a package to create a more inviting learning environment for the child. This study used a multiple-baseline design across children who were minimally or nonverbal to target social communication. It demonstrated that the combination of motivational procedures resulted in more rapid acquisition and generalization of first word use. The study focused on verbal expressive (spoken) social communication and was thus coined "the natural language paradigm," as the procedures more closely resembled natural adult–child interactions compared to the baseline condition, which was highly structured and adult-driven. However, further research showed that the motivational procedures were applicable to many other behaviors, and it was renamed "pivotal response treatment." Since this time, many studies conducted within and outside our laboratories have corroborated the efficacy of PRT (de Kort et al., 2022; Mohammadzaheri et al., 2022; Suhrheinrich et al., 2022). Additionally, studies have replicated the effects targeting different behaviors, different age groups, and with different measures. We will describe a few of these studies.

In a randomized clinical trial implemented in the public schools, Mohammadzaheri et al. (2014) compared the effectiveness of treatment as usual (TAU), consisting of an adult-driven applied behavior analysis (ABA) intervention procedures, with PRT, which included motivational components, on communication skills. Thirty elementary school-aged children with autism, aged 6 to 12 years old, participated in the study. The children were matched based on age, sex, and MLU. Intervention was provided in the public schools by speech and language specialists and graduate students. The data showed that PRT resulted in significantly greater improvements in targeted language areas (lengthening the children's MLU) as well as untargeted areas after 3 months of intervention. Specifically, regarding untargeted areas, the PRT group showed significantly larger improvements on the pragmatic scales on the Children's Communication Checklist (CCC) as reported by both teachers and parents who were naïve to the experimental target behavior and group in which the children participated. The CCC includes measures of pragmatic domains measured on five subscales: (a) inappropriate initiation, (b) coherence, (c) stereotyped language, (d) use of context, and (e) rapport. The sum of these scales is the "pragmatic composite." These results suggest wider overall gains than those specifically targeted, supporting the concept of "pivotal" areas, in this somewhat older group of children.

In a quasi-experimental trial, Duifhuis et al. (2017) investigated the effects of PRT compared with a TAU group on autism symptoms in 24 children aged 3–8 years. In addition to autism symptoms, their study also investigated whether PRT versus a TAU would affect general interfering behaviors, as well as parental stress levels. Eleven children were placed in the PRT group and 13 in the TAU group. The PRT group received twenty 45-minute intervention sessions, focusing on communication goals, over a 6-month period. The TAU group received parent psychoeducation and parent mediation therapy that ranged from a small number of sessions with a psychologist (e.g., 1 hour per week in a group setting for 5 weeks) to a more intensive in-home parent education (e.g., twice weekly 75-minute sessions over 20 weeks). The primary outcome measure in this study was the Autism Diagnostic Observation Schedule (ADOS), and their secondary outcome measures were the Social Responsiveness Scale (SRS), the Child Behavior Checklist (CBCL), and the Nijmegen Parental Stress Inventory–Short Version (NOSI-K). These tests were given before treatment, after 3 months, and again at 6 months. Following intervention, although neither group demonstrated significant differences in the general problem behavior and parental stress levels, the children in the PRT condition improved significantly on the total score on the Autism Diagnostic Observation Schedule compared to the TAU group. That is, following intervention, the PRT group showed significantly fewer characteristics of ASD, whereas those characteristics increased in the TAU group. The results demonstrated a statistically significant interaction between group and time on the total ADOS scores.

Samadi et al. (2019) conducted another quasi-experimental study with a pretest, posttest, and follow-up to compare the effectiveness of PRT with a control group. Measures included diagnostic characteristics and cognitive processing areas. Participants were twenty 6–8-year-old children on the autism spectrum who were described by the authors as "high-functioning." Sessions were conducted twice weekly for 20 sessions. The Cognitive Assessment System (CAS), which assesses cognitive processing; the Trip Task, which assesses feelings and future planning using the participants' descriptions of pictures; and the Autism Spectrum Screening Questionnaire (ASSQ) were used for data collection. The authors reported that 2 months following the completion of intervention, the scores of future thinking on the Trip Test and cognitive processes (planning) on the CAS were significantly improved in the PRT group compared to the control group. This study showed promising results for PRT as an intervention for improving general cognitive areas in children with ASD and suggested that some cognitive components may be malleable through implementation of PRT.

De Korte et al. (2021) conducted a randomized controlled trial with 44 children with ASD, aged 9 to 15 years. In this study, the children were randomly allocated to either a PRT group ($n = 22$), which targeted individually defined social communication areas during a protocol of approximately 12 weekly 45-minute sessions, or a TAU group ($n = 22$) consisting of various interventions for 1.5 hours per week to 1 hour per month. Measurements were obtained after 12 and 20 weeks of intervention and after a 2-month follow-up period. The findings of this study showed positive treatment effects for both groups, with larger gains for children and adolescents in the PRT group. Additionally, significantly larger improvements in parent-rated general social-communicative skills, behavioral, and emotional (particularly regarding attention issues) occurred in the PRT group in comparison to the TAU group. In that study, the PRT group also showed collateral improvements in adaptive socialization skills and attention as rated by parents. Finally, anonymous ratings of global functioning showed larger gains in the PRT group. Regarding severity of ASD characteristics observed on the ADOS-2, no significant group differences were found, and no treatment differential effects were found on parenting stress. Overall, this showed that along with greater improvements in targeted areas, generalization of gains and collateral gains in co-occurring areas, particularly improved attention, were significantly larger following PRT.

Other research regarding the effectiveness of PRT motivational components has been applied to another pivotal area, child initiations. In the context of a multiple baseline across participants design, Koegel et al. (2010) examined the acquisition of conventional language and question asking in three preschool children with autism. At preintervention, participants could say more than 50 words and had begun to combine words based on observational data, tests, language samples, and parent report. Following the PRT intervention, there was a rapid increase in the use of questions in all three children. Generalization of question asking was also observed in these children. This study suggested that the PRT motivational strategies used were helpful in promoting the generalization of question asking. Similar findings were noted in a multiple-baseline design across three participants targeting the child-initiated question "Where?" (Koegel et al., 2010).

In the context of a multiple-baseline design, Koegel et al. (2014) examined the efficacy of using the motivational strategies of PRT to increase social question asking for three young children with autism. The results showed that the number of targeted questions increased following the intervention (10 hours per week and 2 hours of parent training for 10 months). In addition, increases in asking untargeted questions were observed during social interactions. The children also improved their communication and adaptive behavior, and their social initiations increased following intervention for question asking that included the motivational strategies.

Bozkus-Genc and Yucesoy-Ozkan (2021) used a concurrent multiple-baseline design study across four children with ASD to evaluate the effectiveness of PRT on the acquisition, maintenance, and generalization of initiations in the form of question asking. They also measured collateral changes in language development and other areas of development. The results of this study showed significant improvement in initiated question asking across all three children and collateral gains in language and other areas of development. Further, the children in this study were able to generalize the question-asking initiations to natural settings and maintain these gains over time. Again, this points to the benefit of carefully selecting areas to target, while including the motivational components during intervention.

Mohammadzaheri et al. (2021) also investigated the effect of PRT on improving verbal initiations in children with ASD, aged 6 to 12 years, using a randomized clinical trial design. The intervention was conducted in the public schools by speech and language specialists 3 times a week for 2 months, totaling 24 one-hour sessions for each participant. The PRT intervention taught a series of child initiated "wh" questions, and attention and assistance-seeking initiations. The TAU group received standard speech therapy without specifically targeting initiations. The results showed that the PRT group significantly increased in their number of targeted verbal initiations. The PRT group also improved significantly in their general communication skills as measured on structured verbal interactions and pragmatic areas on the CCC as well as MLU compared to the TAU group. Again, this study demonstrated significant gains in both targeted and untargeted areas and again suggested added value when selecting specific pivotal areas, such as child initiations.

An additional strength of PRT is lower levels of interfering behaviors that most likely function as escape or avoidance. For example, Koegel et al. (1992) implemented PRT during language intervention and measured interfering (disruptive) behavior in preschool children diagnosed with autism. Using a multiple-reversals design, they used two language teaching conditions; one condition consisted of a traditional adult-driven intervention, and the other used PRT to target language structures. The results showed that the children rarely engaged in interfering behaviors during the PRT sessions, in contrast to the adult-driven intervention, where considerable disruptive and interfering behaviors were exhibited. This study added to the literature showing concomitant gains in untargeted areas. That is, in addition to greater responding, faster learning, and improved affect, when the PRT motivational procedures were incorporated, interfering aggressive and disruptive behaviors were minimal.

A larger group study using a randomized clinical trial design with intervention implemented by speech and language specialists in public schools with older children also demonstrated improvements in behavior when using PRT. That is, Mohammadzaheri et al. (2015) compared the effectiveness of an adult-driven ABA intervention with PRT on disruptive behavior during language intervention of children with autism, aged 6 to 12 years old. Thirty children participated in the study who were matched based on age, sex, and mean length of utterance. The results showed that PRT resulted in significantly lower levels of disruptive and interfering behaviors.

Related, Ventola et al. (2016) evaluated changes in interfering restricted and repetitive behaviors (RRBs) following a 16-week open trial of PRT (compared to preintervention measures). Fifteen children diagnosed with ASD, ages 4 to 7 years, participated and the intervention focused on social communication and responsiveness. The results showed that RRB symptom severity decreased significantly following the PRT intervention. As well, there were significant decreases in six subdomains of the RBS-R, including repetitive movements and sensory seeking behavior, self-injury, compulsive behaviors, ritualistic behaviors, sameness, and restricted behaviors. Finally, on the Aberrant Behavior Checklist (ABC), significant reductions on the stereotypy subdomain (repetitive movements) occurred. Overall, the results showed a significant reduction in RRB after intervention. Although PRT clearly addressed pivotal social communication skills, it had a secondary effect on reducing RRBs.

Along with more rapid acquisition of a wide variety of target behaviors, greater generalization, and the additional benefit of untargeted behaviors improving, researchers have demonstrated that PRT can be effective when implemented by neurotypical peers in school settings in the context of play. Harper et al. (2008) assessed social skills gains in two elementary school children using a multiple-baseline design. The researchers used the PRT motivational techniques through peer education to improve the social interactions during recess activities. The results showed an improvement in social initiations and turn taking during recess activities, compared to baseline.

Thus, PRT intervention with successful outcomes both in targeted and untargeted areas has been implemented by a variety of providers, including professionals

(Mohammadzaheri et al., 2014, 2021), parents (Symon, 2005), paraprofessionals (Robinson, 2011), and peers (Harper et al., 2008).

In regard to physiological changes, some studies have examined neural correlations and behavioral changes following PRT. For example, Voos et al. (2013) conducted the first functional magnetic resonance imaging (fMRI) study to assess changes in brain activity following 16 weeks (8–10 hours per week) of PRT in two autistic preschoolers who scored in the average or above-average range on standardized cognitive and language tests. In this study, both children showed increased activity in the left ventricular prefrontal cortex, left ventricular peripheral cortex, right amygdala, right posterior superior temporal gyrus, and bilateral gyrus fusiform, and left dorsal peripheral and left ventricular peripheral cortex. The results showed that the nervous systems that are related to social function were affected by implementation of PRT.

In another study, Venkataraman et al. (2016) tested the brain responses using fMRI in 19 school children with ASD (mean age, 5.87 years, ±1.09 years), described as "high-functioning," following 16 weeks of PRT (5 hours of direct intervention with a clinician and 2 hours of weekly parent education in the home). The researchers evaluated the posterior cingulate cortex, which is involved in self-regulation and social cognition, and showed functional changes in response to biological movement. The changes in the posterior cingulate cortex activity were associated with decreased function of the orbitofrontal cortex, which is involved in assessing the level of reward associated with external stimuli, and increased function in the temporal cortex, which is involved in understanding biological movement and facial recognition. The researchers interpreted the functional symmetry that followed the implementation of PRT that resulted in increased recognition of social stimuli and involvement of higher social perception areas, again suggesting improved brain changes following PRT.

Although the specific areas of brain changes are interesting, brain changes are expected to occur with learning. Therefore, the effects of PRT compared to TAU are of interest. This was addressed in a randomized controlled trial study by Mohammadzaheri et al. (2022), who examined the effectiveness of PRT on brain activity in children with ASD compared to a TAU control group. In this study, 20 autistic boys aged 6–12 years were randomly assigned to PRT or TAU groups. Children in both groups were matched based on age and MLU. The intervention consisted of 24 sessions for 60 minutes 3 days a week focusing on child initiations. Questions, general communication skills, MLU, and brain activity were tested before and after the intervention. The results showed that PRT resulted in a significant improvement in behavioral areas in addition to being associated with oscillations in brain activity in several brain regions compared with the TAU group. Thus, collateral neurological changes were observed after PRT compared to the TAU group.

In addition to individual studies, several systematic reviews and meta-analyses regarding PRT have been published and will be discussed in chronological order.

It is important to note that there has been an increase in the number of studies relating to autism interventions (Gitimoghaddam et al., 2022); thus, review articles may not include all relevant PRT studies.

Verschuur et al. (2014) reviewed 39 PRT studies with 420 children published before June 2013. The authors found that in addition to targeted areas, PRT resulted in improvements in communication and play skills and for some children, reductions in interfering behaviors and improvements in affect. No studies reported negative outcomes, with all studies reporting positive or mixed outcomes. This review also found that most caregivers and staff members were able to implement PRT with fidelity. Bozkus-Genc and Vuran (2013) reviewed PRT studies published between 1980 and 2011, related to social communication. Twenty-three studies with 79 participants were included in the study. Targeted social communication areas included play initiations, initiating conversations and social interactions, and initiating and continuing joint attention. The settings included educational (special and general education classrooms), clinic, home, and various play settings (playroom, play garden). Implementers included parents and care providers, peers, teachers, researchers, paraprofessionals, and clinicians, most using one-on-one intervention formats. Although improvements were observed in the various behaviors along with stimulus response and setting generalization, the authors noted that social validity, FoI, and long-term maintenance were measured in fewer than a quarter of the studies, an important consideration that is now being included more frequently in current studies.

Another systematic review by Boudreau et al. (2015) focused on peer-mediated PRT (PM-PRT) interventions with school-age children with ASD. They reviewed five PM-PRT studies that used single-subject designs with 29 participants (eight with ASD and 21 peer trainers). Their review reported that most of the PM-PRT studies demonstrated positive results. However, they concluded that the small existing research base, while highly promising, did not yet meet the criteria to be classified as an evidence-based practice for improving social skill deficits in children with ASD, and that further research is needed.

Using a meta-analysis of outcomes of group-design studies, Tiede & Walton (2019) examined interventions using the more general category of natural developmental behavioral intervention strategies, many of which incorporate PRT components. Their study found the largest effects for social engagement and general cognitive development and some significant positive effects for expressive language, reduction in the characteristics of autism spectrum disorder, and play skills. Small effects were found for joint attention and receptive language.

In another systematic review of five randomized controlled trials, Ona et al. (2020) examined the effectiveness of PRT on social communication, social interaction, and repetitive behavior for children with ASD. Their review indicated that PRT may have a positive effect on expressive language, social interaction, and repetitive behavior. The effects on further outcomes, receptive language, and early learning skills were more uncertain. They suggested the need for further high-quality research in the area.

Forbes et al. (2020) reviewed studies relating only to verbal and linguistic behavior following PRT published between 1987 and 2018. Fifty studies were included in their analysis, including 15 group designs and 35 single-case design studies. The authors pointed out that a limitation of their review was that studies were excluded that did not explicitly report that all the PRT components were used (e.g., articles such as Koegel et al., 2010 were not included) or when strict adherence to PRT procedures was not determined. Nevertheless, the review found that PRT was effective in producing gains in phonology, suprasegmentals, semantics, and syntax as well as word use and vocabulary.

Finally, in an umbrella systematic review, Uljarević et al. (2022) reviewed six systematic reviews covering a time period up to 2018. They also identified 10 randomized clinical trials of PRT. They found that almost all of the studies reported statistically significant improvements in a variety of language and communicative areas. Additionally, their review showed that positive effects were demonstrated by the majority of the children on outcome measures, which ranged from natural observations to standardized tests and parent checklists. They also noted that all studies reported that the primary interventionists (parents and clinicians) were able to meet a >85% FoI.

Thus, publications from case reports, single-case and group studies, randomized controlled trials, systematic reviews, and meta-analyses support PRT as an evidence-based intervention (Hume et al., 2021; Wong et al., 2015), particularly for improving social communication. However, there are still questions that warrant additional research. For example, specific target behaviors have varied across studies. There is a wide range of targeted areas within the PRT research, with some studies targeting first words and functional utterances (Coolican et al., 2010; Koegel et al., 1987), and others, social conversation (Koegel et al., 2014). Although this demonstrates PRT's effectiveness with a wide range of presenting characteristics in the ASD diagnosis, research regarding the relative effectiveness and added value of particular target areas and behavioral characteristics is warranted (Forbes et al., 2020). Additionally, studies have varied greatly in the measures used to assess change from the behavior directly targeted to collateral gains in other areas on standardized tests (Ledbetter-Cho et al., 2017; Uljarovic et al., 2022). This makes it more difficult to compare studies.

Additionally, PRT studies have varied in age of the participants, ranging from infants (Koegel et al., 2014) to adults (Vogler, 2017). Outcome and dependent measures have also varied greatly in the published research (Oljarovic et al., 2022). Further, the length and method of intervention have been different across studies ranging from short-term interventions (Hardan et al., 2015) to relatively longer intervention periods (Duifhuis et al., 2017). Longitudinal studies are lacking as well as research focusing on the ideal age range relating to response to intervention.

Thus, research is warranted regarding the optimal dosage, target behavior, strength of individual components, and participant characteristics to further understand the effectiveness of PRT.

Furthermore, while most studies have focused on the collateral gains of PRT, few have assessed the gains in parents and service providers (Verschuur et al., 2014). As well, studies on the speed of response, cost effectiveness, and maintenance and generalization of goals are also warranted (Verschuur et al., 2014). There have been a large variety of methods and service delivery modalities (e.g., in person, one-on-one, groups, and telehealth) and length of training to fidelity, making it challenging to determine the optimum type and amount of PRT necessary for child and service provider gains (Verschuur et al., 2014). Also, while stress has been shown to decrease in parents while they are providing PRT compared to an adult-driven ABA (Koegel et al., 1996), overall stress levels remain high (Duifhuis et al., 2017), suggesting the need for additional research in this area.

Consistent with other intervention approaches, some children demonstrate greater improvements following PRT intervention than others. Certainly, researchers have been interested in response to intervention and delineating various phenotypes to match interventions to cognitive, language, and behavioral expressions of ASD, especially given the wide heterogeneity in ASD. This area would benefit from additional research. To date, most studies have suggested that the greater the skills at entry to an intervention program, the greater the gains during intervention; however, more emphasis on the type of intervention programs that best match a particular individual's needs based on their characteristics would be beneficial (Koegel et al., 2020).

Mediators and moderators of intervention may also prove to be valuable. For example, while parent education is an integral part of PRT (Koegel & Koegel, 2012), research regarding the effectiveness of parents who do and do not meet FoI and the outcomes for children whose parents provide a high versus low number of opportunities (trials) is critical in understanding the effectiveness of PRT, particularly for training purposes. Similarly, Verschuur and colleagues (2017) trained staff members at an in-patient unit with children aged 7 to 13 years. Although improvement in targeted areas occurred following intervention, improvements on the CCC-2 and the Vineland-II were not evidenced. Because these areas have been shown to improve in other studies with children living at home (Hardan et al., 2015; Mohammadzaheri et al., 2014, 2015), this suggests that parents may be especially important change agents and additional research in this area may be fruitful.

Further, acceptability of the treatment (social validity) has not been assessed in all PRT studies. However, the long-standing motivational components (Koegel et al., 1987) and strength-based approach (Koegel et al., 1997) of PRT have been discussed as valuable and family friendly; as a step toward emphasizing autistic individuals' strengths and quality of life; and as an increasingly acceptable intervention (Kim & Trainor, 2020; Schuck et al., 2021).

These studies suggest that while many interventions result in progress, particular attention to both the targeted areas and the way in which the intervention is implemented (i.e., using motivational components) may result in improved overall gains. However, many areas clearly continue to warrant further research. As well, many similar naturalistic interventions have evolved (e.g., Schreibman et al., 2015) that incorporate some or all the PRT procedures or have reportedly made a slight modification of the original procedures (e.g., PRISM; Vernon et al., 2019). This is encouraging as it suggests the importance of these procedures (Delprato, 2001). However, it makes comprehensive systematic analyses of PRT more challenging, as important articles may be excluded.

15.6 Practice Implications

PRT research has been effectively implemented using a variety of formats. The results of studies suggest that PRT can be integrated into daily routines and educational programs and can be implemented with fidelity by parents, paraprofessionals, teachers, and peers. Additionally, while most studies have provided one-on-one intervention, for time efficiency, the possibility of teaching PRT in-group formats has been assessed. For example, Minjarez and colleagues (2011) compared a PRT small-group intervention format with an individual PRT session format for parents of children with autism aged 2 to 7 years. Seventeen families participated, with eight participating in the group and nine participating individually. The parent education was implemented for 10 weeks with 90-minute sessions per week using a lecture, video examples, reading worksheets, and homework. Additionally, the parents brought in video examples of themselves working with their child for feedback. The results showed that the group intervention was similarly effective to the individual intervention, with all parents showing improvements in their FoI and significant improvements in functional verbal utterances for all children following intervention.

Another study investigating PRTG used a randomized clinical trial (Hardan et al., 2015) to target language areas in 53 children with ASD, aged 2 to 6 years. Families were randomly assigned to a PRTG or a psychoeducational group for 12 weeks. During intervention, the parents in the PRTG learned PRT techniques that promote language development, and families in the psychoeducational group were provided with general information about ASD. The results of this research showed that most of the parents (84%) attending the PRTG format were able to meet FoI, and the children in the PRTG showed significantly greater improvements in the frequency of utterance compared with children in the psychoeducation group. Additionally, adaptive communication on the Vineland-II showed greater improvements in the PRTG condition. These results indicated that parents were able to learn PRT in a group format that positively affected their children's communication during a short-term group PRT intervention format.

Concerning treatment implementation, studies have showed that PRT can be implemented with fidelity by individuals of different educational backgrounds as well as peers. For example, many studies have shown that PRT can effectively be implemented with fidelity by parents (Hardan et al., 2015; Symon, 2005). Verschuur and colleagues (2017) assessed the effectiveness of training staff members to implement PRT with children who were undergoing intervention at an inpatient facility due to either extreme behavior issues or parent inability to manage or cope with parenting their child. Participants were 14 employees and 13 children with ASD between 6 and 14 years of age, and data were collected in the context of a multiple-baseline design. Training consisted of four 6-hour sessions, and staff members were taught to target self-initiated questions. Results showed that all staff members improved in the median number of opportunities they provided to the children for question asking, with 11 showing statistically significant improvements. Eight staff members showed improvement during post intervention and seven during follow-up. Additionally, question asking improved for all 13 children during intervention and remained above baseline measures at post intervention, with eight showing statistically significant improvements.

Some studies have also focused on teaching PRT to teachers. For example, Suhrheinrich et al. (2020) evaluated outcomes of a large, randomized clinical trial with 79 teachers in the control group and 98 in the PRT group. The teachers in the PRT group were taught to use Classroom Pivotal Response Teaching (CPRT). The training consisted of 12 hours of small-group sessions and one 1-on-1 session in each teacher's classroom. Teachers reported that they used CPRT for an average of 47 minutes a day and reported overall satisfaction and high self-confidence in their ability to use CPRT with their students. The study demonstrated the acceptability and feasibility of the CPRT training protocol and indicated that fidelity might be higher during the training year, suggesting the need for booster sessions during subsequent years.

In a multiple-baseline design study across dyads, Kowitt (2018) investigated the effectiveness of PRT on question asking in high school settings with adolescents and young adults with ASD. In this study, two paraprofessionals and one special education teacher (n = 3) were taught to perform PRT with a student with whom they had previously worked. Training was implemented using a PowerPoint presentation, a manual, and handouts with approximately 2 hours of training per provider and video feedback ranging from 19.5 to 35.5 minutes. If FoI fell below 80%, the trainer met with the school provider. The results of the study found that while all three teachers improved in their training of question asking, only one teacher met the 80% FoI criterion. However, following the training, all three students improved in their targeted question asking and two students demonstrated varying levels of generalization to other untargeted questions. Brief PRT trainings may be somewhat helpful for students, but less effective in maintaining skills in the paraprofessionals and teachers.

15.6.1 Treatment Outcomes

Although the bulk of the research has shown that PRT is particularly helpful for social communication, there have been children who did not acquire spoken verbal communication following PRT. To address this issue, Koegel et al. (2009) used a nonconcurrent multiple-baseline across-participants design to examine the application of attentional cues to facilitate the acquisition of first words in nonverbal children with autism. Three nonverbal autistic children participated who had received PRT for 9 to 28 weeks before the 6 to 10 weeks of intervention focusing on expressive verbal words. The addition of an individualized orienting cue to gain the child's attention before presenting a verbal model improved the acquisition of first words. However, one of the three participants made some, but little, progress. Understanding variables that may account for a small percentage of young children not acquiring first words or other target goal with PRT is unclear. PRT studies with other social communication have resulted in various outcomes, with adults who show lower levels of social interaction during baseline making the smallest gains after intervention (Koegel et al., 2021). Again, reviews have suggested that higher performance at entry into an intervention program is frequently associated with higher performance at exit, regardless of the program (Koegel et al., 2019), and may be relevant to PRT interventions.

Another issue relates to the number of opportunities provided to the individual. Preliminary research suggests that the greatest outcomes occur when PRT is implemented when FoI is met and a high frequency of trials is presented (Hardan, 2019). The research suggests that most individuals are able to meet FoI for PRT; however, practice with feedback appears to be important. Participants in the studies that provided regular feedback were quite successful in their implementation of the procedures. Understanding the degree to which providers need to become proficient and the frequency of opportunities provided for optimal child outcomes would provide helpful information for practitioners. Undoubtedly, a combination of incoming characteristics, environmental factors, and implementation of intervention techniques plays a role in outcomes and warrants further investigation.

15.6.2 Practice Implication Guidelines

Case histories, single-subject design studies, and an accumulating number of randomized clinical trials are demonstrating the effectiveness of PRT. Most of the studies have focused on comparing PRT with the treatment as usual, a psychoeducational intervention, or adult-driven behavioral interventions. While intervention can be implemented with FoI by individuals without a background in special education or ASD, collaboration regarding selecting initial and new goals, implementation of the procedures, and coordination of PRT across settings is recommended (Koegel & Koegel, 2019). The increase in naturalistic interventions that incorporate various motivational procedures described in the initial study by Koegel and colleagues (1987) and early incidental teaching studies (McGee et al., 1983, 1985, 1986) suggests ease of implementation and underscores the importance of these variables (Schreibman et al., 2015).

15.7 References

Ashbaugh, K., Koegel, R. L., & Koegel, L. K. (2017). Increasing social integration for college students with autism spectrum disorder. *Behavioral Development Bulletin*, *22*(1), 183.

Boudreau, A. M., Corkum, P., Meko, K., & Smith, I. M. (2015). Peer-mediated pivotal response treatment for young children with autism spectrum disorders: A systematic review. *Canadian Journal of School Psychology*, *30*(3), 218–235. doi: 10.1177/0829573515581156

Bozkus-Genc, G., & Vuran, S. (2013). Examination of studies targeting social skills with pivotal response treatment. *Educational Sciences: Theory and Practice*, *13*(3), 1730–1742.

Bozkus-Genc, G., & Yucesoy-Ozkan, S. (2021). The efficacy of pivotal response treatment in teaching question-asking initiations to young Turkish children with autism spectrum disorder. *Journal of Autism Developmental Disorders*, *51*(11), 3868–3886. https://doi.org/10.1007/s10803-020-04848-y

Bruinsma, Y. E. (2004). Increases in the joint attention behavior of eye gaze alternation to share enjoyment as a collateral effect of pivotal response treatment for three children with autism. [Doctoral dissertation, University of California, Santa Barbara].

Carr, M. E., Moore, D. W., & Anderson, A. (2014). Self-management interventions on students with autism: A meta-analysis of single-subject research. *Exceptional Children*, *81*(1), 28–44.

Cohen, S., Koegel, R., Koegel, L. K., Engstrom, E., Young, K., & Quach, A. (2022). Using self-management and visual cues to improve responses to nonverbal social cues in adults with autism spectrum disorder. *Behavior Modification*, *46*(3), 529–552.

Coolican, J., Smith, I. M., & Bryson, S. E. (2010). Brief parent training in pivotal response treatment for preschoolers with autism. *Journal of Child Psychology and Psychiatry*, *51*(12), 1321–1330.

Delprato, D. J. (2001). Comparisons of discrete-trial and normalized behavioral language intervention for young children with autism. *Journal of Autism and Developmental Disorders*, *31*(3), 315–325.

Dunlap, G. (1984). The influence of task variation and maintenance tasks on the learning and affect of autistic children. *Journal of Experimental Child Psychology*, *37*(1), 41–64.

Dunlap, G., & Koegel, R. L. (1980). Motivating autistic children through stimulus variation. *Journal of Applied Behavior Analysis*, *13*(4), 619–627.

Ebrahim, M. T. E. S. (2019). Effectiveness of a pivotal response training programme in joint attention and social interaction of kindergarten children with autism spectrum disorder. *Psycho-Educational Research Reviews*, *82*(2), 48–56.

Duifhuis, E. A., den Boer, J. C., Doornbos, A., Buitelaar, J. K., Oosterling, I. J., & Klip, H. (2017). The effect of pivotal response treatment in children with autism spectrum disorders: A non-randomized study with a blinded outcome measure. *Journal of Autism and Developmental Disorders*, *47*, 231–242 https://doi.org/10.1007/s10803-016-2916-0.

Forbes, H. J., Travers, J. C., & Vickers Johnson, J. (2020). A systematic review of linguistic and verbal behavior outcomes of pivotal response treatment. *Journal of Autism and Developmental Disorders*, *50*(3), 766–778.

Gengoux, G. W., Abrams, D. A., Schuck, R., Millan, M. E., Libove, R., Ardel, C. M., Phillips, J. M., Fox, M., Frazier, T. W., & Hardan, A. Y. (2019). A pivotal response treatment package for children with autism spectrum disorder: An RCT. *Pediatrics*, *144*(3), e20190178. https://doi.org/10.1542/peds.2019-0178

Gitimoghaddam, M., Chichkine, N., McArthur, L., Sangha, S. S., & Symington, V. (2022). Applied behavior analysis in children and youth with autism spectrum disorders: A scoping review. *Perspectives on Behavior Science*, 45, 1–37.

Hardan, A. Y. (2019). Targeting language deficits in young children with autism: Evidence from two randomized controlled trials. Presentation at the annual Pivotal Response Treatment Conference, Stanford University, Stanford, California.

Hardan, A. Y., Gengoux, G. W., Berquist, K. L., Libove, R. A., Ardel, C. M., Phillips, J., Frazier, T. W., & Minjarez, M. B. (2015). A randomized controlled trial of pivotal response treatment group for parents of children with autism. *Journal of Child Psychology and Psychiatry, 56*(8), 884–892.

Harper, C. B., Symon, J. B., & Frea, W. D. (2008). Recess is time-in: Using peers to improve social skills of children with autism. *Journal of Autism and Developmental Disorders, 38*(5), 815–826. doi: 10.1007/s10803-007-0449-2

Hume, K., Steinbrenner, J. R., Odom, S. L., Morin, K. L., Nowell, S. W., Tomaszewski, B., Szendrey, S., McIntyre, N.S., Yücesoy-Özkan, S. & Savage, M. N. (2021). Evidence-based practices for children, youth, and young adults with autism: Third generation review. *Journal of Autism and Developmental Disorders, 51*(11), 4013–4032.

Kim, S., & Trainor, A. A. (2020). Applicability and feasibility of pivotal response treatment with Korean American children with autism. *Education and Training in Autism and Developmental Disabilities, 55*(1), 75–88.

Koegel, L. K., Ashbaugh, K., Navab, A., & Koegel, R. L. (2016). Improving empathic communication skills in adults with autism spectrum disorder. *Journal of Autism and Developmental Disorders, 46*(3), 921–933.

Koegel, L. K., Bryan, K. M., Su, P., Vaidya, M., & Camarata, S. (2019). Intervention for nonverbal and minimally-verbal individuals with autism: A systematic review. *International Journal of Pediatric Research, 5*(2), 1–16. doi: 10.23937/2469-5769/1510056

Koegel, L. K., Bryan, K. M., Su, P. L., Vaidya, M., & Camarata, S. (2020). Definitions of nonverbal and minimally verbal in research for autism: A systematic review of the literature. *Journal of Autism and Developmental Disorders, 50*(8), 2957–2972.

Koegel, L. K., Harrower, J. K., & Koegel, R. L. (1999). Support for children with developmental disabilities in full inclusion classrooms through self-management. *Journal of Positive Behavior Interventions, 1*(1), 26–34.

Koegel, L. K., Koegel, R. L., & Carter, C. M. (1998). Pivotal responses and the natural language teaching paradigm. *Seminars in Speech and Language, 19*(4), 355–372.

Koegel, L. K., Koegel, R. L., Green-Hopkins, I., & Barnes, C. C. (2010). Brief report: Question-asking and collateral language acquisition in children with autism. *Journal of Autism and Developmental Disorders, 40*(4), 509–515. doi: 10.1007/s10803-009-0896-z

Koegel, L. K., Koegel, R. L., Shoshan, Y., & McNerney, E. (1999). Pivotal response intervention II: Preliminary long-term outcome data. *Research and Practice for Persons With Severe Disabilities, 24*(3), 186–198.

Koegel, L. K., Koegel, R. L., & Smith, A. (1997). Variables related to differences in standardized test outcomes for children with autism. *Journal of Autism and Developmental Disorders, 27*(3), 233–243.

Koegel, L. K., Koplen, Z., Koegel, B., & Koegel, R. L. (2021). Using a question bank intervention to improve socially initiated questions in adolescents and adults with autism. *Journal of Speech, Language, and Hearing Research, 64*(4), 1331–1339.

Koegel, L. K., Park, M. N., & Koegel, R. L. (2014). Using self-management to improve the reciprocal social conversation of children with autism spectrum disorder. *Journal of Autism and Developmental Disorders, 44*(5), 1055–1063.

Koegel, L. K., Singh, A. K., & Koegel, R. L. (2010). Improving motivation for academics in children with autism. *Journal of Autism Developmental Disorders, 40*(9), 1057–1066.

Koegel, R. L., Bimbela, A., & Schreibman, L. (1996). Collateral effects of parent training on family interactions. *Journal of Autism and Developmental Disorders, 26*(3), 347–359.

Koegel, R. L., Bradshaw, J. L., Ashbaugh, K., & Koegel, L. K. (2014). Improving question asking initiations in young children with autism using pivotal response treatment. *Journal of Autism and Developmental Disorders, 44*(4), 816–827. https://doi.org/10.1007/s10803013-1932-6

Koegel, R. L., Camarata, S., Koegel, L. K., Ben-Tall, A., & Smith, A. E. (1998). Increasing speech intelligibility in children with autism. *Journal of Autism and Developmental Disorders, 28*(3), 241–251.

Koegel, R. L., Dyer, K., & Bell, L. K. (1987). The influence of child-preferred activities on autistic children's social behavior. *Journal of Applied Behavior Analysis, 20*(3), 243–252.

Koegel, R. L., & Koegel, L. K. (2012). *The PRT pocket guide: Pivotal response treatment for autism spectrum disorders.* Baltimore: Brookes.

Koegel, R. L., & Koegel, L. K. (2019). *Pivotal response treatment for autism spectrum disorders.* Baltimore: Brookes.

Koegel, R. L., Koegel, L. K., & Surratt, A. (1992). Language intervention and disruptive behavior in preschool children with autism. *Journal of Autism and Developmental Disorders, 22*(2), 141–153.

Koegel, R. L., & Mentis, M. (1985). Motivation in childhood autism: Can they or won't they? *Journal of Child Psychology and Psychiatry, 26*(2), 185–191.

Koegel, R. L., O'Dell, M., & Dunlap, G. (1988). Producing speech use in nonverbal autistic children by reinforcing attempts. *Journal of Autism and Developmental Disorders, 18*(4), 525–538.

Koegel, R. L., O'Dell, M. C., & Koegel, L. K. (1987). A natural language teaching paradigm for nonverbal autistic children. *Journal of Autism and Developmental Disorders, 17*(2), 187–200.

Koegel, R. L., Shirotova L., & Koegel L. K. (2009) Brief report: Using individualized orienting cues to facilitate first-word acquisition in non-responders with autism. *Journal of Autism and Developmental Disorders, 39*(11), 1587–1592.

Koegel, R. L., & Wilhelm, H. (1973). Selective responding to the components of multiple visual cues by autistic children. *Journal of Experimental Child Psychology, 15*(3), 442–453.

Koegel, R. L., & Williams, J. A. (1980). Direct versus indirect response-reinforcer relationships in teaching autistic children. *Journal of Abnormal Psychology, 8*(4), 537–547.

de Korte, M. W., van Dongen-Boomsma, M., Oosterling, I. J., Buitelaar, J., & Staal, W. G. (2022). Pivotal response treatment (PRT) parent group training for young children with autism spectrum disorder: A pilot study. *Scientific Reports, 12*(1), 1–9.

de Korte, M. W. P., van den Berk-Smeekens, I., Buitelaar, J. K., Staal, W.G., & van Dongen-Boomsma, M. (2021). Pivotal response treatment for school-aged children and adolescents with autism spectrum disorder: A randomized controlled trial. *Journal of Autism and Developmental Disorders, 51*(12), 4506–4519. https://doi.org/10.1007/s10803-021-04886-0

de Korte, M. W. P., Kaijadoe, S. P. T., Buitelaar, J. K. et al. (2022). Pivotal response treatment (PRT)—Parent group training for young children with autism spectrum disorder: A qualitative study on perspectives of parents. *Journal of Autism and Developmental Disorders, 52,* 5414–5427. https://doi.org/10.1007/s10803-021-05397-8

Kowitt, J. (2018). Implementing pivotal response treatment to teach question-asking to high school students with autism spectrum disorder: A pilot study. [Doctoral dissertation]. University of California Santa Barbara.

Kuhn, L. R., Bodkin, A. E., Devlin, S. D., & Doggett, R. A. (2008). Using pivotal response training with peers in special education to facilitate play in two children with autism. *Education and Training in Developmental Disabilities, 43*(1), 37–45.

Ledbetter-Cho, K., Lang, R., Watkins, L., & Zamora, C. (2017). Systematic review of collateral effects of focused interventions for children with autism spectrum disorder. *Autism and Developmental Language Impairments, 2,* 1–22.

Lovaas, O. I., Berberich, J. P., Perloff, B. F., & Schaeffer, B. (1966). Acquisition of imitative speech by schizophrenic children. *Focus on Autistic Behavior, 6*(1), 1–5.

Lovaas, O. I., Schreibman, L., Koegel, R., & Rehm, R. (1971). Selective responding by autistic children to multiple sensory input. *Journal of Abnormal Psychology, 77*(3), 211.

Lovaas, O. I., Schreibman, L., & Koegel, R. L. (1974). A behavior modification approach to the treatment of autistic children. *Journal of Autism and Childhood Schizophrenia, 4*(2), 111–129.

Maier, S. F., & Seligman, M. E. (1976). Learned helplessness: Theory and evidence. *Journal of Experimental Psychology: General, 105*(1), 3–46.

McGee, G. G., Krantz, P. J., Mason, D., & McClannahan, L. E. (1983). A modified incidental teaching procedure for autistic youth: Acquisition and generalization of receptive object labels. *Journal of Applied Behavior Analysis, 16*(3), 329–338.

McGee, G. G., Krantz, P. J., & McClannahan, L. E. (1985). The facilitative effects of incidental teaching on preposition use by autistic children. *Journal of Applied Behavior Analysis, 18*(1), 17–31.

McGee, G. G., Krantz, P. J., & McClannahan, L. E. (1986). An extension of incidental teaching procedures to reading instruction for autistic children. *Journal of Applied Behavior Analysis, 19*(2), 147–157.

Minjarez, M. B., Williams, S. E., Mercier, E. M., & Hardan, A. Y. (2011). Pivotal response group treatment program for parents of children with autism. *Journal of Autism and Developmental Disorders, 41*(1), 92–101.

Mohammadzaheri, F., Koegel, L. K., Bakhshi, E., Khosrowabadi, R., & Soleymani, Z. (2022). The effect of teaching initiations on the communication of children with autism spectrum disorder: A randomized clinical trial. *Journal of Autism and Developmental Disorders, 52*(6), 2598–2609. https://doi.org/10.1007/s10803-021-05153-y

Mohammadzaheri, F., Koegel, L. K., Rezaee, M., & Rafiee, S. M. (2014). A randomized clinical trial comparison between pivotal response treatment (PRT) and structured applied behavior analysis (ABA) intervention for children with autism. *Journal of Autism and Developmental Disorders, 44*(11), 2769–2777.

Mohammadzaheri, F., Koegel, L. K., Rezaei, M., & Bakhshi, E. (2015). A randomized clinical trial comparison between pivotal response treatment (PRT) and adult-driven applied behavior analysis (ABA) intervention on disruptive behaviors in public school children with autism. *Journal of Autism and Developmental Disorders, 45*(9), 2899–2907.

Mohammadzaheri, F., Koegel, L. K., Soleymani, Z., Khosrowabadi, R., & Bakhshi, E. (2022). Neural correlates of enhancing question asking and initiations in children with autism spectrum disorders: A randomized clinical trial. *Social Neuroscience, 17*(2), 181–192.

Murphy, A., Robinson, S. E., Cote, D. L., Karge, B. D., & Lee, T. (2016). A teacher's use of video to train paraprofessionals in pivotal response techniques. *Journal of Special Education Apprenticeship, 4*(2), 1–19.

Nefdt, N., Koegel, R., Singer, G., & Gerber, M. (2010). The use of a self-directed learning program to provide introductory training in pivotal response treatment to parents of children with autism. *Journal of Positive Behavior Interventions, 12*(1), 23–32.

Ona, H. N., Larsen, K., Nordheim, L. V., & Brurberg, K. G. (2020). Effects of pivotal response treatment (PRT) for children with autism spectrum disorders (ASD): A systematic review. *Review Journal of Autism and Developmental Disorders, 7*(1), 78–90. https://doi.org/10.1007/s40489-019-00180-z

Pierce, K., & Schreibman, L. (1997). Multiple peer use of pivotal response training to increase social behaviors of classmates with autism: Results from trained and untrained peers. *Journal of Applied Behavior Analysis, 30*(1), 157–160.

Pierce, K. L., & Schreibman, L. (1994). Teaching daily living skills to children with autism in unsupervised settings through pictorial self-management. *Journal of Applied Behavior Analysis, 27*(3), 471–481.

Robinson, S. E. (2011). Teaching paraprofessionals of students with autism to implement pivotal response treatment in inclusive school settings using a brief video feedback training package. *Focus on Autism and Other Developmental Disabilities, 26*(2), 105–118.

Samadi, M., Ghamarani, A., & Faramarzi, S. (2019). Effectiveness of pivotal response treatment on future thinking and PASS processes in children with autism spectrum disorder. *Journal of Research in Behavioural Sciences, 17*(3), 495–507.

Schreibman, L., Dawson, G., Stahmer, A. C., Landa, R., Rogers, S. J., McGee, G. G., Kasari, C., Ingersoll, B., Kaiser, A. P., Bruinsma, Y., McNerney, E., Wetherby, A., & Halladay, A. (2015). Naturalistic developmental behavioral interventions: Empirically validated treatments for autism spectrum disorder. *Journal of Autism and Developmental Disorders, 45*(8), 2411–2428.

Schuck, R. K., Tagavi, D. M., Baiden, K. M., Dwyer, P., Williams, Z. J., Osuna, A., Ferguson, E. F., Muñoz, M. J., Poyser, S. K., Johnson, J. F., & Vernon, T. W. (2021). Neurodiversity and autism intervention: Reconciling perspectives through a naturalistic developmental behavioral intervention framework. *Journal of Autism and Developmental Disorders, 52*(10), 4625–4645.

Southall, C. M., & Gast, D. L. (2011). Self-management procedures: A comparison across the autism spectrum. *Education and Training in Autism and Developmental Disabilities, 46*(2), 155–171.

Stahmer, A. C., Suhrheinrich, J., Reed, S., & Schreibman, L. (2012). What works for you? Using teacher feedback to inform adaptations of pivotal response training for classroom use. *Autism Research and Treatment, 11*(18), 1–11.

Suhrheinrich, J., Rieth, S. R., Dickson, K. S., Roesch, S., & Stahmer, A. C. (2020). Classroom pivotal response teaching: Teacher training outcomes of a community efficacy trial. *Teacher Education and Special Education, 43*(3), 215–234. doi: 10.1177/0888406419850876

Suhrheinrich, J., Wang, T., Chan, J., Holt, T., Stahmer, A. C., Rieth, S. R., Roesch, S., & Sam, A. (2022). Developing an empirically-based adaptation an training model for intervention scale up of classroom pivotal response teaching: A protocol paper. *International Journal of Educational Research Open, 3*, 100107.

Symon, J. B. (2005). Expanding interventions for children with autism: Parents as trainers. *Journal of Positive Behavior Interventions, 7*(3), 159–173.

Tiede, G., & Walton, K. M. (2019). Meta-analysis of naturalistic developmental behavioral interventions for young children with autism spectrum disorder. *Autism, 23*(8), 2080–2095. doi: 10.1177/1362361319836371

Uljarević, M., Billingham, W., Cooper, M. N., Condron, P., & Hardan, A. Y. (2022). Examining effectiveness and predictors of treatment response of pivotal response treatment in autism: An umbrella review and a meta-analysis. *Frontiers in Psychiatry, 12*, 766150. https://doi.org/10.3389/fpsyt.2021.766150.

Venkataraman, A., Yang, D. Y. J., Dvornek, N., Staib, L. H., Duncan, J. S., Pelphrey, K. A., & Ventola, P. (2016). Pivotal response treatment prompts a functional rewiring of the brain amongst individuals with autism spectrum disorder. *Neuroreport, 27*(14), 1081–1085.

Ventola, P. E., Yang, D., Abdullahi, S. M., Paisley, C. A., Braconnier, M. L., & Sukhodolsky, D.G. (2016). Brief report: Reduced restricted and repetitive behaviors after pivotal response treatment. *Journal of Autism and Developmental Disorders, 46*, 2813–2820. https://doi.org/10.1007/s10803-016-2813-6

Vernon, T. W., Holden, A. N., Barrett, A. C., Bradshaw, J., Ko, J. A., McGarry, E. S., Horowitz, E. J., Tagavi, D. M., & German, T. C. (2019). A pilot randomized clinical trial of an enhanced pivotal response treatment approach for young children with autism: The PRISM model. *Journal of Autism and Developmental Disorders, 49*(6), 2358–2373.

Verschuur, R., Didden, R., Lang, R., Sigafoos, J., & Huskens, B. (2014). Pivotal response treatment for children with autism spectrum disorders: A systematic review. *Review Journal of Autism and Developmental Disorders, 1*(1), 34–61.

Verschuur, R., Huskens, B., Verhoeven, L., & Didden, R. (2017). Increasing opportunities for question asking in school-aged children with autism spectrum disorder: Effectiveness of staff training in pivotal response treatment. *Journal of Autism Developmental Disorders, 47*(2), 490–505. https://doi.org/10.1007/s10803-016-2966-3

Vismara, L. A., & Lyons, G. L. (2007). Using perseverative interests to elicit joint attention behaviors in young children with autism: Theoretical and clinical implications for understanding motivation. *Journal of Positive Behavior Interventions, 9*(4), 214–228.

Vogler, J. C. (2017). Increasing self-initiated question asking with adults with autism using pivotal response training strategies and constant time delay. [Master's thesis]. University of California Santa Barbara. https://uknowledge.uky.edu/edsrc_etds/52/

Voos, A. C., Pelphrey, K. A., Tirrell, J., Bolling, D. Z., Vander Wyk, B., Kaiser, M. D., McPartland, J. C., Volkmar, F. R., & Ventola, P. (2013). Neural mechanisms of improvements in social motivation after pivotal response treatment: Two case studies. *Journal of Autism and Developmental Disorders, 43*(1), 1–10. https://doi.org/10.1007/s10803-012-1683-9

Williams, J. A., Koegel, R. L., & Egel, A. L. (1981). Response-reinforcer relationships and improved learning in autistic children. *Journal of Applied Behavior Analysis, 14*(1), 53–60.

Wong, C., Odom, S. L., Hume, K. A., Cox, A. W., Fettig, A., Kucharczyk, S., Brock, M. E., Plavnick, J. B., Fleury, V. P. & Schultz, T. R. (2015). Evidence-based practices for children, youth, and young adults with autism spectrum disorder: A comprehensive review. *Journal of Autism and Developmental Disorders, 45*(7), 1951–1966.

16

Naturalistic Developmental Behavioral Interventions

Kyle M. Frost
University of Massachusetts Chan Medical School

Diondra Straiton
Michigan State University

Sarah R. Edmunds
University of South Carolina

Melissa Maye
Henry Ford Health, Center for Health Policy and Health Services Research; Michigan State University, College of Human Medicine, Pediatrics and Human Development

Katherine Pickard
Emory University School of Medicine

16.1 Technical Abstract

Background: Naturalistic developmental behavioral interventions (NDBIs) are a class of early interventions for young autistic children that blend principles from applied behavior analysis and developmental science. NDBIs involve teaching clinically meaningful skills in the context of motivating, reciprocal, child-led interactions using incidental and natural opportunities for child learning. **Method:** In this chapter, we summarize information from multiple systematic reviews, including clinical practice guidelines and meta-analyses, to describe the empirical support for NDBIs. This material was supplemented with focused literature searches to summarize what is known about how and by whom NDBIs are implemented in the community. **Results:** Multiple meta-analyses suggest that NDBIs yield statistically significant, positive treatment effects for improving children's social communication skills. Implementation-focused literature suggests that NDBIs can be implemented in a variety of formats, delivery modalities, and intensities, and by providers from a variety of training backgrounds. **Discussion:** NDBIs have been studied in many randomized controlled trials; however, outcome measures involving caregiver report represent a source of bias in the research literature. Relatively little is known about the long-term effects and cost-effectiveness of NDBIs, and more research is needed on social validity, particularly

Kyle M. Frost et al., *Naturalistic Developmental Behavioral Interventions*. In: *Lifespan Treatment for Autistic Individuals*. Edited by: Peter Sturmey, Russell Lang, and James K. Luiselli, Oxford University Press. © Oxford University Press (2025).
DOI: 10.1093/oso/9780197635841.003.0016

from the perspective of autistic people. **Practitioner recommendations:** The literature suggests that young autistic children with social communication delays may benefit from NDBIs, and that parents can learn to implement NDBI techniques at home with the support of a skilled practitioner.

16.2 Layperson Summary

NDBIs are a class of early interventions for young autistic children that blend principles from applied behavior analysis and developmental science. NDBIs focus on teaching functional social communication skills (e.g., vocalization, gestures, turn taking, imitation, and play) in the context of fun, child-led activities and daily routines. By embedding opportunities for learning within highly engaging and motivating social interactions, NDBIs seek to maximize opportunities to naturally reward and support emerging social communication skills. NDBIs can be implemented by providers with a variety of training backgrounds, such as psychology, behavior analysis, speech-language pathology, and early childhood education. Parents can also successfully learn and implement NDBIs at home with the help of a trained clinician.

Experimental studies suggest that NDBIs can support children's social communication growth, even when delivered at a relatively low intensity. NDBIs can also be implemented in different ways, including parent coaching models delivered by telehealth, or classroom-based group models, but they have most often been studied in 1:1 interaction. Several programs under the NDBI umbrella are considered evidence-based by the National Clearinghouse on Autism Evidence and Practice. NDBIs are not known to have negative side effects but are not necessarily indicated for children with high-priority goals outside of social communication (e.g., feeding concerns or self-injurious behaviors). Relatively little is known about the long-term effects and cost-effectiveness of NDBIs, and more research is needed on how community members feel about them, particularly from the perspective of autistic people.

16.3 Treatment Summary Table

Treatment summary: Naturalistic Developmental Behavioral Intervention

Treatment description: NDBIs focus on teaching functional social communication skills (e.g., vocalization, gestures, turn taking, imitation, and play) in the context of fun and affectively rich child-led activities and daily routines. By embedding opportunities for learning within highly engaging and motivating social interactions, NDBIs seek to maximize opportunities to naturally reinforce emerging social communication skills.

Expected outcomes: NDBIs have been found to support the development of a variety of social communication skills in early childhood, including social engagement, imitation, play, joint attention, gestures, expressive communication, and receptive communication.

Methods: Adults implementing NDBIs support child motivation and engagement in joint activities by following the child's lead in an affectively rich, playful interaction. Within a joint activity, the adult facilitates natural and incidental learning opportunities through modeling, creating situations likely to elicit communication, and responding to all child attempts to communicate. When appropriate, the adult uses behavioral principles to teach the child a new skill using clear, scaffolded prompts and natural reinforcement (e.g., praise, return to child-led play).

Expertise required to implement treatment: Practitioners from a variety of training backgrounds, including behavior analysis, early childhood education, speech-language pathology, and psychology, can learn to implement NDBIs. In addition, caregivers or other nonspecialists can learn to implement NDBIs with support from a clinician, as many NDBIs are implemented using caregiver-mediated approaches.

Risks and negative side effects: NDBIs are not known to have negative side effects but are not necessarily indicated for children with high-priority service needs outside of social communication.

Additional considerations and limitations: While NDBIs have research support, little is known about their long-term outcomes, cost-effectiveness, and the optimal dose for supporting social communication for children at different ages and developmental levels.

16.4 Introduction

16.4.1 Treatment Description

NDBIs are a class of evidence-based early interventions for young autistic children that blend principles from applied behavior analysis and developmental science. The umbrella term *NDBI* was coined in a seminal publication by Schreibman and colleagues to describe a variety of empirically supported interventions with common features and shared theoretical origins (Schreibman et al., 2015). Though specific NDBI models have distinct procedures and technical differences in their implementation, they all share several common features, including similar goals and objectives, a common theoretical basis and rationale, and overlapping instructional strategies or intervention elements (Bruinsma et al., 2020; Frost et al., 2020; Schreibman et al., 2015). Manualized NDBI interventions include the Early Start Denver model (ESDM; Rogers & Dawson, 2010), enhanced milieu teaching (EMT; Kaiser et al., 2000; Kaiser & Hester, 1994), joint attention, symbolic play, engagement, and regulation (JASPER; Kasari et al., 2021), pivotal response treatment (PRT; Schreibman & Koegel, 2005), Project ImPACT (Ingersoll & Dvortcsak, 2019), social ABCs (Brian et al., 2016, 2017), and others (Bruinsma et al., 2020; Frost et al., 2020; Schreibman et al., 2015) In this chapter, rather than describing one or more treatment packages in detail, we emphasize shared features and common elements of NDBIs and their evidence base to provide a broader description of this class of early interventions.

While individual NDBI models vary in the specific combination of instructional strategies they recommend, there are numerous common treatment elements which are recommended across many NDBIs. These common elements were identified systematically using input from NDBI experts to support the development of an observational rating tool called the *NDBI-Fi*, which measures implementation of common NDBI treatment elements (Table 16.1; Frost et al., 2020). In all NDBIs, intervention techniques are recommended to support children's motivation and engagement in a joint activity with their interaction partner; these include such techniques as sitting in front of and at a similar level to the child (e.g., on the floor or at a child-size table), allowing the child choice in what activity to engage in and how to play (e.g., choosing a toy or activity or picking out a snack), and using positive affect and playful animation (e.g., excited tone of voice, exaggerated gestures). In addition, NDBIs recommend facilitating natural and incidental opportunities for child learning through modeling communication (i.e., describing or narrating the activity), responding meaningfully to the child's communications and actions, and creating or seizing natural opportunities for the child to communicate (e.g., pausing during a tickle game, handing the child a sealed bag of chips that they cannot open on their own). Last, NDBIs use behavioral principles to teach new skills, by using prompting and natural reinforcement tailored to the activity and the child's goals and interests. These teaching episodes are naturally embedded and distributed across a child-led interaction, rather than implemented rapidly in succession during a highly structured interaction.

In addition to sharing several common treatment elements, NDBIs share a variety of other common features (Bruinsma et al., 2020; Schreibman et al., 2015). For example, NDBIs share a basic rationale and objectives consistent with their theoretical origins (see section 16.4.2). They target early social communication skills, and thus tend to be most appropriate for young children (e.g., <7 years old) with social communication delays. NDBIs have clearly specified procedures (e.g., treatment manual) as well as protocols for evaluating practitioner adherence to those procedures (i.e., measurement of treatment fidelity). NDBIs involve setting individualized goals which are subsequently monitored over the course of intervention, with goals often centered on child social communication, broadly construed (see section 16.4.2). Lastly, intervention takes place during daily routines and in play (Schreibman et al., 2015), as learning is thought to be enriched in natural, socially meaningful contexts (Dunst et al., 2001). Consistent with this approach, NDBIs are frequently implemented as caregiver-mediated interventions, in which caregivers are coached by a trained clinician to implement NDBI at home.

Table 16.1 Common treatment elements of NDBIs as identified in the NDBI-Fi

NDBI-Fi Items	Brief Description	Rationale and Target Outcomes
1. Face-to-face and on the child's level	Child and adult are positioned on a similar level and facing each other	Supporting child motivation and social engagement in joint activities
2. Following the child's lead	Child and adult are both active participants in child-chosen activity	
3. Positive affect and animation	Adult uses positive affect; adult matches affect to child's sensory needs	
4. Modeling appropriate language	Adult adjusts language to the child's developmental level	Facilitating natural and incidental learning opportunities to build communication skills
5. Responding to attempts to communicate	Adult verbally responds to child's communication behaviors by repeating, clarifying, or expanding	
6. Using communicative temptations	Adult creates situations to elicit communication from the child followed by a brief period of expectant waiting	
7. Frequency of direct teaching episodes	Adult directs the child to demonstrate new or emerging skills regularly throughout the interaction	Using behavioral principles to teach developmentally appropriate skills
8. Quality of direct teaching episodes	Adult uses high-quality teaching strategies (e.g., clear instructions, when child is motivated, contingent and natural reinforcement)	

NDBI = naturalistic developmental behavioral intervention.
Source: Table reproduced in part from Frost et al. (2020).

16.4.2 Rationale and Objectives

Starting in the 1970s, intervention programs and strategies based in principles of behavioral learning and operant conditioning began to show evidence for increasing the language, adaptive, and cognitive skills of autistic youth (Lovaas, 1987; Schreibman & Carr, 1978; Strain et al., 1979). These early programs, many based in discrete trial training (DTT) or verbal behavior (Lovaas, 1987; Skinner, 1957), were designed to be delivered at high intensity within an adult-directed interaction. In approaches such as DTT, skills were often broken down into component parts and taught in structured, controlled settings (e.g., at a table in a quiet room), using consistent prompting and highly motivating (often primary) reinforcement (Smith, 2001). After a skill was chained together and mastered in these structured and controlled settings, it was then taught in other contexts to promote generalization. Although research has demonstrated that behavioral approaches can support child learning, there was also concern that skills learned through these approaches were not consistently generalized to different settings or more naturalistic interactions (Smith, 2001).

The burgeoning of developmental theory and science emerged in parallel with the behavioral intervention boom. Developmental science was grounded in understanding typical and atypical developmental trajectories. This research helped to inform strategies that could be used to support key differences seen in autistic children's development, including delays or differences in social reciprocity, engagement, and imitation (Dawson & Adams, 1984; Mundy et al., 1990; Rogers & Pennington, 1991). Developmental theory emphasizes that children learn best when they are actively engaged in experiences that are developmentally appropriate, meaningful to the child, and affectively rich (Cicchetti, 1989). A central component of developmental theory is the identification of developmentally appropriate goals and activities for the child, targeting skills that develop next in a typical developmental sequence (Lifter et al., 1993). Such skills are considered within a child's "zone of proximal development" and provide a foundation for the acquisition of subsequent skills. NDBIs also embody developmental theory in their emphasis on teaching within child-led and child-initiated activities. This emphasis allows adults to support a child's social engagement in order to naturally reinforce a variety of developmentally appropriate skills (Prizant et al., 2003).

Although behavioral and developmental strategies were rooted in distinct theories, early research demonstrated that these strategies could be integrated, resulting in interventions that could better impact the generalization of skills in young autistic children (R. L. Koegel et al., 1987; McGee et al., 1985). These NDBI intervention models continued to use principles of learning theory, but supplemented behavioral principles with developmentally informed intervention targets, embedding intervention within naturalistic settings (e.g., play, daily routines), including parents and other family members, emphasizing child-led activities, and focusing on naturally occurring motivation to support new skill development.

More recently, autistic self-advocates as well as autistic and nonautistic researchers have begun to consider whether NDBIs are compatible with the neurodiversity movement, a social justice and civil rights movement which emerged in the 1990s. The neurodiversity movement emphasizes that atypical neurodevelopment should be respected and valued as natural variation in the human experience, much like biodiversity is valued and considered essential for healthy ecosystems (Blume, 1998; Schuck et al., 2021; Singer, 2017). The neurodiversity and autistic self-advocacy movements value the "autistic way of being" and emphasize personal strengths, self-determination, and improving quality of life for neurodivergent individuals (Schuck et al., 2021; Sinclair, 1993). While the neurodiversity movement did not explicitly inform the development of NDBIs, some have argued that aspects of NDBIs align with central tenets of the neurodiversity movement (Schuck et al., 2021). For example, NDBIs focus on improving quality of life by supporting the development of functional and adaptive skills to help children to thrive in their environment, emphasizing social communication development. In addition, NDBIs rely heavily on child motivation, incorporate shared control between the child and interventionist, and require interventionists to respond to *all* communicative attempts as meaningful (Schuck et al., 2021). However, many autistic advocates have argued that any intervention with ties to ABA, NDBIs included, are fundamentally inconsistent with principles of neurodiversity. Overall, the consideration of neurodiversity concepts within early intervention has been limited thus far (Leadbitter et al., 2021), and it is unclear whether NDBIs as a whole are consistent with neurodiversity principles; this is an area ripe for increased attention in the field.

Common goals targeted by NDBIs focus on social communication and related domains, such as social engagement, joint attention, receptive and expressive communication (including verbal and nonverbal communication), imitation, and play skills. Improving social communication is thought to be functional and meaningful for children, and is thus a high-priority treatment goal for autistic people and their families (Roche et al., 2021; Rodger et al., 2004). Moreover, social communication skills are thought to be "pivotal" skills that have a cascading effect on the child's global development (i.e., by providing the child with foundational skills to optimally learn from their social environment; Gengoux et al., 2020; L. K. Koegel et al., 2016). While all NDBIs target social communication skills, some NDBI models are more comprehensive in their focus, targeting an array of developmental outcomes such as communication skills, adaptive behavior, and motor skills (e.g., ESDM), while others target more focused developmental outcomes such as joint attention, play, and social engagement (e.g., JASPER). Regardless of the type of goal, NDBI practitioners structure all goals to follow a developmental sequence by teaching skills that are slightly above a child's current skill level. This approach requires the interventionist to adjust targets over time as the child masters new skills (R. L. Koegel et al., 2001; Masten & Cicchetti, 2010; Schreibman et al., 2020). In NDBIs, new skills are taught in the context of activities tailored to a child's interests in order to support their engagement and motivation to engage with a social interaction partner. After a child attempts a new skill, social behavior (e.g., praise, positive affect) is paired with natural reinforcement embedded within the activity (e.g., access to a preferred item, completion of an exciting play action). Learning skills with a social partner within playful activities is thought to help children learn that social interaction can be fun and can occur on the child's own terms.

NDBIs promote skill generalization by targeting skills across multiple domains concurrently within the same interaction. For example, an NDBI interventionist might simultaneously target turn taking, requesting, initiating social interaction, and fine motor skills in one teaching session. As these skills naturally occur together in real-world situations, this method of direct teaching is thought to support generalization across different daily routines or play activities. This approach is called a "developmental systems approach" (Griffiths & Tabery, 2013) and stands in contrast with more highly structured interventions that focus on discrete skill development in each domain separately (Schreibman et al., 2020).

16.4.3 Mechanisms of Action

While behavioral and developmental theory contribute to our understanding of how and why NDBIs might improve children's social communication, empirical evidence for the purported mechanisms of action for NDBIs is—as of yet—thin. NDBIs are thought to work by increasing children's everyday access to enriched, supported social interactions in a naturalistic setting. Recent research on parent-mediated NDBIs supports this hypothesis. For example, Yoder and colleagues (2021b) found that Project ImPACT improved social communication and language for toddlers at high likelihood of autism *only* as mediated by the extent to which parents used Project ImPACT strategies as intended (i.e., treatment fidelity).

NDBI efficacy has been found to be mediated both by increased adult responsiveness and by growth in children's pivotal skills. First, NDBIs teach interventionists to be more responsive to *all* child communication acts, including less developmentally advanced attempts (e.g., gaze, vocalizations, gestures). This may increase the amount of feedback and reinforcement children receive for communicating and therefore increase children's motivation to continue (Edmunds et al., 2019; Warlaumont et al., 2014). Indeed, increased parental "synchrony" and "mirrored pacing" have been found to mediate treatment effects on child social communication (Aldred et al., 2012; A. C. Gulsrud et al., 2016; Pickles et al., 2015). Second, NDBIs may be a particularly effective early intervention approach because many of them are designed to target "pivotal" skills that facilitate a developmental cascade of skill progression in multiple domains across the first 3 to 5 years of life (e.g., Green et al., 2017). For example, early intervention has been found to be effective at improving child social communication 6 months to 3 years after intervention ends, as mediated by children's pivotal skill growth in imitation, intentional communication (Yoder et al., 2021a), and initiation attempts (Pickles et al., 2015). In addition, recent work demonstrates how supporting social engagement and social communication broadly may provide children with the necessary skills to benefit from adult language input (Clark-Whitney et al., 2022).

16.4.4 Considerations for Implementation

NDBIs are intended to be implemented in a variety of clinical settings and by providers with numerous disciplinary backgrounds, making them particularly well suited for implementation across diverse practice settings. Providers associated with the delivery of NDBIs often include speech language pathologists, psychologists, behavioral clinicians (e.g., Board-Certified Behavior Analysts), occupational therapists, and special educators. While NDBIs were primarily developed within university-affiliated clinics, many research teams have shifted to examining the effectiveness of NDBIs when delivered within diverse service systems, including early intervention systems, school systems, and outpatient clinical settings.

NDBIs have been implemented in the Part C early intervention (EI) system, which provides therapeutic services to children 0–3 years with developmental delays under Part C of the Individuals with Disabilities Education Act. Upward of 10% of children served in EI systems have an increased likelihood of being autistic (Eisenhower et al., 2021). Thus, the EI system is viewed as an entry point to services during a critical window of early development, particularly for children who do not yet have a medical diagnosis of autism spectrum disorder (Maenner et al., 2021). Further, EI systems use a family-centered model (Adams et al., 2013; Tomasello et al., 2010) and are well suited for the implementation of parent-mediated intervention (Pellecchia et al., 2022), including parent-mediated NDBIs. Research suggests that EI providers significantly improve their fidelity to parent coaching in NDBIs when they receive training and ongoing consultation (Rogers et al., 2022; Stahmer et al., 2019). Such training can increase reach, with 6 times the number of children receiving NDBIs 4 years following implementation efforts (Rieth et al., 2022).

Autistic children increasingly receive services from practitioners of applied behavior analysis (ABA), particularly following the expansion of insurance mandates and Medicaid waivers for ABA services (Barry et al., 2017; Kornack et al., 2014). Given that aspects of NDBI are consistent with behavioral principles (e.g., prompting, reinforcement), ABA practitioners may choose to implement NDBIs when working with young autistic children on social communication goals. However, it is important for ABA clinicians to understand that NDBIs are not synonymous with embedded discrete trials in the natural environment (i.e., natural environment teaching; D'Agostino et al., in press). As such, dissemination and training efforts to support ABA clinicians in learning NDBIs must emphasize key principles in developmental psychology such as social learning theory and social constructivism (D'Agostino et al., in press).

Speech-language pathologists (SLPs) focus much of their practice on social communication goals; thus, NDBIs are often highly consistent with SLP services for young children (Rieth et al., 2018). Indeed, some NDBI approaches were co-developed by SLPs (e.g., Project ImPACT; Ingersoll & Dvortcsak, 2019; SCERTS; Prizant et al., 2003). SLPs tend to have foundational training in developmental science and relative strengths in providing developmentally appropriate expansions on children's subtle communication behaviors (Rieth et al., 2018).

NDBIs have also been adapted for group settings in childcare centers and preschools. Given the overlap between NDBI and quality early childhood teaching principles, childcare classrooms and preschools may serve as natural contexts to implement NDBIs in community settings, thus boosting access to total intervention hours for many families (Maye et al., 2020). This is supported by preliminary research suggesting that early childhood education providers are able to provide NDBI interventions with fidelity (Tupou et al., 2019). However, most research has examined NDBIs in 1:1 delivery context, and more research is needed to understand how components of NDBIs may or may not fit in inclusive educational settings (see section 16.5.6).

We hope we have demonstrated that NDBI can be implemented by practitioners from diverse training backgrounds and clinical settings. It is also important to acknowledge that although many NDBIs are packaged and intended to be delivered in a manualized format, providers may be familiar with and use NDBI strategies to some extent in the absence of formal training. Recent research conducted with early intervention providers (Pickard et al., 2021) and ABA providers (Hampton & Sandbank, 2021) demonstrates that practitioners self-report use of select NDBI techniques consistent with their disciplinary background, although it is unclear the extent to which developmental and behavioral techniques are truly integrated. Approaches to NDBI training and dissemination may benefit from tailoring to capitalize on clinicians' strengths and areas of expertise while helping them to meaningfully incorporate additional intervention techniques and theory into their practice.

16.5 Research Background

A relatively large and growing body of literature has examined the efficacy of a variety of manualized NDBIs. Here, we summarize what is known about the efficacy and effectiveness of NDBIs, emphasizing results from the latest evidence-based practice guidelines, systematic reviews, and meta-analyses where applicable. Following this summary, we describe the quality of the research literature surrounding this class of interventions, identifying key limitations and unanswered questions in the field.

16.5.1 Primary Outcomes

The National Clearinghouse on Autism Evidence and Practice denoted a variety of "focused intervention practices" as evidence-based for young children, according to a systematic review of research literature (Hume et al., 2021; Steinbrenner et al., 2020). These practices, found to improve children's communication, joint attention, and play, include several common elements of NDBIs, such as naturalistic intervention, modeling, antecedent-based intervention, prompting, and reinforcement. Moreover, several manualized NDBIs were also characterized as evidence-based in this review, including JASPER (Kasari et al., 2006, 2021), Project ImPACT (Ingersoll & Dvortcsak, 2019), milieu teaching (Kaiser et al., 2000), and pivotal response training (Schreibman & Koegel, 2005).

Recent meta-analyses have also examined summary effects of NDBIs by aggregating across studies. A meta-analysis of 27 group design studies comparing NDBIs to inactive control groups found several significant, positive effects of NDBIs on child outcomes (Tiede & Walton, 2019). Statistically significant, moderate effect sizes were found for social engagement and cognitive development, and small but significant effects were found for expressive communication, autism symptomatology, and play. Researchers found marginal effects on joint attention and receptive language, and nonsignificant effects for adaptive behavior.

Sandbank and colleagues conducted a broader meta-analysis on group design studies of early interventions for autism, including 26 studies of NDBIs (Sandbank et al., 2020). Aggregating results across randomized controlled trials (RCTs), the researchers found significant effects of NDBIs on social communication, language, and play outcomes. When excluding caregiver-reported outcomes, which are susceptible to bias due to caregivers' knowledge of study group assignment, social communication and play outcomes remained significant. However, no studies of any early intervention type, NDBI or otherwise, showed significant effects when excluding all outcomes subject to detection bias (i.e., any assessment involving an individual aware of intervention allocation; Sandbank et al., 2020), suggesting need for improvement in the quality of the early intervention literature.

16.5.2 Long-Term Effects

Although a growing body of evidence suggests that NDBIs may have positive effects on children's social communication development, most studies only examine a short-term follow-up period. As such, less is known about the long-term impacts of NDBIs or whether they affect more generalized life outcomes for children who receive them. One long-term study of ESDM found that children who received two years of intensive ESDM maintained treatment gains relative to a community intervention control group in a variety of domains when evaluated two years later, despite receiving fewer hours of intervention during the follow up period (Estes et al., 2015). This supports the idea that NDBIs can have long-term impacts. However, this study examined more intensive service delivery than many other studies of NDBIs, and findings must be replicated before we can draw strong conclusions about the long-term durability of treatment effects.

16.5.3 Social Validity

The social validity of an intervention is multifaceted and includes: whether or not the intervention outcome is viewed as important and clinically meaningful, whether or not it is time- and cost-effective, whether the procedures are acceptable and satisfactory, and whether the intervention occurs in a "natural" (i.e., typical) context (Reichow et al., 2011). Literature on the social validity of packaged NDBIs is still emerging (Callahan et al., 2017; D'Agostino et al., 2019). NDBIs appear to have high levels of social validity according to providers (D'Agostino et al., 2020). However, NDBI efficacy studies do not always include measures of social validity, and often focus on select aspects of social validity (e.g., clinically meaningful improvement; D'Agostino et al., 2020). With regard to parent-perceived social validity, caregivers view the outcomes and efficacy of NDBIs positively, but they may have concerns about its time-effectiveness, feasibility, and their own self-efficacy (Gevarter et al., 2022; Jurek et al., 2022). Future research on the social validity of NDBIs should consider multiple aspects of social validity and take care to include a greater variety of stakeholders, especially autistic people.

NDBIs can be implemented by clinicians and caregivers alike. They can also be delivered in one-on-one contexts or in group settings—and can be delivered in person and via telehealth.

16.5.4 Parent-Mediated Intervention

While NDBIs are often delivered by clinicians directly with children, NDBIs increasingly emphasize parent-mediated intervention, in which caregivers are taught intervention strategies to support their child's learning across home and community activities. Some NDBIs have been developed as standalone parent-mediated treatment models (e.g., Project ImPACT, Social ABCs), while others incorporate parent coaching to supplement to interventionist-delivered intervention (Dawson et al., 2010). Most parent-mediated NDBIs use coaching models grounded in adult learning theory, which points to specific strategies for motivating and teaching adult learners (Dunst et al., 2010; Rush & Shelden, 2011). Parent-mediated NDBIs capitalize on the role of caregivers in social communication development with the goal of building reciprocal interactions between caregivers and their children that foster social engagement and naturalistic learning opportunities. Despite having a lower intensity, parent-mediated intervention models assume that family's practice NDBI strategies across meaningful daily routines outside of direct therapy sessions. Thus, parent learning and practice of NDBIs are meant to increase the amount of intervention time that children receive (Casagrande & Ingersoll, 2017).

Recent research examining the outcomes of parent-mediated NDBIs has shown that caregivers are just as effective at implementing NDBI strategies as clinicians (Crank et al., 2021) and that parent-mediated NDBIs result in gains in both proximal and distal child social communication skills (Brian et al., 2022; Nevill et al., 2018; Yoder et al., 2021a). Additionally, caregiver participation in parent-mediated NDBIs has been associated with increased capacity for self-reflection and increased report of empowerment and self-efficacy among parents who participate (Pickard et al., 2016; Siller et al., 2018).

16.5.5 Telehealth Delivery

Telehealth delivery of NDBIs has become more common, with empirical studies across a variety of parent-mediated NDBI models showing improvement in parent fidelity and child social communication outcomes, including reciprocal imitation training (Wainer et al., 2021), Project ImPACT (Ingersoll et al., 2016; Ingersoll & Berger, 2015; Sengupta et al., 2020), pivotal response treatment (McGarry et al., 2020), JASPER (Shire et al., 2021), and ESDM (Vismara et al., 2018). Training interventionists via telehealth to achieve fidelity on NDBI models has also become quite common and has clear benefits for increasing accessibility to training (D'Agostino et al., 2020; Neely et al., 2020; Rogers et al., 2022).

16.5.6 Group Delivery

Most research to date has focused on NDBIs in individual contexts, with limited research evaluating group contexts. Studies of parent-mediated PRT suggest that parents can learn NDBI strategies from group sessions with other parents and that child outcomes are favorable even when parents are taught in the group format (Hardan et al., 2015; Minjarez et al., 2011). There is a small body of literature on interventionist-delivered NDBI with groups of children; thus far, studies suggest that improvements in child outcomes are favorable for NDBIs delivered in various small-group early intervention and educational settings (Akshoomoff et al., 2010; Chang et al., 2016; Eapen et al., 2013; A. Gulsrud et al., 2019; Morgan et al., 2018; Stahmer & Ingersoll, 2004; Wong, 2013). To date, NDBI classroom adaptations have generally combined group intervention sessions with individual 1:1 sessions throughout the day (Chang et al., 2016; Engelstad et al., 2020; Sinai-Gavrilov et al., 2020; Vivanti, Paynter, et al., 2014).

Historically, sustainment of NDBI interventions within these settings has largely been limited to duration of grant funding. More recently, researchers have explored barriers to implementation of specific interventions (Wilson & Landa, 2019) and identified barriers to implementation ahead of adaptation to promote sustainability and penetration into the classroom environment (Maye et al., 2020, 2022). Indeed, a classroom adaptation of JASPER was found to be sustainable following removal of grant support in a preschool environment (Shire et al., 2019), suggesting this is a promising direction for future implementation.

16.5.7 Cost-Effectiveness

Few studies have evaluated the relative cost-effectiveness of NDBIs compared to community care as usual. Cidav and colleagues (2017) examined cost in a research trial of ESDM, which included two years of intensive, interventionist-delivered

ESDM supplemented by parent training (Dawson et al., 2010; Estes et al., 2015). Although children who received ESDM had $14,000 higher annual health-related costs than children receiving community care during the intervention period, they used fewer services during the 2-year follow-up period (–$19,000 compared to the control group), representing a full offset of the costs associated with early, intensive ESDM (Cidav et al., 2017).

Low-intensity parent-mediated NDBIs are thought to be cost-effective because they require fewer service hours with a trained clinician (Oono et al., 2013); however, parent-mediated interventions may come at a cost to parents' own time and productivity due to time spent participating in services (Tsiplova et al., 2022). Better understanding the cost of provider training and service delivery of NDBIs relative to usual care is a vital next step when considering whether NDBIs are "shelf-ready" for implementation at scale.

16.5.8 Recommended Dose and Intensity

Historically, the consensus for dosage of behavioral interventions for autistic children has been "more is better." In practice, however, client receipt of NDBI ranges from quite low (e.g., time-limited, parent mediated intervention) to very high (e.g., 30+ hours per week). Some research suggests that more hours of behavioral intervention are indeed predictive of greater treatment gains (e.g., Linstead et al., 2017). However, recent meta-analyses suggest that the total dose of NDBI does not significantly moderate most treatment outcomes (Crank et al., 2021; Tiede & Walton, 2019). Such findings are consistent with a recent randomized trial which directly compared lower- and higher-dose NDBI and behavioral intervention (Rogers et al., 2021), finding that dose did not predict primary outcomes. Yet analysis of the same data found that dose did predict spontaneous communication growth only for children with fewer autism characteristics (Yoder et al., 2020). A limiting factor is that this study compared two relatively high-intensity interventions (15 vs. 25 hours per week); as such, it is not clear whether results would hold with a greater range of treatment intensity. Moreover, the question of dose is particularly complicated in the case of parent-mediated interventions (or those with a parent-mediated component, as was the case in Rogers et al., 2021), in which caregivers implement interventions to a variable degree with regard to both quality and amount. Indeed, caregivers are meant to embed NDBI strategies throughout daily routines, making the idea of "dose" difficult to conceptualize and measure.

Taken together, these meta-analytic and experimental findings challenge conventional clinical wisdom, suggesting that more intensive intervention is necessarily most effective but warrants further investigation. Given limited evidence for an ideal dose/intensity, we agree with others who have argued that recommendations should be individualized to children and families' needs and reevaluated regularly based on child progress, with attention to families' priorities, financial/time resources, and children's developmental level and opportunities for leisure and socialization (Pellecchia et al., 2019; Sandbank, Bottema-Beutel, et al., 2021). Indeed, it seems unlikely that there is an optimal dose, and rather that different children and families present with unique needs.

16.5.9 Rigor and Quality in NDBI Research

Research across NDBIs is characterized by substantial heterogeneity, which complicates our understanding of the magnitude and timing of treatment effects. This includes wide heterogeneity in treatment dose, with one meta-analysis examining studies ranging from 9 to 1,581 professional contact hours (Tiede & Walton, 2019), as well as variation in treatment setting (e.g., home, school, clinic), child characteristics, outcome measures, and who implements the intervention (e.g., parent/caregiver, research staff, teacher). Systematic reviews of specific manualized NDBIs, including ESDM (Waddington et al., 2016) JASPER (Waddington et al., 2021), PRT (Ona et al., 2020), and SCERTS (Yi et al., 2022), also described substantial variation in study characteristics, suggesting that there are considerable differences in how NDBIs are implemented even within the same model. Despite this heterogeneity, a recent meta-analysis of NDBIs found that effect sizes did not vary systematically based on children's chronological age, sex, or language ability, treatment dose (i.e., hours), or implementer type (i.e., clinician, educator, caregiver, combination; Crank et al., 2021).

Compared to other early interventions for autism, the quality of the empirical support for NDBIs is relatively high (Sandbank et al., 2020), with NDBIs often being studied using an RCT design. Compared to studies of other types of early intervention for autism, NDBI studies relied less often on potentially biased reports from parents and teachers to describe child outcomes, relying more on assessors who are naïve to group assignment. NDBIs have also frequently been studied in community settings and/or with the intervention delivery from nonexperts (e.g., caregivers); these effectiveness trials contribute to our understanding of how these interventions may perform in the settings in which children receive routine care (Tiede & Walton, 2019).

However, in the context of NDBI research, child outcomes are frequently measured in the context of naturalistic interactions with caregivers (Sandbank et al., 2020). While this is consistent with the purpose and aims of NDBIs, given their emphasis on the natural environment and involving caregivers in their child's intervention, this represents a potentially significant source of bias in measurement of treatment outcomes, particularly when parents have been involved in the intervention (Sandbank et al., 2020). Indeed, meta-analytic work found that treatment effects for social engagement were significantly larger when measured in interactions with someone involved in the intervention than with an unfamiliar play partner (Tiede & Walton, 2019), suggesting that some of the observed change in child outcomes can be accounted for by the adult play partner's behavior. While this lends support for the hypothesized mechanisms of NDBI, this is a substantial limitation in our understanding of how NDBIs may impact child outcomes outside of the contexts and targets of intervention (Sandbank, Chow, et al., 2021).

16.5.10 Research Summary

NDBIs result in gains in child social communication skills, broadly construed, and these gains exist for various children, across contexts and modalities. However, the research is not without limitations. While we see evidence of gains in child social communication, whether these gains are maintained long term or result in broader downstream benefits (e.g., educational outcomes, quality of life) is not yet known. Furthermore, many studies use outcome measures that involve caregiver or teacher report, which introduces a source of bias in outcome measurement. While NDBI strategies have a clear theoretical rationale, limited empirical work has confirmed their active ingredients and mechanisms of change.

16.6 Practice Implications

16.6.1 Treatment Outcomes

NDBIs are appropriate for young children whose families have identified developmental concerns regarding social communication as important goals for their child. NDBIs have been demonstrated to increase language skills, cognitive skills, and in some cases, even a reduction in autism-related challenges (Bruinsma et al., 2020). While a growing evidence base supports the use of NDBIs, it is important to note that methodological limitations of research still constrain our understanding of any given intervention's true potential impact (Sandbank et al., 2020). Moreover, researchers and clinicians are still unsure of for whom NDBIs work best, and whether there are meaningful variations in which NDBIs may be most effective for a given child (Vivanti, Prior, et al., 2014). Some research indicates that children with a higher level of object interest may have a more robust response to NDBI intervention (Carter et al., 2011; R. L. Koegel et al., 2001; Yoder & Stone, 2006). Some studies have also suggested that (a) children with higher developmental and language scores at baseline may be more likely to respond to NDBI interventions, and (b) children with more autism-related challenges are more likely to be slow responders (Vivanti, Prior, et al., 2014; Yoder et al., 2020) Even so, a recent meta-analysis found that treatment effect sizes did not vary systematically based on children's chronological age, sex, or language ability (Crank et al., 2021).

There are, however, instances in which NDBIs are contraindicated. Clinicians tend to agree that if a child has severe behavior or safety concerns (e.g., self-injury, eloping), those concerns may be more urgent than social communication goals (Ingersoll & Dvortcsak, 2019). Additionally, parents may prioritize other areas (e.g., feeding, dressing, toileting) over social communication, making NDBIs a less appropriate fit. While there are no known side effects, some autistic individuals have indicated that NDBIs may overemphasize spoken language over alternate methods of communication. Additionally, in terms of limitations, NDBIs may not work for all children. In fact, some children have been identified as nonresponders or slow responders to NDBI and it is unclear as to what specific aspect(s) of the child's unique profile contribute to this status.

16.6.2 Practice Implication Guidelines

As discussed in this chapter, NDBIs can be delivered by providers with various backgrounds working in diverse treatment settings. Additional research is needed to understand how to support the wide-scale implementation of NDBIs in existing care systems such as Part C early intervention, Medicaid-funded community mental health, and schools. At present, intensive research and quality improvement initiatives are underway to determine the requisite qualifications for those who will eventually be tasked with providing NDBIs within our communities. Initial research indicates that while contextual adaptation is necessary in fitting the NDBI model to a given setting, it is important to prioritize preservice education about developmental milestones and autism as well as training on specific NDBI strategies (Pickard et al., 2021). Future researchers, clinicians, and policymakers might consider how formal trainings that couple coursework with ongoing coaching and fidelity monitoring and/or inclusion of NDBIs in college-level coursework and practicum opportunities can ensure that clinicians receive sufficient training and experience prior to entering independent practice. Although a combination of preservice and in-service training efforts can build a workforce equipped to deliver NDBIs, attention to policies at the national, state, and local level that support the delivery of and reimbursement for NDBI services is essential for supporting NDBI implementation within community contexts.

16.6.3 Additional Resources

- Bruinsma, Y. E., Minjarez, M. B., Schreibman, L., & Stahmer, A. C. (2020). *Naturalistic developmental behavioral interventions for autism spectrum disorder*. Baltimore: Brookes. https://products.brookespublishing.com/Naturalistic-Developmental-Behavioral-Interventions-for-Autism-Spectrum-Disorder-P1142.aspx
- Early Start Denver model online modules: https://helpisinyourhands.org/course

- Pivotal Response Training AFIRM module: https://afirm.fpg.unc.edu/pivotal-response-training
- Rogers, S. J., Dawson, G., & Vismara, L. A. (2012). *An early start for your child with autism.* New York: Guilford Press. https://www.guilford.com/books/An-Early-Start-for-Your-Child-with-Autism/Rogers-Dawson-Vismara/9781609184704
- Seattle Children's Autism 204 Lecture on NDBI: https://youtu.be/iPTUsaRZplI
- World Health Organization Caregiver Skills Training eLearning modules: https://openwho.org/courses/caregiver-skills-training

16.7 References

Adams, R. C., Tapia, C., Council on Children with Disabilities, Murphy, N. A., Norwood Jr, K. W., Adams, R. C., Burke, R. T., Friedman, S. L., Houtrow, A. J., & Kalichman, M. A. (2013). Early intervention, IDEA Part C services, and the medical home: Collaboration for best practice and best outcomes. *Pediatrics, 132*(4), e1073–e1088.

Akshoomoff, N., Stahmer, A. C., Corsello, C., & Mahrer, N. E. (2010). What happens next? Follow-up from the children's toddler school program. *Journal of Positive Behavior Interventions, 12*(4), 245–253.

Aldred, C., Green, J., Emsley, R., & McConachie, H. (2012). Brief report: Mediation of treatment effect in a communication intervention for pre-school children with autism. *Journal of Autism and Developmental Disorders, 42*(3), 447–454.

Barry, C. L., Epstein, A. J., Marcus, S. C., Kennedy-Hendricks, A., Candon, M. K., Xie, M., & Mandell, D. S. (2017). Effects of state insurance mandates on health care use and spending for autism spectrum disorder. *Health Affairs, 36*(10), 1754–1761.

Blume, H. (1998). Neurodiversity: On the neurological underpinnings of geekdom. *The Atlantic, 30.* https://www.theatlantic.com/magazine/archive/1998/09/neurodiversity/305909/

Brian, J., Drmic, I., Roncadin, C., Dowds, E., Shaver, C., Smith, I. M., Zwaigenbaum, L., Sacrey, L.-A. R., & Bryson, S. E. (2022). Effectiveness of a parent-mediated intervention for toddlers with autism spectrum disorder: Evidence from a large community implementation. *Autism* 26(7), 1882–1897. https://doi.org/10.1177/13623613211068934

Brian, J., Smith, I. M., Zwaigenbaum, L., & Bryson, S. E. (2017). Cross-site randomized control trial of the *Social ABCs* caregiver-mediated intervention for toddlers with autism spectrum disorder: RCT of caregiver-mediated early ASD intervention. *Autism Research, 10*(10), 1700–1711. https://doi.org/10.1002/aur.1818

Brian, J., Smith, I. M., Zwaigenbaum, L., Roberts, W., & Bryson, S. E. (2016). The social ABCs caregiver-mediated intervention for toddlers with autism spectrum disorder: Feasibility, acceptability, and evidence of promise from a multisite study. *Autism Research, 9*(8), 899–912.

Bruinsma, Y., Minjarez, M. B., Schreibman, L., & Stahmer, A. C. (Eds.). (2020). *Naturalistic developmental behavioral interventions for autism spectrum disorder.* Baltimore: Brookes.

Callahan, K., Hughes, H. L., Mehta, S., Toussaint, K. A., Nichols, S. M., Ma, P. S., Kutlu, M., & Wang, H.-T. (2017). Social validity of evidence-based practices and emerging interventions in autism. *Focus on Autism and Other Developmental Disabilities, 32*(3), 188–197.

Carter, A. S., Messinger, D. S., Stone, W. L., Celimli, S., Nahmias, A. S., & Yoder, P. J. (2011). A randomized controlled trial of Hanen's "More Than Words" in toddlers with early autism symptoms: Hanen's "More Than Words" RCT. *Journal of Child Psychology and Psychiatry, 52*(7), 741–752. https://doi.org/10.1111/j.1469-7610.2011.02395.x

Casagrande, K. A., & Ingersoll, B. R. (2017). Parent-mediated interventions for social communication in young children with ASD. In J.B. Leaf (ed.) *Handbook of social skills and autism spectrum disorder* (pp. 285–312). Cham: Springer.

Chang, Y.-C., Shire, S. Y., Shih, W., Gelfand, C., & Kasari, C. (2016). Preschool deployment of evidence-based social communication intervention: JASPER in the vlassroom. *Journal of Autism and Developmental Disorders, 46*(6), 2211–2223. https://doi.org/10.1007/s10803-016-2752-2

Cicchetti, D. (1989). Developmental psychopathology: Some thoughts on its evolution. *Development and Psychopathology*, *1*(1), 1–4.

Cidav, Z., Munson, J., Estes, A., Dawson, G., Rogers, S., & Mandell, D. (2017). Cost offset associated with Early Start Denver model for children with autism. *Journal of the American Academy of Child & Adolescent Psychiatry*, *56*(9), 777–783. https://doi.org/10.1016/j.jaac.2017.06.007

Clark-Whitney, E., Klein, C. B., Hadley, P. A., Lord, C., & Kim, S. H. (2022). Caregiver language input supports sentence diversity in young children with autism spectrum disorder. *Journal of Speech, Language, and Hearing Research*, *65*(4), 1465–1477. https://doi.org/10.1044/2021_JSLHR-21-00458

Crank, J. E., Sandbank, M., Dunham, K., Crowley, S., Bottema-Beutel, K., Feldman, J., & Woynaroski, T. G. (2021). Understanding the effects of naturalistic developmental behavioral interventions: A project AIM meta-analysis. *Autism Research*, 14: 817–834. https://doi.org/10.1002/aur.2471

D'Agostino, S., Douglas, S. N., & Duenas, A. D. (2019). Practitioner-implemented naturalistic developmental behavioral interventions: Systematic review of social validity practices. *Topics in Early Childhood Special Education*, *39*(3), 170–182.

D'Agostino, S., Douglas, S. N., & Horton, E. (2020). Inclusive preschool practitioners' implementation of naturalistic developmental behavioral intervention using telehealth training. *Journal of Autism and Developmental Disorders*, *50*(3), 864–880.

D'Agostino, S., Duenas, A. D., Bravo, A., Tyson, K., Straiton, D., Salvatore, G. L., Pacia, C., & Pellecchia, M. (2023). Toward deeper understanding and wide-scale implementation of naturalistic developmental behavioral interventions. *Autism*, *27*(1):253–258.

Dawson, G., & Adams, A. (1984). Imitation and social responsiveness in autistic children. *Journal of Abnormal Child Psychology*, *12*(2), 209–226.

Dawson, G., Rogers, S., Munson, J., Smith, M., Winter, J., Greenson, J., Donaldson, A., & Varley, J. (2010). Randomized, controlled trial of an intervention for toddlers with autism: The Early Start Denver model. *Pediatrics*, *125*(1), e17–23. https://doi.org/10.1542/peds.2009-0958

Dunst, C. J., Bruder, M. B., Trivette, C. M., Raab, M., & McLean, M. (2001). Natural learning opportunities for infants, toddlers, and preschoolers. *Young Exceptional Children*, *4*(3), 18–25. https://doi.org/10.1177/109625060100400303

Dunst, C. J., Trivette, C. M., & Hamby, W. (2010). Meta-analysis of the effectiveness of four adult learning methods and strategies. *International Journal of Continuing Engineering Education and Lifelong Learning*, *3*(1), 22.

Eapen, V., Črnčec, R., & Walter, A. (2013). Clinical outcomes of an early intervention program for preschool children with autism spectrum disorder in a community group setting. *BMC Pediatrics*, *13*(1), 1–9.

Edmunds, S. R., Kover, S. T., & Stone, W. L. (2019). The relation between parent verbal responsiveness and child communication in young children with or at risk for autism spectrum disorder: A systematic review and meta-analysis. *Autism Research*, *12*(0), 715–731. https://doi.org/10.1002/aur.2100

Eisenhower, A., Martinez Pedraza, F., Sheldrick, R. C., Frenette, E., Hoch, N., Brunt, S., & Carter, A. S. (2021). Multi-stage screening in early intervention: A critical strategy for improving ASD identification and addressing disparities. *Journal of Autism and Developmental Disorders*, *51*(3), 868–883.

Engelstad, A.-M., Holingue, C., & Landa, R. J. (2020). Early Achievements for education settings: An embedded teacher-implemented social communication intervention for preschoolers with autism spectrum disorder. *Perspectives of the ASHA Special Interest Groups*, *5*(3), 582–601.

Estes, A., Munson, J., Rogers, S. J., Greenson, J., Winter, J., & Dawson, G. (2015). Long-term outcomes of early intervention in 6-year-old children with autism spectrum disorder. *Journal of the American Academy of Child & Adolescent Psychiatry*, *54*(7), 580–587. https://doi.org/10.1016/j.jaac.2015.04.005

Frost, K. M., Brian, J., Gengoux, G. W., Hardan, A., Rieth, S. R., Stahmer, A., & Ingersoll, B. (2020). Identifying and measuring the common elements of naturalistic developmental behavioral interventions for autism spectrum disorder: Development of the NDBI-Fi. *Autism*, *24*(8), 2285–2297. https://doi.org/10.1177/1362361320944011

Gengoux, G. W., McNerney, E., & Minjarez, M. B. (2020). Selecting meaningful skills for teaching in the natural environment. In Y. Bruinsma, M. B. Minjarez, L. Schreibman, & A. C. Stahmer (Eds.), *Naturalistic developmental behavioral interventions for autism spectrum disorder* (pp. 45–75). Baltimore: Brookes.

Gevarter, C., Najar, A. M., Flake, J., Tapia-Alvidrez, F., & Lucero, A. (2022). Naturalistic communication training for early intervention providers and latinx parents of children with signs of autism. *Journal of Developmental and Physical Disabilities, 34*(1), 147–169.

Green, J., Pickles, A., Pasco, G., Bedford, R., Wan, M. W., Elsabbagh, M., Slonims, V., Gliga, T., Jones, E., Cheung, C., Charman, T., Johnson, M., & The British Autism Study of Infant Siblings (BASIS) Team. (2017). Randomised trial of a parent-mediated intervention for infants at high risk for autism: Longitudinal outcomes to age 3 years. *Journal of Child Psychology and Psychiatry, 58*(12), 1330–1340. https://doi.org/10.1111/jcpp.12728

Griffiths, P. E., & Tabery, J. (2013). Developmental systems theory: What does it explain, and how does it explain it? In *Advances in child development and behavior* (Vol. 44, pp. 65–94). Amsterdam: Elsevier.

Gulsrud, A., Carr, T., Williams, J., Panganiban, J., Jones, F., Kimbrough, J., Shih, W., & Kasari, C. (2019). Developmental screening and early intervention in a childcare setting for young children at risk for autism and other developmental delays: A feasibility trial. *Autism Research, 12*(9), 1423–1433.

Gulsrud, A. C., Hellemann, G., Shire, S., & Kasari, C. (2016). Isolating active ingredients in a parent-mediated social communication intervention for toddlers with autism spectrum disorder. *Journal of Child Psychology and Psychiatry, 57*(5), 606–613. https://doi.org/10.1111/jcpp.12481

Hampton, L. H., & Sandbank, M. P. (2021). Keeping up with the evidence base: Survey of behavior professionals about naturalistic developmental behavioral interventions. *Autism.*, 26, 875–888. https://doi.org/10.1177/13623613211035233

Hardan, A. Y., Gengoux, G. W., Berquist, K. L., Libove, R. A., Ardel, C. M., Phillips, J., Frazier, T. W., & Minjarez, M. B. (2015). A randomized controlled trial of pivotal response treatment group for parents of children with autism. *Journal of Child Psychology and Psychiatry, 56*(8), 884–892. https://doi.org/10.1111/jcpp.12354

Hume, K., Steinbrenner, J. R., Odom, S. L., Morin, K. L., Nowell, S. W., Tomaszewski, B., Szendrey, S., McIntyre, N. S., Yücesoy-Özkan, S., & Savage, M. N. (2021). Evidence-based practices for children, youth, and young adults with autism: Third generation review. *Journal of Autism and Developmental Disorders, 51*(11), 4013–4032. https://doi.org/10.1007/s10803-020-04844-2

Ingersoll, B., & Berger, N. I. (2015). Parent engagement with a telehealth-based parent-mediated intervention program for children with autism spectrum disorders: Predictors of program use and parent outcomes. *Journal of Medical Internet Research, 17*(10), e227. https://doi.org/10.2196/jmir.4913

Ingersoll, B., & Dvortcsak, A. (2019). *Teaching social communication to children with autism and other developmental delays: The Project ImPACT guide to coaching parents and the Project ImPACT manual for parents* (2nd ed.). New York: Guilford Press.

Ingersoll, B., Wainer, A. L., Berger, N. I., Pickard, K., & Bonter, N. (2016). Comparison of a self-directed and therapist-assisted telehealth parent-mediated intervention for children with ASD: A pilot RCT. *Journal of Autism and Developmental Disorders, 46*(7), 2275–2284. https://doi.org/10.1007/s10803-016-2755-z

Jurek, L., Leadbitter, K., Falissard, B., Colin, C., Touzet, S., & Geoffray, M.-M. (2022). Parental experience of parent-mediated intervention for children with ASD: A systematic review and qualitative evidence synthesis. *Autism, 27*(3):647–666.

Kaiser, A. P., Hancock, T. B., & Nietfeld, J. P. (2000). The effects of parent-implemented enhanced milieu teaching on the social communication of children who have autism. *Early Education & Development, 11*(4), 423–446. https://doi.org/10.1207/s15566935eed1104_4

Kaiser, A. P., & Hester, P. P. (1994). Generalized effects of enhanced milieu teaching. *Journal of Speech, Language, and Hearing Research, 37*(6), 1320–1340.

Kasari, C., Freeman, S., & Paparella, T. (2006). Joint attention and symbolic play in young children with autism: A randomized controlled intervention study: Joint attention and symbolic play in young children with autism. *Journal of Child Psychology and Psychiatry, 47*(6), 611–620. https://doi.org/10.1111/j.1469-7610.2005.01567.x

Kasari, C., Gulsrud, A. C., Shire, S. Y., & Strawbridge, C. (2021). *The JASPER model for children with autism: Promoting joint attention, symbolic play, engagement, and regulation.* New York: Guilford.

Koegel, L. K., Ashbaugh, K., & Koegel, R. L. (2016). Pivotal response treatment. In R. Lang, T. B. Hancock, & N. N. Singh (Eds.), *Early intervention for young children with autism spectrum disorder* (pp. 85–112). Cham: Springer. https://doi.org/10.1007/978-3-319-30925-5_4

Koegel, R. L., Koegel, L. K., & McNerney, E. K. (2001). Pivotal areas in intervention for autism. *Journal of Clinical Child & Adolescent Psychology, 30*(1), 19–32. https://doi.org/10.1207/S15374424JCCP3001_4

Koegel, R. L., O'Dell, M. C., & Koegel, L. K. (1987). A natural language teaching paradigm for nonverbal autistic children. *Journal of Autism and Developmental Disorders, 17*(2), 187–200.

Kornack, J., Persicke, A., Cervantes, P., Jang, J., & Dixon, D. (2014). Economics of autism spectrum disorders: An overview of treatment and research funding. In J. Tarbox, D. R. Dixon, P. Sturmey, & J. L. Matson (Eds.), *Handbook of early intervention for autism spectrum disorders: Research, policy, and practice* (pp. 165–178). New York: Springer. https://doi.org/10.1007/978-1-4939-0401-3_9

Leadbitter, K., Buckle, K. L., Ellis, C., & Dekker, M. (2021). Autistic self-advocacy and the neurodiversity movement: Implications for autism early intervention research and practice. *Frontiers in Psychology, 12*, 635–690. https://doi.org/10.3389/fpsyg.2021.635690

Lifter, K., Sulzer-Azaroff, B., Anderson, S. R., & Cowdery, G. E. (1993). Teaching play activities to preschool children with disabilities: The importance of developmental considerations. *Journal of Early Intervention, 17*(2), 139–159.

Linstead, E., Dixon, D., Hong, E., Burns, C., French, R., Novack, M., & Granpeesheh, D. (2017). An evaluation of the effects of intensity and duration on outcomes across treatment domains for children with autism spectrum disorder. *Translational Psychiatry, 7*(9), e1234–e1234.

Lovaas, O. I. (1987). Behavioral treatment and normal educational and intellectual functioning in young autistic children. *Journal of Consulting and Clinical Psychology, 55*(1), 3–9.

Maenner, M. J., Shaw, K. A., Bakian, A. V., Bilder, D. A., Durkin, M. S., Esler, A., Furnier, S. M., Hallas, L., Hall-Lande, J., & Hudson, A. (2021). Prevalence and characteristics of autism spectrum disorder among children aged 8 years—Autism and developmental disabilities monitoring network, 11 sites, United States, 2018. *MMWR Surveillance Summaries, 70*(11), 1.

Masten, A. S., & Cicchetti, D. (2010). Developmental cascades. *Development and Psychopathology, 22*(3), 491–495.

Maye, M., Edmunds, S., Stone-MacDonald, A., & Carter, A. S. (2022). Preparation for adaptation of intensive early intervention for toddlers with ASD: Childcare providers' perspectives on training approach. *Early Childhood Education Journal, 51*(7), 1181–1188.

Maye, M., Sanchez, V. E., Stone-MacDonald, A., & Carter, A. S. (2020). Early Interventionists' Appraisals of Intervention Strategies for Toddlers with Autism Spectrum Disorder and Their Peers in Inclusive Childcare Classrooms. *Journal of Autism and Developmental Disorders*. https://doi.org/10.1007/s10803-020-04456-w

McGarry, E., Vernon, T., & Baktha, A. (2020). Brief report: A pilot online pivotal response treatment training program for parents of toddlers with autism spectrum disorder. *Journal of Autism and Developmental Disorders, 50*(9), 3424–3431.

McGee, G. G., Krantz, P. J., & McClannahan, L. E. (1985). The facilitative effects of incidental teaching on preposition use by autistic children. *Journal of Applied Behavior Analysis, 18*(1), 17–31.

Minjarez, M. B., Williams, S. E., Mercier, E. M., & Hardan, A. Y. (2011). Pivotal response group treatment program for parents of children with autism. *Journal of Autism and Developmental Disorders, 41*(1), 92–101.

Morgan, L., Hooker, J. L., Sparapani, N., Reinhardt, V. P., Schatschneider, C., & Wetherby, A. M. (2018). Cluster randomized trial of the classroom SCERTS intervention for elementary students with autism spectrum disorder. *Journal of Consulting and Clinical Psychology, 86*(7), 631.

Mundy, P., Sigman, M., & Kasari, C. (1990). A longitudinal study of joint attention and language development in autistic children. *Journal of Autism and Developmental Disorders, 20*(1), 115–128. https://doi.org/10.1007/BF02206861

Neely, L., Hong, E. R., Kawamini, S., Umana, I., & Kurz, I. (2020). Intercontinental telehealth to train Japanese interventionists in incidental teaching for children with autism. *Journal of Behavioral Education, 29*(2), 433–448.

Nevill, R. E., Lecavalier, L., & Stratis, E. A. (2018). Meta-analysis of parent-mediated interventions for young children with autism spectrum disorder. *Autism, 22*(2), 84–98. https://doi.org/10.1177/1362361316677838

Ona, H. N., Larsen, K., Nordheim, L. V., & Brurberg, K. G. (2020). Effects of pivotal response treatment (PRT) for children with autism spectrum disorders (ASD): A systematic review. *Review Journal of Autism and Developmental Disorders, 7*(1), 78–90. https://doi.org/10.1007/s40489-019-00180-z

Oono, I. P., Honey, E. J., & McConachie, H. (2013). Parent-mediated early intervention for young children with autism spectrum disorders (ASD). *Cochrane Database of Systematic Reviews*. https://doi.org/10.1002/14651858.CD009774.pub2

Pellecchia, M., Iadarola, S., & Stahmer, A. C. (2019). How meaningful is more? Considerations regarding intensity in early intensive behavioral intervention. *Autism, 23*(5), 1075–1078. https://doi.org/10.1177/1362361319854844

Pellecchia, M., Mandell, D. S., Beidas, R. S., Dunst, C. J., Tomczuk, L., Newman, J., Zeigler, L., & Stahmer, A. C. (2022). Parent coaching in early intervention for autism spectrum disorder: A brief report. *Journal of Early Intervention, 45*(2), 185–197. https://doi.org/10.1177/10538151221095860

Pickard, K., Mellman, H., Frost, K., Reaven, J., & Ingersoll, B. (2021). Balancing fidelity and flexibility: Usual care for young children with an increased likelihood of having autism spectrum disorder within an early intervention system. *Journal of Autism and Developmental Disorders.* https://doi.org/10.1007/s10803-021-04882-4

Pickard, K., Wainer, A. L., Bailey, K. M., & Ingersoll, B. (2016). A mixed-method evaluation of the feasibility and acceptability of a telehealth-based parent-mediated intervention for children with autism spectrum disorder. *Autism, 20*(7), 845–855. https://doi.org/10.1177/1362361315614496

Pickles, A., Harris, V., Green, J., Aldred, C., McConachie, H., Slonims, V., Le Couteur, A., Hudry, K., Charman, T., & the PACT Consortium. (2015). Treatment mechanism in the MRC preschool autism communication trial: Implications for study design and parent-focussed therapy for children. *Journal of Child Psychology and Psychiatry, 56*(2), 162–170. https://doi.org/10.1111/jcpp.12291

Prizant, B. M., Wetherby, A. M., Rubin, E., & Laurent, A. C. (2003). The SCERTS model: A transactional, family-centered approach to enhancing communication and socioemotional abilities of children with autism spectrum disorder. *Infants & Young Children, 16*(4), 296–316.

Reichow, B., Doehring, P., Cicchetti, D. V., & Volkmar, F. R. (2011). *Evidence-based practices and treatments for children with autism.* Cham: Springer.

Rieth, S. R., Dickson, K. S., Ko, J., Haine-Schlagel, R., Gaines, K., Brookman-Frazee, L., & Stahmer, A. C. (2022). Provider perspectives and reach of an evidence-based intervention in community services for toddlers. *Autism, 26*(3), 628–639.

Rieth, S. R., Haine-Schlagel, R., Burgeson, M., Searcy, K., Dickson, K. S., & Stahmer, A. C. (2018). Integrating a parent-implemented blend of developmental and behavioral intervention strategies into speech-language treatment for toddlers at risk for autism spectrum disorder. *Seminars in Speech & Language, 39*(02), 114–124.

Roche, L., Adams, D., & Clark, M. (2021). Research priorities of the autism community: A systematic review of key stakeholder perspectives. *Autism, 25*(2), 336–348. https://doi.org/10.1177/1362361320967790

Rodger, S., Braithwaite, M., & Keen, D. (2004). Early intervention for children with autism: Parental priorities. *Australasian Journal of Early Childhood, 29*(3), 34–41.

Rogers, S. J., & Dawson, G. (2010). *Early start Denver model for young children with autism: Promoting language, learning, and engagement.* New York: Guilford Press.

Rogers, S. J., & Pennington, B. F. (1991). A theoretical approach to the deficits in infantile autism. *Development and Psychopathology, 3*, 26.

Rogers, S. J., Stahmer, A., Talbott, M., Young, G., Fuller, E., Pellecchia, M., Barber, A., & Griffith, E. (2022). Feasibility of delivering parent-implemented NDBI interventions in low-resource regions: A pilot randomized controlled study. *Journal of Neurodevelopmental Disorders, 14*(1), 3. https://doi.org/10.1186/s11689-021-09410-0

Rogers, S. J., Yoder, P. J., Estes, A., Warren, Z., McEachin, J., Munson, J., Rocha, M., Greenson, J., Wallace, L., Gardner, E., Dawson, G., Sugar, C. A., Hellemann, G., & Whelan, F. (2021). A multisite randomized controlled trial comparing the effects of intervention intensity and intervention style on outcomes for young children with autism. *Journal of the American Academy of Child & Adolescent Psychiatry, 60*(6), 710–722. https://doi.org/10.1016/j.jaac.2020.06.013

Rush, D. D., & Shelden, M. L. (2011). *The early childhood coaching handbook.* Baltimore: Brookes.

Sandbank, M., Bottema-Beutel, K., Crowley, S., Cassidy, M., Dunham, K., Feldman, J. I., Crank, J., Albarran, S. A., Raj, S., Mahbub, P., & Woynaroski, T. G. (2020). Project AIM: Autism intervention meta-analysis for studies of young children. *Psychological Bulletin, 146*(1), 1–29. https://doi.org/10.1037/bul0000215

Sandbank, M., Bottema-Beutel, K., & Woynaroski, T. (2021). Intervention recommendations for children with autism in light of a changing evidence base. *JAMA Pediatrics, 175*(4), 341–342.

Sandbank, M., Chow, J., Bottema-Beutel, K., & Woynaroski, T. (2021). Evaluating evidence-based practice in light of the boundedness and proximity of outcomes: Capturing the scope of change. *Autism Research, 14*, 1536–1542. https://doi.org/10.1002/aur.2527

Schreibman, L., & Carr, E. G. (1978). Elimination of echolalic responding to questions through the training of a generalized verbal response. *Journal of Applied Behavior Analysis, 11*(4), 453–463.

Schreibman, L., Dawson, G., Stahmer, A. C., Landa, R., Rogers, S. J., McGee, G. G., Kasari, C., Ingersoll, B., Kaiser, A. P., Bruinsma, Y., McNerney, E., Wetherby, A., & Halladay, A. (2015). Naturalistic developmental behavioral interventions: Empirically validated treatments for autism spectrum disorder. *Journal of Autism and Developmental Disorders, 45*(8), 2411–2428. https://doi.org/10.1007/s10803-015-2407-8

Schreibman, L., Jobin, A., & Dawson, G. (2020). Understanding NDBI. In Y. Bruinsma, M. B. Minjarez, L. Schreibman, & A. C. Stahmer (Eds.), *Naturalistic developmental behavioral interventions for autism spectrum disorder*. Baltimore: Brookes.

Schreibman, L., & Koegel, R. L. (2005). Training for parents of children with autism: Pivotal responses, generalization, and individualization of interventions. In E.D. Hibbs & P. S. Jensen (Eds.), *Psychosocial treatments for child and adolescent disorders: Empirically based strategies for clinical practice* (pp. 605–631). Washington DC: American Psychological Association.

Schuck, R. K., Tagavi, D. M., Baiden, K. M. P., Dwyer, P., Williams, Z. J., Osuna, A., Ferguson, E. F., Jimenez Muñoz, M., Poyser, S. K., Johnson, J. F., & Vernon, T. W. (2021). Neurodiversity and autism intervention: Reconciling perspectives through a naturalistic developmental behavioral intervention framework. *Journal of Autism and Developmental Disorders, 52*, 4625–4645. https://doi.org/10.1007/s10803-021-05316-x

Sengupta, K., Mahadik, S., & Kapoor, G. (2020). Glocalizing project ImPACT: Feasibility, acceptability and preliminary outcomes of a parent-mediated social communication intervention for autism adapted to the Indian context. *Research in Autism Spectrum Disorders, 76*, 101585. https://doi.org/10.1016/j.rasd.2020.101585

Shire, S. Y., Shih, W., Chang, Y.-C., Bracaglia, S., Kodjoe, M., & Kasari, C. (2019). Sustained community implementation of JASPER intervention with toddlers with autism. *Journal of Autism and Developmental Disorders, 49*(5), 1863–1875.

Shire, S. Y., Worthman, L. B., & Arbuckle, S. (2021). A technology-enabled adaptation of face-to-face caregiver-mediated JASPER intervention: Preliminary examination of video conferenced caregiver coaching. *American Journal on Intellectual and Developmental Disabilities, 126*(5), 421–434.

Siller, M., Hotez, E., Swanson, M., Delavenne, A., Hutman, T., & Sigman, M. (2018). Parent coaching increases the parents' capacity for reflection and self-evaluation: Results from a clinical trial in autism. *Attachment & Human Development, 20*(3), 287–308.

Sinai-Gavrilov, Y., Gev, T., Mor-Snir, I., Vivanti, G., & Golan, O. (2020). Integrating the Early Start Denver model into Israeli community autism spectrum disorder preschools: Effectiveness and treatment response predictors. *Autism, 24*(8), 2081–2093.

Sinclair, J. (1993). Don't mourn for us. *Our Voice, 1*(3). http://www.autreat.com/dont_mourn.html

Singer, J. (2017). *Neurodiversity: The birth of an idea.* Self-published.

Skinner, B. F. (1957). *Verbal behavior.* Crows Nest, NSW: Appleton-Century-Crofts. https://doi.org/10.1037/11256-000

Smith, T. (2001). Discrete trial training in the treatment of autism. *Focus on Autism and Other Developmental Disabilities, 16*(2), 86–92. https://doi.org/10.1177/108835760101600204

Stahmer, A. C., & Ingersoll, B. (2004). Inclusive programming for toddlers with autism spectrum disorders: Outcomes from the children's toddler school. *Journal of Positive Behavior Interventions, 6*(2), 67–82.

Stahmer, A. C., Rieth, S. R., Dickson, K. S., Feder, J., Burgeson, M., Searcy, K., & Brookman-Frazee, L. (2019). Project ImPACT for toddlers: Pilot outcomes of a community adaptation of an intervention for autism risk. *Autism, 24*(3), 617–632. https://doi.org/10.1177/1362361319878080

Steinbrenner, J. R., Hume, K., Odom, S. L., Morin, K. L., Nowell, S. W., Tomaszewski, B., Szendrey, S., McIntyre, N. S., Yücesoy-Özkan, Ş., & Savage, M. N. (2020). *Evidence-based practices for children, youth, and young adults with autism.* Chapel Hill: The University of North Carolina at Chapel Hill, Frank Porter Graham Child Development Institute, National Clearinghouse on Autism Evidence and Practice Review Team.

Strain, P. S., Kerr, M. M., & Ragland, E. U. (1979). Effects of peer-mediated social initiations and prompting/reinforcement procedures on the social behavior of autistic children. *Journal of Autism and Developmental Disorders, 9*(1), 41–54.

Tiede, G., & Walton, K. M. (2019). Meta-analysis of naturalistic developmental behavioral interventions for young children with autism spectrum disorder. *Autism*, 23(8), 2080–2095. https://doi.org/10.1177/1362361319836371

Tomasello, N. M., Manning, A. R., & Dulmus, C. N. (2010). Family-centered early intervention for infants and toddlers with disabilities. *Journal of Family Social Work, 13*(2), 163–172.

Tsiplova, K., Jegathisawaran, J., Mirenda, P., Kalynchuk, K., Colozzo, P., Smith, V., & Ungar, W. J. (2022). Parent coaching intervention for children with suspected autism spectrum disorder: Cost analysis. *Research in Autism Spectrum Disorders, 93*, 101949. https://doi.org/10.1016/j.rasd.2022.101949

Tupou, J., van Der Meer, L., Waddington, H., & Sigafoos, J. (2019). Preschool interventions for children with autism spectrum disorder: A review of effectiveness studies. *Review Journal of Autism and Developmental Disorders, 6*(4), 381–402.

Vismara, L. A., McCormick, C. E., Wagner, A. L., Monlux, K., Nadhan, A., & Young, G. S. (2018). Telehealth parent training in the Early Start Denver model: Results from a randomized controlled study. *Focus on Autism and Other Developmental Disabilities, 33*(2), 67–79.

Vivanti, G., Paynter, J., Duncan, E., Fothergill, H., Dissanayake, C., & Rogers, S. J. (2014). Effectiveness and feasibility of the Early Start Denver model implemented in a group-based community childcare setting. *Journal of Autism and Developmental Disorders, 44*(12), 3140–3153.

Vivanti, G., Prior, M., Williams, K., & Dissanayake, C. (2014). Predictors of outcomes in autism early intervention: Why don't we know more? *Frontiers in Pediatrics, 2*. https://doi.org/10.3389/fped.2014.00058

Waddington, H., van der Meer, L., & Sigafoos, J. (2016). Effectiveness of the Early Start Denver model: A systematic review. *Review Journal of Autism and Developmental Disorders, 3*(2), 93–106. https://doi.org/10.1007/s40489-015-0068-3

Waddington, H., Reynolds, J. E., Macaskill, E., Curtis, S., Taylor, L. J., & Whitehouse, A. J. (2021). The effects of JASPER intervention for children with autism spectrum disorder: A systematic review. *Autism, 25*(8), 2370–2385. https://doi.org/10.1177/13623613211019162

Wainer, A. L., Arnold, Z. E., Leonczyk, C., & Valluripalli Soorya, L. (2021). Examining a stepped-care telehealth program for parents of young children with autism: A proof-of-concept trial. *Molecular Autism, 12*(1), 1–14.

Warlaumont, A. S., Richards, J. A., Gilkerson, J., & Oller, D. K. (2014). A social feedback loop for speech development and its reduction in autism. *Psychological Science, 25*(7), 1314–1324.

Wilson, K. P., & Landa, R. J. (2019). Barriers to educator implementation of a classroom-based intervention for preschoolers with autism spectrum disorder. *Frontiers in Education, 4*, 1–10.

Wong, C. S. (2013). A play and joint attention intervention for teachers of young children with autism: A randomized controlled pilot study. *Autism, 17*(3), 340–357.

Yi, J., Kim, W., & Lee, J. (2022). Effectiveness of the SCERTS Model–based interventions for autistic children: A systematic review. *Journal of Speech, Language, and Hearing Research, 65*(7), 2662–2676. https://doi.org/10.1044/2022_JSLHR-21-00518

Yoder, P. J., Rogers, S., Estes, A., Warren, Z., Munson, J., Hellemann, G., & McEachin, J. (2020). Interaction of treatment intensity and autism severity on frequency and maturity of spontaneous communication in toddlers with autism spectrum disorder. *Autism Research, 13*(11), 1902–1912. https://doi.org/10.1002/aur.2416

Yoder, P. J., & Stone, W. L. (2006). A randomized comparison of the effect of two prelinguistic communication interventions on the acquisition of spoken communication in preschoolers with ASD. *Journal of Speech Language Hearing Research, 49*, 698–711. https://doi.org/10.1044/1092-4388(2006/051).

Yoder, P. J., Stone, W. L., & Edmunds, S. R. (2021a). For which younger siblings of children with autism spectrum disorder does parent-mediated intervention work? *Autism, 25*(1), 58–69. https://doi.org/10.1177/1362361320943373

Yoder, P. J., Stone, W. L., & Edmunds, S. R. (2021b). Parent utilization of ImPACT intervention strategies is a mediator of proximal then distal social communication outcomes in younger siblings of children with ASD. *Autism, 25*(1), 44–57. https://doi.org/10.1177/1362361320946883

17
LEAP Preschool

Phillip S. Strain, and Edward Bovey
PELE Center, University of Denver

17.1 Technical Abstract

Background: LEAP Preschool is a comprehensive treatment model that relies on both groups of providers and nondisabled, same age-peers as intervention agents. Peers play a major role in supporting the communication and social skills of 3–5-year-old classmates with autism. **Method:** Operating in transdisciplinary teams, teachers, their assistants, and related services providers primarily employ embedded and naturalistic teaching techniques to address all the identified developmental needs of children with autism. Supplementing the half-day preschool, adult family members are coached in basic behavioral strategies to make home and community routines as enjoyable as possible. **Results:** LEAP Preschool has been shown to make large improvements in children's social, language, cognitive, and adaptive skills and to reduce the severity of autism symptoms. **Discussion:** The success of the model is dependent upon very high levels of implementation fidelity and replication sites typically need 2 years to reach fidelity. Quality implementation of LEAP Preschool requires a strong commitment not just from practitioners but administrative personnel as well. There is no evidence that children's entering level of behavior is predictive of success in LEAP. Currently, there are over 150 certified LEAP sites in the United States.

17.2 Layperson Summary

LEAP Preschool is an early childhood inclusion model comprised of a half-day preschool and in-home/community coaching for adult family members to acquire skills needed to make daily routines run as smoothly and enjoyably as possible. What distinguishes LEAP from other models based upon behavior analytic principles is the reliance on neurotypical peers to facilitate the social and communicative skills of classmates with autism. LEAP has been the subject of dozens of peer-reviewed studies, including the largest school-based randomized trial to date. LEAP outcomes are also unique in the sense that data show improvements in all developmental domains. LEAP has been recognized as a comprehensive treatment model by multiple professional sources as have the discrete intervention

Phillip S. Strain, and Edward Bovey, *LEAP Preschool*. In: *Lifespan Treatment for Autistic Individuals*.
Edited by: Peter Sturmey, Russell Lang, and James K. Luiselli, Oxford University Press.
© Oxford University Press (2025). DOI: 10.1093/oso/9780197635841.003.0017

components used in the overall model. Information about LEAP and how to start a replication site is available at https://morgridge.du.edu/pele-center.

17.3 LEAP Treatment Summary Table

Treatment summary: LEAP Preschool Model

Treatment description: LEAP Preschool is a comprehensive treatment model that relies on groups of providers in educational settings and neurotypical age peers as intervention agents. Operating as a true transdisciplinary team, educators (early childhood educators [ECEs] and early childhood special educators [ECSEs]), paraeducators, and related services personnel (speech language pathologists, occupational therapists, physical therapists, Board-Certified Behavioral Analysts) collaboratively plan and deliver instruction within the context of typical preschool routines. Class peers play a key role in facilitating the social and communicative skills of children with autism, and they serve as continuous models of desired behavior during embedded instructional opportunities facilitated by adults. The LEAP model also includes coaching for adult family members in routines at home and in the community that they perceive to be most stressful.

Expected outcomes: Based upon extant research findings, we observe that high-fidelity LEAP sites achieve consistent positive outcomes in the communicative, social, cognitive, and adaptive domains. Similarly, we also observe reductions in autism symptomology. Social validity and maintenance data generally show that LEAP participants maintain gains into elementary school and beyond. This effect is enhanced when children continue to be educated in inclusive classrooms. Direct observational comparisons between typical preschool children and LEAP participants with autism show that the social and engagement behaviors between these two groups are very similar after 2 years of intervention.

Methods: LEAP utilizes a wide variety of evidence-based instructional strategies that can be easily incorporated into a typical set of preschool routines while ensuring maximum social and instructional inclusion. Transdisciplinary teams of adults primarily use some version of child-initiated learning strategies focused on the goals and objectives identified in children's individualized education plans (IEPs). Extensive use is also made of visual supports throughout the day, maximizing the predictability of each daily routine, embedding hundreds of learning opportunities across the preschool day, and reviewing child data at the end of each day. The coaching provided to the adult family members and other caregivers is based upon their selection of home and community routines that are most challenging for them. Coaches provide direct support during these routines to enhance their predictability and ensure that adult directions are simple and clear, that children's approximations toward appropriate engagement is consistently reinforced, and that adults identify when they feel confident and comfortable with less support.

Expertise required: A wide range of practitioners and peers have been successful at implementing LEAP. In fact, we have found no correlation between degree status and years of experience as predictors of LEAP replication success. However, studies have shown a very powerful and direct linear relationship between scores on our fidelity measure, the LEAP quality program indicators (LEAP QPI), and child outcomes.

Risks and negative side effects: There have been no adverse effects reported in any studies on LEAP. However, it is essential to note that across both group and single-case studies, very high levels of treatment fidelity have been achieved. Where no or poor fidelity data are available, it is a risk to assume that positive child and family outcomes will accrue.

Additional considerations and limitations: In most cases, establishing a high-fidelity LEAP replication site requires 2 years of coaching. In addition, because of the requirements to have at least three adults in a class at all times, to have a minimum ratio of two typically developing peers for each child with autism, and to provide regular opportunities for all providers to plan together to deliver instruction during typical preschool routines, many programs need time and new resources to create these conditions.

17.4 Introduction

17.4.1 Intervention Description

The LEAP Preschool model is a fully inclusive, transdisciplinary model of service delivery used to remediate the core social, communication, and behavior deficits in children with autism and other developmental disabilities. LEAP is grounded in the principles of applied behavior analysis delivered within the context of an inclusive classroom setting.

The LEAP Preschool model began in 1981 as a model demonstration program funded by the Handicapped Children's Early Education Program, US Department of Education. LEAP was initially funded to demonstrate the efficacy of inclusion for young children with autism. In the 40-plus-year history of LEAP, the classrooms have been the site for extensive research and training activities. LEAP research initiatives have focused on demonstrating the unique contributions of specific program components to child and family behavior change. Over 30 peer-reviewed studies have demonstrated the efficacy of the LEAP model as a comprehensive program as well as the strategies used for teaching peer-related social skills, communication skills, and cognitive and preacademic skills. Additional studies have demonstrated parents' skill acquisition and subsequent changes in child behavior in home settings that are attributable to LEAP's family skill training.

LEAP classrooms are operated through partner local education agencies (LEAs), including school districts, Head Start grantees, and private childcare programs. Because of the variation in lead agencies, the size of LEAP classrooms varies from site to site and has included classrooms with as few as 12 and as many as 22 students. This variability in class size means it is important that classrooms maintain an appropriate ratio of young children with autism or other developmental disabilities and typically developing preschoolers. Our research and years of implementation experience have demonstrated that maintaining a ratio of at least two nondisabled children for each child with autism is crucial to implementation fidelity, and a classroom should have no more than six children with IEPs. Children with autism should start as close to 3 years old as possible and, based on the importance of peers in the inclusive classroom, we recommend mixed-age preschool classrooms (3-, 4-, and 5-year-olds).

Staffing of LEAP classrooms varies by LEA but with a standard that includes at least three adults present in LEAP classrooms each day. The most common staffing is with an ECSE teacher and two instructional assistants, but classrooms led by ECE teachers and co-teaching arrangements (ECSE & ECE teachers collaborating together) are also common. Related service providers such as speech and language specialists, occupational therapists, and physical therapists are also included as members of the transdisciplinary team. This will be addressed in more detail below. In the service of promoting child skill generalization, LEAP teams practice a transdisciplinary model of service delivery. That is, all staff engage in role exchange on a planned, daily basis, taking on a variety of classroom responsibilities.

LEAP classrooms vary in length and number of days children attend per week based on the structure of the LEA operating the classroom. The most common format consists of two half-day sessions with children attending school 4 days per week. This format provides approximately 11 hours of classroom time per week (2 hours 45 minutes per day for 4 days) with the fifth day used by the classroom team to engage in crucial teaming activities, including curriculum planning, individualized planning, collaboration, and family visits/communication, which is part of LEAP's broader family skill training component. Family skill training begins with staff delivering the nine modules of behavior teaching strategies, resulting in families delivering intervention throughout the day in home and community settings. Families determine the contexts in which training occurs by nominating routines that are of a particular level of difficulty.

17.4.2 Rationale and Objectives

Before discussing specific strategies that are foundational to the implementation of LEAP, it is important to understand that the LEAP model has a number of guiding principles that form the foundation of the model, all of which are consistent with broad early childhood best practice guidelines. These specific principles are as follows: (a) Inclusion begins full-time from day one. Children with autism and other developmental disabilities are provided with the necessary level of prompting and individualized support to participate in all classroom activities. (b) The design of LEAP classrooms begins with establishing a high-quality setting for typically developing children. LEAP has been implemented effectively in classrooms utilizing a variety of early childhood models and preschool/pre-K curricula. (c) Typically developing children play a major intervention role in LEAP. The children are provided with comprehensive, daily instruction to facilitate the social and communicative behaviors of peers with autism. (d) Learning objectives are written so that teaching continues until generalized behavior change is achieved. Learning objectives are further described according to relevant prompting hierarchies. Thus, individualized data are collected on children's behavioral movement toward independent performance, not in terms of percentage of correct responses, trials accomplished, or similar indices. (e) Skill training for families focuses on providing adult family members with the behavioral teaching strategies sufficient for them to experience less stress and more pleasure in daily routines such as meals, bedtime, dressing, and community outings. Specifically, parents are coached in home and community settings of their choice to master skills around understanding and shaping child behaviors, giving effective directions, using reinforcement, teaching new skills, and encouraging language and communication. (f) Intensity in the LEAP model is not defined by hours per week that individuals are paid to deliver service. The algorithm defining intensity is far more complex and includes, for each developmental domain of concern, the following factors: (a) number of opportunities to respond; (b) the functionality of objectives chosen; (c) the selection of an instructional method that maximizes children's engagement and minimizes errors; (d) the coaching of staff to deliver the chosen intervention with fidelity; and (e) the use of data systems and decision-making rules that minimize children's exposure to less-than-optimal interventions; (f) LEAP utilizes a *variety* of evidence-based intervention approaches that lend themself to fidelity implementation within an inclusive early childhood environment.

17.4.3 Considerations for Implementation

This section provides a brief overview of key intervention elements of the LEAP model including peer-mediated instruction, embedded instruction, incidental teaching, systematic data collection, and family support.

Peer-Mediated Instruction. The social skill deficits of young children with autism are well established (Strain, 1990). In fact, one of the defining characteristics of the diagnosis is the atypical ways these children interact with peers, family members, and others with whom they come into contact. However, we also know that social skills deficits occur in many children both with and without disabilities. As such, promoting the social development of children with autism and nondisabled children is one of the primary goals of the LEAP model. While a significant amount of preschool inclusion research has concluded that young children with social delays engage in social interactions more frequently in inclusive settings than in noninclusive settings, mere placement in an inclusive environment does not automatically result in increased social acceptance or the modeling of desired peer behavior (Gresham & Gresham, 1982; Guralnick, 1990; Guralnick & Groom, 1988; Peck & Cooke, 1983; Schultz & Turnbull, 1983; Striefel et al., 1991). To address these significant social delays and maximize the positive impact of the inclusive early childhood environment, LEAP classrooms implement a four-part approach to the implementation of a peer-mediated social skills package.

Direct Instruction of Key Social Behaviors. Instruction in peer-mediated social skills focuses on five simple behaviors that previous research has indicated are important for social participation and the development of friendships. They are

(a) initiating an interaction; (b) giving a toy or item; (c) asking for a toy or item; (d) giving a play direction; and (e) giving a complement.

Instruction in these core skills is taught to the entire class, one at a time, during a planned social skills instruction lesson during Large Group/Circle Time. Instruction follows a specific scope and sequence that includes (a) describing the skills, (b) demonstrating the skill correctly adult to adult, (c) demonstrating the skill incorrectly (doing it wrong) adult to adult and then correcting the mistake, (d) having a child demonstrate with adult, and (e) having a child demonstrate with another child. Instruction continues daily until classroom teachers are observing children use the targeted skill across the day. Unlike most curricula, the length of time spent teaching each skill is specific to the children in the class instead of tied to a specific number of days or weeks of instruction. Some skills might be mastered quickly, in just a couple weeks, while others might require a month or longer of repeated, daily instruction before children begin using the skill across the day.

Embedding Peer Social Opportunities Across the Day. Since instruction is occurring during daily Circle Time, the classroom team plans for child-to-child interactions to occur as part of planned, ongoing daily classroom routines. These embedded peer social interactions are instrumental in ensuring children are practicing the targeted social behavior(s) with enough intensity to ensure the skills are learned, and eventually generalized to other less structured times of the day. Planned, embedded social interactions can include routines like a child acting as the classroom greeter, a child inviting the next child to a consistent daily routine like signing in, using a child to give their peers the "5-Minute Warning" before clean-up, having a child pass out and collect Circle props or materials, a child inviting a peer to line up for outside time, and/or a child inviting a child to a special art project or activity. In fact, we would suggest that all of these examples would be consistent peer social routines that would be important in creating sufficient practice opportunities to master peer social interactions.

Adult Prompting of Peer Social Interactions. Building on the planned, embedded social opportunities described above, teachers look for naturally occurring opportunities for children to interact during child-directed/child-choice activities across the day such as Center/Free Play Time and Outside Time. During these times, adults focus on children's play and ask themselves, "Are peer social interactions occurring?" And, if not, what could they do to promote and support interactions during play. One important tip is that if adults are active in children's play (e.g., in the Dramatic Play area with the children sitting at the table), then children's social bids and interactions tend to be directed toward the adult in that area. Thus, teachers in LEAP classrooms learn to monitor and observe children's play and only step into play when optimum "teachable" moments occur. For example, if an adult is watching children play in the Dramatic Play area and sees that children are primarily engaged in parallel play, the adult can step in, model social interactions, and/or prompt the children to interact using the targeted social skill.

Systematic Reinforcement of Targeted Social Behaviors. The final component of the LEAP social skills package is developing a system to reinforce children when they utilize the targeted peer social skill. Reinforcers can take many forms, but our standard strategy is the use of Super Stars, simple star necklaces made by the children in the classroom. During the social skills lesson, the teacher will remind children that if the teachers "catch them" using the specific, targeted social skill to play with their friends, they might receive a Super Star. It is important to recognize that because children may have varying social skills to begin with, the Super Stars are reserved for what the teachers determine to be "effortful" behavior. So, if two nondisabled "best friends" are observed using the targeted skill, teachers might respond with positive descriptive feedback, a high five, and encouragement to use the skill with another child. Similarly, if a peer uses the targeted skill with a child with social delays, and they respond appropriately, the teacher can give Super Stars to both children. After Centers, when the class comes back together for the next Large Group time, the classroom teacher takes a moment to reflect on the targeted Social Skill and recognize the children that earned a Super Star using songs, cheers, or even items from the classroom Treasure Chest.

Embedded Instruction. Also known as embedded learning opportunities (ELOs), embedded instruction involves incorporating opportunities for children to learn and use specific, targeted skills within planned, consistently occurring classroom routines. To best understand how these skills are embedded into the classroom day, one first has to understand how LEAP breaks a typical classroom day down into Routines^3 or, Routines within Routines within Routines. This starts with a predictable classroom schedule that is then broken down into the specific activities that children do across the day. For clarity's sake, we have adopted the following terms to describe the different levels of routines: *Events*, *Activities*, and *Routines.*

Events (Routine^1) are the primary parts of the daily schedule that would be represented on the visual schedule in the classroom, for example (a) Arrival; (b) Table Time; (c) Circle Time; (d) Centers/Play Time; (e) Story Circle; (f) Snack; (g) Outside, Small Groups; (h) Goodbye Circle; and (i) Departure.

Activities (Routines^2) are the specific components of the Event, or said another way, they are the consistent activities within the Event. Each Activity within the Event ideally happens every day. For example, Arrival could include (a) saying goodbye to parents; (b) finding your cubby, (c) taking out your snack and home folder and putting them in the appropriate place; (d) hanging up your coat and backpack; (e) washing hands; (f) emotions check-in; and (g) choosing a table to play.

Every classroom will have its own unique daily schedule (Events) and its own sets of Activities. Remember, *only* activities that take place *every day* as part of the Event count when creating Routines^3. If an Activity only happens occasionally it does not work well for creating predictable routines.

Finally, Routines (Routines^3) are the steps that a child will engage in to complete each Activity. These are the specific steps (or task analysis) for the Activity and the level at which embedded instruction occurs. Using the example above, we can choose one of the Activities and further define the steps the child will undertake to complete the Activity. Just like with the Events and the Activities, these Routines should happen in a consistent way every day. So for *Emotions Check In* the child needs to (a) initiate to helper (get their attention); (b) ask for their name/picture (show helper which one is yours if needed); (c) accept their name/picture when it is offered; (d) respond to the helpers prompt of "How do you feel today?"; and (e) put their name/picture in the pocket associated with how they are feeling (see Table 17.1).

It is at this level, the level of Routines, that embedded instruction occurs. In this example the embedded instruction goals could be recognizing/identifying their name or picture, initiating to a peer, and demonstrating emotional literacy or expressing how they are feeling. With these Routines[3] and ELOs carefully planned and incorporated across the classroom day, it is possible to provide children with hundreds of planned instructional opportunities in a single day that focus on supporting the child's active engagement and participation in the classroom.

Incidental Teaching. As LEAP serves children diagnosed with autism in a fully inclusive environment from day one, it is crucial to have a primary instructional strategy that allows teachers to provide individualized instruction to all students and to capitalize on the numerous teachable moments that can and do occur across the day. To do this effectively, LEAP classrooms utilize incidental teaching as a primary instructional strategy in the classroom. Incidental teaching has been used

Table 17.1 Routines[3]

Event (Routine[1])	Activity (Routine[2])	Routine (Routine[3])
Arrival	Say Goodbye to Parents	Parent says goodbye to child, child says goodbye to parent, gives hug or high five
	Find Cubby	Walk to cubby, find cubby by referencing name and/or picture
	Unpack Backpack	Unzip backpack, take out snack, put in snack bin, take out home folder, put in folder bin
	Put Things in Cubby	Hang up backpack, hang up coat
	Wash Hands	Get soap, turn on water, wash hands, turn off water, dry hands, throw away towel
	Emotions Check-In	Initiate interaction with helper (get their attention), ask for their name/picture (show helper which one is theirs if needed), accept their name/picture from helper, respond to helper's prompt, "How do you feel today?," put picture/name in associated pocket
	Pick a Table Activity	Pick a table picture, walk to table, put picture in box, sit down, play

effectively to teach language and communication, play skills, self-help skills, and cognitive skills to children with autism, children diagnosed with other developmental disabilities, and neurotypical children (Hart & Risley, 1975; Kohler et al., 1997; McGee et al., 1999; Strain & Bovey, 2011). Incidental teaching differs from other teaching methodologies in that it includes an intentional step in which adults encourage and wait for the child to initiate the teaching episode/interaction. This simple step has proved valuable in teaching a variety of skills to children with autism and, in the generalization of skills, as incidental teaching also helps support the development of social initiations. The comprehensive use of incidental teaching also provides (a) the ability to provide instruction across people and settings; (b) the flexibility to utilize a variety of instructional stimuli based on the child's interest; (c) the use of natural reinforcers; and (d) the enhanced generalization of skills to new environments.

17.4.4 Systematic Data Collection and Data-Based Decision-Making

The LEAP model utilizes a continuous and dynamic assessment process to maximize developmental gains for children with IEPs. This starts with learning objectives that are written such that instruction continues until generalized behavior change is achieved. Learning objectives are described according to relevant prompting hierarchies, and data are collected on children's behavioral movement toward the rigorous standard of independent, generalized performance, not in terms of percent correct, trials accomplished, or other similar indices. To accomplish these outcomes, LEAP's data system has evolved over the last 40 years with four core principles in mind.

The data system must be useable. One of the biggest barriers to the successful use of data systems is that they are cumbersome for teachers and staff. In over 40 years of working with inclusive classrooms, we have repeatedly seen classroom teams that collect data, file it away, and do not look at it until it is time for quarterly, 6-month, or annual reviews. Or we have seen situations when classrooms are understaffed or stressed by child behaviors and data systems are abandoned because they were too difficult or time consuming to implement—exactly the opposite of what teachers need in these circumstances. So the development of a data system that is intuitive; easy to use for teachers, instructional assistants, and related service providers; and is useable in assessing behavior change over time has been a priority.

The data system must be linked to instructional strategies. As described earlier, the majority of instruction in LEAP classrooms is delivered through incidental teaching and embedded teaching episodes. Developing a data system that supports teachers' documentation of what is occurring during these brief teaching episodes has been the priority. Thus, it made sense to develop a system that tracks the levels (or amount) of prompting and/or assistance related to children's successful participation across the classroom day.

The system must be accurate (enough). With the LEAP data system, we have moved away from trying to track data on a trial-by-trial basis. Instead, we use a (relatively) subjective system that assigns a single data point for each goal that best represents the child's generalized performance across all instructional opportunities for that skill over the course of the day. This system helps us assess the child's overall performance and participation, not just how they did in one activity, with one set of materials or with one adult. As instruction occurs across the day, teachers use tic marks to represent the prompting level or assistance needed at that time. Ideally, by the end of the day, there are numerous tic marks for each individualized goal and the teacher can then circle the number that best represents the child's overall performance across the day.

The system must be responsive to changes in child behavior. One of the primary functions of a data system is to show behavior change over time. Data in LEAP classrooms are collected daily to help show these changes in behavior but perhaps even more importantly to help teachers provide instruction and prompting at the correct level to drive progress. Providing instruction/prompting at the correct level, within the Zone of Proximal Development, is ever changing, and our data system helps us make these important instructional decisions. So what happened today informs how one prompts tomorrow, and what happens tomorrow will drive instruction on the next day.

Using these principles, LEAP's data system has proven to be an effective tool not just for showing progress over time but also for helping teachers identify how to provide instruction at the right level, within the Zone of Proximal Development (Vygotsky, 1978), and to support the child's continued movement toward independent and generalized use of the targeted skill(s).

17.4.5 Family Support

The final core strategy is behavioral skill training for the families of the young children attending LEAP classrooms. LEAP's policies and practices related to working with families of young children with disabilities reflect (a) a family-centered approach to early intervention that respects families as decision-makers, (b) is responsive to the needs of families, (c) conforms with families values and beliefs, (d) builds on families strengths, and (e) focuses on the development of functional skills across environments.

This behavioral skill training component focuses on teaching parents and/or caregivers the basic principles of behavior management as well as strategies for teaching children new skills. Training activities can include didactic instruction (i.e., a behavior skill training curriculum for parents has been developed and field-tested over the last 40 years) as well as individual "practice sessions" in home and community settings. Practice sessions focus on family-identified outcomes, both for their child and family. Specific intervention strategies for achieving desired outcomes (e.g., child will remain seated at the dinner table and eat a variety of food items) are modeled (by the family service coordinator) for the family in the natural environment. Family members then "practice" these skills with their child, with the family service coordinator providing encouragement and positive/corrective feedback.

17.5 Research Background

17.5.1 Search Procedures

This research description section is comprised of four distinct parts: (a) initial randomized controlled trial (RCT) and related follow-up studies; (b) single-case design studies to examine individual active ingredients of LEAP; (c) clustered RCT and 4-year follow-up; and (d) sustainability measurement development and evaluation. These studies represent a complete portrayal of all studies funded to document the overall efficacy of the LEAP model as well as its discrete components. In the interest of full disclosure, this chapter's first author was the principal investigator on all studies.

17.5.2 Overview of Studies Identified

In 1981, simultaneous with the initiation of LEAP, we were funded by the National Institutes of Mental Health (NIMH) to conduct an RCT of LEAP. The study called for the diagnosis of children 3 to 5 years of age by licensed child psychiatrists and the subsequent random assignment to attend LEAP or the only available community site at the time in Pittsburgh, Pennsylvania. At the end of Year 2 of the 5-year project, the NIMH conducted a preplanned site review. At that time the site visit team reviewed preliminary data specific to children's changes in cognitive growth, social interactions, language acquisition, and autism symptoms. In each case, there were very large, nonoverlapping differences favoring LEAP classroom participants. The site visit panel concluded that the study, as designed, should be halted because of ethical concerns with continuing random assignments. Instead, the panel recommended that we continue to enroll children in LEAP and utilize single-case designs to assess the impact of discrete LEAP components on specific child and family outcomes. The site visit team also suggested that we continue to follow LEAP graduates and report on the preliminary findings from the RCT. The results from those follow-ups and preliminary data reporting were as follows: (1) Children in LEAP generally showed significant reductions in autistic symptoms after 2 years of intervention, whereas comparison children did not (Strain & Cordisco, 1993); (2) children in LEAP made marked developmental progress on intellectual and language measures, whereas comparison children did not (Hoyson et al., 1985; Strain & Hoyson, 2000); (3) on observational measures taken in school and at home, LEAP children were far more socially engaged and appropriate (Strain et al., 1996); (4) no negative and some positive (e.g., better social skills, fewer disruptive behaviors) outcomes accrued to typical children in the LEAP model (Strain, 1987); (5) gains for LEAP children maintained following program participation with 24 of 51 children enrolled in regular education classes (oldest cohort in college at the time) with no signs of developmental regression (Strain & Hoyson, 2000); and (6) adult family members who participated in LEAP were significantly less likely than comparison families to show signs of significant stress and depression following the early intervention experience (Strain, 1987).

In addition to these enrollment-specific results enumerated above, we have considered it to be ethically and scientifically necessary to conduct various substudies to demonstrate the efficacy of key model components that represent specific replication training content. These include (a) teaching typical children to facilitate the social and communicative competence of their class peers with autism, (b) teaching IEP objectives within routine class activities, and (c) providing extensive skill training for family members in order to address child behavior issues in home and community settings. The summarized results from these areas of study follow: (1) Typically developing peers as young as 36 months can be taught to utilize facilitative social and communicative initiations with their peers with autism (Goldstein & Wickstrom, 1986; Strain & Danko, 1995). (2) Peers' use of facilitative strategies results in higher rates of communicative interaction for preschoolers with autism (Goldstein & Wickstrom, 1986; Kohler et al, 1997; Strain, 1987). (3) The peer facilitative strategies produce "day one" effects, suggesting that the delayed social and communicative abilities of many young children with autism may be attributable, in part, to the socially nonresponsive, developmentally segregated settings in which they are most often educated (Kohler & Strain, 1992; Strain & Odom, 1986). (4) For many children who receive the peer-mediated intervention, their eventual level of social participation falls within the typical range for their age cohorts (Strain, 1987). (5) The potency of the peer-mediated intervention extends across both settings (Strain, 1987; Strain & Hoyson, 2000) and time (Strain et al., 1996). (6) The naturalistic or incidental teaching used at LEAP to influence cognitive outcomes yields approximately 2 months developmental gain for each month enrolled (Hoyson et al., 1985; Strain & Cordisco, 1993). (7) When compared to one-to-one, tutorial instruction, the LEAP incidental teaching model yields more active engagement and more complex developmental skills by children with autism *and* their typical peers (Kohler et al., 1997). (8) LEAP's parent skill training component produces broad-based and long-lasting effects, including (a) generalized use of skills in naturalistic contexts; (b) child behavior improvements in active engagement and challenging behaviors; (c) high levels of family satisfaction with the training program; and (d) decreased levels of stress and depression, especially as families exit the intervention program and move to what they perceive to be less supportive service programs (Strain, 1985, 1987). Together, over 28 peer-reviewed component analysis studies far exceed the "efficacious" intervention criteria for within-subject designs as established by Division 12 of the American Psychological Association (Lonigan et al., 1998). Specifically, the peer social initiation component has been replicated across 88 participants; the incidental teaching component has been replicated across 24 participants; and the family component has been replicated across 50 participants. Across all single-case design studies, children were between 36 and 54 months of age when enrolled and all had received an autism diagnosis by at least one child psychiatrist. Their Childhood Autism Rating Scale (CARS) scores placed them in the "moderate" to "severe" range.

In 2006, we instituted a clustered randomized comparison design study in which preschool classrooms were assigned, via a table of random numbers, to either the full-scale LEAP replication training or to a comparison condition in which preschool staff were provided LEAP intervention manuals only. We elected to employ this particular comparison group arrangement for the following reasons. First, our prior experience using a general community standard of practice versus the LEAP model suggested that similar comparisons may be trivial, providing little useful data. Second, our prior experience establishing over 150 replications across the United States suggested that child outcome data closely matched that of our original experimental cohort. Third, since the LEAP intervention occurs at the classroom level, it followed logically to randomly assign classrooms. Finally, since our treatment manuals have been commercially available, over 1000 districts have purchased these materials and only a handful have been involved in formal replication. Thus, we believe that using our treatment manuals without follow-along training was a logical standard for comparison purposes.

In this study we recruited on a nationwide basis to promote maximum generalization of findings (address external validity issues). In our recruitment we included large metropolitan districts, suburban districts, rural districts, geographic areas where all staff have advanced degrees, geographic areas where personnel shortages were critical, districts that primarily provide inclusionary services, and districts where very few children with autism were in inclusive settings.

Prior to random assignment to study groups, we "over-recruited" classrooms that were *willing and able* to be LEAP replication sites. Having this unique universe of potential sites was crucial for the following reasons. First, we strongly support Kazdin's (2003) position that willingness or implementation commitment must be equivalent across groups in any psychosocial trial. Second, restricting ourselves to "able" sites alleviated a number of potential confounds. Specifically, "able" sites shared these commonalities: (a) intensity of services provided; (b) enrollment of children with autism in inclusive settings; (c) set ratio of adults to children (at least 1:4) and a minimum of three adults in the classroom; and (d) minimum ratio of nondisabled peers to children with autism (2:1). Each of these variables has been related to developmental outcomes for children with autism (Lovaas, 1982; McGee et al., 1999; Strain & Hoyson, 2000; Strain et al., 1998). To provide data to address a number of generalization issues, we let variables of provider education and experience vary as they might.

During Year 1, we recruited 30 classrooms from which we randomly assigned 15 to our full replication protocol and 15 to receive treatment manuals only. Because of uncontrollable decisions specific to district-related child placements, we ended up with 12 classrooms in the manuals-only comparison condition. Specifically, three of the designated comparison classes did not ultimately have children with autism enrolled as planned.

In Year 3, we recruited 26 additional classrooms and randomly assigned 13 classrooms to the intervention protocol and 13 classrooms to the manuals-only comparison condition. Again, as a result of district decision-making around child placement, two of the assigned comparison classes did not have children enrolled with autism as planned. Across all sites and all years, we had the following study participants: (a) 123 experimental teachers and 107 comparison teachers and (b) 177 experimental children with autism and 117 comparison children with autism.

Preschools assigned to the comparison condition were provided LEAP's intervention manuals and training presentation materials (PowerPoint presentations) for (a) family skill training; (b) social skills training; and (c) design and operation of the inclusive classroom.

Study outcome highlights are as follows: (a) both groups were equivalent on all child measures prior to intervention; (b) teacher experience and training was equivalent across groups; (c) we experienced less than 3% attrition in both groups between initial assessment and year 2 follow-up measures (we detected no initial differences between participants who stayed versus those who did not and following Hedges [2007], we "estimated" the treatment effects for attrition Ss by using a "worst case" scenario, thereby biasing against finding group differences); (d) on our direct observation, fidelity of intervention measure (LEAP QPI) intervention classes were implementing over 90% of all program components after 2 years, whereas comparison classes were implementing less than 50% of practices; (e) on standardized measures of cognitive development (Mullen) and language development (PLS-4), children in intervention classes made, on average, twice the developmental gain as comparison class children; (f) on a standardized measure of autism symptom severity (CARS), children in the treatment classes showed an average reduction in severity of 6.1 points as compared to an average reduction of 2.8 points for comparison class children; (g) on a standardized measure of social behavior growth (SSRS), children in intervention classes showed an average positive percentile change of 28.6 points versus 11.9 points for comparison class children; and (h) on the problem behavior scale of this same measure (SSRS), children in treatment classes showed an average positive percentile change of 7.0 versus 4.3 points for the comparison cohort. Multivariate repeated-measures analysis of variance showed all differences between groups to be significant at the .05 level and beyond. This analytic method was chosen because we had (a) no "missing data"; (b) the assessment schedule was consistent across all participants; and (c) this analytic method was appropriate to the basic study design, and multivariate repeated-measures analysis of variance has been used in all prior early childhood autism RCTs. Following Hedges's (2007) recommendation, we adjusted student's t and degrees of freedom in line with total sample size, cluster size, and intraclass correlations (.22 in this study) prior to conducting these statistics. The significant group differences represent effect sizes ranging from .59 to .92. Effect sizes were based on Glass's estimator (Hedges, 1981) and all reached statistical significance. In effect, then, the resulting data represent an appropriately conservative estimate of group difference. Additional methods used to mitigate bias included (a) keeping assessors naïve to study hypotheses; (b) having a personnel "firewall" separating staff who were working with sites to reach fidelity and those collecting outcome data; (c) having data collection, scoring, and storage subject to multiple reliability/accuracy checks; and (d) having outcome data processed independent of the principal investigator.

In addition to the analyses discussed above, we were able to detect important correlations between our fidelity (LEAP QPI) measure scores and child outcomes in our treatment group. Put simply, "best outcome" was associated with the highest levels of fidelity on each outcome index (gain score) (ranged from $r = .67$ for SSRS data to $r = .86$ for PLS-4 data). These significant positive correlations, when combined with the lack of significant correlation between initial child performance and ultimate outcomes and the lack of significant correlation between teacher characteristics and outcomes, speak to the essential focus in autism studies on fidelity of treatment (Dunlap & Carr, 2007). This clustered RCT (Strain & Bovey, 2011) was reviewed by the US Department of Education's What Works Clearinghouse and given its highest methodological rating.

The 4-year follow-up to the clustered RCT was designed to answer three broad questions, as described next.

What Is the Stability of Classroom Placement Across 4 Years (K–3)? One of the more interesting data points from this follow-up study is the absolute consistency in placement options across time. We observed *no* examples of children (total N = 108) moving from an "autism" labeled setting to an inclusive environment nor did we see any examples of children being placed in a more restrictive setting once they were originally in an inclusive kindergarten program. Interestingly enough, a majority of sites that enrolled study graduates from both study arms in "autism" classes at kindergarten had adopted brand-named curricula and instructional practices that aimed to prepare children for inclusive settings. At least through third grade, this hoped-for outcome was not observed. Based on prior research on K–12 placements, these results should not be surprising (McNulty et al., 1988). Moreover, the factor that apparently controlled many initial kindergarten decisions, namely the district's unilateral policy regarding an appropriate setting for children with autism, is consistent with our team's prior analysis of placement decisions in ECSE classes in Pennsylvania (Miller et al., 1991).

What Is Driving Initial Kindergarten Placement Decisions? We found what must be considered a disturbing pattern of "child-independent" decisions for individuals in both arms of the study. Simply put, where children were placed was driven by a district-level decision conditioned on opinions about "other" individuals with autism and/or historical precedent. Operational policies varied widely. For example, several districts placed children from both arms of the study in "autism" classes because those children had, at least at one point, that diagnosis. A couple of districts essentially argued that children had made progress in an inclusive preschool and therefore they should be enrolled in a similar kindergarten. On occasion, assertive action by parents altered these policy positions.

What Do Children in LEAP RCT Look Like 4 Years Away From Intervention? To examine this question, we assessed original RCT participants in both study arms using a battery of measures, including (a) Kaufman Brief Achievement Test; (b) Test of Oral Language Development—4; (c) Childhood Autism Rating System; (d) Leiter Brief IQ Test; (e) Vineland Adaptive Behavior Scales; and (f) Social Skills Improvement System (Prosocial Behavior).

From 1 to 4 years of this follow-up study, we experienced an overall attrition rate of 32%, evenly divided between children from LEAP and comparison preschool classes.

Mean group differences on the Kaufman of 86 versus 95 for LEAP graduates were not statistically significant using a two-tailed t-test. Similarly, mean TOLD-4 differences of 81 versus 88 for LEAP graduates were not statistically significant using a two-tailed t-test. Leiter mean differences favoring LEAP graduates of 76 versus 93 were statistically significant at .05, $t = 2.12$, $df = 177$. The effect size for this finding was .42. Finally, mean group differences on the Vineland of 94 for comparison children and 98 for LEAP graduates were not statistically significant.

Considering the Social Skills Improvement System, higher scores represent greater perceived social skills by teachers. Differences favoring LEAP participants (31 versus 39.8) were highly statistically significant ($t = 2.99$, $df = 180$, $p < .01$). The effect size for this finding was .52.

Overall, these data indicate that *both* groups of children were doing quite well 4 years away from intervention with all measures favoring LEAP graduates. In the course of this analysis we came to notice a very interesting trend in the data as they relate to class placement. We noticed that children with very similar CARS scores were often in different placements at kindergarten and their subsequent scores on the CARS and other measures were profoundly different 4 years post.

To examine this trend, we went into the database and collected as many pairs of children, regardless of study group, who left preschool with CARS scores within three points of each other and where one member of the pair was subsequently placed in a kindergarten with 80% or greater inclusion or less. We were able to detect 21 such pairs. Our rationale for creating pairs based upon the CARS is that severity of symptoms is generally considered to be the key to determining a child's appropriate placement in a more inclusive environment (Handleman & Harris, 2008; Harris & Handleman, 1993).

For each outcome measure, large differences that were statistically significant at $p < .01$ using two-tailed t-tests were observed (Kaufman, $t = 2.92$, $df = 20$; TOLD, $t = 2.96$, $df = 20$; Leiter, $t = 3.11$, $df = 20$; Vineland $t = 2.99$, $df = 20$). The effect sizes for these findings were Kaufman, .72; TOLD, .66; Leiter, .71; and Vineland, .81. The mean CARS score difference post 4 years were significantly different in favor of the included member of the pairs (two-tailed $t = 2.99$, $df = 20$, $p < .01$). The effect size for this finding was .68.

Data on the Social Skills Improvement System revealed large differences of 43.4 versus 24.5 in favor of included children. This difference was highly significant ($t = 3.44$, $df = 20$, $p < .05$). The effect size for this finding was .48.

Since we collected multiple data points across years of the follow-up study, we were able to judge the stability of behavioral differences across school years. Looking at the data set specific to comparable children enrolled in more specialized versus inclusive settings, we can report that differences were evident at the end of the first follow-up year. Using growth curve analysis, we can further report that *no* significant trends were evident across follow-up years. In other words, behavioral differences at the end of the initial follow-up year remained consistent across all subsequent years. Therefore, one can consider the strong differences across placement years at Grade 3 as reflective of maintenance of behavior outcome difference across 4 years. In this regard, our follow-up data closely align with other early intervention follow-up studies (e.g., Abcedarian and Perry studies) where repeated assessment across years yielded stable patterns of outcome.

Taken together, the results specific to placement and outcome indicate to us that placement might better be considered as an independent rather than a dependent variable in outcome studies. To further explore these stark differences in outcome, we did follow-up interviews with study data collectors to get some indication of what might be at play to account for these differences. From these open-ended interviews, several themes emerged when these individuals talked about other than the measured differences between placements.

The first theme centered on curriculum, a variable we did not directly measure. In the inclusive settings the study children in these classes were full participants in the regular education curriculum. By contrast, in the more segregated settings, districts had often adopted remedial curricula, "autism" curricula, or developed their own "autism" curricula. These curricula, for the most part, were not focused on age- or grade-level academic content and in many ways actually mimicked content that children were exposed to at preschool (e.g., shapes, object names, colors, etc.). Put simply, data collectors felt that many children in less than fully inclusive settings were not challenged developmentally at school. Moreover, the observers could not recall that children in these settings were ever required to do work outside of school, namely, homework. In other words, children were apparently exposed to a very different curriculum at a very different dosage.

The second theme that emerged was related to the specific instructional supports offered by paraeducators in both types of settings. In the segregated contexts, paraeducator activities could be classified in two general ways, either (1) they were providing extremely high levels of support to children, which discouraged children's independent participation, or (2) they were seldom seen to provide direct instruction to children and instead spent most of their time doing housekeeping kinds of chores. Alternatively, in inclusive settings, paraeducators were regularly seen assisting children with academic assignments and particularly providing additional cues (e.g., models, partial physical prompts, prompts to peers) such that children completed tasks accurately and as independently as possible. Again, this observation perhaps speaks to a different "dosage" and quality of instruction.

The final theme that emerged involved the often talked about (but never directly measured!) concept in education of high expectations. This theme was manifest as follows. In segregated settings, observers noted that teachers rarely recognized, commented on, or praised children for correct responding related to preacademic or academic tasks. In contrast, the majority of their feedback to children was reflective of behavior management, encouraging compliance with requests, and general task engagement. Relatedly, when children were not correct in responding, they seldom received corrective feedback. In inclusive settings, teaching staff regularly gave children feedback on their class work, grading activities, suggesting correct answers, and generally holding all children to a standard of accuracy.

One of our greatest challenges in the early intervention field is closing the gap between what is known about effective instructional practices and the sustained use of those practices in public school settings (Stain et al., 2012). Tremendous strides have been made over the last 30 years in identifying discrete instructional tactics and in the development of comprehensive intervention programs at the early childhood level for children with autism (Odom, Boyd, et al., 2010; Odom, Collet-Klingenberg et al., 2010). All too often, however, evidence-based interventions get adopted, were haphazardly supported at an administrative level, and ultimately dropped. The sustained use of evidence-based interventions by public school teachers has largely gone unstudied in the autism field. Yet we can draw some vital lessons as a conceptual starting point from the relatively long history of sustainability research in other areas of education and child mental health. For example, we know that sustainability is not guaranteed by better child outcomes; that sustainability efforts must be planned, purposeful, and targeted; that sustainability practices occur at the individual teacher level *and* at the larger policy and program levels; and that the factors that influence sustainability are, by and large, malleable (Aarons et al., 2011; Chambers, 2014; Saldana & Chamberlain, 2012). With these lessons in mind, this 4-year project had three overarching goals in the service of understanding the conditions under which teachers reach and sustain high levels of intervention fidelity across time: (a) to examine the use of a previously developed measure of sustainability in a large and diverse sample of LEAP replication sites; (b) to identify specific sustainability factors that predict teachers' initial and sustained fidelity; and (c) to lay the empirical foundation for building a professional development intervention package that can be used to enhance sustainability efforts across settings.

Over a 4-year period, we collected both treatment fidelity data (LEAP QPI) and data on the LEAP-Fidelity and Sustainability Tool (LEAP-FAST) Sustainability Measure across 150 replication sites. These sites ranged from 1 to 27 years after achieving initial fidelity. Thirty of the 150 sites were launched during the study period and thus we were able to determine if the LEAP-FAST would also predict time to reach initial treatment fidelity.

The LEAP-FAST is a nine-factor interview protocol consisting of these general factors: (1) functional leadership team, (2) staff readiness and buy-in, (3) family involvement, (4) strategies for promoting and sustaining program-wide implementation, (5) core LEAP features emphasized, (6) procedures for individualization in place, (7) staff capacity building in place, (8) implementation and outcome measures in place, and (9) personnel policies and fiscal policies in place.

In brief, the results show that (a) the LEAP-FAST factor structure was confirmed, (b) raters reach agreement levels above 85% on the LEAP-FAST and QPI, (c) programs that scored above 90% on the LEAP-FAST met fidelity criteria of 90% an average of 3 months quicker than lower scoring replication sites, and (d) regardless of years away from initial training and coaching to reach fidelity, replication sites maintained high fidelity when their LEAP-FAST scores were 90% or higher.

17.6 Practice Implications

17.6.1 Treatment Outcomes

Overall, LEAP outcome studies show that children with autism make significant development gains in cognition, communication, social skills, and adaptive skills and that these gains generalize to new settings and maintain across time, most particularly when future settings are fully inclusive.

17.6.2 Practice Implications Guidelines

On occasion, the expansion of evidence-based, service delivery options for young children with autism presents a dilemma for families. How does one choose an approach in the present-day situation where comparative outcome data are lacking? Service delivery systems, and in particular, public education entities, are presented with a similar dilemma when they try to make a choice around which early intervention model to adopt.

Over the last 40 plus years of research in the LEAP model, several data points can be useful to both families and service delivery systems. Each of these is briefly described next.

To the best of our knowledge, there is no known relationship between child outcomes in LEAP and children's initial cognitive, language, social and autism symptoms (Strain & Bovey, 2011). In fact, the correlation between these indices and outcome approaches zero! What does predict outcome then? Across both single-case designs and group studies, the fidelity with which the designated intervention is delivered has a direct and linear relationship with outcome (Strain et al., 2021), and the age at which children first access a LEAP classroom is correlated with outcomes in that the younger a child is when they start LEAP the better the outcome (Strain & Bovey, 2011). Considering these data, the major practice implications are these. One, when considering LEAP, the child's initial level of performance should not be of primary concern. Two, what needs to be in place in all LEAP sites is the quarterly use of our fidelity measure, the LEAP QPI, and practice-based coaching to ensure fidelity and sustainability of practices.

A second data point for consideration is the accumulated research on peers as agents of intervention for young children with autism. Four decades of research has shown that peers are at least as effective and often more effective agents of social skills intervention as are well-trained adults (Steed et al., 2021). Additionally, the mere presence of nondisabled peers has been shown to be a potent and cost-effective mechanism for promoting the maintenance and generalization of social skills by young children autism (Bryant & Fox, 1995; Hecimovic et al., 1985; Strain, 1984, 1985). Considering that deficits in the social relationship domain are a primary defining feature of autism, intervention approaches that provide no or only sporadic access to nondisabled peers and peer-mediated intervention may be precluding children with autism from arguably the most effective means of addressing this core deficit area. Our research also demonstrates that access to nondisabled peers alone may not produce significant outcomes, so it is considered a necessary, but not sufficient, model component. LEAP is certainly not the only inclusive model of early intervention, but research conducted at LEAP highlights the importance of nondisabled peers to any considerations around best practices.

17.7 References

Aarons, G. A., Hurlburt, M., & Horwitz, S. M. (2011). Advancing a conceptual model of evidence-based practice implementation in public service sectors. *Administration and Policy in Mental Health, 38*(1), 4–23. https://doi.org/10.1007/s10488-010-0327-7

Bryant, S. E., & Fox, S. K. (1995). Behavior modeling training and generalization: Interaction of learning point type and number of modeling scenarios. *Psychological Record, 45*(3), 495–503. https://doi.org/10.1007/BF03395157

Chambers, D. A. (2014). Guiding theory for dissemination and implementation research: A reflection on models used in research and practice. In R.S. Beida, & P.C. Kendall (Eds.), *Dissemination and implementation of evidence-based practices in child and adolescent mental health* (pp. 38–62). New York: Oxford University Press.

Dunlap, G., & Carr, E.G. (2007). Positive behavior support and developmental disabilities: A summary and analysis of research. In S. L. Odom, R. H. Horner, M. Snell, & J. Blacher (Eds.), *Handbook of developmental disabilities* (pp. 469–482). New York: Guilford.

Goldstein, H., & Wickstrom, S. (1986). Peer intervention effects on communicative interaction among handicapped and nonhandicapped preschoolers. *Journal of Applied Behavior Analysis, 19*, 209–214. https://psycnet.apa.org/doi/10.1901/jaba.1986.19-209

Gresham, F. M., & Gresham, G. N. (1982). Interdependent, dependent, and independent group contingencies for controlling disruptive behavior. *The Journal of Special Education, 16*(1), 101–110. https://doi.org/10.1177/002246698201600110

Guralnick, M. J. (1990). Social competence and early intervention. *Journal of Early Intervention, 14*(1), 3–14. https://doi.org/10.1177/105381519001400101

Guralnick, M. J., & Groom, J. M. (1988). Peer interactions in mainstreamed and specialized classrooms: A comparative analysis. *Exceptional Children, 54*(5), 415–425. https://doi.org/10.1177/001440298805400504

Harris, S., & Handleman, J. (Eds.). (1993). *Preschool education programs for children with autism.* Austin, TX: Pro-Ed.

Handleman, J., & Harris, S. (Eds.). (2008). *Preschool education programs for children with autism* (3rd ed.). Austin, TX: Pro-Ed.

Hart, B., & Risley, T. R. (1975). Incidental teaching of language in the preschool. *Journal of Applied Behavior Analysis, 8*(4), 411–420. https://doi.org/10.1901%2Fjaba.1975.8-411

Hecimovic, A., Fox, J. J., Shores, R. E., & Strain, P. S. (1985). An analysis of developmentally integrated and segregated free play settings and the generalization of newly-acquired social behaviors of socially withdrawn preschoolers. *Behavioral Assessment, 7*(4), 367–388.

Hedges, L. V. (1981). Distribution theory for Glass's estimator of effect size and related estimators. *Journal of Educational Statistics, 6*, 107–128. https://doi.org/10.2307/1164588

Hedges, L. V. (2007). Correcting a significance test for clustering. *Journal of Educational and Behavioral Statistics, 32*, 151–179. https://doi.org/10.3102/1076998606298040

Hoyson, M., Jamieson, B., & Strain, P.S. (1985). Individualized group instruction of normally developing and autistic-like children: The LEAP curriculum model. *Journal of the Division for Early Childhood, 8*, 157–172. https://doi.org/10.1177/105381518400800209

Kazdin, A. E. (Ed.). (2003). *Methodological issues and strategies in clinical research* (3rd ed.). Washington, DC: American Psychological Association.

Kohler, F. W., & Strain, P. S. (1992). Applied behavior analysis and the movement to restructure schools: Compatibility and opportunities for collaboration. *Journal of Behavioral Education, 2*, 367–390. https://doi.org/10.1007/BF00952355

Kohler, F. W., Strain, P. S., Hoyson, M., & Jamieson, B. (1997). Merging naturalistic teaching and peer-based strategies to address the IEP objectives of preschoolers with autism: an examination of structural and child behavior outcomes. *Focus on Autism and Developmental Disabilities, 12*(4), 196–206. https://doi.org/10.1177/108835769701200402

Lonigan, C. J., Elbert, J. C., & Johnson, S. B. (1998). Empirically supported psychosocial interventions for children: An overview. *Journal of Clinical and Child Psychology, 27*, 138–145. https://doi.org/10.1207/s15374424jccp2702_1

Lovaas, O. I. (1982, August). An overview of the young autism project. Paper presented at the meeting of the American Psychological Association, Washington, DC.

McGee, G. G., Morrier, M. J., & Daly, T. (1999). An incidental teaching approach to early intervention for toddlers with autism. *Journal of the Associate for Persons with Severe Handicaps, 24*(3), 133–146. https://doi.org/10.2511/rpsd.24.3.133

McNulty, B., Widerstrom, A. H., Goodwin, L. D., & Campbell, S. (1988). Who should be served, where and why: Local special education administrators' views. *Topics in Early Childhood Special Education, 8*, 51–60. https://doi.org/10.1177/027112148800800305

Miller, L. J., Boyd, K., Hunsicker, S., McKinley, J., Strain, P. S., & Wu, A. (1991). Effectiveness of integrated programming in early childhood. *PF/CEC Newsletter/Journal, 30*, 2–4.

Odom, S. L., Boyd, B. A., Hall, L. J., & Hume, K. (2010). Evaluation of comprehensive treatment models for individuals with autism spectrum disorders. *Journal of Autism and Developmental Disorders, 40*, 425–436. https://doi.org/10.1007/s10803-009-0825-1

Odom, S. L., Collet-Klingenberg, L., Rogers. S. J., & Hatton, D. D. (2010). Evidence-based practices in interventions for children and youth with autism spectrum disorders. *Preventing School Failure: Alternative Education for Children and Youth, 54*(4), 275–282. https://doi.org/10.1080/10459881003785506

Peck, C. A., & Cooke, T. P. (1983). Benefits of mainstreaming at the early childhood level: How much can we expect: *Analysis and Intervention in Developmental Disabilities, 3*, 1–22. https://doi.org/10.1016/0270-4684(83)90023-X

Saldana, L., & Chamberlain, P. (2012), Supporting implementation: The role of community development teams to build infrastructure. *American Journal of Community Psychology, 50*, 334–346. https://doi.org/10.1007/s10464-012-9503-0

Schultz, J. B., & Turnbull, A. P. (1983). *Mainstreaming handicapped students: A guide for classroom teachers* (2nd ed.). Boston: Allyn & Bacon.

Steed, E., Barton, E. E., & Strain, P. (2021). Instructional approaches that promote positive social outcomes for young children: A historical literature review. *Journal of Positive Behavior Interventions, 23*(3), 201–213. https://doi.org/10.1177/1098300720916717

Strain, P. S. (1984). Social behavior patterns of nonhandicapped and developmentally disabled friend pairs in mainstream preschools. *Analysis and Intervention in Developmental Disabilities, 4*, 15–28. https://doi.org/10.1016/0270-4684(84)90015-6

Strain, P. S. (1985). Social and non-social determinants of acceptability in handicapped preschool children. *Topics in Early Childhood Special Education, 4*, 47–58. https://doi.org/10.1177/027112148500400406

Strain, P. S. (1987). Parent training with young autistic children: A report on the LEAP model. *Zero to Three, 7*, 7–12.

Strain, P. S. (1990). LRE for preschool children with handicaps: What we know, what we should be doing. *Journal of Early Intervention, 14*, 305–311. https://doi.org/10.1177/105381519001400401

Strain, P. S., & Bovey, E. H. (2011). Randomized, controlled trial of the LEAP model of early intervention for young children with autism spectrum disorders. *Topics in Early Childhood Special Education, 31*(3), 133–154. https://doi.org/10.1177/0271121411408740

Strain, P. S., & Cordisco, L. (1993). The LEAP preschool model. In S. Harris & J. Handleman (Eds.), *Preschool programs for children with autism* (pp. 115–126). Austin, TX: Pro-Ed.

Strain, P. S., & Danko, C. (1995). Caregivers' encouragement of positive interaction between preschoolers' with autism and their siblings. *Journal of Emotional and Behavioral Disorders, 3*, 12–12. https://doi.org/10.1177/106342669500300101

Strain, P. S., Fox, L., & Barton, E. E. (2021). On expanding the definition and use of procedural fidelity. *Research and Practice for Persons with Severe Disabilities, 46*(3), 173–183. https://doi.org/10.1177/15407969211036911

Strain, P. S., Goldstein, H., & Kohler, F. W. (1996). LEAP: Peer-mediated intervention for young children with autism. In E. Hibbs & P. Jensen (Eds.), *Psychosocial treatments for child and adolescent disorders* (pp. 573–587). Washington, DC: APA.

Strain, P. S., & Hoyson, M. (2000). The need for longitudinal, intensive social skills Intervention: LEAP follow-up outcomes. *Topics in Early Childhood Special Education, 20*, 116–122. https://doi.org/10.1177/027112140002000207

Strain, P. S., & Odom, S. L. (1986). Peer social initiations: An effective intervention for social skill deficits of exceptional children. *Exceptional Children, 52*, 543–551. https://doi.org/10.1177/001440298605200607

Strain, P. S., Schwartz, I., & Barton, E. (2012). Providing intervention for young children with autism spectrum disorders: What we still need to accomplish. *Journal of Early Intervention, 33*, 321–332. https://doi.org/10.1177/1053815111429970

Strain, P. S., Wolery, M., & Izeman, S. (1998). Considerations for administrators in the design of service options for young children with autism and their families. *Young Exceptional Children, 1*, 8–16. https://doi.org/10.1177/109625069800100202

Striefel, S., Killoran, J., & Quintero, M. (1991). *Functional integration for success: Preschool intervention*. Austin, TX: Pro-Ed.

Vygotsky, L. S.(1978). *Mind in society: The development of higher psychological processes*. Cambridge, MA: Harvard University Press.

18

Promoting the Emergence of Advanced Knowledge

Relational Training System (PEAK)

Jordan Belisle
Missouri State University

Yi Zhihui, Meredith Matthews, and Mark R. Dixon
University of Illinois, Chicago

18.1 Technical Abstract

Background: The PEAK relational training system (PEAK) is a comprehensive language and cognitive assessment and training curriculum. PEAK utilizes advances in verbal behavior, stimulus equivalence, and relational frame theories. Research on PEAK has amassed data at both the subject and population level supporting the psychometrics of the various assessments and implementation of the curriculum across clinical settings. This chapter summarizes the PEAK curriculum to date. **Method:** The authors review the history of relational frame theory as it extends from earlier work in behavior analysis using verbal behavior theory as the primary model, suggesting that new theories are needed to advance practice. The following sections detail how each PEAK module assesses and develops programming designed across operant response categories and summarizes research to date on each component of the curriculum. Finally, suggestions are provided for the use of PEAK in therapeutic and special education settings and links to other curricula extending from these same essential theories. **Results:** The results of this review suggest that PEAK integrates traditional and contemporary theories of language and cognition within the field of behavior analysis. In so doing, four curricula have been developed to target the learning processes of direct training, generalization, equivalence, and relational framing. There is considerable evidence of the efficacy of PEAK, primarily in application with autistic learners, although more research is needed from multiple labs and at the population level. PEAK can be implemented in both healthcare settings and in special education. **Discussion:** Users are cautioned against adopting a strictly medical model and should adapt the curriculum. Clear links are evident with similar technologies, such as the LIFE and AIM programs that aspire to target daily living and social emotional skills, respectively. In this way, PEAK may be best viewed as one element of a comprehensive training

Jordan Belisle et al., *Promoting the Emergence of Advanced Knowledge.* In: *Lifespan Treatment for Autistic Individuals.*
Edited by: Peter Sturmey, Russell Lang, and James K. Luiselli, Oxford University Press. © Oxford University Press (2025).
DOI: 10.1093/oso/9780197635841.003.0018

system for autistic learners. **Practitioner recommendations:** Practitioners who are interested in targeting language and cognitive skills as a broad construct may consider PEAK as an evidence-based treatment option.

18.2 Layperson Summary

The PEAK is a comprehensive language and cognitive assessment and training curriculum that can be used with autistic learners. This chapter reviews the theory underlying PEAK, each of the four PEAK modules (direct training, generalization, equivalence, and transformation), and research underlying the various elements of PEAK. The program has been used in research and in practice within healthcare and special education settings. In healthcare settings, the purpose of PEAK is primarily to support core deficits associated with a diagnosis, such as autism spectrum disorder (ASD) and intellectual disabilities. In special education settings, the purpose of PEAK is to support the attainment of learning objectives in a school setting. The chapter concludes by discussing the importance of flexibility and individuation in programming and links to other curricula extending from the same foundational theories and procedures, including LIFE and AIM programs.

18.3 Treatment Summary Table

Treatment summary: PEAK Relational Training System

Treatment description: PEAK is an assessment and curriculum designed to support language and cognitive learning. The program integrates elements of verbal behavior, stimulus equivalence, and relational frame theory. Each of these approaches is integrated throughout four PEAK learning modules that target core learning processes, and several studies have evaluated elements of PEAK across settings and populations.

Expected outcomes: At the subject level of analysis, PEAK assessments provide a list of developmentally appropriate skill targets, and improvements in the target skills should emerge through training. Several studies have also demonstrated the emergence of untrained skills through generalization and relational framing processes that are at the core of the curriculum. At the population level of analysis, improvements in intelligence test scores have been demonstrated within randomized control trial evaluations with autistic learners.

Methods: PEAK is implemented by conducting the PEAK Comprehensive Assessment (PCA), a 2-hour direct assessment of learning across the learning processes of direct training, generalization, equivalence, and relational learning. Scores on the PCA are then used along with clinical judgement to select training programs that correspond to assessment items. Each training program contains a detailed task analysis to implement the program, and the implementer determines stimuli that can be tailored to the learner's needs and interests. Programs are trained to mastery criteria, and once mastered, new stimuli can be introduced to the program or new programs that build on previous programs can be introduced to the curriculum. Implementers continue to add new and more complex programs to shape language and cognitive development as a broad construct.

Expertise required to implement treatment: PEAK was designed for use by multiple professionals and parents, although expertise and training may influence the approach and depth of training. PEAK is most often implemented by behavior technicians, teachers, or paraprofessionals, and programming is developed by a behavior analyst. Support from other professionals such as speech and language pathologists, psychologists, and others can even further the development of comprehensive assessments, evaluation of learning outcomes, and individuation of programming.
Risks and negative side effects: PEAK primarily utilizes a discrete trial training arrangement that, if implemented incorrectly and without guidance of a trained professional, can lead to fatigue or burnout for both learners and implementers. PEAK programming may also need to be adjusted to achieve mastery to avoid implementing programming in a way that is not effective for each learner.
Additional considerations and limitations: Practitioners should utilize their knowledge of the learning processes underlying the curriculum and their educational expertise to individualize programming. PEAK is best viewed as an assessment and curricular tool to support the development of programming that is highly individualized. Further research is also needed at the population level and is currently underway. PEAK is best viewed as an assessment and curricular tool to support the development of programming that is highly individualized. Further research is also needed at the population level and is currently underway.

18.4 Introduction

18.4.1 Treatment Description

At the turn of the century, the field of behavior analysis established itself as a professional practicing discipline. Applied behavior analysis (ABA) rapidly moved from a set of skills someone working in a variety of clinical environments might possess in a certain degree, to a prescribed intervention approach that rose in demand across the globe. Much of that demand was driven by an interest in improving the language and behavioral abilities of persons with autism and a professional regulation to ensure effective practicing standards. At the beginning of the decade, there were an estimated 392 certified behavior analysts that exponentiated to 6,948 by 2010 (Behavior Analysis Certification Board, 2022a). In the United States, this growth occurred along with licensing in many states protecting the professional designation of "applied behavior analyst" that has grown to include over 34 states (Behavior Analysis Certification Board, 2022b). This time also saw the development of a first wave of assessment tools that could measure language learning of autistic children that were developed from Skinner's verbal behavior theory (1957; see also Carnett et al., 2019, for summary of impacts of this framework in disability intervention). Several assessment tools emerged as criterion referenced assessments designed for use with children whose language was below typically developing peers to systematically guide intervention programming (e.g., the *Verbal Behavior Milestones Assessment and Placement Program*, VB MAPP, Sundberg, 2008; the *Assessment of Basic Language and Learning Skills—Revised*, Partington, 2006) and, at least in the United States' insurance-funded healthcare system, provided evidence for a need for behavioral services with autistic populations targeting language and communication deficits.

In our own field, the development of these assessment tools and others provided an outline for an exponentially growing body of behavior analysts to guide behavioral services; however, significant limitations in this first wave of assessment and intervention surfaced in the preceding decade. Whereas the theoretical foundation of these instruments and others may be solidly grounded in Skinner's theory of language learning, psychometric research supporting the validity and reliability of the assessments was not immediately forthcoming (Ackley et al., 2019). By 2020, only five studies were published that evaluated the construction of the two most commonly used assessments by behavior analysts (Padilla, 2020). Psychometric evaluations are a staple in fields like clinical psychology, speech and language pathology, and social work, and in the fields of education and special education they and are critical for population-level comparison (Belisle et al., 2021).

For philosophical reasons, behavior analysts may simply value psychometric research to a lesser extent than other disciplines, instead favoring intervention outcome research that is consistent with the pragmatic tradition of the applied subfield, captured under the core dimension of *effective* (Baer et al., 1968). However, effectiveness research also failed to emerge, with no studies suggesting that developing an intervention program guided by the progression of many of these tools leads to any demonstrable change in language and cognition of learners. Finally, a growing body of research beginning in the early 1980s and exponentiating within behavior analytic research between 2000 and 2020 (Belisle et al., 2020) suggested that language learning may occur through a process called derived relational responding in the absence of direct reinforcement (Barnes-Holmes et al., 2018; Critchfield et al., 2018). Thus, the traditional Skinnerian account of language learning—around which much of our applied subfield evolved—was in the process of being usurped by more contemporary language learning models that were both more theoretically consistent with other fields interested in the study language, such as psycholinguistics, and simultaneously yielding hundreds of basic and early translational studies. Today, derived relational responding is recognized as an empirical fact. This has led the field to reconsider many of the foundational traditions and assumptions of the first-wave movement that operated as the focal point of much of the graduate-level training of behavior analysts and paved a path for innovation in the assessment and support of language learning of autistic children.

The *Promoting the Emergence of Advanced Knowledge: Relational Training System* (PEAK Relational Training System, or PEAK; Dixon, 2014a, 2014b, 2015, 2016) developed from within this second-wave movement along with other applied technologies (e.g., *Strengthening Mental Abilities Through Relational Training*, SMART; Cassidy et al., 2011). The theoretical basis of PEAK integrates three learning paradigms: Skinner's verbal operant theory, stimulus equivalence (Sidman, 1971; Sidman & Tailby, 1982), and relational frame theory (RFT; Hayes et al., 2001). The latter two theoretical models incorporate derived relational response repertoires for a more complete account of language learning—moving beyond the direct teaching of content (e.g., number of tacts or mands in a learner's repertoire)—to "learning how to learn" as the main focus of training (Dixon, 2014a). Assessment in PEAK is completed using a combination of standardized direct assessment across different learning modalities and types of relational learning, indirect analyses completed by practitioners or caregivers familiar with the learner, and clinical judgement. Results from assessments are then used to develop training targets that are developmentally appropriate and can support core learning deficits experienced by children and adults with disabilities, including those with a diagnosis of autism.

Whereas psychometric research on earlier assessments was slow to emerge, research on PEAK assessments began in 2014 along with the release of the first PEAK module (Dixon, 2014a). This research established convergent validity through strong correlations between existing language and communication assessments and intellectual functioning (see Dixon, Belisle, et al., 2017). The reliability of the assessment strategy in PEAK was also supported through test-retest and interrater agreement analyses (Dixon, Belisle, et al., 2017). As for intervention programs guided by the PEAK curriculum, several single-case experimental designs have established that the training strategies described in PEAK are efficacious in teaching the target skills, including those that have generally been considered outside of the reach of practicing behavior analysis (e.g., perspective taking, e.g., Barron et al., 2019; categorical relating, Dixon et al., 2017). Beyond these single-subject outcomes, randomized control trial data have also established that training can lead to skill acquisition beyond training as usual (McKeel et al., 2015) and can significantly improve intelligence test performance in autistic children and with less training duration than traditional programming that can involve 20 or more hours of intervention each week (i.e., 4 hours per week; Dixon et al., 2021)—and these results have been replicated by multiple research laboratories throughout the United States (e.g., May & St. Cyr, 2021).

The growth of PEAK corresponded with an overall growth in behavior analytic research incorporating derived relational responding within training. This work that extends far beyond PEAK began to exponentiate around 2010 (Belisle, Paliliunas, Lauer, et al., 2020) to the present day, and a considerable amount of this work was based on programs contained within PEAK itself. In many ways, this represents a revolution (as defined by Kuhn, 1962) in the areas of ABA concerned with interventions for autistic learners. The revolution is one of multiple research and analytic strategies, guided by data and experimental methodologies, and incorporating the vast basic experimental literature on how language learning actually emerges. The revolution extends beyond PEAK as the total number of Board-Certified Behavior Analysts increases to over 55,000 in the year 2022, over 20 years from when this work first started—and it is to the broader relational learning movement happening within the field of behavior analysis that we now turn.

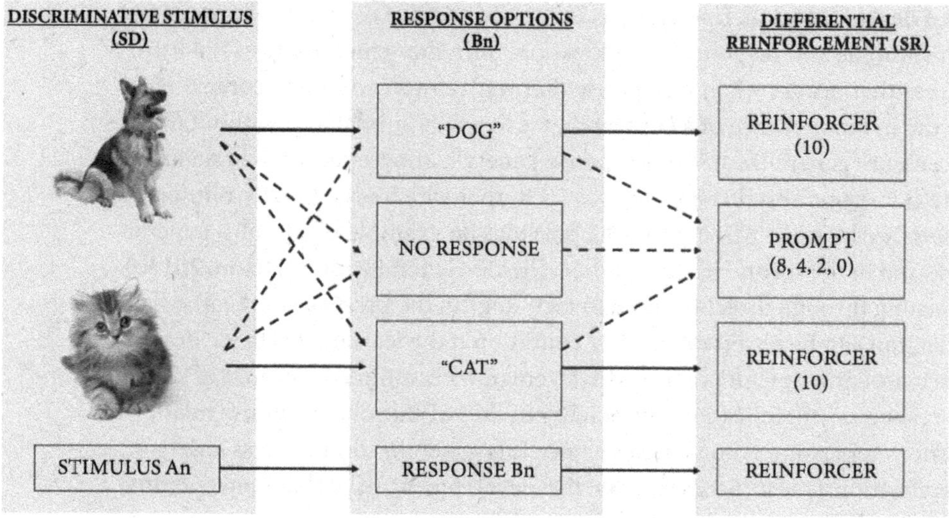

Figure 18.1 Visual representation of a direct reinforcement language learning model used in the PEAK-DT module

18.4.2 Rationale and Objectives

Verbal behavior training was predicated on a simple premise: We engage in verbal behavior because doing so has been directly reinforced by the verbal community that serves as the listener. This basic model is shown in Figure 18.1. For example, if a learner is presented with the visual image of a dog or sees a dog in the natural environment, the utterance "dog" is reinforced and other potential responses are not reinforced, such as "cat." This process is called differential reinforcement (see Chapter 3), and this specific example can functionally operate as a tact if reinforcement is general (e.g., praise for saying the right thing), a mand if reinforcement is specific (e.g., access to the dog), or other verbal operants depending on the context and reinforcer functions. Additional stimuli may be present that make the correct response more likely, such as a parent priming the response by saying "That is a d . . . " to evoke the response "dog," serving as a prompt. Within PEAK, verbal behavior programming includes both prompting and reinforcement and independent correct responses are scores higher (i.e., 10) than prompted or incorrect responses (i.e., 0, 2, 4, or 8) depending on the amount of assistance needed for the learner to respond correctly. This same strategy can be used to teach several verbal responses (Bn) occasioned by different stimulus arrangements (discriminative stimuli, SDs), such as a cat or any other animal or stimulus, where the response is directly reinforced (SR). This training method is familiar to many practicing behavior analysts and is a staple in discrete trial and naturalistic environment training strategies with autistic learners (Kane et al., 2010). This direct training approach is used exclusively in the PEAK Direct Training module (Dixon, 2014a).

A great deal of learning, however, occurs in the absence of direct reinforcement through stimulus and response generalization. Stimulus generalization is a learning process that occurs when a response that was reinforced in one context (SD) also occurs in the presence of a context that is formally similar and without direct reinforcement (generalized SD). Response generalization occurs when a similar response (i.e., generalized response) occurs to that which was directly reinforced in response to the same SD. Figure 18.2 provides an example of stimulus generalization found in the second PEAK module, PEAK-Generalization (Dixon, 2014b). After learning through direct training to tact "dog" in the presence of the first dog, generalization can be observed in a test condition if the learner also tacts "dog" in the presence of other pictures of dogs that were never reinforced. Because of stimulus and response generalization, the actual number of stimulus-response relations in a learner's repertoire is considerable once this generalization process emerges.

Generalization is also necessary for the development of verbal concepts that include both generalization and discrimination. For example, correct responding in Figure 18.2 necessitates saying "dog" only in the presence of objects that resemble dogs and not in the presence of other objects that may be formally similar along other dimensions, such as in the presence of cats. At the same time, the concept "cat" requires both generalization of the "cat" response and discrimination when other objects are present (e.g., dogs). Because prompting and reinforcement are never used under test conditions, test trials can only be scored a 10 (independent correct response) or a 0 (incorrect response) within the PEAK scoring system. By implementing a train and test strategy, behavior analysts and technicians can see generalized learning occurring alongside direct training targets. When generalization is not occurring, strategies are provided such as introducing more similar stimuli to "bridge the gap" to the directly trained targets or reinforcing subsets of generalized behavior and testing the remaining behaviors (Dixon, 2014b). Ultimately, this module is not about the generalized content of any given program but encouraging generalizing itself as a generalized operant (i.e., an operant that occurs across contexts and situations).

Generalization is not a novel concept but is necessary within verbal behavior training. For example, research by Dixon et al. (2015) demonstrated that scores on the PEAK-DT modules and scores on the VB-MAPP were linearly correlated at lower PEAK-DT values (100 or below out of 184); however, once participants scored above 5 out of 184 on the PEAK-G assessment, they were likely to receive the highest possible score on the VB-MAPP (170). Moreover, whereas the programming targets in PEAK-DT represent skills expected of typically developing children aged 1 to 8 years (Dixon et al., 2014) based on normative analyses, PEAK-G targets range from age 5 to 13 years using this same analytic strategy (Dixon, Rowsey, et al., 2017).

Both processes (direct reinforcement and generalization) were described over a half-century ago by Skinner (1957) and appear within multiple behavior analytic technologies (Ackley et al., 2019). At the same time, mounting evidence is emerging

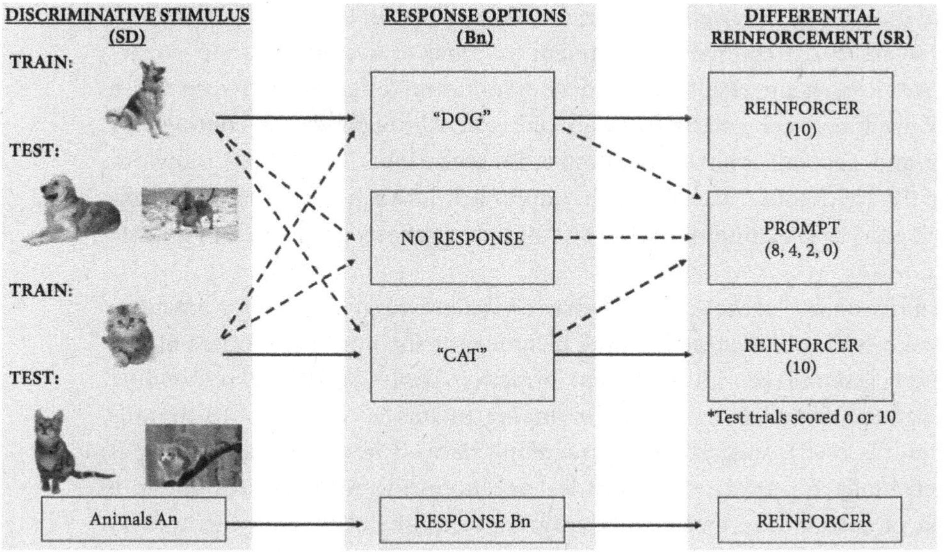

Figure 18.2 Visual representation of a generalization language learning model used in the PEAK-G module

suggesting that these processes may be necessary but are not sufficient within a comprehensive language training program. The first reason is theoretical and has been established as an empirical fact in the basic experimental literature—people learn in ways that occur in the absence of direct reinforcement and cannot be explained through stimulus or response generalization alone. Although attempts have been made to account for more complex language topographies by introducing verbal mediational occurring somewhere within the skin (e.g., Michael et al., 2011; Sundberg et al., 2018), these approaches have more so resembled stimulus-organism-response (S-O-R) psychology. In S-O-R psychology, a molecular or efficient cause is placed somewhere inside the organism without explicit consideration of the external context within which these behaviors take place. As well, technologies have yet to emerge from these explanatory constructs with sufficient outcome data to suggest that these approaches offer any greater utility than strictly focusing on those verbal response patterns that are directly observable and measurable (i.e., derived relational responding).

The second reason is practical. Based on a large-scale analysis of ABA service outcomes with autistic populations (US Department of Defense, report on insurance beneficiaries from one company, published in 2019), outcomes of traditional language training guided by any number of verbal behavior technologies have not produced outcomes resembling those reported in the highly controlled experimental literature. These results correspond with outcomes reported by Dixon et al. (2021) where a control group of participants received training guided by verbal behavior models alone (PEAK-DT, PEAK-G, and VB-MAPP targets) and outcomes did not significantly deviate from those of a control group who received no intervention services. In a larger-scale analysis (Dixon et al., 2023) comparing treatment as usual to a control group receiving no services, again results showed no significant difference between those who received services and those who did not. Although direct contingency learning and generalization are undoubtedly efficacious in teaching individualized skills (McKeel et al., 2015), that approach alone has not been demonstrated to lead to meaningful changes in broader learner repertoires of autistic children.

A third reason is that the scope of behavior analytic services narrows considerably when models of language learning include only the most basic forms of discrimination, generalization, and concept formation. Derived relational responding has been documented in typically developing infants as young as 18 months (Pelaez et al., 2000), suggesting that targeting derived relational responding is developmentally appropriate for most learners accessing ABA services due to a diagnosis of autism. The inclusion of relational learning also opens the door to other intervention approaches that are grounded in RFT such as acceptance and commitment therapy (ACT) and curricula designed to promote greater independence and autonomy, both contained in the recent *Accept. Identify. Move.* curriculum (AIM; Dixon & Paliliunas, 2018) and *LIFE skill emergent system* (LIFE; Dixon, 2021) described at the end of this chapter.

In terms of the inclusion of stimulus equivalence and relational framing within PEAK, stimulus equivalence was a major breakthrough in understanding human language and cognition (Critchfield et al., 2018). In its basic preparation, if a learner is taught that a stimulus A is the same as a stimulus B (A-B), the learner may derive that B is also the same as A (B-A, symmetry). If the learner is also taught that the stimulus B is the same as a stimulus C (B-C), the learner may also derive the symmetrical C-B relation. We may also expect the derivation of the untrained transitive A-C relation and the equivalence C-A relation to emerge without direct reinforcement. This bidirectional equivalence relation has been documented in hundreds of studies with human participants across numerous stimulus arrangements (Hayes et al., 2021; O'Connor et al., 2017); yet this same behavior has not occurred without considerable direct training in a nonhuman animal. A reasonable conclusion is that humans may be especially capable of forming complex equivalence classes and to teach *human* language necessitates targeting symmetrical, transitive, and equivalence relational responding.

An example of how this is accomplished within the third PEAK module, PEAK Equivalence (PEAK-E), is provided in Figure 18.3 (note that this example is only one of 184 total programs). The image of the dog is the A stimulus of our first equivalence class and can be labeled A1. Images of other animals such as cats or frogs would operate as A2 and A3 stimuli, and the total number of classes is at the discretion of the program developer. First, responding "dog" (B1) is reinforced in the presence of the image of the dog (A1) as an initial tact response (A1-B1). Second, when provided an array containing the text stimuli D-O-G (C1), C-A-T

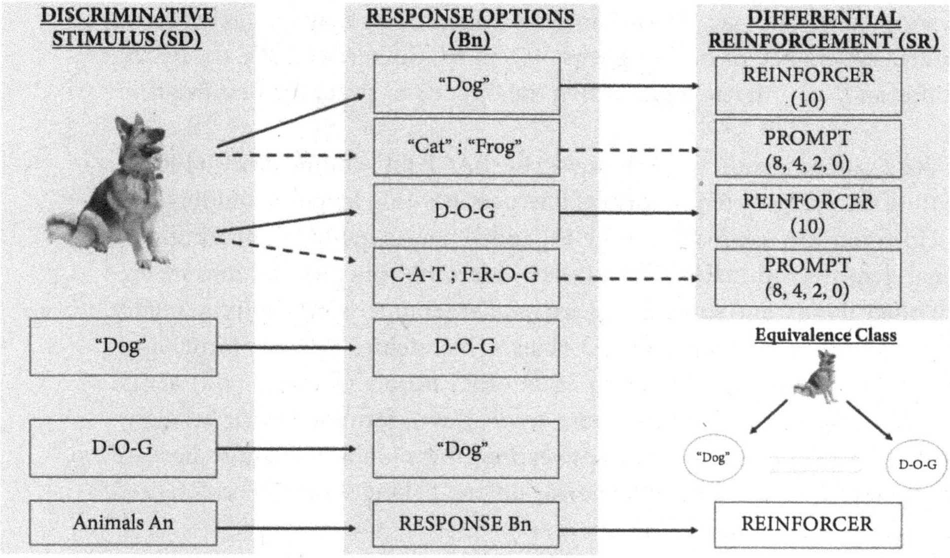

Figure 18.3 Visual representation of the equivalence language learning model used in the PEAK-E module

(C2), and F-R-O-G (C3), selecting the D-O-G text is reinforced in the presence of the image of the dog (A1) (A1-C1). Prompting and reinforcement are used during direct training of this subset of relations, and the implementers utilize the same scoring system. For this program, the equivalence relations are also tested (scored as either a 10 or 0 because no prompts are used in testing). For the B1-C1 test, the text array is presented, and the implementer asks, "Which spells dog?" For the C1-B1 test, D-O-G is presented, and the implementer asks, "What does this spell?" When correct responding occurs regularly across all relations, the image, the word, and the text form an equivalence class that is shown in the bottom right of the image.

As in PEAK-G, the actual content of the training in PEAK-E is secondary to the opportunity to practice derived relational responding. Earlier programs begin with simple identity matching that does not involve derived relations but may occasion their occurrence. Programs then progress to simple symmetry programs using only visual and auditory stimuli, but eventually programs involve other sense modes such as taste, smell, and touch. In human language, experience involves every possible sense mode. Describing and understanding these experiences is part of deeper human connection and involvement with the verbal community. For example, Dixon et al. (2017) evaluated a PEAK-E program using jellybeans, where the participants were directly taught to taste the jellybean and to select a corresponding image representing the flavor (A-B), and when provided the image to state the name of the flavor (B-C). After training these two relations across multiple jellybean flavors, the participants were able to taste the jellybean and describe the flavor verbally (A-C, transitive relation) and use the name to request their favorite jellybean (i.e., derived mand). This process may be analogous to the familiar experience of deciding what to eat for dinner: verbally describing the options and, at a private level, tasting the options to select the best available option.

As of 2022, stimulus equivalence is now in the BACB fifth edition task list (2022), highlighting the necessity of this form of instruction within language training programs. However, this approach can be expanded considerably by incorporating additional elements within RFT. Not all relations are the same. Some things are *bigger* than other things, and some things are *smaller* (comparison). Objects *contain* other objects and are *contained by* other objects (hierarchies/category formation). People also perceive things differently from other people (I versus you) across space (here versus there) and time (now versus then), forming deictic relations. The term "equivalence" is not adequate to express these kinds of relations because they are not equal. They are simultaneously different along some dimensions and the same along other dimensions.

This can be seen in the example provided in Figure 18.4, building off our earlier examples and adapted from the fourth PEAK module, PEAK-Transformation (PEAK-T). In this case, all of the relational classes (dog, bear, and rabbit) are animals. The learner is first taught that the dog (A1) is "bigger than" a rabbit (B1) and the dog (A1) is smaller than a bear (C1). Scoring is the same as the other PEAK modules representing the needed prompting levels within direct training of this relational subset. Testing may then establish that the learner can identify that the rabbit is also "smaller than" the dog and that the bear is "bigger than" the dog. We call this mutual entailment because symmetry assumes that these stimuli are the same. In addition, the relational terms "bigger than" and "smaller than" are called contextual cues, because they function to describe the type of relation, in this case comparison along the dimension of relative size. The implementer may also test for the combinatorially entailed relations by asking, "Which is bigger, a bear or a rabbit?" and "Which is smaller, a bear or a rabbit?" Successfully answering the question relies on the shared relation with both bear and rabbit to the initial dog stimulus. Once again, scoring of the test relation can only be 10 (independent correct response) or 0 (incorrect response). This same arrangement can occur with any sets of animals or any objects that differ along the dimension of relative size, and this same framework is used throughout PEAK-T across different kinds of comparisons (e.g., speed) and different relational frame families (i.e., coordination, comparison, distinction, opposition, hierarchies, and deictics).

Two other assumptions within RFT are critical in developing comprehensive language programming. The first is the concept of transformation of stimulus function. The amount of learning that can take place through derived relational responding is vast, and we are only just beginning to scratch the surface of this complexity (Belisle, 2020). Given these verbal relations, behavior in novel contexts may emerge consistent with these relations—that is, the function of the

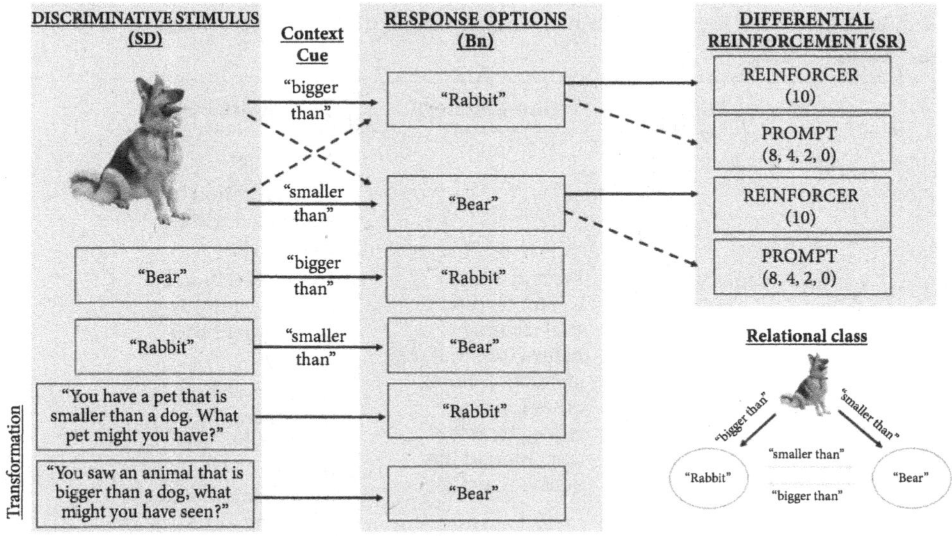

Figure 18.4 Visual representation of the RFT language learning model used in the PEAK-T module

context has transformed consistent with relational behavior. The figure provides an example that could be developed within PEAK-T in a transformation test, where given knowledge that a rabbit is smaller than a dog and presented with the question, "You have a pet that is smaller than a dog. What pet might you have seen?" the learner may respond by saying "a rabbit." The potential interaction of multiple frames could also be assessed; for example, both a rabbit and a frog are animals that are smaller than a dog, but a rabbit is a common pet and a frog is not, illustrating again the potential complexity of relational behavior that participates in more complex language topographies. Within PEAK-T, transformation tests include problem-solving questions like in the provided example or more naturalistic behavior in common children's games like playing Twister or engaging in word searches (Dixon et al., 2016; Belisle, Paliliunas, Stanley et al., 2021).

The second assumption in RFT is that relational responding itself is a generalized operant, much like generalized imitation (Healy et al., 2000). At some point, a learner does not need to be taught to imitate every single topography, and new topographies do not need to resemble old ones. Imitating itself becomes topographically boundless. Deriving relations appears to work in much the same way, where once the operant of relating is occurring, it can be applied to any given stimulus relation, and through shaping, expands in complexity throughout development. For those whose language and communicating do not occur at an age-typical developmental rate, programs like those contained in PEAK-E and PEAK-T can help shape and develop this skill (Dixon et al., 2021).

Table 18.1 Summary of the four modules in PEAK, the underlying theory, and the training and testing strategy

Module	Underlying Theory	Training Strategy	Testing Strategy
Direct training	Verbal behavior		No testing
Generalization			Generalization tests embedded within trial blocks
Equivalence	Stimulus equivalence	Prompt and reinforce; discrete trial training; naturalistic training; gamified training; other training strategies at the discretion of the behavior analyst	Derived relational tests operating as independent trial blocks
Transformation	Relational frame theory		Derived relational tests operating as independent trial blocks Transformation tests operating as independent trial blocks

18.4.3 Developing Comprehensive Training Using PEAK

The four PEAK modules were published independently and in sequence, mirroring the progression of our scientific understanding of how language learning develops. Each of the four modules is summarized in Table 18.1.

Although the modules were published sequentially, the content is designed for simultaneous implementation. For example, a learner may complete two programs from each of the four modules, whereas another learner who has mastered most of the programs in PEAK-DT and PEAK-G may exclusively focus on programs from the PEAK-E and PEAK-T modules. The relative distribution of programming and the content embedded within each program are selected by the behavior analyst based on their knowledge of language learning, their knowledge of the PEAK program, and other sources of clinical expertise and education. To assist in program selection, the PCA (Dixon 2020) was developed as a fully standardized test that contains test items from all four of the PEAK modules. The test is administered one on one by the program developer with the learner, and materials and a script are provided. Research comparing the results of the PCA with the other PEAK assessment options supports strong convergent validity (Sutton et al., 2021), linking this assessment to the existing research base on the PEAK assessments.

The PCA serves two primary purposes. First, the test operates as an objective pre-post analysis of improvements across each of the four learning modalities within PEAK. Items in the PCA are adapted from a subset of items in PEAK and are not explicitly targeted in the curriculum to avoid training to the test. Second, the PCA aligns with PEAK curricular programming and offers an expedited method for selecting individualized program targets. There are 184 programs in each of the PEAK modules, for a total of 736 potential programs to select from for each learner. Moreover, each program allows for embedding between 1 and 30 stimuli and multiple relations in the later modules for a total of 736 to 22,080 or more total skill targets. To directly test each of these components would take far longer than any actual training that could occur. The PCA provides an estimated score within each of the modules so that programs can be selected immediately upon completion of the test. Once programs are selected, then training proceeds as described above that encompasses the now multiple ways that we know language is acquired and expanding well beyond traditional language training approaches.

Since the initial publication of the PEAK curricula and earlier laboratory-based research, we have seen the emergence of PEAK programming within two primary intervention contexts, including within insurance-funded ABA services and within special education. There are specific considerations in both domains that practitioners should consider when developing and individualizing PEAK that we briefly summarize below.

18.4.4 Considerations for Implementation in Healthcare Systems

Within the healthcare system of multiple countries, including the United States, psychological and behavioral services involve information obtained through diagnostic criteria established in the *Diagnostic and Statistical Manual of Mental Disorders*, fifth edition (*DSM-V*; American Psychiatric Association, 2013) and more recently the *Diagnostic and Statistical Manual of Mental Disorders*, fifth edition, text revision (*DSM-V-TR*; American Psychiatric Association, 2022). The *DSM-V* was initially created as a tool for mental health professionals to have a common language when diagnosing individuals with a variety of different intellectual or neurodiverse profiles. In the *DSM-V-TR*, autism is defined by deficits in social communication and interaction and restricted and repetitive behavior. A diagnosis of autism and intellectual disability is frequently co-occurring. PEAK in healthcare systems is designed to train new language and cognitive skills that participate in social interaction and may expand the repertoire of interests for those receiving services. That is, PEAK programming is designed to directly support specific challenges autistic people may experience in communication and problem solving that necessitate derived relational responding.

Traditionally, language learning programs have been designed by borrowing procedures from previously published curriculum (Love et al., 2009). The PCA provides the necessary information to begin to construct age-norm estimates in the areas of direct contingencies learning, generalization learning, and derived relational responding across the many relational frame families that may affect communication and broader repertoire expansion. Results from the PCA, when combined with other information such as results from functional assessment of challenging behavior, adaptive response inventories, intelligence test results, and information about autism symptoms, are used to inform the scope and duration of ABA services. Scores in each module (and within each factor of each module) provide a list of program targets that are age and developmentally appropriate and build in complexity to shape language and cognitive skills.

For example, deictic programs in the PEAK-T module target pivotal behaviors involved in taking the perspective of others. Successful social communication and interaction involves much more than regurgitating a social script or any other directly trained social behavior; rather, it involves taking the perspective of the other person, considering their interests, and referencing both their vocal and non-vocal behaviors. By strengthening deictic relating, we may expect improvements in social interaction and communication by addressing the core deficit (i.e., relational responding). Moreover, deictic relating may increase the learner's repertoire of interests as they begin attending to the interests of others. Deictic responding is also contained directly within creative play, for example when acting out scenes from a movie with dolls or action figures that can expand the array of play options that were otherwise inaccessible without deictic responding.

Within healthcare services, programming must be individualized to meet the needs of the learner and will require the behavior analyst to understand the underlying principles and recent advances in the literature. Whereas novice implementers may simply use PEAK as described within the modules, advanced implementers may use a variety of strategies to customize PEAK for more individualized learning experiences. For example, Belisle et al. (2022) developed a method to gamify receptive identification PEAK programs in a way that is similar to playing a video game and captures elements of responding like response rate in addition to response accuracy. Additional digital adaptations have begun design ranging from PEAK worksheets and applications. Modifying stimulus targets to contain elements of already established interests of the learners may also improve rates of mastery, and including elements found in the learner's natural environment may promote generalization of new skills. When combined with behavioral interventions developed from a functional assessment, PEAK programs can also be modified to establish alternative behaviors that are more dynamic and flexible than those that emerge through direct training of only a singular response topography. Moreover, each PEAK module contains a blank program template in which behavior analysts can create program content if the content is not contained in the curriculum. It is critically important that the content match the behavior complexity of current PEAK programs to continue to shape complex response repertoires.

PCA outcomes can also be combined with other assessment information that can provide even greater insight, especially when outcomes on those assessment scores have established convergent validity with PEAK outcomes. For example, research has reported convergent outcomes between PEAK assessments and the VB-MAPP (Dixon et al., 2015), the VABS-II and ABLLS-R (Malkin et al., 2017), expressive and receptive language tests like the EOWPVT-4 and the ROWPVT-4 (McKeel et al., 2015), measures of vocabulary such as the PPVT (Dixon, Carman et al., 2014), and even measures of intellectual functioning and autism severity (Sutton et al., 2021). Evaluating the specific results within these other assessment relative to outcomes reported in the PCA can lead to even greater individualization and may help to directly support language and communication and repetitive behaviors of autistic learners. Established correlations between PEAK and other outcomes of interest within healthcare services also help to establish the relationship from each of the learning modalities contained in PEAK and the outcomes of interest to families receiving services.

18.4.5 Considerations for Implementation in Special Education Settings

Unlike traditional outpatient behavior health settings, special education settings within schools require unique considerations. National and local laws often drive policies and resources available in special education settings. In the United States, for example, practices are heavily influenced by legislation such as the No Child Left Behind Act of 2001 and the Individuals with Disabilities Education Act of 1990. Several key differences exist when providing behavior analytic services in special education programs, and practitioners should carefully consider them when implementing PEAK in school settings.

First, are the resources available when implementing ABA programs, including staffing, space, and time? This consideration is not unique to PEAK, and it speaks broadly to ABA overall. Unlike traditional ABA settings, where clinicians usually have several hours a day dedicated to structured teaching, the dosage in special education settings can be significantly lower as time is allocated to teaching educational content. In this case, PEAK is designed to strengthen important learning behaviors in each module that can augment academic performance and learning within core content areas in the classroom as determined by the classroom teacher. It is not uncommon for a student to receive only a few hours of language training per day at school using tools such as PEAK. Moreover, staff may not be familiar with behavior analytic terms and procedures, and time necessary to provide adequate staff training and supervision should be considered when implementing PEAK in schools. PEAK intentionally avoids using technical terms when describing program implementation, and early research has established that staff unfamiliar with behavior analytic terms can successfully implement PEAK procedures at school. For example, Hahs and Jarynowski (2019) successfully used behavior skill training techniques to train six school paraprofessionals to implement PEAK Direct Training programs accurately over 6 weeks, and learners' performance in these PEAK programs improved with accurate implementation by paraprofessionals maintained at follow-up.

A second consideration is determining the appropriate dosage of intervention. Although very few studies have studied the impact of dosage on students' outcomes, studies have suggested that intervention based on PEAK can produce socially significant outcomes at a smaller dosage than programs that exclusively use direct training targets. For example, Mckeel et al. (2015) reported favorable outcomes within the special educational settings where 40 students were randomly assigned to the PEAK intervention group and the treatment-as-usual group. Participants in the treatment-as-usual group continued to receive routine special education services, while those in the PEAK intervention group received instructions based on the PEAK curriculum in several 25-minute sessions for 1 month. Results showed that those receiving PEAK-based interventions made significantly more improvements in language skills. In a recent study, Belisle, Clark, et al. (2021) reported the outcome of implementing PEAK-based instructions among five autistic students in special education settings. For 3 months, participants on average received 1.5 hours of PEAK-based instructions daily, and results showed improved performance during standardized testing, acquisition of novel verbal operants, and generalization to home and other settings. Although a relatively small dosage of PEAK intervention seems to produce socially significant outcomes in schools, behavior analysts should also be cautious when defaulting to a lower dosage for convenience and instead base decisions on progress monitoring data collection focused on the educational performance of the student and on collaboration with educators. Often within special education settings, those with the most substantial needs receive more support, either in the form of one-on-one aid or longer duration within specialized classrooms, as well as other services such as occupational therapy, physical therapy, and speech and language. Behavior analysts should attempt to work closely to integrate PEAK programming within these existing services, leveraging the flexibility of the PEAK curriculum and their knowledge of the basic principles underlying language learning as described in PEAK.

A third consideration is to use relational training procedures in addressing academic skills directly. As mentioned earlier, PEAK is not unique in the list of 736 skills identified across its four modules. It is unique in its conceptualization of how learning occurs, the different underlying behavior processes, and the use of relational training procedures in accelerating learning. Many PEAK programs can be adapted to match the Common Core standards and potentially contribute to the learner's academic success. For example, Dixon et al. (2016) demonstrated the effectiveness of teaching geometry skills among autistic students using protocols adapted from the PEAK Equivalence module. In a similar study, geography skills were taught to two autistic students in special education settings using methods adapted from the same PEAK module (Dixon, Stanley, et al., 2017). Many contents covered in the PEAK Direct Training module can be easily adapted to match English Language and Art (ELA) Common Core standards. Many skills outlined in the Generalization module also match routine activities and scenarios a learner might encounter at school. Once again, some of the considerations are not unique to PEAK. Practitioners should carefully evaluate the learner's context and identify intervention goals that address both the learner's academic and clinical needs. It is also critically important that behavior analysts in school settings understand their role in supporting, not replacing, the education that is occurring within regular education and specialized education that has been tailored to meet the specific needs of the learner.

18.4.6 Expanding on the PEAK Curriculum: LIFE and AIM

Each of the four different learning modalities (direct contingency, generalization, stimulus equivalence, and relational framing) constitutes a complete picture of developing complex language and cognitive skills. However, these four different processes are not explicitly combined into one single instance of teaching, which might prevent the learner from benefiting more fully when PEAK is not combined with other tools. For example, the *LIFE Skill Emergence System* (LIFE; Dixon, 2021) represents an extension of PEAK in areas of daily living and vocational training. LIFE addresses various adaptive life skills that would significantly promote autonomy and independence by empowering the learner with not only *what to* learn but also *how to* learn. The first of its series, the Functional module, contains 250 skills that cover various topographies of behavior needed for an individual to achieve value-driven independent living. These skills are categorized into four factors of performance complexity (essential skills, foundations skills, independent skills, and liberating skills) and across content domains (performance, personal care, social, home, and leisure). Program targets in LIFE are constructed similar to PEAK programs by including directly trained targets achieved through chaining of complex topographies, generalization of the skills in new contexts and with disruption that necessitates problem solving, and verbal flexibility that augments this training. However, in contrast to PEAK, the LIFE curriculum integrates all four of the teaching modalities on every curricula program.

For example, LIFE Program I 61: Conversate About Future or Past Events from the Functional module sets the overall goal for the learner to engage in conversation about future or past events. The direct training objective resembles the traditional instructional methods for life skills, wherein the clinician directly reinforces successful links in a conversational chain naturalistically or in a contrived conversational event. For example, toward the end of the session, the clinician might ask the learner what they did during the session and reinforce a series of variable intraverbal exchanges that contain accurate information about the session. Although there is value in the topography of such responding, targeting skills in this way runs the risk of requiring the learner to simply remember these responses without truly understanding the question (i.e., engaging in a series of scripted responses). To decrease the likelihood of this risk, a generalization objective is immediately introduced after or concurrent to the direct training objective to promote the learner's response in other contexts. For example, the clinician might ask the learner what they did the morning before the session began or what they are planning to do that evening. This is a higher-level skill that requires the learner to derive relations among events happening in the past or probabilistic events in the future. To assist in this, verbal flexibility training that closely mirrors PEAK program may be developed to teach the deictic verbal relations needed to perform this skill. For example, the instructor may present a verbal statement and ask the learner if the statement describes a past or future event, such as "I have a book club meeting next week. Is that in the past or the future?" and the correct response is "the future." A more complex example would occur if the clinician asks, "Pretend today is Thursday and there is a movie on Wednesday of the same week. Is movie night in the past or future?" and the correct response will be "the past." Research is currently underway to evaluate the relationship between verbal flexibility elements of LIFE and the training targets contained in the curriculum.

Another interesting extension of PEAK is its connection with language-based interventions such as those rooted in ACT. In short, ACT is a language-based treatment model where six different behavior processes are targeted in order to improve the learner's psychological flexibility. Evidence has suggested that ACT-based behavior analytic intervention can promote parental adherence to ABA caregiver training protocols (Yi & Dixon, 2021), increase psychological flexibility and mindfulness among caregivers of autistic children (Hahs et al., 2019), and improve mental health status and prosocial behavior among autistic individuals (Pahnke et al., 2014). What is less clear is whether there exist certain prerequisite skills in order for an autistic individual to benefit from ACT. Given that the therapeutic approach of ACT requires frequent use of language and metaphors, deficits in language and analogical reasoning would potentially negatively impact its outcome. This might be particularly challenging because autistic individuals often experience difficulties in relational framing. Existing protocols in ACT might need significant adaptation in order to be effective among individuals with developmental delays. Curriculums such as the AIM might be especially beneficial given its tiered adaptation with emerging research supporting its effectiveness in school settings (e.g., Issen et al., 2021), clinical settings (Gilsenan et al., 2021), and psychometric properties of measures used (Bachmann et al., 2021). What is particularly of interest is that the PEAK Transformation module contains programs explicitly overlapping with processes captured in the psychological flexibility model. Emerging evidence has shown improved outcomes of ACT-based interventions when relational training is provided simultaneously.

For example, in the study by Gilsenan et al. (2021), the research team evaluated the impact of relational training on learners' performance during ACT sessions among three autistic teenagers. A concurrent multiple baseline across participant design was used where participants were exposed to ACT, ACT + relational training, and, subsequently, the maintenance phase. In the first phase, ACT protocols adapted from the AIM curriculum were used as a stand-alone intervention for all three participants. In the second phase, all three participants were exposed to six to eight PEAK Transformation module programs using relational training procedures targeting psychological flexibility processes. In the maintenance phase, participants were exposed to ACT-based protocols only. All three participants' engagement during ACT sessions showed significant improvement during relational training and maintained a higher level of engagement during ACT sessions after completing the relational training protocol. Similar to LIFE programs, AIM lessons and contingency systems may be strengthened through use of the PEAK curriculum, although more research is needed to understand this relationship more completely. Nonetheless, developing complex relational abilities opens up an array of interventions options that have been historically inaccessible to behavior analysts and, as a consequence, to people served using behavior analytic technologies.

18.5 Research Background and Future Directions

The empirical footprint of PEAK overshadows all other behavior analytic language and verbal behavior assessment and training programs. Table 18.2 displays a summary of the total number of publications, journals, and research type that have been reported on PEAK to date. Currently PEAK has amassed 62 peer-reviewed publications in the professional literature. Of this body of work, three have been randomized controlled trials, 26 have been single-case experimental designs, and 12 have been conceptual, critique, or literature reviews. There have been three book chapters, including this current installment. PEAK has been shown to converge or correlate with 13 different existing testing instruments or assessments and has documented positive behavior change for clients in 31 different studies. There are no other behavior analytic tools designed to either assess or treat language limitations in persons with disabilities that share this degree of empirical support. However, these data are a fraction of the totality of research that PEAK stands to benefit from in order to ensure its longevity and importance within and beyond the behavior analytic community. Larger randomized trials, longitudinal analyses, dosage comparisons, technology transfer, scalability, and ecological validity studies are necessary to better buttress and inform the existing research base.

When a radically advanced technology such as PEAK enters both the scientific community and the commercial marketplace, a careful and critical evaluation of utility should occur. Over the past decade, some researchers have expressed concerns regarding PEAK (Witts, 2018). However, entangled in such commentaries have often been criticisms of RFT, group design research, convergent validity measures, data analysis selection procedures, and overall appraisal of PEAK's impact from traditional treatment as usual (Beaujean & Farmer, 2021). PEAK authors have responded to concerns and have enjoyed the intellectual debates that such dialogue has spurred. However, what remains lacking in the literature is an empirical body of

Table 18.2 Number of peer-reviewed publications on different content area of PEAK

Content Area	Number of Peer-Reviewed Publications*
Clinical outcome of systematic implementation of PEAK	5
Psychometric properties of PEAK-based assessments	19
Skill-specific gains produced by PEAK-based instructions	26
Referencing PEAK in other areas	6
Review and critiques of PEAK	6

* The numbers reported were indexed in May 2022.

work revealing limitations of PEAK beyond those noted by the authors themselves who have published PEAK's empirical findings.

18.6 Conclusions and Practice Implications

In conclusion, the field of ABA is growing exponentially, and with it, modern technologies are emerging emphasizing derived relational responding from an RFT account. PEAK is one such technology that emphasizes language and cognitive training that can participate within comprehensive behavioral programming for autistic learners. The empirical necessity to embed language learning beyond that established through direct contingencies or generalization has now been well established, yet our field is still catching up. As noted by Enoch and Nicholson. (2020), few behavior analysts have been exposed to relational training technologies within their graduate coursework that may create a barrier to adopting PEAK or other similar technologies. Despite unambiguous evidence of the advantages of these strategies to promote generalizable learning, more traditional assessments created during a first wave at the initial conditions of the field are still commonplace (Padilla, 2020). PEAK represents a first attempt to streamline RFT technologies into a comprehensive program that does not necessitate deep understanding of RFT or its empirical basis but adopts a sufficiently flexible structure such that practitioners with this knowledge can create programming that exceeds the basic structure of the curriculum. An aggressive research strategy at the early conditions of PEAK established experimental evidence of its utility early on using multiple analytic strategies, including correlational comparisons with existing assessments, single-case experimental evaluation of selected programs, and randomized control trial evaluations of the totality of the curriculum against more traditional approaches.

As the research continues to expand, this chapter will likely become dated. And, like the first wave, empirical analysis may reveal critical flaws in PEAK and more advanced conceptualizations of relational learning will likely emerge. These advances may be observed in future iterations of PEAK or other technologies that extend from it, or they may not. If not, it is our hope that what we have discovered in using and evaluating PEAK has paved the way for the next wave of new technologies that will take its place. Ultimately, learners served by PEAK and other technologies are the benefactors of this current revolution and the next one. We must remain self-critical and self-correcting, and we must never become satisfied or satiated with the status quo of our applied subfield. There is still more to learn than is currently known. There is still more to do than is currently done. Such is the nature of progressive science and scientific revolutions within it (Kuhn, 1962). We make no explicit or implied claims that PEAK is the final chapter of a scientific revolution in the way we treat language and cognitive deficits in persons with disabilities. PEAK is merely the current iteration that is demonstrating increased success beyond previous methods. However, what remains at the forefront is the needs of a child that sits in front of the practicing behavior analyst and what can be done today to help that child, given all available options. The burden of learning new tools and their underlying behavioral mechanisms is real; however, when data do exist suggesting that PEAK has considerable utility, it appears that the burden should be embraced to support the futures of countless children.

18.7 References

Ackley, M., Subramanian, J. W., Moore, J. W., Litten, S., Lundy, M. P., & Bishop, S. K. (2019). A review of language development protocols for individuals with autism. *Journal of Behavioral Education, 28*(3), 362–388. https://doi.org/10.1007/s10864-019-09327-8

American Psychiatric Association. (2013). *Diagnostic and statistical manual of mental disorders* (5th ed.). Washington, DC: Author.

American Psychiatric Association. (2022). *Diagnostic and statistical manual of mental disorders* (5th ed., text revision). Washington, DC: Author.

Bachmann, K., Hinman, J. M., Yi, Z., & Dixon, M. R. (2021). Evaluating the convergent and divergent validity of the Children's Psychological Flexibility Questionnaire (CPFQ) among children with autism. *Advances in Neurodevelopmental Disorders, 5*(3), 298–303. https://doi.org/10.1007/s41252-021-00206-w

Baer, D. M., Wolf, M. M., & Risley, T. R. (1968). Some current dimensions of applied behavior analysis. *Journal of Applied Behavior Analysis, 1*(1), 91–97. https://doi.org/10.1901/jaba.1968.1-91

Barnes-Holmes, D., Finn, M., McEnteggart, C., & Barnes-Holmes, Y. (2018). Derived stimulus relations and their role in a behavior-analytic account of human language and cognition. *Perspectives on Behavior Science, 41*(1), 155–173. https://doi.org/10.1007/s40614-017-0124-7

Barron, B. F., Verkuylen, L., Belisle, J., Paliliunas, D., & Dixon, M. R. (2019). Teaching "then-later" and "here-there" relations to children with autism: An evaluation of single reversals and transformation of stimulus function. *Behavior Analysis in Practice, 12*(1), 167–175. https://doi.org/10.1007/s40617-018-0216-1

Beaujean, A. A., & Farmer, R. L. (2021). Conceptual and methodological concerns: A commentary on "randomized controlled trial evaluation of ABA content on IQ gains in children with autism." *Journal of Behavioral Education, 30*(3), 479–488. https://doi.org/10.1007/s10864-020-09408-z

Behavior Analysis Certification Board (BACB). (2022a). BACB certificant data. https://www.bacb.com/bacb-certificant-data/

Behavior Analysis Certification Board (BACB). (2022b). U.S. state licensure of behavior analysts. https://www.bacb.com/u-s-licensure-of-behavior-analysts/

Belisle, J. (2020). Model dependent realism and the rule-governed behavior of behavior analysts: Applications to derived relational responding. *Perspectives on Behavior Science, 43*(2), 321–342. https://doi.org/10.1007/s40614-020-00247-x

Belisle, J., Burke, R., & Dennis, L. (2022). An initial evaluation of a gamified program to teach conditional discriminations within curricular programming. *Behavior Analysis: Research and Practice*. https://doi.org/10.1037/bar0000253

Belisle, J., Clark, L., Welch, K., McDonald, N., Dennis, L., & Sickman, E. (2021). Evaluation of broad skill repertoire changes over 3 months of PEAK implementation in a special education classroom. *Behavior Analysis in Practice, 15*, 324–329. https://doi.org/10.1007/s40617-021-00657-6

Belisle, J., Paliliunas, D., Lauer, T., Giamanco, A., Lee, B., & Sickman, E. (2020). Derived relational responding and transformations of function in children: A review of applied behavior-analytic journals. *The Analysis of Verbal Behavior, 36*(1), 115–145. https://doi.org/10.1007/s40616-019-00123-z

Belisle, J., Paliliunas, D., Stanley, C. R., Barron, B. F., & Dixon, M. R. (2021). Top-down attentional processing and relational density evident in word search performance of children. *Behavior Analysis in Practice*, 15, 684–697. https://doi.org/10.1007/s40617-021-00614-3

Belisle, J., Stanley, C. R., & Dixon, M. R. (2021). *Research methods for the practicing behavior analyst*. Carbondale, Illinois: Emergent Press.

Carnett, A., Raulston, T. J., & Charpentier, J. (2019). The application of Skinner's analysis of verbal behavior for teaching communication skills to persons with developmental disabilities. *Current Developmental Disorders Reports, 6*(3), 131–137. https://doi.org/10.1007/s40474-019-00170-0

Cassidy, S., Roche, B., & Hayes, S. C. (2011). A relational frame training intervention to raise intelligence quotients: A pilot study. *The Psychological Record, 61*(2), 173–198. https://doi.org/10.1007/BF03395755

Critchfield, T. S., Barnes-Holmes, D., & Dougher, M. J. (2018). What Sidman did—Historical and contemporary significance of research on derived stimulus relations. *Perspectives on Behavior Science, 41*(1), 9–32. https://doi.org/10.1007/s40614-018-0154-9

Dixon, M. R. (2014a). *PEAK: Direct training module*. Carbondale, Illinois: Emergent Press.

Dixon, M. R. (2014b). *PEAK: Generalization module*. Carbondale, Illinois: Emergent Press.

Dixon, M. R. (2015). *PEAK: Equivalence module*. Carbondale, Illinois: Emergent Press.

Dixon, M. R. (2016). *PEAK: Transformation module*. Carbondale, Illinois: Emergent Press.

Dixon, M. R. (2020): *Comprehensive assessment*. Carbondale, Illinois: Emergent Press.

Dixon, M. R. (2021). *LIFE skill emergent system: Functional module*. Carbondale, Illinois: Emergent Press.

Dixon, M. R., Belisle, J., McKeel, A., Whiting, S., Speelman, R., Daar, J. H., & Rowsey, K. (2017). An internal and critical review of the PEAK relational training system for children with autism and related intellectual disabilities: 2014–2017. *The Behavior Analyst, 40*(2), 493–521. https://doi.org/10.1007/s40614-017-0119-4

Dixon, M. R., Belisle, J., Stanley, C., Rowsey, K., Daar, J. H., & Szekely, S. (2015). Toward a behavior analysis of complex language for children with autism: Evaluating the relationship between PEAK and the VB-MAPP. *Journal of Developmental and Physical Disabilities, 27*(2), 223–233. https://doi.org/10.1007/s10882-014-9410-4

Dixon, M. R., Belisle, J., Stanley, C. R., Daar, J. H., & Williams, L. A. (2016). Derived equivalence relations of geometry skills in students with autism: An application of the PEAK-E curriculum. *The Analysis of Verbal Behavior, 32*(1), 38–45. https://doi.org/10.1007/s40616-016-0051-9

Dixon, M. R., Belisle, J., Stanley, C. R., Speelman, R. C., Rowsey, K. E., Kime, D., & Daar, J. H. (2017). Establishing derived categorical responding in children with disabilities using the PEAK-E curriculum. *Journal of Applied Behavior Analysis, 50*(1), 134–145. https://doi.org/10.1002/jaba.355

Dixon, M. R., Belisle, J., Whiting, S. W., & Rowsey, K. E. (2014a). Normative sample of the PEAK relational training system: Direct training module and subsequent comparisons to individuals with autism. *Research in Autism Spectrum Disorders, 8*(11), 1597–1606. https://doi.org/10.1007/s40614-017-0119-4

Dixon, M. R., Carman, J., Tyler, P. A., Whiting, S. W., Enoch, M. R., & Daar, J. H. (2014b). PEAK relational training system for children with autism and developmental disabilities: Correlations with Peabody picture vocabulary test and assessment reliability. *Journal of Developmental and Physical Disabilities, 26*(5), 603–614. https://doi.org/10.1007/s10882-014-9384-2

Dixon, M. R., & Paliliunas, D. (2018). *Accept. Identify. Move.: A behavior analytic curriculum for social-emotional development in children*. Carbondale, Illinois: Emergent Press.

Dixon, M. R., Paliliunas, D., Barron, B. F., Schmick, A. M., & Stanley, C. R. (2021). Randomized controlled trial evaluation of ABA content on IQ gains in children with autism. *Journal of Behavioral Education, 30*(3), 455–477. https://doi.org/10.1007/s10864-019-09344-7

Dixon, M. R., Rowsey, K. E., Gunnarsson, K. F., Belisle, J., Stanley, C. R., & Daar, J. H. (2017). Normative sample of the PEAK relational training system: Generalization module with comparison to individuals with autism. *Journal of Behavioral Education, 26*(1), 101–122. https://doi.org/10.1007/s10864-016-9261-4

Dixon, M. R., Speelman, R. C., Rowsey, K. E., & Belisle, J. (2016). Derived rule-following and transformations of stimulus function in a children's game: An application of PEAK-E with children with developmental disabilities. *Journal of Contextual Behavioral Science, 5*(3), 186–192. https://doi.org/10.1016/j.jcbs.2016.05.002

Dixon, M. R., Stanley, C., Belisle, J., Galliford, M. E., Alholail, A., & Schmick, A. M. (2017). Establishing derived equivalence relations of basic geography skills in children with autism. *The Analysis of Verbal Behavior, 33*(2), 290–295. https://doi.org/10.1007/s40616-017-0084-8

Dixon, M. R., Yi, Z., Sutton, A., & Pikula, A. (2023). Randomized-controlled trial examining differing content of ABA therapy delivered to autistic children. *Journal of Contextual Behavioral Science, 28*, 169–179.

Enoch, M. R., & Nicholson, S. L. (2020). Acceptance and commitment therapy and relational frame theory in the field of applied behavior analysis: The acceptability and perspective of the practicing BCBA. *Behavior Analysis in Practice, 13*(3), 609–617. https://doi.org/10.1007/s40617-020-00416-z

Gilsenan, C. M., Yi, Z., Hinman, J. M., Barron, B. F., & Dixon, M. R. (2021). Using relational training to improve performance during acceptance and commitment training sessions. *Behavior Analysis in Practice, 15*, 1–13. https://doi.org/10.1007/s40617-021-00574-8

Hahs, A. D., Dixon, M. R., & Paliliunas, D. (2019). Randomized controlled trial of a brief acceptance and commitment training for parents of individuals diagnosed with autism spectrum disorders. *Journal of Contextual Behavioral Science, 12*, 154–159. https://doi.org/10.1016/j.jcbs.2018.03.002

Hahs, A. D., & Jarynowski, J. (2019). Targeting staff treatment integrity of the PEAK relational training system using behavioral skills training. *Behavior Analysis in Practice, 12*(1), 209–215. https://doi.org/10.1007/s40617-018-00278-6

Hayes, S. C., Barnes-Holmes, D., & Roche, B. (2001). *Relational frame theory: A post-Skinnerian account of human language and cognition.* Amsterdam: Kluwer Academic/Plenum.

Hayes, S. C., Law, S., Assemi, K., Falletta-Cowden, N., Shamblin, M., Burleigh, K., Olla, R., Forman, M. & Smith, P. (2021). Relating is an operant: A fly over of 35 years of RFT research. *Perspectivas em Análise do Comportamento, 12*(1), 5–32. https://doi.org/10.18761/PAC.2021.v12.RFT.02

Healy, O., Barnes-Holmes, D., & Smeets, P. M. (2000). Derived relational responding as generalized operant behavior. *Journal of the Experimental Analysis of Behavior, 74*(2), 207–227. https://doi.org/10.1901/jeab.2000.74-207

Issen, T., Hinman, J. M., & Dixon, M. R. (2021). Utilizing the AIM curriculum to improve job performance in an educational setting for children with autism and related disabilities. *Behavior Analysis in Practice, 15*, 172–178. https://doi.org/10.1007/s40617-020-00528-6

Kane, M., Connell, J. E., & Pellecchia, M. (2010). A quantitative analysis of language interventions for children with autism. *The Behavior Analyst Today, 11*(2), 128.

Kuhn, T. S. (1962). *The structure of scientific revolutions.* Chicago: University of Chicago Press.

Love, J. R., Carr, J. E., Almason, S. M., & Petursdottir, A. I. (2009). Early and intensive behavioral intervention for autism: A survey of clinical practices. *Research in Autism Spectrum Disorders, 3*(2), 421–428. https://doi.org/10.1016/j.rasd.2008.08.008Get

Malkin, A., Dixon, M. R., Speelman, R. C., & Luke, N. (2017). Evaluating the relationships between the PEAK relational training system–direct training module, assessment of basic language and learning skills–revised, and the Vineland adaptive behavior scales–II. *Journal of Developmental and Physical Disabilities, 29*(2), 341–351. https://doi.org/10.1007/s10882-016-9527-8

May, B. K., & St Cyr, J. (2021). The impact of the PEAK curriculum on standardized measures of intelligence: A systems level randomized control trial. *Advances in Neurodevelopmental Disorders, 5*(3), 245–255. https://doi.org/10.1007/s41252-021-00199-6

McKeel, A., Rowsey, K., Dixon, M. R., & Daar, J. H. (2015). Correlation between PEAK relational training system and one-word picture vocabulary tests. *Research in Autism Spectrum Disorders, 12*, 34–39. https://doi.org/10.1016/j.rasd.2014.12.007

McKeel, A. N., Dixon, M. R., Daar, J. H., Rowsey, K. E., & Szekely, S. (2015). Evaluating the efficacy of the PEAK relational training system using a randomized controlled trial of children with autism. *Journal of Behavioral Education, 24*(2), 230–241. https://doi.org/10.1007/s10864-015-9219-y

Michael, J., Palmer, D. C., & Sundberg, M. L. (2011). The multiple control of verbal behavior. *The Analysis of Verbal Behavior, 27*(1), 3–22. https://doi.org/10.1007/BF03393089

O'Connor, M., Farrell, L., Munnelly, A., & McHugh, L. (2017). Citation analysis of relational frame theory: 2009–2016. *Journal of Contextual Behavioral Science*, *6*(2), 152–158. https://doi.org/10.1016/j.jcbs.2017.04.009

Padilla, K. L. (2020). Global assessment use and practices in applied behavior analysis: Surveying the field. *Research in Autism Spectrum Disorders*, *79*, 101676. https://doi.org/10.1016/j.rasd.2020.101676

Pahnke, J., Lundgren, T., Hursti, T., & Hirvikoski, T. (2014). Outcomes of an acceptance and commitment therapy-based skills training group for students with high-functioning autism spectrum disorder: A quasi-experimental pilot study. *Autism*, *18*(8), 953–964. https://doi.org/10.1177/1362361313501091

Partington, J. W. (2006). *Assessment of Basic Language and Learning Skills–Revised (ABLLS-R)*. Davie: Behavior Analysis, Inc.

Pelaez, M., Gewirtz, J. L., Sanchez, A., & Mahabir, N. M. (2000). Exploring stimulus equivalence formation in infants. *Behavioral Development Bulletin*, *9*(1), 20–25. https://doi.org/10.1037/h0100534

Sidman, M. (1971). Reading and auditory-visual equivalences. *Journal of Speech and Hearing Research*, *14*(1), 5–13.

Sidman, M., & Tailby, W. (1982). Conditional discrimination vs. matching to sample: An expansion of the testing paradigm. *Journal of the Experimental Analysis of Behavior*, *37*(1), 5–22. https://doi.org/10.1901/jeab.1982.37-5

Skinner, B. F. (1957). *Verbal behavior*. Brattleboro, Vermont: Echo Point Books & Media.

Sundberg, C. T., Sundberg, M. L., & Michael, J. (2018). Covert verbal mediation in arbitrary matching to sample. *Journal of the Experimental Analysis of Behavior*, *109*(3), 600–623. https://doi.org/10.1002/jeab.434

Sundberg, M. L. (2008). *Verbal Behavior Milestones Assessment and Placement Program (VB-MAPP)*. Concord, CO: AVB Press.

Sutton, A., Pikula, A., Yi, Z., & Dixon, M. R. (2021). Evaluating the convergent validity of the PEAK Comprehensive Assessment (PCA): Intelligence, behavior challenges, and autism symptom severity. *Journal of Developmental and Physical Disabilities*, 34, 549–570. https://doi.org/10.1007/s10882-021-09814-9

US Department of Defense. (2019). *The Department of Defense Comprehensive Autism Care Demonstration Quarterly Report to Congress Second Quarter, Fiscal Year 2019*. https://www.altteaching.org/wp-content/uploads/2019/11/TRICARE-Autism-Report.pdf

Witts, B. N. (2018). An external review of the conclusions regarding the peak direct training module. *Journal of Applied Behavior Analysis*, *51*(3), 719–737. https://doi.org/10.1002/jaba.491

Yi, Z., & Dixon, M. R. (2021). Developing and enhancing adherence to a telehealth ABA parent training curriculum for caregivers of children with autism. *Behavior Analysis in Practice*, *14*(1), 58–74. https://doi.org/10.1007/s40617-020-00464-5

19

Social Skills Training

Erin Kang
Montclair State University

Mary Isaac Cargill
Montclair State University

Sadaf Khawar
Montclair State University

Britney Jeyanayagam
Montclair State University

Rachel G. McDonald
Montclair State University

Matthew D. Lerner
Stony Brook University

19.1 Technical Abstract

Background: Social skills trainings (SSTs) aim to address differences in social functioning that are associated with autism spectrum disorder. Knowledge-based SSTs promote social skills acquisition through didactic teaching of "social knowledge" and structured opportunities for skills rehearsal. Performance-based SSTs aim to facilitate implicit learning of social behaviors through spontaneous peer interactions via games and drama- and theater-based activities. **Method:** To review and synthesize research on SSTs, we examined empirical studies and review articles examining SSTs with autistic individuals. **Results:** SSTs are generally effective for improving social knowledge and competence, communication skills, and relational skills in autistic individuals, and they may be adapted to address social demands across the lifespan. **Discussion:** Research suggests promising effects of SSTs on social functioning in autistic individuals. However, most existing literature evaluating SSTs has focused on White, male autistic adolescents without co-occurring intellectual disabilities, necessitating more robust investigation of the efficacy of these treatments. **Practitioner recommendations:** SSTs can be delivered by a range of practitioners in various settings. Rather than expecting autistic individuals to change their social behaviors or to conform to social norms,

Erin Kang et al., *Social Skills Training*. In: *Lifespan Treatment for Autistic Individuals*. Edited by: Peter Sturmey, Russell Lang, and James K. Luiselli, Oxford University Press. © Oxford University Press (2025).
DOI: 10.1093/oso/9780197635841.003.0019

it may be more effective to understand communication differences and provide opportunities for building upon skills to promote social competence.

19.2 Layperson Summary

Social skills training is a commonly used intervention that seeks to assist with the difficulties in social communication and interaction commonly experienced by autistic individuals. SSTs use a variety of approaches to provide autistic individuals opportunities to learn and practice social skills, including a combination of direct teaching and roleplay activities, games, and theater- or acting-based activities. Treatment may occur in an individual capacity or in group settings. Most SSTs consist of 60–90-minute sessions that take place weekly; some more intensive programs consist of 5–6-hour sessions that take place 5 days a week for several weeks. These interventions may be led by a number of professionals, including clinical, school, and other support personnel, granted they have taken specialized training courses about the intervention, typically delivered by the developer to ensure treatment fidelity. Empirical evaluation supports the effectiveness of SSTs at improving the overall social skills of autistic individuals, particularly those with average or above-average intelligence, when compared to those not receiving treatment. More specifically, SSTs lead to gains in understanding social behavior and situations, and improvements in communication skills, peer relationships, and overall social competence. These advances in social skills are also often associated with decreases in anxiety, loneliness, and peer victimization. No risks or negative side effects of SSTs have been reported in the extant literature; however, autistic self-advocates and other stakeholders in the neurodiversity movement have voiced concerns about SSTs. While SST has focused mostly on working with autistic individuals, some SST programs can facilitate meetings and community-based activities to bring caregivers and families together to share experiences.

19.3 Treatment Summary Table

Treatment summary: Social Skills Training

Treatment description: SST seek to address challenges in social functioning experienced by autistic individuals, namely challenges in social-emotional reciprocity, verbal and nonverbal communication, and in developing and maintaining peer relationships. SSTs may use various strategies, including direct teaching, role-play activities, games, or play, to provide opportunities for autistic individuals to learn and practice social skills. SSTs may take individual or group formats and may be effective for individuals across the lifespan.

Expected outcomes: SSTs generally lead to improvements in social knowledge, social competence, conversational and nonverbal communication skills, and skills associated with making and keeping reciprocal friendships.

Methods: SSTs take on a variety of forms, differing in duration, intensity, structure, and specific treatment targets depending on the intended treatment population and goals. Knowledge-based SSTs involve the explicit teaching of social rules through direct instruction and provide opportunities for in vivo practice of skills during structured activities supervised by instructors available to provide feedback and reinforcement. Performance-based SSTs allow for the implicit learning of social skills by providing natural opportunities for peer interaction through game-, theater-, and drama-based activities.

Expertise required to implement treatment: SSTs may be delivered by a variety of professionals, including clinical, school, and other support personnel, contingent upon receiving training in delivery of the SSTs, typically by the intervention's developer.

Risks and negative side effects: There are no significant risks or negative side effects reported in SSTs literature. However, there have been some anecdotal concerns around unintended negative consequences (e.g., inauthenticity, increases in social anxiety) with prescriptive approaches in teaching social skills.

Additional considerations and limitations: SSTs are designed to treat autistic individuals with average or above-average IQs; however, some treatments are inclusive of all cognitive abilities. Additionally, most evaluations of treatment effectiveness have been conducted with White, upper-class males. As such, knowledge of the effectiveness of SSTs across areas of socioeconomic, gender, and racial diversity is unclear.

19.4 Introduction

19.4.1 Treatment Description

Autism spectrum disorder (ASD), henceforth referred to as autism,[1] is characterized by differences in social communication in tandem with the presence of restricted or repetitive behaviors or interests (American Psychiatric Association, 2013). SSTs aim to promote skill acquisition in social context that will help enable autistic individuals to navigate their social environment, interact with others, and build meaningful relationships (Bishop-Fitzpatrick et al., 2015; McMahon et al., 2013; Wong et al., 2015). SSTs are one of the widely used intervention approaches for autistic youth (McMahon et al., 2013; Wolstencroft et al., 2018). There are different types of SST approaches. Knowledge-based SSTs have a more structured and didactic approach in which specific, predetermined social skills topics are reviewed per session (Gates et al., 2017). Conversely, performance-based social skills trainings (PBSSTs) promote implicit learning of facets of social skills by spontaneous peer interactions through theater/drama or game-based activities (e.g., Marro et al., 2019; McDonald et al., 2022).

[1] The language utilized herein is congruent with suggestions from Bottema-Beutel and colleagues (2021) in the hopes of limiting stigmatization. These suggestions include, but are not limited to, the use of identity-first rather than person-first language, nonmedicalized language (e.g., minimizing pathologizing language such as "disorder"), and references to "nonautistic" people rather than "typically developing" or "neurotypical" people. However, when referencing the specific *DSM-5* disorder rather than the person, autism spectrum disorder (ASD) will be used.

19.4.2 Rationale and Objectives

Social skills development is a critical domain for autistic individuals, as these abilities impact several important domains of functioning, including academic (Elliot et al., 2001) and psychological functioning (Coie et al., 1995; Rodriguez et al., 2021). For example, knowing how to engage with peers enables autistic people to make and maintain friendships, and this has been shown to buffer against stressful life events and peer victimization and to reduce bullying (Estell et al., 2009; Miller & Ingham, 1976). Contrary to the prevailing belief that differences in friendship making underlie the inability and disinterest of autistic individuals to form social relationships, autistic children do want friends (Mendelson et al., 2016). However, compared to neurotypical children, the quantity of friends is less and the quality of friendship is poorer, according to self- and peer-report (Chang & Dean, 2022; Mendelson et al., 2016). Additional secondary gains of social competence are improvement in emotion regulation and decrease in anxiety and repetitive behaviors, including self-injurious behaviors (Tse et al., 2007). The impact of the differences in social skills is palpable for many autistic children and adolescents, and SSTs seek to equip them with relevant skills to improve their overall quality of life across the lifespan (Tse et al., 2007).

Various theories suggest there may be differences in how autistic and nonautistic individuals acquire social problem-solving skills, and SSTs are designed to address these core differences in social functioning in autistic people (Reichow & Volkmar, 2010). Social cognition concerns the myriad of socio-cognitive processes (e.g., perception, attention, memory, action planning) which underpin social knowledge (i.e., the knowing what to do in social situations) that in turn promotes social behavior. Facets of social cognition that are often targeted in SSTs include differences in theory of mind development (Frith, 2008; Senju, 2013), facial emotion recognition (Lozier et al., 2014), and memory for faces (Corbett et al., 2016). Further, differences in social information processing in autistic individuals can relate to challenges in attending to environmental stimuli efficiently as well as socio-emotional reciprocity which lead to compromised social competence in autistic individuals (Lerner & Mikami, 2012; Mendelson et al., 2016). Therefore, SST approaches for individuals that address these differences are likely to be most conducive in addressing core autistic differences due to the interplay of domains of functioning.

14.4.3 Considerations for Implementation

Traditionally, many SSTs for autistic people have been based in structured learning. Many of these knowledge-based SSTs take a didactic approach wherein an instructor explicitly teaches various social skills (Goldstein & McGinnis, 1997; Gunning et al., 2019; Herbrecht et al., 2009; Lopata et al., 2013; Vernon et al., 1996;

Wolstencroft et al., 2018). Knowledge-based SSTs target skills related to academic and social success, such as nonverbal communication, emotion regulation, effective listening, perspective taking, and emotion recognition (Derosier et al., 2011). These skills are intended to help individuals on the autism spectrum adjust to increased social demands (Reichow & Volkmar, 2010). Knowledge-based SSTs are grounded in the belief that autistic people may require additional support when learning social skills, as they may not obtain these skills from observing their environment (Gralinski & Kopp, 1993). Therefore, the in vivo practice component of SSTs is vital because it allows participants to actively engage with the target skills while the instructor is present to provide feedback as necessary. This SST format allows for immediate reinforcement when autistic participants use the targeted skill rather than relying on social reinforcement since it is unclear whether this is a sufficient reinforcer for autistic people (Reichow et al., 2012). Providing autistic children and adolescents with immediate reinforcement for displaying desired social skills should increase the likelihood of the skill being used again, thereby creating additional repetitions and opportunities for practice.

These knowledge-based SSTs also utilize various activities to explicitly teach the aforementioned skills. One common activity in knowledge-based SSTs is role playing, in which group members act out social skills in pairs while other members and trainers observe and provide performance feedback. Another common activity, modeling, is closely associated with role playing, and involves the trainers demonstrating a social skill so that group members can later reproduce it in their role plays (Goldstein & McGinnis, 1997; Lopata et al., 2010; Thomeer et al., 2019; Waugh & Peskin, 2015). Modeling and role playing work in conjunction to facilitate group members' practice of their learned social knowledge. Another common strategy in group sessions is utilizing social stories, which describe specific activities and situational behavior (Gray & Garand, 1993). Additional strategies include video modeling, wherein autistic children watch a video demonstration of a skill and are then encouraged to act it out themselves (Bellini & Akullian, 2007), and incorporating nonautistic siblings and peers into the intervention to model skills and tutor participants (Kohler & Strain, 1990; Radley et al., 2020). In addition to the modeling and role-playing activities that pervade most knowledge-based SSTs, some interventions such as the Secret Agent Society (Beaumont, 2010) utilize additional strategies such as computerized games aimed at teaching emotion recognition, appropriate emotional expression, and skills to solve common social problems.

In contrast to knowledge-based SSTs, PBSSTs do not utilize explicit, didactic instruction and rather allow participants to implicitly learn social skills through spontaneous interactions with their autistic and typically developing peers in supported, enriched environments (Marro et al., 2019; McDonald et al., 2022). Intervention leaders still provide support to participants as necessary, but PBSSTs do not utilize the traditional didactic approach to teaching social skills and instead rely more heavily on the in vivo practice component. The activities utilized in

PBSSTs are adaptable and capitalize on motivating participants to make the peer interactions more reinforcing. Many autistic people have special interests that can be motivating; therefore, integrating these special interests into PBSST activities may increase the intervention's effectiveness. PBSSTs therefore aim to provide autistic people with an enriched environment that successfully promotes social skill acquisition and reinforces naturalistic peer interactions (McDonald et al., 2022).

Recent work has been conducted to develop treatments utilizing virtual reality (VR) and computer-based intervention approaches (CBI) to target social skills (McCoy et al., 2016; Mesa-Gresa et al., 2018). Interventions using VR provide a simulated environment in which participants practice their social skills with either a confederate/preprogrammed robot or enter scenarios that are preprogrammed to elicit the skill. The goal of these treatments is to provide a realistic space for children to practice elicited social communication behaviors in a simulated naturalistic environment, which may be advantageous for generalization of skills and may aid in the general improvements in social cognition (Bekele et al., 2013; Cheng et al., 2015; Ip et al., 2018). CBI approaches provide a similar electronic environment where social interactions are simulated to mimic naturalistic social settings that provide space for practicing skills. While many of these programs use confederates or interactive characters, some allow participants to play computer-based games with other peers (Bauminger-Zviely et al., 2013; Beaumont & Sofronoff, 2008; Bernard-Opitz et al., 2001; Cheng & Ye, 2010).

As people develop and mature across the lifespan, they are met with increasing social demands and are expected to communicate in more socially complex ways (Tantam, 2003). Autistic people's differences in social abilities are often highlighted by these increased demands, and differences in these areas can result in peer rejection, loneliness, and poorer friendship quality (Bauminger & Kasari, 2000; Cresswell et al., 2019). Although many SSTs focus primarily on autistic adolescents, the target age range for these interventions ranges widely from 2 to 45 years old (Gorenstein et al., 2020; Pickles et al., 2016) to respond to the increased social demands across the lifespan. Furthermore, SSTs allow opportunities for autistic or otherwise neurodivergent youth to meet, interact, and develop friendships with one another, which has been shown to protect against the deleterious impact of social struggles, reduce perceived loneliness and mental health struggles, and increase self-worth (Bauminger et al., 2004; Mazurek, 2014; Whitehouse et al., 2009).

19.5 Research Background

Knowledge-based, performance-based, and computer-based SSTs have demonstrated the ability to address social and communicative differences commonly associated with autism. These SSTs vary widely in terms of content, duration, and targeted skills, and as such, they also reflect a wide variety of promising outcomes related to social communication and social cognition. Several interventions have demonstrated efficacy through rigorous research, including randomized controlled trials (RCTs; Afsharnejad et al., 2021; Corbett et al., 2016, 2023; Laugeson et al., 2009; Lerner & Mikami, 2012; Lopata et al., 2010; Thomeer et al., 2019). Furthermore, these SSTs were carried out in a variety of contexts, including schools, clinics, and other community settings (Beadle-Brown et al., 2018; Guli et al., 2013; Marro et al., 2019), and several have demonstrated reliable results through replication studies (Lerner & Mikami, 2012; Schohl et al., 2014; Thomeer et al., 2012).

19.5.1 Knowledge-Based SSTs

Among the myriad of knowledge-based SSTs, PEERS, KONTAKT, Skillstreaming, and summerMAX appear to have the most empirical support (Afsharnejad et al., 2021; Laugeson, 2017; Laugeson et al., 2012; Lopata et al., 2010; Thomeer et al., 2012, 2019). In addition to practicing the social skills in vivo with other participants, researchers have identified other elements of effective SSTs, including a small group format, concurrent parent training, reinforcement, and homework assignments (Moody & Laugeson, 2020). There is some variability in the duration and intensity among these knowledge-based interventions. Although most consist of weekly 60–90-minute sessions for 8 to 22 weeks (Begeer et al., 2015; McMahon et al., 2013), other formats are emerging, such as a more intensive multiweek summer camp format (Lopata et al., 2010). It is presently unclear whether intensity/duration of SST differentially impacts acquisition of social skills. For example, one study suggests that these factors are not related to intervention outcomes (Tyminski et al., 2008), and another suggests that longer interventions are positively related to certain social outcomes such as peer interaction and friendship making (McMahon et al., 2013). Given these inconsistent results, more research is needed to explore differences in this area.

Overall, these SSTs seem to consistently improve social competence, friendship quality, and loneliness in this age group, with less consistent improvements related to social communication and emotion recognition (Reichow et al., 2012). These interventions seem to promote positive changes in social communication, social reciprocity, social motivation, peer engagement (e.g., play behaviors and friendship-making skills), and level of autistic traits, with several of these changes being sustained for up to 5 years post intervention (Ichikawa et al., 2013; Pickles et al., 2016; Tripathi et al., 2021). A recent review of the literature in this area reported largely positive results from SST involvement and suggested that underpowered studies with too few participants could explain differences in results across studies (Cappadocia & Weiss, 2011).

19.5.2 Example Intervention: Program for the Education and Enrichment of Relational Skills

One of the most extensively tested social skills interventions for autistic adolescents is the Program for the Education and Enrichment of Relational Skills (PEERS; Laugeson & Frankel, 2011). The PEERS intervention targets autistic adolescents between 12 to 17 years of age, and it consists of 90-minute sessions, typically delivered once a week over the course of 14 to 16 weeks. This intervention is unique in that two groups run concurrently: a social skills group for autistic adolescents and a parent group. In the adolescent group, autistic adolescents learn and practice social skills, while in the parent group, parents learn how to coach their adolescents to help them apply their newly acquired social skills. Some of the areas targeted by PEERS include conversational skills, appropriate use of humor, electronic communication, responding to bullying, politely exiting conversations, and planning social get-togethers with friends.

Results from RCTs indicate that the PEERS intervention improved parent-reported social skills, and autism symptoms related to social responsiveness, as well as social knowledge, friendship quality, and social engagement (Laugeson et al., 2009, 2012). One study found that most of these improvements were maintained at a 14-week follow-up, except for social knowledge. Encouragingly, problematic behaviors (e.g., hyperactivity and inattention, externalizing behaviors, internalizing behaviors) continued to decrease after the intervention, seemingly due to parental coaching post intervention (Laugeson et al., 2012). Furthermore, it seems that many of these improvements are durable and may even continue to improve for up to 5 years after completing PEERS, as demonstrated by autistic adolescents' maintenance of gains in social skills knowledge and frequency of peer interactions, as well as their further improvement in social functioning and social responsiveness post intervention (Mandelberg et al., 2014). Despite the fact that the social skills targeted in SSTs for older children are more complex, the evidence suggests that PEERS and other interventions are nonetheless effective.

19.5.3 Developmental Considerations

Younger, preschool-aged children can participate in certain knowledge-based SSTs to develop age-appropriate social skills. One option for this age group that has a substantive evidence base is the PEERS for Preschoolers program (P4P; (Laugeson et al., 2016). The PEERS intervention has been adapted for young autistic children between the ages of 4 and 6 years to include (1) social skill content delivery via puppet shows; (2) mock playdates during the final 20–30 minutes of each session to practice the targeted social skills; and (3) weekly homework assignments, including completing playdates with children not involved in the PEERS for Preschoolers intervention to promote skill generalizability to other social contexts (Park et al.,

2022). Traditional PEERS for Preschoolers intervention is associated with significant improvements in social responsiveness, social engagement with peers, cooperation, self-control, responsibility, and problem behaviors (e.g., hyperactivity and inattention, bullying, and externalizing behaviors; Tripathi et al., 2021), while an abbreviated 8-week version of the intervention improved overall social skills, social behavior, and social communication (Factor et al., 2022), with some of these improvements maintained at follow-up.

Just as the shift from childhood to adolescence is fraught with different environments and increased social demands that may require increased support for autistic people, the transition from adolescence to adulthood is also challenging. The PEERS intervention has been further adapted for use with young adults 18 to 24 years of age (Laugeson, 2017), with reconfiguration of the initial modules to better reflect adult experiences, as well as the addition of three modules pertaining to romantic relationships. The evidence indicates that PEERS for Young Adults significantly improved overall social skills, frequency of social engagement, social skills knowledge, empathy, and social responsiveness (Gantman et al., 2012; Laugeson et al., 2015; McVey et al., 2016). Additionally, one study also reported a reduction in restricted and repetitive behaviors as well as sustained treatment effects and novel improvements in social communication, assertion, responsibility, and empathy at a 16-week follow-up, perhaps suggesting a delayed effect in some areas (Laugeson et al., 2015). The current body of research provides limited but promising evidence that autistic individuals ranging from preschoolers to young adults can benefit from knowledge-based SSTs.

19.5.4 Performance-Based SSTs

There is substantial variation in the activities and strategies utilized in PBSSTs, which include game-based activities, music, dance, and drama- or theater-based approaches (Aithal et al., 2021; Lagasse, 2017; Lerner et al., 2011; Lindsay et al., 2017). These interventions are most commonly delivered via weekly sessions of 60–90-minute duration, but a few are more intensive, consisting of 5- to 6-hour sessions each weekday over the course of several months in the summer (McMahon et al., 2013). There is a wide range of specific approaches utilized in PBSSTs, and we describe them thematically.

19.5.5 Drama- or Theater-Based PBSSTs

There has been a recent increase in drama- or theater-based PBSSTs (McDonald et al., 2022). These SSTs provide participants with training in various acting techniques that naturally provide opportunities for social interaction with others. Activities associated with these PBSSTs include rehearsing scenes from well-known plays, crafting and narrating novel stories, working with peers and intervention leaders to develop characters, and improvising scenes and dialogue with other autistic participants and nonautistic peer mentors (Beadle-Brown et al., 2018; Corbett et al., 2016; Guli et al., 2013; Mehling et al., 2017). Across different interventions, these PBSSTs tend to target autistic children and adolescents. There is also great variability in the implementation and dosage of such interventions. Many consist of weekly 45–90-minute sessions that span 10 to 16 weeks, while others are more intensive and entail multihour sessions each weekday over the course of multiple weeks (e.g., summer camp format). Although exact approaches differ between interventions, drama- and theater-based PBSSTs seek to target social skills related to theory of mind, flexible thinking, perspective taking, verbal and nonverbal communication, cooperation, emotion recognition, eye contact, and interactive play (Beadle-Brown et al., 2018; Corbett et al., 2016; Guli et al., 2013; Lerner et al., 2007; Mehling et al., 2017). The activities require participants to receive, interpret, and respond to information from others, and they may also increase participants' imaginative abilities.

19.5.6 Example Drama- or Theater-Based Intervention: SDARI

One drama- and theater-based PBSST with substantial empirical support is sociodramatic affective relational intervention (SDARI; Lerner et al., 2007). This approach utilizes acting games and strong age-appropriate motivators to facilitate intrinsic motivation, and it is grounded in naturalistic skill building via positive social reinforcement and relationship building (Kang et al., 2020; Lerner et al., 2007). SDARI has been successfully delivered in both lab-based and community-based settings and has been flexibly and effectively implemented (Lerner et al., 2011; Lerner & Mikami, 2012; Marro et al., 2019). Across different studies, autistic children and adolescents aged 11 to 17 years completed four 90-minute sessions (Lerner & Mikami, 2012), ten 90-minutes sessions (Marro et al., 2019), or a 6-week summer camp where they completed 5-hour sessions each weekday (Lerner et al., 2011). Although results are mixed across different intervention designs, SDARI appears effective at improving social assertion, emotion recognition, social problems, reciprocal friendships, and theory of mind, with evidence of sustained improvement in some of these areas post intervention (Lerner et al., 2011; Lerner & Mikami, 2012; Marro et al., 2019). It seems that SDARI is generally effective for improving social skills in autistic children and adolescents, and that gains may be linked to factors such as intervention setting, duration, and intensity. Relatedly, SDARI seeks to strengthen autistic people's existing social skills by incorporating special interests and practicing skills in a safe, supportive environment, rather than encouraging adaptation to nonautistic standards of social behavior.

19.5.7 Game-Based PBSSTs

Game-based PBSSTs capitalize on children's natural interest in game play to help impart social skills, while also providing a safe environment for children to practice their skills with peers. One of the most established game-based PBSSTs is LEGO™ Club, which is typically geared toward autistic children and adolescents between the ages of 6 and 16 years (Legoff, 2004). The logistics of LEGO™ Club vary widely, with weekly sessions lasting between 20 and 90 minutes and spanning anywhere from 4 weeks to several years in a variety of settings, including clinics, schools, and participants' homes (Lindsay et al., 2017), with individual and collaborative group-based activities (Legoff, 2004). During LEGO™ Club, different roles and responsibilities (e.g., "engineer," "supplier," 'builder') are assigned to group members (Legoff et al., 2014; Legoff, 2004). This approach emphasizes verbal and nonverbal communication, joint attention, attentional control, collaborative problem solving, sharing, and turn taking (Legoff & Sherman, 2006).

Results from various studies about LEGO™ Club reflect improvement in participants' social competence, communication skills, and ability to establish and maintain friendships, as well as their adaptive behaviors, belonging, coping skills, and time spent playing alone (Legoff & Sherman, 2006; Lindsay et al., 2017). The most effective LEGO™ Club interventions were those conducted by clinicians or educators in clinic- or school-based settings and that consisted of weekly sessions lasting at least an hour. Notably, many of the most effective interventions were relatively short term (3 to 18 hours of total intervention time), suggesting that social skill gains eventually plateau; however, more work is needed to explore the effects of dosage in this PBSST (Lindsay et al., 2017). Furthermore, participants with better verbal abilities tended to demonstrate more improvement than those with less-developed verbal abilities (Legoff & Sherman, 2006). In sum, LEGO™ Club seems to have a positive impact on various social abilities in autistic children and adolescents. LEGO™ Club takes a similar approach to SDARI in that the goal is to strengthen existing social skills by incorporating special interests and naturally reinforcing their social skills in a supported setting.

Overall, PBSSTs seem to promote positive changes in a variety of social skills, including social communication, social awareness, social interaction, assertion, emotion recognition, social knowledge, theory of mind, and adaptive behaviors (Beadle-Brown et al., 2018; Corbett et al., 2016; Guli et al., 2013; Legoff et al., 2014; Lerner & Mikami, 2012; Mehling et al., 2017). A recent review of the literature in this area reflected largely positive results from involvement in drama- or theater-based PBSSTs (McDonald et al., 2022), but more research is needed to corroborate these promising findings and explore PBSSTs in more depth. Furthermore, most PBSSTs are geared toward autistic children and adolescents, so future research should aim to address the effectiveness of such interventions in an adult population.

19.5.8 Computer-Based/Virtual Reality Approaches

These computer-based/virtual reality programs are intended to provide spaces for participants to interact with their peers without the pressure of an in vivo experience, in hopes of allowing them to gradually get more comfortable with these skills prior to using them more fluidly in their daily lives. Recent reviews on these interventions have demonstrated effectiveness in treating targeted skills such as emotion recognition, social communication, and emotional reciprocity, among other social skills (Karami et al., 2021; McCoy et al., 2016; Mesa-Gresa et al., 2018). While these interventions have displayed some effectiveness and efficacy in positively impacting social communication and emotion recognition, many of these projects have not been replicated and include small sample sizes of children (Karami et al., 2021). Further, while many studies have been published on the topic, there is a lack of cohesiveness in the approach to treatment and a lack of consistent targets posing difficulty in specific treatment recommendations. For instance, while not originally intended to be a CBI, many SSTs have been adapted to a Zoom- or computer-based format over the course of the COVID-19 pandemic (i.e., Secret Agent Society; MacEvilly & Brosnan, 2020). However, this area displays promising results and should be closely monitored for replication of effects and emerging treatment approaches.

19.5.9 SSTs and Anxiety

Autistic individuals experience high rates of anxiety disorders, which often exacerbate challenges in peer relationships and increase fear in social settings (McVey et al., 2016; Simonoff et al., 2008). Previous research suggests anxiety symptoms may contribute to reductions in positive experiences and improvements during and following SSTs (Gerber et al., 2022; Hillier et al., 2018; Spain et al., 2017; Spain & Blainey, 2015; White et al., 2013), and secondary anxiety-related improvements following SSTs are variable across participants (Kang et al., 2020). Given this, few SSTs have dedicated targets for anxiety symptoms.

The multimodal anxiety and social skills intervention (MASSI) utilizes a combined approach to treatment, where anxiety disorders are addressed in simultaneous individual therapy using adapted cognitive-behavioral approaches and social skills are addressed using group SST approaches. MASSI evinced improvements in social responsiveness and global functioning, as well as trends toward improvements in dimensional parent- and clinician-reported anxiety symptoms (White et al., 2013, 2018). This suggests MASSI may be effective in treating both social skills difficulties and anxiety symptoms in autistic adolescents. Another intervention examined the effects of an unstructured group performance-based approach to both social skills and anxiety components, paired with individual therapy sessions to supplement anxiety management in autistic adults (Spain et al., 2017). This intervention displayed effectiveness in improving social anxiety and avoidance; however, other facets of social functioning were not examined, and the effectiveness of the treatment protocol in improving areas of social functioning is unclear. In general, combined anxiety social skills treatments show some evidence in improving both anxiety and social skills in autistic individuals. However, they have not been extensively examined in large groups of individuals. Further, both interventions involved participants in older age ranges with IQs greater than 70, and research should be extended to evaluate effects across developmental levels.

19.5.10 Maintenance and Generalization of Effects

One of the key criticisms of the current empirical literature base around SSTs via reviews and meta-analyses of SSTs is the minimal examination of maintenance and generalization of effects (Gates et al., 2017; White et al., 2007). For instance, gains in social skills via SSTs may not necessarily translate into peer interactions in naturalistic settings (e.g., playground interactions, playdates) and/or do not relate to improvements in the quality of peer interactions (Chang & Dean, 2022). Therefore, those SSTs that have a practice component in the community (MacKay et al., 2007; Tse et al., 2007) and/or have regular parental involvement (Hillier et al., 2007) can be effective in generalizing and maintaining treatment gains outside of the initial setting. A recent systematic review examined generalization and maintenance effects in SSTs for preschool-aged autistic children (Gunning et al., 2019), and fortunately, the number of studies that assessed generalization and/or maintenance has increased in recent decades. The Gunning at al. review emphasizes that employing naturalistic intervention strategies and targeting social behaviors can contribute to the successful generalization of outcomes, with factors such as duration and setting potentially playing a role (Gunning et al., 2019).

19.5.11 Limitations

Despite substantial support for the effectiveness of SSTs, the existing literature has predominantly concentrated on White male adolescents from upper-middle class backgrounds and IQs greater than 70 (Corbett et al., 2016; Happe, 1995; Hoogenhout & Malcolm-Smith, 2017; Lerner & Mikami, 2012; Marro et al., 2019; Safer-Lichtenstein et al., 2019). This lack of diversity limits the ability to appraise the impact of cultural and socioeconomical factors on treatment outcomes. Assessing the effectiveness and feasibility of cultural adaptations, such as translating manuals and modeling videos to other languages or modification of specific targets to be congruent with cultural norms, has similarly been largely neglected (Davenport et al., 2018). Therefore, these findings should not be assumed to generalize to individuals from underrepresented communities.

Notable methodological limitations include small and poorly characterized study samples. Additionally, the majority of the studies did not have a control group, which is often necessary to identify a cause-and-effect relationship between intervention and skill acquisition (Bauminger, 2007; MacKay et al., 2007; Tse et al., 2007). Additionally, while some of these SSTs have reported promising replications (Lerner & Mikami, 2012; Schohl et al., 2014; Thomeer et al., 2012), others are still in need of replication to corroborate promising initial findings (Beadle-Brown et al., 2018; Guli et al., 2013; Mehling et al., 2017), including examination of the degree to which learned skills generalize and are maintained. Many SSTs require replication to establish efficacy across a broader range of participant characteristics, promoting inclusivity and generalizability. Moreover, most SSTs with documented efficacy require training from the intervention developers to ensure treatment fidelity, thus limiting accessibility to community stakeholders. Furthermore, there is a need to use multimodal assessment methods and more sensitive measures to assess constructs in intervention research, including multiple informants and direct observations (Bauminger, 2007). Additionally, while SSTs for older autistic individuals have shown positive effects on social responsiveness (Dubreucq et al., 2022), future research should focus on older autistic adults' specific social challenges (e.g., romantic relationships; employment; Hillier et al., 2007).

19.6 Practice Implications

19.6.1 Treatment Outcomes

Overall, the research supports promising results of SSTs for autism in improving social functioning in autistic individuals, with several thorough reviews and clinical guidance on individual SSTs (Leaf, 2017; White et al., 2007) and group-based SSTs (Gates et al., 2017; Wolstencroft et al., 2018). There is evidence for SSTs across the lifespan, with programs adapted for autistic preschoolers (e.g., Park et al., 2022) to adults demonstrating large positive effects on social responsiveness (Dubreucq et al., 2022). Hence, it is expected that autistic individuals will show some improvement in social functioning outcomes following SSTs. However, it is also important to recognize that many of these effects may not consistently generalize, and there are notable methodological limitations of the current literature base, such as relying predominantly on parent- or self-report measures and lack of active control conditions.

19.6.2 Practice Implication Guidelines

Although every SST is distinct, many knowledge- and performance-based SSTs have substantial and rigorous research supporting their positive effects on autistic individuals. Several factors warrant consideration when implementing SSTs.

First, while some programs provide services for young autistic children and adults, many provide trainings for those between the ages of 8 and 17 years. For example, although SSTs for adolescents may be geared toward developing friendships and understanding social cues, they often may not address other social information necessary during adulthood (e.g., workplace boundaries, professionalism). For young children, providing opportunities for social skills development early in life may reduce the effects of peer rejection and bullying in new school-based environments. Therefore, it is particularly important that SSTs focus on expanding these approaches to include other developmental periods outside of late childhood and adolescents.

Relatedly, many of these trainings exclude individuals with intellectual disabilities, which results in a large portion of children without social skills treatment options. Individuals with co-occurring ASD and intellectual disabilities experience more social difficulties, reduced friendships, and increased mental health difficulties compared to same-aged autistic peers (Carter et al., 2010; Hughes et al., 2012; Matson & Shoemaker, 2009; Taheri et al., 2016).

It is also imperative that SSTs seek to understand the impact of these interventions in more accessible settings to reduce parental burden and improve access to care. Some SSTs have established combined effects on mental health conditions, which provide a reduction in treatment burden for families. Future treatments should seek to continue this trend of combining treatment methods to reduce mental health difficulties, improve quality of life, and reduce the need for mental health intervention.

Although no harmful side effects have been reported in the literature, SSTs have faced increasing criticism regarding the potential unintended negative consequences associated with using explicit rules to teach implicit social processes (Bottema-Beutel et al., 2018). In addition, some autistic self-advocates have expressed concerns regarding certain SST approaches potentially causing emotional harm by fostering an increase in camouflaging and masking behaviors (Hull et al., 2017), instead of embracing and celebrating the unique qualities of autistic individuals. Future SST development should include input from autistic self-advocates to ensure that their perspectives and priorities are appropriately reflected in these interventions (Monahan et al., 2023). Practitioners should seek to focus on understanding social communication differences in autistic individuals and using these insights to flexibly facilitate opportunities to develop social support networks and establish meaningful social relationships, rather than trying to teach autistic individuals to change their communication styles and comply with explicit social rules. Moreover, effects of SSTs may lie in tapping into motivation and special interests through games, drama-based activities, and/or use of naturalistic settings (e.g., playground, playdates), which may be inherently more rewarding. In sum, the extant literature regarding SSTs offers promising evidence supporting their use with autistic individuals across the lifespan, as each SST targets distinct areas related to social cognition and social communication, enabling tailored support based on individual needs.

19.7 References

Afsharnejad, B., Falkmer, M., Black, M. H., Alach, T., Lenhard, F., Fridell, A., Coco, C., Milne, K., Bölte, S., & Girdler, S. (2021). KONTAKT® social skills group training for Australian adolescents with autism spectrum disorder: A randomized controlled trial. *European Child and Adolescent Psychiatry, 31*, 1695–1713. https://doi.org/10.1007/s00787-021-01814-6

Aithal, S., Karkou, V., Makris, S., Karaminis, T., & Powell, J. (2021). A dance movement psychotherapy intervention for the wellbeing of children with an autism spectrum disorder: A pilot intervention study. *Frontiers in Psychology, 12*, 1–15. https://doi.org/10.3389/FPSYG.2021.588418/FULL

American Psychiatric Association. (2013). *Diagnostic and statistical manual of mental disorders.* Washington, DC: Author. https://doi.org/10.1176/appi.books.9780890425596

Bauminger, N. (2007). Brief report: Group social-multimodal intervention for HFASD. *Journal of Autism and Developmental Disorders, 37*(8), 1605–1615. https://doi.org/10.1007/s10803-006-0246-3

Bauminger, N., & Kasari, C. (2000). Loneliness and friendship in high-functioning children with autism. *Child Development, 71*(2), 447–456.

Bauminger, N., Shulman, C., & Agam, G. (2004). The link between perceptions of self and of social relationships in high-functioning children with autism. *Journal of Developmental and Physical Disabilities, 16*(2), 193–214.

Bauminger-Zviely, N., Eden, S., Zancanaro, M., Weiss, P. L., & Gal, E. (2013). Increasing social engagement in children with high-functioning autism spectrum disorder using collaborative technologies in the school environment. *Autism, 17*(3), 317–339. https://doi.org/10.1177/1362361312472989

Beadle-Brown, J., Wilkinson, D., Richardson, L., Shaughnessy, N., Trimingham, M., Leigh, J., Whelton, B., & Himmerich, J. (2018). Imagining autism: Feasibility of a drama-based intervention on the social, communicative and imaginative behaviour of children with autism. *Autism, 22*(8), 915–927. https://doi.org/10.1177/1362361317710797

Beaumont, R. (2010). *Secret agent society: Solving the mystery of social encounters—Facilitator manual.* Brisbane, Australia: The Social Skills Training Institute.

Beaumont, R., & Sofronoff, K. (2008). A multi-component social skills intervention for children with Asperger syndrome: The Junior Detective Training Program. *Journal of Child Psychology and Psychiatry and Allied Disciplines, 49*(7), 743–753. https://doi.org/10.1111/j.1469-7610.2008.01920.x

Begeer, S., Howlin, P., Hoddenbach, E., Clauser, C., Lindauer, R., Clifford, P., Gevers, C., Boer, F., & Koot, H. M. (2015). Effects and moderators of a short theory of mind intervention for children with autism spectrum disorder: A randomized controlled trial. *Autism Research, 8*(6), 738–748. https://doi.org/10.1002/aur.1489

Bekele, E., Zheng, Z., Swanson, A., Crittendon, J., Warren, Z., & Sarkar, N. (2013). Understanding how adolescents with autism respond to facial expressions in virtual reality environments. *IEEE Transactions on Visualization and Computer Graphics, 19*(4), 711–720. https://doi.org/10.1109/TVCG.2013.42

Bellini, S., & Akullian, J. (2007). A meta-analysis of video modeling and video self-modeling interventions for children and adolescents with autism spectrum disorders. *Exceptional Children, 73*(3), 264–287.

Bernard-Opitz, V., Sriram, N., & Nakhoda-Sapuan, S. (2001). Enhancing social problem solving in children with autism and normal children through computer-assisted instruction. *Journal of Autism and Developmental Disorders, 31*(4), 377–384. https://doi.org/10.1023/A:1010660502130

Bishop-Fitzpatrick, L., Mazefsky, C. A., Minshew, N. J., & Eack, S. M. (2015). The relationship between stress and social functioning in adults with autism spectrum disorder and without intellectual disability. *Autism Research, 8*(2), 164–173. https://doi.org/10.1002/aur.1433

Bottema-Beutel, K., Kapp, S. K., Lester, J. N., Sasson, N. J., & Hand, B. N. (2021). Avoiding ableist language: Suggestions for autism researchers. *Autism in Adulthood, 3*(1), 18–29.

Bottema-Beutel, K., Park, H., & Kim, S. Y. (2018). Commentary on social skills training curricula for individuals with ASD: Social interaction, authenticity, and stigma. *Journal of Autism and Developmental Disorders, 48*(3), 953–964. https://doi.org/10.1007/s10803-017-3400-1

Cappadocia, M. C., & Weiss, J. A. (2011). Review of social skills training groups for youth with Asperger syndrome and high functioning autism. *Research in Autism Spectrum Disorders, 5*(1), 70–78. https://doi.org/10.1016/j.rasd.2010.04.001

Carter, E. W., Sisco, L. G., Chung, Y.-C., & Stanton-Chapman, T. L. (2010). Peer interactions of students with intellectual disabilities and/or autism: A map of the intervention literature. *Research and Practice for Persons with Severe Disabilities, 3*, 63–69.

Chang, Y.-C., & Dean, M. (2022). Friendship interventions and measurements in children with ASD: A systematic review. *Research in Autism Spectrum Disorders, 93*. https://doi.org/10.1016/j.rasd.2022.101947

Cheng, Y., Huang, C. L., & Yang, C. S. (2015). Using a 3D immersive virtual environment system to enhance social understanding and social skills for children with autism spectrum disorders. *Focus on Autism and Other Developmental Disabilities, 30*(4). https://doi.org/10.1177/1088357615583473

Cheng, Y., & Ye, J. (2010). Exploring the social competence of students with autism spectrum conditions in a collaborative virtual learning environment: The pilot study. *Computers and Education, 54*(4), 1068–1077. https://doi.org/10.1016/j.compedu.2009.10.011

Coie, J., Terry, R., Lenox, K., Lochman, J., & Hyman, C. (1995). Childhood peer rejection and aggression as predictors of stable patterns of adolescent disorder. *Development and Psychopathology, 7*, 697–713.

Corbett, B. A., Key, A. P., Qualls, L., Fecteau, S., Newsom, C., Coke, C., & Yoder, P. (2016). Improvement in social competence using a randomized trial of a theatre intervention for children with autism spectrum disorder. *Journal of Autism and Developmental Disorders, 46*(2), 658–672. https://doi.org/10.1007/s10803-015-2600-9

Corbett, B. A., White, S., Lerner, M., Preacher, K. J., Klemencic, M. E., Simmons, G. L., Pilkington, J., Gable, P., Gioia, A., & Key, A. P. (2023). Peers, play, and performance to build social salience in autistic youth: A multisite randomized clinical trial. *Journal of Consulting and Clinical Psychology., 91, 411–425.* https://doi.org/10.1037/ccp0000821

Cresswell, L., Hinch, R., & Cage, E. (2019). The experiences of peer relationships amongst autistic adolescents: A systematic review of the qualitative evidence. *Research in autism spectrum disorders, 61*, 45–60. https://doi.org/10.1016/j.rasd.2019.01.003

Davenport, M., Mazurek, M., Brown, A., & McCollom, E. (2018). A systematic review of cultural considerations and adaptation of social skills interventions for individuals with autism spectrum disorder. *Research in Autism Spectrum Disorders, 52*(April), 23–33. https://doi.org/10.1016/j.rasd.2018.05.003

Derosier, M. E., Swick, D. C., Davis, N. O., McMillen, J. S., & Matthews, R. (2011). The efficacy of a social skills group intervention for improving social behaviors in children with high functioning autism spectrum disorders. *Journal of Autism and Developmental Disorders, 41*(8), 1033–1043. https://doi.org/10.1007/s10803-010-1128-2

Dubreucq, J., Haesebaert, F., Plasse, J., Dubreucq, M., & Franck, N. (2022). A systematic review and meta-analysis of social skills training for adults with autism spectrum disorder. *Journal of Autism and Developmental Disorders, 52*(4), 1598–1609. https://doi.org/10.1007/s10803-021-05058-w

Elliot, S., Malecki, C., & Demaray, M. (2001). New directions in social skills assessment and intervention for elementary and middle school students. *Exceptionality*, 9, 19–32.

Estell, D. B., Farmer, T. W., Irvin, M. J., Crowther, A., Akos, P., & Boudah, D. J. (2009). Students with exceptionalities and the peer group context of bullying and victimization in late elementary school. *Journal of Child and Family Studies, 18*(2), 136–150. https://doi.org/10.1007/s10826-008-9214-1

Factor, R. S., Rea, H. M., Laugeson, E. A., & Scarpa, A. (2022). Examining feasibility and outcomes of the PEERS® for Preschoolers program. *Journal of Autism and Developmental Disorders*. https://doi.org/10.1007/s10803-022-05502-5

Frith, C. D. (2008). Social cognition. *Philosophical Transactions of the Royal Society B: Biological Sciences, 363*(1499), 2033–2039. https://doi.org/10.1098/rstb.2008.0005

Gantman, A., Kapp, S. K., Orenski, K., & Laugeson, E. A. (2012). Social skills training for young adults with high-functioning autism spectrum disorders: A randomized controlled pilot study. *Journal of Autism and Developmental Disorders, 42*(6), 1094–1103. https://doi.org/10.1007/s10803-011-1350-6

Gates, J. A., Kang, E., & Lerner, M. D. (2017). Efficacy of group social skills interventions for youth with autism spectrum disorder: A systematic review and meta-analysis. *Clinical Psychology Review, 52*, 164–181. https://doi.org/10.1016/j.cpr.2017.01.006

Gerber, A. H., Kang, E., Nahmias, A. S., Libsack, E. J., Simson, C., & Lerner, M. D. (2022). Predictors of treatment response to a community-delivered group social skills intervention for youth with ASD. *Journal of Autism and Developmental Disorders*. https://doi.org/10.1007/s10803-022-05559-2

Goldstein, A., & McGinnis, E. (1997). *Skillstreaming the adolescent: New strategies and perspectives for teaching prosocial skills.* Champaign: Research Press.

Gorenstein, M., Giserman-Kiss, I., Feldman, E., Isenstein, E. L., Donnelly, L., Wang, A. T., & Foss-Feig, J. H. (2020). Brief report: A Job-Based Social Skills Program (JOBSS) for adults with autism spectrum disorder: A pilot randomized controlled trial. *Journal of Autism and Developmental Disorders, 50*(12), 4527–4534. https://doi.org/10.1007/s10803-020-04482-8

Gralinski, J. H., & Kopp, C. B. (1993). Everyday rules for behavior: Mothers' requests to young children. *Developmental Psychology, 29*, 573–584.

Gray, C. A., & Garand, J. D. (1993). Social stories: Improving responses of students with autism with accurate social information. *Focus on Autistic Behavior, 8*(1), 1–10.

Guli, L. A., Semrud-Clikeman, M., Lerner, M. D., & Britton, N. (2013). Social Competence Intervention Program (SCIP): A pilot study of a creative drama program for youth with social difficulties. *Arts in Psychotherapy, 40*(1), 37–44. https://doi.org/10.1016/j.aip.2012.09.002

Gunning, C., Holloway, J., Fee, B., Breathnach, Ó., Bergin, C. M., Greene, I., & Ní Bheoláin, R. (2019). A systematic review of generalization and maintenance outcomes of social skills intervention for preschool children with autism spectrum disorder. *Review Journal of Autism and Developmental Disorders, 6*(2), 172–199. https://doi.org/10.1007/s40489-019-00162-1

Happe, F. G. E. (1995). The role of age and verbal ability in the theory of mind task performance of subjects with autism. *Child Development, 66*(3), 843. https://doi.org/10.2307/1131954

Herbrecht, E., Poustka, F., Birnkammer, S., Duketis, E., Schlitt, S., Schmötzer, G., & Bölte, S. (2009). Pilot evaluation of the Frankfurt social skills training for children and adolescents with autism spectrum disorder. *European Child and Adolescent Psychiatry, 18*(6), 327–335. https://doi.org/10.1007/s00787-008-0734-4

Hillier, A., Fish, T., Cloppert, P., & Beversdorf, D. Q. (2007). Outcomes of a social and vocational skills support group for adolescents and young adults on the autism spectrum. *Focus on Autism and Other Developmental Disabilities, 22*(2), 107–115. https://doi.org/10.1177/10883576070220020201

Hillier, A., Goldstein, J., Murphy, D., Trietsch, R., Keeves, J., Mendes, E., & Queenan, A. (2018). Supporting university students with autism spectrum disorder. *Autism, 22*(1), 20–28. https://doi.org/10.1177/1362361317699584

Hoogenhout, M., & Malcolm-Smith, S. (2017). Theory of mind predicts severity level in autism. *Autism, 21*(2), 242–252. https://doi.org/10.1177/1362361316636758

Hughes, C., Kaplan, L., Bernstein, R., Boykin, M., Reilly, C., Brigham, N., Cosgriff, J., Heilingoetter, J., & Harvey, M. (2012). Increasing social interaction skills of secondary school students with autism and/or intellectual disability: A review of interventions. *Research & Practice for Persons with Severe Disabilities, 37*(4), 288–307.

Hull, L., Petrides, K. V., Allison, C., Smith, P., Baron-Cohen, S., Lai, M. C., & Mandy, W. (2017). "Putting on my best normal": Social camouflaging in adults with autism spectrum conditions. *Journal of Autism and Developmental Disorders, 47*(8), 2519–2534. https://doi.org/10.1007/s10803-017-3166-5

Ichikawa, K., Takahashi, Y., Ando, M., Anme, T., Ishizaki, T., Yamaguchi, H., & Nakayama, T. (2013). TEACCH-based group social skills training for children with high-functioning autism: A pilot randomized controlled trial. *BioPsychoSocial Medicine, 7*(1), 1–8. https://doi.org/10.1186/1751-0759-7-14

Ip, H. H. S., Wong, S. W. L., Chan, D. F. Y., Byrne, J., Li, C., Yuan, V. S. N., Lau, K. S. Y., & Wong, J. Y. W. (2018). Enhance emotional and social adaptation skills for children with autism spectrum disorder: A virtual reality enabled approach. *Computers and Education, 117*, 1–15. https://doi.org/10.1016/j.compedu.2017.09.010

Kang, E., Gioia, A., Pugliese, C. E., Islam, N. Y., Martinez-Pedraza, F. de L., Girard, R. M., McLeod, B. D., Carter, A. S., & Lerner, M. D. (2020). Alliance-outcome associations in a community-based social skills intervention for youth with autism spectrum disorder. *Behavior Therapy, 52*, 324–337. https://doi.org/10.1016/j.beth.2020.04.006

Karami, B., Koushki, R., Arabgol, F., Rahmani, M., & Vahabie, A. H. (2021). Effectiveness of virtual/augmented reality–based therapeutic interventions on individuals with autism spectrum disorder: A comprehensive meta-analysis. *Frontiers in Psychiatry, 12*, 1–8. https://doi.org/10.3389/fpsyt.2021.665326

Kohler, F. W., & Strain, P. S. (1990). Peer-assisted interventions: Early promises, notable achievements, and future aspirations. *Clinical Psychology Review, 10*(4), 441–452.

Lagasse, A. B. (2017). Social outcomes in children with autism spectrum disorder: A review of music therapy outcomes. *Patient Related Outcome Measures, 8*, 23–32. https://doi.org/10.2147/PROM.S106267

Laugeson, E. A. (2017). *PEERS® for young adults: Social skills training for adults with autism spectrum disorder and other social challenges.* London: Routledge.

Laugeson, E. A., Frankel, F., Gantman, A., Dillon, A. R., & Mogil, C. (2012). Evidence-based social skills training for adolescents with autism spectrum disorders: The UCLA PEERS program. *Journal of Autism and Developmental Disorders, 42*(6), 1025–1036. https://doi.org/10.1007/s10803-011-1339-1

Laugeson, E. A., Frankel, F., Mogil, C., & Dillon, A. R. (2009). Parent-assisted social skills training to improve friendships in teens with autism spectrum disorders. *Journal of Autism and Developmental Disorders, 39*(4), 596–606. https://doi.org/10.1007/s10803-008-0664-5

Laugeson, E. A., Gantman, A., Kapp, S. K., Orenski, K., & Ellingsen, R. (2015). A randomized controlled trial to improve social skills in young adults with autism spectrum disorder: The UCLA PEERS® Program. *Journal of Autism and Developmental Disorders, 45*(12), 3978–3989. https://doi.org/10.1007/s10803-015-2504-8

Laugeson, E. A., Park, M. N., Bolton, C., Bolourian, Y., & Sanderson, J. (2016). A randomized controlled trial of a parent-assisted social skills treatment: The UCLA PEERS® for Preschoolers program. Poster abstract presented at the International Meeting for Autism Research, Baltimore, MD.

Laugeson, P., & Frankel, F. (2011). *Social skills for teenagers with developmental and autism spectrum disorders: The PEERS treatment manual.* London: Routledge.

Leaf, J. B. (Ed.). (2017). *Handbook of social skills and autism spectrum disorder: Assessment, curricula, and intervention.* Cham: Springer.

LeGoff, D.B. (2004). Use of LEGO as a therapeutic medium for improving social competence. *Journal of Autism and Developmental Disorders, 34*(5), 557–571.

LeGoff, D. B., de la Cuesta, G. G., Krauss, G.W., & Baron-Cohen, S. (2014). *LEGO®-based therapy: How to build social competence through LEGO®-based clubs for children with autism and related conditions.* London: Jessica Kingsley.

LeGoff, D. B. & Sherman, M. (2006). Long-term outcome of social skills intervention based on interactive LEGO© play. *Autism, 10*(4), 317–329. https://doi.org/10.1177/1362361306064403

Lerner, M. D., Girard, R., Culp, M., Cruwys, S., & Levine, K. (2007). *Spotlight program manual.* Danvers, MA: North Shore Arc.

Lerner, M. D., & Mikami, A. Y. (2012). A preliminary randomized controlled trial of two social skills interventions for youth with high-functioning autism spectrum disorders. *Focus on Autism and Other Developmental Disabilities, 27*(3), 147–157. https://doi.org/10.1177/1088357612450613

Lerner, M. D., Mikami, A. Y., & Levine, K. (2011). Socio-dramatic affective-relational intervention for adolescents with Asperger syndrome & high functioning autism: Pilot study. *Autism, 15*(1), 21–42. https://doi.org/10.1177/1362361309353613

Lindsay, S., Hounsell, K. G., & Cassiani, C. (2017). A scoping review of the role of LEGO® therapy for improving inclusion and social skills among children and youth with autism. *Disability and Health Journal, 10*(2), 173–182. https://doi.org/10.1016/j.dhjo.2016.10.010

Lopata, C., Thomeer, M. L., Volker, M. A., & Lee, G. K. (2013). A manualized summer program for social skills in children with high-functioning ASD. In A. Scarpa, S. W. White, & T. Attwood (Eds.), *CBT for Children and Adolescents with High-Functioning Autism Spectrum Disorders*, 199–225, New York: Guilford Press.

Lopata, C., Thomeer, M. L., Volker, M. A., Toomey, J. A., Nida, R. E., Lee, G. K., Smerbeck, A. M., & Rodgers, J. D. (2010). RCT of a manualized social treatment for high-functioning autism spectrum disorders. *Journal of Autism and Developmental Disorders, 40*(11), 1297–1310. https://doi.org/10.1007/s10803-010-0989-8

Lozier, L. M., Vanmeter, J. W., & Marsh, A. A. (2014). Impairments in facial affect recognition associated with autism spectrum disorders: A meta-analysis. *Development and Psychopathology, 26*(4pt1), 933–945. https://doi.org/10.1017/S0954579414000479

MacEvilly, D., & Brosnan, G. (2020). Adapting an emotional regulation and social communication skills group programme to teletherapy, in response to the Covid-19 pandemic. *Irish Journal of Psychological Medicine, 39*, 423–428. https://doi.org/10.1017/ipm.2020.109

MacKay, T., Knott, F., & Dunlop, A. (2007). Developing social interaction and understanding in individuals with autism spectrum disorder: A groupwork intervention. *Journal of Intellectual & Developmental Disability, 32*(4), 279–290. https://doi.org/10.1080/13668250701689280

Mandelberg, J., Laugeson, E. A., Cunningham, T. D., Ellingsen, R., Bates, S., & Frankel, F. (2014). Long-term treatment outcomes for parent-assisted social skills training for adolescents with autism spectrum disorders: The UCLA PEERS program. *Journal of Mental Health Research in Intellectual Disabilities, 7*(1), 45–73. https://doi.org/10.1080/19315864.2012.730600

Marro, B. M., Kang, E., Hauschild, K. M., Normansell, K. M., Tamara Abu-Ramadan, B. M., & Matthew Lerner, B. D. (2019). Social performance-based interventions promote gains in social knowledge in the absence of explicit training for youth with autism spectrum disorder. *Bulletin of the Menninger Clinic, 83*(3), 301–325. https://doi.org/10.1521/bumc.2019.83.3.301.

Matson, J. L., & Shoemaker, M. (2009). Intellectual disability and its relationship to autism spectrum disorders. *Research in Developmental Disabilities, 30*(6), 1107–1114. https://doi.org/10.1016/j.ridd.2009.06.003

Mazurek, M. O. (2014). Loneliness, friendship, and well-being in adults with autism spectrum disorders. *Autism, 18*(3), 223–232. https://doi.org/10.1177/1362361312474121

McCoy, A., Holloway, J., Healy, O., Rispoli, M., & Neely, L. (2016). A systematic review and evaluation of video modeling, role-play and computer-based instruction as social skills interventions for children and adolescents with high-functioning autism. *Review Journal of Autism and Developmental Disorders, 3*(1), 48–67. https://doi.org/10.1007/s40489-015-0065-6

McDonald, R. G., Khawar, S., Yacoub, N., Cargill, M. I., Lerner, M. D., & Kang, E. (2022). Performance- and theater-based interventions for supporting social cognition and social communication in autistic youth: A review and theoretical synthesis. *Seminars in Speech and Language, 43*(4), 255–276. https://doi.org/10.1055/s-0042-1750763

McMahon, C. M., Vismara, L. A., & Solomon, M. (2013). Measuring changes in social behavior during a social skills intervention for higher-functioning children and adolescents with autism spectrum disorder. *Journal of Autism and Developmental Disorders, 43*(8), 1843–1856. https://doi.org/10.1007/s10803-012-1733-3

McVey, A. J., Dolan, B. K., Willar, K. S., Pleiss, S., Karst, J. S., Casnar, C. L., Caiozzo, C., Vogt, E. M., Gordon, N. S., & Van Hecke, A. V. (2016). A replication and extension of the PEERS® for Young Adults social skills intervention: Examining effects on social skills and social anxiety in young adults with autism spectrum disorder. *Journal of Autism and Developmental Disorders, 46*(12), 3739–3754. https://doi.org/10.1007/s10803-016-2911-5

Mehling, M. H., Tassé, M. J., & Root, R. (2017). Shakespeare and autism: An exploratory evaluation of the Hunter Heartbeat Method. *Research and Practice in Intellectual and Developmental Disabilities, 4*(2). https://doi.org/10.1080/23297018.2016.1207202

Mendelson, J. L., Gates, J. A., & Lerner, M. D. (2016). Friendship in school-age boys with autism spectrum disorders: A meta-analytic summary and developmental, process-based model. *Psychological Bulletin, 142*(6), 601–622. https://doi.org/10.1037/bul0000041

Mesa-Gresa, P., Gil-Gómez, H., Lozano-Quilis, J. A., & Gil-Gómez, J. A. (2018). Effectiveness of virtual reality for children and adolescents with autism spectrum disorder: An evidence-based systematic review. *Sensors (Switzerland), 18*(8), 1–15. https://doi.org/10.3390/s18082486

Miller, P. M., & Ingham, J. G. (1976). Social psychiatry friends, confidants and symptoms. *Social Psychiatry, 11,* 51–58. https://doi.org/10.1007/BF00578738.

Monahan, J., Freedman, B., Pini, K., & Lloyd, R. (2023). Autistic input in social skills interventions for young adults: A systematic review of the literature. *Review Journal of Autism and Developmental Disorders, 10*(1), 1–21. https://doi.org/10.1007/s40489-021-00280-9

Moody, C. T., & Laugeson, E. A. (2020). Social skills training in autism spectrum disorder across the lifespan. *Child and Adolescent Psychiatric Clinics of North America, 29*(2), 359–371. https://doi.org/10.1016/j.chc.2019.11.001

Park, M. N., Moulton, E., & Laugeson, E. (2022). Parent-assisted social skills training for children with autism spectrum disorder: PEERS® for preschoolers. *Focus on Autism and Other Developmental Disabilities, 38*(2), 80–89.

Pickles, A., Le Couteur, A., Leadbitter, K., Salomone, E., Cole-Fletcher, R., Tobin, H., Gammer, I., Lowry, J., Vamvakas, G., Byford, S., Aldred, C., Slonims, V., McConachie, H., Howlin, P., Parr, J. R., Charman, T., & Green, J. (2016). Parent-mediated social communication therapy for young children with autism (PACT): Long-term follow-up of a randomised controlled trial. *The Lancet, 388*(10059), 2501–2509. https://doi.org/10.1016/S0140-6736(16)31229-6

Radley, K. C., Dart, E. H., Brennan, K. J., Helbig, K. A., Lehman, E. L., Silberman, M., & Mendanhall, K. (2020). Social skills teaching for individuals with autism spectrum disorder: A systematic review. *Advances in Neurodevelopmental Disorders, 4*(3), 215–226. https://doi.org/10.1007/s41252-020-00170-x

Reichow, B., Steiner, A. M., & Volkmar, F. (2012). Social skills groups for people aged 6 to 21 with autism spectrum disorders (ASD). *Campbell Systematic Reviews, 8*(1), 1–76. https://doi.org/10.4073/csr.2012.16

Reichow, B., & Volkmar, F. R. (2010). Social skills interventions for individuals with autism: Evaluation for evidence-based practices within a best evidence synthesis framework. *Journal of Autism and Developmental Disorders, 40*(2), 149–166. https://doi.org/10.1007/s10803-009-0842-0

Rodriguez, G., Drastal, K., & Hartley, S. L. (2021). Cross-lagged model of bullying victimization and mental health problems in children with autism in middle to older childhood. *Autism, 25*(1), 90–101. https://doi.org/10.1177/1362361320947513

Safer-Lichtenstein, J., Hamilton, J. C., & McIntyre, L. L. (2019). Examining demographics in randomized controlled trials of group-based social skills interventions for individuals with autism spectrum disorder. *Journal of Autism and Developmental Disorders, 49*(8), 3453–3461. https://doi.org/10.1007/s10803-019-04063-4

Schohl, K. A., Van Hecke, A. V., Carson, A. M., Dolan, B., Karst, J., & Stevens, S. (2014). A replication and extension of the PEERS intervention: Examining effects on social skills and social anxiety in adolescents with autism spectrum disorders. *Journal of Autism and Developmental Disorders, 44*(3), 532–545. https://doi.org/10.1007/s10803-013-1900-1

Senju, A. (2013). Atypical development of spontaneous social cognition in autism spectrum disorders. *Brain and Development, 35*(2), 96–101. https://doi.org/10.1016/j.braindev.2012.08.002

Simonoff, E., Pickles, A., Charman, T., Chandler, S., Loucas, T., & Baird, G. (2008). Psychiatric disorders in children with autism spectrum disorders: Prevalence, comorbidity, and associated factors in a population-derived sample. *Journal of the American Academy of Child and Adolescent Psychiatry, 47*(8), 921–929. https://doi.org/10.1097/CHI.0b013e318179964f

Spain, D., & Blainey, S. H. (2015). Group social skills interventions for adults with high-functioning autism spectrum disorders: A systematic review. *Autism, 19*(7), 874–886. https://doi.org/10.1177/1362361315587659

Spain, D., Blainey, S. H., & Vaillancourt, K. (2017). Group cognitive behaviour therapy (CBT) for social interaction anxiety in adults with autism spectrum disorders (ASD). *Research in Autism Spectrum Disorders, 41*, 20–30. https://doi.org/10.1016/j.rasd.2017.07.005

Taheri, A., Perry, A., & Minnes, P. (2016). Examining the social participation of children and adolescents with intellectual disabilities and autism spectrum disorder in relation to peers. *Journal of Intellectual Disability Research, 60*(5), 435–443. https://doi.org/10.1111/jir.12289

Tantam, D. (2003). The challenge of adolescents and adults with Asperger syndrome. *Child & Adolescent Psychiatric Clinics of North America, 12*, 143–163. https://doi.org/10.1016/s1056-4993(02)00053-6.

Thomeer, M. L., Lopata, C., Donnelly, J. P., Booth, A., Shanahan, A., Federiconi, V., McDonald, C. A., & Rodgers, J. D. (2019). Community effectiveness RCT of a comprehensive psychosocial treatment for high-functioning children with ASD. *Journal of Clinical Child and Adolescent Psychology, 48*(1), S119–S130. https://doi.org/10.1080/15374416.2016.1247359

Thomeer, M. L., Lopata, C., Volker, M. A., Toomey, J. A., Lee, G. K., Smerbeck, A. M., Rodgers, J. D., Mcdonald, C. A., & Smith, R. A. (2012). Randomized clinical trial replication of a psychosocial treatment for children with high-functioning autism spectrum disorders. *Psychology in the Schools, 49*(10), 942–954. https://doi.org/10.1002/pits.21647

Tripathi, I., Estabillo, J. A., Moody, C. T., & Laugeson, E. A. (2021). Long-term treatment outcomes of PEERS® for Preschoolers: A parent-mediated social skills training program for children with autism spectrum disorder. *Journal of Autism and Developmental Disorders*. https://doi.org/10.1007/s10803-021-05147-w

Tse, J., Strulovitch, J., Tagalakis, V., Meng, L., & Fombonne, E. (2007). Social skills training for adolescents with Asperger syndrome and high-functioning autism. *Journal of Autism and Developmental Disorders, 37*(10), 1960–1968. https://doi.org/10.1007/s10803-006-0343-3

Tyminski, R. F., Philip, D. M. H., & Moore, J. (2008). The impact of group psychotherapy on social development in children with pervasive developmental disorders. *International Journal of Group Psychothapy, 58*(3), 363–379.

Vernon, S., Schumaker, J. B., & Deshler, D. D. (1996). *The SCORE skills: Social skills for cooperative groups*. Lawrence: Edge Enterprises.

Waugh, C., & Peskin, J. (2015). Improving the social skills of children with HFASD: An intervention study. *Journal of Autism and Developmental Disorders, 45*(9), 2961–2980. https://doi.org/10.1007/s10803-015-2459-9

White, S. W., Keonig, K., & Scahill, L. (2007). Social skills development in children with autism spectrum disorders: A review of the intervention research. *Journal of Autism and Developmental Disorders, 37*(10), 1858–1868. https://doi.org/10.1007/s10803-006-0320-x

White, S. W., Ollendick, T., Albano, A. M., Oswald, D., Johnson, C., Southam-Gerow, M. A., Kim, I., & Scahill, L. (2013). Randomized controlled trial: Multimodal anxiety and social skill intervention for adolescents with autism spectrum disorder. *Journal of Autism and Developmental Disorders, 43*(2), 382–394. https://doi.org/10.1007/s10803-012-1577-x

White, S. W., Simmons, G. L., Gotham, K. O., Conner, C. M., Smith, I. C., Beck, K. B., & Mazefsky, C. A. (2018). Psychosocial treatments targeting anxiety and depression in adolescents and adults on the autism spectrum: Review of the latest research and recommended future directions. *Current Psychiatry Reports, 20*(10), 1–17. https://doi.org/10.1007/s11920-018-0949-0

Whitehouse, A. J. O., Durkin, K., Jaquet, E., & Ziatas, K. (2009). Friendship, loneliness and depression in adolescents with Asperger's syndrome. *Journal of Adolescence, 32*(2), 309–322. https://doi.org/10.1016/j.adolescence.2008.03.004

Wolstencroft, J., Robinson, L., Srinivasan, R., Kerry, E., Mandy, W., & Skuse, D. (2018). A systematic review of group social skills interventions, and meta-analysis of outcomes, for children with high functioning ASD. *Journal of Autism and Developmental Disorders, 48*(7), 2293–2307. https://doi.org/10.1007/s10803-018-3485-1

Wong, C., Odom, S. L., Hume, K. A., Cox, A. W., Fettig, A., Kucharczyk, S., Brock, M. E., Plavnick, J. B., Fleury, V. P., & Schultz, T. R. (2015). Evidence-based practices for children, youth, and young adults with autism spectrum disorder: A comprehensive review. *Journal of Autism and Developmental Disorders, 45*(7), 1951–1966. https://doi.org/10.1007/s10803-014-2351-z

20

Exposure Therapy for Anxiety or Obsessive-Compulsive Disorders Adapted for Autism Spectrum Disorder

Johann M. D'Souza
University of Houston; Baylor College of Medicine

Allie N. Townsend
Baylor College of Medicine; The Chicago School of Professional Psychology

Kristen H. Erps
University of Houston; Baylor College of Medicine

Leandra N. Berry
Baylor College of Medicine; Texas Children's Hospital

Sophie C. Schneider, Andrew G. Guzick, and Eric A. Storch
Baylor College of Medicine

20.1 Technical Abstract

Background: Exposure therapy, a core component of cognitive-behavioral therapy, is the gold standard psychotherapeutic treatment for anxiety and obsessive-compulsive disorders. **Method:** We summarize the results of meta-analyses, reviews, and randomized controlled trials that study exposure therapy for anxiety and obsessive-compulsive disorders in people with autism spectrum disorder (ASD). **Results:** Exposure therapy is highly effective in treating anxiety and obsessive-compulsive disorders in people with ASD, although it is important to adapt the delivery of exposure therapy for ASD clients, such as through increased parental involvement, length of treatment, rewards, and communication with teaching aids. **Discussion:** Future research should attempt to isolate the effect of exposure therapy from other cognitive-behavioral components, as well as study exposure therapy in both autistic people with lower IQ and adults with ASD. **Practitioner recommendations:** People with co-occurring ASD and anxiety or obsessive-compulsive disorders greatly benefit from exposure therapy that is adapted to address their unique challenges.

Johann M. D'Souza et al., *Exposure Therapy for Anxiety or Obsessive-Compulsive Disorders Adapted for Autism Spectrum Disorder*. In: *Lifespan Treatment for Autistic Individuals*. Edited by: Peter Sturmey, Russell Lang, and James K. Luiselli, Oxford University Press. © Oxford University Press (2025). DOI: 10.1093/oso/9780197635841.003.0020

20.2 Layperson Summary

Exposure therapy is effective for treating anxiety and obsessive-compulsive disorders. When people gradually face their fears, they learn that their feared outcomes are unlikely to come true, or if they do, they can handle them. Exposure therapy is usually conducted by trained therapists as part of a broader form of therapy called "cognitive-behavioral therapy." Scientific research has shown that exposure therapy helps most people with anxiety and related disorders feel less anxious and live improved lives. This has been shown to be the case for people with and without ASD. Despite the apprehension some feel in the face of exposure therapy, there is little risk of negative side effects.

20.3 Treatment Summary Table

Treatment summary: Exposure Therapy

Treatment description: Exposure therapy involves patients approaching and engaging with anxiety-producing stimuli in a gradual and supported manner. This treatment is done with objectively safe stimuli, meaning that the feared items, activities, or situations pose no additional risk beyond typical daily living. The overall goal of the treatment is to teach the individual that their fears are not dangerous, and they can, in fact, tolerate them.

Expected outcomes: Reduction in anxiety and avoidance, as well as improved tolerance toward feeling anxious.

Methods: Identify feared stimuli. Encounter feared stimuli from least feared to most feared, whether in the imagination or real life, and prevent avoidance and safety behavior.

Expertise required to implement treatment: Training during graduate school and continuing education under the supervision of an experienced therapist.

Risks and negative side effects: A short-term but temporary increase in anxiety is common.

Additional considerations and limitations: It is important to adapt traditional exposure therapy to clients with ASD through increased parental involvement, length of treatment, rewards, and communication and teaching aids.

20.4 Introduction

20.4.1 Treatment Description

Exposure therapy is a highly effective, transdiagnostic treatment for anxiety and obsessive-compulsive disorder (OCD), including for those with ASD, which is a core component of cognitive-behavioral therapy (CBT; Arch et al., 2012; Foa, 2011; McGuire & Storch, 2018). Exposure therapy specifically involves systematically approaching and engaging with anxiety-producing stimuli without rituals or safety behaviors (Abramowitz et al., 2019; Kaczkurkin & Foa, 2015). Fears can be faced in real life or by imagining them. In either case, the exposure is conducted in a way that is objectively safe, meaning that the feared items, activities, or situations pose little or no additional risk beyond typical daily living. The overall goal of the treatment is to teach the individual that their fears are not dangerous, and they can, in fact, tolerate them (Craske et al., 2014). Exposure therapy can be done in many formats. Treatment proceeds from psychoeducation to a functional assessment, hierarchy development, exposure and response prevention, and finally relapse prevention. For those with ASD, exposure therapy is adapted through increased parental involvement, length of treatment, rewards, and communication and teaching aids. However, it is important to note at the outset that much of the ASD and anxiety literature, including most of the studies reported in this chapter, focuses on those with higher functioning ASD.

20.4.2 Rationale and Objectives

20.4.2.1 ASD and Anxiety

Individuals with ASD often have co-occurring emotional and psychiatric disorders (Richa et al., 2014). ASD often co-occurs with anxiety, with over 40% of autistic youth and adults diagnosed with at least one anxiety disorder (Hollocks et al., 2019; van Steensel et al., 2011). For children and adolescents with ASD, the most common co-occurring anxiety disorders include specific phobias (30–44%), OCD (17–37%), separation anxiety disorder (9–38%), and generalized anxiety disorder (15–35%; van Steensel et al., 2011; White et al., 2009). Some of the most common co-occurring anxiety disorders for adults include social phobia (29%), generalized anxiety disorder (26%), panic/agoraphobia (28%), and OCD (22%; Hollocks et al., 2019). There are a number of reasons why people with ASD may experience elevated anxiety. For instance, social skills deficits can lead to social avoidance for fear that one will not know how to act. Also, a core symptom of ASD is preference for sameness and rigidity. This can lead to anxiety when encountering a situation that requires psychological flexibility. More broadly, those with ASD exhibit emotion regulation challenges, which can lead to a greater internalizing response in the face of a stressor.

The prevalence of co-occurring anxiety appears not only to vary with age but also with gender and some ASD-related clinical features (Gotham et al., 2015). A study examining co-occurring anxiety disorders in autistic individuals found that children with ASD and intellectual impairment (i.e., IQ < 70) are less likely to have co-occurring anxiety compared to autistic individuals without an intellectual impairment (Kerns et al., 2021). Of note, autistic children with intellectual impairment and co-occurring anxiety are predominately diagnosed with specific phobias (Kerns et al., 2020). One study examined autistic individuals across the lifespan and found that both higher ASD symptom severity and female gender were associated with heightened anxiety symptoms (Uljarević et al., 2020). This finding is consistent with literature suggesting that female gender uniquely predicts the presence of mood disorders in autistic individuals (Lever & Geurts, 2016).

Anxiety disorders can negatively impact various aspects of an individual's life, including physical health, socialization, and academic or professional success (Adams and Emerson, 2021; de Lijster et al., 2018). Studies have shown that autistic individuals with co-occurring anxiety suffer from poorer quality of life compared to those with ASD without anxiety disorders (Smith et al., 2019; van Steensel et al., 2012). Moreover, anxiety disorders appear to be a stronger predictor of overall quality of life than ASD characteristics for autistic youth and, for adults with ASD, anxiety moderates the relationship between ASD severity and quality of life (Adams and Emerson, 2021; Smith et al., 2019). However, it is not clear to what extent these results would hold true for those with higher levels of ASD severity. In addition to poorer quality of life, autistic youth with anxiety disorders experience significantly greater negative impact on both parent life and life outside the home than those without ASD (Adams and Emerson, 2021). This may be due in part to the interaction of autistic characteristics and anxious symptoms, which, when combined, lead to greater interference with a child's daily life (Adams and Emerson, 2021).

Compared to typically developing individuals, individuals with ASD also experience heightened suicidal ideation and attempt (Zahid & Upthegrove, 2017). In the general population, the presence of an anxiety disorder is a well-established risk factor for suicidal ideation and attempt (Nepon et al., 2010; Wiebenga et al., 2021). Similarly, anxiety disorders appear to be positively associated with suicidality for those with ASD (Hedley and Uljarević, 2018; Horowitz et al., 2018).

20.4.2.2 Theoretical Model of Exposure Therapy

Before discussing the mechanisms of change for exposure therapy, we will discuss the onset and maintenance of fears. Fears typically develop via classical conditioning, a process wherein a neutral stimulus becomes associated with a stimulus that naturally provokes a fear response (Mowrer, 1960). This association results in the previously neutral stimulus provoking the same fear response as the naturally feared stimulus. This can be done through direct experience, observational learning, or informational transmission. For example, someone with ASD may develop a fear of talking to new people, because he experienced awkward silences during previous encounters with strangers.

Once the fear has developed, it is maintained through the operant conditioning principle of avoidance (Abramowitz et al., 2019; Kaczkurkin & Foa, 2015; Mowrer, 1960). Avoidance perpetuates the fear through multiple pathways. First, avoidance (or engagement in rituals) prevents the individual from new, corrective learning that could provide alternative experiences and reactions to the stimuli (Blakey & Abramowitz, 2016). Second, avoidance is negatively reinforced, given that the removal/prevention of anxiety increases the likelihood the individual will use avoidance in the future (Blakely & Abramowitz, 2016). Although a short-term solution, repeated avoidance commonly generalizes to objects/situations beyond the originally feared stimuli, which results in increased functional impairment. Avoidance can be more or less obvious. Safety behaviors can be conceptualized as a subtle form of avoidance that prevents full contact with, or exposure to, the feared stimuli.

Safety behaviors often allow the individual to confront feared stimuli; however, the individual develops the belief that such confrontation is only possible when safety behaviors are present. For someone with ASD, a safety behavior could include asking for reassurance or only going to social events if a close caregiver or friend is present. For those with OCD, compulsive rituals, such as excessive handwashing, are often a more obvious form of avoidance than safety behaviors. Taken together, classical conditioning may develop a fear, yet avoidance and operant conditioning serve to maintain, and oftentimes generalize, the fear and associated anxiety response.

In addition to the behavioral components detailed above, fear and anxiety are associated with maladaptive cognitions (Abramowitz et al., 2019; Kaczkurkin & Foa, 2015). These dysfunctional beliefs generally stem from interpreting harmless stimuli as highly threatening and dangerous. Such maladaptive cognitions include emotional reasoning, black-and-white thinking, overgeneralizing, discounting the positive, catastrophizing, and labeling. For example, someone could believe "Everyone thinks I'm bad at sports" and therefore get discouraged from participating. Maladaptive cognitions reinforce the idea that a neutral stimulus is dangerous, which in turn leads the individual to seek safety through avoidance. In this way, maladaptive thoughts and avoidant behaviors reinforce one another and exacerbate the fear response, ultimately leading to fear of the experience of anxiety itself (Abramowitz et al., 2019).

The effectiveness of exposure therapy is explained by two theories: habituation and inhibitory learning. The theories hold in common that exposure therapy works because new, corrective learning occurs when facing a feared situation without experiencing a subsequent negative outcome or, alternatively, handling the negative outcome better than anticipated. According to the habituation theory, the body experiences reduced reactivity to a feared stimulus after repeated exposure to it as long as safety behaviors are not performed (Rankin et al., 2009). According to this theory, the fear association gets weaker over time and exposure is maximized by achieving habituation in and across sessions (Benito et al., 2018). According to the inhibitory learning theory (or safety learning theory), exposure does not necessarily weaken a fear association, but rather creates and strengthens new associations that are neutral or even positive when the individual learns that the feared consequence does not occur. Over time, new neutral or even positive memories are created with the previously feared stimuli. According to this theory, exposure is maximized by highlighting the discrepancy between the individual's predicted feared consequence and the actual consequence (or lack thereof) after exposure (Craske et al., 2014).

20.4.3 Considerations for Implementation

Exposure therapy begins with psychoeducation, which is imperative in setting the foundation for treatment. Psychoeducation includes providing information to the patient on the nature of the patient's disorder and the rationale for how and why exposure treatment works and is appropriate. Psychoeducation is also important in communicating the fact that exposures are safe and effective (Schneider et al., 2020). Patient comprehension of treatment fosters engagement and treatment compliance and clears up common misunderstandings such as that exposure therapy can be harmful.

Exposure therapy is an individualized treatment that requires a clear understanding of unique patient factors that contribute to disorder maintenance and onset, which are used to optimize the design and implementation of exposure exercises for each patient (Abramowitz et al., 2019). A functional assessment is completed to gather and conceptualize the patient-specific antecedents and consequences associated with the patient's anxiety. Given the highly heterogeneous nature of anxiety and related disorders, it is imperative to understand the patient's specific fears and associated behaviors. The main areas of interest in a functional assessment include fear cues, feared consequences of being exposed to fear cues, and avoidance and safety-seeking behaviors. Fear cues include any external or internal triggers (thoughts, images, bodily sensations) that incite anxiety responses. The feared consequences are typically influenced by the patient's maladaptive cognitions. A deep understanding of these factors, the specific fears, antecedents, consequences, and links among them, allow for the development of an appropriate, patient-specific treatment plan.

Once the functional assessment has been completed, a fear hierarchy is collaboratively created by the therapist and patient (Abramowitz et al., 2019). The fear hierarchy is a numeric ranking of severity for various actions and stimuli that would provoke anxiety. A typical hierarchy is constructed on a 0–10 or 0–100 scale, but this can be adapted to suit the needs of each patient. For example, ratings can be simplified: Use a picture of a ladder and assign each rung to a fear in an ascending fashion; use an easy, medium, hard scale; or use forced choice by providing two options and asking which one is easier. The ranking system has a number of advantages; for example, it allows for easier entry into exposures by starting with a less feared exposure. It also serves as a treatment roadmap that guides the treatment plan and fosters a sense of progress in and out of sessions. Like the functional assessment, the exposure hierarchy should be tailored to the patient's specific fears and avoidance behaviors. A patient can complete multiple hierarchies, with a different hierarchy for each set of related fears, or one hierarchy that includes representative examples of different kinds of fears.

Once the hierarchy has been completed, exposures begin in earnest. In general, this is at the highest point of the hierarchy that the patient is willing and able to endure without engaging in avoidance or safety behaviors, but clinical consideration should be given so that the first exposure is not too difficult. There are multiple types of exposures that can be implemented, including in vivo, imaginal, and interoceptive exposures (Kaczkurkin & Foa, 2015). In vivo exposure requires direct confrontation with the feared stimuli. In vivo exposure is not always possible, given lack of accessibility. In these circumstances, imaginal exposure may be indicated wherein the patient imagines confrontation with the feared stimuli in real time. Interoceptive exposure has the patient intentionally induce the physiological symptoms of anxiety, such as increased heart rate, dizziness, and sweating. Regardless of the type of exposure utilized, all forms seek to have the patient approach, rather than avoid, feared stimuli.

Exposures generally proceed from easiest to hardest, a procedure known as graduated exposure (Zoellner et al., 2008). Typically, exposures are completed from low to higher distress ratings to build confidence. However, proceeding in a nonlinear fashion may increase generalization and therefore the effectiveness of treatment (Craske et al., 2014). Patients are usually recommended to remain exposed to the feared stimuli until their distress ratings decrease by 50%, although this may not be necessary for producing beneficial treatment outcomes (Craske et al., 2014). This guideline remains useful in ensuring that exposures are conducted for enough time to allow for corrective learning and increase the probability a patient will not engage in safety behaviors after the exposure has ended (Benito et al., 2018).

Cognitive techniques can be used to enhance the outcomes of exposure therapy. One such technique is expectancy violation, which entails preparing the exposure by asking the patient to identify his or her feared consequences of engaging in the exposure and following the exposure by asking if the feared consequence occurred. If the predicted outcome is one that is not easily evaluated (e.g., going to hell), highlighting the patient's ability to tolerate the distress is indicated. Further, if the feared outcome does occur (e.g., peers noticing anxiety symptoms), assessing the severity of the consequences can illustrate a discrepancy between the predicted and actual ability to cope in an anxiety-provoking situation. In sum, this portion of treatment consists of repeated and prolonged exposure to feared stimuli, the concurrent prevention of avoidance and safety behaviors, and violating feared expectations.

Once the exposure component of treatment has been completed and the patient is functioning at the desired level, the final portion of treatment consists of relapse prevention. Relapse prevention includes identifying and consolidating the most helpful and effective strategies learned in treatment. Predicting challenges and highlighting the patient's ability to independently implement applicable strategies is indicated to foster confidence and self-efficacy. Lastly, self-reflection and self-monitoring are encouraged, alongside identifying warning signs that would suggest returning to treatment.

20.5 Research Background

20.5.1 Exposure Therapy in General

Robust literature supports exposure therapy as an effective and efficacious treatment for anxiety and related disorders (DiMauro et al., 2013; Hofmann et al., 2012; Olatunji et al., 2013). Treatments that utilize exposure have been empirically validated for diagnoses including, but not limited to, generalized anxiety disorder, social anxiety disorder, specific phobia, panic disorder, OCD, and posttraumatic stress disorder (Carpenter et al., 2018).

As the name suggests, generalized anxiety disorder is characterized by worries in multiple domains rather than a single identifiable fear. Therefore, exposure is one of multiple CBT components used to treat generalized anxiety disorder. The exposures utilized are often imaginal exposure of worst-case scenarios, although in vivo exposures can be utilized as well (Kaczkurkin & Foa, 2015). There is little research isolating the effect of exposure therapy for generalized anxiety disorder, although meta-analytic research has found CBT to be more advantageous than treatments that do not include exposure therapy for generalized anxiety disorder (Cuijpers et al., 2014). Symptoms of generalized anxiety and worry can overlap with symptoms of ASD, for example, seeking certainty about the upcoming schedule and sensitivity to changes in the expected routine. Planned and unplanned exposures can enhance flexibility by incorporated changes in the routine.

CBT for social anxiety disorder has demonstrated superiority compared to waitlist, placebo, and non-exposure-based treatments (Mayo-Wilson et al., 2014). Initial studies of CBT for social anxiety disorder showed that exposure did not add benefit to cognitive therapy. However, more recent research has shown the combination of cognitive and exposure behavioral treatments to be superior to monotherapy (Feske & Chambless, 1995; Mayo-Wilson et al., 2014). In vivo exposures are commonly used and include participation in various social situations. For those with ASD, this may initially require social skills support, for example, by prepping the patient with strategies for starting conversation and facilitating nonverbal communication such as eye contact and gestures.

Exposure therapy is considered the first-line treatment for specific phobias (Kaczkurkin & Foa, 2015). Meta-analytic research demonstrates exposure to be superior to placebo, no treatment, and non-exposure-based therapies (Wolitzky-Taylor et al., 2008). Conducting exposure to the phobic stimuli in varied contexts results in superior treatment outcomes (Bandarian-Balooch et al., 2015; Vansteenwegen et al., 2007). Some research has demonstrated that single-session exposure treatment can be effective for treating specific phobia. However, treatment outcomes are superior for multiple sessions (Vika et al., 2009). Specific phobias for those with ASD may be idiosyncratic and include fear of certain sensory stimuli such as places with loud noises.

Given that panic disorder is characterized by a pathological fear of anxiety symptoms, interoceptive exposures are the primary focus of exposure treatment. Although panic disorder treatment can include multiple forms of exposures, interoceptive exposures have been associated with superior outcomes compared to in vivo exposures (Craske et al., 2003; Pompoli et al., 2018). Additional research has shown in-person exposure therapy to be more effective compared to self-help or therapist-guided online exposure therapy for panic disorder (Cuijpers et al. 2010; Olthuis et al. 2015; Pompoli et al., 2018).

Empirical literature has clearly and consistently demonstrated exposure and response prevention as the front-line treatment for OCD. Exposure and response prevention has been found to be superior to waitlist, medication, and other psychological therapies (Foa et al., 2005; Janardhan-Reddy et al., 2020; Romanelli et al., 2014; Skapinakis et al., 2016). Exposure and response prevention for OCD involves both in vivo and imaginal exposures to the feared obsession while preventing the accompanying compulsion, including avoidance and safety behaviors (McGuire et al., 2014). OCD often includes a desire for reassurance. To address this, it is important for therapists and caregivers to clearly state an intended reduction in reassurance giving and accommodations to anxiety so that the patient grows in self-efficacy over time (Lebowtiz et al., 2020).

Prolonged exposure is a gold-standard treatment for posttraumatic stress disorder (Powers et al., 2010). As the name suggests, treatment consists of lengthy and frequent exposure to the feared memory. While cognitive processing therapy is similarly efficacious for treating posttraumatic stress disorder, therapists may find cognitive work more difficult to communicate with someone with ASD as opposed to the behavioral exercises in prolonged exposure because of the intellectual disability and communication challenges often associated with ASD (Hagopian et al., 2017; Powers et al., 2010; Rosen et al., 2016). Taken together, exposure therapy is a critical treatment component for anxiety and related disorders, and the supplementation of additional CBT techniques required varies by diagnosis.

20.5.2 Exposure Therapy in ASD

A large body of literature shows that treatments that use exposure therapy are also effective in those with ASD (Johnco & Storch, 2015; Kester & Lucyshyn, 2018; Zaboski & Storch, 2018). While there have been few studies that have isolated the effect of exposure therapy versus other CBT components for those with ASD, there is strong support for CBT treatments for ASD which incorporate exposure therapy (Guzick et al., 2021). Most of these studies have sampled children and adolescents rather than adults (Slaughter et al., 2020). Below, we highlight the results of multicomponent CBT interventions adapted for ASD, which include exposure therapy as a central intervention. First, we will report studies with children and adolescents and then studies with adults. Afterward, we will explain in what way these interventions were adapted to better suit those with ASD.

BIACA, or *Behavioral Interventions for Anxiety in Children with Autism* (Wood et al., 2009), is a CBT intervention tailored to an ASD population. This treatment was adapted from standard CBT by allowing the therapist and parents to choose which treatment modules are most appropriate for the child, addressing ASD-specific concerns such as social skills and restricted interests, increasing parental involvement, increasing session length, and providing differential reinforcement of approach and avoidance behavior during exposure. Building on pilot studies demonstrating efficacy in children (Wood et al., 2009) and adolescents (Storch et al., 2015; Wood et al., 2015), a more recent study used a larger sample size to compare *Modified BIACA* with the most well-supported CBT intervention for typically developing children (*Coping Cat*) and treatment as usual for autistic children with anxiety (Wood et al., 2020). The *Coping Cat* intervention included emotion recognition, reappraisal, modeling, rehearsal, exposure, and reinforcement. *Modified BIACA* included similar components as well as social communication, self-regulation, and perspective taking. Those in the *Modified BIACA* group showed significantly lower anxiety scores than those in standard CBT or treatment as usual. A subsequent study on the same data found that greater internalizing problems and ASD severity predicted poorer outcome across treatments, but the effect was less pronounced for those who received *BIACA* versus *Coping Cat* or treatment as usual (Storch et al., 2021).

Discussing + Doing = Daring is based on a CBT protocol used to treat children with anxiety and is modified for children with autism by incorporating parental involvement (Van Steensel & Bögels, 2014). One study found this intervention to be more effective than treatment as usual for remitting anxiety disorders in autistic children (Van Steensel et al., 2014).

Facing Your Fears is a group CBT protocol for children with ASD and anxiety (Reaven et al., 2012). Like *BIACA*, it is longer and includes greater parental involvement than similar programs for typically developing children. An early trial of this treatment found that participants in the CBT group were about 5 times more likely to have a clinically meaningful positive treatment response than those in the treatment-as-usual condition (Reaven et al., 2009).

Multimodal Anxiety and Social Skills Intervention (*MASSI*) is a CBT program utilizing exposure which addresses both anxiety and social skills deficits in adolescents with autism (White et al., 2010). It uses a modular approach and combines individual therapy, group therapy, and parent education. One study found that adolescents treated with *MASSI* showed reduced ASD social impairment and anxiety as compared to waitlist, although the reduction in anxiety was not statistically significant (White et al., 2013).

Finally, the established *Cool Kids* manual for child anxiety was adapted for those with ASD by increasing the total treatment time, including more time dedicated to relaxation and exposure exercises, using more visual aids, reducing the cognitive component, and adding a parent manual (Chalfant et al., 2007). One study found that *Adapted Cool Kids* outperformed waitlist in self-, parent-, and teacher-reported measures of anxiety. In sum, the above studies support the effectiveness of exposure-based CBT interventions adapted to treat children with ASD.

Unfortunately, there are far fewer controlled trials on exposure-based CBT for adults with ASD (Spain et al., 2015). One study adapted exposure and response prevention for autistic adolescents and adults with anxiety by taking greater care in explaining information over more sessions, including more visual aids, and providing more structure in sessions (Russell et al., 2013). The study compared adapted ERP with anxiety management and found that both groups demonstrated significant reductions in OCD symptoms with no significant between-group differences.

However, the adapted ERP group had a stronger effect size for treatment improvement, as well as about twice as many treatment responders.

Another study for autistic adults focused on quality of life rather than anxiety and compared CBT with a socializing control group which consisted in participating in group activities (Hesselmark et al., 2014). The CBT intervention was adapted to adults with ASD by accommodating lower executive functioning and social skills. Participants in both groups reported a statistically significant increase in quality of life with no difference between groups. The positive effect of the control group could be due to its similarity to exposure therapy, given that it consisted of participation in social activities on a weekly basis, which can be seen as an ecologically valid in vivo exposure. Furthermore, CBT is primarily used to target reduction in anxiety rather than increase quality of life.

There is comparatively weaker evidence for exposure-based therapy in adults versus children and adolescents with ASD, with fewer studies and smaller sample sizes. However, based on the strong research support for exposure-based CBT in adults without ASD and the strong support for youth with ASD and co-occurring anxiety, it is reasonable to believe a similar pattern of findings would emerge for adults if rigorous, large-scale studies were conducted, though this is an important empirical question that might be explored in future research.

20.6 Practice Implications

20.6.1 Treatment Outcomes

While many studies have tested the effectiveness of CBT for anxiety among individuals with ASD, there is limited research isolating the effect of exposure therapy, either alone or within another treatment (Slaughter et al., 2020). One such study found that the exposure phase of a CBT treatment for youth with ASD and anxiety corresponded with more rapid symptom reduction as compared to the psychoeducation and cognitive therapy phases (Guzick et al., 2021). Of interest, this finding held both for standard CBT and CBT adapted for youth with ASD. The study also found that participants improved during the initial psychoeducation phase, but improvement slowed down during the cognitive skills phase. These findings could be explained by the cognitive and communication deficits consistent with ASD and support the idea of focusing on behavioral components such as exposure (Ryan et al., 2017). Future studies could replicate this method by directly comparing treatment components.

Most of the studies reported in this review have excluded participants with significant intellectual disability. It is possible that improvements would be less pronounced in those with lower intellectual functioning due to the difficulty of communicating concepts (Hagopian et al., 2017; Rosen et al., 2016). If this is the case, it would be interesting to study the extent to which these decrements can be improved simply through increasing treatment dose versus further adapting strategies to meet the needs of this population. Finally, there is much less research on exposure therapy for adults with ASD as compared to children and adolescents with ASD.

Lastly, research could explore how to facilitate access to exposure therapy for those with ASD. Options include telehealth, iCBT, parent-led therapy, and stepped-care approaches. Telehealth, in which treatment is conducted virtually, is an increasingly popular option, and research can clarify the benefits and drawbacks as compared to in-person therapy. A telehealth version of *Facing Your Fears* was found to reduce parent-reported anxiety as compared to waitlist (Hepburn et al., 2016). While virtual sessions may make it much easier for the patient and parent to attend, they also limit the depth of communication such as nonverbal communication and use of visual aids. Furthermore, in-person sessions provide a naturalistic in vivo exposure to socializing and other challenges that come with leaving the home, which could be particularly helpful for this population. Internet-based CBT, or iCBT, is much more cost-effective than in-person therapy or telehealth, because it utilizes online programming, which requires little to no therapist involvement. A recent study on iCBT for adolescent youth with ASD and OCD found that iCBT resulted in clinically significant anxiety reduction (Wickberg et al., 2022). Although the iCBT condition did not show the same treatment gains as the in-person CBT condition, the iCBT condition was much more cost-effective because therapist involvement was limited to asynchronous messages from time to time.

Parent-led therapy can also be done with reduced therapist involvement. A recent pilot study of parent-led CBT for children with ASD and anxiety found that 38% of children were free of their primary diagnosis by the end of treatment (Byrne et al., 2022). The intervention included group sessions for parents led by a trained therapist. The parents then implemented the treatment to their children on their own. The group format allowed for less therapist time. The stepped-care model utilizes lower intensity interventions such as parent-led therapy as a first line of treatment (Ramirez et al., 2020). If treatment goals are not achieved in the first step of treatment, then the patient is elevated to standard therapist-led CBT.

20.6.2 Practice Implication Guidelines

While exposure-based CBT is effective for children, adolescents, and adults with anxiety and ASD, it does show more attenuated levels of anxiety improvement over time as compared to typically developing individuals (van Steensel & Bögels, 2015). People with ASD may exhibit clinical characteristics that impact treatment engagement such as rigidity, social skills deficits, lower intrinsic motivation, lower insight, verbal deficits, and resistance to change (Kerns et al., 2016). Therapists have reported rigidity in thinking as the greatest challenge in treating people with

ASD (Cooper et al., 2018). Given the challenges that people with ASD face, it is important to adapt exposure therapy to this population. First, care must be taken in the case conceptualization phase to understand the patient's challenges and develop the appropriate treatment plan. Then, the common challenges listed above can be addressed by greater parental involvement, length of treatment, rewards, communication, and/or teaching aids.

20.6.2.1 Case Conceptualization and Treatment Plan

Identification of the functional level of the patient is imperative from the onset of treatment to know to what extent adaptations should be provided. On the one hand, adaptations are helpful when addressing a specific deficit; on the other hand, unnecessary adaptions could artificially restrict the patient's growth. During the case conceptualization, it is also important to distinguish between anxiety symptoms and symptoms of ASD that may seem to overlap. For example, rigid adherence to rules may be a symptom of OCD or it may be due to ASD (Nadeau et al., 2011). Likewise, lack of eye contact may be a symptom of social anxiety, or it may be due to ASD. A functional analysis (FA) can provide a differential diagnosis and help elucidate treatment targets (Vasa et al., 2016). When creating the hierarchy, keep in mind that common anxiety triggers for people with ASD include changes in routine, novel situations, socializing, and sensory stimuli (Ramirez et al., 2021). Furthermore, sensory sensitivity may lead to elevated baseline levels of anxiety and anxiety provoked by otherwise normal circumstances such as the amount of light or noise in the therapy room. Finally, recognize that adherence to treatment may improve indirectly by providing more structure in the patient's life generally, such as utilizing a schedule and to-do lists, having routines and attainable goals, and teaching problem-solving strategies (Kerns et al., 2016).

20.6.2.2 Parental Involvement

A recent meta-analysis of 23 studies found that greater parental involvement in treatment is associated with better treatment outcomes for youth with ASD (Perihan et al., 2020). Given that cognitive and social deficits due to ASD persist into adulthood, it would seem reasonable that the benefits of parental involvement would apply to working with adults with ASD as well (Van Steensel et al., 2017). Parents can assist the therapist in understanding the patient's particular challenges and can facilitate exposure practice at home (Salloum et al., 2018; Storch et al., 2020). Parents also facilitate attendance to sessions by remembering appointments, arranging transportation, and providing encouragement or incentives when the participant does not feel like attending. However, parents are not only important for what they do but also for what they do not do. Parents can often give reassurance and accommodate undesirable behavior out of empathy, not knowing that reassurance and accommodations only serve to maintain restricted, repetitive, or disruptive behaviors and anxiety (Abramowitz et al., 2019; Feldman et al., 2019;

Frank et al., 2020; Koller et al., 2021; Storch et al., 2015). Therefore, psychoeducation for parents and involvement in exposure exercises is very important so that they understand the vicious cycle that reassurance and accommodations foster and actively develop new patterns of interaction. In reducing and eliminating accommodations, parents provide the patient with a sort of natural exposure to everyday, real-life challenges. In fact, one treatment for childhood anxiety that has been shown to be equally effective as individual child CBT is based almost exclusively on reducing parental accommodations (Lebowitz et al., 2020).

20.6.2.3 Treatment Dose

Outcomes are better for treatments that include more sessions and have longer session length (Kerns et al., 2016). A recent meta-analysis of 23 studies of youth with anxiety and ASD found that, in general, short-term interventions (less than 12 sessions) were much less effective than standard-term interventions (12–14 sessions), which were a little less effective than long-term interventions (16 sessions or more; Perihan et al., 2020). One outlier was a 12-session program that was much more effective than all other interventions, including the long-term interventions (Chalfant et al., 2007). Of note, each session was 2 hours long. In addition, the parents were involved in group sessions. Also, the program met weekly for nine sessions and then met monthly for three booster sessions, so the extended follow-up over time may have provided an added benefit.

20.6.2.4 Rewards

Rewards can be used to shape the participant's behavior over time by incentivizing desired behavior and disincentivizing undesired behavior. Rewards may include attention, praise, high-fives, playtime, or prizes. Whether in-session with the therapist or out-of-session with the parent, tangible and intangible rewards can be used to incentivize attendance to sessions, engagement in exposures, and adherence to homework. For example, the client can be rewarded for facing each rung of the fear hierarchy, with rewards increasing in value as the hierarchy advances. This approach is used for neurotypical children with anxiety (Rapee et al., 2008). It is important to tailor the rewards to the audience, especially when considering that restricted interests is a feature of ASD. Some propose a systematic preference assessment to identify the participant's preferences (Hagopian et al., 2004).

20.6.2.5 Communication and Teaching Aids

Communication deficits are a salient feature of ASD and can interfere with any treatment, including exposure therapy (Kerns et al., 2016). The first step is to identify the severity of deficits and then implement strategies and aids that account for the deficits. Such teaching aids include prompting, modeling, and visual tools. Prompting is based on the memory principle that recognition is easier than recall.

When the individual appears to be struggling to come up with an answer, the therapist or parent can provide a visual or vocal prompt to help the individual recall the answer. This facilitates more learning than if the individual were simply told the answer. Visual aids can facilitate learning by appealing to multiple senses. Visual aids can include body language, gestures, signs, pictures, and objects for demonstration. For example, the hierarchy ladder can be a picture of a ladder with a description next to each rung. Another way to facilitate understanding is to simplify language and use concrete tasks and activities rather than abstract or theoretical descriptions. Keep in mind that ideas may have to be repeated multiple times both during and across sessions. Finally, it may be helpful if the sessions themselves are clearly structured, so the individual knows what to expect when. Regardless of the strategy, it is important that teaching aids are developmentally appropriate and only used when necessary, so that they enhance rather than impede the development and participation of the individual.

20.7 References

Abramowitz, J. S., Deacon, B. J., & Whiteside, S. P. H. (2019). Involving significant others in treatment. In *Exposure therapy for anxiety: Principles and practice* (2nd ed., pp. 337–352). New York: Guilford Press.

Adams, D., & Emerson, L.-M. (2021). The impact of anxiety in children on the autism spectrum. *Journal of Autism and Developmental Disorders,51*(6), 1909–1920. https://doi.org/10.1007/s10803-020-04673-3

Arch, J. J., Eifert, G. H., Davies, C., Vilardaga, J. C. P., Rose, R. D., & Craske, M. G. (2012). Randomized clinical trial of cognitive behavioral therapy (CBT) versus acceptance and commitment therapy (ACT) for mixed anxiety disorders.*Journal of Consulting and Clinical Psychology,80*(5), 750–765. https://doi.org/10.1037/a0028310

Bandarian-Balooch, S., Neumann, D. L., & Boschen, M. J. (2015). Exposure treatment in multiple contexts attenuates return of fear via renewal in high spider fearful individuals. *Journal of Behavior Therapy and Experimental Psychiatry,47*, 138–144. https://doi.org/10.1016/j.jbtep.2014.12.006

Benito, K. G., Machan, J., Freeman, J. B., Garcia, A. M., Walther, M., Frank, H., Wellen, B., Stewart, E., Edmunds, J., Kemp, J., Sapyta, J., & Franklin, M. (2018). Measuring fear change within exposures: Functionally-defined habituation predicts outcome in three randomized controlled trials for pediatric OCD. *Journal of Consulting and Clinical Psychology, 86*(7), 615–630. https://doi.org/10.1037/ccp0000315

Blakey, S. M., & Abramowitz, J. S. (2016). The effects of safety behaviors during exposure therapy for anxiety: Critical analysis from an inhibitory learning perspective. *Clinical Psychology Review, 49*, 1–15. https://doi.org/10.1016/j.cpr.2016.07.002

Byrne, G., Ghráda, Á. N., & O'Mahony, T. (2022). Parent-led cognitive behavioural therapy for children with autism spectrum conditions: A pilot study. *Journal of Autism and Developmental Disorders*, 53(1), 263–274. https://doi.org/10.1007/s10803-022-05424-2

Carpenter, J. K., Andrews, L. A., Witcraft, S. M., Powers, M. B., Smits, J. A., & Hofmann, S. G. (2018). Cognitive behavioral therapy for anxiety and related disorders: A meta-analysis of randomized placebo-controlled trials. *Depression and Anxiety, 35*(6), 502–514. https://doi.org/10.1002/da.22728

Chalfant, A. M., Rapee, R., & Carroll, L. (2007). Treating anxiety disorders in children with high functioning autism spectrum disorders: A controlled trial. *Journal of Autism and Developmental Disorders, 37*(10), 1842–1857. https://doi.org/10.1007/s10803-006-0318-4

Cooper, J. O., Heron, T. E., & Heward, W. L. (2007). Applied behavior analysis. Upper Saddle River, NJ: Pearson.

Cooper, K., Loades, M. E., & Russell, A. (2018). Adapting psychological therapies for autism. *Research in Autism Spectrum Disorders, 45*, 43–50. https://doi.org/10.1016/j.rasd.2017.11.002

Craske, M. G., DeCola, J. P., Sachs, A. D., & Pontillo, D. C. (2003). Panic control treatment for agoraphobia. *Journal of Anxiety Disorders,17*(3), 321–333. https://doi.org/10.1016/s0887-6185(02)00203-7

Craske, M. G., Treanor, M., Conway, C. C., Zbozinek, T., & Vervliet, B. (2014). Maximizing exposure therapy: An inhibitory learning approach. *Behaviour Research and Therapy,58*, 10–23. https://doi.org/10.1016/j.brat.2014.04.006

Cuijpers, P., Donker, T., van Straten, A., Li, J., & Andersson, G. (2010). Is guided self-help as effective as face-to-face psychotherapy for depression and anxiety disorders? A systematic review and meta-analysis of comparative outcome studies. *Psychological Medicine,40*(12), 1943–1957. https://doi.org/10.1017/s0033291710000772

Cuijpers, P., Sijbrandij, M., Koole, S., Huibers, M., Berking, M., & Andersson, G. (2014). Psychological treatment of generalized anxiety disorder: A meta-analysis. *Clinical Psychology Review,34*(2), 130–140. https://doi.org/10.1016/j.cpr.2014.01.002

DiMauro, J., Domingues, J., Fernandez, G., & Tolin, D. F. (2013). Long-term effectiveness of CBT for anxiety disorders in an adult outpatient clinic sample: A follow-up study. *Behaviour Research and Therapy,51*(2), 82–86. https://doi.org/10.1016/j.brat.2012.10.003

Feldman, I., Koller, J., Lebowitz, E. R., Shulman, C., Ben Itzchak, E., & Zachor, D. A. (2019). Family accommodation in autism spectrum disorder. *Journal of Autism and Developmental Disorders, 49*(9), 3602–3610. https://doi.org/10.1007/s10803-019-04078-x

Feske, U., & Chambless, D. L. (1995). Cognitive behavioral versus exposure only treatment for social phobia: A meta-analysis. *Behavior Therapy,26*(4), 695–720. https://doi.org/10.1016/s0005-7894(05)80040-1

Foa, E. B. (2011). Prolonged exposure therapy: Past, present, and future. *Depression and Anxiety, 28*, 1043–1047. https://doi.org/10.1002/da.20907

Foa, E. B., Liebowitz, M. R., Kozak, M. J., Davies, S., Campeas, R., Franklin, M. E., Huppert, J. D., Kjernisted, K., Rowan, V., Schmidt, A. B., Simpson, H. B., & Tu, X. (2005). Randomized, placebo-controlled trial of exposure and ritual prevention, clomipramine, and their combination in the treatment of obsessive-compulsive disorder. *American Journal of Psychiatry,162*(1), 151–161. https://doi.org/10.1176/appi.ajp.162.1.151

Frank, H. E., Kagan, E. R., Storch, E. A., Wood, J. J., Kerns, C. M., Lewin, A. B., Small, B. J., & Kendall, P. C. (2020). Accommodation of anxiety in youth with autism spectrum disorder: Results from the TAASD study. *Journal of Clinical Child & Adolescent Psychology, 51*(2), 219–229. https://doi.org/10.1080/15374416.2020.1759075

Gotham, K., Brunwasser, S. M., & Lord, C. (2015). Depressive and anxiety symptom trajectories from school age through young adulthood in samples with autism spectrum disorder and developmental delay. *Journal of the American Academy of Child & Adolescent Psychiatry, 54*(5), 369–376. https://doi.org/10.1016/j.jaac.2015.02.005

Guzick, A. G., Schneider, S. C., Kendall, P. C., Wood, J. J., Kerns, C. M., Small, B. J., Park, H., Cepeda, S. L. & Storch, E. A. (2021, June). Change during cognitive and exposure phases of cognitive-behavioral therapy for youth with anxiety and autism spectrum disorders. Poster presented at the 2021 Journal of Clinical Child and Adolescent Psychology (JCCAP) Future Directions Forum.

Hagopian, L. P., Lilly, M., & Davis, T. E. (2017). Behavioral treatments for anxiety in minimally verbal children with ASD. In C. M. Kerns, P. Renno, E. A. Storch, P. C. Kendall, & J. J. Wood (Eds.), *Anxiety in children and adolescents with autism spectrum disorder* (pp. 193–210). New York: Academic Press. https://doi.org/10.1016/B978-0-12-805122-1.00010-7

Hagopian, L. P., Long, E. S., & Rush, K. S. (2004). Preference assessment procedures for individuals with developmental disabilities. *Behavior Modification, 28*(5), 668–677. https://doi.org/10.1177/0145445503259836

Hedley, D., & Uljarević, M. (2018). Systematic review of suicide in autism spectrum disorder: Current trends and implications. *Current Developmental Disorders Reports,5*(1), 65–76. https://doi.org/10.1007/s40474-018-0133-6

Hepburn, S. L., Blakeley-Smith, A., Wolff, B., & Reaven, J. A. (2016). Telehealth delivery of cognitive-behavioral intervention to youth with autism spectrum disorder and anxiety: A pilot study. *Autism, 20*(2), 207–218. https://doi.org/10.1177/1362361315575164

Hesselmark, E., Plenty, S., & Bejerot, S. (2014). Group cognitive behavioural therapy and group recreational activity for adults with autism spectrum disorders: A preliminary randomized controlled trial. *Autism, 18*(6), 672–683. https://doi.org/10.1177/1362361313493681

Hofmann, S. G., Asnaani, A., Vonk, I. J. J., Sawyer, A. T., & Fang, A. (2012). The efficacy of cognitive behavioral therapy: A review of meta-analyses. *Cognitive Therapy and Research,36*(5), 427–440. https://doi.org/10.1007/s10608-012-9476-1

Hollocks, M. J., Lerh, J. W., Magiati, I., Meiser-Stedman, R., & Brugha, T. S. (2019). Anxiety and depression in adults with autism spectrum disorder: A systematic review and meta-analysis. *Psychological Medicine, 49*(4), 559–572. https://doi.org/10.1017/s0033291718002283

Horowitz, L. M., Thurm, A., Farmer, C., Mazefsky, C., Lanzillo, E., Bridge, J. A., Greenbaum, R., Pao, M., Siegel, M., Autism and Developmental Disorders Inpatient Research Collaborative (ADDIRC). (2018). Talking about death or suicide: Prevalence and clinical correlates in youth with autism spectrum disorder in the psychiatric inpatient setting. *Journal of Autism and Developmental Disorders,48*(11), 3702–3710. https://doi.org/10.1007/s10803-017-3180-7

Janardhan-Reddy, Y., Sudhir, P., Manjula, M., Arumugham, S., & Narayanaswamy, J. (2020). Clinical practice guidelines for cognitive-behavioral therapies in anxiety disorders and obsessive-compulsive and related disorders. *Indian Journal of Psychiatry,62*(8), 230. https://doi.org/10.4103/psychiatry.indianjpsychiatry_773_19

Johnco, C., & Storch, E. A. (2015). Anxiety in youth with autism spectrum disorders: Implications for treatment. *Expert Review of Neurotherapeutics,15*(11), 1343–1352. https://doi.org/10.1586/14737175.2015.1111762

Kaczkurkin, A., & Foa, E. (2015). Cognitive-behavioral therapy for anxiety disorders: An update on the empirical evidence. *Anxiety,17*(3), 337–346. https://doi.org/10.31887/dcns.2015.17.3/akaczkurkin

Kerns, C. M., Roux, A. M., Connell, J. E., & Shattuck, P. T. (2016). Adapting cognitive behavioral techniques to address anxiety and depression in cognitively able emerging adults on the autism spectrum. *Cognitive and Behavioral Practice, 23*(3), 329–340. https://doi.org/10.1016/j.cbpra.2016.06.002

Kerns, C. M., Winder-Patel, B., Iosif, A. M., Nordahl, C. W., Heath, B., Solomon, M., & Amaral, D. G. (2021). Clinically significant anxiety in children with autism spectrum disorder and varied intellectual functioning. *Journal of Clinical Child & Adolescent Psychology,50*(6), 780–795. https://doi.org/10.1080/15374416.2019.1703712

Kester, K. R., & Lucyshyn, J. M. (2018). Cognitive behavior therapy to treat anxiety among children with autism spectrum disorders: A systematic review. *Research in Autism Spectrum Disorders, 52*, 37–50. https://doi.org/10.1016/j.rasd.2018.05.002

Koller, J., David, T., Bar, N., & Lebowitz, E. R. (2021). The role of family accommodation of RRBs in disruptive behavior among children with autism. *Journal of Autism and Developmental Disorders, 52*(6), 2505–2511. https://doi.org/10.1007/s10803-021-05163-w

Lebowitz, E. R., Marin, C., Martino, A., Shimshoni, Y., & Silverman, W. K. (2020). Parent-based treatment as efficacious as cognitive-behavioral therapy for childhood anxiety: A randomized non-inferiority study of supportive parenting for anxious childhood emotions. *Journal of the American Academy of Child & Adolescent Psychiatry, 59*(3), 362–372. https://doi.org/10.1016/j.jaac.2019.02.014

Lever, A. G., & Geurts, H. M. (2016). Psychiatric co-occurring symptoms and disorders in young, middle-aged, and older adults with autism spectrum disorder. *Journal of Autism and Developmental Disorders,46*(6), 1916–1930. https://doi.org/10.1007/s10803-016-2722-8

de Lijster, J. M., Dieleman, G. C., Utens, E. M., Dierckx, B., Wierenga, M., Verhulst, F. C., & Legerstee, J. S. (2018). Social and academic functioning in adolescents with anxiety disorders: A systematic review. *Journal of Affective Disorders,230*, 108–117. https://doi.org/10.1016/j.jad.2018.01.008

Mayo-Wilson, E., Dias, S., Mavranezouli, I., Kew, K., Clark, D. M., Ades, A. E., & Pilling, S. (2014). Psychological and pharmacological interventions for social anxiety disorder in adults: a systematic review and network meta-analysis. *The Lancet Psychiatry,1*(5), 368–376. https://doi.org/10.1016/s2215-0366(14)70329-3

McGuire, J. F., Lewin, A. B., & Storch, E. A. (2014). Enhancing exposure therapy for anxiety disorders, obsessive-compulsive disorder and post-traumatic stress disorder. *Expert Review of Neurotherapeutics,14*(8), 893–910. https://doi.org/10.1586/14737175.2014.934677

McGuire, J. F., & Storch, E. A. (2018). An inhibitory learning approach to cognitive-behavioral therapy for children and adolescents. *Cognitive and Behavioral Practice.* https://doi.org/10.1016/j.cbpra.2017.12.003

Mowrer, O. (1960). *Learning theory and behavior.* New York: John Wiley and Sons. https://doi.org/10.1037/10802-000

Nadeau, J., Sulkowski, M. L., Ung, D., Wood, J. J., Lewin, A. B., Murphy, T. K., May, J. E., & Storch, E. A. (2011). Treatment of comorbid anxiety and autism spectrum disorders. *Neuropsychiatry, 1*(6), 567. doi: 10.2217/npy.11.62

Nepon, J., Belik, S. L., Bolton, J., & Sareen, J. (2010). The relationship between anxiety disorders and suicide attempts: Findings from the National Epidemiologic Survey on Alcohol and Related Conditions. *Depression and Anxiety,27*(9), 791–798. https://doi.org/10.1002/da.20674

Olatunji, B. O., Davis, M. L., Powers, M. B., & Smits, J. A. J. (2013). Cognitive-behavioral therapy for obsessive-compulsive disorder: A meta-analysis of treatment outcome and moderators. *Journal of Psychiatric Research,47*(1), 33–41. https://doi.org/10.1016/j.jpsychires.2012.08.020

Olthuis, J. V., Watt, M. C., Bailey, K., Hayden, J. A., & Stewart, S. H. (2015). Therapist-supported Internet cognitive behavioural therapy for anxiety disorders in adults. *Cochrane Database of Systematic Reviews.*, *3*(3), 1–141. https://doi.org/10.1002/14651858.cd011565

Perihan, C., Burke, M., Bowman-Perrott, L., Bicer, A., Gallup, J., Thompson, J., & Sallese, M. (2020). Effects of cognitive behavioral therapy for reducing anxiety in children with high functioning ASD: A systematic review and meta-analysis. *Journal of Autism and Developmental Disorders, 50*(6), 1958–1972. https://doi.org/10.1007/s10803-019-03949-7

Pompoli, A., Furukawa, T. A., Efthimiou, O., Imai, H., Tajika, A., & Salanti, G. (2018). Dismantling cognitive-behaviour therapy for panic disorder: A systematic review and component network meta-analysis. *Psychological Medicine,48*(12), 1945–1953. https://doi.org/10.1017/s0033291717003919

Powers, M. B., Halpern, J. M., Ferenschak, M. P., Gillihan, S. J., & Foa, E. B. (2010). A meta-analytic review of prolonged exposure for posttraumatic stress disorder. *Clinical Psychology Review, 30*(6), 635–641. https://doi.org/10.1016/j.cpr.2010.04.007

Ramirez, A. C., Grebe, S. C., McNeel, M. M., Limon, D. L., Schneider, S. C., Berry, L. N., Goin-Kochel, R. P., Cepeda, S. L., Voigt, R. G., Salloum, A., & Storch, E. A. (2020). Parent-led, stepped-care cognitive-behavioral therapy for youth with autism and co-occurring anxiety: Study rationale and method. *Brazilian Journal of Psychiatry, 42*, 638–645. https://doi.org/10.1590/1516-4446-2020-0897

Ramirez, A. C., Perez, M. I., Limon, D., Storch, E. A., & Schneider, S. C. (2021). Cognitive behavioral therapy for anxiety in children with autism spectrum disorders. In *Diagnosis, management and modeling of neurodevelopmental disorders* (pp. 447–455). New York: Academic Press. https://doi.org/10.1016/B978-0-12-817988-8.00040-3

Rankin, C. H., Abrams, T., Barry, R. J., Bhatnagar, S., Clayton, D. F., Colombo, J., Coppola, G., Geyer, M. A., Glanzman, D. L., Marsland, S., & McSweeney, F. K. (2009). Habituation revisited: An updated and revised description of the behavioral characteristics of habituation. *Neurobiology of Learning and Memory,92*(2), 135–138. https://doi.org/10.1016/j.nlm.2008.09.012

Rapee, R., Wignall, A., Spence, S., Lyneham, H., & Cobham, V. (2008). *Helping your anxious child: A step-by-step guide for parents.* Oakland, CA: New Harbinger.

Reaven, J., Blakeley-Smith, A., Nichols S., Dasari M., Flanigan E., Hepburn, S. (2009). Cognitive behavioral group treatment for anxiety symptoms in children with high-functioning autism spectrum disorders: A pilot study. *Focus on Autism and Other Developmental Disabilities, 24*(1), 27–37. https://doi.org/10.1111/j.1469-7610.2011.02486.x

Reaven, J., Blakeley-Smith, A., Leuthe, E., Moody, E., & Hepburn, S. (2012). Facing your fears in adolescence: Cognitive-behavioral therapy for high-functioning autism spectrum disorders and anxiety. *Autism Research and Treatment., 2012*, 1–13. https://doi.org/10.1155/2012/423905

Richa, S., Fahed, M., Khoury, E., & Mishra, B. (2014). Suicide in autism spectrum disorders. *Archives of Suicide Research, 18*(4), 327–339. https://doi.org/10.1080/13811118.2013.824834

Romanelli, R. J., Wu, F. M., Gamba, R., Mojtabai, R., & Segal, J. B. (2014). Behavioral therapy and serotonin reuptake inhibitor pharmacotherapy in the treatment of obsessive-compulsive disorder: a systematic review and meta-analysis of head-to-head randomized controlled trials. *Depression and Anxiety, 31*(8), 641–652. https://doi.org/10.1002/da.22232

Rosen, T. E., Connell, J. E., & Kerns, C. M. (2016). A review of behavioral interventions for anxiety-related behaviors in lower-functioning individuals with autism. *Behavioral Interventions, 31*(2), 120–143. https://doi.org/10.1002/bin.1442

Russell, A. J., Jassi, A., Fullana, M. A., Mack, H., Johnston, K., Heyman, I., Murphy, D. G., & Mataix-Cols, D. (2013). Cognitive behavior therapy for comorbid obsessive-compulsive disorder in high-functioning autism spectrum disorders: A randomized controlled trial. *Depression and Anxiety, 30*(8), 697–708. https://doi.org/10.1002/da.22053

Ryan, P. M., Kaskas, M. M., & Davis, T. E. (2017). *Cognitive-behavioral principles and their applications within autism spectrum disorder.* Amsterdam: Elsevier. https://doi.org/10.1016/B978-0-12-805122-1.00006-5

Salloum, A., Andel, R., Lewin, A. B., Johnco, C., McBride, N. M., & Storch, E. A. (2018). Family accommodation as a predictor of cognitive-behavioral treatment outcome for childhood anxiety. *Families in Society: The Journal of Contemporary Social Services, 99*(1), 45–55. https://doi.org/10.1177/1044389418756326

Schneider, S. C., Knott, L., Cepeda, S. L., Hana, L. M., McIngvale, E., Goodman, W. K., & Storch, E. A. (2020). Serious negative consequences associated with exposure and response prevention for obsessive-compulsive disorder: A survey of therapist attitudes and experiences. *Depression and Anxiety, 37*(5), 418–428. https://doi.org/10.1002/da.23000

Skapinakis, P., Caldwell, D. M., Hollingworth, W., Bryden, P., Fineberg, N. A., Salkovskis, P., Welton, N. J., Baxter, H., Kessler, D., Churchill, R., & Lewis, G. (2016). Pharmacological and psychotherapeutic interventions for management of obsessive-compulsive disorder in adults: A systematic review and network meta-analysis. *The Lancet Psychiatry,3*(8), 730–739. https://doi.org/10.1016/s2215-0366(16)30069-4

Slaughter, A. M., McNeel, M. M., Storch, E. A., & Mire, S. S. (2020). Where should we go from here? Identified gaps in the literature in psychosocial interventions for youth with autism spectrum disorder and comorbid anxiety. *Children's Health Care, 49*(4), 435–471.

Smith, I. C., Ollendick, T. H., & White, S. W. (2019). Anxiety moderates the influence of ASD severity on quality of life in adults with ASD. *Research in Autism Spectrum Disorders,62*, 39–47. https://doi.org/10.1016/j.rasd.2019.03.001

Spain, D., Sin, J., Chalder, T., Murphy, D., & Happe, F. (2015). Cognitive behaviour therapy for adults with autism spectrum disorders and psychiatric co-morbidity: A review. *Research in Autism Spectrum Disorders, 9*, 151–162. https://doi.org/10.1016/j.rasd.2014.10.019

Van Steensel, F. J., Bögels, S. M., & Perrin, S. (2011). Anxiety disorders in children and adolescents with autistic spectrum disorders: A meta-analysis. *Clinical Child and Family Psychology Review,14*(3), 302–317. https://doi.org/10.1007/s10567-011-0097-0

Van Steensel, F. J. A., & Bögels, S. M. (2014). CBT for anxiety disorders in children with and without autism spectrum disorders. *Journal of Consulting and Clinical Psychology, 83*(3), 512–523. https://doi.org/10.1037/a0039108

Van Steensel, F. J. A., & Bögels, S. M. (2015). CBT for anxiety disorders in children with and without autism spectrum disorders. *Journal of Consulting and Clinical Psychology, 83*(3), 512. https://doi.org/10.1037/a0039108

Van Steensel, F. J. A., Bögels, S. M., & Dirksen, C. D. (2012). Anxiety and quality of life: Clinically anxious children with and without autism spectrum disorders compared. *Journal of Clinical Child & Adolescent Psychology,41*(6), 731–738. https://doi.org/10.1080/15374416.2012.698725

Van Steensel, F. J. A., Dirksen, C. D., & Bögels, S. M. (2014). Cost-effectiveness of cognitive-behavioral therapy versus treatment as usual for anxiety disorders in children with autism spectrum disorder. *Research in Autism Spectrum Disorders, 8*(2), 127–137. https://doi.org/10.1016/j.rasd.2013.11.001

Van Steensel, F. J. A., Zegers, V. M., & Bögels, S. (2017). Predictors of treatment effectiveness for youth with ASD and comorbid anxiety disorders: It all depends on the family? *Journal of Autism and Developmental Disorders,47*(3), 636–645. https://doi.org/10.1007/s10803-016-2956-5

Storch, E. A., Arnold, E. B., Lewin, A. B., Nadeau, J. M., Jones, A. M., De Nadai, A. S., Mutch, P. J., Selles, R. R., Ung, D., & Murphy, T. K. (2013). The effect of cognitive-behavioral therapy versus treatment as usual for anxiety in children with autism spectrum disorders: A randomized, controlled trial. *Journal of the American Academy of Child & Adolescent Psychiatry, 52*(2), 132–142. https://doi.org/10.1016/j.jaac.2012.11.007

Storch, E. A., Lewin, A. B., Collier, A. B., Arnold, E., De Nadai, A. S., Dane, B. F., Nadeau, J. M., Mutch, P. J., & Murphy, T. K. (2015). A randomized controlled trial of cognitive-behavioral therapy versus treatment as usual for adolescents with autism spectrum disorders and comorbid anxiety. *Depression and Anxiety, 32*(3), 174–181. https://doi.org/10.1002/da.22332

Storch, E. A., Schneider, S. C., De Nadai, A. S., Selles, R. R., McBride, N. M., Grebe, S.C., Bergez, K. C., Ramirez, A., Viana, A. G., & Lewin, A. B. (2020). A pilot study of family-based exposure-focused treatment for youth with autism spectrum disorder and anxiety *Child Psychiatry & Human Development, 51*(2), 209–219. https://doi.org/10.1007/s10578-019-00923-3

Storch, E. A., Wood, J. J., Guzick, A. G., Small, B. J., Kerns, C. M., Ordaz, D. L., Schneider, S. C., & Kendall, P. C. (2021). Moderators of response to personalized and standard care cognitive-behavioral therapy for youth with autism spectrum disorder and comorbid anxiety. *Journal of Autism and Developmental Disorders, 52*, 950–958. https://doi.org/10.1007/s10803-021-05000-0

Storch, Zavrou, S., Collier, A. B., Ung, D., Arnold, E. B., Mutch, P. J., Lewin, A. B., & Murphy, T. K. (2015). Preliminary study of family accommodation in youth with autism spectrum disorders and anxiety: Incidence, clinical correlates, and behavioral treatment response. *Journal of Anxiety Disorders, 34*, 94–99. https://doi.org/10.1016/j.janxdis.2015.06.007

Uljarević, M., Hedley, D., Rose-Foley, K., Magiati, I., Cai, R. Y., Dissanayake, C., Richdale, A., & Trollor, J. (2020). Anxiety and depression from adolescence to old age in autism spectrum disorder. *Journal of Autism and Developmental Disorders,50*(9), 3155–3165. https://doi.org/10.1007/s10803-019-04084-z

Vansteenwegen, D., Vervliet, B., Iberico, C., Baeyens, F., Van den Bergh, O., & Hermans, D. (2007). The repeated confrontation with videotapes of spiders in multiple contexts attenuates renewal of fear in spider-anxious students. *Behaviour Research and Therapy,45*(6), 1169–1179. https://doi.org/10.1016/j.brat.2006.08.023

Vasa, R. A., Mazurek, M. O., Mahajan, R., Bennett, A. E., Bernal, M. P., Nozzolillo, A. A., Arnold, L. E., & Coury, D. L. (2016). Assessment and treatment of anxiety in youth with autism spectrum disorders. *Pediatrics, 137*(Suppl. 2), S115–S123. https://doi.org/10.1542/peds.2015-2851J

Vika, M., Skaret, E., Raadal, M., Öst, L.-G., & Kvale, G. (2009). One- vs. five-session treatment of intra-oral injection phobia: a randomized clinical study. *European Journal of Oral Sciences,117*(3), 279–285. https://doi.org/10.1111/j.1600-0722.2009.00628.x

White, S. W., Albano, A. M., Johnson, C. R., Kasari, C., Ollendick, T., Klin, A., Oswald, D., & Scahill, L. (2010). Development of a cognitive-behavioral intervention program to treat anxiety and social deficits in teens with high-functioning autism. *Clinical Child and Family Psychology Review, 13*(1), 77–90. https://doi.org/10.1007/s10567-009-0062-3

White, S. W., Ollendick, T., Albano, A. M., Oswald, D., Johnson, C., Southam-Gerow, M. A., Kim, I., & Scahill, L. (2013). Randomized controlled trial: Multimodal anxiety and social skill intervention for adolescents with autism spectrum disorder. *Journal of Autism and Developmental Disorders, 43*(2), 382–394. https://doi.org/10.1007/s10803-012-1577-x

White, S. W., Oswald, D., Ollendick, T., & Scahill, L. (2009). Anxiety in children and adolescents with autism spectrum disorders. *Clinical Psychology Review, 29*(3), 216–229. https://doi.org/10.1016/j.cpr.2009.01.003

Wickberg, F., Lenhard, F., Aspvall, K., Serlachius, E., Andrén, P., Johansson, F., Silverberg-Mörse, M., & Mataix-Cols, D. (2022). Feasibility of internet-delivered cognitive-behavior therapy for obsessive-compulsive disorder in youth with autism spectrum disorder: A clinical benchmark study. *Internet Interventions, 28*, 1–8. https://doi.org/10.1016/j.invent.2022.100520

Wiebenga, J. X., Dickhoff, J., Mérelle, S. Y., Eikelenboom, M., Heering, H. D., Gilissen, R., ... & Penninx, B. W. (2021). Prevalence, course, and determinants of suicide ideation and attempts in patients with a depressive and/or anxiety disorder: A review of NESDA findings. *Journal of Affective Disorders, 283*, 267–277. https://doi.org/10.1016/j.jad.2021.01.053

Wolitzky-Taylor, K. B., Horowitz, J. D., Powers, M. B., & Telch, M. J. (2008). Psychological approaches in the treatment of specific phobias: A meta-analysis. *Clinical Psychology Review,28*(6), 1021–1037. https://doi.org/10.1016/j.cpr.2008.02.007

Wood, J. J., Drahota, A., Sze, K., Har, K., Chiu, A., & Langer, D. A. (2009). Cognitive behavioral therapy for anxiety in children with autism spectrum disorders: A randomized, controlled trial. *Journal of Child Psychology and Psychiatry, 50*(3), 224–234. https://doi.org/10.1111/j.1469-7610.2008.01948.x

Wood, J. J., Ehrenreich-May, J., Alessandri, M., Fujii, C., Renno, P., Laugeson, E., Piacentini, J. C., De Nadai, A. S., Arnold, E., Lewin, A. B., Murphy, T. K., & Storch, E. A. (2015). Cognitive behavioral therapy for early adolescents with autism spectrum disorders and clinical anxiety: A randomized, controlled trial. *Behavior Therapy, 46*(1), 7–19. https://doi.org/10.1016/j.beth.2014.01.002

Wood, J. J., Kendall, P. C., Wood, K. S., Kerns, C. M., Seltzer, M., Small, B. J., Lewin, A. B., & Storch, E. A. (2020). Cognitive behavioral treatments for anxiety in children with autism spectrum disorder: A randomized clinical trial. *JAMA Psychiatry, 77*(5), 474–483. doi:10.1001/jamapsychiatry.2019.4160

Zaboski, B. A., & Storch, E. A. (2018). Comorbid autism spectrum disorder and anxiety disorders: A brief review. *Future Neurology,13*(1), 31–37. https://doi.org/10.2217/fnl-2017-0030

Zahid, S., & Upthegrove, R. (2017). Suicidality in autistic spectrum disorders. *Crisis,38*(4), 237–246. https://doi.org/10.1027/0227-5910/a000458

Zoellner, L. A., Abramowitz, J. S., Moore, S. A., & Slagle, D. M. (2008). Flooding. In W. T. O'Donohue, & J. E. Fisher (Eds.), *Cognitive behavior therapy: Applying empirically supported techniques in your practice*(pp. 202–210). Hoboken, NJ: John Wiley & Sons.

21

Acceptance and Commitment Training

Thomas G. Szabo, and Celia Heyman
Capella University

21.1 Technical Abstract

Background: Acceptance and commitment training (ACTr; Hayes et al., 2004) has been researched with both clinical trials and single-case design research methods as a treatment that helps reduce the impact of verbal behavior that persistently interferes with relevant direct contingencies. When used in applied behavior analysis (ABA), ACTr expands otherwise narrowly constricted verbal repertoires to reorient overt behavior toward less salient but important, larger positive reinforcers. The aim of ACTr is to improve psychological flexibility—the capacity to persist in difficult tasks or pivot to new activities that contact larger reinforcers that are not immediately available. Six core repertoires may be isolated and targeted in ACTr interventions as verbal aids used to sharpen contingency control over socially significant, observable, measurable behavior. **Method:** A review of the literature was conducted using the PsycINFO® database with keywords that included acceptance and commitment training or acceptance and commitment therapy, ABA, and autism. Other related keywords included relational frame theory and verbal behavior. Single-case design research investigating ACTr as an intervention in contexts common to ABA practice are summarized and treatment recommendations are presented. **Results:** The evidence supporting ACTr in ABA is mounting and strategies for using ACTr with autistic individuals are consistently evolving. Although it is early to argue that ACTr could be a routine part of everyday ABA, the flurry of current research suggests the value of ACTr as an intervention strategy to be used with autistic individuals, caregivers, stakeholders, and human service staff. **Discussion:** ACTr appears to be a viable ABA treatment with broad applicability among those possessing nascent to well-established verbal skills. Methods for teaching practitioners to use function-based, person-centered ACTr approaches are currently in development. However, in the absence of such practitioner training, ACTr specialists often reach for manualized approaches that have been described in the literature. Although this would seem to assure that the exercises are based on existing evidence, the result may be cookie-cutter applications of ACTr. Since this would be as antithetical to the aim of psychological flexibility as it is to ABA more broadly, future research should focus on practitioner training in methods of ACTr functional assessment and the design of unique,

Thomas G. Szabo, and Celia Heyman, *Acceptance and Commitment Training*. In: *Lifespan Treatment for Autistic Individuals*. Edited by: Peter Sturmey, Russell Lang, and James K. Luiselli, Oxford University Press. © Oxford University Press (2025). DOI: 10.1093/oso/9780197635841.003.0021 personalized treatments. **Practitioner recommendations:** When the behavior of persons with verbal abilities is insensitive to direct contingency management, consider assessing the six component repertoires of psychological flexibility and treating those that appear to be excessive or deficient.

21.2 Layperson Summary

To help individuals with autism decrease or increase socially important behavior, the most empirically supported of available treatments is ABA, which involves changing relevant contextual variables such as antecedents and consequences. A vast body of empirical literature supports the use of ABA procedures in the treatment of behaviors associated with autism. Nevertheless, treatment failures have been documented, resurgence occurs, and at times, those with verbal skills either do not offer or withdraw their assent for common ABA treatments. Of additional concern is that ABA strategies helpful in supporting those with minimal verbal skills may lose their social validity with those who are older and have acquired verbal skills. Strategies are needed to promote successful behavior among these individuals, and additional ABA strategies may be needed to help caregivers and support staff.

In recent years, ABA researchers have turned their attention in these matters to strategies that improve psychological flexibility, which can be defined as the capacity to persist in difficult tasks or pivot to new activities associated with improved life outcomes. ACTr (Hayes et al., 2004) involves the assessment and differential treatment of six functionally distinct classes of verbal behavior that together comprise psychological flexibility.

ACTr is of particular value because it may be implemented by virtually anyone who has learned the basic strategy. Although initially developed by and for psychotherapists as acceptance and commitment therapy (ACT; Hayes et al., 1999), ACTr has been developed for use by coaches, pastoral counselors, teachers, behavior analysts, and others that help individuals aiming to improve their performance. Over 1,000 randomized controlled trials document the effectiveness of ACT for a wide variety of ailments, and an emerging single-case design research program is now underway supporting the use of an iteration of this kind of psychological flexibility training geared to the needs of practitioners who do not conduct psychotherapy.

The measure of success in ACTr is successful working; that is, when ACTr has been effective, those receiving services begin engaging in important behaviors that have a high probability of contacting positive reinforcement. In other words, when prevailing methods for changing a person's behavior have not gained sufficient traction, ACTr can help improve their grip and generate behavioral momentum. Yet despite these advantages, there are risks associated with ACTr. The most notable of these is the possibility that ACTr practitioners will step over the line and engage in psychotherapy. A second risk worthy of mention is that practitioners could attempt ACTr strategies for which they have not received adequate training or supervision. Graduate courses in ACTr are no longer uncommon; nevertheless, until the empirical ABA literature on ACTr advances further, these courses will remain electives.

Fortunately, there are a number of BCBAs with advanced training in ACTr who currently offer continuing education courses and consultation; many of these courses are publicized on social media and are easily found with standard Internet searches for professional training in ACT and ACTr. A wide variety of publicly available resources are also available to families and practitioners for learning about ACT and ACTr. The most accessible of these is the website of the Association for Contextual Behavior Science (ACBS; www.contextualscience.org). ACBS is an international membership organization comprised of academic and practice professionals seeking to lessen human suffering and improve human well-being through the advancement of contextual behavior science. Many resources are available to nonmembers, but membership is not cost prohibitive. Membership dues are values based; that is, those joining are allowed to offer dues based on their ability to pay and the extent to which they foresee using resources available to members. ACBS and other science organizations, such as the Association for Behavior Analysis International and the Association for Positive Behavior Support, regularly host conferences at which advancements are discussed in invited talks, symposia, panels, and workshops. Books on ACT and ACTr are widely available from major publishing houses.

21.3 Treatment Summary Table

Treatment summary: Acceptance and Commitment Training

Treatment description: ACTr involves a wide variety of exercises that improve contingency control over behavior by weakening unhelpful verbal relations. In situations where direct contingency management produces less than criterion changes in behavior, interfering verbal behavior can be assessed and addressed. Treatment usually involves (a) practicing outside relevant social contexts, (b) collecting data on the frequency, duration, or latency of practice as well as on the use of newly acquired skills in real-world situations, and (c) reinforcement.

Expected outcomes: ACTr is usually part of an ongoing course of ABA treatment; thus, the relevant outcomes are changes in the frequency, duration, or latency of socially useful behaviors that can be observed and measured.

Methods: Methods may vary from physical activities, guided meditations, to writing, and they may be done privately, in dyads, small groups, or large groups. As a general rule, the mechanism of action in ACTr is verbal extinction. That is, during ACTr, participants are verbally exposed to challenging situations in a somewhat playful format. They are invited to do what they have done in the past but without reinforcement until the unworkability of their attempts to solve these problems in characteristic ways becomes apparent. Unlike other ABA approaches, in ACTr, the therapist does not offer solutions; rather, the therapist assists by asking the participant what else they might do in situations where the strategies they have tried in the past no longer work.

Expertise required to implement treatment: Unlike other ABA approaches, the ACTr stance is that of a fellow traveler. Said differently, the ACTr practitioner's expertise is that of being another person who regularly gets stuck in verbal traps but who has found a few ways to get unstuck. Human verbal traps are varied and idiosyncratic; thus, the best ACTr interventionists are skilled at designing individualized treatments tailored to the unique verbal behaviors of the persons involved.

Risks and negative side effects: The line between ACT and ACTr requires formal training to properly distinguish. As a generality, ACT therapists elicit challenging emotions, thoughts, memories, and bodily sensations, whereas ACTr practitioners generally neither elicit nor do they avoid these difficulties. An inherent risk in walking this razor's edge is that practitioners will not back off when approaching content for which they have insufficient training, skill, or credentials. Another risk is that therapists will use strategies that seem to make light of difficulties that are hard for clients and thereby invalidating their experiences. In these situations, it is possible that clients may become agitated or otherwise adversely affected by the treatment.

Additional considerations and limitations: ACTr practitioners are encouraged to seek formal training, ongoing consultation, and to regularly ask themselves if their procedures are consistent with the seven dimensions of ABA, as articulated in Baer et al. (1968).

21.4 Introduction

21.4.1 Treatment Description

ACTr is a framework for treatment that addresses rigid verbal behavior that obstructs contingency control over socially important behavior. The topography of ACTr interventions can vary extensively. One widely employed modality of treatment is self-reflection. Not to be confused with introspection, the tool by which cognitive therapies seek to help an individual find the sources of their malaise within their psyches, self-reflection involves describing one's verbal behavior about contingencies of reinforcement and evaluating the effectiveness of these statements at tacting, or identifying, behavior that produces real-world reinforcement. Behavior analysts classify behavior that labels nonverbal parts of the world as tacts, or labels that are reinforced by praise from others. When an individual identifies deficiencies in these tacts, they are asked to develop new statements that more closely fit the existing contingencies. As individuals improve at precisely identifying contingencies, they are asked to describe differences in variables across a variety of conditions. The aim is to induce response variability that is under sharper gradients of stimulus control.

Another widely used modality of treatment is guided meditation. Meditations guided by a facilitator also should not be confused with relaxation exercises or self-soothing activities. On the contrary, guided meditations often involve verbal exposure to difficult situations. Participants are asked to allow themselves to feel, think, remember, and even to experience physical sensations associated with circumstances that are difficult for them to navigate. Although it is possible that ACT therapists might use this modality to explore events from the distant past, ACTr practitioners are more likely to draw upon current situations that are difficult for their clients.

ACTr practitioners frequently draw upon metaphors to help clients expand verbal knowledge of their overt behavior in common situations they face. Skinner (1957) described metaphorical extensions of tact relations as useful when the concrete details of a relation are difficult to observe directly. In ACTr, using metaphor helps clients to see their experience from a distance, or to do what Hayes refers to as "seeing seeing" (Hayes, 1984, p. 102). Similarly, Skinner explained that with verbal behavior, a person learns to report that they are behaving, and in so doing, they demonstrate self-knowledge (Skinner, 1974) but that defective self-knowledge needing psychological intervention may ensue when people react incongruently to stimuli generated by their own behavior (Skinner, 1953). For example, when a person's behavior is cowardly but they describe it as being compassionate, they escape punishment from others and aversive self-stimulation (self-shaming) but lose knowledge of themselves in the process. Many ACTr practitioners rely upon "classic" ACT metaphors that were described in the 1999 book to address such behavior, and many others use stock metaphors found in protocols and books. More advanced ACTr practitioners learn to listen for figurative speech in the verbal repertoires of their clients. Even those with more nascent verbal skills engage in pretend actions and use figures of speech that might easily be overlooked. Captured by a skilled practitioner, these can be used in experiential exercises in which clients do what they have been doing and observe the way what they commonly do works in shallow ways but fails at deeper, more important aims.

Experiential exercises may involve writing, closed-eye visualization, or physical action. Physicalized metaphors are powerful because when bodily exertion, adrenaline, perspiration, emotion, and operant reinforcement are combined, they produce more memorable events. If all this emerges from a metaphor or figure of speech that the client emitted, it is that much more memorable because it is "theirs." When later asked to reproduce this activity as a home practice exercise, the individual is more likely to follow through with the assignment if the event was paired with many sources of reinforcement, including the release of endogenous reinforcers such as adrenaline and social reinforcers in the forms of praise and humor. When reinforced for doing so, autistic individuals and others who otherwise appear to relate to their experiences in a notable "concrete" manner may engage in metaphor construction and exploration. Although the setup that clinicians use will need to vary when working with individuals of diverse verbal and developmental backgrounds, the general treatment framework of an experience that is playful and challenging remains consistent regardless of client skillset.

Many clinicians use self-report questionnaires to conduct ACTr functional assessments. Common among these are the Acceptance and Action Questionnaire-II (AAQ; Bond et al., 2011); the White Bear Suppression Inventory (WBSI; Wegner & Zanakos, 1994), used to assess thought suppression; the Parenting Stress Index Short Form (PSI-SF; Abidin, 1995); the Frieburg Mindfulness Inventory (FBI; Walach et al., 2006); and the Mindful Attention Awareness Scale (MAAS; Brown & Ryan, 2003), used to evaluate the extent to which individuals dispassionately observe the believability of their thoughts. It is important to note that authoritative texts have recommended exercising caution when interpreting results from self-report measures because these are easily faked or the questions may be misunderstood and answered imprecisely (Cooper et al., 2020). Fortunately, other assessment procedures may be used, such as the ACT matrix (Polk et al., 2016), described below.

The ACT matrix is a discrimination aid that helps clients view their repertoire in terms of covert and overt classes of positively and negatively reinforced behavior. A grid composed of two intersecting lines that form a Cartesian plane is drawn, forming four boxes into which a therapist or client adds statements about why a particular domain of concern matters to them, what they have been doing that has not paid off well, what that experience is like, and what actions they engage in that appear to work better for them. Although some use the ACT matrix as an intervention, the ACT matrix may be particularly useful at helping practitioners identify patterns of interfering verbal behavior to be targeted in subsequent ACTr interventions. In this way, the ACT matrix serves as both an indirect and as a descriptive functional assessment (Cooper et al., 2020).

Coding statements a person makes when exposed to the ACT matrix may be the equivalent of an indirect functional assessment if the person talks about verbal behavior they engaged in during previous circumstances. Consider the statement "I used to think I was stupid if I didn't know all the details of a conversation topic, so I'd go full-on Geek Master whenever I talked to people I was attracted to." Coding this involves classifying current verbal behavior about past verbal behavior; thus, the assessment is indirect and, as when conducting any indirect assessment, should be done with the utmost of caution. In contrast, coding the statement "I just want to geek out with you because I figure if I don't, you'll think I don't know my stuff" involves coding verbal behavior that is currently being emitted as a tact about the immediate contingencies. Assessing verbal behavior for its quality as a tact of the existing current contingencies is a kind of ACTr descriptive functional assessment.

Whether using the ACT matrix to conduct indirect or descriptive functional assessment of verbal behavior, it is important to collect enough samples from which to quantitatively evaluate the frequency, duration, latency, and even the magnitude of these responses. Evaluating verbal behavior that describes or qualifies other verbal behavior, which Skinner (1957) termed autoclitics, is important, too, because although some samples might not occur with great frequency, they may be emitted with emphasis compared to other utterances that occur more frequently but without much weight. Factoring in autoclitic responses such as changes in voice volume, tone, pitch, bodily posture, and use of facial or hand expressions is important in conducting this kind of ACTr functional assessment. Taken together, the topographies of verbal utterances and paralinguistic cues offer a rich ensemble of behavior from which to generate hypotheses about the way a person's verbal behavior could be obstructing the effects of direct contingencies. Given this as a general strategy, the next step is to identify relevant classes of inflexible verbal interfering behaviors and their counterpart flexible behaviors.

Patterns of verbal behavior addressed in ACTr can be broken into the following six overarching classes: (a) fusion/defusion, (b) experiential avoidance/acceptance, (c) loss of situational awareness/present moment awareness, (d) inflexible/flexible perspective taking, (e) loss of contact with values/valuing, and (f) values-incongruent behavior/committed action. Psychologists refer to these as processes, but it may be more parsimonious to conceptualize them as repertoires of behavior under supplemental sources of control. For example, fusion is behavior under the control of rules that describe weak or nonoptimal contingencies of reinforcement. When verbal rules are tightly bound to behavior, there is little room for variation in the context of subtle changes in circumstances. For instance, the rule "Person-first language is more respectful than disability-first language" was commonly invoked long after members of the disability community began to challenge assumptions that undergird it. Disability rights advocates indicated that person-first language is used to describe children with disabilities far more frequently than it is used to describe children or adults without disabilities (Gernsbacher, 2016). Differential application of person-first language in scholarly writing that pertains to those with severely stigmatized life circumstances further stigmatizes them (Gernsbacher, 2017). Despite this outcry from advocates dating as far back as 1999 (St. Louis, 1999), it wasn't until the most recent Publication Manual of the American Psychological Association (American Psychological Association, 2020) that scholars have been asked to consider using disability-first language. In this case and more broadly, defusion work would involve procedures that help to disconnect behavior from unworkable rules so that new, more contextually sensitive rules can be formulated. Writers that reflect upon ways to change their use of person-first language (or other common conventions that no longer function to convey respect) are practicing defusion.

Experiential avoidance involves behavior that is tightly constricted in the presence of aversive contingencies. When a person hides from emotions, memories, thoughts, or bodily sensations that occur in the context of doing things that matter to them, they are engaging in experiential avoidance. Skinner described behavior that might well be termed experiential avoidance when discussing the way a child avoids sitting in the dentist's waiting room. The child is not avoiding the drill at this moment, but rather, the emotional components of anxiety that occur because the dentist's office itself elicits these complex emotions (Skinner, 1953). Whereas it may be said that humans avoid people, places, and things due to a history of negative reinforcement for doing so, humans may also avoid *thinking about* people, places, and things; thus, experiential avoidance is different from direct contingency avoidance. By way of illustration, you may recall times when you or someone you know said, "I just don't care to think about all that" when asked to consider the possible downsides of a course of action. Whereas fusion is a failure to *disconnect* action from difficult thoughts, rules, or emotions, experiential avoidance is failure to *connect with* challenging content. In contrast, acceptance is the willingness to approach pain as a source of information about the world and behavior that would be successful in a current set of circumstances.

Loss of situational awareness can be defined as behavior under the control of past and future contingencies of reinforcement. Perhaps all human behavior should be influenced by past and future contingencies because without attending to such determinants, we would be unable to learn from the past or plan for the future. But a person whose behavior is not adequately oriented to what is going on in the present is at risk of missing important opportunities. Consider the self-isolating behaviors of Ronan, a young adult autistic person who identifies as a man and who was ridiculed extensively during high school by kids his own age. Currently away at college in new surroundings, Ronan might be considered attractive by many young people in the dorm, but he withdraws from others and tells himself, "They always say they're your friend, but they never are." If Ronan makes many such statements, it would be a fair hypothesis to say that his verbal behavior temporally distorts the contingencies of reinforcement. Although what he says might have been true to some degree in another context, the words "always" and "never" suggest that he is blind to potential sources of friendship and intimacy in the current context. Were he to learn to say, "Some people in the past said they were my friends and didn't mean it, but maybe not all people will do the same," Ronan might subsequently look for people and activities in the present moment that would make a difference in his life.

Inflexible perspective taking about self or others may be characterized as behavior framed in terms of a single view of one's own or another person's behavioral repertoire without regard to the contingency demands of the current context. When a person relates to themselves or others in a rigid way, they may affix a label to themselves that they apply irrespective of circumstance. Such self-limiting categorizations serve as harmful bars that keep them from trying new modes of behavior. The developers of ACT found it helpful to distinguish between self-as-content, self-as-process, and self-as-context (Hayes et al., 1999). Self-as-content involves seeing self in terms of verbal labels. "I am a loser" serves as a global label that may be an accurate tact of one or more events but inaccurate as a general statement because it is emitted devoid of context. "I was a loser in today's game because I played too aggressively, so tomorrow I'm playing with a more nuanced approach" shows flexible attention to variables that could result in more effective performance. Self-as-process is a repertoire that involves seeing one's experience over a long period of time. When a person reflects about the consistency between ways they saw themselves as a child and ways they see themselves as an adult, they are viewing their lives from an unfolding but stable locus of perspective. A sense of self-as-process such as this can be quite helpful; yet overextended, it can be the source of great suffering. "I was the kid who cried at every siren and dog bark; I think I'll always be that kid" exemplifies the kind of rigid process focus that could impede the quest for growth and change. The third of these selfing repertoires, self-as-context, involves seeing self as a mode of action under the control of relevant environmental variables. This is perhaps closest to Skinner's concept of self (Skinner, 1953). From an ACT perspective, even self-as-context can be overextended. For example, "I can be whatever you want me to be" is a statement that shows sensitivity to context but lacks grounding in long-term patterns of self-identification that lead to stability and a sense of direction in life. Taken together, flexible perspective taking involves balancing three repertoires related to the content, process, and context of life experiences.

Loss of contact with values might be defined as behavior under the control of rigid or poorly articulated rules organizing a limited set of actions that lead mostly to smaller, immediately available reinforcers. In plain language, a lost sense of values involves failing to articulate what matters most in life. Losing sight of cherished life aims and settling for smaller payoffs gained from less effortful behavior may result from the behaviors of describing weak contingencies and subsequently establishing impoverished goals. Skinner (1979) suggested that this failure to adequately examine upcoming contingencies is predictable; evolution generally prepares our bodies for an environment several generations past, and similarly, reinforcement prepares us to do today what worked for us yesterday. He argued that verbal behavior allows humans to turn to the future, predict coming changes in the environment based on broad trends in immediate and remote data, and set goals to ensure long-term positive outcomes. Because natural and behavioral selection processes orient humans toward the past, Skinner suggested we need special training to learn to act with respect to our future survival needs. For Skinner, the ultimate value was survival, but he suggested that other values, such as scholarly, artistic, leisure, and health-related values, are related to long-term survival.

ACTr values work can hasten the shift from looking backward to peering into a future that has not yet occurred. In an ACTr intervention, working with a younger autistic person might involve placing things of importance to the child in front of them and asking them to place the ones they like most near them and others in line behind those that are most valued. This version of a multiple stimulus with replacement preference assessment (DeLeon & Iwata, 1996) is a starting point from which to build in abstract replacements. For example, if the child places dolls of a mother and child bear close to her, a subsequent task might involve placing photos of her own mother and herself among other items. The aim is to help the child respond to an increasingly arbitrary equivalence class from which the concept of valuing will later emerge. In contrast, helping an adult autistic person who says, "I care about family; after all, I live with them" to sharpen their picture of this value might involve asking the individual to describe special times that they shared with particular members of the family, list things that matter to them about their interactions with family, and identify those they would be most willing to work hard to help were they to ask.

The ultimate aim of ACTr is to orient a person's behavior to be in better alignment with their stated values. When a person's behavior is incongruent with their overarching priorities, they may do things that feel good in the moment but that offer little long-term benefit. They may appear to wander from one task to the next without a plan, with limited goals, and without a clear direction of travel. In contrast, putting one foot in front of the next in service of broad life aims is committed action. By way of example, consider the behavior of Marge, an autistic 10th-grade girl. High school years can be challenging for most teenagers and for autistic teens in particular. The simple ratio and interval schedules of primary reinforcement during elementary school are supplanted with an assortment of compound schedules that vary from class to class, each with delayed, conditioned reinforcement. Marge cared what her teachers thought of her in grade school. She yearned to become a biochemist, and with help from her teachers, she set goals throughout elementary school for extra projects that put her in position to go to a good prep school. Come high school though, she no longer had opportunity to connect individually with each of her teachers. Tests and assignments were spread out across the month in ways that did not make sense to her. Other kids related to one another with increasingly sophisticated social rules that she found difficult to decipher. She wished to pursue her interest in biochemistry, but without encouragement and without explicit instruction in where to find opportunities, she sank into a world of online gaming that offered her friendships in a virtual community but disconnected her from science and math learning for which she secretly longed. During an ACTr session, asked to close her eyes and see herself doing the most important thing she could imagine, Marge burst into tears. She had moved very far from her values, and the exercise spotlighted the distance from her life aims she had traveled. Fortunately, the behavior analyst helped her set small, achievable goals, established reliable schedules of meaningful reinforcement, and together, they shifted her daily behavior in a new direction toward the future that Marge wanted her life to be about. This brief intervention focused on increasing committed behavior had a profound effect upon Marge.

21.4.2 Rationale and Objectives

A central concern among those who use ABA principles to right their own lives is that changing behavior by manipulating antecedents and consequences works magnificently when you manage the contingencies for other people but less reliably when you manage contingencies for yourself. At least one of the issues is something that Skinner described in *Science and Human Behavior* (Skinner, 1953). He said that it is easy enough to set goals and arrange antecedents to evoke behavior, but when you have set aside reinforcers for completing tasks that you do not finish, there is little stopping you from taking the stimuli that had been earmarked as reinforcers. ACTr is designed to address this fundamental issue by helping orient behavior toward larger, later reinforcers when smaller, sooner ones that are less useful in the long run are easily accessible.

But ACTr has deeper roots; it is a way of addressing the kind of human suffering that is unique to those with verbal repertoires. Consider this illustration. Barron and Caleb are 22-year-old autistic brothers. Barron is medically fragile and does not engage in any form of verbal behavior. He relies on staff members of a group home to assist him with adult daily living skills. Caleb lives independently and attends college. Caleb has friends but at times notices that he does not understand the things that others are laughing at when socializing in groups. When Barron cries, his care providers examine the environment to identify whether he is hot, cold, hungry, or thirsty. Barron's wailing ceases when the right stimuli have been identified. Caleb, on the other hand, will worry at times about his disability. He regularly wonders if he has he said something foolish and if others might be distancing themselves from him because he is autistic. Of even deeper concern to Caleb are the times when others seem to sincerely appreciate him. He worries that the next words out of his mouth might be the ones that end his friendships with the others. That has never happened, but he imagines that it could, and the more he appraises this thought and tries to dismiss it, the more he finds himself saying "Don't blow it—you're going to ruin everything" to himself.

Of course, there are moments when Caleb forgets to worry about these things. These are delightful fragments of time, but they are upended by another worry: "What if I start worrying again and then I blow it?" In other words, Caleb begins worrying about worrying. The more he attempts to control this by distracting himself, focusing on his friends, assuring himself he is okay, thinking positively, the more his worrying rebounds. Like a beachball he is holding under water, at some point the ball pushes to the surface. When Barron's needs are met, his suffering ends. When Caleb's needs are met, his most potent suffering is just beginning. Because to avoid such worrying, the next solution is to avoid seeing friends, avoid going places his friends might go, and avoid doing things that he has in the past discussed doing with friends, even though he has never done these things before.

The kind of suffering Caleb experiences is unique to those with verbal repertoires. It may be resistant to treatments such as contingent and noncontingent reinforcement. This kind of suffering is the product of overextended verbal behavior in which things arbitrarily related, such as activities he has talked about doing and worrying, are connected with rule statements, such as "If you do this, you will . . . " In other words, Caleb says, "If I go to the street fair my friends and I talked about going to, I will worry horribly, the way I do when I'm with them."

In some less emotionally charged circumstances, disputing thoughts such as these may help. But more recalcitrant thoughts, emotions, and memories may not succumb to reason. Bodily issues such as physical disabilities or overresponsiveness to sound do not yield. Persistent symptoms associated with autism do not end, even after years of ABA therapy. Humans have evolved remarkable skills for solving problems. Ours is the only species that uses equipment to alternately fly in the air and travel under the water across vast distances. Moreover, we appear to be the only species capable of using symbolic means to communicate about things in a distant future and remote past that we ourselves have not experienced. But we are at a loss when we apply the same strategies that solve engineering problems to the problems of thinking about dying, feeling bereaved, or simultaneously wishing others well and wanting them to experience pain.

ACTr uses paradoxical means to address suffering of this nature. Rather than trying to eliminate pain, the ACTr approach is to acknowledge it, observe it, and perhaps even invite it to the dinner table, so to speak. From an ACTr perspective, pain is the gateway to purpose. Suffering is the bitter taste of sustenance. Equally paradoxical is the notion that problem solving itself is the very problem that needs to be solved; that is, by relinquishing efforts to remove unmanageable pain, pain becomes more manageable.

Treatment objectives in ACTr are equally paradoxical. The general method involves exercises such as the guided meditations, writing, and physicalized metaphors (described above) that elicit curiosity about the experience. Rather than a person that offers solutions, the ACTr facilitator serves as another pilgrim on the quest. When a client demands that the ACTr practitioner proposes a solution, the practitioner suggests that the solution is in experiencing the full weight of the problem.

This aspect of ACTr is difficult for practitioners because the ABA field has evolved in the traditional model of practitioner-as-expert. Behavior analysts are trained to come to meetings with a plan, to offer a rationale, model, or practice, and to reinforce successive approximations of an effective behavior. The fellow pilgrim stance of ACTr stance involves the therapist's willingness to walk into session without a plan. Instead, the therapist explains that the psychological flexibility model involves experiencing all thoughts and emotions just as they are. The therapist must be intimately, personally familiar with both the unworkable avoidance of such difficulties and the more paradoxically helpful approach toward them. Sitting beside clients without an immediate solution (or at least being willing to delay offering one) is a difficult pivot for ABA practitioners. Yet this is merely an extension of the modeling we have always done. When an ACTr practitioner models the willingness to sit with discomfort, they are showing their client that this is a pathway to reinforcement.

The mechanism of action in ACTr is exposure. In classical behavior therapy, clients are exposed either through systematic desensitization or flooding to a conditioned stimulus (CS) that has been paired in the client's past with an unconditioned stimulus (US). Repeated or intense exposures to the CS without the aversive effects of the US result in respondent extinction. For example, a boy that has been bitten by a dog and trembles uncontrollably in the presence of his grandma's dogs is exposed to black-and-white pictures of dogs, colorful pictures of dogs, recordings of dogs, a furry doll, a dog in a cage at the other end of the room, a dog on a leash, and so on. In operant behavior therapy, the boy is asked to approach the CS and engage in behavior that is incompatible with the undesirable avoidance responses for which he has come to address. Continuing the previous example, the client would be asked to pet fur on a three-dimensional picture of a dog, pet a stuffed dog, talk to a dog in a cage, talk to a dog on a leash, walk toward the dog on a leash, and so on. In each case, avoidance is placed on extinction and approach is reinforced. The result in this procedure is operant extinction.

ACTr is similarly based in exposure that involves both respondent and operant extinction, but the procedure involves *verbal* exposure. No dogs are brought into the therapy context. Instead, dogs are discussed in detail. The discussion evokes details that bear out specific verbal relations that repeat excessively in the client's verbal behavior. The practitioner listens for an ensemble of relational cues that lead to a hypothesis about the most important of the inflexible repertoires described above (fusion, experiential avoidance, etc.) to target. For example, if the boy makes numerous statements suggesting that they "see no point in going near dogs," that "there's no reason his grandma should have dogs," and the therapist observes the boy's jaw tightening when he talks about the physical sensations, one hypothesis could be that the boy has lost connection with the value of honoring his grandma's lifestyle choices.

After this, the therapist arranges a role play that involves verbal exposure in which the boy and the therapist do what the boy has been doing—they complain together about grandma having useless dogs in her house. During their gripe session, the therapist observes that they are spending all their time complaining, and not talking to grandma, not seeing her, not helping her out with her shopping, not playing games with her. When the client observes that all this complaining isn't working for him, the ACTr practitioner asks, "What else can you do?" and brainstorms with the boy until extinction induces behavioral variability related to valuing grandma and her chosen lifestyle. At this point, the therapist asks the boy if he would pick up the phone, call his grandma, and arrange a way that they might meet.

To fully understand the way verbal exposure works in this example requires a brief introduction to relational frame theory (RFT; Hayes et al., 2001). RFT emerged somewhat simultaneously with ACT and supplies a basic human operant account of the phenomena involved in psychological flexibility. It is beyond the scope of this chapter to provide an in-depth analysis of RFT, but book-length treatments regarding RFT and ABA have recently been advanced (Ming et al., 2021, 2022), and readers are encouraged to examine these materials.

Nevertheless, as a brief introduction to the way that RFT informs ACTr, consider that Sidman and Tailby (1982) reported an unexpected finding in which conditional discrimination procedures used to teach verbal skills to cognitively disabled children resulted in the acquisition of both symmetrical and transitive relations without explicit instruction or reinforcement. In lay terms, these authors showed that new relations emerge between stimuli that bear no formal similarity to one another (picture of an object, spoken word for the object, and written word for the object) without direct training. The work showed that by using a simple matching to sample procedure similar to many children's games today, literacy skills can be rapidly and successfully acquired. Although these findings were predicted by mathematical set theory, they were unanticipated in the operant learning paradigm and provided evidence that *verbal* stimulus classes can be taught. Hundreds of studies followed, further demonstrating this phenomenon of stimulus equivalence and its utility in teaching basic literacy skills in which spoken words, objects, pictures, and written symbols share meaning, even though they are physically dissimilar.

A decade later, Steele and Hayes (1991) advanced a theoretical account of the equivalence phenomenon. This theory posits that the equivalence phenomenon is a result of relational responding learned through multiple exemplar training applied to increasingly arbitrary stimuli such as spoken or written words and using arbitrary relational cues, such as "equal to" or the conventional symbol "=." The account, later dubbed RFT, suggested that equivalence relations are but one of many different families of relations, such as distinction, opposition, hierarchy, spatiality, temporality, causality, and perspective (formally referred to as deixis, or the meld of person, place, and time). Steele and Hayes exposed college-bound high school students to nonarbitrary stimuli (related along topographical or formal dimensions). Some were pretrained to select relations of sameness, opposition, and difference; others received no pretraining. After that, the participants were exposed to arbitrary stimuli in the form of unfamiliar geometric shapes and taught some of the relations between them. Some participants were taught that A is SAME as B, B is OPPOSITE to C, but others were taught that B is DIFFERENT from C. Participants taught the SAME and OPPOSITE relations for AB and BC easily derived relations about BA, CB, AC, and CA, but relations were ambiguous when B is DIFFERENT from C was taught, so responses to these questions showed variability. In a second experiment, the investigators brought all three types of relations under stimulus control, thus demonstrating that arbitrarily applicable relational responding—that is, responding to physically dissimilar stimuli on the basis of arbitrary cues, such as the words opposite, same, and different—can be taught in ways that exceed the simple on/off character of equivalence/nonequivalence relations. That arbitrarily applicable relational responding may be the basic unit of verbal behavior was an extension of Skinner's functional account of verbal behavior. Thus, from its inception, RFT sought to explain and offer new avenues for research into the phenomena described earlier in the chapter, namely the unique troubles humans with verbal skills have regarding time, emotions, rules, self, values, and action.

The earliest application of ACTr with autistic people was conducted by Eilers and Hayes (2015) in a component analysis comprised of two studies. In the first, defusion (rules repeated in a silly voice) plus exposure (experimenter enforced new rules) was used to reduce tantrums surrounding rules in three young autistic children. In the second study, defusion plus exposure was compared to exposure alone. Both studies showed that defusion plus exposure worked to reduce unwanted tantrums and increase engagement with tasks and the second demonstrated that defusion plus exposure worked better than exposure alone. From an RFT perspective, the rule "everyone MUST FOLLOW my rules" involves two arbitrary relata, or things being related—*everyone* and *rules*. Their connection is specified by the relational cue MUST FOLLOW. Defusion served to transform the stimulus function of the relational cue; that is, its strength was weakened when the participants were asked to playfully repeat the rule in a silly voice. From an RFT lens, ACTr works when stimuli transform in function from being aversive to being appetitive, thus facilitating the move from avoidance to approach.

21.4.3 Considerations for Implementation

ACTr is a framework for treating psychological rigidity; it is not a prescribed sequence of procedures. There are countless ways to organize an ACTr intervention, limited only by the therapist's imaginative use of metaphor, humor, movement, art, and willingness to be present to difficult thoughts and emotions. Nevertheless, some essential ingredients ought to permeate all ACTr interventions across their various topographies. Below is a brief list.

21.4.3.1 Consenting

Researchers are admonished to consider the consent process as an ongoing set of procedures, but practitioners seldom receive the same advice. Given that ACTr bears some resemblance to psychotherapy, it is wise to conduct ongoing consent procedures. Simply checking in and asking if the procedures are acceptable is a wise practice. Formal social validity assessment serves a similar function and will be discussed below (see section 21.4.3.6). In particular, when a client has a longer history of difficulties, if the behavior the practitioner is assisting with is suitable for ACTr, more frequent requests to verify that it is okay to proceed are useful.

21.4.3.2 Functional Assessment

Functional assessment is the hallmark of behavior analysis. Although prevention and acquisition interventions can be conducted without formal evaluation of behavioral function, behavior reduction ought to involve careful attention to behavior–environment relations. The current state of the literature (see section 21.5) suggests that the most economical approach is to conduct functional behavior assessment and, where possible, experimental functional analysis of direct contingencies that maintain the unwanted response class, defined as social positive, social negative, automatic positive, automatic negative relations (Cooper et al., 2020). If an individual with verbal skills is not responding to direct contingency management procedures and multiple attempts have been made to clarify ambiguities in the functional assessment or analysis, a fair preliminary hypothesis is that the individual is engaging in interfering verbal behavior. From there, the practitioner should use the ACT matrix or some other assessment approach to generate a hypothesis regarding the most likely class of interfering verbal repertoire.

21.4.3.3 Intervention

ACTr interventions aim to generate socially important, observable, measurable behavior that is resistant to direct contingency management. The general strategy is to undermine entrenched verbal patterns via verbal exposure to the unworkability of problem-solving strategies that a client is currently using. Practitioners induce variability in verbal behavior during multiple exemplar training, role play, practice, and home practice assignments. Conventional exercises include writing, closed-eye visualization, or physical action (physicalized metaphors).

21.4.3.4 Home Practice and Data Collection

Clients should be asked to practice at home and to collect data on their practice. When stressful situations arise in life, clients should be asked to use these strategies, track the outcomes, and collect data. Practitioners ought to develop systems by which to reinforce daily practice and real-world use of these strategies. With clients unable to collect their own data, parents and other mediators can assist. Data may include video, audio, writing, or art products of practice sessions. Real-world data may simply include self-collected data. Practitioners may ask some clients to complete ACT matrices as part of their home practice.

21.4.3.5 Generalization and Maintenance

ACTr does not end when a client's verbal behavior changes; the treatment is considered complete when the client changes their overt behavior and that change is durable over time and across new situations. When ACTr has been successful, behavior comes back under the control of direct contingencies of reinforcement after which the ACTr treatment can be faded. However, given the ubiquity of social training and reinforcement for emotional problem solving, it is likely that clients will need to use ACTr for some time to come, perhaps forever. Preparing clients for this should begin early in treatment to dispel any potential misunderstandings. For most people, undermining verbal rigidity is a lifelong affair.

21.4.3.6 Social Validity

Risks associated with ACTr described above include the possibility that practitioners will cross the line into psychotherapy, practice beyond their scope of competence, or attempt to use humor in ways that clients experience as invalidating. One way that practitioners can monitor the quality of their work and their development of skills is to ask clients to complete social validity surveys. As with any other ABA programming, assessing social validity before, during, and after treatment regarding the importance of the goals, acceptability of the procedures, and strength of the outcomes respectively is an important part of an ACTr intervention.

21.5 Research Background

For the purposes of this volume, a selective review of the literature was conducted using the PsycINFO® database with keywords that included acceptance and commitment training or acceptance and commitment therapy, ABA, and autism or ASD. Other related keywords included relational frame theory and verbal behavior. Studies were included only if they used single-case design methods with procedures for ensuring experimental control, such as the use of multiple baseline across participants design strategies. Thus, group design studies and case reports were excluded from this report. Single-case design research investigating ACTr as an intervention in contexts common to ABA practice are summarized below, and a few rigorously designed studies are described in detail. Because mindfulness is a substantial component of ACTr that comprises four of the six repertoires (acceptance, defusion, present moment awareness, and flexible perspective), studies that evaluated mindfulness and did not refer to their work as ACTr were included.

An initial search turned up 173 studies, after which any studies that did not meet the inclusion criteria were removed. In all, 23 studies met the criteria described above and are included in this review. These papers were further classified into four primary population categories of child, adult, parent, and staff participants. Because our interest in this paper is to shed light on the current state of the literature regarding ACTr across the lifespan of autistic people, we further separated the studies into those with participants under the age of 13 and those 13 or older.

Studies were evaluated for their overall rigor on the basis of eight criteria, each weighted equally, though in the narrative below, we will offer some cautions regarding the quality of some that met the initial criteria. The initial eight criteria are described in Table 21.1. To calculate rigor, we counted the number of criteria that were satisfied, divided the total by the number of categories (eight), and multiplied by 100. The overall rigor of the 23 studies reviewed was 63%, as depicted in Table 21.2.

Although initially this may seem to be a weak score, it is important to note that ACTr is a relatively new topic for ABA investigation that has been in development

Table 21.1 Criteria for evaluating overall rigor

Criteria	Description
Direct measurement of behavior	An investigator, parent, staff member, or the participant observed and measured rate, duration, latency, or percentage of intervals during which a behavior occurred.
Functional assessment or analysis (FBA)	Researchers assessed either the function of an overt behavior slated for reduction and/or the function of an ACTr repertoire hypothesized to be interfering with direct contingency management.
External validity (EV)	The study was a replication and extension of previous work or lent support to previous findings.
Interobserver agreement (IOA)	Quality of data was evaluated by comparing a secondary observer's data to that of a primary coder.
Treatment integrity (TI)	Fidelity of implementation was formally evaluated by an observer.
Social validity (SV)	Stakeholder satisfaction with goals, methods, and/or outcomes was formally assessed with Likert scale rating forms.
Speed of response	An intervention was coded as efficient if it was completed in four sessions or less and produced nonoverlapping data after the fourth session.
Durability	An intervention was coded as durable if desired results were obtained in formal efforts to assess maintenance (sustained results over time) and/or generalization (transfer of results to new situations).

only during the last 18 years. During the first 11 of those years, there was only one active research team headed by Nirbhay Singh, who did not publish findings in flagship ABA journals of the era such as *Journal of Applied Behavior Analysis*, *Psychological Record*, and *The Behavior Analyst*. As illustrated in Figure 21.1, beginning in 2015, other investigators began publishing ACTr studies and the average rate of publication began to rise, most notably in the *Journal of Contextual Behavior Science* (N = 8) and *Behavior Analysis in Practice* (N = 3).

Four studies (Eilers & Hayes, 2015; Gilsenan et al., 2022; Szabo, 2019; Wilson et al., 2022) examined ACTr in young autistic children. Eilers and Hayes (2015, fully described above) worked with three young children with ASD and evaluated the effects of a cognitive defusion exercise to address their repetitive and restrictive behaviors. Wilson et al. (2022) assessed the effects of individualized ACT intervention for several male students from 10 to 11 years old. Gilsenan et al. (2022) examined the effects of relational training to improve engagement with ACTr sessions for three young children with ASD.

Table 21.2 Rigor ratings for all studies (N = 23)

Population	Team	Overall Rigor	Direct Measure	FBA	EV	IOA	TI	SV	Speed	Durability
Young Children										
	Eilers & Hayes, 2015	0.63	1	0	0	1	1	1	1	0
	Gilsenan et al. 2022	0.63	1	0	1	1	0	0	1	1
	Szabo 2019	1.0	1	1**	1	1	1	1	1	1
	Wilson 2022	0.75	1	0	1	1	1	1	0	1
Adolescent										
	Singh 2018	0.36	1	1	0	1	0	0	0	0
	Singh 2011a	0.63	1	1	1	1	0	0	0	1
	Singh 2011b	0.75	1	1	1	1	0	0	1	1
	Szabo et al. 2019	0.75	1	0	0	1	1	1	1	1
Adult										
	Brazeau 2017	0.75	1	0	0	1	1	1	1	1
	Hutchinson 2019	0.88	1	0	1	1	1	1	1	1
Parent										
	Gould 2018	0.63	1	0	1	1	0	0	0	1
	Raulston 2019	0.88	1	1	1	1	1	1	1	0
	Singh 2006a	0.25	1	0	0	1	0	0	0	0
	Singh 2007	0.75	1	0	1	1	0	1	1	1
	Singh 2010	0.63	1	0	1	1	0	1	0	1
Staff										
	Castro 2016	0.5	1	0	1	1	0	1	0	0
	Little 2020	0.36	1	0	0	1	0	0	0	1
	Pingo 2019	0.36	1	0	0	1	0	0	1	0
	Chancey 2019	0.75	1	0	1	1	0	1	1	1
	Singh 2017	0.63	1*	0	1	1	1	0	0	1
	Singh 2006b	0.5	1*	0	1	1	0	1	0	0
	Singh 2009	0.5	1*	0	1	1	0	0	0	1
	Singh 2004	0.36	1*	0	1	1	0	0	0	0
Total		0.63	1.0	0.78	0.57	1.0	0.35	0.52	0.48	0.65

Note. Scores assigned in each category were either 1 (met criterion) or 0 (did not meet criterion). Four studies, depicted with a single asterisk (1*), met criterion for direct measurement but displayed frequency data for nonstandard units of time (per day, week shift, or percent of intervals per week). One study, depicted with two asterisks (1**), met criterion for functional behavior assessment and conducted an additional experimental functional analysis.

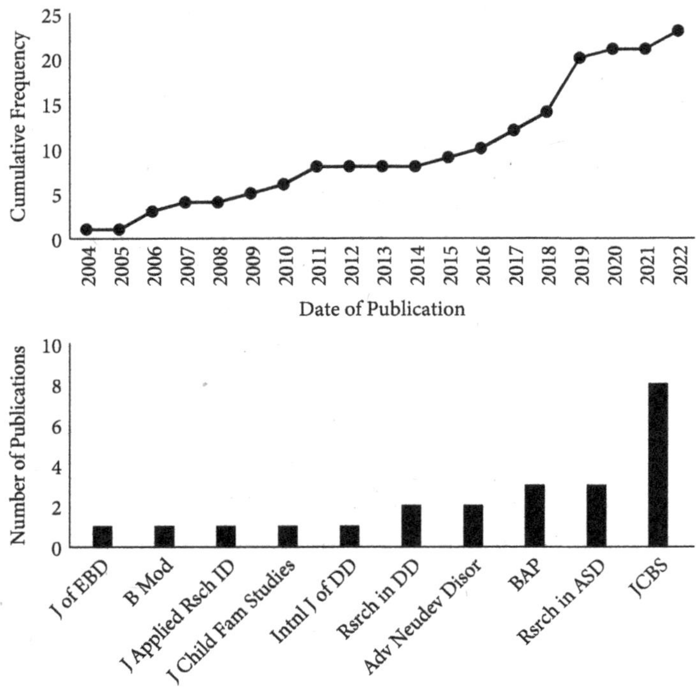

Figure 21.1 Cumulative frequency of publications and number of publications per journal

Note. Cumulative frequency by year (upper panel) and number of publications by journal (lower panel).

Szabo (2019) employed a nonconcurrent multiple-probe design across participants to evaluate ACTr on treatment-resistant tantrums in the presence of rule changes for three young children from 8 to 10 years old. To date, this was the most carefully constructed ABA study on ACTr based on the evaluation criteria required for this volume, so we will offer a more detailed description. The dependent measures included rate per hour of inflexible behaviors and requests for rule changes. A single contingency functional analysis (Iwata et al., 1994) was conducted prior to baseline data collection. For all three participants, the function of the inflexible behavior identified was escape from a new game rule. Participants were taught a function-based replacement behavior of manding (i.e., requesting) to maintain the old rules or for sameness. Discrimination training was then used to teach when mands for rule change will be and will not be reinforced. To help participants transfer the acquired skills to more naturalistic settings, training for generalization took place 2 weeks after discrimination training was applied to random games at various times and locations in the homes. Even after training for generalization and maintenance took place, resurgence of inflexible behaviors was evident under challenging situations. To address these treatment-resistant overt behaviors, researchers conducted a second functional assessment of indirect-acting contingencies that might have been maintaining private interfering behavior, such as privately repeating an inflexible rule. This second functional assessment involved (a) coding the frequency of certain classes of verbal responses described and (b) hypothesizing a verbal consequence. The intervention consisted of an individualized 4-hour training of the six ACTr repertoires skills with emphasis on playful manding for rule changes. It is important to note that this study did not introduce ACTr initially. The participants first underwent a functional analysis to determine the direct contingencies influencing their behavior. Due to slow progress for all three participants after having contacted a function-based treatment of differential reinforcement plus extinction, a secondary functional assessment was conducted to reveal the covert interfering behaviors responsible for the inadequate progress. The ACTr intervention helped all three participants change socially relevant overt behavior and was the first of a new generation of ACTr studies showing that the model was a framework from which novel iterations of ACTr can be developed based on individuals and their unique needs.

Four published studies meeting criteria for inclusion in this volume focused on the behavior of autistic adolescents. With three different teams, Singh et al. (2018, 2011b, 2011a) evaluated mindfulness for reducing aggressive behavior among autistic adolescents. In one of these studies, participants reduced their use of psychotropic medications. Two of the three studies showed sustained improvements at follow-up, one of the three met the speed of response criterion, and all three superimposed ACTr methods on function-based treatments established after FBAs. The fourth adolescent study, conducted by Szabo et al. (2019), evaluated a novel ACTr protocol to increase athletic engagement in three older autistic adolescents that were members of a rock climbing team. First, a behavior analyst assisted the team's coach in restructuring direct contingencies. This was enough to bring one participant's behavior under effective stimulus control. For the remaining two participants, the ACTr protocol served to bring practice and competition performance back under direct contingency control. The intervention was efficient, showed durability, and the effects generalized to novel environments.

Two studies (Brazeau et al., 2017; Hutchinson et al., 2019) conducted with adults met criteria for inclusion in this review. These studies both focused on the use of ACTr to manage interfering anxiety during job interviews. Both studies met the efficiency criterion and showed evidence of durability; the second served as a systematic replication of the first, thus demonstrating external validity.

Five studies offered evidence of ACTr effects with parents of autistic children. Gould et al. (2018) taught parents strategies for increasing values-based behavior that each participant said they wanted to engage in more frequently. Participants turned in photographs of themselves engaging in valued activities as permanent product evidence of their behavior. Raulston et al. (2019) delivered an efficient intervention for parent–child dyads. Of particular note, these researchers used a stringent concurrent randomized multiple baseline across parent–child dyads and evaluated the strengths of their findings using a between-cases standardized mean difference analysis in addition to performing visual analysis of the data. This was among the three most rigorously designed studies in the sample included in this review. Three additional studies conducted by Singh et al. (2006a, 2007, 2010) involved multiple baseline across parent–child dyads. In these studies, investigators asked whether parents would respond to child aggression more effectively after mindfulness training, and by doing so, help their children to access reinforcement using more socially appropriate behaviors. One these studies (Singh et al. 2007) met the speed of response criterion, and two (Singh et al., 2007, 2010) showed positive long-term results.

The largest group of included studies (N = 8) addressed the needs of staff people working with autistic clients of varying ages. Castro et al. (2016) evaluated values exercises pertinent to direct care workers. Outcomes from a multiple baseline across participants design showed that staff members emitted 11–16 more engagement responses with clients following ACTr relative to baseline. Of note, the authors suggested that variables such as parents' demographic backgrounds, family dynamics, and mental health ought to be considered when programming for dosage and individualizing components of the ACTr intervention. Little et al. (2020) used ACTr to improve staff delivery of behavioral skills training. Their results showed durability at follow-up. BST by itself did not achieve desired results, but when followed with ACTr, all participants met criterion. Nevertheless, it remains unclear whether the intervention could have been more efficient had BST and ACTr been delivered together as a package intervention. In a similar study, Pingo et al (2019) evaluated feedback only and feedback plus ACTr. As was the case in Castro et al., the addition of ACTr improved active treatment. This team's method offered a slight improvement over Little et al. in that the feedback plus ACTr condition followed feedback alone, thereby demonstrating that the salient intervention component was ACTr. Chancey et al. (2019) improved caregiver interactions with clients using ACTr. Of importance, this intervention was quite brief (two 15-minute sessions) and produced effects that maintained at follow-up.

Four studies by Singh et al. (2004, 2006b, 2009, 2017) evaluated changes in staff and client performance following staff training in mindfulness components of ACTr. Participants in Singh et al. (2017) reduced client aggression and in Singh et al. (2004) increased indices of happiness, such as smiling and laughter. Of note, Singh et al. (2017) was the one study included in this review that delivered telehealth instruction to the staff members. Singh et al. (2006b) successfully reduced staffing ratios along with aggression after mindfulness training. Singh et al. (2009) showed reductions in several socially important secondary measures, such as physical restraints, stat medications, injuries to peers, and injuries to staff. Although each of the four studies used multiple-baseline designs, the measurement strategies involved nonstandard metrics such as frequency per day, per week, per shift, and percent of intervals per week. Nonstandard measurement tactics are easier for teachers and paraprofessionals to collect in their milieus, but the data obtained are less interpretable because it is unclear whether the counting time was consistent across days during these observation periods. Of additional note, none of these studies met the efficiency criterion for this review.

Many of the studies reviewed herein evaluated teaching the mindfulness components of ACTr exclusively. Taken together, results of mindfulness-only studies show smaller effect sizes (more overlapping data points, longer time to respond to treatment) than ACTr studies that included mindfulness plus values and action strategies. The most rigorous ACTr studies (Hutchinson et al., 2019; Raulston et al., 2019; Szabo, 2019) each showed strong results, met the efficiency criterion, showed maintenance effects, and extended previous findings. That these studies focusing on all six ACTr repertoires should show stronger effects is not surprising. Villatte et al. (2016) showed that psychosocial treatment with mindfulness components of ACT were effective, but less so than treatment with mindfulness plus values and action components.

In summary, the literature base for ACTr as a component of ABA treatment is beginning to congeal into a firm body of evidence. Taken together, the overall rigor of the 23 studies reviewed was 63%, and nine of the studies (39% of the sample) showed an overall rigor of 75% or higher. Many topics have yet to be investigated, such as the conditions under which it is better to begin with direct contingency management plus ACTr and the best functional assessment procedures for identifying important ACTr repertoires for efficient, effective intervention. An additional topic that should be investigated is the development of procedures for conducting experimental functional analysis of ACTr repertoires.

21.6 Practice Implications

21.6.1 Treatment Outcomes

Similar to ACT conducted as psychotherapy, ACTr aims to help improve overt behavior emitted in socially relevant contexts. However, psychotherapists are not bound by the same limits to scope of practice that govern work performed by behavior analysts and other nonpsychotherapist practitioners. Whereas psychotherapists may elect to rely exclusively on self-report measures or even verbal reports delivered in session, ACTr practitioners assure that clients change and maintain behavior to meet their long-term needs. In fact, reinforcement for steps taken toward larger rewards that are available later is a pivotal strategy in teaching others to delay gratification. The natural organismic tendency to discount rewards for which there is a delay by orienting toward smaller rewards available sooner has been demonstrated in many species that emit operant behavior. Most can be trained to delay gratification by shaping successive approximations of desired behavior and progressive schedules of reinforcement, but humans can acquire this repertoire faster than other species with verbal mediation strategies—ACTr generates relatively rapid results when role plays and other methods reveal the relationship among valued outcomes, psychological flexibility repertoires, and overt behavior.

An interesting outcome of ACTr is that those who regularly practice it learn the folly of trying to feel *better* and the wisdom of aiming to *feel* better. In other words, one important outcome of ACTr is the development of skills for experiencing all there is to experience in life—the good and the bad—with equanimity. It is not that pain lessens so much as that pain becomes more a source of information about life and how to live it. More technically, extinction in ACTr does not remove aversive stimuli; rather, like any other extinction procedure, it results in new behavior with a higher likelihood of contacting reinforcement.

The line between ACTr and ACT or some other form of psychotherapy may be difficult to discern. As a general rule, if a behavior that a client wishes to address is not socially significant, observable, and measurable, then it may not be a suitable target for ACTr. Additionally, some behaviors clients ask to address are deeply painful and connected to a history of trauma for which a behavior analyst or other ACTr practitioner may not have received formal training and supervision. Practitioners should be on the lookout for matters that require additional training, consultation, or referral to another expert. At the very least, practitioners should proceed with caution and have a background in culturally responsive, trauma-informed care. A final caution is that if an ACTr functional assessment is inconclusive and shows excesses across many or all of the six repertoires, consider referring to a psychotherapist who would have more time to address each of these matters. Although it is possible to construct exercises that address many or all of the ACTr repertoires, it is better to err on the side of caution and at the very least work with another professional.

ACTr can only be conducted with clients whose verbal repertoires include intraverbal responding or back-and-forth speaker–listener interaction that does not correspond point to point (Skinner, 1957). Despite this limitation, it can be surprising just how easily a skillful practitioner can adapt ACTr to meet the needs of individuals with quite limited skills. Pretend play, music, art, and dance can all be used to generate flexibility. For example, Szabo (2019) conducted a 4-hour ACTr intervention for young autistic children with limited verbal skills using a commercially available non-identity-conditional discrimination game, balls of various sizes, colored pens, sticky notes, bandanas, a bowl of ice, and other items that promoted a sense of play and excitement.

Many ACTr interventions such as the one above include activities that are lighthearted. The aim is to induce a sense of play and curiosity toward otherwise aversive events. In the context of fun, stimulus functions may shift from aversive to appetitive. At the same time, it is possible that poking fun at emotionally difficult material could be experienced as invalidating. ACTr practitioners are thus cautioned to make use of an ongoing consenting process (see section 21.4.3.1 for details).

21.6.2 Practice Implication Guidelines

Based on the literature reviewed above, following is a list of practice recommendations.

1. Obtain consent before beginning and frequently throughout treatment.
2. Conduct direct contingency functional assessment or analysis and exhaust all options for intervening with direct contingency management before beginning ACTr. It is possible that at some point in the future, investigators will explore the effectiveness and efficiency of beginning treatment with both direct and indirect (ACTr) contingency management. Until such dismantling studies have been conducted, use ACTr sparingly.
3. Conduct ACTr functional assessment before beginning and continuously throughout ACTr treatment. Function-based treatment is the foundation of ABA and should be a standard for the design of ACTr interventions.
4. Interventions should range across writing, guided meditation, metaphor development, physicalized metaphor, game, and other modalities. Overuse of guided meditations or any other topography of treatment suggests inflexible practitioner behavior.
5. Listen for metaphor or other figurative speech from which to design interventions. In particular, listen for "dead metaphors," or metaphors and figures of speech so commonplace that they are easily overlooked (Lakoff & Johnson, 1980). For example, should a client say, "I'm falling to pieces," it would be easy to miss the opportunity to turn this into an intervention. Physicalizing the fall and breaking into pieces would be both fun and challenging.
6. Along the lines of fun and challenging, interventions constructed from the in vivo speech of clients offer rich opportunities for practitioners to evolve a treatment in the moment with the client, not knowing how it will proceed or reach its endpoint. Practitioner willingness to venture into the unknown beside the client is the heart of ACTr; it is fun and challenging for both members of the dyad.
7. An activity is most valuable when the client says something like "What I'm doing isn't working and I don't know what else to do." Hayes et al. (1999) referred to this as creative hopelessness, the point from which response variability is on the verge of occurring.
8. In the above circumstance, practitioners are best to offer compassion and the willingness to be as perplexed and without an expert solution as is the client. The practitioner's expertise is in understanding the model, which requires getting stuck in real time before getting unstuck to have meaning to the client. There are no breakthroughs without breakdowns.
9. Role play is as challenging for practitioners as it is for clients. Many practitioners avoid role plays when they are unsure of their skills. Yet properly

acquainted with the model and the mechanism of action in ACTr, practitioners ought to be willing to try. Clients often say that they appreciate therapists that are nervous and willing to try.

10. Assign home practice and data collection. Home practice should be brief; it often requires no more than a minute of concerted behavior. Data collection should include permanent products where possible. Data may be collected on frequency, duration, or latency measures and may be collected by clients or their stakeholders.
11. Program for generalization and maintenance. As Stokes and Baer (1977) commented, the most frequently used method of programming for generalization, "train and hope," is also the least analytical. It is no more helpful in ACTr than in any other topography of ABA treatment.
12. Assess social validity of the goals, procedures, and outcomes before, during, and after ACTr, respectively. A recent selective review appears to show a substantial increase in social validity assessment in empirical studies over previous years between 2019 and 2020 (Huntington et al., 2022). This was a selective review of eight ABA journals over a 10-year period (2010–2020) that showed of 899 empirical studies that met their inclusion criteria, 47% (422) included social validity assessments of some kind. This is a substantial increase from earlier assessments (e.g., Ferguson et al., 2019). However, Huntington et al. did not evaluate the type of social validity assessments that were conducted. It is possible that some studies included in the final count merely discussed the investigators' impressions of the social validity of the goals, outcomes, or procedures, without formal quantitative or qualitative procedures evaluating stakeholder impressions. The authors rightly point out, though, that the effort to ongoingly solicit feedback from those receiving services has important implications for the client, the intervention, and, given the recent critical feedback that ABA has received, for the entire field of ABA. ACTr interventions should be subjected to the same rigorous standard.
13. Consider trauma history, power, privilege, race, ethnicity, socioeconomic status, gender, sexual orientation, language, and dialect. These variables have not been adequately addressed in evaluations of ABA treatments, no more so in research on ACTr. Practitioners may be able to lead the way by asking clients to consider the way social arrangements in ACTr help to reduce or increase marginalization that results from intersecting aspects of social stratification. Practitioners may collect preliminary data and use their data to challenge investigators to rigorously pursue the development of culturally humble and responsive ACTr.
14. Design research and practice using participatory procedures. It is likely that researchers and participants operate under different contingencies. That is, participants seek help with problems, whereas researchers seek generalizable knowledge). Likewise, it bears scrutiny that practitioners

also operate under different contingencies—they seek to help and receive reimbursement for services. To the extent possible, it seems important to collaborate and equalize relationships during these endeavors. A less than perfect but honest example is this manuscript, which was developed in collaboration with autistic self-advocates. Fawcett (1991) called for this type of community-based participatory research in which social inequalities and injustices are remediated via collaboration. Recently, Pritchett et al. renewed the call. To the extent that ACTr practitioners construct interventions with their clients, they are living up to this standard. When succumbing to the urge to drive treatment as an infallible expert, the practitioner is falling back on what has been called paternalistic practices. The autistic community deserves more. The ACTr model described herein is in position to help ABA move toward greater participatory practice.

21.7 References

Abidin, R. R. (1995). *Parenting stress index professional manual* (3rd ed.). Washington, DC: Psychological Assessment Resources.

American Psychological Association. (2020). *Publication manual of the American Psychological Association* (7th ed.). Washington, DC: APA. https://doi.org/10.1037/0000165-000

Baer, D. M., Wolf, M. M., & Risley, T. R. (1968). Some current dimensions of applied behavior analysis. *Journal of Applied Behavior Analysis, 1*(1), 91–97. https://doi.org/10.1901%2Fjaba.1968.1-91

Bond, F. W., Hayes, S. C., Baer, R. A., Carpenter, K. M., Guenole, N., Orcutt, H. K., Waltz, T., & Zettle, R. D. (2011). Preliminary psychometric properties of the Acceptance and Action Questionnaire-II: A revised measure of psychological inflexibility and experiential avoidance. *Behavior Therapy, 42*(4), 676–688. https://doi.org/10.1016/j.beth.2011.03.007

Brazeau, K., Rehfeldt, R. A., Mazo, A., Smalley, S., Krus, S., & Henson, L. (2017). On the efficacy of mindfulness, defusion, and behavioral skills training on job interviewing skills in dually-diagnosed adults with developmental disorders. *Journal of Contextual Behavioral Science, 6*(2), 145–151. https://doi.org/10.1016/j.jcbs.2017.04.002

Brown, K. W., & Ryan, R. M. (2003). The benefits of being present: Mindfulness and its role in psychological well-being. *Journal of Personality and Social Psychology, 84*(4), 822–848. https://doi.org/10.1037/0022-3514.84.4.822

Castro, M., Rehfeldt, R. A., & Root, W. B. (2016). On the role of values clarification and committed actions in enhancing the engagement of direct care workers with clients with severe developmental disorders. *Journal of Contextual Behavioral Science, 5*(4), 201–207. https://doi.org/10.1016/j.jcbs.2016.09.003

Chancey, C., Weihl, C., Root, W. B., Rehfeldt, R. A., McCauley, D., Takeguchi, K., & Pritchard, J. (2019). The impact of mindfulness skills on interactions between direct care staff and adults with developmental disabilities. *Journal of Contextual Behavioral Science, 12*, 160–169. https://doi.org/10.1016/j.jcbs.2018.07.004

Cooper, J. O., Heron, T. E., & Heward, W. L. (2020). *Applied behavior analysis* (3rd ed.). Hoboken, NJ: Pearson Education.

DeLeon, I. G., & Iwata, B. A. (1996). Evaluation of a multiple-stimulus presentation format for assessing reinforcer preferences. *Journal of Applied Behavior Analysis, 29*(4), 519–533. https://doi.org/10.1901/jaba.1996.29-519

Eilers, H. J., & Hayes, S. C. (2015). Exposure and response prevention therapy with cognitive defusion exercises to reduce repetitive and restrictive behaviors displayed by children with autism spectrum disorder. *Research in Autism Spectrum Disorders, 19*, 18–31. https://doi.org/10.1016/j.rasd.2014.12.014

Fawcett, S. B. (1991). Some values guiding community research and action. *Journal of Applied Behavior Analysis, 24*(4), 621–636. https://doi.org/10.1901/jaba.1991.24-621

Ferguson, J. L., Cihon, J. H., Leaf, J. B., Van Meter, S. M., McEachin, J., & Leaf, R. (2019). Assessment of social validity trends in the journal of applied behavior analysis. *European Journal of Behavior Analysis, 20*(1), 146–157. https://doi.org/10.1080/15021149.2018.1534771

Gernsbacher, M. A. (2016). Analyses of person-first language in scholarly writing: Technical report. Open Science Framework. doi: 10.17605/OSF.IO/982AJ

Gernsbacher, M. A. (2017). Editorial perspective: The use of person-first language in scholarly writing may accentuate stigma. *Journal of Child Psychology and Psychiatry, 58*(7), 859–861. https://doi.org/10.1111/jcpp.12706

Gilsenan, C. M., Yi, Z., Hinman, J. M., Barron, B. F., & Dixon, M. R. (2022). Using relational training to improve performance during acceptance and commitment training sessions. *Behavior Analysis in Practice, 15*(1), 179–191. https://doi.org/10.1007/s40617-021-00574-8

Gould, E. R., Tarbox, J., & Coyne, L. (2018). Evaluating the effects of acceptance and commitment training on the overt behavior of parents of children with autism. *Journal of Contextual Behavioral Science, 7*, 81–88. https://doi.org/10.1016/j.jcbs.2017.06.003

Hayes, S. C. (1984). Making sense of spirituality. *Behaviorism, 12*(2), 99–110.

Hayes, S. C., Barnes-Holmes, D., & Roche, B. (Eds.). (2001). *Relational frame theory: A post-Skinnerian account of human language and cognition*. New York: Kluwer Academic.

Hayes, S. C., Bissett, R., Roget, N., Padilla, M., Kohlenberg, B. S., Fisher, G., Masuda, A., Pistorello, J., Rye, A. K., Berry, K., & Niccolls, R. (2004). The impact of acceptance and commitment training and multicultural training on the stigmatizing attitudes and professional burnout of substance abuse counselors. *Behavior Therapy, 35*(4), 821–835. https://doi.org/10.1016/S0005-7894(04)80022-4

Hayes, S. C., Strosahl, K. D., & Wilson, K. G. (1999). *Acceptance and commitment therapy: An experiential approach to behavior change*. Reno, NV: Context Press.

Hutchinson, V. D., Rehfeldt, R. A., Hertel, I., & Root, W. B. (2019). Exploring the efficacy of acceptance and commitment therapy and behavioral skills training to teach interview skills to adults with autism spectrum disorders. *Advances in Neurodevelopmental Disorders, 3*, 450–456. https://doi.org/10.1007/s41252-019-00136-8

Huntington, R. N., Badgett, N. M., Rosenberg, N. E., Greeny, K., Bravo, A., Bristol, A. M., Byun, Y. H., & Park, A. S. (2022). Social validity in behavioral research: A selective review. *Perspectives in Behavioral Science*. https://doi.org/10.1007/s40614-022-00364-9

Iwata, B. A., Dorsey, M. F., Slifer, K. J., Bauman, K. E., & Richman, G. S. (1994). Toward a functional analysis of self-injury. *Journal of Applied Behavior Analysis, 27*(2), 197–209. https://doi.org/10.1901/jaba.1994.27-197

Lakoff, R., & Johnson, M. (1980). *Metaphors we live by*. Chicago: University of Chicago Press.

Little, A., Tarbox, J., & Alzaabi, K. (2020). Using acceptance and commitment training to enhance the effectiveness of behavioral skills training. *Journal of Contextual Behavioral Science, 16*, 9–16. https://doi.org/10.1016/j.jcbs.2020.02.002

Ming, S., Gould, E., & Fiebig, J. H. (2022). *Understanding and applying relational frame theory: Mastering the foundations of complex language in our work and lives as behavior analysts*. Oakland, CA: New Harbinger.

Ming, S., Stewart, I., & McElwee, J. (2021). *Using RFT to promote generative language: Volume 1*. Orlando, FL: Hedgehog.

Pingo, J. C., Dixon, M. R., & Paliliunas, D. (2019). Intervention enhancing effects of acceptance and commitment training on performance feedback for direct support professional work performance, stress, and job satisfaction. *Behavior Analysis in Practice, 13*, 1–10. 10.1007/s40617-019-00333-w

Polk, K. L., Schoendorff, B., Webster, M., & Olaz, F. O. (2016). *The essential guide to the ACT matrix: A step-by-step approach to using the ACT matrix model in clinical practice*. Oakland, CA: New Harbinger.

Raulston, T. J., Zemantic, P. K., Machalicek, W., Hieneman, M., Kurtz Nelson, E., Barton, H., Hansen, S. G., & Frantz, R. J. (2019). Effects of a brief mindfulness-infused behavioral parent training for mothers of children with autism spectrum disorder. *Journal of Contextual Behavioral Science, 13*, 42–51. https://doi.org/10.1016/j.jcbs.2019.05.001

Sidman, M., & Tailby, W. (1982). Conditional discrimination vs. matching to sample: An expansion of the testing paradigm. *Journal of the Experimental Analysis of Behavior, 37*(1), 5–22. https://doi.org/10.1901/jeab.1982.37-5

Singh, N. N., Chan, J., Karazsia, B. T., McPherson, C. L., & Jackman, M. M. (2017). Telehealth training of teachers to teach a mindfulness-based procedure for self-management of aggressive behavior to students with intellectual and developmental disabilities. *International Journal of Developmental Disabilities, 63*(4), 195–203. https://doi.org/10.1080/20473869.2016.1277841

Singh, N. N., Lancioni, G. E., Karazsia, B. T., Myers, R. E., Kim, E., Chan, J., Jackman, M. M., McPherson, C. L., & Janson, M. (2018). Surfing the urge: An informal mindfulness practice for the self-management of aggression by adolescents with autism spectrum disorder. *Journal of Contextual Behavioral Science, 12*, 170–177. https://doi.org/10.1016/j.jcbs.2018.10.003

Singh, N. N., Lancioni, G. E., Manikam, R., Winton, A. S. W., Singh, A. N. A., Singh, J., & Singh, A. D. A. (2011b). A mindfulness-based strategy for self-management of aggressive behavior in adolescents with autism. *Research in Autism Spectrum Disorders, 5*(3), 1153–1158. https://doi.org/10.1016/j.rasd.2010.12.012

Singh, N. N., Lancioni, G. E., Singh, A. D. A., Winton, A. S. W., Singh, A. N. A., & Singh, J. (2011a). Adolescents with Asperger syndrome can use a mindfulness-based strategy to control their aggressive behavior. *Research in Autism Spectrum Disorders, 5*(3), 1103–1109. https://doi.org/10.1016/j.rasd.2010.12.006

Singh, N. N., Lancioni, G. E., Winton, A. S. W., Curtis, W. J., Wahler, R. G., Sabaawi, M., Singh, J., & McAleavey, K. (2006a). Mindful staff increase learning and reduce aggression in adults with developmental disabilities. *Research in Developmental Disabilities, 27*(5), 545–558. 10.1016/j.ridd.2005.07.002

Singh, N. N., Lancioni, G. E., Winton, A. S. W., Fisher, B. C., Wahler, R. G., McAleavey, K., Singh, J., & Sabaawi, M. (2006b). Mindful parenting decreases aggression, noncompliance, and self-injury in children with autism. *Journal of Emotional and Behavioral Disorders, 14*(3), 169–177. https://doi.org/10.1177/10634266060140030401

Singh, N. N., Lancioni, G. E., Winton, A. S. W., Singh, A. N., Adkins, A. D., & Singh, J. (2009). Mindful staff can reduce the use of physical restraints when providing care to individuals with intellectual disabilities. *Journal of Applied Research in Intellectual Disabilities, 22*, 194–202. https://doi.org/10.1111/j.1468-3148.2008.00488.x

Singh, N. N., Lancioni, G. E., Winton, A. S. W., Singh, J., Curtis, W. J., Wahler, R. G., & McAleavey, K. M. (2007). Mindful parenting decreases aggression and increases social behavior in children with developmental disabilities. *Behavior Modification, 31*(6), 749–771. 10.1177/0145445507300924

Singh, N. N., Lancioni, G. E., Winton, A. S. W., Wahler, R. G., Singh, J., & Sage, M. (2004). Mindful caregiving increases happiness among individuals with profound multiple disabilities. *Research in Developmental Disabilities, 25*(2), 207–218. 10.1016/j.ridd.2003.05.001

Singh, N. N., Singh, A. N., Lancioni, G. E., Singh, J., Winton, A. S. W., & Adkins, A. D. (2010). Mindfulness training for parents and their children with ADHD increases the children's compliance. *Journal of Child and Family Studies, 19*, 157–166. https://doi.org/10.1007/s10826-009-9272-z

Skinner, B. F. (1953). *Science and human behavior.* New York: Macmillan.

Skinner, B. F. (1957). *Verbal behavior.* Crows Nest, NJ: Appleton–Century–Crofts. https://doi.org/10.1037/11256-000

Skinner, B. F. (1974). *About behaviorism.* New York: Alfred A. Knopf.

Skinner, B. F. (1979). *The shaping of a behaviorist.* New York: Knopf.

St. Louis, K.O. (1999). Person-first labeling and stuttering. *Journal of Fluency Disorders, 24*, 1–24.

Steele, D., & Hayes, S. C. (1991). Stimulus equivalence and arbitrarily applicable relational responding. *Journal of the Experimental Analysis of Behavior, 56*(3), 519–555. https://doi.org/10.1901/jeab.1991.56-519

Stokes, T. F., & Baer, D. M. (1977). An implicit technology of generalization. *Journal of Applied Behavior Analysis, 10*(2), 349–367. https://doi.org/10.1901/jaba.1977.10-349

Szabo, T. (2019). Acceptance and commitment training for reducing inflexible behaviors in children with autism. *Journal of Contextual Behavioral Science, 12*, 178–188. https://doi.org/10.1016/j.jcbs.2019.03.001

Szabo, T. G., Willis, P. B., & Palinski, C. J. (2019). Watch me try: ACT for improving athletic performance of young adults with ASD. *Advances in Neurodevelopmental Disorders, 3*, 434–449. https://doi.org/10.1007/s41252-019-00129-7

Villatte, J. L., Vilardaga, R., Villatte, M., Plumb Vilardaga, J. C., Atkins, D. C., & Hayes, S. C. (2016). Acceptance and commitment therapy modules: Differential impact on treatment processes and outcomes. *Behaviour Research and Therapy, 77*, 52–61. https://doi.org/10.1016/j.brat.2015.12.001

Walach, H., Buchheld, N., Buttenmüller, V., Kleinknecht, N., & Schmidt, S. (2006). Measuring mindfulness—The Freiburg Mindfulness Inventory (FMI). *Personality and Individual Differences, 40*(8), 1543–1555. https://doi.org/10.1016/j.paid.2005.11.025

Wegner, D. M., & Zanakos, S. (1994). Chronic thought suppression. *Journal of Personality, 62*(4), 615–640. https://doi.org/10.1111/j.1467-6494.1994.tb00311.x

Wilson, A. N., Dzugan, E., & Hutchinson, V. D. (2022). Using a nonconcurrent multiple-baseline across-participants design to examine the effects of individualized ACT at school. *Behavior Analysis in Practice, 15*, 141–154. https://doi.org/10.1007/s40617-021-00558-8

22

Mindfulness and Mindfulness-Based Interventions

Yoon-Suk Hwang
The University of Queensland

Nirbhay N. Singh
Medical College of Georgia, Augusta University

22.1 Technical Abstract

Background: Autistic people commonly experience psychological and behavioral challenges that may compromise their quality of life as well as that of their families. Mindfulness-based interventions (MBIs) have been used to address such challenges. We reviewed the characteristics and quality of the extant studies using MBIs with autistic people. **Method**: We searched three databases using a combination of two key terms, autis* and mindful*, in the abstract field to identify relevant studies. This yielded 151 abstracts in ProQuest, 190 in PsycINFO via Ovid, and 114 in PubMed. We then screened the 455 abstracts based on the following inclusion criteria: (1) published in a peer-reviewed journal; (2) reported empirical data; (3) participants were autistic people; (4) mindfulness-based practices formed the main component of the intervention; (5) written in English; and (6) full text of the study was available. This resulted in the selection of 44 abstracts which met the inclusion criteria, and full text analyses of these abstracts resulted in the selection of 27 studies for further review. **Results:** Most studies investigated the effects of MBIs on psychological and behavioral challenges typically experienced by autistic individuals. Overall, some studies reported statistically significant intervention effects on depression, anxiety, rumination, stress, emotion regulation, and general quality of life. No statistically significant changes were reported in the core symptoms of autism, chronic sleep problems, and autism-specific quality of life. Overall, the review indicated an emerging literature that is promising in terms of the effects of the MBIs in specific areas but somewhat compromised in terms of the quality of this research. No adverse effects of MBIs were reported for autistic people. **Discussion:** The evidence is mostly mixed in terms of effectiveness, and there are some inconsistent findings between and within MBIs. A range of factors may explain such discrepancies, including participant learning profiles, conceptual framework of mindfulness and intervention content, measurement, settings, and instructional methods. **Practitioner recommendations:** The review highlights specific MBIs

Yoon-Suk Hwang, and Nirbhay N. Singh, *Mindfulness and Mindfulness-Based Interventions*. In: *Lifespan Treatment for Autistic Individuals*. Edited by: Peter Sturmey, Russell Lang, and James K. Luiselli, Oxford University Press.
© Oxford University Press (2025). DOI: 10.1093/oso/9780197635841.003.0022

and their effects on psychological and behavioral challenges of autistic individuals. While the outcomes are not always robust, there is enough research evidence on which professionals and families can base their choice of MBIs when providing services to autistic children, adolescents, and adults. The need for professionals using MBIs to be authentic and to embody mindfulness through their own personal practice of mindfulness meditation cannot be emphasized enough as a key factor in treatment outcomes. Family members need to balance their choice of MBIs against alternative evidence-based interventions that are currently available in order to provide the most effective treatments for their autistic children.

22.2 Layperson Summary

Mindfulness meditation is a contemplative practice. A core part of mindfulness practice is keeping attention and awareness on the here and now. Engaging in this practice as frequently and continuously as possible will help a practitioner to become knowledgeable concerning her inner experience (e.g., breath, feelings, and thoughts) and external stimuli (e.g., sounds, smells, and actions) that can influence her way of living. This knowledge will help mindfulness practitioners to respond to life difficulties more skillfully. Potential mindfulness teachers of autistic people need to have conceptual and practical knowledge of mindfulness, autistic individuals, and teaching skills. In other words, potential MBI instructors need to know what they teach, who they teach, and how they teach. All of these come with time and practice.

Our review of current MBI studies suggests mindfulness practice may support autistic people in addressing their psychological and behavioral challenges, such as depression, anxiety, rumination, quality of life, stress, emotion regulation, and their behaviors that others may find challenging to deal with. The studies provide some support for using MBIs with autistic individuals, but the data are not very robust and await independent replication. There were inconsistencies in the findings both within and between studies; the causes of these inconsistencies remain to be investigated. None of the studies reported negative side effects of practicing mindfulness. Professionals and family members should carefully discern which MBIs may be appropriately used with autistic children, adolescents, and adults in their care.

22.3 Treatment Summary Table

Treatment summary: Mindfulness-Based Interventions

Treatment description: MBIs are a family of evidence-based interventions that seek to alleviate health and mental health problems in neurodiverse populations. Mindfulness-based stress reduction (MBSR) is the prototypic first-generation program that is taught in eight weekly sessions, typically 2.5 hours long, and an all-day retreat usually held in the weekend between the sixth and seventh weeks. The second-generation programs differ somewhat in terms of program components and include varying degrees of Buddhist teachings that enhance mindfulness in daily life.

Expected outcomes: Outcomes typically involve changes in levels of state and trait mindfulness, and in the variables targeted by the specific intervention. For example, interventions may target the following variables: stress, anxiety, and depression; trauma and suicidal ideation; eating behavior or weight reduction; reduction in pain due to medical or physical conditions; emotional regulation and executive functioning; challenging behaviors; and so on.

Methods: The methods used for implementing the interventions vary with the type of program. For example, the Four Noble Truths provide a useful framework for developing and implementing appropriate practices. The Buddha based his teachings on his own path to awakening and presented them in terms of his personal experience. He explicitly noted that each practitioner should test whether the same practices are effective for them. Briefly, the Four Noble Truths are (1) suffering, which is understood not as suffering per se in the Western sense, but that life is "unsatisfactory"; (2) that what arises from unsatisfactoriness of life is "craving," which is the wanting of conditions of life to be other than what they are; (3) that the craving can be overcome; and (4) that the practice of the Noble Eightfold Path provides the way for the cessation of suffering and achievement of liberation. In terms of MBIs, the Four Noble Truths can be implemented as requiring the individual to (1) understand and acknowledge suffering; (2) see the craving as our automatic responses to the transient conditions that pervade our life; (3) understand how letting go of our habitual (automatic) responses to life events leads to cessation of reactivity; and (4) engage in practices that develop nonreactive awareness of life as it unfolds, and with discernment to engage in wholesome responses, as needed. Another approach is to base the practices on the Four Foundations of Mindfulness as explicated in the *Satipaṭṭhāna Sutta.* Regardless of the actual approach adopted in MBIs, all provide explicit descriptions of the steps used to teach clients how to change their relationship to events that unfold in their life by skillfully managing their responses to these events.

Expertise required to implement treatment: The MBI instructor needs to have adequate training, practice, and personal attributes. Beyond having cognitive knowledge of Buddhism, mindfulness, and outcome research, the instructor must embody mindfulness through developing and maintaining a consistent personal mindfulness meditation practice (almost) daily. The capacity to embody mindfulness is evidenced only with long-term mindfulness practice. It is a bottom-up process where wisdom is generated through meditation practice instead of knowledge acquired through reading relevant texts and research, which is a top-down process. Embodied mindfulness is reflected in the instructor's daily behavior, which includes acceptance, beginner's mind, curiosity, letting go, nonjudging, nonstriving, and patience. These attitudes and attributes are not learned but are outcomes of mindfulness meditation. The instructor with these characteristics can be considered "authentic" and can present the intervention based on lived experience. In addition, the instructor should be fully versed in the training protocol and curriculum of the specific MBI being taught.

Risks and negative side effects: The limited literature on risks and negative side effects of MBIs suggest that there is little risk and very low occurrence of side effects of using MBIs clinically to manage psychological and psychiatric problems. Measuring side effects of MBIs is a complex task because the intervention itself is expected to reveal unpleasant emotions, feelings, and thoughts that are part of life. Well-trained instructors prepare the participants to anticipate these experiences and to work with these effects in their meditation practice so that they can skillfully deal with difficult emotions, cognitions, and other adversities of daily life. Clinicians should be alert to potential sources of risks and harm for their clients that may include aspects of the program, client, and instructor (therapist or mindfulness teacher), and to provide appropriate remedies or antidotes as needed.

Additional considerations and limitations: There is a mistaken belief among some clinicians that mindfulness is an easy intervention to deliver without a personal investment in training and practice. Often the unstated question is "How hard can it be to teach a client to focus on their breath?" and an honest answer would be "Quite hard." Not unlike any accredited clinical intervention (e.g., dialectical behavior therapy), it requires a great deal of personal training in mindfulness-based practices and expertise to effectively teach MBIs to anyone, including clients with psychological, psychiatric, and medical conditions. Delivering an MBI may look simple, but it is not easy.

22.4 Introduction

The concept of mindfulness has existed in different forms across indigenous cultures, and it is typically grounded in spiritual practices. Western interest in mindfulness is primarily based on the teachings of the Buddha. Even from the time of the Buddha, mindfulness has been defined and practiced in different ways. In research studies, it is commonly defined as the "awareness that emerges through paying attention on purpose, in the present moment, and nonjudgmentally to the unfolding of experience moment by moment" (Kabat-Zinn, 2003, p. 145). The first mindfulness-based program, MBSR, integrated insight meditation, other contemplative practices (e. g., Zen, yoga), psychological theories of stress, and mindful ways of coping with stress in health and mental healthcare (Kabat-Zinn, 1990). This seminal program provided the foundation for mindfulness-based cognitive therapy (MBCT) that encompasses mindfulness-based practices and cognitive therapy for depression (Segal et al., 2002). These MBIs formed the basis of what has been termed mindfulness-based programs (MBPs), which include "systematic and sustained training in formal and informal mindfulness meditation practices for both teacher and participants" (Crane et al., 2017, p. 991). Based on these two MBPs, several client- and behavior-specific programs have been developed (e.g., Bardacke, 2012; Bowen et al., 2010; Kristeller & Wolever, 2011) that form the "first generation of mindfulness-based programs." Numerous MBIs, which have been adapted from MBSR and MBCT but do not incorporate the same teacher-training process and other MBP standards, have been and continue to be developed and tested for their effectiveness. Some of these programs, which are more spiritual in nature, with explicit Buddhist teachings, are examples of the "second generation of mindfulness-based programs" (Van Gordon et al., 2015). Except for a single study that used MBSR (Beck et al., 2020), most of intervention research with autistic individuals has used MBIs either derived from MBSR and MBCT or developed independently but incorporate various aspects of the two MBPs.

22.5 Research Background

We reviewed the extant literature on MBIs for autistic individuals. There are two groups of studies, those presented first are group-design studies and those that follow are single-subject design studies.

In a pre-post waitlist control group study, Spek et al. (2013) provided a modified MBCT program to 42 Dutch autistic adults. Program modifications included an extra weekly session, removed metaphors and ambiguous/imaginative sentences, and provided individual support while delivering group training to 10–11 participants at a time. The program was delivered by a psychologist and a clinical psychologist who attended the 8-day MBCT educational program for therapists. The average age of the intervention group was 44.4 years (*SD* = 11.1), and the average age of the control group was 40.1 years (*SD* = 11). The effects of the modified MBCT on the autistic adults, compared to those on the waitlist control group, included statistically significant reduction in depression, anxiety, and rumination, along with increased positive affect. These self-reported improvements on psychological measures showed medium to large effect sizes. This was a methodologically robust feasibility study that had a serious limitation, namely the use of a waitlist control, which essentially showed that the modified MBCT intervention was more effective than doing nothing and that the intervention effects could have resulted from several nonspecific factors, including expectation bias.

Kiep et al. (2015) reported a study that included 20 participants from the Spek et al. (2013) study and 30 additional autistic adults. The outcomes were similar to those reported by Spek et al. That is, there were significant reductions in psychological problems and psychopathology symptoms (e.g., anxiety, fear, depression, agoraphobia) and significant increases in positive mood maintained at 9-week follow-up. Again, a limitation of this study was the lack of a control condition, which precludes drawing any causal conclusions about the effects of the modified MBCT intervention. Given that the Spek et al. and Kiep et al. studies used multiple rating scales for measuring outcomes, the interpretation of the overall effects may have been tainted by common method bias (Podsakoff et al., 2012).

In an adaptation of the MBCT program specifically for adolescents, de Bruin et al. (2015) used the MYmind program with 23 autistic adolescents (mean age = 15.8 years, *SD* = 2.7). In addition, parents of these adolescents participated in a parallel mindful parenting program. MBCT was adapted by including highly structured sessions, concrete language, and reductions in verbal guidance and inquiry, along with an extra training session. A total of nine weekly 1.5-hour group training sessions were delivered in a group training format by mental healthcare professionals who had completed MYmind teacher training. Results based on parent report showed a significant increase in quality of life at posttest and 9-week follow-up, and a significant decrease in rumination at 9-week follow-up. No significant effects were reported by the participating adolescents on levels of mindfulness, autism symptoms, and worry. This study suffered from a lack of a control group and likely common method bias.

The effects of the MYmind program were also evaluated in subsequent studies. For example, Ridderinkhof et al. (2018) investigated short-, middle-, and long-term effects of MYmind with 45 autistic children (mean age = 13.03 years, *SD* = 2.7). Child and family mental healthcare professionals trained in MYmind provided the training. When compared to baseline, the autistic children's self-reports showed reductions in externalizing symptoms and attention problems at 2-month and 1-year follow-up, reductions in stress at 2-month follow-up, and increases in emotional well-being at 1-year follow-up. No significant changes were reported in levels of mindfulness and chronic sleep problems. Parent reports, however, showed significant improvements in children's social communication, and emotional and behavioral functioning on all occasions. The differences between self-ratings and parental ratings point to one of the limitations of self-ratings because there is no control for how well the children understand the intent of the questions included in the rating scales, and if there is differential response bias between the self-ratings and parental ratings.

In a qualitative study, Ridderinkhof et al. (2019) explored the effects of MYmind from the perspective of the autistic children. Interviews with 14 participating children and adolescents (age range = 9–17 years) yielded eight themes suggesting change processes. They included connecting with peers, being aware, being in the here and now, letting be, determining a strategy, being calm, and attuning to others. A further quantitative study by Ridderinkhof et al. (2020) assessed the effects of MYmind on the attention of autistic children (mean age = 12.9 years, *SD* = 3.2) when compared to those without autism (mean age = 13 years; *SD* = 3.1). The child version of the Attention Network Test was administered to measure alerting, orienting, and executive attention. The findings showed no statistically significant changes in attention of the 49 autistic children when compared to the 50 children without autism.

Ridderinkhof et al. (2021) conducted a multiple baseline study that examined whether individually provided MYmind training improved mental health goals over time of the five autistic adolescents (aged 14 to 19 years) with clinically elevated internalizing symptoms. Of the five autistic adolescents, four showed medium-sized improvements in some of their personal goals (e.g., decreased negative thoughts, feeling bodily relaxed) and one adolescent showed a deterioration in goal achievements during intervention and at the 2-month follow-up phase.

In a within-subject repeated measures design study, Salem-Guirgis et al. (2019) evaluated the effects of MYmind with 23 autistic adolescents (mean age = 15.7 years, *SD* = 2.6) on a battery of measures. The findings showed similar patterns as those reported by Ridderinkhof et al. (2018). Self-reported improvements were reported for ruminative response reflection and depression at 10-week follow-up, but not in mindfulness and internalizing and externalizing behavior at any time point. Parents reported improvements in their children's behavioral symptoms at postintervention, and adaptive skills and social motivation at postintervention and 10-week follow-up.

Ho et al. (2021) investigated the effects of MYmind on Chinese autistic children when compared to children without autism within a randomized controlled trial with a waitlist control group. The instructors were clinical psychologists and social workers with experience in providing services to autistic people, training in teaching the MYmind program, and had a minimum of 4 years of practicing mindfulness meditation. When compared to within-group baseline and the 18 waitlist control group children (mean age = 12.5, *SD* = 2.1), parental reports showed no statistically significant difference in the 19 intervention group children (mean age = 13.7, *SD* = 2.3) on social responsiveness, internalizing and externalizing behavior, and executive function.

Conner and White (2018) in a purported feasibility study evaluated the effects of a modified MBCT program in which the standard eight weekly, 2.5-hour group sessions were reduced to six weekly 1-hour individual sessions, meditation sessions were shortened from 1 hour to 20 minutes, and metaphors and idiomatic speech were reduced. A master's-level therapist with training and clinical experience with autistic adults and mindfulness delivered the program. All nine autistic adults (mean age = 19.6 years old, *SD* = 2.2) who participated in this study completed individual training without reporting adverse events. Four of the nine participants reported reliable decreases in difficulties with impulse control and increases in access to emotion regulation strategies, and three participants reported increases in emotional acceptance. In addition, the program was rated by the participants as being helpful. One of the limitations of this study is that it was a small underpowered outcome study rather than a true feasibility study. Ideally, feasibility studies focus on critical parameters that are needed to design the main study such as a willingness of participants to be randomized, clinicians' recruitment of participants, number of people eligible, and follow-up, response, and adherence/compliance rates (Bowen et al., 2009).

One randomized controlled study by Sizoo and Kuiper (2017) compared the effects of a modified MBSR program with 32 autistic adults in the experimental group, and cognitive behavior therapy (CBT) with 27 autistic adults in the active control condition on anxiety and depression. The standard eight weekly 2.5-hour MBSR sessions were changed to 13 weekly 90-minute sessions and included mindful eating, body scan, mindful breathing, walking, movement and sitting, physical reactions to stress, and observation of thoughts. Experienced therapists trained in MBSR or CBT techniques provided the programs. The results showed a significant time effect on anxiety, depression, autistic symptoms, and general mood. Overall, both MBSR and CBT were effective in reducing anxiety, depressive symptoms, autistic symptoms and rumination, and in increasing global mood at postintervention. Both programs had a sustained effect at 3-month follow-up.

A three-arm randomized controlled trial by Gaigg et al. (2020) compared the effects of MBT and CBT against a waitlist control. Training was delivered online as self-guided programs with videos and audio files explaining core concepts and exercises of MBT and CBT. A total of 54 autistic adults (age range = 23.7 to 66.3) were randomly assigned to one of the three groups. When compared to the control condition, self-report results showed significant improvements in anxiety and depression for both experimental groups. In addition, about 78% of the MBT group and 100% of the CBT group showed reliable reductions in anxiety at 3-month follow-up. Over 50% of each experimental group maintained the intervention effects at 6-month follow-up. The completion rate of MBT was 88% compared to the 64% for CBT.

Kemeny et al. (2022) compared the effectiveness of the three intervention conditions, HeartMath (HM) mindfulness-based techniques, therapeutic horse riding (THR), and no intervention control, in a within-subject crossover design study. A group of 27 autistic children and adolescents (age range = 12 to 21 years) were randomly assigned to each of the three conditions for 10 weeks with a 2-month washout period between conditions. An individual 1-hour HM session included heart-focused breathing, stress education, positive feeling and energy activation, and emotion identification. The single THR session consisted of one-half hour of groundwork and one-half hour of riding. A HM coach and a certified therapeutic recreation specialist administered the programs, respectively. Results showed reductions in stress as indicated by cortisol levels immediately following HM and THR sessions, but this effect was not found a week following the termination of either intervention. The HM had more impact on heart-rate variability, whereas the THR had more impact on decreasing some self-reported stressors. Ratings by the participants and their parents regarding stress and social responsiveness showed no changes due to the intervention, although some individual items of the measures showed statistically significant change for HM from baseline to follow-up. However, the significance of changes in individual items in a rating scale is not psychometrically meaningful. Furthermore, there is some question regarding how much mindfulness meditation and other contemplative practices were included in the HM intervention.

Pagni et al. (2019) compared the effects of a modified MBSR program with 15 autistic adults (mean age = 32.3 years, *SD* =13.7) to an active control group with 13 autistic adults (mean age = 31.6 years, *SD* = 13.2). The modified MBSR program included mindfulness of breathing, eating, walking, conversing, body scan, and other practices, and the active control group included stress reduction tips and techniques. The modified MBSR program was co-implemented by an experienced, certified MBSR trainer and a speech-language pathologist with long-standing experience in autism. Findings based on self-report measures and functional magnetic resonance imaging (fMRI) showed significant improvements in the MBSR group only. These included reductions in depression, increased activity of right middle cingulate cortex (MCC) during self-reflection, and increased functional connectivity between right MCC and pre/postcentral. No change was found in anxiety and in ventromedial prefrontal CORTEX (vmPFC) for both groups. fMRI findings suggested MBSR may increase primary sensorimotor input to higher-order cognitive brain regions. The study was likely underpowered because of the small group sizes and the uncertain relationship of the modified MBSR program to the standard version. It must be remembered that modified versions of any standard program do not have the evidence base of the full program.

Braden et al. (2022) reported a randomized controlled trial that compared a modified MBSR program against an active control that provided social and relaxation supports. Twenty-eight autistic adults (mean age =30.3 years, *SD* =11.7) were randomly assigned to the modified MBSR group and 27 autistic adults (mean age = 32.6 years, *SD* =14.8) to the active control group. The experimental group was taught by a certified MBSR instructor and the active control group by a clinician experienced in providing autism services. Based on self- and proxy-reports, both groups showed improvements in mental health–related quality of life but no improvements in autism-specific quality of life. Improvements in disability-related quality of life were reported only for the MBSR group.

In a feasibility study, Lunsky et al. (2022) modified the MBSR program in collaboration with autistic advisors. The standard eight weekly 2.5-hour in-person sessions were changed to six weekly 1-hour online sessions with shortened guided meditations and home practice recordings. All meditation practices and activities were presented as optional, and multiple communication alternatives were provided during online sessions along with technical and practical support 15 minutes prior to commencing each of the weekly sessions. A mindfulness instructor, technical support facilitator, and an autistic advisor formed the teaching team. Of 57 autistic adults (mean age = 31 years, *SD* = 8.75), 37 completed the intervention. Within-group comparison showed reductions in self-ratings of depression, anxiety, and stress, and increases in levels of mindfulness and self-compassion. One of the strengths of this study was the inclusion of autistic advisors to customize the intervention specifically for this population for online training. A related strength was the inclusion of the autistic advisor as a member of the teaching team. While the study had methodology limitations, it provided a pathway for further exploration of variables that may enable autistic people to better engage in MBIs in a more meaningful manner.

In contrast to the modified MBSR studies, Beck et al. (2020) delivered the standard MBSR program to 12 autistic adults (mean age = 37.6 years, *SD* = 14) without changing its content and instructional method. The instructor was a MBSR teacher with an extensive history of providing autism services. The study met fidelity standards as assessed on the MBI-TAC criteria (Griffith et al., 2021), including participant satisfaction with the intervention. In terms of initial outcomes, the participants' self-reports indicated enhanced positive outlook but not in mindfulness, quality of life, well-being, and life satisfaction. This study was useful in providing initial data showing that the standard MBSR program could be implemented with fidelity with autistic adults, albeit with very limited positive outcomes. As well, the study questions the requirement for a priori modifications made to the standard

MBSR program used in other studies in the absence of data supporting its need. Of course, this was a small study that should be replicated before we can say more about the need for modified MBSR programs.

A few studies investigated the effects of newly developed MBIs that are not derivatives of the standard MBSR or MBCT programs. For example, Drüsedau et al. (2022) introduced a structured group psychotherapy mindfulness-infused program (i.e., TuTASS: Mindful perception of body and emotion) with the aim of helping autistic children to understand their emotions and body, and the body language of others. The program teaches individuals how to (1) distinguish individual senses, along with emotions and physical responses connected to these senses, and (2) characterize and cope with perception of emotions and body, and perception of oneself and others. The program was taught in small groups of five to eight children, using verbal instruction, role plays, board games, and group discussion. Parent-rated outcomes from a single group of 25 autistic children (mean age = 10.1, *SD* =1.3) showed improvements in social motivation, external, social, thought and attention problems, rule breaking and aggressive behavior, and emotional symptoms. Both children and parents rated the program as highly beneficial. Although methodologically weak (e.g., no control group), the results are encouraging in that a mindfulness-infused psychotherapy program with young children may produce a broad spectrum of positive effects. It would be critical to understand what aspects of standard MBIs were infused in this program and how much variance in the outcomes can be attributed to the mindfulness component.

Juliano et al. (2020) evaluated the effects of a new school-based MBI (i.e., Mindful Schools, which included instructions on breathing, bodies, listening, thoughts, and emotions) for improving inhibition and selective attention in 27 autistic children (mean age = 13.6 years, *SD* = 1.7) with co-occurring attention-deficit hyperactivity disorder and anxiety. A 30-minute session of this program was delivered by a mindfulness instructor twice a week for 8 consecutive weeks. Neuropsychological measures indicated significant improvements in inhibition and interference control, with medium effect sizes and overall selective attention with large effect size. Using three experimental assessments instead of the usual rating scales was a strength of this study that could be incorporated in other school-based MBIs. Although the data are suggestive of positive outcomes, the research did not include a control group, and a replication of this study is needed to verify that similar outcomes can be evidenced from a randomized controlled study.

Hatfield et al. (2022) evaluated the effects of the Mindful Movers group program with 14 autistic children (mean age = 11.1, *SD* = 1.5), taught in 10 weekly 75-minute sessions with emotion check, mindful movement, breathing and guided meditation for bodily sensations, and strategies that can be used outside of the group sessions. Two occupational therapists with yoga and mindfulness teaching qualifications developed and administered the program. Self-ratings showed no significant quantitative change in the children's levels of mindfulness, anxiety, and well-being. Interviews with children and their parents noted that breathing and yoga helped them feel calmer, and parents observed reduced anxiety in their children. Qualitative findings addressed the need for more support for children as well as challenges and benefits of group intervention. A strength of this MBI is that it is group-based because children tend to do better in groups when engaging in mindfulness-based practices, but the lack of self-rated positive effects may outweigh the qualitative findings of enhanced calmness and reduced anxiety due to expectation bias.

Another recent study by Hartley et al. (2022) examined the feasibility of a new self-guided mindfulness app, Smiling Mind, for autistic children and their parents in a planned randomized controlled study. Recruitment problems reduced the study to just five autistic children and their 11 caregivers. While several lessons were learned, the key issue that can be highlighted from this study is the need for feasibility studies of new MBIs. Noted earlier, a good feasibility study provides data on key variables such as recruitment issues, willingness of participants to be randomized, dropout rates, adherence to protocol rates, acceptance of the intended intervention, consideration of target population needs and fit of the new MBI, sustainability, and so on. Undertaking a randomized controlled trial of a new intervention, including MBIs, without supporting feasibility data may be unethical.

Finally, Hwang et al. (2015) reported a pre-post and 12-month follow-up study that provided mother-mediated MBI to six autistic children (aged 8 to 15 years) with challenging behavior. Upon completion of an 8-week mindfulness-based group training for the six mothers, a mindfulness teacher with over 20 years of teaching experience and a researcher with extensive experience in mindfulness and autism services assisted the mothers by making three weekly home visits to teach their children mindfulness exercises developed from the individual interviews with their children. The exercises were designed to ground attention and awareness over time using body movements, sounds, and breathing. The mothers continued to practice the exercises with their children for 12 months. At the conclusion of mindfulness training for mothers, significant reductions were reported in the levels of children's challenging behavior. A further significant reduction was reported by the mothers in anxiety and thought problems at the conclusion of mother-mediated mindfulness training for their children. This study highlighted the importance of ongoing support for practice engagement such as online and offline group meetings during the yearlong practice period. In addition, one of the six mothers did not complete the training to her child. This showed that a child's learning opportunities may be determined by the availability and readiness of a parent as a teacher.

In addition to multicomponent MBIs, a small group of single-case research design studies used simple, informal MBIs that can be taught to autistic children, adolescents, and adults as inhibitory control practices for behaviors that prove challenging to their parents and caregivers. These are behaviors that people with or without autism sometimes engage in to obtain social attention and tangibles or to avoid or escape from demand (aversive) situations. The behaviors often are thought to be unacceptable in family and social contexts, but teaching alternative functionally equivalent behaviors that result in the same outcomes for autistic individuals can be daunting. Until recently, behavior analytic methods have been the only evidence-based techniques that have proven successful, though not always effective when used in daily life by parents and caregivers.

The most commonly used MBI for this purpose has been the Soles of the Feet (SoF) practice, an evidence-based manualized MBI used with multiple populations across the lifespan (Felver et al., 2022). The SoF practice includes (a) teaching individuals to recognize the antecedents that occasion their challenging behavior, (b) having them disengage their attention from those antecedents, (c) moving their attention to a neutral point on the body (i.e., somatic sensations of their feet), thereby discontinuing the escalation of the challenging behavior, and (d) returning calmly to the current activity (Felver & Singh, 2020). In addition, the individuals are encouraged to practice the SoF skills in different contexts, thereby supporting generalization across settings and people (Felver et al., 2014; Singh et al., 2003).

Singh et al. (2011) taught mothers of three autistic adolescents (aged 14, 16, and 17 years) to use SoF for themselves so they could teach their children to apply this practice when anger begins to arise. Once they achieved competence in using the SoF practice, the mothers taught the adolescents to use the SoF for their challenging behavior within a multiple-baseline design across participants. The baseline phase lasted 3, 5, and 10 weeks, respectively, across the three adolescents. Training was 30 minutes daily for 5 consecutive days and then the adolescents used it for 23 to 31 weeks. The results were clinically significant reductions in individually operationalized aggressive behavior from 14, 20, and 16 events per week, respectively, during the baseline phase to 0, 0, and 0 during the last 4 weeks of using it in daily life. In addition, the three adolescents engaged in 4, 3, and 3 aggressive behaviors, respectively, during the 3-year follow-up phase.

Subsequent studies replicated the effectiveness of SoF with different trainers, in different settings, and using a different instructional mode. For example, Ahemaitijiang et al. (2020) replicated SoF with three Chinese autistic adolescents (aged 14, 15, and 17 years) who had aggressive and destructive behavior and limited expressive language. Training for the mothers began with daily 30-minute focused meditation followed by four 30-minute training sessions on teaching SoF. The mothers then taught SoF to their children in 24, 15-minute,sessions over 3 weeks, and the autistic adolescents used the SoF practice in their daily lives for 29 to 34 weeks. Results showed reductions in physical aggression and destructive behavior across all three adolescents that were close to zero at the termination of intervention phase and at 1-year follow-up. The three mothers rated the social validity of the SoF practice at 4.6, 4.2, and 4.6 out of 5, respectively.

In a recent study, Shah et al. (2022) used a multiple-baseline design across participants to assess the effects of teaching the SoF practice to three autistic children (aged 9, 10, and 9 years) with challenging behaviors who were students at a private special school. An intern with a master's in mental health counseling at the school who was trained in the SoF practice taught the children individually in 20- to 30-minute sessions for 5 consecutive days. The results were mixed. Teacher reports suggested an increase in two students' challenging behavior from baseline to postintervention and a decrease in one student's challenging behavior. However, independent direct observations showed reductions in all three adolescents' individually defined challenging behavior from baseline to postintervention by 65%, 57%, and 56%, respectively. The average score of teacher-rated social validity of SoF (4.27 out of 5) was much higher than that of student-rated social validity (3.04 out of 5). One of the strengths of this study was having an independent observer collect behavioral data of the adolescents' challenging behaviors, especially in view of the qualitative observations of the teachers typically being unreliable.

In a telehealth study, Singh et al. (2021) provided consultation to a community-based mental health agency treatment team for three autistic adolescents (aged 17, 19, and 13 years) with severe self-injurious behavior (SIB). The consultation in real time included advising the team on developing and implementing behavior support plans and SoF intervention for their clients' SIB. When the treatment team implemented the behavior support plans for the three autistic adolescents, there were minor reductions in the frequency of SIB from 13.7, 7.2, and 10.1 at baseline to 12.4, 6.1, and 9.8, respectively, following behavioral intervention. Data were collected for a new baseline, and the team's behavior analyst taught the SoF practice to the three autistic adolescents for self-management of their SIB. Their mean baseline rates of SIB were 14, 9.6, and 10.4, respectively, which decreased to 3.8, 3.9, and 4.6 during the SoF intervention, attesting to statistical and clinical significance of the decreased SIB due to the SoF intervention. The treatment team's members and the autistic adolescents rated the social validity of the SoF intervention much more highly when compared to the behavioral intervention. One of the strengths of this study was that the agency's treatment team was able to use the real-time consultation to good effect in learning about a new clinical intervention and using it to assist their clients to self-manage their SIB. Such consultation models may enhance the ability of treatment teams to provide effective services to clients who typically would not have access to high-level clinical services.

Another informal MBI reported by Singh et al. (2019) taught Surfing the Urge to three autistic adolescents (aged 16, 17, and 17 years) for self-management of their physical aggression. Surfing the Urge was developed in the context of addiction treatment based on the Buddhist teaching of impermanence—the momentary arising, abiding, and dissolution of all conditioned phenomena (Marlatt & Gordon, 1985). In this study, an experienced mindfulness trainer taught this practice to the three autistic adolescents in 30-minute training sessions during 6 nonconsecutive days. Following training, the adolescents used the practice in their daily lives for 31, 29, and 26 weeks, respectively, whenever they had the urge to engage in verbal or physical aggression. Statistically significant reductions from baseline to intervention for verbal aggression (from 15.8, 5.5, and 12.0 at baseline to 2.2, 1.8, and 3.7 during intervention, respectively) and physical aggression (from 3.5, 2.8, and 7.7 at baseline to 1.1, 1.3, and 3.2 during intervention, respectively) resulted from the use of this practice. In addition, the three adolescents' psychopharmacological treatment for physical aggression was terminated by the family physician during the 19th week, 23rd week, and 25th week of intervention at the adolescents' regular medical checkup. Surfing the Urge may be a useful strategy for self-control of a range of challenging behaviors, but it requires a high level of cognitive self-awareness of the arising of urges (i.e., antecedents) to engage in socially undesirable behaviors and self-control by putting the urges on an extinction schedule.

22.6 Discussion and Practice Implementations

22.6.1 Treatment Outcomes

The use of mindfulness as an intervention with the general population is about 40 years old. It has been used in the field of developmental disabilities for almost 20 years, and about 10 years specifically with autistic children, adolescents, and adults. Thus, we may have more enthusiasm than evidence for its utility as an evidence-based intervention at the present time. This chapter presented a descriptive assessment of the breadth and quality of current evidence for its effectiveness as a viable intervention for a range of issues in autistic individuals. Undoubtedly, the data are suggestive of the potential of MBIs for enhancing quality of life by enabling autistic people to self-manage their clinical (e.g., anxiety, depression) and behavioral issues (e.g., verbal and physical aggression, disruptive behavior), as well as for personal growth as a human being.

There is a certain commonality in the current research on MBIs and MBIs with autistic individuals. The MBIs used in this population are based mainly on two standard evidence-based programs (i.e., MBSR and MBCT). However, except for one small study (Beck et al., 2020), some investigators seem to have assumed that an a priori adaptation of these programs is needed because autistic people may not be able to fully utilize them for some unstated reason or because of the practical exigences of the research or clinical setting. Indeed, virtually all group-design studies included adaptations and modifications of the two standard programs, or they have designed new programs specifically for the study, often without presenting a theoretical or clinical rationale for such programs. This is to be expected in an emerging field where there is much jostling for academic preeminence, but is it in the best interest of autistic people who need assistance in dealing with their clinical and behavioral issues? One of the implications is that practitioners should be wary of using MBIs if the supportive data come from a single study. Until such findings are independently rated as evidence-based on predefined, standard criteria, they are merely suggestive and should not be accepted as anything but that.

In general, our review indicated that there is suggestive evidence of the utility of some MBIs for a range of issues often seen in autistic people. MYmind is probably the most promising MBI, especially considering the various replications across cultures and countries. While there are still too few studies available to qualify it as evidence based, it is perhaps one of the most effective based on current research. In terms of future research, what is needed to establish MYmind as evidence based includes preregistration of prospective studies by independent researchers, tighter methodology, larger sample sizes based on adequate power analysis, an active control condition that is evidence based, multiple methods for assessing outcomes, and intent-to-treat analyses. In the meantime, clinicians and families should feel reasonably confident in using MYmind to assess its effectiveness in community and family settings.

Of all the MBIs used in the single-case design studies we reviewed, the SoF is the only one that has been rated as evidence based (Felver et al., 2022). While there are only a limited number of studies attesting to the effectiveness of the SoF practice with autistic individuals, there is a larger pool of studies with individuals with developmental disabilities, regular school children without disabilities, and in other populations such as Alzheimer's disease, Prader-Willi syndrome, and adolescents with conduct disorder. Also, SoF often is used adjunctively with many MBIs, such as in mindful parenting studies (e.g., Lo et al., 2022). In addition to SoF, other MBIs have been evaluated in single-case design studies but only as test balloon studies of new interventions, such as Surfing the Urge (Singh et al., 2019), SOBER (Singh et al., 2018), and shenpa and calm abiding (Singh et al., 2014). Clinicians and families can use the SoF practice with confidence for treating behaviors that are based on lack of inhibitory control of challenging behaviors arising from negative emotional arousal. However, the SoF intervention may need extensive adaptations depending on the individual's level of intellectual impairment (Singh et al., 2007). Also, alternative evidence-based interventions, such as positive behavior support, should be considered when making a choice of interventions for specific individuals.

Our review identified certain clinical areas as being amenable to change through MBIs, including depression, anxiety, rumination, general quality of life, stress, and emotion regulation. In contrast, other areas were identified that appeared to be immune to the effects of current MBIs, for example, specific symptoms of autism, chronic sleep problems, and autism-specific quality of life. Furthermore, inconsistent effects were reported for mindfulness, attention, and internalizing and externalizing behavior. The discrepancies in the results were found within and between programs. Participant learning profiles, intervention content, settings, instructional methods, and measurement may explain such discrepancies. A discussion of these factors may be instructive for researchers to assist in contextualizing further research, and for professionals and families in translating the research into practice.

Diverse learning preferences in autistic individuals may play a role. For example, attending a group session to learn and practice mindfulness with peers was anxiety provoking, annoying, and boring for some participants as this learning arrangement put them into crowded and noisy environments, whereas the same activity was pleasant for others as they could meet new people and have a sense of community (Hatfield et al., 2022). Positive psychological change was more consistently reported in studies that provided MBIs to autistic adults than to autistic children. The existing psychological and socioeconomic resources may affect autistic people's capacity to commit to ongoing practice engagement. For example, anxiety motivates or even necessitates autistic people to learn to practice mindfulness, but it may be difficult for them to attend a mindfulness training session (Hartley et al., 2022).

Impairments due to autism also may influence individuals' capacity to engage in mindfulness practice and therefore the effectiveness of MBIs may be compromised. However, information on impairments was documented only in a few studies either as information on the participants or as outcome variables. For example, Ahemaitijiang et al. (2020) reported reductions in externalizing behavior of autistic children at support level 1. Braden et al. (2022) reported improved health- and disability-related quality of life for a group of autistic adults with an average ADOS total score of 11.86, and de Bruin et al. (2015) reported no statistically significant effects of MYmind on the core symptoms of autism. It would behoove researchers to include sufficient participant information that may elucidate which MBIs are effective for which subgroup of autistic participants. This kind of information would be valuable for professionals and families to have when deciding which interventions may be optimal for specific clients or family members.

Intervention content, settings, and instructional methods warrant more attention in research reports. Several studies implemented modified MBPs (e.g., MBSR and MBCT). The variability of modified instructional format (e.g., change from eight weekly 2.5-hour group sessions to six weekly 50-minute individual sessions) seems greater than that of modified content (e.g., removal of metaphors). Newly developed MBIs provided mindfulness training to enhance emotion and attention regulation through shorter and more frequent sessions than previously implemented MBIs. Researchers need to provide their rationale for making these changes to ensure that they are theory- or data-based and not just on situational ease of implementing an MBI.

Insufficient or little information about the conceptual framework of mindfulness and mindfulness trainers was noted in several studies. Mindfulness was sometimes not defined in these studies. The reason for clearly defining the nature of mindfulness used in a study is because there needs to be a strong correlation between the chosen definition and the tool used to measure mindfulness. For example, if the Bishop et al. (2004) definition of mindfulness is used, then the Philadelphia Mindfulness Scale (Cardaciotto et al., 2008) would be the measure of choice because this scale maps well with this definition, whereas the more commonly used Five Facet Mindfulness Questionnaire (Baer et al., 2006) does not. Forming a positive and nourishing relationship with teachers is important for any learners. It is, however, particularly important for people on the spectrum, as it can easily influence the nature and level of their learning engagement (Saggers et al., 2011). Implementation of an MBI in the field of autism requires not only specific knowledge and teaching skills for autistic people but also cognitive and experiential understanding of mindfulness practice (Hwang & Kearney, 2015). All of these come with practice.

Group versus individual training and in-person versus online training constitute an MBI instructional method quadrant. In-person group training was most frequently adopted in the reviewed studies and has been diversified to online individual and group training. Different instructional methods present a different set of benefits and challenges for autistic persons. In-person group training can provide a sense of community, but it also exposes them to adverse stimuli, such as noise and crowded physical and psychological environments (e.g., Hatfield et al., 2022). In-person individual training enables customized learning but inevitably limits the number of training recipients at a time (e.g., Conner & White, 2018). Online group training was feasible when technological and individual learning supports were in place, but it had relatively high attrition rates (e.g., Lunsky et al., 2022). Online individual training resulted in contrasting findings. For example, a study that provided 10 mindfulness exercises through videos and audio files reported completion rates of MBI higher than those of CBT (i.e., 88% vs. 64%, respectively), with self-reported improvements in anxiety and depression (Gaigg et al., 2020). In contrast, data analysis was compromised in another study using a self-guided app because of high attrition (Hartley et al., 2022).

An apparent failure in executing a study as initially planned provided crucial information about barriers to participation in MBIs and engagement in ongoing practice. Online app-based training may work for some but not for others, especially those who require ongoing regular support and practice reminders, are time poor and highly anxious, or prefer in-person practice with a trusted teacher. A major difference between the Gaigg et al. (2020) and Hartley et al. (2022) studies was regular checking in for practice engagement, because weekly contact was provided in the study with high completion rate (Gaigg et al., 2020).

How to measure change may matter. Intervention effects were frequently measured through subjective report (i.e., rating scales). When used together, parent reports of intervention effects tend to be more positive than self-reports (e.g., Ridderinkhof et al., 2018; Salem-Guirgis et al., 2019). Furthermore, it is likely that studies suffered from common method bias because two or more constructs were measured in the same survey, which is likely to produce spurious correlations among the items measuring these constructs owing to response styles, social desirability, and priming effects which are independent from the true correlations among the constructs being measured (Podsakoff et al., 2012). A limited number of studies used objective neurological testing, and their findings were generally positive. However, mixed findings were reported as well. For example, no significant training effects were found in alerting, orienting, and executive attention of autistic children and adolescents as measured with the child version of the attention network test (Ridderinkhof et al., 2020). In contrast, significant improvements were reported in children's inhibition, interference control, and selective attention as measured with the Walk/Don't Walk test, Color-Word Interference test, and Cancellation test (Juliano et al., 2020). The most consistent intervention effects were reported in studies using direct behavioral observations (e.g., Ahemaitijiang et al., 2020; Singh et al., 2011, 2019).

22.6.2 Practice Implication Guidelines

Unlike clinical interventions that require students to attend coursework and pass practicum exams, mindfulness requires long-term daily practice of mindfulness meditation so that the instructor can embody what they are teaching. The issue is one of authenticity of the instructor—one can teach only what has been personally experienced. Many researchers appear to base their knowledge of mindfulness on an intellectual understanding of the concepts and even of Buddhist teachings by reading texts and research articles. Intellectual knowledge is good as far as it goes, but mindfulness is totally experiential; it can be acquired only by single mindedly meditating for long periods on the meditation cushion, and then practicing in daily life away from the cushion. The instructor needs to know the effects and side effects of meditation so that they can prepare clients should they react similarly. There are program, client, and instructor variables that may contribute to outcome effects, including unintended or unpleasant effects. The instructor must have an awareness and appreciation of unpleasant experiences that their clients may encounter and be able to teach them how to work skillfully with the unpleasant emotions, negative thoughts and cognitions, and physical discomforts that arise during and following meditation but are also part of life itself. Professionals and family members should be wary of mindfulness instructors who do not have a long-standing personal practice of mindfulness, are overly positive about the effects of MBIs, or see an MBI only as "clinical" intervention and not as a transformative mind-body practice.

When choosing an MBI to implement with a client or family member, it is critical to know the evidence base as well as the specific training steps required of the instructor and client. As we have emphasized, while the evidence base is growing rather rapidly, there are large gaps in our knowledge about specific MBIs. With regard to autism, although there is a small but growing research literature on old and new MBIs, professionals and families must cast a critical eye on the evidence base for each one, which currently is meager and rarely independently replicated. Furthermore, there is an extensive research literature on alternative evidence-based interventions, notably early intervention programs, intensive behavioral treatments, positive behavior support, and cognitive-behavioral therapy CBT) that should be considered as first-line proven practices. Also, there is a large selection of controversial therapies for autism to be avoided in the best interest of autistic children, adolescents, and adults (Foxx & Mulick, 2015). To ensure informed decisions, professionals and family members should read the research literature with an open but critical awareness of what alternatives are available.

When an MBI has been selected, professionals and family members should get some training in the specifics of the MBI either through certified instructors or from the developers of the MBI. Typically, these MBIs are task analyzed and manualized with detailed instructions and great ideas for implementation. While it is critical to digest all the information in the manuals, remember that the manuals are like a finger pointing to the moon. They serve as a guide and are not meant to bind you to rigid adherence to each step in the process. As a professional or family member, you should feel free to adjust the teachings to the needs of the autistic individual you are working with and to present the material in the idiom and culture that the person prefers or is used to. Contextualize the information and ensure the individual's participation by giving plenty of choices so that the recipient is always the "north star" of the teaching process. After all, your instructions are supposed to enhance the quality of life of the individual as the ultimate outcome rather than total adherence to the intervention manual. Be authentic to the teachings specified in the manual but flexible in your teaching methods. Mindfulness instruction is best experienced when there is acceptance, authenticity, calmness, compassion, kindness, warmth, and no power differential between the instructor and the individual.

22.7 References

Ahemaitijiang, N., Hu, X., Yang, X., & Han, Z. R. (2020). Effects of meditation on the Soles of the Feet on the aggressive and destructive behaviors of Chinese adolescents with autism spectrum disorders. *Mindfulness, 11*, 230–240. https://doi.org/10.1007/s12671-019-01246-z

Amaro, A., & Singh, N. N. (2021). Mindfulness: Definitions, attributes, and mechanisms. In N. N. Singh & S. D. Singh Joy (Eds.), *Mindfulness-based interventions with children and adolescents: Research and practice* (pp. 11–33). London: Routledge.

Baer, R. A., Smith, G. T., Hopkins, J., Krietemeyer, J., & Toney, L. (2006). Using self-report assessment methods to explore facets of mindfulness. *Assessment, 13*, 27–45. https://doi.org/10.1177/1073191105283504

Bardacke, N. (2012). *Mindful birthing: Training the mind, body, and heart for childbirth and beyond.* New York: HarperCollins.

Beck, K. B., Greco, C. M., Terhorst, L. A., Skidmore, E. R., Kulzer, J. L., & McCue, M. P. (2020). Mindfulness-based stress reduction for adults with autism spectrum disorder: Feasibility and estimated effects. *Mindfulness, 11*, 1286–1297. https://doi.org/10.1007/s12671-020-01345-2

Bishop, S. R., Lau, M., Shapiro, S., Carlson, L., Anderson, N. D., Carmody, J., Segal, Z. V., Abbey, S., Speca, M., Velting, D., & Devins, G. (2004). Mindfulness: A proposed operational definition. *Clinical Psychology: Science and Practice, 11*(3), 230–241. https://doi.org/10.1093/clipsy.bph077

Bowen, D. J., Kreuter, M., Spring, B., Cofta-Woerpel, L., Linnan, L., Weiner, D., Bakken, S., Kaplan, C., Squiers, L., & Fernandez, M. (2009). How we design feasibility studies. *American Journal of Preventive Medicine, 36*(5), 452–457. https://doi.org/10.1016/j.amepre.2009.02.002

Bowen, S., Chawla, N., & Marlatt, G. A. (2010). *Mindfulness-based relapse prevention for addictive behaviors: A clinician's guide.* New York: Guilford Press.

Braden, B. B., Pagni, B. A., Monahan, L., Walsh, M. J. M., Dixon, M. V., Delaney, S., Ballard, L., & Ware Jr., J. E. (2022). Quality of life in adults with autism spectrum disorder: influence of age, sex, and a controlled, randomized mindfulness-based stress reduction pilot intervention. *Quality of Life Research, 31*, 1427–1440. https://doi.org/10.1007/s11136-021-03013-x

de Bruin, E. I., Blom, R., Smit, F. M., van Steensel, F. J., & Bögels, S. M. (2015). MYmind: Mindfulness training for youngsters with autism spectrum disorders and their parents. *Autism, 19*(8), 906–914. https://doi.org/10.1177/1362361314553279

Cardaciotto, L., Herbert, J. D., Forman, E. M., Moitra, E., & Farrow, V. (2008). The assessment of present-moment awareness and acceptance: The Philadelphia Mindfulness Scale. *Assessment, 15*(2), 204–223. https://doi.org/10.1177/1073191107311467

Conner, C. M., & White, S. W. (2018). Brief report: Feasibility and preliminary efficacy of individual mindfulness therapy for adults with autism spectrum disorder. *Journal of Autism and Developmental Disorders, 48*, 290–300. DOI: 10.1007/s10803-017-3312-0

Crane, R. S., Brewer, J., Feldman, C, Kabat-Zinn, J., Santorelli, S., Williams, J. M. G., & Kuyken, W. (2017). What defines mindfulness-based programs? The warp and the weft. *Psychological Medicine, 47*, 990–999. DOI: 10.1017/S0033291716003317

Druüsedau, L., Schoba, A., Conzelmann, A., Sokolov, A., Hautzinger, M., Renner, T. J., & Barth, G. M. (2022). A structured group intervention (TüTASS) with focus on self-perception and mindfulness for children with autism spectrum disorder, ASD. A pilot study. *European Archives of Psychiatry and Clinical Neuroscience, 272*, 177–185. https://doi.org/10.1007/s00406-021-01281-9

Felver, J. C., Clawson, A. J., Ash, T. L., Martens, B. K., Wang, Q., & Singh, N. N. (2022). Meta-analysis of mindfulness-based program soles of the feet for disruptive behaviors. *Behavior Modification, 46*(6), 1488–1516. https://doi.org/10.1177/01454455211073738

Felver, J. C., Frank, J. L., & McEachern, A. D. (2014). Effectiveness, acceptability, and feasibility of the Soles of the Feet mindfulness-based intervention with elementary school students. *Mindfulness, 5*, 589–597. DOI: 10.1007/s12671-013-0238-2

Felver, J. C., & Singh, N. N. (2020). *Mindfulness in the classroom: An evidence-based program to reduce disruptive behavior and increase academic engagement.* Oakland, CA: New Harbinger.

Foxx, R. M., & Mulick, J. M. (2015). *Controversial therapies for autism and intellectual disabilities: Fad, fashion, and science in professional practice* (2nd ed.). London: Routledge.

Gaigg, S. B., Flaxman, P. E., McLaven, G., Shah, R., Bowler, D. M., Meyer, B., Roestorf, A., Haenschel, C., Rodgers, J., & South, M. (2020). Self-guided mindfulness and cognitive behavioural practices reduce anxiety in autistic adults: A pilot 8-month waitlist-controlled trial of widely available online tools. *Autism, 24*(4), 867–883. https://doi.org/10.1177/1362361320909184

Van Gordon, W., Shonin, E., & Griffiths, M. D. (2015). Towards a second generation of mindfulness-based interventions. *Australian and New Zealand Journal of Psychiatry, 49*, 591–592. https://doi.org/10.1177/0004867415577437

Griffith, G. M., Crane, R. S., Baer, R., Fernandez, E., Giommi, F., Herbette, G., & Koerbel, L. (2021). Implementing the Mindfulness-Based Interventions: Teaching Assessment Criteria (MBI-TAC) in mindfulness-based teacher training. *Global Advances in Health and Medicine.* DOI: 10.1177/2164956121998340.

Hartley, M., Dorstyn, D., & Due, C. (2022). Challenges encountered with a mindfulness app: Lessons learnt from a pilot randomized trial involving caregivers and individuals with autism. *Research in Autism Spectrum Disorders, 96*, 1–9. DOI: 10.1016/j.rasd.2022.101991

Hatfield, M. K., Ashcroft, E., Maguire, S., Kershaw, L., & Ciccarelli, M. (2022). "Stop and just breathe for a minute": Perspectives of children on the autism spectrum and their caregivers on a mindfulness group. *Journal of Autism and Developmental Disorders, 53*(9), 3394–3405. https://doi.org/10.1007/s10803-022-05542-x

Ho, R. Y. F., Zhang, D., Chan, S. K. C., Gao, T. T., Lee, E. K. P., Lo, H. H. M., Yeung, P. A., Lai, K. Y. C., Bögels, S. M., Bruin, E. I. d., & Wong, S. Y. S. (2021). Brief report: Mindfulness training for Chinese adolescents with autism spectrum disorder and their parents in Hong Kong. *Journal of Autism and Developmental Disorders, 51*, 4147–4159. https://doi.org/10.1007/s10803-020-04729-4

Hwang, Y.-S., & Kearney, P. (2015). *A mindfulness intervention for children with autism spectrum disorder: New directions in research and practice.* Cham: Springer.

Hwang, Y.-S., Kearney, P., Klieve, H., Lang, W., & Roberts, J. (2015). Cultivating mind: Mindfulness interventions for children with autism spectrum disorder and problem behaviours, and their mothers. *Journal of Child and Family Studies, 24*, 3093–3106. DOI: 10.1007/s10826-015-0114-x

Juliano, A. C., Alexander, A. O., DeLuca, J., & Genova, H. (2020). Feasibility of a school-based mindfulness program for improving inhibitory skills in children with autism spectrum disorder. *Research in Developmental Disabilities, 101*, 1036–1041. https://doi.org/10.1016/j.ridd.2020.103641

Kabat-Zinn, J. (1990). *Full catastrophe living. Using the wisdom of your body and mind to face stress, pain, and illness.* New York: Dell.

Kabat-Zinn, J. (2003). Mindfulness-based interventions in context: Past, present, and future. *Clinical psychology: Science and Practice, 10*, 144–156. https://doi.org/10.1093/clipsy.bpg016

Kemeny, B., Burk, S., Hutchins, D., & Gramlich, C. (2022). Therapeutic riding or Mindfulness: Comparative effectiveness of two recreational therapy interventions for adolescents with autism. *Journal of Autism and Developmental Disorders, 52*, 2438–2462. https://doi.org/10.1007/s10803-021-05136-z

Kiep, M., Spek, A. A., & Hoeben, L. (2015). Mindfulness-based therapy in adults with an autism spectrum disorder: Do treatment effects last? *Mindfulness, 6*, 637–644. https://doi.org/10.1007/s12671-014-0299-x

Kristeller, J. L., & Wolever, R. Q. (2011). Mindfulness-based eating awareness training for treating binge eating disorder: The conceptual foundation. *Eating Disorders, 19*(1), 49–61. https://doi.org/10.1080/10640266.2011.533605

Lo, H. H., Lau, E. N. S., Tam, C. H. L., Ngai, S., Chan, S. H. W., Leung, F. H., Wong, E. T., Wong, E. W. Y., Wong, G. O. C., Tsang, A. W. K., & Singh, N. N. (2022). Effects of a mindful parenting workshop for parents of adolescents following social unrest in Hong Kong. *Mindfulness, 13*(1), 248–261. https://doi.org/10.1007/s12671-021-01790-7

Lunsky, Y., Redquest, B., Albaum, C., Hutton, S., Share, M., Share-Strom, D., & Weiss, J. (2022). Virtual group–based mindfulness intervention for autistic adults: A feasibility study. *Mindfulness, 13*, 1706–1718. https://doi.org/10.1007/s12671-022-01909-4

Marlatt, G. A., & Gordon, J. R. (1985). *Relapse prevention: Maintenance strategies in the treatment of addictive behaviors*. New York: Guilford Press.

Pagni, B. A., Walsh, M. J. M., Foldes, E., Sebren, A., Dixon, M. V., Guerithault, N., & Braden, B. B. (2019). The neural correlates of mindfulness-induced depression reduction in adults with autism spectrum disorder: A pilot study. *Journal of Neuroscience Research, 98*, 1150–1161. https://doi.org/10.1002/jnr.24600

Podsakoff, P. M., MacKenzie, S. B., & Podsakoff, N. P. (2012). Sources of method bias in social science research and recommendations on how to control it. *Annual Review of Psychology, 63*, 539–569. https://doi.org/10.1146/annurev-psych-120710-100452

Ridderinkhof, A., Bruin, E. I. d., Blom, R., & Bögels, S. M. (2018). Mindfulness-based program for children with autism spectrum disorder and their parents: Direct and long-term improvements. *Mindfulness, 9*, 773–791. DOI: 10.1007/s12671-017-0815-x

Ridderinkhof, A., Bruin, E. I. d., Blom, R., Singh, N. N., & Bögels, S. M. (2019). Mindfulness-based program for autism spectrum disorder: A qualitative study of the experiences of children and parents. *Mindfulness, 10*, 1936–1951. https://doi.org/10.1007/s12671-019-01202-x

Ridderinkhof, A., Bruin, E. I. d., Driesschen, S. v. d., & Bögels, S. M. (2020). Attention in children with autism spectrum disorder and the effects of a mindfulness-based program. *Journal of Attention Disoders, 24*(5), 681–692. https://doi.org/10.1177/108705471879742

Ridderinkhof, A., Elmose, M., Bruin, E. I. d., Blom, R., Salem-Guirgis, S., Weiss, J. A., Meer, P. v. d., Singh, N. N., & Bögels, S. M. (2021). A person-centered approach in investigating a mindfulness-based program for adolescents with autism spectrum disorder. *Mindfulness, 12*, 2394–2414. https://doi.org/10.1007/s12671-021-01668-8

Saggers, B., Hwang, Y.-S., & Mercer, K. L. (2011). Your voice counts: Listening to the voice of high school students with autism spectrum disorder. *Australasian Journal of Special Education, 35*(2), 173–190. DOI: https://doi.org/10.1375/ajse.35.2.173

Salem-Guirgis, S., Albaum, C., Tablon, P., Riosa, P. B., Nicholas, D. B., Drmic, I. E., & Weiss, J. A. (2019). MYmind: A concurrent group-based mindfulness intervention for youth with autism and their parents. *Mindfulness, 10*, 1730–1743. https://doi.org/10.1007/s12671-019-01107-9

Segal, Z. V., Williams, J. M. G., & Teasdale, J. D. (2002). *Mindfulness-based cognitive therapy for depression: A new approach to preventing relapse*. New York: Guilford Press.

Shah, M., Moskowitz, L. J., & Felver, J. C. (2022). Soles of the Feet mindfulness-based program for students with autism spectrum disorder and challenging behavior. *Mindfulness, 13*, 1342–1353. https://doi.org/10.1007/s12671-022-01887-7

Singh, N. N., Lancioni, G. E., Karazsia, B. T., Myers, R. E., Kim, E., Chan, J., Jackman, M. M., McPherson, C. L., & Janson, M. (2019). Surfing the urge: An informal mindfulness practice for the self-management of aggression by adolescents with autism spectrum disorder. *Journal of Contextual Behavioral Science, 12*, 170–177. https://doi.org/10.1016/j.jcbs.2018.10.003

Singh, N. N., Lancioni, G. E., Karazsia, B. T., Winton, A. S. W., Singh, J., & Wahler, R. T. (2014). Shenpa and compassionate abiding: mindfulness-based practices for anger and aggression by individuals with schizophrenia. *International Journal of Mental Health and Addiction, 12*, 138–152. DOI: 10.1007/s11469-013-9469-7

Singh, N. N., Lancioni, G. E., Manikam, R., Winton, A. S. W., Singh, A. N. A., Singh, J., & Singh, A. D. A. (2011). A mindfulness-based strategy for self-management of aggressive behaviour in adolescents with autism. *Research in Autism Spectrum Disorders*, *5*, 1153–1158. https://doi.org/10.1016/j.rasd.2010.12.012

Singh, N. N., Lancioni, G. E., Medvedev, O. N., Hwang, Y.-S., & Myers, R. E. (2021). Real-time telehealth treatment team consultation for self-injury by individuals with autism spectrum disorder. *Advances in Neurodevelopmental Disorders*, *5*, 170–182. https://doi.org/10.1007/s41252-021-00192-z

Singh, N. N., Lancioni, G. E., Myers, R. E., Karazsia, B. T., McPherson, C. L., Jackman, M. M., Kim, E., & Thompson, T. (2018). Effects of SOBER Breathing space on aggression in children with autism spectrum disorder and collateral effects on parental use of physical restraints. *Advances in Neurodevelopmental Disorders*, *2*, 362–374. https://doi.org/10.1007/s41252-018-0073-5

Singh, N. N., Lancioni, G. E., Winton, A. S. W., Adkins, A. D., Singh, J., & Singh, A. N. (2007). Mindfulness training assists individuals with moderate mental retardation to maintain their community placements. *Behavior Modification*, *31*, 800–814. https://doi.org/10.1177/0145445507300925

Singh, N. N., Wahler, R. G., Adkins, A. D., Myers, R. E., & The Mindfulness Research Group. (2003). Soles of the feet: a mindfulness-based self- control intervention for aggression by an individual with mild mental retardation and mental illness. *Research in Developmental Disabilities*, *24*, 158–169. https://doi.org/10.1016/S0891-4222(03)00026-X

Sizoo, B. B., & Kuiper, E. (2017). Cognitive behavioural therapy and mindfulness based stressreduction may be equally effective in reducing anxiety anddepression in adults with autism spectrum disorders. *Research in Developmental Disabilities*, *61*, 47–55. https://doi.org/10.1016/j.ridd.2017.03.004

Spek, A. A., van Ham, N. C., & Nyklicek, I. (2013). Mindfulness-based therapy in adults with an autism spectrum disorder: A randomized controlled trial. *Research in Developmental Disabilities*, *34*(1), 246–253. https://doi.org/10.1016/j.ridd.2012.08.009

23

Anger Management and Autism Spectrum Disorders

Peter Sturmey
The Graduate Center and Department of Psychology, Queens College, City University of New York

23.1 Technical Abstract

Background: Anger management is a package of cognitive and behavioral strategies used to decrease anger and aggression; increase emotional regulation, alternative adaptive skills, and coping abilities; and improve quality of life for children and adults with autism spectrum disorder (ASD) and their parents. **Method:** The literature was searched with Google Scholar using terms "autism" and "anger management" with supplementary searches for specific forms of anger management. References and citations were searched for empirical articles evaluating anger management with individuals with ASD. **Results:** Since there were three randomized controlled trials (RCTs) for anger management reporting various positive outcomes with children with ASD and their parents, it can be concluded that anger management is an evidence-based approach for children and anger and aggression problems. **Discussion:** There is now preliminary evidence for the effectiveness of anger management with children with ASD. Additionally, the involvement of parents is a positive feature which may have benefits for the parents, such as increased confidence. The number of experimental studies of anger management with individuals with ASD and the range of populations with ASD, however, is limited. Thus, we should be cautious regarding the confidence in these conclusions. No studies were located with adults with ASD, and no experimental studies were located for common forms of anger management such as aggression replacement training (ART), Novaco's approach, or relaxation training alone. Future research should attend to the following issues: (a) the preliminary results should be replicated by independent groups of researchers; (b) the evaluations should be extended to other groups, especially adults with ASD; (c) future research should conduct evaluations of standard approaches to anger management such as ART, Novaco's approach, relaxation training, and so on to children and adults with ASD; (d) attention should be paid to defining and measuring the independent variable explicitly and comprehensively; (e) consider controlling and explicitly manipulating anger triggers during evaluations of anger management; and (f) explore the

Peter Sturmey, *Anger Management and Autism Spectrum Disorders*. In: *Lifespan Treatment for Autistic Individuals*. Edited by: Peter Sturmey, Russell Lang, and James K. Luiselli, Oxford University Press. © Oxford University Press (2025). DOI: 10.1093/oso/9780197635841.003.0023 distinction between angry and nonangry aggression and its treatment implications. **Practitioner recommendations:** When working with children and young people with ASD and anger/aggression, consider using anger management as one treatment option. Currently the Stress and Anger Management Program (STAMP) (Scarpa et al., 2012) has a treatment manual available for practitioner use. For practitioners working with adults with ASD, consider other evidence-based practices for anger/aggression and/or adopt versions of anger management that have been evaluated for children and young persons with ASD for adults.

23.2 Layperson Summary

Children and adults with ASD often have problems recognizing and controlling their negative emotions, such as anger. They can learn other ways to think and behave in situations that are challenging for them. Anger management is a treatment package to teach several important skills, such as changing the way one thinks. The skills also include behavior, such as being assertive or walking away from anger-provoking situations. Anger management includes the use of reward (reinforcement) and time-out at home and in school. Anger management also includes parental involvement, including education about anger, observing their child's behavior, and helping their child to control their emotions and behavior more effectively. This is often done with groups of parents while their children receive anger management. Anger management is one credible among several options in managing angry and aggressive behavior in children and adults with ASD.

23.3 Treatment Summary Table

Treatment summary: Anger Management

Treatment description: Anger management is a cognitive-behavioral package of skills training that addresses thoughts, feelings, and behavior related to angry emotions and overt behavior such as aggression. It usually identifies triggers for anger and thoughts, feeling, and behavior that lead to anger and aggression. It then teaches the person to think, feel, and behave more effectively in provocative situations or to minimize, remove, or otherwise manage the triggers for anger. It is often combined with traditional behavioral interventions such as time-out, functional behavioral assessment, and behavioral parent training, as well as contemporary treatment strategies such mindfulness and dialectic behavior therapy.

Expected outcomes: Three RCTs conducted with children and adolescents with ASD have found reductions in anger and aggression, improvements in child and adolescent coping strategies, and increase in parent confidence in handling their children's angry behavior.

Methods: Anger management can be delivered individually or in small groups. It often incorporates parallel parent education and training and support groups. It can be delivered in 6–10 weekly groups. Some forms of anger management such as STAMP have accompanying treatment manuals and are very structured. Anger management usually involves child groups that are designed to be fun, includes practice of anger management skills in role play, and specifies homework assignments done in coordination with parents.

Expertise required to implement treatment: There is no formal statement that specifies the expertise and skills and/or licenses required and/or research knowledge to conduct anger management adequately. Hence, anger management has been conducted by a range of therapists with master's- and doctoral-level training, graduate students supervised by professors, appropriately trained and supported behavior technicians, and parents and other family members. In one or two papers, there are cursory descriptions of use of a therapy manual and supervision of therapists or graduate students from more experienced practitioners or educators, but the descriptions are insufficiently detailed to guide practice and professional training. The availability of manuals for some forms of anger management may be of assistance to specify what skills are needed, but the extent of training required to implement anger management accurately and flexibly has not been specified.

Risks and negative side effects: There are no known and documented risks and negative side effects. Some treatments incorporated within anger management might include operant extinction that could occasion child and parent distress and temporary emotional side effects. The parent groups, which require attendance at weekly meetings, may be disruptive to parents' work, daily activities, and attending to other family members.

Additional considerations and limitations: The literature supporting anger management with individuals with ASD is moderate and limited to three experimental studies of children and adolescents, two of which were with higher functioning ASD with average IQ mostly with families with average or above-average incomes and nondiverse samples of families. No experimental evaluations of anger management with adults with ASD were located. Future research should extend the literature to adults, conduct component analyses or dismantling studies of these treatment packages, clarify and measure the independent variable more comprehensively, and determine the place of anger management in the array of evidence-based practices for aggression and related behavioral issues.

23.4 Introduction

23.4.1 Treatment Description

Anger is a commonly identified human emotion and experienced by many if not all humans. Novaco (1976) described anger as follows: "The arousal of anger, in an elementary sense, can be viewed as an emotional response to provocation that has identifiable autonomic . . . , central nervous system . . . , and cognitive . . . components. Whether or not anger leads to aggressive behavior depends on the magnitude and appraisal of the provocation, situational constraints, expected outcomes, and the person's preferred style of coping" (p. 1124). Hence, in Novaco's view, a provocation triggers an emotional response with autonomic, central nervous system, and cognitive components, which may or may not be expressed behaviorally, depending upon the person's learning history and environmental factors. This definition does not distinguish among adaptive, nonproblematic, and problematic forms of anger requiring intervention.

Anger seems quite useful in many contexts in that it energizes behavior and is expressive of the angry person's emotional state to others. It is also useful to the individual in getting their needs met, sometimes more quickly and efficiently than otherwise might have occurred (Novaco, 1976). Angry or aggressive behavior can be quite effective in obtaining a range of consequences for the angry person, such as attention from others, tangibles, and termination of aversive stimulation (DiGiuseppe et al., 2023). Skinner (1953), in a discussion of angry emotional behavior, noted that an angry person's behavior also appears to be reinforced in part by the suffering of others, for example, as shown by their interest in violent sports and other forms of human suffering or the desire of the angry person for revenge against the perpetrator of their injustice. Cognitive accounts of anger emphasize that anger often appears to be shown in response to rule violation by others who treat the angry person with disrespect when they are worthy of such respect. Indeed, angry people—in contrast to previous speculation to the contrary—often have *high* self-esteem (Kernis et al., 1989). It is not merely that another person disrespected the angry person, but rather that of all the people deserving of respect and esteem, the other person disrespected *me*, an especially worthy person!

Everyday anger turns into problematic anger when there are negative consequences for the angry person, their friends, family, coworkers, and society generally, and when it becomes pervasive. The angry person may manage their angry behavior through ineffective methods, such as avoidance, rumination, and alcohol and drug use. They may also be overly vigilant for insults and have a weak repertoire of dealing with everyday situations effectively, such as responding to minor triggers and stressors with extreme anger and aggression. The people around them may avoid them and/or the triggers for the angry person's anger. They seem to "walk on eggshells" in case they trigger an angry episode. Society pays a large penalty for anger in terms of prevention, treatment, and legal protections for family (Sturmey, 2023), work, and other forms of angry violence through societal structures, such as schools, the law, mental health, and the penal system (Sturmey, 2022).

Individuals with ASD, like other people, also experience both daily and problematic anger. Given that anger is mediated by covert verbal behavior concerning other people and that individuals with ASD have challenges related to a wide range of aspects of social and verbal behavior, including expressing and understanding emotions, it is not surprising that some individuals with ASD experience problematic anger.

23.4.2 Rationale and Objectives

Given the challenges that individuals with ASD have with emotional and angry behavior, anger management has been adapted and extended from its applications in other contexts, such as adult outpatient and forensic applications. These applications have included identifying the triggers for angry emotions, the inappropriate covert and overt behaviors that may occur, and the alternate effective and appropriate behavioral repertoires that can be taught to replace inappropriate angry behavior. These strategies have included removal or better management of triggers for angry behavior, learning other covert and overt responses to triggers for angry behavior, and modification of contingencies of reinforcement and punishment to change relevant adaptive and maladaptive behavioral repertoires. This is often done by a therapist working in collaboration with parents, school practitioners, and residential staff. Thus, the objectives of anger management are increasing adaptive covert and overt behavior in the face of provocation, reducing problematic anger behavior, improving parenting skills, and enhancing the quality of life for all concerned. These strategies are often combined with a variety of typical behavioral strategies and more contemporary cognitive-behavioral therapy (CBT) strategies. (See below.)

23.4.3 Considerations for Implementation

Anger management has been delivered both individually and in group formats and supplemented by parent support groups that parallel groups for children. At least one standardized and evaluated treatment manual exists (Scarpa et al., 2012) that may be a useful resource to practitioners.

An important consideration in anger management that has not received sufficient attention is the identification and management of discriminative stimuli ("triggers") for angry behavior. Although both definitions of anger and treatment procedures acknowledge that this is an essential step in anger management, the procedures for comprehensive assessment and management are not spelled out in sufficient detail for practitioners. When assessing the discriminative stimuli for angry behavior, a pretreatment probe or brief baseline may be inadequate to identify all the relevant discriminative stimuli because caretakers typically avoid problematic situations that evoke child aggression. One solution to the problem of assessing discriminative stimuli is to conduct a comprehensive functional behavioral assessment. For example, in a study on anger management with adults who had mild intellectual disability, Travis and Sturmey (2013) reviewed 12 months of token economy data for each individual to identify potential discriminative stimuli for anger/aggression and then presented those stimuli systematically approximately every 10 minutes to observe if they evoked aggression/angry behavior on at least 20% of trials. Five identified triggers were used during anger management groups and five triggers as generalization probes to assess the effects of treatment on untrained stimuli in the natural environment.

The assessment and management of discriminative stimuli are also important during treatment evaluation. Although most studies of anger management have been quite positive, a question remains as to how these effects occurred. The presence of caretakers during training is a good pragmatic strategy that might promote generalization from a therapy group, but it is unclear if the subsequent reduction in anger or aggression is due to caretakers learning about and avoiding presenting discriminative stimuli rather than promoting skills use when triggers occur. Thus, the changes reported in anger management studies might be due to removing provocative stimuli rather than learning to behave appropriately in their presence. One solution is to systematically present the provocative stimuli at baseline, during, and after intervention (Travis & Sturmey, 2013). Practitioners and family member might balk at this suggestion, but during treatment they can consider the safest and appropriate way to present triggers for anger progressively while balancing implementing treatment with safety.

23.5 Research Background

There is relatively limited research on anger management and individuals with ASD. For example, systematic reviews by Ho et al. (2010, 2018) identified only one experimental evaluation of anger management with individuals with Asperger syndrome (i.e., Sofronoff et al., 2007). Further, the amount of research since the publication of that systematic review has been limited, although there have been reports on nonexperimental case studies with positive outcomes (e. g., Carter, 2010; Greig et al., 2019; Holland, 2015).

As noted above, the earliest RCT to evaluate anger management with individuals with ASD comes from Sofronoff et al. (2007). The authors recruited 52 children aged 9–14 years with Asperger syndrome in metropolitan Brisbane. The children were systematically screened for the presence of Asperger syndrome and anger using standard psychometric instruments, a brief IQ test, parental and child interviews, and behavior diaries. Two children were excluded because they did not meet diagnostic criteria for Asperger syndrome during initial screening, and five families withdrew their children from the study on assignments to the condition. (The authors did not report which condition these children were assigned to.) There were 23 boys and one girl in the treatment condition and 20 boys and one girl in the control group. The average IQs in each group were 105 and 109, respectively, and the minimum IQ for the entire sample was 95. No children were excluded due to comorbid attention-deficit/hyperactivity disorder.

Anger management had two components: a CBT child group and a parent group. The child CBT consisted of six 2-hour weekly sessions, which included fun sessions, a workbook for each child, and weekly homework assignments. The material was presented using the metaphor of being a space explorer and a toolbox of strategies, including recognizing positive and negative emotions, different aspects of anger, how to restore positive feelings, social stories, and a final treatment plan. The program was delivered by trained and supervised graduate students with adherence checks for 25% of videotaped sessions. Children worked in pairs with two therapists. Parents also worked in parallel groups on the same material as their children, and therapists encouraged the parents to work with their children on assignments related to the content of each session. In the waitlist control, children and parents completed the pre- and postassessments.

The authors collected data at preintervention, postintervention, and a 6-week follow-up. There was good evidence of the effectiveness of anger management. Only parents in the treatment group reported an overall reduction in anger and on two of four subscales and an anger measure. Similar results were found for parental reports of anger, as well as their own and their children's confidence in dealing with anger. When asked to generate solutions to vignettes of anger, children in the CBT group reported an increased number of appropriate solutions to anger-provoking situations. Of the 75% of parents who responded, most reported finding the program highly valuable, including positive changes in their children. These differences were maintained at 6-week follow-up. Of 18 teachers who could be contacted by phone, 16 reported improvements in child behavior at school.

In a second RCT, Clifford et al. (2022) evaluated a slightly different approach to anger management. Their approach included elements of traditional anger management as well as elements of dialectic behavior therapy and mindfulness; thus, the authors emphasized that their approach highlighted attentional aspects of anger management. The study included 51 children with ASD (8 to 13 years old) and average IQ in mainstream schools who were predominantly from middle- and high-income, nonimmigrant Dutch families. The authors randomized the children to either the "anger can go!" treatment or an active control condition. The treatment consisted of (1) teaching use of an anger management thermometer, (2) functional behavior assessment, (3) time-out for low-level anger, (4) shifting attention away from anger-provoking stimuli, and (5) creating solutions for anger-provoking situations, including dialectic behavior therapy strategies. The treatment was highly structured and manualized with workbooks for the children. One parent attended the last 10 minutes of each session, and a therapist also visited school to introduce and practice time-out in that setting. There was also an active parent education group which met for three sessions which paralleled the content of the children's sessions. The treatment was delivered in nine, 60-minute weekly sessions while the active control group received only the parent sessions.

The outcomes were evaluated using multiple psychometric measures of anger, aggression, and coping skills. Outcomes on measures of aggression, tantrums, and arguing were mixed with statistically significant effects on some scales and not others. Parents reported more use of some but not all adaptive anger coping strategies, but there was no reduction in parental maladaptive strategies and rumination. There was no difference in secondary measures, such as quality of life and parental stress. Teachers did not report a reduction in aggression, perhaps due to lack of treatment implementation. Thus, the authors concluded that intervention has some effects on anger, aggression, and coping skills, but not on broader measures, such as quality of life.

Finally, the STAMP program (Scarpa et al., 2012) emphasizes teaching children emotional regulation skills to recognize and manage both labile and negative affect, such as retraining child attributions. Intervention includes identifying and understanding emotions; social, thinking, and special interest tools; and appropriate and inappropriate emotional, cognitive, and behavioral aids. It also includes some fairly typical behavioral interventions, such as behavioral monitoring of aggression and tantrums; contingency management for inappropriate behavior in the group, such as removing aggressive children from the group sessions; behavior support plans;

teaching teachers to use time-out; and behavioral parent training. Finally, STAMP emphasizes and enhances the role of parents in providing assistance with these challenges. There is a parallel parent group that covers the same material as the child group, with observation of the children's sessions, handouts, and homework assignments with children. Thus, STAMP is a multicomponent package of cognitive and behavioral interventions adapted to the developmental level of young children with ASD (Scarpa et al., 2009).

In an initial pilot study, Scarpa and Reyes (2011) reported a pre-post comparison of STAMP anger management for children with ASD confirmed with the *Autism Diagnostic Observation Schedule*. There were 11 children aged 4.5–7 years from predominantly high-income families. The authors randomized the children to treatment or delayed treatment. When comparing the pre- and postdata for both groups combined, there were statistically significant reductions in parents' reports of the frequency and duration of aggression, improved emotional regulation and negative emotions, more child responses to appropriate solutions to a vignette concerning anger, and improved parental self-confidence and parental perceptions of child confidence. This pilot study suggested that the STAMP anger management program was a promising treatment.

Subsequently, Factor et al. (2019) reported an extension of this pilot study in a small-scale RCT of the STAMP program. The authors randomized 23 children aged 4–7 years with ASD, of whom 19 were boys, and their parents to the STAMP program or a waitlist control. Four children were dropped, one because he did not meet eligibility criteria and three families decided not to participate. This sample was constituted from the participants in the original pilot study plus 12 new families; thus, this sample overlaps substantially with the pilot data. Using standardized psychometric measures, Factor et al. found that child emotional regulation, parent confidence, and child problem behavior improved post training only in the experimental group.

Little or no evidence was found regarding several commonly used and researched approaches to anger management. The historically classic approach to anger has been ART (Glick & Goldstein, 1987). ART has an extensive literature in other contexts and with other populations (Brännström et al., 2016) and recently has been modified and enhanced in various ways. However, the application specifically to individuals with ASD is limited, notwithstanding a few studies of ART in this area, and those that have been published absent an experimental design (Moynahan, 2003; Moynahan & Strømgren, 2005). There was little research on the highly influential and well-researched approach to anger from Novaco (1975, 1976) explicitly with individuals with ASD, although some nonexperimental studies included some individuals with ASD (Kellner & Tutin, 1995), and some studies that focused on intellectual disabilities and anger management may well have included some individuals with ASD (see Hamelin et al., 2013; Nicoll et al., 2013). Similarly, no studies were identified that used relaxation training alone as an anger management strategy for individuals with ASD.

Applying Chambless and Hollon's (1998) criteria for evidence-based practices allows for only limited confidence in conclusions due primarily to the very limited quantity of experimental evidence. We may conclude, based on three RCTs on anger management with children and adolescents aged up to 14 years, two of which were with children with average IQs, that anger management is an evidence-based practice. It should be noted that the treatments in each of these studies, while sharing some features, were substantially different; therefore, we need replications of all three of these experiments. Second, there were no experimental evaluations of anger management with other populations, such as individuals with autism rather than Asperger syndrome, individuals with intellectual disabilities, and adults with ASD. Again, research is needed to extend the earlier results to these other populations. Third, each of these individual programs is classified as a promising approach because there is currently only one RCT and no replication studies for each of these three treatment packages. Fourth, there was no experimental evidence evaluating several traditional cognitive-behavioral approaches to anger (e.g., ART and Novaco's program) for individuals with ASD; hence, these anger management packages are not evidence-based practices for individuals with ASD at this time due to the lack of experimental evidence.

An important issue in evaluating the literature on anger management and ASD is one that has been observed elsewhere in the psychotherapy outcome literature, namely the proliferation of varied, multicomponent treatment packages often with labels that are difficult to understand because the treatment labels are imprecise or incomplete. This problem makes it difficult to address the key issue of independent replication of the effects of a particular approach to anger management. For example, two treatment packages might be labeled "cognitive behavior therapy" or "anger management." One might be a narrow version of CBT, whereas another treatment package also labeled "cognitive behavior therapy" or "anger management" might be broad and eclectic, including functional assessment, graded exposure to anger triggers, dialectic behavior therapy, and mindfulness strategies, in addition to traditional CBT anger management strategies.

Another challenge in this literature is defining and measuring the independent variable. Although anger management is relatively well described and, in some cases, commercially available, manuals exist that specify the topics and activities of each session, but assessment of the independent variable has been limited, although at least one study reported some form of checks on treatment integrity (Sofronoff et al., 2007). The anger management literature often defines the treatment as the number of sessions or as the percentage of elements of sessions therapists delivered correctly. However, this literature rarely reports on what the participants do and learn in the group. For example, although a participant might attend all sessions, it is usually unclear if they learned and applied any of the skills reviewed in the session either in the group or in the natural environment. Future research could attend both to the conceptual issue of what constitutes treatment and the practical issue of what the participant must do to show that they learned anger management skills (Hamelin et al., 2013).

Finally, the term "anger" is used throughout this literature. Yet the distinction between anger as a covert behavior, anger as covert behavior that results in overt angry behavior, and overt nonangry aggressive behavior is not made either in the definition or measurement of anger. If these distinctions are meaningful, then the challenge for both researchers and practitioners is to assess these differences reliably and to select the treatment for each individual that matches the kind of aggressive behavior the person shows. For example, a researcher or practitioner might ask if we can reliably assess angry and nonangry aggression and use this to predict the best treatment. Pertinent questions might be these: Does angry aggression respond more to anger management than operant-based treatment based on the function of the person's overt aggressive behavior, and does nonangry, operant aggression respond better to function-based treatment than anger management?

23.6 Practice Implications

23.6.1 Treatment Outcomes

Anger management with children and adolescents with ASD may be effective in teaching them better coping skills and reduce their aggressive behavior. It may also benefit parents to become more confident in handling their children's problem behavior and be pleased with their children's progress. There is little research on children with ASD and intellectual disabilities and no studies with adults with ASD. Practitioners should be cautious in extending anger management to these populations as practitioners may need to modify anger management, such as simplifying or removing metaphorical language (e.g., individuals being "a space explorer").

There is currently no evidence outlining the limitations to using anger management with individuals with ASD, but the literature on CBT and intellectual disabilities may be relevant. Often therapies should be modified by having sessions delivered more slowly over more sessions, making the content more concrete and involving caretakers. Some individuals with ASD may not learn essential anger management skills in the current format; hence, practitioners should monitor skill acquisition in each person. Providing additional sessions and/or in collaboration with parents to ensure the acquisition and generalization of individual skills appears warranted.

A final consideration for practitioners is isolating where anger management lies within the array of treatments for problem behavior. There are now a number of potentially effective treatments for problem behavior, some of which have a much greater evidence base than anger management with individuals with ASD. Practitioners must decide where anger management lies within this array of treatment options.

23.6.2 Practice Implication Guidelines

Based on the three RCTs, practitioners should consider anger management for children and adolescents with ASD and anger/aggression. It should be noted that anger management is one option for these problems, and other treatment methods such as functional communication training have a more extensive and robust outcomes (Gerow et al., 2018; Gregori et al., 2020). For adults with ASD, there are no experimental studies for anger management; hence, practitioners should be cautious in extending anger management to adults with ASD when there are alternatives, such as functional communication training, available (Gregori et al., 2020).

When considering implementation of anger management, practitioners should adhere to an established treatment manual, such as Scarpa et al. (2012). They should also receive initial supervision from a more experienced practitioner who can observe implementation and give feedback on their implementation skills, preferably on multiple and varied clients. This feedback could gradually be faded contingent on practitioner competence.

A final consideration noted above is that practitioners should actively assess and manage antecedent stimuli in the use of anger management. This requires careful initial evaluation of all the relevant antecedents for anger/aggression, including those that practitioners usually avoid and subsequent careful introduction of antecedents for anger/aggression as intervention proceeds. Evaluation should not only include rates of anger/aggression but should also include probes on all relevant antecedents as intervention progresses.

23.7 References

Brännström, L., Kaunitz, C., Andershed, A. K., South, S., & Smedslund, G. (2016). Aggression replacement training (ART) for reducing antisocial behavior in adolescents and adults: A systematic review. *Aggression and Violent Behavior, 27*, 30–41.

Carter, S. (2010). Cognitive behavioural intervention for anger in adolescents diagnosed with Asperger syndrome: A report on the use of the "Exploring Feelings" programme with two adolescent young men. *Good Autism Practice (GAP), 11*(2), 13–17.

Chambless, D. L., & Hollon, S. D. (1998). Defining empirically supported therapies. *Journal of Consulting and Clinical Psychology, 66*(1), 7–18.

Clifford, P., Gevers, C., Jonkman, K. M., Boer, F., & Begeer, S. (2022). The effectiveness of an attention-based intervention for school-aged autistic children with anger regulating problems: A randomized controlled trial. *Autism Research, 15*(10), 1971–1984.

DiGiuseppe, R., Cannella, C., & Kelter, J. (2023). Effective anger treatments require a functional analysis of the anger response. In T. A. Cavell, & K. T. Malcolm (Eds.), *Anger, aggression, and interventions for interpersonal violence* (pp. 55–76). London: Routledge.

Factor, R. S., Swain, D. M., Antezana, L., Muskett, A., Gatto, A. J., Radtke, S. R., & Scarpa, A. (2019). Teaching emotion regulation to children with autism spectrum disorder: Outcomes of the Stress and Anger Management Program (STAMP). *Bulletin of the Menninger Clinic, 83*(3), 235–258.

Gerow, S., Hagan-Burke, S., Rispoli, M., Gregori, E., Mason, R., & Ninci, J. (2018). A systematic review of parent-implemented functional communication training for children with ASD. *Behavior Modification, 42*(3), 335–363.

Glick, B., & Goldstein, A. P. (1987). Aggression replacement training. *Journal of Counseling & Development, 65*(7), 356–362.

Gregori, E., Wendt, O., Gerow, S., Peltier, C., Genc-Tosun, D., Lory, C., & Gold, Z. S. (2020). Functional communication training for adults with autism spectrum disorder: A systematic review and quality appraisal. *Journal of Behavioral Education, 29*, 42–63.

Greig, A., MacKay, T., & Ginter, L. (2019). Supporting the mental health of children and young people: A survey of Scottish educational psychology services. *Educational Psychology in Practice, 35*(3), 257–270.

Hamelin, J., Travis, R., & Sturmey, P. (2013). Anger management and intellectual disabilities: A systematic review. *Journal of Mental Health Research in Intellectual Disabilities, 6*(1), 60–70.

Ho, B. P., Stephenson, J., & Carter, M. (2018). Cognitive-behavioral approaches for children with autism spectrum disorder: A trend analysis. *Research in Autism Spectrum Disorders, 45*, 27–41.

Ho, B. P. V., Carter, M., & Stephenson, J. (2010) Anger management using a cognitive-behavioural approach for children with special education needs: A literature review and meta-analysis. *International Journal of Disability, Development & Education, 57*(3), 245–265. DOI: 10.1080/1034912X.2010.501169

Holland, B. (2015). Using the Exploring Feelings programme to address anger with two adolescents with autism. *Good Autism Practice (GAP), 16*(1), 53–60.

Kellner, M. H., & Tutin, J. (1995). A school-based anger management program for developmentally and emotionally disabled high school students. *Adolescence, 30*(120), 813–826.

Kernis, M. H., Grannemann, B. D., & Barclay, L. C. (1989). Stability and level of self-esteem as predictors of anger arousal and hostility. *Journal of Personality and Social Psychology, 56*(6), 1013.

Moynahan, L. (2003). Enhanced aggression replacement training with children and youth with autism spectrum disorder. *Reclaiming Children and Youth, 12*(3), 174.

Moynahan, L., & Strømgren, B. (2005) Preliminary results of aggression replacement training for Norwegian youth with aggressive behaviour and with a different diagnosis, *Psychology, Crime & Law, 11*(4), 411–419.

Nicoll, M., Beail, N., & Saxon, D. (2013). Cognitive behavioural treatment for anger in adults with intellectual disabilities: A systematic review and meta-analysis. *Journal of Applied Research in Intellectual Disabilities, 26*(1), 47–62.

Novaco, R. W. (1975). *Anger control: The development and evaluation of an experimental treatment.* Lexington, MA: D.C. Heath & Co.

Novaco, R. W. (1976). The functions and regulation of the arousal of anger. *American Journal of Psychiatry, 133*(10), 1124–1128.

Scarpa, A., Reyes, N., & Attwood, T. (2009). Cognitive-behavioral therapy for stress and anger management in young children with ASD. In A. Scarpa, S. W., White, & T. Attwood (Eds.), *CBT for children and adolescents with high-functioning autism spectrum disorders* (pp. 147–172). New York: Guilford Press.

Scarpa, A., & Reyes, N. M. (2011). Improving emotion regulation with CBT in young children with high functioning autism spectrum disorders: A pilot study. *Behavioural & Cognitive Psychotherapy, 39*(4), 495–500.

Scarpa, A., Wells, A., & Attwood, T. (2012). *Exploring feelings for young children with high-functioning autism or Asperger's disorder: The STAMP treatment manual.* London: Jessica Kingsley.

Skinner, B. F. (1953). *Science and human behavior.* New York: Simon and Schuster.

Sofronoff, K., Attwood, T., Hinton, S., & Levin, I. (2007). A randomized controlled trial of a cognitive behavioural intervention for anger management in children diagnosed with Asperger syndrome. *Journal of Autism & Developmental Disorders, 37*, 1203–1214.

Sturmey, P. (2022). *Violence and aggression: Integrating theory, research, and practice.* Cham: Springer.

Sturmey, P. (Ed.). (2023). *Violence in families: Integrating research into practice.* Cham: Springer Nature.

Travis, R. W., & Sturmey, P. (2013). Using behavioural skills training to treat aggression in adults with mild intellectual disability in a forensic setting. *Journal of Applied Research in Intellectual Disabilities, 26*(5), 481–488.

24

Robotics and Virtual Learning

Matthew Roberts and An-An Chang
California State University, Northridge (CSUN)

Eric McCoy
California State University, Northridge (CSUN) and Easterseals Southern California

Hunter King and Aaron J. Fischer
University of Utah

Ellie Kazemi
California State University, Northridge (CSUN)

24.1 Technical Abstract

This chapter reviews three emerging technologies and their ability to support individuals on the autism spectrum, specifically virtual reality (VR), telepresence robots, and programmable robots. Studies relevant to each technology's intervention capabilities were collected via online databases. The findings and implications of these studies are discussed. Studies on VR demonstrated strong training abilities for supporting individuals on the autism spectrum, particularly for those practicing social skills. Research on telepresence robots showed promise in assisting educators with behavior assessment procedures and revealed increased compliance and improved academic skills for students. Despite limited research highlighting the role of programmable robots in autism intervention, studies have shown great potential for teaching social and occupational skills. Strengths, limitations, and future directions for each technology are discussed in detail. Important take-home messages for practitioners are also reviewed, with the most important being increased access to care.

24.2 Layperson Summary

VR, telepresence robots, and programmable robots are three emerging technologies in the field of autism intervention. The extent to which each technology has been incorporated into treatments for individuals on the autism spectrum varies. The evidence behind each treatment also varies, with research on VR and telepresence robots in autism intervention surpassing that of programmable

Matthew Roberts et al., *Robotics and Virtual Learning*. In: *Lifespan Treatment for Autistic Individuals*. Edited by: Peter Sturmey, Russell Lang, and James K. Luiselli, Oxford University Press. © Oxford University Press (2025).
DOI: 10.1093/oso/9780197635841.003.0024

robots. Regardless of their status in the field, each technology holds great potential. VR tightens the reliability of intervention delivery and has been used to provide immediate feedback for training in areas like social skills. With the ability to create and utilize a wide range of contingencies, VR reduces the need for controlled settings, such as classrooms. Whereas a social skills intervention may normally require several trainers, a virtual world only needs to be programmed to represent those trainers and other relevant contingencies. Telepresence robots allow practitioners to broaden their reach and increase access to care for marginalized populations, especially those living in more rural areas. By using telepresence technology, a practitioner or trainer can broadcast an intervention instantly, eliminating travel costs and boosting efficiency for both the client and practitioner. Similar to VR technology, programmable robots provide the opportunity to increase reliability by programming specific intervention contingencies to be delivered in a precise manner. Instead of displaying training through a screen, however, robots have a humanlike presence and can deliver an intervention as such.

24.3 Introduction

In 2018, the Center for Disease Control estimated that autism spectrum disorder (ASD) impacts 1 in 54 individuals—a 100% increase since 2006 when the rate was 1 in 110 individuals. This rapid increase calls for greater efforts by service providers to offer individualized care to a high volume of individuals across the lifespan, living in various geographical areas, despite shortages in qualified staff. Fortunately, the technological age in which we live has brought with it new methods of harnessing technology to bring valid and reliable interventions to individuals on the autism spectrum. Moreover, technological efficiency enables the provision of treatment to an increased number of individuals, particularly those who may not have previously had the means to access the care they need.

Individuals on the autism spectrum experience difficulties in social-emotional reciprocity, nonverbal communication, and developing and maintaining relationships, along with particularities in interest and motor skills (Zoder-Martell et al., 2021). Years of experimental and clinical research have resulted in the development of various behavioral interventions that have been shown to help individuals on the autism spectrum meet their treatment goals (Rodgers et al., 2021). In the current digital age, practitioners and researchers have increasingly focused on how technology can be leveraged to develop more effective and accessible training programs. For instance, technologies such as VR and telepresence robots can enable remote service provision, reducing the need for direct practitioner contact, eliminating the burden of travel, and expanding the reach of practitioners trained to deliver ASD interventions (Ashburner et al., 2016).

24.3.1 Degree of Immersion: What Is the Simplest Technology Needed for Behavior Change?

Dechsling et al. (2021) categorized the different kinds of VR simulation hardware used in research into (a) desktop/laptop/monitor, (b) handheld devices (e.g., tablets, smartphones), (c) CAVE/Kinect (e.g., motion sensors), (d) head-mounted displays (HMDs) (e.g., VR goggles, augmented reality/smart glasses). Depending on the simulation hardware, the participants experience varying degrees of immersion. A simple way to look at immersion is to ask how much of the real world versus the virtual environment the participant can see.

24.3.1.1 Nonimmersive Hardware

On the low end of the spectrum, the less immersive hardware includes desktop/laptop monitors. Participants using traditional screen monitors can typically see both the virtual environment on the screen and the real world. Researchers have found that participants have preconceived notions about nonimmersive hardware. When surveyed, participants expressed that regular desktop/laptop monitors are less interesting than modern HMDs. However, there is insufficient evidence to rule that more immersive VR training is more effective than training with nonimmersive hardware. One may even argue that "nonimmersive" is a misnomer. Although the learner is limited in their physical ability to manipulate the virtual environment (i.e., point-and-click interactions), there are extensive tools and strategies around how to increase the learner's interest and engagement in the content and increase the feeling of immersion despite the technical limitations. A highly realistic, nonimmersive simulation can still elicit strong emotional responses from some learners (Diemer et al., 2015).

24.3.1.2 Semi-immersive Hardware

Hardware like smart glasses, simulation caves, and robots is developed to bring the users halfway between the virtual and digital world. Users can engage with the virtual environment through motion sensors or webcams. While using these technologies, users can experience the virtual world without losing touch with the physical world around them. These technologies often require advanced programming software with some level of AI recognition to adapt to the user's immediate environment or to read the user's body language (see Proud et al., 2003, for a full rubric evaluating the level of autonomy for an AI).

24.3.1.3 Fully Immersive Hardware

The most visually immersive hardware is HMDs, given that they completely block out any view of the real world and other potential distractions. In most cases, users would engage with the virtual environment using handheld controllers, but mice and webcams can be used as replacements. A notable advantage over semi-immersive hardware is that immersive technology allows the developers full control of what the users can see. With immersive technology, developers can help users experience completely new realities they have never experienced before or cannot physically access.

24.3.2 Purpose of the Chapter

This chapter reviews three emerging and promising technologies for supporting individuals on the autism spectrum: VR, telepresence robots, and programmable robots. The degree to which each technology can support consultation, supervision, and training will be discussed, in addition to the potential of each technology for supporting autism intervention delivery.

One such technology which has recently seen an increased presence in practice and in societies around the world is VR (Huygelier et al., 2019). VR involves experiencing the sensory world through a virtual lens via some form of a digital display (e.g., monitors, projectors, HMDs) and controllers (e.g., keyboard, mouse, handheld controllers, motion caption camera). Virtual desktop and laptop simulations are common examples of less immersive VR training tools. Over recent years, immersive VR with HMDs has entered the broader culture as a popular way to experience entertainment, particularly video games (Pallavicini et al., 2019). This increase in demand brings with it faster improvements and efforts to promote accessibility. For these reasons, VR has become a valuable asset for other modes of utilization. When it comes to interventions for individuals on the autism spectrum, practitioners have found ways to incorporate VR technology into existing methodologies to strengthen reliability and increase efficiency and accessibility (Moon & Ke, 2021).

Telecommunication through telepresence robots has also witnessed an increased use among practitioners (King et al., 2021). The term *telepresence* has been defined as "the sense of being in another environment" (Kristoffersson et al., 2013, p. 1). Although difficult to achieve through traditional videoconferencing, several functional characteristics of mobile telepresence robots (MTRs) can enhance the perception of being physically present in a classroom during remote service delivery (Fischer, Bloomfield, et al., 2019). Such features lend themselves well to the interpersonal nature of direct instruction and indirect consultative support, offering educators and consultants a feasible option for ensuring the unabated delivery of student support.

Many telepresence robots include a docking system that incorporates video conferencing software (e.g., Zoom, GoMeet, Skype) onto a stationary or mobile robot device that can be operated from a remote location (Kristoffersson et al., 2013). In this fashion, a consultant or interventionist can control the functioning of the robot for purposes of direct/indirect service provision. In addition, there are two general types of telepresence robots. The first type is an MTR (e.g., Double Robot), where an individual moves the robot around the physical environment in which it is positioned (e.g., classroom, clinic). The second type is a stationary robot (e.g., Kubi Robot) that allows an individual to remotely alter the position of the camera's pane of view (i.e., left, right, up, down). Despite their functional differences, both robot types permit social interaction between two or more people located in geographically distant locations, lending to their applied value in supporting the behavioral outcomes of individuals on the autism spectrum.

The third technology with great potential for supporting individuals on the autism spectrum includes what are most known as robots. These lifelike entities can be programmed to display several human or animal-like behaviors. Many features of programmable robots are beneficial for training, research, and practice related to supporting individuals on the autism spectrum (Dautenhahn, 2003). These robots are typically humanoid in appearance and can behave in a human-like manner. For instance, they can move their limbs, speak, and react to voices and faces. The ability for these robots to be programmed to exhibit behavior based on what they see or hear in their environment grants robots large amounts of utility in a number of fields and, in our case, health and psycho-diagnostic intervention delivery.

An ongoing line of research continues to underscore the feasibility of integrating the technologies into ASD treatment programs and, furthermore, their potential to produce socially important outcomes (e.g., King et al., 2021; Lakatos et al., 2021; Smith et al., 2014). VR, telepresence robots, and programmable robots vary in their presence in practice today and in the amount of supporting research, and this chapter will discuss the current trends of each technology and highlight the existing literature. Additionally, the strengths and limitations inherent to each technology will be discussed. One of the most important strengths, and a key takeaway from this chapter, is how the flexibility afforded by technology can be harnessed to increase access to care. Due to recent advances in technology-informed ASD treatment programming, previously underserved communities (i.e., families with geographical or financial barriers) may now find quality treatment to be more accessible.

24.4 Virtual Reality

Treatment summary: Virtual Reality

Treatment description: VR utilizes preprogrammed contingencies to deliver training (i.e., social skills) to individuals on the autism spectrum. In its most immersive form, users wear a headset through which a training program is broadcasted, allowing the user to interact with the training and receive immediate feedback.

Expected outcomes: Research on using VR to deliver autism interventions has demonstrated positive outcomes for individuals on the autism spectrum in occupational and social skill areas.

Methods: Preprogrammed training programs deliver a training intervention through a screen. Interactive controllers allow users to respond and interact with the training and receive direct feedback. This process can be repeated as many times as necessary. Teachers and practitioners can now employ methods such as behavior skills training without the burden of obtaining resources such as additional trainers or controlled environments that are difficult to access.

Expertise required to implement treatment: Some knowledge of VR is recommended for any service providers wishing to incorporate this technology into their interventions. It is also recommended that practitioners are familiar with existing virtual training programs available to them. A background in autism intervention delivery is also strongly recommended.

Risks and negative side effects: Cybersickness, or motion sickness induced by a mismatch between the experienced virtual environment and the real outside world, is a common side effect of engaging with VR technology. Users can avoid cybersickness by taking frequent breaks. Users should also take the necessary precautions by making themselves aware of their surroundings before using VR technology.

Additional considerations and limitations: Anyone planning to use VR to deliver autism interventions should be aware of their client's personal preferences and capacities. Conditions that increase susceptibility to motion sickness (e.g., brain injuries, vertigo, or visual impairments) should be noted. Such considerations should be taken into account when planning a virtual training session.

Perhaps the most popular and accessible form of technology capable of supporting the implementation of ASD interventions is VR (Huygelier et al., 2019). VR has become a cornerstone of the technological world: changing the landscape of the videogame world and reinventing the way we experience our surroundings (Pallavicini et al., 2019). A virtual setting, or world, is a simulation of real-world environments containing various entities. Both the entities and the environment in which they exist are often manipulable by the player or user (Bartle, 2003). This feature renders VR ideal for interventions for which contingencies may need to be precisely altered. Furthermore, because some interventions require specific settings and multiple personnel, such simulations can be advantageous when the desired setting or personnel are unavailable. Schools, for instance, are full of bustling, tightly synchronized activity, making spare staff and empty classrooms difficult to come by. Such scarcity can be overcome by utilizing VR in educational settings, allowing the interventionist to customize the environment experienced by the student. This advantage can be particularly beneficial for students on the autism spectrum who may need to practice social skills in a highly structured environment.

Scholars have also explored the feasibility and effectiveness of providing direct instruction through VR with behavior skills training (BST). From daily living to social and safety skills, BST is effective for teaching complex skills to individuals on the autism spectrum (Leaf et al., 2015; Morgan & Wine, 2018). After providing instruction and modeling appropriate target behaviors, behavior analysts and technicians provide feedback to individuals on their performance (DiGennaro Reed & Henley, 2005; Shaprio & Kazemi, 2017). Although BST often leads to high levels of skill acquisition and treatment integrity (Schaefer & Andzik, 2021), it can be impractical to implement due to its high recurring cost of operation, such as the presence of an expert trainer to provide ongoing, individualized feedback on the learner's performance. As computers became more advanced and user-friendly, trainers were able to create self-directed asynchronous learning tools called computer-based instructions (CBIs) (Ramdoss et al., 2011). By incorporating CBIs into training, trainers were able to excuse themselves from the instruction, model portions of the training, and turn their focus toward the practice and feedback portions to deliver individualized performance feedback. With new immersive technology like VR becoming more accessible, behavior analysts have new mediums to explore and utilize to create engaging and effective interventions.

24.4.1 Practical Applications

Research on the clinical applications of VR technology has largely focused on teaching social skills to people on the autism spectrum in various settings. For instance, Ip et al. (2018) taught 94 children on the autism spectrum (age 6–12) emotional and social adaptation skills for daily living by having the learners engage with the virtual world projected onto large screens; learners' behaviors were tracked using a nonintrusive motion detection camera. For late-adolescent/adult learners who are in transition (i.e., from educational to professional settings), social skills in professional settings become an essential part of life. Smith et al. (2014) developed a nonimmersive VR job interview training to teach 16 adults on the autism spectrum how to appropriately navigate and answer interview questions using scripted video responses. The implications of this study cannot be understated. If practitioners working with transition-aged individuals can find a way to integrate VR into their toolkit, countless doors will be opened for prospective individuals on the autism spectrum.

In the tech industry, role plays digitally replicated in a virtual environment are referred to as "simulations." Arthur Glenberg, a cognitive psychology professor studying theory of cognition, described simulation as "thinking about possible consequences based on learning history." In his 2019 ABAI conference lecture, he stated that people learn through doing, especially complex verbal skills such as processing emotions and communication. In 2004, Glenberg and colleagues found that children who can manipulate items during story time are able to better infer questions. Then later, Davidson (2010) published an article on his observations of how an inability to physically express negative emotions by frowning can lead to longer latency to vocally communicate negative emotions. And to further confirm that simulations are helpful for teaching complex skills, Kontra et al. (2015) taught angular momentum and vector addition to college students and replicated it with children with disabilities. They found that learners who got to experience the physical sensations performed better on the posttest.

With the demand for autism treatment services on the rise, it is critical for behavior analysts to leverage VR simulations to improve patient care. Behavior analysts have the background necessary to set up real-world environments for skill development. By applying the same behavioral principles to the digital space, behavior analysts can create innovative learning experiences that support skill growth.

24.4.1.1 Nonimmersive Technology

Setting out to make training programs more accessible, Smith et al. (2014) developed a highly autonomous artificial intelligence (AI) conversation partner that plays the role of a job recruiter interviewing a candidate for a position. After demonstrating positive outcomes for individuals on the autism spectrum, the authors replicated these findings in other populations, including individuals with schizophrenia (Smith et al., 2015a), posttraumatic stress disorder (Smith et al., 2015b), and substance abuse disorder (Smith et al., 2016). Importantly, Ward and Esposito (2018) replicated Smith et al.'s (2014) findings with another cohort of adolescents on the autism spectrum, further contributing to the growing literature on VR-informed ASD treatment.

During the instruction portion of the simulation, learners have access to digital resources that inform them about common interview questions and etiquettes. Models of appropriate responses are also provided in both written and spoken form. When the learner is ready to begin the rehearsal by starting the simulation, they will first be greeted by a female job recruiter AI named Molly Porter®. Through branching conversation, learners can practice navigating interview questions ranging in difficulty from low to high. On the low difficulty, Smith and colleagues programmed Molly to be friendlier and more forgiving of mistakes made by the learners. However, on a higher difficulty setting, Molly is programmed to openly display her disdain for the user's incorrect response with head shakes and changes in her tone of voice. High-difficulty Molly is designed to test for generalization of skills and would put users in unexpected scenarios like asking them illegal interview questions (i.e., What is your age or religious background?).

One important takeaway from the VR-JIT project is that advanced technology is not always necessary to create an effective asynchronous simulation. Using nonimmersive technology like desktops and laptops can achieve performance improvement without requiring extensive financial investment in the early development stages. Especially with new online no-code software builders, trainers with little or no programming experience can recreate effective in-person role plays into asynchronous simulations.

24.4.1.2 Immersive Technology

Yuan and Ip (2018) used VR to teach emotional and social skills to children on the autism spectrum in Hong Kong. A total of 72 students (average age 8) on the autism spectrum were divided into two groups. Half of the students were presented with a VR training, while the other half acted as the control group and received the same training at a later time. During the training, a group of three to four students would first review what they learned about the targeted skills in previous lessons and then individually enter the Cave Automatic Virtual Environment (CAVE) for practice, in which the virtual environment is projected onto the walls and the participant can interact by moving freely in the space, in front of motion sensors. Each training session lasted an hour and ended with a discussion session to review the lessons learned and ways to apply them to real life. The authors designed six learning scenarios to best replicate a typical day of a primary school–aged child in Hong Kong.

24.4.2 VR Simulation: Stand-Alone Training or Supplement Material?

VR simulations can be presented in a synchronous, asynchronous, or hybrid format. In a synchronous format, human trainers hide behind a virtual avatar and model social and natural consequences of participants' behavior. With asynchronous VR training programs, human trainers are not required to be present at all. The trainer would need to preprogram the AI with a decision-making tree, but the AI will independently respond accordingly, contingent on the participant's behavior. Hybrid formats are typically involved asynchronous training programs combined with in-person probes and optional feedback reviews (Chang et al., 2022).

24.4.3 Strengths and Limitations of Virtual Reality

Summarizing the results of their systematic literature review of VR training with autonomous AI between 2010 and 2020, Chang et al. (2020) found that VR training is not only effective but also popular among participants, parents, teachers, and trainers. For instance, users found VR training to be more engaging and fun, while parents and teachers witnessed participants display newly acquired skills in natural settings. Further, lower rates of attrition occurred for participants who were trained with VR compared to traditional learning methods (e.g., in-person lectures). Another strength of VR training is its capability to accurately capture a participant's live performance. Data can be collected, reviewed, and used as feedback to improve performance over time.

Despite the documented benefits of VR, a notable limitation of this technology regards its potential to elicit motion sickness. Whether from wearing a VR headset, riding on a roller coaster, or rocking about on a boat out at sea, the physical discomforts induced by motion sickness can affect almost anyone and must be considered when implementing ASD interventions using VR technology. Motion sickness caused by extended VR usage is called cybersickness. Existing full-immersive

VR hardware is not built for users to use for extended periods of time (del Cid et al., 2020). Yuan and Ip (2018) mentioned that due to previous bad experiences with VR technology, some participants were initially reluctant to participate, but all reported habituation to wearing the technology within three training sessions. Similarly, in a more recent study, Palmisano and Constable (2022) found that some people can habituate to cybersickness over time, but switching to a different simulation requires the user to habituate to the new training. Existing computer-based instructions (e.g., Relias, SmarterU) tend to string multiple short modules together for one extended training session. If VR is to become a common tool for services providers working with individuals on the autism spectrum, it is important that they consider these limitations and continue to find promising solutions.

24.4.4 Practical Recommendations and Future Directions

As we have discussed, VR technology, when applied correctly, can have numerous benefits for ASD-focused interventions. The alleviation of concerns related to social abilities and professional skills can help ease the stress of childhood and pave the path to success for transition-aged individuals on the autism spectrum. Customizing environments, amplifying accessibility, and pinpointing contingency control are all ways that VR contributes to preexisting interventions, and bringing those advantages into practice helps alleviate the concerns posed by ASD, allowing individuals to discover their capacities and utilize their strengths out in the world. In the future, practitioners must be diligent in their efforts to integrate VR into their work. By the same token, researchers and practitioners examining interventions for ASD should direct their attention toward better understanding the consequences of combining VR technology with ASD interventions.

24.4.4.1 Direct Service Provision

There is growing evidence supporting the use of VR simulations to increase skill acquisition among people with and without disabilities (Chang et al., 2022; Mosher & Carreon, 2021; Rebelo et al., 2012). Scholars argue that several unique attributes of simulated environments are likely implicated in the effectiveness of VR treatment, such as (a) unlimited opportunities to practice newly learned skills, (b) breadth of role-playing scenarios, (c) accurate and continuous performance measurement, (d) controlled yet customizable learning environment, (e) freedom from harmful social and natural consequences, and (f) affordable and accessible learning opportunities (Chang et al., 2022; Rebelo et al., 2012). Researchers have been using VR simulations to teach skills for more than a decade, with a heavy focus on teaching social skills (Chang et al., 2022). For instance, Lorenzo et al. (2016) used VR to teach children ages 7–12 how to identify emotions, identify emotions, initiate a conversation, and respond to peer interactions. Similarly, Ke and Moon (2018) used a 3D virtual playground with a social-gaming component to improve prosocial interactions among eight children ages 10–14 on the autism spectrum. Lastly, safety skills have been tested; for instance, Parish-Morris et al. (2018)used Floreo Police Safety Modules to teach 28 adolescents and adults on the autism spectrum how to interact with police.

24.5 Telepresence Robots

Treatment summary: Telepresence Robots

Treatment description: Consultants successfully used telepresence robots to remotely train educators to support the behavioral and academic needs of individuals on the autism spectrum. To date, these indirect supports occurred in schools and specifically focused on educators' adherence to functional analysis procedures, student compliance with educator requests, and increasing students' ability to discriminate numbers.

Expected outcomes: Previous research has shown that training delivered via telepresence robots successfully increased educators' adherence to evidence-based behavior assessment procedures, students' compliance with educators' requests, and students' ability to accurately discriminate numbers.

Methods: Using telepresence robots, consultants met with educators across several sessions to conceptualize student needs, deliver behavioral skills training until a training-based criterion was met, explore environmental considerations for treatment delivery, provide ongoing performance feedback to educators based on their adherence to treatment components, and measure students' response to treatment.

Expertise required to implement treatment: It is recommended that consultants, who plan to deliver support through telepresence robots, increase their knowledge of and experience with videoconferencing software, privacy laws respective to the state in which remote supports will be delivered, and strategies to maintain a strong working alliance with team members during remote service provision.

Risks and negative side effects: An unstable Internet connection can negatively impact the fluidity of communication during videoconferencing, clarity of video and audio, and the consultant's ability to remotely access the telepresence robot's functions. In addition, the ability of the MTR to traverse environments is partially limited by its maximum speed capability, indicating that it may fall short of capturing all occurrences of behavior. Lastly, the novelty of a telepresence robot may result in reactivity until the client becomes accustomed to its presence. An unstable Internet connection can negatively impact the fluidity of communication during videoconferencing, clarity of video and audio, and the consultant's ability to remotely access the telepresence robot's functions. In addition, the ability of the MTR to traverse environments is restricted by its maximum speed capability, indicating that it may fall short of capturing all occurrences of behavior. Lastly, the novelty of telepresence robots may result in some reactivity until individuals acclimate to its presence.

Additional considerations and limitations: Clinicians most often use telepresence robots to indirectly support individuals on the autism spectrum through educator and caregiver consultation. While a growing literature supports the use of this technology for purposes of indirect service delivery, scholars have yet to explicate best practices for the direct provision of ASD support via telepresence robots. Thus, it will be helpful to consider who most often works with the client and whether it would be more feasible and socially valid to remotely provide that individual(s) with the knowledge and skills needed to support their delivery of a respective ASD treatment program.

Individuals with ASD often present with complex social-communicative impairments that limit their ability to form close relationships and benefit from academic instruction (Bellini et al., 2007; Zoder-Martell et al., 2021). These impairments can be quite pervasive and are unlikely to diminish over time (Tantam, 2003), underscoring the need for early and effective intervention. Traditionally delivered in-person, evidence-based strategies that have shown to effectively target some of the core deficits of ASD can be comprehensive and time-intensive (Tachibana et al., 2017), indicating that ongoing training and performance feedback is often necessary to support a clinician's adherence to treatment procedures. Considering some of the well-known barriers to in-person service provision (e.g., travel, time, expenses), scholars have increasingly recognized the importance of ensuring the unabated, remote delivery of these supports via technological means, such as videoconferencing and telepresence robots. While empirical evaluations of telepresence robots are sparse within the behavioral and educational literature, they are emerging (King et al., 2021). This line of study has focused primarily on evaluating the feasibility, acceptability, and efficacy of delivering school psychology services through telepresence robots to engender socially significant changes in individuals on the autism spectrum, as well as their educators.

24.5.1 Teleconsultation and Telepresence Robots

In the field of education, consultants are privy to several models of consultation when working with students and educators. Of those models (e.g., conjoint-behavioral; Sheridan & Kratochwill; consultee-centered; Caplan, 1970; instructional; Rosenfield, 1987), problem-solving consultation (PSC) has the strongest empirical support for supporting student and staff behavior in school settings (Erchul & Ward, 2016). The theoretical underpinnings of PSC are grounded in the principles of applied behavior analysis, lending itself to a structured yet collaborative process that places emphasis on the attainment of targeted outcomes (e.g., compliance, work completion, social engagement). While traditionally delivered in person, [tele]consultants have increasingly relied on technology as a medium through which to deliver PSC, which is generally referred to as teleconsultation. This mode of indirect service delivery allows consultants to work with their consultees irrespective of geographic location and other constraints associated with in-person service delivery. Consequently, the flexibility afforded by teleconsultation is primarily realized in its ability to increase access to care for those in need (Fischer et al., 2017). In addition, teleconsultation has not only shown to result in reductions in travel time and travel costs but also improvements in a consultee's adherence to the components of a treatment program and the social and behavioral outcomes of individuals on the autism spectrum (Gibson et al., 2010; Young & Ireson, 2003).

24.5.2 Practical Applications

To better understand the overall status of the school-based teleconsultation literature, King et al. (2021) summarized the outcomes of 13 studies that reported the use of telecommunication technologies to deliver school psychology services. Of those studies, only three used telepresence robots and provided a clear demonstration of how this technology can be incorporated into the PSC model to support the outcomes of students on the autism spectrum and their respective special educators (Bloomfield et al., 2020; Fischer, Bloomfield, et al., 2019; Fischer, Clark, et al., 2019). As such, each study is described below in terms of the interventions used, primary and secondary outcomes, and the type of technology used to facilitate support to students on the autism spectrum and their support staff.

24.5.2.1 Academic Intervention

Fischer, Bloomfield et al. (2019) used the Kubi Robot to coach educators on a stimulus-fading intervention designed to increase a student's ability to expressively discriminate three numbers (e.g., 7, 8, and 9). Stimulus fading is a strategy used to gradually increase one's ability to independently complete a difficult task. For example, in the present study, the researchers targeted the student's vocal expression of numbers. They approached this by first presenting the student with a flashcard that included seven printed dots overlaid with the numerical image of the number seven. Over time, and contingent upon expressing the correct number, researchers gradually decreased the opacity of the number so that only the dot configuration remained. Following the gradual fading of the number's visibility, the student successfully recognized and vocally indicated the numerical value of only the dot configuration.

This study included three distinct phases, all of which were conducted via the Kubi Robot. The first phase was an assessment of the student's baseline number discrimination performance, during which the robot was positioned in view of the work area, allowing the consultant to directly observe the educator's delivery of several number discrimination tasks. Next, the consultant and educator collaboratively developed a behavior intervention plan followed by one virtual training session to ensure that the educator felt comfortable in their abilities to implement the plan. During the implementation phase of their study, the educator demonstrated high levels of treatment integrity and endorsed commensurate levels of technological acceptability. In terms of student outcomes, the stimulus fading procedures effectively increased the student's ability to vocally discriminate the numerical value of each dot formation associated with three distinct numbers.

24.5.2.2 Behavior Assessment

Bloomfield et al. (2020) used the Double MTR to train four educators on functional analysis (FA) procedures and the stationary Kubi Robot to directly observe educators' delivery of such procedures to three students with an educational classification of autism. FA is a systematic procedure for identifying the environmental variables that reliably evoke and reinforce the occurrence of a behavior. Although FA is generally considered to be a more intrusive method of assessment relative to indirect and descriptive procedures, it is the most precise method for identifying the environmental variables surrounding the occurrence of a behavior. This underscores the importance of training educators on FA procedures (Nesselrode et al., 2022).

During educators' delivery of the FA, the Kubi Robot was positioned in the corner of the room, allowing for a clear view of the assessment area. Using videoconferencing, the consultants interacted with educators via a tablet that was positioned on top of the Kubi Robot, which allowed for immediate performance feedback during role-play scenarios. The results of their study showed that educators demonstrated moderate to high levels of FA procedural integrity and reported high levels of acceptability for the use of telepresence robots to facilitate training.

24.5.2.3 Behavior Intervention

In response to limited resources in a rural school district, Fischer, Bloomfield, et al. (2019) examined the feasibility of telepresence robots to increase compliance in three students with an educational classification of traumatic brain injury, intellectual disability, and autism. Following one on-site meeting to describe the nature of the study and obtain informed consent, teleconsultation procedures were conducted remotely via two telepresence robots, the mobile Double Robot and the stationary Kubi Robot. Consultants remotely trained each educator on data collection procedures and a three-step prompting compliance intervention (Wilder et al., 2012) until they reached mastery criteria. Following training, educators positioned the telepresence robot in a location within their classroom that allowed the remote consultant to observe the educator's adherence to intervention components and the student's response to intervention.

The results of Fischer, Bloomfield, et al.'s study showed that, with ongoing performance feedback, teachers successfully adhered to the three-step prompting intervention that successfully resulted in moderate increases in compliance for all three students (omnibus Tau-U effect size of .70; Vannest & Ninci 2015). Furthermore, teachers endorsed high levels of technology acceptability with receiving behavioral support via telepresence robots.

24.5.3 Strengths and Limitations of Telepresence Robots

Despite the limited available evidence on the use of telepresence robots to facilitate teleconsultation, the above studies underscore their potential to support not only the outcomes of students on the autism spectrum but also educators' capacity to implement behaviorally focused assessment and intervention strategies.

Furthermore, across these studies, educators endorsed high levels of technology acceptability, which is a noteworthy outcome as previous research shows that individuals who reside in underserved communities tend to endorse limited access to and knowledge of technology applications (Mitchell et al., 2019). In the current digital age, technology has undoubtedly resulted in more convenient and, in some cases, efficient modes of service provision (Fallon et al., 2020; von Hagen et al., 2021). While consultants are encouraged to familiarize themselves with telecommunication technologies to broaden their service delivery repertoire, they should also remain aware of others' (e.g., consultees, clients) comfort with technology use. Thus, for consultants who support the outcomes of children and youth on the autism spectrum through telepresence robots, ongoing collaboration on technology use should be a staple throughout the consultation process.

In addition, the practical value of telepresence robots hinges on the degree to which their functional properties remain viable in certain treatment contexts. With regard to teleconsultation, the Double and Kubi Robots allow the consultant to remotely alter the camera's pane of view to ensure continued observation of the client and/or consultee in the treatment setting. Indeed, this function should suffice in most environments; however, events may arise during school-based teleconsultation that test the capabilities of a stationary telepresence robot (i.e., camera mobility; Bice-Urbach & Kratochwill, 2016). For instance, previous research indicates that elopement is one of the most challenging behaviors that students on the autism spectrum exhibit (Scheithauer et al., 2021). In the absence of adult supervision, elopement can expose the student to dangerous situations both within and outside the classroom setting. This is an important consideration, given that the "stationary" Kubi Robot remains effective so long as individuals remain physically present within the observation area. While this is a notable limitation of the Kubi Robot, the Double Robot does afford the luxury of physical movement, yet at the expense of greater cost for purchase.

Indeed, there are some noteworthy limitations to MTRs, such as the speed at which they can traverse environments. While no study has empirically evaluated the necessary speed to effectively use MTRs in treatment contexts that involve physical movement, the manufacturing specifications of the Double Robot, for example, specify a mobility speed comparable to that of a slow/moderate walking pace (e.g., 2–3 miles per hour; Barreira et al., 2010). Thus, while the Double Robot presumably would allow individuals to engage in conversation when transitioning from room to room, its maximum speed capability may limit [tele]consultants' ability to remain in proximity to students on the autism spectrum who have a history of "bolting" (i.e., running away from adults; Scheithauer et al., 2021).

24.5.4 Practical Recommendations and Future Directions

The recency of stationary robots and MTRs leaves much to be said in terms of empirical guidance for harnessing their capabilities in certain treatment contexts.

For instance, to our knowledge, literature on the use of telepresence robots for supporting students on the autism spectrum has primarily focused on indirect service delivery within the field of education (King et al., 2021). While special educators and support staff often engage in interdisciplinary collaboration to coordinate services for their students, their primary role involves the direct implementation of academic and behavior support (Billingsley & Bettini, 2019). Unfortunately, health issues, weather conditions, structural barriers, or personal matters may arise that prevent educators from being physically present within the classroom setting (Lee et al., 2015). With assistance from on-site staff, the mobility function of telepresence robots may accommodate special educators' ability to directly interact with their students through telepresence (i.e., virtual presence via the telepresence robot). The use of MTRs in this context could have socially valid implications for the remote delivery of behavior support.

24.5.4.1 Direct Service Provision

Antecedent manipulations have been shown to effectively reduce different forms of disruptive behavior among children and youth on the autism spectrum, such as elopement (Boyle & Adamson, 2017; Conroy et al., 2004). Previous research indicates that staff attention, in the form of redirection, is often provided to students who elope from a teacher-designated area (Boyle et al., 2017; Piazza et al., 1997). Thus, in the case of attention-maintained elopement, the delivery of noncontingent reinforcement and proximity control via MTRs may provide educators with a feasible method for preventing instances of elopement and other behaviors maintained by attention. For instance, the videoconferencing and mobility features of MTRs bolster the educator's telepresence, allowing them to traverse the classroom environment and engage in face-to-face interaction with their students. In this fashion, the proximity of the MTR and periodic delivery of verbal praise, or otherwise positive statements, may effectively decrease students' need to engage in disruptive behavior maintained by attention.

Nonetheless, the formal characteristics of an MTR may pose unique considerations for facilitating classroom management strategies. For example, because ASD is characterized by deficits in social communication, the absence of anatomically correct human features on an MTR and the two-dimensional presentation of facial features on a screen may negatively impact the social perception and visual attention of students on the autism spectrum. Consequently, hindrances to social perception and visual attention may depress the validity and clarity of "remotely delivered" praise statements. Furthermore, students with developmental disabilities may experience a lack of habituation to and sensory overstimulation from the novel features of an MTR, even in light of continued exposure (Jarvinen et al., 2013; Vivanti et al., 2018). Thus, one potential solution to this issue may involve the development of a telepresence robot equipped with humanlike features, such as manipulation-capable robot arms (Cha et al., 2017). While yet to be substantiated in K-12 settings with those on the autism spectrum, exploring this line of study would represent a fruitful addition to the literature on telepresence robots.

24.6 Programmable Robots

Treatment summary: Programmable Robots

Treatment description: Lifelike entities called robots can be programmed to deliver interventions for teaching skills to individuals on the autism spectrum. Without the need for a direct practitioner, interventions can be programmed to reliably teach occupational and social skills to a vast number of individuals with fewer time constraints.

Expected outcomes: Robot-mediated interventions have been shown to successfully teach skills relevant to challenges associated with autism. Although research directly examining responses for individuals on the autism spectrum is limited, research would suggest that such individuals would respond positively to robot-mediated training.

Methods: Robot-mediated service provision involves programming robots to deliver interventions with previously demonstrated effectiveness. Recipients and providers can customize delivery based on personal preference to maximize engagement.

Expertise required to implement treatment: Some familiarity with the mechanisms of action for robot-mediated intervention is necessary for effective delivery. This includes an understanding of how delivery translates from a human teacher/practitioner to a robotic service provider.

Risks and negative side effects: Given their fully robotic nature, robot utilization may lack the adult supervision necessary to manage challenging behavior. Additionally, technical difficulties may arise when using robots to deliver interventions, calling for increased precaution when engaging in intervention delivery.

Additional considerations and limitations: The flexibility and versatility of robots make them ideal for delivering a wide array of autism interventions.

Programmable robots are what most of us think of when we hear the term "robots." These are typically physical entities that interact with the environment. Consequently, programmable robots can be designed and programmed to imitate skills training normally provided by an interventionist. Humanoid robots are the most commonly used robots for applications in autism services (Ismail et al., 2017) and are characterized by their humanlike shape or features. There are two classes of humanoid robots: animatronics and robotics. Animatronics and robotics are both machines that can be operated by humans or preprogrammed using computers. Robots and animatronics are distinguished by their appearance, such that robots appear more "machine-like," whereas animatronics are developed to resemble living beings (e.g., electronic toy dogs). The lifelike appearance of animatronic robots offers a unique social component that has the potential to bolster the acceptability and efficacy of robot-informed therapy. For example, the KASPAR robot) looked strikingly similar to a human child and was designed to be a therapeutic toy for children with autism (Ismail et al., 2018).

The key feature of the robots used in research surrounding autism services compared to other robots (i.e., NAO, PROBO, KASPAR) is that they are usually social robots. This means that their AI systems are designed to specifically interact with humans, rather than being designed to complete simple motor tasks, such as mechanically working in a factory setting or lifting large objects. These robots are designed in a way that makes their primary function involve human interaction. This can range from making facial expressions to talking and dancing in front of a human audience. However, not all social robots are humanoid robots. For example, the Keepon Pro is a small yellow robot with a snowman-like appearance that has been used with children who have difficulty with interpersonal communication (Ismail et al., 2017).

Most social robots, specifically humanoid ones, can move their limbs, speak, and react to voices and faces. The ability for these robots to be programmed to exhibit behavior based on what they see or hear in their environment gives them a lot of utility. The NAO (pronounced "now") robot by SoftBank Robotics is an excellent example and one of the most popular programmable robots used today.

There are two ways programmable robots can be used. One way is with a human operator actively controlling the robot from a distance using a computer. The other way is by preprogramming the robot to engage in different behaviors based on what it is seeing or hearing, often referred to as "autonomous" control. Both methods are often used and have their own benefits and weaknesses. A human controlling the robot from a distance often referred to as "Wizard-of-Oz" control, is beneficial because it is easy to modify the robot's behavior in real time and react to unexpected circumstances or technical difficulties. The downside to this kind of control is that it reduces the value of the robot's demonstration. The value is reduced because if the robot requires a human operator, the human could perform the procedures the robot attempts to demonstrate. The alternative, autonomous control, is the ideal method of utilization for robot-mediated intervention. However, it is extremely difficult to program robots to autonomously engage in and react to a lot of the environmental variables present during therapy sessions for individuals on the autism spectrum. For example, if a robot was designed to conduct a round of discrete trial training trials, it could reliably provide praise as a reinforcer after a correct response, but there is no way to program the robot to autonomously address escape-maintained problem behavior that may arise due to these trials.

Researchers have been creative in the development of these robots to support children with autism in other ways. One way is teaching necessary skills to teachers and practitioners. Robots, simulating clients, can be helpful for training because the trainees are exposed to real-life scenarios and challenges (e.g., a client experiencing a breakdown of emotions), access new or rare experiences (e.g., a client engaging in self-injury in the form of hitting their own head), obtain immediate performance feedback from the robot or a trainer standing by, and repeatedly practice in a safe environment. Kazemi and Stedman-Falls (2016) demonstrated this utility by using an NAO robot as a simulated client to teach students to conduct two different types of preference assessments. The study demonstrated that people perform preference assessments with actual children similarly regardless of whether they had a human actor or a robot present for their training.

Another use for these robots in practice is to serve as a reinforcer for appropriate behavior. Social robots typically have the capability to sing and dance to children's favorite songs and dances, and their humanlike appearance does offer a social component. Playing with these robots can be very reinforcing (Hudson & Lewis, 2020). Additional studies have shown that many individuals on the autism spectrum are more enthusiastic when interacting with robots instead of people (Begum et al., 2016). The benefits do not cease with merely increased enthusiasm. Social robots have contributed to increases in valuable activities such as increased attention, imitation, verbal utterances, and social activities (Begum et al., 2016; Kim et al., 2013; Wainer et al., 2014). Additionally, social robots have been used as tools attractors, mediators, and measurement tools in autism services (Pennisi et al., 2016). They have been effective at motivating children with autism who are receiving services to attend to different activities. A common pattern in many of the studies in the area of robotics and autism is the primary emphasis on the domains of social interaction and communication skills (DiPietro et al., 2019). Although this might be the case, some researchers have also begun to explore the utility of social robots when teaching more complicated skills like theory of mind and visual perspective-taking skills (Lakatos et al., 2021).

As researchers are gathering more information and building on previous work, one study has taken this area of literature further than many may have thought possible and utilized a robot in the position of a therapist to teach skills (Korneder et al., 2021). Korneder et al. (2021) used a NAO robot to teach children with autism intraverbal skills. The robot was able to implement a very simple procedure using prompt delays to teach children to answer WH- questions. While prompt delays are simple and straightforward procedures to implement, the robot's ability to implement the procedure and achieve significant results highlights the potential of these robots in these spaces.

Although the results are mixed, we are seeing autonomy move toward a position wherein research will begin to evaluate whether robots can support teaching skills. One study utilized a robot as an assistive tool to teach listener responding skills. Rather than instructing the participant to touch specific stimuli, the child was instructed to send the robot over to the correct stimuli (Chaldi & Mantzanidou, 2021). The researchers found that children were actually more willing to participate when using the robot compared to when only using action cards. This research supports other studies, such as one by Hudson and Lewis (2020), which demonstrated that play with robots can be used as a reinforcer to increase appropriate behavior.

The literature surrounding the increasing robot presence in ASD services continues to grow today. At Easterseals Southern California, in a collaborative effort with California State University, Northridge, behavior analysts are conducting experiments in which a robot will serve as an actual therapist to conduct a reinforcer assessment. Rather than being an assistive tool or playing a supportive role, a robot will actually be conducting the assessment across from an actual child and collecting data. These behavior analysts are also conducting another experiment utilizing a robot to provide feedback to new behavior interventionists on their ability to teach listener responding skills.

Ideally, the utilization of robots for robot-mediated intervention would reduce the cost of direct service provision and increase the accessibility of behavioral services to low-income and low-population areas. However, this is not yet the current reality due to the novelty of robotics research in the field of behavior analysis. Robots are not yet at a level where they can implement all of the necessary programs required for socially significant behavior change. Barriers include lack of research, empirical demonstrations, and support in public opinion. It is difficult to argue the benefits of a robot therapist when a trained human is likely to do the job much better, gain more support, and build stronger rapport.

A robot is able to complete tasks with pinpoint consistency that is difficult for a human to achieve. Additionally, they are able to make data-based decisions using data they gather in real time. If programmed effectively, a robot could demonstrate the skills necessary to conduct many different procedures. However, research continues to demonstrate that people generally perform better in human-mediated sessions rather than in robot-mediated alternatives (Begum et al., 2016; Bekele et al., 2014; Duoquette et al., 2008).

24.6.1 Strengths and Limitations of Programmable Robots

If you are planning to use programmable robots in areas like schools, homes, or clinics, proceed with caution. First, be sure that you know the robot's role, and be aware of its proven capabilities. It is not ethical to consider a session fully implemented by a robot without supervision to be in the best interest of the client. However, using a programmable robot as a reinforcer is acceptable. Given the current literature in robotics and behavior analysis, this is the most acceptable position for a robot to be currently when in an applied setting. Not every client will find the robot's participation reinforcing. However, for clients that do, a programmable robot can be extremely effective. Its ability to perform preferred activities can be tailored specifically for the client's individual interests. This ability limits satiation that can occur with more mundane toys or activities.

Accessibility is a limitation of programmable robots when applied to interventions. Whereas virtual technology can be broadcast anywhere with a reliable Internet connection, the use of programmable robots requires face-to-face contact. Consequently, either the client must travel to the programmable robot, or the programmable robot must be transported to the client. Such efforts may be expensive for the client and/or practitioner and could complicate the logistics of service delivery. In particular, rural populations living in remote areas may find it more difficult to access the services made available by programmable robots.

24.6.2 Practical Recommendations and Future Directions

In the future, robots may serve as behavior intervention implementers, trainers, or simulated clients for training purposes. However, to get there, more research will need to be established. Specifically, in order for a robot to implement one or more parts of an intervention, the robot-mediated portion of that intervention must become evidence-based. Robots are moving quickly to the role of trainers and simulated clients. They have already been applied to play these roles, although it is not widespread or common in practice.

There are a few barriers to the establishment of robot-mediated interventions as evidence-based practices that need to be addressed by robotics researchers. Two of the primary reasons that robot-mediated interventions have not been more widespread in a clinical space are a lack of research reporting demonstrating experimental control and a lack of replicability. The description of the materials used in robot-mediated intervention studies is often insufficient for replication. Researchers need to be more explicit in the description of the software and strategies used in the programming of their robots so other researchers can replicate their methods (Begum et al., 2016).

We may also begin to see an intersection of different types of technologies. If a robot is programmed to work as a trainer, it is possible that there can be an augmented reality component in the training environment. This could be beneficial for programming common stimuli into the teaching procedure, promoting the generalization of skills learned in the teaching environment to the natural environment.

24.6.2.1 Direct Service Provision

Few instances exist in which a robot has provided direct services to individuals on the autism spectrum, but a study by Korneder et al. (2021) demonstrated a robot's utility in teaching a new skill to a child. They recruited three children with ASD who had a history of using WH- questions (i.e., questions that begin with what, who, and where), but could not demonstrate the skill in the baseline phase. Using a multiple-baseline design, they demonstrated that a robot could teach children to answer WH- questions by implementing a simple intraverbal teaching procedure using a time-delay prompt hierarchy. Although researchers delivered social praise for correct responding and closed incorrect trials by saying things like "Let's try again," the robot delivered instructions and prompts. Each participant in the study showed improvement only when the robot-mediated intervention was introduced. Although the robot is capable of presenting reinforcers, in this particular study, the researchers presented the reinforcers. Although research is in the process of demonstrating the utility of programmable robots in providing services for individuals with autism, it is still highly unethical to use a robot to provide direct services outside of an experimental setting due to the lack of research needed to establish robot-mediated intervention as an evidence-based practice.

24.7 Conclusion

The possibilities for AI-mediated ASD interventions are bountiful, offering numerous benefits to the increasing number of individuals and their families. When we harness the power of technology to support intervention implementation, we can bring better, faster training to the hands of people who need it most. With the incorporation of technology, training no longer needs to be one-size-fits-all but rather suits the individual based on their unique needs. Technology is highly customizable yet still consistent and standardized. It does not experience fatigue or drift. The ability to design and program virtual worlds, AI-conversational partners, and robots further enhances the fidelity with which treatment is delivered and evaluated across large user bases without significantly increasing the cost of operation. Lastly, and perhaps most importantly, technologically bolstered interventions help facilitate widespread access to treatment. Individuals and families who may have lacked the resources to access quality care now have the ability to connect remotely. With the incidence and prevalence of ASD diagnoses rapidly increasing in recent years, rendering high-quality interventions readily available to the broadest possible populations should be the primary goal of ASD researchers and practitioners.

24.7.1 Newer Is Not Always Better

While it is highly advantageous to explore new technology (e.g., HMDs, augmented reality glasses), it is just as important to find innovative ways to combine the technology that is already available to us. Technology is not and should not be mutually exclusive. The intersection of VR technology, telepresence robots, and programmable robots in practice can be greatly beneficial to its recipients. This intersection falls into the realms of mixed reality or extended reality. Recall hardware's degree of immersion, as discussed in previous sections. AI-powered learning experiences come in varying degrees of immersion, with different benefits and limitations. For instance, during the pandemic, behavioral services were difficult to provide via telehealth because there were no trained intervention implementers present with the participants. However, if an agency has the resources to provide animatronic companions to participants, then there may be less disruption to services. In this example, the behavior analyst can combine a virtual world with a telepresence robot whereby the practitioner broadcasts a virtual world directly to the client and provides remote access to combined instruction through a virtual lens. By using common hardware (e.g., webcam, projectors) with newer technology (e.g., animatronics), behavior analysts can create learning experiences of varying degrees of immersion.

In this chapter, we have discussed three emerging technologies, all of which have shown promise in supporting individuals on the autism spectrum. In the years ahead, as technology becomes more available to various populations, we will likely see further utilization of technology in supporting individuals seeking psychological care. Service providers should pay close attention to these trends and constantly be on the lookout for ways to incorporate technology into their practice. Doing so will help providers stay at the forefront of intervention delivery, ensure that their clients are receiving the most up-to-date services, and promote the greatest level of accessibility. Researchers can support this process by improving our understanding of how technology impacts treatment delivery. Understanding this process is critical for making sure that both providers and recipients are fully aware of the risks that emerge when moving from a traditional, hands-on model to a technology-mediated model of intervention delivery.

24.8 References

Ashburner, J., Vickerstaff, S., Beetge, J., & Copley, J. (2016). Remote versus face-to-face delivery of early intervention programs for children with autism spectrum disorders: Perceptions of rural families and service providers. *Research in Autism Spectrum Disorders, 23*(1), 1–14. https://doi-org.ezproxy.shsu.edu/10.1016/j.rasd.2015.11.011

Barreira, T. V., Rowe, D. A., & Kang, M. (2010). Parameters of walking and jogging in healthy young adults. *International Journal of Exercise Science, 3*(1), 4–13. https://digitalcommons.wku.edu/ijes/vol3/iss1/2

Bartle, R. A. (2003). *Creating virtual worlds.* Creative Commons Licence 4.0

Begum, M., Serna, R. W., & Yanco, H. A. (2016). Are robots ready to deliver autism interventions? A comprehensive review. *International Journal of Social Robotics, 8*(2), 157–181. DOI: 10.1007/s12369-016-0346-y

Bekele, E., Crittendon, J. A., Swanson, A., Sarkar, N., & Warren, Z. E. (2014). Pilot clinical application of an adaptive robotic system for young children with Autism. *Autism, 18*(5), 598–608. https://doi.org/10.1177/1362361313479454

Bellini, S., Peters, J. K., Benner, L., & Hopf, A. (2007). A meta-analysis of school-based social skills interventions for children with autism spectrum disorders. *Remedial and Special Education, 28*(3), 153–162. https://doi.org/10.1177/07419325070280030401

Bice-Urbach, B. J., & Kratochwill, T. K. (2016). Teleconsultation: The use of technology to improve evidence-based practices in rural communities. *Journal of School Psychology, 56*, 27–43. https://doi.org/10.1016/j.jsp.2016.02.001

Billingsley, B., & Bettini, E. (2019). Special education teacher attrition and retention: A review of the literature. *Review of Educational Research, 89*(5), 697–744. https://doi.org/10.3102/0034654319862495

Bloomfield, B. S., Fischer, A. J., King, H. C., Lehman, E. L., & Clark, R. R. (2020). Exploring implementor error during remotely conducted school-based functional analysis telehealth training package. *Journal of Applied School Psychology, 36*(4), 1–29. https://doi.org/10.1080/15377903.2020.1749204

Boyle, M. A., & Adamson, R. M. (2017). Systematic review of functional analysis and treatment of elopement (2000–2015). *Behavior Analysis and Practice, 10*(4), 375–385. https://link.springer.com/article/10.1007/s40617-017-019

Boyle, S., McCoy, A., McNaughton, D., & Light, J. (2017). Effects of &"Transition to Literacy&" software on the sight word recognition skills of children with speech/language delays and their typically developing peers. Presentation at the annual Conference of the Council for Exceptional Children, Boston, MA.

Caplan, G. (1970). *The theory and practice of mental health consultation.* New York: Basic Books.

Cha, E., Chen, S., & Mataric, M. J. (2017). Designing telepresence robots for K-12 education. In *6th IEEE International Symposium on Robot and Human Interactive Communication* (pp. 683–688, Lisbon, Portugal.). https://doi.org/10.1109/ROMAN.2017.8172377

Chaldi, D., & Mantzanidou, G. (2021). Improving listener responding skill using Bee-Bot® in autism spectrum disorder: Case study. *European Journal of Special Education Research, 7*(2), 161–169. http://dx.doi.org/10.46827/ejse.v7i2.3823

Chang, A., Kazemi, E., Esmaeili, V., & Davis, M. (2022). The effectiveness of virtual reality training: A systematic review. *Journal of Organizational Behavior Management, 44*(3), 214–232. https://doi.org/10.1080/01608061.2023.2240767

Conroy, M. A., Asmus, J. M., Ladwig, C. N., Sellers, J. A., & Valcante, G. (2004). The effects of proximity on the classroom behaviors of students with autism in general education settings. *Behavioral Disorders, 29*(2), 119–129. https://doi.org/10.1177/019874290402900201

Dautenhahn, K. (2003). Roles and functions of robots in human society: Implications from research in autism therapy. *Robotica Cambridge, 21*(4), 443–452.

Davidson, R. J. (2010). Empirical explorations of mindfulness: conceptual and methodological conundrums. *Emotions, 10*(1), 8–11. https://doi.org/10.1037/a0018480

Dechsling, A., Orm, S., Kalandadze, T., Sütterlin, S., Øien, R. A., Shic, F., & Nordahl-Hansen, A. (2021). Virtual and augmented reality in social skills interventions for individuals with autism spectrum disorder: A scoping review., *52*(11), 4692–4707. *Journal of Autism and Developmental Disorders.* https://doi.org/10.1007/s10803-021-05338-5

Del Cid, D. A., Larranaga, D., Leitao, M., Mosher, R. L., Berzenski, S. R., Gandhi, V., & Drew, S. A. (2020). Exploratory factor analysis and validity of the Virtual Reality Symptom Questionnaire and computer use survey. *Ergonomics, 64*(1), 69–77. https://doi.org/10.1080/00140139.2020.1820083

Diemer, J., Alpers, G. W., Peperkorn, H. M., Shiban, Y., & Mühlberger, A. (2015). The impact of perception and presence on emotional reactions: A review of research in virtual reality. *Frontiers in Psychology, 6*, 1–9. https://doi.org/10.3389/fpsyg.2015.00026

DiGennaro Reed, F. D., & Henley, A. J. (2015). A survey of staff training and performance management practices: The good, the bad, and the ugly. *Behavior Analysis in Practice*, 8, 1626. https://doi.org/10.1007/s40617-015-0044-5

DiPietro, J., Kelemen, A., Liang, Y., & Sik-Lanyi, C. (2019). Computer-and robot-assisted therapies to aid social and intellectual functioning of children with autism spectrum disorder. *Medicina, 55*(8), 440. https://doi.org/10.3390/medicina55080440

Duquette, A., Michaud, F., & Mercier, H. (2008). Exploring the use of a mobile robot as an imitation agent with children with low-functioning autism. *Autonomous Robots, 24*(2), 147–157. https://doi.org/10.1007/s10514-007-9056-5

Erchul, W. P., & Ward, C. S. (2016). Problem-solving consultation. In S. R. Jimerson, M. K. Burns, & A. M. VanDerHeyden (Eds.), *Handbook of response to intervention: The science and practice of multi-tiered systems of support* (2nd ed., pp. 73–86). Springer Science + Business Media. https://doi.org/10.1007/978-1-4899-7568-3_6

Fallon, L. M., Collier-Meek, M. A., Kurtz, K. D., & DeFouw, E. R. (2020). Emailed implementation supports to promote treatment integrity: Comparing the effectiveness and acceptability of prompts and performance feedback. *Journal of School Psychology, 68*, 113–128. https://doi.org/10.1016/j.jsp.2018.03.001

Fischer, A. J., Bloomfield, B. S., Clark, R. R., McClelland, A. L., & Erchul, W. P. (2019). Increasing student compliance with teacher instructions using telepresence robot problem-solving teleconsultation. *International Journal of School & Educational Psychology, 7*(Suppl. 1), 158–172. https://doi.org/10.1080/21683603.2018.1470948

Fischer, A. J., Clark, R. R., Bloomfield, B. S., Askings, D. C., & Erchul, W. (2019). Using teleconsultation to teach expressive number discrimination through stimulus fading and reinforcement. *Journal of Applied School Psychology, 35*(4), 339–356. https://doi.org/10.1080/15377903.2019.1587803

Fischer, A. J., Dart, E. H., Radley, K, C., Richardson, D., Clark, R., & Wimberly, J. (2017). An evaluation of the effectiveness and acceptability of teleconsultation. *Journal of Educational and Psychological Consultation, 27*(4), 437–458. https://doi.org/10.1080/10474412.2016.1235978

Gibson, J. L., Pennington, R. C., Stenhoff, D. M., & Hopper, J. S. (2010). Using desktop videoconferencing to deliver interventions to a preschool student with autism. *Topics in Early Childhood Special Education, 29*(4), 214–225. https://doi.org/10.1177/0271121409352873

von Hagen, A., Muller, B., Sedlak, A., Bachmann, G., Herbert, J., & Buttner, G. (2021). Efficacy of remote as compared to in-person school psychology services: A rapid systematic evidence review. *Journal of Educational and Psychological Consultation, 32*(2), 210–238. https://doi.org/10.1080/10474412.2021.1963267

Hudson, C., & Lewis, L. (2020). Social robots as reinforcement in applied behavior analysis. In *Companion of the 2020 ACM/IEEE International Conference on Human-Robot Interaction* (pp. 266–268), Cambridge, UK. https://doi.org/10.1145/3371382.3378233

Huygelier, H., Schraepen, B., van Ee, R., Vanden Abeele, V., & Gillebert, C. (2019). Acceptance of immersive head-mounted virtual reality in older adults. *Scientific Reports, 9*(1), 1–12.

Ip, H. S. H., Simpson, W. L. Wong, Chan, D. F. Y., Byrne, J., Li, C., Yuan, V. S. N., Lau, K. S. Y., & Wong, J. Y. W. (2018). Enhance emotional and social adaptation skills for children with autism spectrum disorder: A virtual reality enabled approach. *Computers and Education, 117,* 1–15. https://doi.org/10.1016/j.compedu.2017.09.010

Ismail, L., Verhoeven, T., Dambre, J., & Wyffels, F. (2018). Leveraging robotics research for children with autism: a review. *International Journal of Social Robotics, 11*(3), 389–410. http://doi.org/10.1007/s12369-018-0508-1

Ismail, M., Azamon, N., & Khalid, N. (2017) Application of robots to improve social and communication skills among autistic children. *Journal of Manufacturing Technology, 12*(1), 421–430.

Jarvinen, A., Korenberg, J. R., & Bellugi, U. (2013). The social phenotype of Williams syndrome. *Current Opinion in Neurobiology, 23*(3), 414–422. https://doi.org/10.1016/j.conb.2012.12.006

Kazemi, E., & Stedman-Falls, L. M. (2016). Can humanoid robots serve as patient simulators in behavior analytic research and practice? *Behavior Analysis: Research and Practice, 16*(3), 135–146. http://dx.doi.org/10.1037/bar0000046

Ke, F., & Moon, J. (2018). Virtual collaborative gaming as social skills training for high-functioning autistic children: Virtual gaming for autistic children. *British Journal of Educational Technology, 49*(4), 728–741. https://doi.org/10.1111/bjet.12626

Kim, E. S., Berkovits, L. D., Bernier, E. P., Leyzberg, D., Shic, F., Paul, R., & Scassellati, B. (2013). Social robots as embedded reinforcers of social behavior in children with autism. *Journal of Autism and Developmental Disorders, 43*(5), 1038–1049. https://doi.org/10.1007/s10803-012-1645-2

King, H. C., Bloomfield, B., Wu, S., & Fischer, A. J. (2021). A systematic review of school teleconsultation: Implications for research and practice. *School Psychology Review, 51*(2), 237–256. https://doi.org/10.1080/2372966X.2021.1894478

Kontra, C., Lyons, D. J., Fischer, S. M., & Beilock, S. L. (2015). Physical experience enhances science learning. *Psychological Science, 26*(6), 737–749. https://doi.org/10.1177/0956797615569355

Korneder, J., Louie, W. G., Pawluk, C. M., Abbas, I., Brys, M., & Rooney, F. (2021). Robot-mediated interventions for teaching children with ASD: A new intraverbal skill. *Assistive Technology, 34*(6), 707–716. https://doi.org/10.1080/10400435.2021.1930284

Kristoffersson, M., Gu, L., & Zhang, Y. (2013). Home-School Collaboration in Sweden and China. *US-China. Education Review B, 3*(3), 188–201. ISSN 2161-6248

Lakatos, G., Wood, L., Syrdal, D., Robins, B., Zaraki, A., & Dautenhahn, K. (2021). Robot-mediated intervention can assist children with autism to develop visual perspective taking skills. *Paladyn, Journal of Behavioral Robotics, 12*(1), 87–101. https://doi.org/10.1515/pjbr-2021-0007

Leaf, J. B., Townley-Cochran, D., Taubman, M., Cihon, J. H., Oppenheim-Leaf, M. L., Kassardjian, A., Leaf, R., McEachin, J., & Pentz, T. G. (2015). The teaching interaction procedure and behavioral skills training for individuals diagnosed with autism spectrum disorder: A review and commentary. *Review Journal of Autism and Developmental Disorders, 2*(4), 402–413. https://doi.org/10.1007/s40489-015-0060-y

Lee, M., Goodman, C., Dandapani, N., & Kekahio, W. (2015). Review of international research on factors underlying teacher absenteeism. National Center for Education and Regional Assistance. Institute of Educational Sciences. https://files.eric.ed.gov/fulltext/ED555740.pdf

Lorenzo, G., Lledó, A., Pomares, J., & Roig, R. (2016). Design and application of an immersive virtual reality system to enhance emotional skills for children with autism spectrum disorders. *Computers & Education, 98,* 192–205. https://doi.org/10.1016/j.compedu.2016.03.018

Mitchell, U. A., Chebli, P. G., Ruggiero, L., & Muramatsu, N. (2019). The digital divide in health-related technology use: The significance of race/ethnicity. *The Gerontologist, 59*(1), 6–14. https://doi.org/10.1093/geront/gny138

Moon, J., & Ke, F. (2021). Exploring the treatment integrity of virtual reality-based social skills training for children with high-functioning autism. *Interactive Learning Environments,* 29(6), 939–953. https://doi-org.ezproxy.shsu.edu/10.1080/10494820.2019.1613665

Morgan, C. A., & Wine, B. (2018). Evaluation of behavior skills training for teaching work skills to a student with autism spectrum disorder. *Education and Treatment of Children, 41*(2), 223–232. https://doi.org/10.1353/etc.2018.0009

Mosher, M. A., & Carreon, A. C. (2021). Teaching social skills to students with autism spectrum disorder through augmented, virtual and mixed reality. *Research in Learning Technology, 29*, 1–22. https://doi.org/10.25304/rlt.v29.2626

Nesselrode, R., Falcomata, T. S., Hills, L., & Erhard, P. (2022). Functional analysis in public school settings: A systematic review of the literature. *Behavior Analysis in Practice, 15*(3), 958–970. https://doi.org/10.1007/s40617-022-00679-8

Pallavicini, F., Pepe, A., & Minissi, M. E. (2019). Gaming in virtual reality: What changes in terms of usability, emotional response and sense of presence compared to non-immersive video games? *Simulation & Gaming, 50*(2), 136–159. https://doi-org.ezproxy.shsu.edu/10.1177/1046878119831420

Palmisano, S., & Constable, R. (2022). Reductions in sickness with repeated exposure to HMD-based virtual reality appear to be game-specific. *Virtual Reality, 26*(6), 1373-1389. https://doi.org/10.1007/s10055-022-00634-6

Parish-Morris, J., Solorzano, R., Ravindran, V., Sazawal, V., Turnacioglu, S., Zitter, A., Miller, J. S., & Mccleery, J. P. (2018). Immersive virtual reality to improve police interaction skills in adolescents and adults with autism spectrum disorder: Preliminary results of a phase I feasibility and safety trial. Proc of the 23rd Annual CyberPsychology, CyberTherapy & Social Networking Conference, Gatineau, Canada.

Pennisi, P., Tonacci, A., Tartarisco, G., Billeci, L., Ruta, L., Gangemi, S., & Pioggia, G. (2016). Autism and social robotics: A systematic review. *Autism Research, 9*(2), 165–183. https://doi.org/10.1002/aur.1527

Piazza, C. C., Hanley, G. P., Bowman, L. G., Ruyter, J. M., Lindauer, S. E., & Saiontz, D. M. (1997). Functional analysis and treatment of elopement. *Journal of Applied Behavior Analysis, 30*(4), 653–672. https://doi.org/10.1901/jaba.1997.30-653

Proud, R. W., Hart, J. J., & Mrozinski, R. B. (2003). Methods for determining the level of autonomy of design into a human spaceflight vehicle: A function specific approach. NASA Johnson Space Center. https://ntrs.nasa.gov/api/citations/20100017272/downloads/20100017272.pdf

Ramdoss, S., Mulloy, A., Lang, R., O'Reilly, M., Sigafoos, J., Lancioni, G., Didden, R., & El Zein, F. (2011). Use of computer-based interventions to improve literacy skills in students with autism spectrum disorders: A systematic review. *Research in Autism Spectrum Disorders, 5*(4), 1306–1318. https://doi.org/10.1016/j.rasd.2011.03.004

Rebelo, F., Noriega, P., Duarte, E., & Soares, M. (2012). Using virtual reality to assess user experience. *Human Factors, 54*(6), 964–982. https://doi.org/10.1177/0018720812465006

Rodgers, M., Simmonds, M., Marshall, D., Hodgson, R., Stewart, L. A., Rai, D., Wright, K., Ben-Itzchak, E., Eikeseth, S., Eldevik, S., Kovshoff, H., Magiati, I., Osborne, L. A., Reed, P., Vivanti, G., Zachor, D., & Couteur, A. L. (2021). Intensive behavioral interventions based on applied behavior analysis for young children with autism: An international collaborative individual participant data meta-analysis. *Autism, 25*(4), 1137–1153. https://doi.org/10.1177/1362361320985680

Rosenfeld, H. (1987). Impasse and interpretation: Therapeutic and anti-therapeutic factors in the psychoanalytic treatment of psychotic, borderline, and neurotic patients. Tavistock/Routledge.

Shapiro, M., & Kazemi, E. (2017). A review of training strategies to teach individuals implementation of behavioral interventions. *Journal of Organizational Behavior Management, 37*(1), 32–62. https://doi.org/10.1080/01608061.2016.1267066

Schaefer, J. M., & Andzik, N. R. (2021). Evaluating behavioral skills training as an evidence-based practice when training parents to intervene with their children. *Behavior Modification, 45*(6), 887–910. https://doi.org/10.1177/0145445520923996

Scheithauer, M., Call, N. A., Mevers, J. L., McCracken, C. E., & Scahill, L. (2021). A feasibility randomized clinical trial of a structured function-based intervention for elopement in children with autism spectrum disorder. *Journal of Autism and Developmental Disorders, 51*, 2866–2875. https://doi.org/10.1007/s10803-020-04753-4

Smith, M. J., Bell, M. D., Wright, M. A., Humm, L. B., Olsen, D., & Fleming, M. F. (2016). Virtual reality job interview training and 6-month employment outcomes for individuals with substance use disorders seeking employment. *Journal of Vocational Rehabilitation, 44*(3), 323–332. https://doi.org/10.3233/JVR-160802

Smith, M. J., Boteler Humm, L., Fleming, M. F., Jordan, N., Wright, M. A., Ginger, E. J., Wright, K., Olsen, D., & Bell, M. D. (2015). Virtual reality job interview training for veterans with posttraumatic stress disorder. *Journal of Vocational Rehabilitation*, *42*(3), 271–279. https://doi.org/10.3233/JVR-150748

Smith, M. J., Ginger, E. J., Wright, K., Wright, M. A., Taylor, J. L., Humm, L. B., Olsen, D. E., Bell, M. D., & Fleming, M. F. (2014). Virtual reality job interview training in adults with autism spectrum disorder. *Journal of Autism and Developmental Disorders*, *44*(10), 2450–2463. https://doi.org/10.1007/s10803-014-2113-y

Tachibana, Y., Miyazaki, C., Ota, E., Mori, R., Hwang, Y., Kobayashi, E., Terasaka, A., Tang, J., & Kamio, Y. (2017). A systematic review and meta-analysis of comprehensive interventions for preschool children with autism spectrum disorder. *PLOS ONE*, *12*(12), 1–28. https://doi.org/10.1371/journal.pone.0186502

Tantum, D. (2003). The challenge of adolescents and adults with Asperger syndrome. Child and Adolescent Psychiatry Clinics, *12*(1), 143–163. https://psycnet.apa.org/doi/10.1016/S1056-4993(02)00053-6

Vannest, K. J., & Ninci, J. (2015). Evaluating intervention effects in single-case research designs. *Journal of Counseling and Development*, *93*(4), 403–411. https://doi.org/10.1002/jcad.12038

Vivanti, G., Hocking, D. R., Fanning, A. J., Uljarevic, M., Postorino, V., Mazzone, L., & Dissanayake, C. (2018). Attention to novelty versus repetition: Contrasting habituation profiles in autism and Williams syndrome. *Developmental Cognitive Neuroscience*, *29*, 54–60. https://doi.org/10.1016/j.dcn.2017.01.006

Wainer, J., Robins, B., Amirabdollahian, F., & Dautenhahn, K. (2014). Using the humanoid robot kaspar to autonomously play triadic games and facilitate collaborative play among children with autism. *Autonomous Mental Development*, *6*(3), 183–199. https://doi.org/10.1109/TAMD.2014.2303116

Ward, D. M., & Esposito, M. C. (2018). Virtual reality in transition program for adults with Autism: Self-efficacy, confidence, and interview skills. *Contemporary School Psychology*, *23*(4), 423–431. https://doi.org/10.1007/s40688-018-0195-9

Wilder, D. A., Meyers, K., Fischetti, A., Leon, Y., Nicholson, K., & Allison, J. (2012). An analysis of modifications to the three-step guidance compliance procedure necessary to achieve compliance among preschool children. *Journal of Applied Behavior Analysis*, *45*(1), 121–130. https://doi.org/10.1901/jaba.2012.45-121

Young, T. L., & Ireson, C. (2003). Effectiveness of school-based telehealth care in urban and rural elementary schools. *Pediatrics*, *112*(5), 1088–1094. https://doi.org/10.1542/peds/112.5.1088

Yuan, S. N. V., & Ip, H. H. S. (2018). Using virtual reality to train emotional and social skills in children with autism spectrum disorder. *London Journal of Primary Care*, *10*(4), 110–112. https://doi.org/10.1080/17571472.2018.1483000

Zoder-Martell, K. A., Flores, M. T., Schiuchetti, M. B., Markelz, A. M., & Sayyeh, L. (2021). Teachers' willingness to use a telepresence robot for consultation with students with autism spectrum disorder. *Contemporary School Psychology*, 26(2), 263–277. https://doi.org/10.1007/s40688-021-00359-4

25

Movement-Based Interventions

Sudha M. Srinivasan, and Deborah J. Bubela
Physical Therapy Program, Department of Kinesiology, University of Connecticut;
Institute for Health, Intervention and Policy (InCHIP), University of Connecticut;
The Connecticut Institute for the Brain and Cognitive Sciences (IBACS),
University of Connecticut

25.1 Technical Abstract

Background: Recently, there has been growing recognition of sensorimotor impairments being present in a majority of children with autism spectrum disorder (ASD), with movement-related challenges persisting in adolescence and adulthood. This chapter discusses the role of movement and physical activity–based interventions in the treatment of individuals with ASD across the lifespan. We provide a summary of the effects of movement and physical activity interventions on motoric and physical fitness–related outcomes in individuals with ASD. In addition, we present existing evidence on the effects of movement interventions in managing core autism-related symptoms in persons with ASD. **Method:** We conducted an extensive narrative review of the literature to date on conventional exercise interventions and novel, creative modes of movement implemented in individuals with ASD across the lifespan. We reviewed relevant systematic reviews, meta-analyses, and individual experimental and quasi-experimental studies in this area to provide recommendations and evidence-based guidelines for clinicians working with individuals with ASD. **Results:** There is consistent evidence that engagement in moderate-to-vigorous exercise can lead to a reduction in repetitive behaviors and improvements in social, cognitive, and motor skills as well as physical fitness-related outcomes in individuals with ASD. Evidence is most promising for improvements in cognitive function following exergaming and martial arts interventions; in socio-emotional skills following music therapies, aquatic interventions, and horseback riding; and in motor and behavioral outcomes following engagement in aerobic exercise, martial arts, and yoga practice. Most of the studies to date have sampled children and adolescents, with few studies conducted in adults in ASD. **Discussion:** The existing literature is limited by small

Sudha M. Srinivasan, and Deborah J. Bubela, *Movement-Based Interventions*. In: *Lifespan Treatment for Autistic Individuals*. Edited by: Peter Sturmey, Russell Lang, and James K. Luiselli, Oxford University Press. © Oxford University Press (2025).
DOI: 10.1093/oso/9780197635841.003.0025

sample sizes, lack of rigor in study designs contributing to medium-to-high risk of bias, variability in the samples recruited, variation in exercise modalities chosen and treatment dosing provided, lack of reporting of size of treatment effects, and lack of long-term follow-up assessments of treatment effects. Future studies should address these limitations by conducting larger randomized controlled trials with strict controls of confounding factors to provide strong evidence for the inclusion of movement interventions in the standard-of-care treatment of individuals with ASD across the lifespan. **Practitioner recommendations:** There is sufficient evidence to recommend the use of movement and physical activity interventions to address core symptoms associated with a diagnosis of ASD as well as to improve physical health and well-being in individuals with ASD. Clinicians should work collaboratively with the individual and their family as well as other specialized healthcare providers to design exercise programs adapted to the unique needs, skill level/capacities, and intrinsic interests/preferences of individuals with ASD to ensure maximum benefits from the training and long-term adherence with the program.

25.2 Layperson Summary

We experience the world around us through movements of our body. Movement is essential for basic life functions such as breathing, eating, talking, walking, managing hygiene, and other daily activities. Moreover, early exploratory bodily movements of young children provide them with opportunities for the development of more sophisticated motor skills that may also contribute to social, communication, and cognitive advancements. Individuals with ASD face movement challenges from early childhood that negatively impact their ability to engage in daily activities and also have consequences for their overall development. Movement and physical activity interventions aim to address these challenges faced by individuals with ASD. Evidence in this area suggests that movement and exercise interventions are effective in promoting gross motor skills, improving physical fitness levels, reducing repetitive behaviors, and improving social and cognitive skills in individuals with ASD. Currently, the strongest evidence of efficacy exists for exercise forms such as aerobic exercise (e.g., jogging, running, and cycling), aquatic interventions, music and movement activities, martial arts practice, yoga, horseback riding, and exergames. There are no known negative side effects of engagement in exercise other than temporary muscle soreness and fatigue that may be experienced by novices unaccustomed to regular exercise. Clinicians and families should obtain medical clearance for the individual with ASD from a physician prior to beginning an exercise program. The program should be tailored to the needs, capacities, and inherent interests of the individual with ASD to ensure sustained engagement and long-term adherence with the training program.

25.3 Treatment Summary Table

Treatment summary: Movement Interventions

Treatment description: Structured and unstructured physical activity that involves active movement of the body, requires effort from large muscles of the arms, legs, and/or trunk, and makes the heart beat faster and the person breathe harder.

Expected outcomes:

- Improvements in core impairment domains for individuals with ASD, including social communication skills, repetitive behaviors, and cognitive/attentional abilities
- Acquisition of motor skills/milestones and improvements in motor proficiency
- Improvements in sensory modulation and arousal
- Improvements in physical activity levels and outcomes related to physical fitness
- Improvements in performance of activities of daily living and levels of functional participation
- Improvements in quality of life and well-being

Methods:

- Movement interventions for acquisition of critical milestones and development of fundamental movement skills in infancy and early childhood
- Conventional exercise involving aerobic exercise, resistance training, and flexibility exercises
- Creative and alternative forms of movement, such as music, dance, yoga, martial arts, horseback riding, and technology-based, whole-body movement games

Expertise required to implement treatment:

- Exercise programs may be designed by well-trained movement clinicians, including physical therapists and occupational therapists in collaboration with the individual with ASD and their families.
- For specialized forms of exercise like dance, music, horseback riding, yoga, martial arts, and so on, programs should be designed and delivered by certified/licensed professionals.

Risks and negative side effects:

- No risks are associated with engagement in movement or exercise programs, provided that prior medical clearance is obtained from a physician for the individual to engage in physical activity/exercise.
- For specialized exercise like martial arts, horseback riding, dance, and so on, exercises must be performed under supervision of a licensed or certified expert to ensure appropriate form and avoid risk of injuries.
- For individuals beginning to exercise, temporary muscle soreness and fatigue are expected for the first few days of the training. It is recommended that the program include warm-up and cool-down components to reduce risk of injuries. The program should also be tailored to progress gradually based on the needs and physical capacities of the individual.

Additional considerations and limitations:

- It is important to identify exercise modalities that are aligned with intrinsic interests/preferences of individuals to ensure long-term adherence with the program.
- The individual's healthcare team must work closely with the individual and their family to develop a family-centric exercise program that is aligned with their goals and priorities.

- It is crucial to tailor the program to the needs and capacities of individual clients to ensure maximum success.
- Sustained engagement with exercise/movement programs is required for long-term benefits.
- The exercise program should incorporate existing behavior management strategies that are effective for the individual with ASD to ensure successful engagement in the program.

25.4 Introduction

25.4.1 Importance of Movement in Childhood and Across the Lifespan

Movement is fundamental to our existence. Evidence of the earliest limb and trunk movements are seen in human fetuses by 10 weeks of gestation, and they increase in quantity and intensity over the course of gestation until the confined space in the womb dampens fetal movements near the end of the pregnancy (Prechtl, 1985, 1986). Newborn babies enter the world crying. This action requires a newborn to take their first big breath, which involves movements of their respiratory and oral muscles (Barlow, 2009; Van Der Meer et al., 2005). Similarly, sucking and swallowing, which are among the earliest motoric behaviors, are essential for sustaining life (Adolph & Berger, 2011). Although early arm and leg movements of infants seem chaotic and reflexive, these movements provide infants opportunities to explore their surrounding physical and social world and learn about the affordances of their body with respect to the environment (Hadders-Algra & Prechtl, 1992; Thelen, 1979, 1981). These early, uncontrolled movements are precursors to more complex, controlled, and precise behaviors such as reaching, crawling, and walking that emerge within the first year through the infant's repeated practice of moving their body against gravity (Adolph & Berger, 2011; McGraw, 1945; Peiper, 1963).

As infants gain upright postural control, their ability to control movements of their arms and legs improves, which in turn is linked to their advancements within other developmental domains (Adolph & Franchak, 2017; Adolph & Hoch, 2019; Needham et al., 2002; Soska et al., 2010; Thelen & Smith, 1996). For example, improvements in gross and fine motor skills allow infants to engage in exploratory object play, which in turn facilitates infants' understanding of cause-effect and means-end relationships, as well as object properties and affordances (Amiel-Tison & Grenier, 1986; Bourgeois et al., 2005; Fontenelle et al., 2007; Gibson, 1988; Rochat & Goubet, 1995; Spencer et al., 2000; Von Hofsten, 1993). Developing the ability to crawl and learning to walk allows infants to independently access distal physical spaces and objects, changes their interactions with caregivers, and fosters a sense of autonomy (Adolph & Robinson, 2013; Anderson et al., 2013; Clearfield, 2011; Franchak et al., 2011; Karasik et al., 2011, 2014; Kretch et al.,

2014). Finally, verbal communication requires a child to precisely synchronize movements of over 80-odd muscles across the face and the throat and coordinate these movements with respiration (Adolph & Berger, 2011; Iverson, 2010). Overall, body movements serve as the means for infants to explore their surrounding world, and they in turn also facilitate advancements in multiple interrelated developmental domains over the course of childhood.

From a physiological standpoint, gross motor play is instrumental in fostering musculoskeletal development, inclusive of bone and muscle growth in young children (Gunter et al., 2012). Active play involving weight-bearing activities such as hopping, running, jumping, skipping, and tumbling is crucial for accrual of bone mass and bone mineralization from toddlerhood all the way to adolescence (Boreham & McKay, 2011; Hind & Burrows, 2007). Similarly, structured and unstructured activities that involve moving against one's own body weight (for preschoolers) or against external resistance (for older children and adolescents) help build muscle strength throughout the core and extremity musculature (Piercy et al., 2018). Children's play activities can often serve as a means of strengthening; climbing on playground equipment, pushing-pulling, and performing anti-gravity postures are all fun ways to explore while strengthening trunk and extremity musculature. Participating in running-based sports provides opportunities to develop lower-body strength as well as improve cardiorespiratory capacity. A majority of these whole-body activities that require sustained effort in the major large muscle groups of the body also help build cardiorespiratory capacity and endurance in children (Bar-Or, 1983; Cohen et al., 2015; Katch, 1983; Rowland, 1981; Sallis et al., 1988).

In addition to promoting anatomical development within the musculoskeletal and cardiorespiratory systems, increasingly challenging movement experiences help children acquire critical motor milestones and develop balance and coordination (Adolph & Berger, 2011; de Boer, 2012; Getchell & Whitall, 2003; Haywood & Getchell, 2021). Within the first year, infants' exploration of their body's movement repertoire paves the way for the acquisition of motor milestones such as neck control, rolling, sitting, crawling, standing, cruising, and walking (Assaiante, 1998; Gesell, 1946; Shirley, 1933; Woollacott et al., 1987). During this formative period, infants discover properties of their own bodies (mass, size, body composition, movements possible at different joints, etc.) as well as those of the surrounding environment (gravity, friction, inertia). They learn to exploit constraints within their bodies and their surrounding physical and social environments to engage in purposeful, goal-directed behaviors (Adolph & Berger, 2011; Adolph & Hoch, 2019; Adolph & Robinson, 2013, 2015). Motor skill acquisition also facilitates the development of bilateral coordination, balance, and imitation/praxis skills (Adolph & Berger, 2011; Dewey, 1993, 1995; Jones, 2007; Vanvuchelen et al., 2011). The increasing repertoire of movements and the association of movement with its effect on the environment allow children to learn how to effectively plan and perform activities to serve a purpose/goal. This motor planning, termed "praxis," helps children deal with a variety of novel tasks and motor-based challenges (Dewey, 1995; Kools & Tweedie, 1975; Mostofsky et al., 2006). A child's ability to accurately imitate will enhance motor learning (Hayes et al., 2007; Murata & Tan, 2009; Shumway-Cook & Woollacott, 2007). Moreover, motor learning processes continue across the lifespan (Haibach et al., 2011; Haywood & Getchell, 2021); learning a new movement skill such as a new sport, dancing, or driving, at any age, requires the individual to learn new and efficient strategies of organizing movements of their body in relation to task and environmental constraints. Although prerequisite fundamental movement skills are mastered in early childhood, motor learning requires a degree of relearning, problem solving, and refinement of existing movement patterns depending on the task and the environmental situation (Shumway-Cook & Woollacott, 2007).

Movement working in conjunction with the body's sensory system is also integral to the child's interpretation of the environment and their ability to act within that environment. For instance, as an infant crawls through their playroom, they constantly receive and are required to process visual input called optic flow. Optic flow provides information on the changing relative state between the infant and their environment that in turn helps guide their movements in the room (Campos et al., 2000; Gibson, 1979). In fact, classical experiments by Campos and colleagues show that movement, or crawling experience, is crucial for the development of depth perception in infants (Anderson et al., 2013; Campos et al., 2000). Moreover, movements of various joints produced by muscular contractions also activate special receptors within the muscles and joints called "proprioceptors," that inform us about where our body is in space even in the absence of vision (Elliot et al., 1988; Hay et al., 2005; Sigmundsson et al., 2000). Finally, linear and angular movements of the head activate the vestibular system located within the inner ear, which plays a crucial role in maintaining balance, developing postural control, modulating alertness, controlling eye movements, and registering the body's movement and orientation in space (Jouen, 1990; Shumway-Cook & Woollacott, 2007). In typically developing infants and children, active experiences of moving in the real world also facilitate mapping and integration across multiple sensory modalities called intermodal perception (Bushnell, 1981; Bushnell & Boudreau, 1993; Gibson & Walker, 1984; Rose & Ruff, 1987; Spelke, 1987). To summarize, bodily movements contribute to our experience of the surrounding physical and social world. Movement plays a crucial role in an individual's physical, psychosocial, mental, and emotional health and well-being throughout the lifespan.

25.4.2 Treatment Description

In this chapter, we define movement interventions as physical activity (PA) that involves large movements of the body in a way that requires muscular effort, expends energy, makes the heart beat faster, and makes the individual breathe harder. Movement-based interventions could involve either structured or unstructured activities (Clevenger et al., 2018; Kinder et al., 2019, 2020). Structured activities are planned, have set objectives, and are organized in a way that the participant is provided ongoing instructions and guidance from an instructor. However, unstructured activities include leisure-time activities where participants have greater autonomy and there are minimal restrictions on the activity (Clevenger et al., 2018; Kinder et al., 2019). Unlike structured contexts, there is no instructor who determines the activity parameters such as the rules and pace of the activities. For instance, physical education (PE) lessons at school qualify as structured PA, whereas PA during recess is an example of unstructured PA (Kinder et al., 2020).

Structured movement/PA contexts are typically organized as well-defined routines with a clear set of expectations and learning objectives for participants. Such activities include extensive guidance and feedback provided during the learning process and maximize opportunities for fostering skill development and PA engagement (Kinder et al., 2020). Structured movement-based interventions may include therapeutic contexts that encourage motor skill development, conventional exercise programs that promote cardiorespiratory and musculoskeletal health, and novel creative movement interventions that foster multisystem development. Structured PA may be provided by therapists, coaches, or community-based program instructors.

Structured movement experiences may be provided to individuals within a therapeutic context to promote fundamental motor skills. For example, infants and toddlers with ASD frequently have delayed acquisition of gross motor milestones such as head control, independent sitting, standing, and walking (Bhat et al., 2012; Flanagan et al., 2012; Iverson et al., 2019; Lloyd et al., 2013; MacDonald et al., 2013; Nickel et al., 2013). Moreover, children with ASD often continue to face movement difficulties through childhood, including poor static and dynamic balance, incoordination, clumsy gait patterns, poor postural control skills, impaired imitation, poor interpersonal synchrony, and difficulties with motor planning and praxis skills (Dewey et al., 2007; Fournier et al., 2010; Gandotra et al., 2020; Green et al., 2009; Kindregan et al., 2015; Lim et al., 2016; Manicolo et al., 2019; Marsh et al., 2009; Minshew et al., 2004; Mostofsky et al., 2006; Paquet et al., 2016; Provost et al., 2007; Rinehart et al., 2006; Whyatt & Craig, 2012). Early movement interventions for infants and toddlers with ASD are targeted toward structuring the environment and setting up tasks in a way to maximize and diversify movement experiences provided to infants to help broaden their movement repertoire (Bhat et al., 2011). For example, to promote the acquisition of rolling, caregivers may be trained to provide the infant's favorite toys on one side of the body slightly out of reach, thereby requiring the infant to roll to play with the toy. Similarly, placing enticing toys at a height on a firm couch/chair may be used to encourage a child to practice floor-to-stand transitions while holding onto a supporting surface. For older children with ASD, movement-based physical therapy interventions are focused on training motor skills within functional contexts to ensure transfer of learning to meaningful everyday contexts and activities of daily living (Downey & Rapport, 2012; Ketcheson et al., 2017; Mieres et al., 2012; Ruggeri et al., 2020). For instance, a physical therapist may address upper-extremity strengthening by pushing and pulling activities and follow up with functional carryover as a child carries his lunch tray in the cafeteria and independently carries his backpack in school. Similarly, they may work with a child with dynamic balance challenges during PE class to train the child to navigate different types of surfaces he may encounter in the community.

Conventional exercise programs, however, are typically designed to target components of an individual's physical fitness and movement control, including measures of body composition, aerobic capacity, muscular strength and endurance, flexibility, balance, and movement speed (Caspersen et al., 1985; Healy et al., 2018; Piercy et al., 2018). Exercise programs may include activities such as brisk walking, running, cycling, swimming, resistance training, or participating in intramural or extramural sports such as tennis, basketball, and soccer (Bremer et al., 2016; Hynes & Block, 2022; Lang et al., 2010; Sowa & Meulenbroek, 2012). Specialized programs such as Unified Sports and Special Olympics have also been designed for children with developmental disabilities, including those with ASD (www.specialolympics.org; Dykens & Cohen, 1996; Tint et al., 2017; Weiss et al., 2003). For children with ASD, conventional exercise programs have been used to promote cardiovascular endurance, skill-related fitness, social functioning, and cognitive/academic skills, manage behavioral impairments, and regulate sensory issues (see details in section on treatment rationale; Bremer et al., 2016; Ferreira et al., 2018; Healy et al., 2018; Howells et al., 2019; Hynes & Block, 2022; Liang et al., 2022; Ruggeri et al., 2020; Tan et al., 2016).

In contrast to conventional exercise programs that use traditional modes of PA, creative movement interventions incorporate novel modalities such as music, dance, yoga, martial arts, equine therapies, and technology-based approaches such as exergaming to promote skills in multiple domains of development (Amonkar et al., 2021; Davis et al., 2015; Jiménez-Muñoz et al., 2022; Morris et al., 2022; Nieforth et al., 2021; Srinivasan & Bhat, 2013; Srinivasan et al., 2018). Creative movement modalities provide opportunities for improvisation, creativity, and playful exploration and are thus perceived as being more intrinsically motivating and enjoyable for participants compared to traditional exercise programs. For individuals with ASD, creative movement therapies have been used to enhance gross motor, social communication, behavioral-affective, cognitive, and participation-related outcomes (Amonkar et al., 2021).

Unstructured PA/movement interventions lack the structure and routine that are characteristic of structured PA contexts and are instead inclusive of self-selected free play, recreational/leisure activities, and unguided and informal activities (Kinder et al., 2020). Similar to creative movement opportunities, unstructured activities typically foster creativity and independence in participants (Kinder et al.,

2020; Theobald et al., 2015). Unstructured movement opportunities within school settings include recess time, before and after school activities, and leisure events (Beighle et al., 2006; Tudor-Locke et al., 2006; Woods et al., 2015). Moreover, for adolescents and adults, unstructured PA may take the form of chores, physically active life skills, and work-related movement/PA (Piercy et al., 2018). Examples of unstructured activities include indoor and outdoor chores as well as recreational activities. Home chores that present a physical demand include yard work, gardening, shoveling snow, vacuuming, washing/cleaning, and walking pets. Recreational activities may include playing yard games, participating in recreational sports, hiking, and rock climbing. PA is also an inherent component of the work demands for construction workers, carpenters, mechanics, nurses, flight attendants, and firefighters, to name a few examples. In the subsequent sections, we discuss the need for and the purported mechanisms underlying the effects of movement/exercise interventions in individuals with ASD. We will then present evidence in support of movement-based interventions for individuals with ASD across the lifespan.

25.4.3 Rationale and Objectives

Bodily movement and regular PA are crucial for maintaining and promoting optimal physical, metabolic, and psychological health, well-being, and quality of life throughout the lifespan. There is abundant research suggesting that regular PA improves cardiometabolic and bone health, helps maintain healthy weight, and reduces the risk of chronic health conditions such as Type 2 diabetes, cardiovascular disease, hypertension, certain types of cancers, and dementia. PA may also reduce anxiety and depression, improve functional abilities, reduce risk of falls and fall-related injuries, improve sleep and sense of well-being, improve cognitive function, and reduce overall mortality due to multiple causes (Piercy et al., 2018; Reiner et al., 2013; Warburton & Bredin, 2017). In view of these health benefits, the PA guidelines for Americans recommend regular PA for individuals with and without disabilities 3 years and above (Piercy et al., 2018). Broadly, it is recommended that preschoolers (3–5 years) stay active throughout the day, 6–17-year-olds accumulate at least 60 minutes of moderate-to-vigorous PA per day, and adults over 18 years engage in at least 150–300 minutes/week of moderate intensity PA for sustained health benefits (Piercy et al., 2018).

Compared to their typically developing peers, individuals with ASD are more likely to be overweight and obese and suffer from medical and cardiovascular conditions such as heart disease and diabetes (Courtney-Long et al., 2015; de Vinck-Baroody et al., 2015; Grondhuis & Aman, 2014; McCoy et al., 2016; Rimmer et al., 2007). For instance, the prevalence of obesity in a sample of children with ASD was 30.4% compared with 23.6% in age-matched children without ASD (Curtin et al., 2010). Individuals with ASD also have lower levels of cardiovascular endurance, muscular function, and flexibility compared to typically developing peers (Pan et al., 2016). On an average, young adults with ASD spend around 13 hours per day sitting (Eaves & Ho, 2008). According to the National Survey of Child Health (2016)(www.childhealthdata.org), only 17% of children with ASD meet the recommended PA guidelines issued by the US Department of Health and Human Services. This trend of inactivity increases with growing age in individuals with ASD (Macdonald et al., 2011; McCoy & Morgan, 2020; Ratcliff et al., 2018). Given the significant disparity between PA engagement in individuals with ASD and their typically developing peers, it is all the more crucial that efforts be made to provide targeted movement/PA-based interventions to improve overall health and well-being and reduce risk of secondary comorbidities in this population across the lifespan.

A clear understanding of the determinants of PA in ASD is foundational to developing effective interventions and opportunities that promote PA in individuals with ASD (Sallis & Hovell, 1990; Sallis et al., 1992; Trost et al., 2002). Several barriers at the individual and environmental levels have been associated with lower participation in movement-based interventions in individuals with ASD (Bandura, 1977, 1986, 2004; Epstein, 1998; McLeroy et al., 1988; Rosenstock, 1974; Tint et al., 2017; Van der Ploeg et al., 2004; Welk, 1999). At the personal level, an individual's existing sensorimotor, social, cognitive, and behavioral skills, perceived movement-related self-efficacy, and motivation to exercise influence PA engagement (Van der Ploeg et al., 2004). Around 87% of children in a large cohort of over 11,000 children with ASD between 5 and 15 years failed on a screening tool for coordination impairments, indicating that they are likely to demonstrate significant motor challenges (Bhat, 2020). Moreover, these movement difficulties were significantly linked to their core symptomatology associated with an ASD diagnosis, including social communication skills, restricted and repetitive behaviors, cognition, and functional skills (Bhat, 2021). The motor challenges present in childhood often persist into adulthood, thereby significantly limiting PA choices for adults with ASD (Bhat, 2020). For example, individuals with ASD with motor incoordination, poor dynamic balance, and impaired motor planning skills may face significant challenges in learning and participating in sports and may in turn prefer seated tasks or activities that do not involve dynamic interactions or require quick or unpredictable motor responses (Chonchaiya et al., 2011; Russell, 2018).

In addition to challenges related to the movement system, impaired social communication, behavioral-cognitive, and sensory modulation abilities in individuals with ASD may also influence their ability to engage in PA (Nichols et al., 2019; Obrusnikova & Miccinello, 2012; Srinivasan et al., 2014). For instance, difficulties in initiating and sustaining conversations, poor joint attention, and impaired social reciprocity may limit an individual's ability to engage in group-based movement activities (Chita-Tegmark, 2016). Similarly, sensory modulation difficulties (i.e., hypo- or hyper-responsiveness to specific sensory stimuli), repetitive stereotypies, and highly restricted and inflexible interests may limit an individual's activity choices for PA (Robertson & Baron-Cohen, 2017; Schauder & Bennetto, 2016). Along the same lines, deficits in executive function and observational learning may also pose challenges for individuals with ASD to learn novel motor skills and activities (Craig et al., 2016; Plavnick & Hume, 2014).

When considering environmental influences, a child's participation in PA will be influenced by negative family beliefs and values toward PA, accessibility and affordability of the PA opportunities, as well as family schedules and financial constraints. Scarcity of appropriate programs and trained staff are also factors limiting individuals' engagement in PAs (Frey et al., 2005; Heller et al., 2002; Mahy et al., 2010; Menear, 2007; Nichols et al., 2019; Pitchford et al., 2016; Shields et al., 2012; Temple, 2009; Temple & Walkley, 2007; Welk, 1999; Yazdani et al., 2013). Overall, it is clear that individuals with ASD engage in low levels of PA compared to age-matched peers and are at higher risk of developing health conditions secondary to sedentary behaviors and reduced PA engagement. They also face additional barriers to PA engagement as a result of their unique sensorimotor and behavioral profiles and limited availability of appropriate programs in some situations.

Movement-based interventions for individuals with ASD have been documented since the 1980s as a means to address repetitive and stereotyped behaviors, reduce frequencies of problem behaviors, and improve academic focus (Srinivasan et al., 2014). It has been found that engaging in brief bouts of moderate-to-vigorous exercise leads to a reduction in stereotyped behaviors as well as an increase in on-task behaviors and engagement in academic lessons among individuals with ASD (Bremer et al., 2016; Ferreira et al., 2018, 2019; Olin et al., 2017; Tarr, 2019; Tarr et al., 2020). A recent meta-analysis of 22 studies involving 274 children with ASD found medium-to-large reductions in stereotyped behaviors following physical exercise intervention. They also found that exercise intensity moderated this effect, with higher exercise intensity sessions leading to greater improvements in stereotypies demonstrated by individuals with ASD (Teh et al., 2022). Several mechanisms have been proposed to explain these treatment effects. Although there is a lack of substantial research to support this hypothesis, physical fatigue associated with exercise may lead to a reduction in problem behaviors (Lang et al., 2010; Rosenthal-Malek & Mitchell, 1997). Others have proposed that exercise may serve as a functional substitute for stereotyped behaviors. To elaborate, exercise helps regulate arousal levels to achieve homeostasis, and it also provides similar sensory input (visual, auditory, tactile-proprioceptive, and/or vestibular) and physical stimulation that is intrinsically pleasurable and reinforcing for an individual with ASD (Lang et al., 2010; Rapp & Vollmer, 2005; Teh et al., 2022). Moreover, with a reduction in stereotypies, there is a concurrent increase in engagement in academic opportunities within the classroom (Neely et al., 2015; Nicholson et al., 2011; Oriel et al., 2011).

Over the last couple of decades, the study of the effects of PA and exercise interventions in individuals with ASD has expanded to include a wide variety of domains/skills. Research has evaluated outcomes related to (a) physical fitness (measures of body composition, cardiovascular capacity, muscular strength and endurance, and flexibility), (b) movement control (balance, body coordination, locomotor skills, object control and manipulation skills, response speed, and agility), (c) social-emotional skills (social responsiveness, social interactions, communication, and emotional regulation), (d) cognitive skills (executive function, attention, working memory, and task-switching abilities), and (e) overall participation in activities of daily living (adaptive functioning, quality of life, well-being, and stress levels) (Bremer et al., 2016; Fang et al., 2019; Healy et al., 2018; Howells et al., 2019; Hynes & Block, 2022; Liang et al., 2022; Ruggeri et al., 2020; Sam et al., 2015; Sowa & Meulenbroek, 2012; Tan et al., 2016).

Exercise has been proposed to be a cost-effective modality that can easily be performed in a variety of settings such as home, school, playground, and community with little to no need for equipment, and without constant supervision/facilitation by highly trained specialists/therapists, compared to other conventional behavioral therapies (Bremer et al., 2016). Moreover, given the evidence for relationships between motor skills, on one hand, and social communication skills, cognitive abilities, repetitive behaviors, and functional skills, on the other, it is not surprising that movement-based interventions may potentially lead to improvements in interrelated multiple domains beyond the motor system (Bhat, 2021; Howells et al., 2019; MacDonald et al., 2013; Rinehart et al., 2018; Zeliadt, 2017). For instance, group exercise programs afford abundant opportunities for turn taking, imitation, shared attention, initiating conversations, and responding to social bids. Therefore, such experiences may be effective in facilitating social understanding and building relationships with coaches, peers, and siblings for individuals with ASD (Healy et al., 2018; Howells et al., 2019; Özer et al., 2012; Sam et al., 2015; Trevarthen & Delafield-Butt, 2013). There is also substantial evidence that regular exercise engagement can boost an individual's cognition/executive function especially in terms of on-task behaviors, cognitive flexibility, and inhibitory control (Liang et al., 2022; Tan et al., 2016). These effects may be a result of direct changes in neural activation patterns, cerebral blood flow patterns, and changes in neurobiological processing involving neurotropic factors, catecholamines, and growth factors. There may also be indirect effects secondary to improved self-efficacy, mood, and other psychosocial functions (Diamond, 2000; Diamond & Ling, 2016; Liang et al., 2022; Machado et al., 2015; Ratey & Loehr, 2011; Tan et al., 2016; Tomporowski et al., 2011; Wegner et al., 2014; Wigal et al., 2013).

The downstream effects of exercise on multiple systems may be related to the type of exercise modality itself (Bremer et al., 2016; Hynes & Block, 2022). Different exercise modes may offer unique physical experiences that may lead to specific effects. For instance, aquatic activities allow practice of motor skills in a gravity-eliminated setting and provide a multisensory experience while avoiding sensory overload, thus allowing individuals to focus on the external environment, which in turn may lead to improved social skills (Heyn, 2003; Mooventhan &

Nivethitha, 2014). Similarly, yoga practice is shown to have a calming effect by reducing hyperactivity and helps improve balance skills (Hynes & Block, 2022). Sports-specific training and aerobic activities are ideally suited to challenge an individual's cardiovascular and musculoskeletal systems (Hynes & Block, 2022). Equine therapies have also been linked to improved social skills in individuals with ASD, possibly due to multiple opportunities for building connections with the horses and the instructors during horse-riding sessions, thereby breaking the social isolation faced by many individuals with ASD (Healy et al., 2018; Srinivasan et al., 2018). However, exergaming activities, which require participants to respond optimally to visual feedback, plan actions strategically, understand constraints of spatial layouts, and map out their actions to that of the gameplay, have led to improved cognitive performance, including memory, spatial awareness, attention, and time on task (Anderson-Hanley et al., 2011; Caro et al., 2017; Hilton et al., 2014; Staiano & Calvert, 2011). These effects are in line with Diamond and Ling (2016), who propose that PA designed with inbuilt complexity, diversity, and novelty will inherently promote cognition (Diamond & Ling, 2016).

Overall, the effects of movement and PA interventions are widespread and span multiple systems that overlap with the core symptomatology in ASD. In the next section, we systematically review the evidence on different types of movement interventions in individuals with ASD across the lifespan.

25.5 Research Background

Research on the effects of movement and PA interventions in the last decade has increased exponentially. While a detailed and historic review of this literature to date in this area is beyond the scope of this chapter, in the current section, we aim to provide readers with a comprehensive summary of the salient literature highlighting key findings relating to PA for individuals with ASD. Wherever available, we will also provide information on effect sizes for reported outcomes. Effect size represents a family of indices that provide an estimate of the magnitude of a treatment effect and typically involve calculations of either a standardized difference between two means (e.g., between the experimental and control groups or from pretest to posttest) or as a correlation between the independent and dependent variables. There are standard guidelines available to qualitatively interpret the size of the effect as being "small," "medium," or "large" in magnitude (Cohen, 1988; Rosenthal & Rosnow, 2008). We will provide readers with a descriptive label (small, medium, or large) for effect sizes reported in individual studies/reviews to aid interpretation of the reported improvements in measured outcomes following movement/PA interventions.

A majority of the comprehensive reviews on structured PA programs report on the combined effects of different types of PA interventions, including conventional exercise and creative movement, irrespective of exercise modality. A few reviews focused exclusively on the effects of specific creative and alternative modes of movement/exercise such as exergaming, creative movement interventions, and animal-assisted interventions. Reviews on movement/PA interventions have measured the effectiveness of interventions as they relate to multiple domains in which individuals with ASD commonly experience challenges, including repetitive behaviors, social communication, cognition, and motor outcomes. While unstructured PA is recognized by stakeholders, including family members, clinicians, and special educators, as being very important to promote active living in individuals with ASD (Athreya et al., 2022; Srinivasan et al., 2022), presently there is sparse systematic research exploring the effects of programs aimed at increasing unstructured PA through gross motor play, chores, and physically active work schedules in individuals with ASD.

25.5.1 Effects of Structured PA Interventions on Outcomes Relating to Challenge Areas for Individuals With ASD

*Repetitive behaviors.*As mentioned in the preceding section, structured movement/PA gained attention as a potential therapeutic modality for individuals with ASD since the early 1980s when researchers started using antecedent aerobic exercise such as jogging or walking as a way to address repetitive and stereotyped behaviors as well as improve academic responses and on-task behaviors following the exercise session in children with ASD (Celiberti et al., 1997; Kern et al., 1982, 1984; Levinson & Reid, 1993; Powers et al., 1992; Rosenthal-Malek & Mitchell, 1997; Watters & Watters, 1980). For instance, brief 5–20-minute bouts of mildly strenuous jogging activities led to a decrease in subsequent frequencies of self-stimulatory behaviors as well as increase in academic responding, classroom on-task behaviors, and appropriate play behaviors in seven children with ASD with high levels of self-stimulatory behaviors (Kern et al., 1982). Thereafter, several more recent studies and reviews have also confirmed the beneficial effects of antecedent exercise on repetitive and maladaptive behaviors and academic responses in individuals with ASD (Ferreira et al., 2019; Morrison et al., 2011; Neely et al., 2015; Nicholson et al., 2011; Olin et al., 2017; Petrus et al., 2008; Teh et al., 2022).

Ferreira and colleagues (2019) in their meta-analysis assessed whether the stereotyped behaviors of 129 children with ASD were affected by nine different types of movement/PA programs, including jogging, trampoline jumping, stationary biking, obstacle course navigation, exergaming, coordination and strength exercises, ball playing, treadmill training, and martial arts "kata" training. Their review results from one randomized and seven nonrandomized intervention trials suggested that PA led to a reduction in occurrences of stereotypies following the physical exercise session, especially if the exercise mechanics were matched with the bodily location of the stereotypy. For example, practice of ball throwing exercises led to diminished hand-flapping stereotypies. While individual studies assessed maintenance of effects at differing time intervals (40, 90, or 120 minutes post exercise, or 30 days after completion of training), the review found some evidence that beneficial effects were maintained even after completion of the exercise session (Ferreira et al., 2019). Similarly, another review reported large effect sizes for reductions in stereotypic behaviors based on three studies of structured programs inclusive of martial arts, horseback riding, and jogging interventions (Bremer et al., 2016). Overall, short bouts of movement/exercise of moderate-to-vigorous intensity seem to help address repetitive behaviors and improve on-task engagement in individuals with ASD.

Social communication skills. Movement interventions have also been used to address social communication difficulties, a hallmark core diagnostic impairment in individuals with ASD. In the very first meta-analysis in this area, Sowa and Meulenbroek (2012) set out to assess the effects of exercise on motor as well as social and communication skills in individuals with ASD. They found insufficient studies specifically addressing communication skills; therefore, they only reported on the effects of PA on social and motor skills based on 16 studies with 133 individuals with ASD (average age: 13.6 years; range 4–41 years). Overall, PA interventions such as swimming, jogging, horseback riding, cycling, weight training, walking, and other leisure PAs led to an average improvement of 40% in motor skills and around 39% in social skills in individuals with ASD (Sowa & Meulenbroek, 2012).

In their review paper, Bremer et al. (2016) focused on the effects of exercise on behavioral symptoms of individuals with ASD up to 16 years of age. Seven studies assessed outcomes pertaining to the social-emotional domain. Effect size calculations from five out of the seven studies that reported sufficient data suggested large variation in effect size estimates ranging from small to large based on the outcome assessed, with an average medium-to-large effect size across studies (Bremer et al., 2016). A more recent meta-analysis by Howells et al. (2019) of the effects of group-based organized PA interventions (including horseback riding, martial arts, soccer, outdoor adventure program, and a multisport summer camp) on social outcomes in children with ASD found 11 studies that reported on outcomes related to social functioning and/or communication. While there was medium-to-high risk of bias in 8 out of the 11 reviewed studies, qualitative analyses suggested that 8 out of the 10 studies reported beneficial effects on social function, and three out of six studies found improved communication following PA interventions. Quantitative meta-analytic procedures based on seven studies, however, suggested a significant small-to-medium effect size for improvements in overall social function, but no significant effects on levels of communication following participation in group-based organized PA compared to a control group (Howells et al., 2019).

It is clear that these findings are preliminary at best, given the poor-to-fair methodological quality of reviewed studies and considering the few numbers of studies per type of exercise modality. Moreover, at present there are no studies that compare the differential effects of different exercise modalities on social function within the same study. Overall, across multiple reviews there is promising low-level scientific evidence for improvements in social skills in children and youth with ASD following participation in swimming, horseback riding, sports, and martial arts interventions (Bremer et al., 2016; Howells et al., 2019; Hynes & Block, 2022; Sam et al., 2015).

Cognition. Although cognitive impairments are not recognized as part of the diagnostic criteria in ASD, it is well-established that individuals with ASD have challenges in cognitive function, especially executive functioning (Hill, 2004). "Executive function" is an umbrella term that includes multiple abilities underlying goal-directed, purposeful behaviors, including planning, task initiation, task shifting, cognitive flexibility, working memory, problem solving, monitoring, response inhibition, and self-control (Craig et al., 2016; Demetriou et al., 2018; Pennington & Ozonoff, 1996). There is evidence that exercise and PA, especially cognitively challenging and enjoyable activities, lead to improvements in executive function (Diamond & Ling, 2016). A meta-analysis of 22 studies that assessed the efficacy of PA interventions in promoting cognitive skills in 128 children and youth with ASD and attention-deficit/hyperactivity disorder (ADHD) suggested small-to-medium improvements in on-task behaviors and simple learning tasks following exercise interventions such as jogging, cycling, exergaming, and creative movement in children with ASD. Specifically, exercise cognitively benefitted around 76.30% individuals with ASD included in the review. The effects of exercise on executive function specifically were not well studied, therefore precluding definitive conclusions on the effects of exercise on executive function (Tan et al., 2016).

In a more recent review, Liang and colleagues (2022) reviewed 14 studies to assess the acute and chronic effects of exercise interventions, including exergaming, martial arts, cycling, jogging, and ball games on cognitive outcomes in individuals with ASD. Their meta-analysis based on a subset of seven studies found an overall small-sized improvement in executive functions following chronic exercise interventions, with small-to-moderate improvements in cognitive flexibility and inhibitory control, but not on working memory. All studies with one exception in this review were randomized controlled or crossover trials and fared as having medium-to-high quality with low risk of bias (Liang et al., 2022). Overall, there is mounting positive evidence for the beneficial effects of aerobic exercise on cognitive function in ASD, although this area warrants further systematic research to replicate the presented findings.

Physical fitness and motor outcomes. In light of the mounting evidence for the pervasive nature of motor impairments and lower levels of PA and physical fitness in individuals with ASD compared to age-matched peers, several research groups have evaluated the effects of exercise and movement-based interventions on PA, physical fitness, and motoric outcomes (see reviews by Healy et al., 2018; Hynes & Block, 2022; Lang et al., 2010; Ruggeri et al., 2020; Sorensen & Zarrett, 2014). A recent review assessed the effects of 34 movement-based and PA intervention studies on motor outcomes in 1,173 individuals with ASD between 3 and 19 years (Ruggeri et al., 2020). The interventions included motor activity interventions (e.g., gymnastics, sports camp, table tennis, soccer, Tai chi, Greek dance, trampoline jumping), motor skill training (e.g., balance, throwing, catching, running, jumping), equine-assisted therapies (hippotherapy and therapeutic horseback riding), aquatic interventions, exergaming, and physical education-based interventions conducted as part of the children's academic programming. The authors reported effects on body structure and function, activity levels, and participation-related outcomes in accordance with the framework of the International Classification of Functioning, Disability, and Health for Children and Youth (ICF-CY). Results from the reviewed small randomized controlled trials and nonrandomized clinical trials intervention studies suggested (a) improved body structure and function (balance, body and manual coordination, reaction time, speed and agility, strength, and cardiovascular fitness) following aquatic, exergaming, motor activity, motor skill, and simulated horseback riding interventions, (b) positive changes in activity outcomes (swim skills, locomotor skills, and manipulative skills) after aquatic, motor activity, motor skill, and simulated horseback riding interventions, and (c) improved quality of life following a physical education intervention. Although promising, the authors commented on the overall low quality and rigor of the reviewed studies and called for more systematic research using large, well-controlled study designs to assess movement-related outcomes, especially at the participation level, following engagement in PA interventions (Ruggeri et al., 2020).

Similar results were also reported in a meta-analysis of 29 PA intervention studies involving 1,009 participants with ASD between 2 and 22 years that suggested an overall medium-sized effect of PA interventions on motor performance of individuals with ASD (Healy et al., 2018). Large effect sizes were found specifically for improvements in manipulative skills (based on three studies), locomotor skills (based on six studies), skill-related fitness (based on 12 studies), and muscular strength/endurance (based on seven studies), with nonsignificant effects on social function (based on six studies) and body composition (based on five studies).

Although limited, some research has also evaluated strategies employed by providers of PA interventions to promote motor learning in individuals with ASD (Ruggeri et al., 2020; Sorensen & Zarrett, 2014). Specifically, frequently used methods to promote learning are based on principles of motor learning (Shumway-Cook & Woollacott, 2007) and conventional treatments for individuals with ASD (Bondy & Frost, 2003; Mesibov et al., 2004). These training methods include (a) strategies to promote practice such as repetitive task practice, contextual practice, task modifications per participant needs; (b) instructional methods, including modeling, verbal guidance, and physical guidance; (c) feedback through tangible positive reinforcement, encouragement, and feedback on task performance; (d) promotion of autonomy through goal-setting and self-monitoring; and (e) structured teaching practices based on behavioral training methodologies to provide predictable activity schedules, structured environments, and visual supports (Ruggeri et al., 2020; Sorensen & Zarrett, 2014). Overall, there is consistent evidence for improvements in gross motor function, fundamental movement skills, and components of physical fitness following movement and exercise interventions.

25.5.2 Effects of Creative and Alternative Movement-Based Interventions in ASD

In contrast to the comprehensive reviews discussed above that reported on the combined effects of conventional exercise and alternative forms of PA, some reviews exclusively focused on assessing the effects of creative and alternative forms of movement in individuals with ASD. We define creative movement therapies as novel whole-body movement interventions that are frequently categorized as alternative and integrated behavioral treatment approaches. Such approaches are distinguished from conventional approaches in that they are child-led and also promote playful exploration, individual creativity, self-expression, and improvisation (Amonkar et al., 2021; Srinivasan & Bhat, 2013). Typically, by their very nature, creative movement interventions integrate multiple domains within the individual, including sensorimotor, social, emotional, and cognitive systems. We include music-based, dance, yoga, martial arts, equine therapies, and whole-body technology-based interventions such as exergaming, active video games, virtual reality, and robotic interventions, within our definition of creative movement therapies. Creative movement interventions harness an individual's interests and may therefore be highly enjoyable and intrinsically motivating for participants, possibly leading to higher compliance compared to standard ASD interventions (Amonkar et al., 2021; Fang et al., 2019; Srinivasan & Bhat, 2013; Srinivasan, Eigsti, Gifford, et al., 2016; Srinivasan, Eigsti, Neelly, et al., 2016; Srinivasan, Kaur, et al., 2015; Srinivasan, Park, et al., 2015).

A recent systematic review of 72 studies (25 music-based, 16 martial arts-based, 12 theater-based, 11 yoga-based, 7 dance-based, and 1 combined music-dance-based interventions) conducted between 1994 and 2021 that employed non-technology-based creative movement therapies in 1939 individuals with ASD between 3 and 65 years suggested positive effects of such interventions on multiple domains (Amonkar et al., 2021). The review included 34 randomized controlled trials, 17 controlled clinical trials, 2 cross-over designs, 18 pre-post designs, and 1 reversal design. To assess risk of bias, the authors used the PEDro scale for clinical trials and the NIH quality assessment tool for single group, pre-post designs. Their assessment indicated that 50% of the clinical trials and 65% of pre-post designs had a moderate-to-high risk of bias, indicating that study rigor in the reviewed literature was poor-to-fair at best. The authors were able to calculate effect size estimates based on data provided in the original report for 89% of the studies (i.e., 64 studies), and around 45% (i.e., 29 studies) of these studies showed significant non-zero effect sizes following creative movement interventions. The review suggested medium-to-large effect sizes for improvements in social communication, motor, and cognitive skills, and medium effect sizes for improvements in behavioral skills following creative movement therapies. Specifically, there is substantial evidence from high-quality studies for improvements in social communication skills through music therapies, limited yet promising evidence for improvements in motor, cognitive, and social communication skills following martial arts therapies, and for improvements in motor and cognitive skills following yoga training.

Amonkar et al. (2021) found both inconclusive and scant evidence for the effects of creative movement on affective and sensory skills as well as functional participation in individuals with ASD. The authors recommended that clinicians work collaboratively with certified creative movement instructors/professionals to design programs tailored to the needs and activity preferences/interests of their clients with ASD (Amonkar et al., 2021).

Animal-assisted intervention (AAI) is another umbrella alternative intervention approach that has gained popularity over recent times for addressing the multisystem difficulties associated with ASD (Fine et al., 2015). It has been postulated that animals may serve as nonjudgmental, nonthreatening, safe, and comforting interaction partners for individuals with ASD, thereby reducing their stress and anxiety, and may also serve as a bridge to foster interactions with other humans (Beetz, 2017; Davis et al., 2015; McNicholas & Collis, 2006; Sams et al., 2006). Such therapies typically involve a component of caring for the animal and building a connection with them, followed by more goal-oriented activities based on targeted skills (Charry-Sánchez et al., 2018; Srinivasan et al., 2018). Equine therapies include both *hippotherapy* (use of the horse and its movement as a therapy tool for improving skills such as balance, postural control, gross motor skills, sensory modulation, and arousal levels) and *therapeutic horseback riding* (sessions that teach students riding skills to promote overall physical, cognitive, emotional, and social well-being of individuals) (Srinivasan et al., 2018). Most commonly assessed outcomes following animal-assisted interactions are social skills followed by other domains such as repetitive and problem behaviors, language and communication skills, ASD severity, positive emotions, motor skills, and stress levels (Nieforth et al., 2021; O'Haire, 2013, 2017; Srinivasan et al., 2018).

Several recent systematic reviews summarizing the effects of animal-assisted interventions in ASD suggest promising, proof-of-concept improvements in social interaction, communication skills, and stress levels with mixed results for repetitive and problem behaviors, positive emotions, and motor skills (Charry-Sánchez et al., 2018; Davis et al., 2015; O'Haire, 2017; O'Haire et al., 2014; Srinivasan et al., 2018). Specifically, with regard to the motor domain, only a handful of studies have evaluated the use of animal assistance, namely, horses, dogs, and dolphins, to facilitate motor outcomes and PA in individuals with ASD (Nieforth et al., 2021; O'Haire, 2017). The results are mixed with some studies reporting improvements in postural control, gait, balance skills, gross motor skills, and PA engagement (Ashtari & Sheikh, 2018; Borgi et al., 2016; Carlisle et al., 2018; De Milander et al., 2016; Jenkins & Reed, 2013; Steiner & Kertesz, 2015), whereas other studies reporting no improvements in outcomes as assessed using standardized motor assessments (Ajzenman et al., 2013; Gabriels et al., 2015). Although there has been a steady increase in the number of studies in this area over the last several years, the consensus across multiple reviews is that these findings are limited by methodological flaws in the reviewed studies, including the lack of large sample sizes and controlled study designs, use of anecdotal observations, issues with study reporting affecting replicability of findings, use of only researcher-constructed measurement systems for assessing outcomes, lack of assessment of treatment fidelity, poor control over confounding variables, and high risk of bias (Charry-Sánchez et al., 2018; Davis et al., 2015; Nieforth et al., 2021; O'Haire, 2017; Srinivasan et al., 2018). Overall, although promising, the evidence on the use of AAI to promote multisystem development in individuals with ASD is presently limited.

Technology-based interventions have gained attention especially over the last decade as potential therapeutic tools for individuals with ASD. This trend stems from the increased reliance on technology by both typically developing individuals and individuals with ASD (Wass & Porayska-Pomsta, 2014). Notably, individuals with ASD are more likely to engage in video or computer-based games compared to other populations, and engagement in online gaming actually increases with age from childhood to adolescence (Engelhardt et al., 2017; Mazurek & Wenstrup, 2013; Mazurek et al., 2012). Videogames are particularly enticing for this population since they are perceived as playful, highly enjoyable, consistent and predictable, less menacing compared to other interventions, have lower social demands, and provide individuals opportunities to exercise active control and autonomy over the nature of the interaction, including pace and difficulty levels. Therefore, such activities afford high levels of sustained motivation and greater adherence to training compared to conventional treatment approaches (Jiménez-Muñoz et al., 2022; Keshavan et al., 2014; Lima et al., 2020; Morris et al., 2022). Moreover, such interactions are relatively safe, promote engagement in whole-body activity within confined environments, afford opportunities for social collaboration with other players, are relatively low-cost and easily accessible for families, and may therefore serve as an adjunct to traditional modes of PA interventions (Fang et al., 2019; Foran & Cermak, 2013; Granic et al., 2014; Lima et al., 2020).

Exergaming is a popular technology-based approach that has gained attention within the research community in ASD. Exergames (exercise + video games) are defined as gaming technologies that require physical exertion or movements; may include components of strength, balance, and flexibility activities; and ultimately motivate PA among individuals or groups (Bogost, 2010; Kappen et al., 2019; Oh & Yang, 2010). Effects of exergaming on individuals with ASD have been studied on physical outcomes such as engagement in moderate-to-vigorous PA, physical fitness levels, and motor skill proficiency, as well as behavioral outcomes such as social communication skills, emotional regulation, frequencies of repetitive behaviors, and executive function skills involved with working memory, task switching, and metacognition (Fang et al., 2019; Lima et al., 2020; Morris et al., 2022).

Fang et al. (2019) conducted a systematic review of 10 studies (5 pre-post designs, 3 case-control studies, 1 randomized controlled trial, and 1 case study) to assess the effects of exergaming on cognitive and physical outcomes in individuals with ASD. The review used the PEDro scale to assess methodological quality of reviewed studies and found that three studies were of high quality, whereas all other studies were of low-to-moderate quality. Around 50% of the reviewed articles did not report any data that could allow effect size estimation. Results suggested that for individuals between 5 and 21 years of age, there is preliminary evidence that exergaming leads to improvements in physical fitness measures (body mass index, speed and agility, aerobic capacity, and muscular strength and endurance), perceived motor skill competence, and cognitive-behavioral outcomes (executive function, task-switching skills, number of repetitive behaviors, and behavioral regulation) (Dickinson & Place, 2014; Fang et al., 2019; Hilton et al., 2014, 2015). Exergaming also led to increased participation in moderate-to-vigorous PA. However, the review found insufficient evidence for improvements in motor skills, emotional regulation, and communication skills following exergaming interventions (Fang et al., 2019).

In another recent review, Morris et al. (2022) assessed the effects of 10 exergaming studies on non-fitness-related outcomes of executive function and motor skills in children (<18 years of age) with ASD (Morris et al., 2022). Similar to the results reported in Fang et al., this review also reported promising improvements in executive function skills. The results for motoric skills were mixed, with three studies reporting improvements in motor coordination and strength and agility skills and two studies suggesting lack of improvements in motor skills. The review also found equivocal results for changes in social communication skills (Morris et al., 2022). Both Fang et al. (2019) and Morris et al. (2022) reported high rates of enjoyment and participant adherence with exergaming activities. Overall, although technology-based active gaming interventions can serve as useful adjuncts to conventional ASD interventions by increasing participant motivation and promoting cognitive skills, evidence for these approaches is presently limited by small sample sizes, lack of rigorous study designs, poor-to-fair study methodological quality, unclear effect size magnitudes for measured outcomes, variability in reported effects based on types of exergames chosen and skill levels of instructors, and lack of sufficient evidence on treatment dosing for therapeutic effects. Future studies should address these concerns prior to inclusion of technology-based interventions into the routine care of individuals with ASD.

25.5.3 Summary of Research Background and Recommendations for Future Research

In the preceding section, we summarized the research evidence to date on both conventional exercise and creative movement interventions in individuals with ASD. There is a growing evidence base for the use of exercise/movement interventions to address both motor and physical fitness–related issues in individuals with ASD as well as their multisystem core impairments in social communication, behavior-affective, and cognitive domains. Conventional exercise interventions such as aerobic exercise, resistance training, and motor skills training were previously the mainstay of movement interventions for individuals with ASD. However, more recently, creative movement/exercise interventions provide intrinsically rewarding opportunities for individuals with ASD to engage in whole-body movement by responding to and incorporating their strengths and preferences/interests. It is important to note that the majority of the research has been conducted in children and adolescents with only a handful of studies evaluating efficacy of movement/PA interventions in adulthood (Barak et al., 2019; Bested et al., 2021; Boso et al., 2007; Duffy et al., 2017; Garcia-Villamisar et al., 2017; Garcia-Villamisar & Dattilo, 2010; Hildebrandt et al., 2016; Hillier et al., 2011; Koch et al., 2015; Mastrominico et al., 2018; Nabors et al., 2021; Pitetti et al., 2007; Savage et al., 2022; Shields et al., 2019). Thus, generalization into effective strategies to address the needs of adults with ASD is limited. Given the evidence for the persistence of motor impairments into young adulthood as well as the trend for increase in levels of inactivity with growing age, there is a dire need for more research to develop PA/movement programs for adults with ASD. Moreover, as discussed in this section, conclusions drawn from studies conducted in this field to date need to be interpreted with caution, given the moderate-to-high risk of bias in a majority of the studies (Ruggeri et al., 2020; Sorensen & Zarrett, 2014). Future studies should involve large sample randomized controlled trials with careful control of confounding factors to collect definitive evidence in support of movement interventions in persons with ASD of all ages (Healy et al., 2018).

Several reviews also discussed difficulties associated with drawing definitive conclusions from the present literature due to factors related to the diversity of recruited participants across studies, variation in treatment dosage provided, and lack of details on exercise intensity of the training programs employed (Bremer et al., 2016; Howells et al., 2019). The scientific merit and ability to draw conclusions would improve if researchers provide more details pertaining to the recruited samples, including IQ levels, measures of ASD severity, and overall adaptive function to better characterize the sample. Additional moderating factors related to participants include existing sensorimotor skills, motivation levels, sensory sensitivities, motor planning abilities, and social skill levels, all of which may impact PA engagement. Some of the variability with the research results may also occur because of factors that cannot be controlled within the research study. Attempts to identify mediators and moderators during the time of the study may help explain results. Researchers should also describe treatment characteristics thoroughly in order to conduct a systematic assessment of dose-response effects (Healy et al., 2018; Sorensen & Zarrett, 2014). Studies could use heart rate monitors or accelerometers to better document exercise intensity and progression during training and allow replicability of study findings (Bremer et al., 2016). Finally, a majority of the studies did not conduct any follow-up tests to assess carryover effects of training after completion of the program (Bremer et al., 2016; Howells et al., 2019; Sorensen & Zarrett, 2014). Assessment of training carryover to better understand the long-term effects of movement interventions in individuals with ASD would surely add to our understanding of what programs will be of most benefit to these individuals as they progress into adulthood.

Furthermore, it would be crucial for studies to implement the interventions as part of community/naturalistic settings and obtain stakeholder input while designing interventions to ensure that the programs are aligned with stakeholder needs, thereby facilitating the research-to-practice transition (Dillon et al., 2017). Based on our literature review, we also recommend that future systematic reviews and meta-analyses conduct separate analyses of studies evaluating the effects of conventional exercise versus creative forms of movement to aid a better understanding of the differential effects of different exercise modalities and the underlying mechanisms of action of unique exercise modes. Although this literature is limited by these methodological issues, preliminary evidence suggests promise for the use of movement interventions to address core impairments and to improve physical, mental, and psychosocial health and well-being in individuals with ASD. Moreover, novel creative movement interventions may serve as adjuncts to conventional modes of exercise/movement delivery to boost adherence and sustained motivation to engage in movement/PA.

25.5.4 Modes of Intervention Delivery: Role of Telehealth in Delivering Movement Interventions

Movement interventions have conventionally been provided face to face to individuals with ASD. However, recently, virtual or telehealth modes of intervention delivery have been increasingly explored by several groups, especially over the past 2 years, in light of the COVID-19 pandemic (Narzisi, 2020; Simacek et al., 2020; Srinivasan et al., 2021; Tohidast et al., 2020; Unholz-Bowden et al., 2020). Telehealth delivery has the advantage of allowing healthcare access to geographically remote families, is cost efficient, affords provision of interventions in the child's naturalistic environments thereby facilitating carryover into the child's routines, and also reduces costs of transportation for family and clinicians (Pickard et al., 2016; Simacek et al., 2020). However, telehealth delivery requires a stable internet connection, may demand greater involvement from caregivers to support online interactions of clinicians with individuals with ASD, and poses challenges especially for more severely affected individuals with ASD who need hand-on-hand assistance or in-person therapist guidance (Bhat et al., 2021; Cleffi et al., 2022; Srinivasan et al., 2021). Telehealth-based interventions in ASD have primarily focused on providing training to caregivers/parents to facilitate their child's development, including social communication and behavioral skills (de Nocker & Toolan, 2021; degli Espinosa et al., 2020; Ferguson et al., 2019; Knutsen et al., 2016; Wainer & Ingersoll, 2015). A recent systematic review of 16 telehealth interventions for persons with ASD reported on both structured and naturalistic behavioral interventions implemented through telehealth to improve skills such as social engagement, joint attention, symbolic play, imitation, and communication skills in children with ASD (de Nocker & Toolan, 2021). All study procedures included providing coaching to caregivers to implement interventions commonly used for persons with ASD. Results indicated that in a majority of studies, there were no significant differences between in-person and telehealth modes of intervention delivery, and telehealth was well-accepted by stakeholders as a mode of intervention delivery (de Nocker & Toolan, 2021; Nohelty et al., 2021).

Few movement intervention studies have used telehealth-based modes to deliver movement/PA interventions to individuals with ASD (Healy & Marchand, 2020; Ketcheson & Pitchford, 2021; Wainer & Ingersoll, 2015). For instance, Healy and Marchand (2020) conducted a 4-week Facebook-delivered, parent-mediated PA intervention based on elements of the social cognitive theory for children with ASD and found positive results for feasibility of implementation, participant engagement, effectiveness of individual components, and PA participation in children with ASD following the intervention (Healy & Marchand, 2020). Similarly, Ketcheson and Pitchford (2021) have proposed a protocol for project PLANE (Physical Literacy and Nutrition Education), a 52-week-long virtual intervention that will provide training to both children with ASD and their caregivers on PA engagement and motor skill development as well as nutritional education through a combination of synchronous and asynchronous sessions. The authors hypothesize that the PLANE training will lead to improvements in body composition, PA levels, and quality of life of individuals with ASD and will be associated with high levels of training fidelity and feasibility of implementation (Ketcheson & Pitchford, 2021).

Similarly, our own research has shown promising results from the implementation of clinician-caregiver co-delivered, telehealth-based, whole-body movement interventions in children with ASD (Bhat et al., 2021; Cleffi et al., 2022; Srinivasan et al., 2021). Although telehealth has its own technical challenges related to Internet connectivity, inherent limitations of teleconferencing software, and need for dedicated hardware, this mode of intervention delivery is a valuable adjunct to conventional in-person modes of delivery, especially in case of clinician/staffing shortages and difficulty accessing care in remote settings. In our experience, the success of telehealth for delivering movement interventions to children with ASD depends heavily on caregiver buy-in and involvement to help set up the technology, provide ongoing support and troubleshooting aid as needed, and to foster engagement/rapport between the child and the clinician during online interactions. Parents may need to be the "therapist in the room" during such interactions to provide demonstrations, prompting, assistance, and feedback as required by the child. This increased involvement may exacerbate parental stress and child frustration in some cases (Srinivasan et al., 2021). Overall, despite some challenges associated with initial setup and subsequent implementation, the telehealth mode of intervention delivery is likely to become more common in years to come, in view of the many advantages of this approach. Accordingly, more research in this area is needed to systematically compare in-person and telehealth modes of intervention delivery for exercise/movement interventions and to develop clear clinical practice guidelines for clinicians using telehealth interventions for their clients with ASD.

25.6 Practice Implications

It is clear from evidence presented in this chapter that movement and exercise/PA-based interventions lead to promising beneficial effects in individuals with ASD. Such interventions not only help enhance physical health and fitness to avoid comorbidities secondary to inactivity (similar to effects in typically developing individuals) but also have far-reaching effects on the core social communication, behavioral, and cognitive impairments central to the diagnosis. Movement-based interventions can provide opportunities for individuals with ASD to socialize with peers, improve attentional focus, regulate their sensory systems, attention, and arousal levels, and reduce stereotypical behaviors. Given these widespread positive effects of whole-body movement and exercise, exercise/PA interventions are indicated across the lifespan with no known contraindications for individuals with ASD.

25.6.1 Developing Adapted and Individually Tailored Movement and PA Programs

The exercise intervention should be designed bearing in mind the interests, preferences, and sensory needs of individuals with ASD, to stimulate interest, and to promote long-term adherence with the prescribed program (Amonkar et al., 2021; Sorensen & Zarrett, 2014; Srinivasan et al., 2014). For example, the predictable and repetitive nature of martial arts might be preferred by a child who desires structure and fixed routines, whereas another child with an interest in technology might be more inclined toward exergaming interventions. Given the heterogeneity in the presentation of individuals with ASD, no "one-size-fits-all" approach can be adopted while designing movement interventions for this population. Instead, it is crucial that the intervention be tailored to the needs of individual clients with ASD to ensure maximum benefits and promote carryover outside the training contexts (Bremer et al., 2016; Sorensen & Zarrett, 2014).

We recommend that whole-body movement/PA interventions be designed and implemented by a team of people with knowledge regarding the unique characteristics of individuals with ASD, and with adequate training to work with individuals with ASD, including experience in implementing behavior management strategies. The team may include families of individuals with ASD, special educators, PE teachers/coaches, licensed physical, occupational, and recreational therapists, and certified, specialized instructors, especially, for implementing creative movement interventions such as dance movement therapies, martial arts, music therapy, and yoga (Amonkar et al., 2021; Srinivasan et al., 2014).

The content of the training program will depend on both the preferences/interests of individuals with ASD (as discussed above) and the intended effects of the interventions. As discussed in the preceding section, certain types of exercise lead to beneficial effects on specific domains of function. For instance, there is evidence for improvements in cognitive function following exergaming and martial arts interventions (Amonkar et al., 2021; Hynes & Block, 2022; Liang et al., 2022; Tan et al., 2016), in socio-emotional skills following music therapies, aquatic interventions, and horseback riding (Amonkar et al., 2021; Bremer et al., 2016; Healy et al., 2018; Srinivasan & Bhat, 2013; Srinivasan et al., 2018), and in motor and behavioral outcomes following martial arts, yoga, and aerobic exercises (Amonkar et al., 2021; Hynes & Block, 2022). These findings do not suggest definitively that the effects of specific exercise modalities are restricted exclusively to specific domains (Bremer et al., 2016). For instance, aquatic interventions may also improve cognitive skills or martial arts training may lead to improved social-emotional functioning; however, there is presently no research evaluating these effects. More research is needed to tease apart the differential effects of different exercise modalities.

We recommend that individuals with ASD should obtain medical clearance from a physician for engagement in PA prior to commencement of the exercise program. Irrespective of the exercise modality chosen, individuals with ASD should follow known principles for participating in healthy, progressive exercise/movement-based programs. To assure maximal benefit and diminish the risk of injury, the program should include a warm-up prior to and cool-down following the main part of the exercise session. These guidelines are applicable to both conventional exercise and creative movement training (Piercy et al., 2018; Srinivasan et al., 2014). It is expected that individuals who are unaccustomed to regular exercise are likely to experience temporary muscle soreness and fatigue associated with commencement of an exercise program.

25.6.2 Training Parameters for Movement and PA Programs

A review of the evidence in support of movement and PA interventions in individuals with ASD indicates significant variability in the dosing of training provided by different studies. For both conventional and creative movement interventions, studies varied widely in terms of the frequency of sessions per week, the overall duration of the training program, and the duration of each individual session (Amonkar et al., 2021; Bremer et al., 2016; Teh et al., 2022). Since no study has systematically varied training dosing parameters and assessed the effects of such variations on measured outcomes, there are presently no clear guidelines for movement and PA interventions for persons with ASD. Instead, we recommend that clinicians follow the age-appropriate guidelines for PA/exercise laid out in the *Physical Activity Guidelines for Americans* (2nd ed.) that apply to individuals with and without chronic disabilities (Piercy et al., 2018). Specifically, it is recommended that preschoolers (3–5 years) stay active throughout the day by engaging in both unstructured play and structured activities such as riding a tricycle, throwing activities, playing tag, and so on. It is also recommended that they engage in activities such as hopping, skipping, jumping, and tumbling, to strengthen their bones. Although guidelines on the specific amount of activity are not available for this age range, a ballpark estimate is around 3 hours/day of all intensities of activity (light, moderate, and vigorous PA).

For school-age children and adolescents (6–17 years), it is recommended that they engage in at least 60 minutes of moderate-to-vigorous PA, with most of this activity being aerobic exercise of vigorous intensity, preferably daily or at least 3 days/week. Similarly, on at least 3 days/week, muscle- and bone-strengthening exercises should be part of the 60 minutes/day PA schedule. For adults (18+ years), 150 to 300 minutes/week of moderate-intensity aerobic PA or 75 to 150 minutes/week of vigorous-intensity aerobic PA per week is recommended. Moreover, as part of PA routine, on at least 2 days/week, adults should engage in moderate or higher intensity of muscle-strengthening exercises. Finally, for older adults (≥65 years), it is recommended that they include components of balance training as part of their regular PA in addition to aerobic and muscle-strengthening activities. In terms of progression, training can be made progressively challenging by increasing the session duration, training frequency, and/or by increasing the difficulty of the tasks practiced. Table 25.1 summarizes our recommendations for conventional exercise and creative movement based on the evidence to date in this area. The present state of evidence is conflicted in terms of the ideal intervention setting for individuals with ASD, specifically, individual versus group exercise programs, with evidence supporting both approaches (Bremer et al., 2016; Healy et al., 2018; Howells et al., 2019; Sowa & Meulenbroek, 2012; Teh et al., 2021).

Table 25.1 Recommendations for prescription of movement-based interventions in individuals with ASD

Characteristics of Movement Interventions	Suggested Initial Prescription	Suggested Progression
Preschoolers (3–5 years)		
Frequency	7 days/week	• Increase variety of activities • Increase bout duration • Increase intensity of activities
Intensity	Light, moderate, and vigorous activity	
Time	3 hours/day accumulated in short bouts	
Type	Active play, structured body weight activities involving aerobic exercise and bone- and muscle-strengthening components • Catching, throwing, and kicking games • Rough and tumble play • Bicycle or tricycle rides, playing tag, swimming, climbing • Hopping, skipping, jumping, running, gymnastics	
School-aged children (6–17 years)		
Frequency	3–5 days/week	• Increase frequency (6–7 days/week) of PA • Increase exercise intensity • Increase duration per bout
Intensity	Moderate to vigorous activity	
Time	≥60 minutes/session (can be accumulated in short bouts)	
Type	Aerobic activity (at least 3 days/week) as well as age-appropriate muscle- and bone-strengthening activities (at least 3 days/week) • *Aerobic*—Running, hopping, skipping, jumping, swimming, dancing, cycling, hiking, riding a manual scooter, playing tag, martial arts, exergaming, playing sports like baseball and softball, house and yard work like sweeping, pushing a lawn mower, etc. • *Muscle strengthening*—using playground equipment, climbing, playing tug-of-war, lifting weights or using weight machines, using resistance bands, yoga • *Bone strengthening*—weight-bearing activities like running, playing jump rope, playing sports like tennis, basketball, etc. involving jumping or rapid change in direction	
Adults (18–65 years)		
Frequency	3–5 days/week	• Increase frequency (6–7 days/week) of PA • Increase intensity of exercise

Characteristics of Movement Interventions	Suggested Initial Prescription	Suggested Progression
Intensity	Moderate to vigorous activity	• Increase duration per bout • Increase no. of sets and weight for resistance training
Time	≥60 minutes/session (can be accumulated in short bouts)	
Type	Moderate aerobic activity (150–300 minutes/week) or vigorous aerobic activity (75–150 minutes/week) spread over the week and muscle strengthening (≥2 days/week) • *Aerobic*—Jogging, running, brisk walking, swimming, water aerobics, dancing, hiking, playing sports like tennis, basketball, etc., high-intensity interval training, kickboxing, step aerobics, exergames, active transportation (walking, biking), physically active occupations, active forms of yoga, Tai chi, yard work or home chores • *Muscle strengthening*—lifting weights, using resistance bands, yoga, calisthenics using body weight (push-ups, pull-ups, planks, etc.), carrying heavy loads, heavy gardening (8–12 repetitions/set; 2–3 sets/exercise) • *Flexibility activities*—yoga, stretching exercises	
Older Adults (65 + years)		
Frequency	3–5 days/week	• Increase frequency (6–7 days/week) of PA • Increase intensity of exercise • Increase duration per bout • Increase no. of sets and weight for resistance training
Intensity	Moderate to vigorous activity	
Time	≥60 minutes/session (can be accumulated in short bouts)	
Type	Guidelines similar to adults (Moderate aerobic activity (150–300 minutes/week) or vigorous aerobic activity (75–150 minutes/week) spread over week and muscle strengthening (≥2 days/week) *Additional considerations*: Perform multicomponent PA inclusive of balance training as well as aerobic and muscle-strengthening activities • *Aerobic*—Jogging, running, brisk walking, swimming, water aerobic exercise class, cycling (stationary or outdoors), dancing, hiking, playing sports like tennis or basketball, active forms of yoga, yard work or home chores	

continued

Table 25.1 *continued*

Characteristics of Movement Interventions	Suggested Initial Prescription	Suggested Progression
	• *Muscle strengthening*—lifting weights, using resistance bands, weight machines, yoga postures, Tai chi, calisthenics using body weight (push-ups, pull-ups, planks, squats, lunges, etc.), gardening (digging, lifting, carrying), carrying groceries, climbing stairs, carrying heavy loads, heavy gardening, shoveling snow (8–12 repetitions/set; 2–3 sets/exercise) • *Balance activities* for fall prevention • *Gait, coordination, and physical function training* as needed • *Flexibility activities*—yoga, stretching exercises	

ASD = autism spectrum disorder; PA = physical activity.

25.6.3 Designing Family-Centric Movement and PA Interventions

While designing interventions for individuals with ASD, it is important to include inputs from key stakeholders, namely self-advocates with ASD, their caregivers/family members, special educators, clinicians, and paraprofessionals (Fletcher-Watson et al., 2019; McDonald et al., 2021). Our recent work that has involved focus group discussions with key stakeholder groups to understand trends and needs related to PA engagement in youth with developmental disabilities (including ASD) as they transition out of school settings revealed key insights (Athreya et al., 2022; Srinivasan et al., 2022). Stakeholders emphasized that children and adolescents primarily receive PA interventions as part of academic programming (PE, sports) and through after-school activities. However, there are few interventions for individuals once they transition out of school settings, with families having to take responsibility of finding programs to engage their adult family member with disability. Specifically, stakeholder groups indicated the need for accessible and affordable community-based programs with well-trained and empathetic instructors for individuals with disabilities across the lifespan. They recommended the need for structured programs with a predictable schedule that provide individuals with multiple options to engage in noncompetitive, enjoyable, and self-paced activities that promote autonomy and independence. Moreover, stakeholders suggested that programs providing individuals with disabilities opportunities to exercise with typically developing peers would be enjoyable for them and promote long-term program adherence. They also indicated the need for tailored programs adapted to the individual's abilities, including sensorimotor, social, and cognitive skills. To promote functional carryover and lifelong active habits, stakeholders recommended integration of PA into age-appropriate activities and regular routines, including as part of chores at home (Athreya et al., 2022; Lang et al., 2010; Sorensen & Zarrett, 2014; Srinivasan et al., 2022; Srinivasan et al., 2014).

25.6.4 Recommendations for Behavioral Strategies to Promote PA Engagement

Working with individuals with ASD can be challenging, given their multisystem impairments. We recommend that clinicians use strategies based on treatment approaches commonly used for individuals with ASD, including applied behavior analysis (ABA, Lovaas, 2003), Teaching and Education of Autistic and Communication Handicapped Children (TEACHH, Mesibov et al., 2004), and Picture Exchange Communication System (PECS, Bondy & Frost, 2003). For instance, effective ABA-based strategies include the use of incremental least-to-most prompting (verbal and gestural prompts followed by manual prompts), fading strategies (reduce amount of prompting as movement skills improve), modeling/demonstrations, structured teaching, and reinforcement schedules with tangible items, tokens, and verbal praise (Lovaas, 2003). Individuals with ASD also greatly benefit from predictable environments, structured routines, and consistency in people, props/exercise equipment, and places of exercise, which is in line with TEACHH principles (Mesibov et al., 2004). Picture schedules provide structure to training sessions and facilitate transitions between activities (Bondy & Frost, 2003). Other strategies that are effective in individuals with ASD are based on principles of sensory integration, motor learning, and self-determination theory (Ayres, 1972; Ryan & Deci, 2000; Shumway-Cook & Woollacott, 2007). Clinicians should choose activities that address the sensory needs of individuals at the start of the movement intervention and through sensory breaks in an ongoing manner, as needed, during the intervention based on the sensory profile (hypo- or hypersensitivity to different sensory stimuli) of their clients (Ayres, 1972). Motor learning principles such as part-whole practice, variable and distributed practice, discovery learning, and appropriate modifications to the task and/or environment to set the "*just right*" challenge for the individual with ASD are critical to ensure success in motor skill acquisition (Shumway-Cook & Woollacott, 2007; Srinivasan et al., 2014). Moreover, intervention strategies based on self-determination theory such as goal setting, promoting autonomy, self-monitoring, and self-efficacy have also been successfully used in individuals with ASD and may be incorporated to improve training efficacy (Pan et al., 2011; Ryan & Deci, 2000; Sorensen & Zarrett,

2014; Srinivasan et al., 2014; Todd & Reid, 2006; Todd et al., 2010). Overall, we recommend that clinicians tailor movement and PA interventions to the individual needs and preferences of their clients and their families to promote lifelong active habits as well as overall health and well-being in individuals with ASD.

25.7 References

Adolph, K. E., & Berger, S. E. (2011). Physical and motor development. In M. H. Bornstein & M. E. Lamb (Eds.), *Developmental science: An advanced textbook* (6th ed., pp. 241–302). Mahwah, NJ: Erlbaum.

Adolph, K. E., & Franchak, J. M. (2017). The development of motor behavior. *Wiley Interdisciplinary Reviews: Cognitive Science, 8*(1–2), e1430. https://doi.org/10.1002/wcs.1430

Adolph, K. E., & Hoch, J. E. (2019). Motor development: Embodied, embedded, enculturated, and enabling. *Annual Review of Psychology, 70*, 141–164. https://doi.org/10.1146/annurev-psych-010418-102836

Adolph, K. E., & Robinson, S. R. (2013). The road to walking: What learning to walk tells us about development. In P. Zelazo (Ed.), *The Oxford handbook of developmental psychology* (pp. 403–443). New York: Oxford University Press.

Adolph, K. E., & Robinson, S. R. (2015). Motor development. In W. Damon & R. Lerner (Series Eds.) & D. Kuhn & R. S. Siegler (Vol. Eds.), *Handbook of child psychology: Cognition, perception, and language* (pp. 161–213). Hoboken, NJ: Wiley. https://doi.org/10.1002/9781118963418.childpsy204

Ajzenman, H. F., Standeven, J. W., & Shurtleff, T. L. (2013). Effect of hippotherapy on motor control, adaptive behaviors, and participation in children with autism spectrum disorder: A pilot study. *The American Journal of Occupational Therapy, 67*(6), 653–663. https://doi.org/10.5014/ajot.2013.008383

Amiel-Tison, C., & Grenier, A. (1986). *Neurological assessment during the first year of life*. New York: Oxford University Press.

Amonkar, N., Su, W. C., Bhat, A. N., & Srinivasan, S. M. (2021). Effects of creative movement therapies on social communication, behavioral-affective, sensorimotor, cognitive, and functional participation skills of individuals with autism spectrum disorder: A systematic review. *Frontiers in Psychiatry, 12*. https://doi.org/10.3389/fpsyt.2021.722874

Anderson, D. I., Campos, J. J., Witherington, D. C., Dahl, A., Rivera, M., He, M., Uchiyama, I., & Barbu-Roth, M. (2013). The role of locomotion in psychological development. *Frontiers in Psychology, 4*, 440. https://doi.org/10.3389/fpsyg.2013.00440

Anderson-Hanley, C., Tureck, K., & Schneiderman, R. L. (2011). Autism and exergaming: Effects on repetitive behaviors and cognition. *Psychology Research and Behavior Management, 4*, 129–137. https://doi.org/10.2147/PRBM.S24016

Ashtari, M., & Sheikh, M. (2018). The effect of swimming with dolphins on the selected balance and strength gross motor skills of eight-yearold children with autism spectrum disorder. *Sport Science, 11*(1), 131–137. https://www.researchgate.net/publication/328699095_The_effect_of_swimming_with_dolphins_on_the_selected_balance_and_strength_gross_motor_skills_of_eight-yearold_children_with_autism_spectrum_disorder

Assaiante, C. (1998). Development of locomotor balance control in healthy children. *Neuroscience & Biobehavioral Reviews, 22*(4), 527–532. https://doi.org/10.1016/S0149-7634(97)00040-7

Athreya, A., Kaba, M., Glenney, S., Bubela, D., & Srinivasan, S. (2022). *Perspectives of clinicians and special educators on physical activity in youth with developmental disabilities: A qualitative study* [Poster presentation]. 2022 Annual Meeting of the International Society for Autism Research (INSAR). Austin, TX. https://www.autism-insar.org/page/INSAR2022Archives

Ayres, A. J. (1972). Improving academic scores through sensory integration. *Journal of Learning Disabilities, 5*(6), 338–343. https://doi.org/10.1177/002221947200500605

Bandura, A. (1977). Self-efficacy: Toward a unifying theory of behavioral change. *Psychological Review, 84*(2), 191. https://doi.org/10.1037/0033-295X.84.2.191

Bandura, A. (1986). The explanatory and predictive scope of self-efficacy theory. Journal of Social and Clinical Psychology, 4(3), 359–373. https://doi.org/10.1521/jscp.1986.4.3.359

Bandura, A. (2002). Social foundations of thought and action. In D. F. Marks (Ed.), *The health psychology reader* (pp. 94–106). Thousand Oaks, CA: Sage. https://dx.doi.org/10.4135/9781446221129.n6

Bandura, A. (2004). Health promotion by social cognitive means. *Health Education & Behavior, 31*(2), 143–164. https://doi.org/10.1177/1090198104263660

Barak, S., Oz, M., Dagan, N., & Hutzler, Y. (2019). The game of life soccer program: Effect on skills, physical fitness and mobility in persons with intellectual disability and autism spectrum disorder. *Journal of Applied Research in Intellectual Disabilities, 32*(6), 1401–1411. https://doi.org/10.1111/jar.12620

Barlow, S. M. (2009). Oral and respiratory control for preterm feeding. *Current Opinion in Otolaryngology & Head and Neck Surgery, 17*(3), 179. https://doi.org/10.1097/MOO.0b013e32832b36fe

Bar-Or, O. (1983). Physiologic responses to exercise of the healthy child. *Pediatric sports medicine for the practitioner* (pp. 1–65). Cham: Springer. https://doi.org/10.1007/978-1-4612-5593-2

Beetz, A. M. (2017). Theories and possible processes of action in animal assisted interventions. *Applied Developmental Science, 21*(2), 139–149. https://doi.org/10.1080/10888691.2016.1262263

Beighle, A., Morgan, C. F., Le Masurier, G., & Pangrazi, R. P. (2006). Children's physical activity during recess and outside of school. *Journal of School Health, 76*(10), 516–520. https://doi.org/10.1111/j.1746-1561.2006.00151.x

Bested, S. R., Carr, K., Sutherland, C. A., Horton, S., & Azar, N. R. (2021). Improving upper extremity motor control in adults with autism spectrum disorder and an intellectual disability through participation in an adapted physical exercise intervention. *Journal on Developmental Disabilities, 26*(1), 1–15. https://doi.org/10.5281/zenodo.4958958

Bhat, A., Galloway, J., & Landa, R. (2012). Relation between early motor delay and later communication delay in infants at risk for autism. *Infant Behavior and Development, 35*(4), 838–846. https://doi.org/10.1016/j.infbeh.2012.07.019

Bhat, A., Landa, R., & Galloway, J. C. (2011). Current perspectives on motor functioning in infants, children, and adults with autism spectrum disorders. *Physical Therapy, 91*(7), 1116–1129. https://doi.org/10.2522/ptj.20100294

Bhat, A., Su, W. C., Cleffi, C., & Srinivasan, S. (2021). A hybrid clinical trial delivery model in the COVID-19 era. *Physical Therapy, 101*(8). https://doi.org/10.1093/ptj/pzab116

Bhat, A. N. (2020). Is motor impairment in autism spectrum disorder (ASD) distinct from developmental coordination disorder (DCD)? A report from the SPARK study. *Physical Therapy, 100*(4), 633–644. https://doi.org/10.1093/ptj/pzz190

Bhat, A. N. (2021). Motor impairment increases in children with autism spectrum disorder as a function of social communication, cognitive and functional impairment, repetitive behavior severity, and comorbid diagnoses: A SPARK study report. *Autism Research, 14*(1), 202–219. https://doi.org/10.1002/aur.2453

de Boer, B. (2012). *Stabilizing bimanual coordination: Changes in interlimb interactions* [Unpublished thesis, VU University Amsterdam, The Netherlands].

Bogost, I. (2010). *Persuasive games: The expressive power of videogames.* Cambridge, MA: MIT Press.

Bondy, A., & Frost, A. (2003). Communication strategies for visual learners. In O. I. Lovaas (Ed.), *Teaching individuals with developmental delays: Basic intervention techniques* (pp. 291–304). Austin, TX: Pro-Ed.

Boreham, C. A., & McKay, H. A. (2011). Physical activity in childhood and bone health. *British Journal of Sports Medicine, 45*(11), 877–879. http://dx.doi.org/10.1136/bjsports-2011-090188

Borgi, M., Loliva, D., Cerino, S., Chiarotti, F., Venerosi, A., Bramini, M., Nonnis, E., Marcelli, M., Vinti, C., & De Santis, C. (2016). Effectiveness of a standardized equine-assisted therapy program for children with autism spectrum disorder. *Journal of Autism and Developmental Disorders, 46*(1), 1–9. https://doi.org/10.1007/s10803-015-2530-6

Boso, M., Emanuele, E., Minazzi, V., Abbamonte, M., & Politi, P. (2007). Effect of long-term interactive music therapy on behavior profile and musical skills in young adults with severe autism. *Journal of Alternative and Complementary Medicine, 13*(7), 709–712. https://doi.org/10.1089/acm.2006.6334

Bourgeois, K. S., Khawar, A. W., Neal, S. A., & Lockman, J. J. (2005). Infant manual exploration of objects, surfaces, and their interrelations. *Infancy, 8*(3), 233–252. https://doi.org/10.1207/s15327078in0803_3

Bremer, E., Crozier, M., & Lloyd, M. (2016). A systematic review of the behavioural outcomes following exercise interventions for children and youth with autism spectrum disorder. *Autism, 20*(8), 899–915. https://doi.org/10.1177/1362361315616002

Bushnell, E. W. (1981). The ontogeny of intermodal relations: Vision and touch in infancy. *Intersensory perception and sensory integration* (pp. 5–36). Cham: Springer. https://doi.org/10.1007/978-1-4615-9197-9_1

Bushnell, E. W., & Boudreau, J. P. (1993). Motor development and the mind: The potential role of motor abilities as a determinant of aspects of perceptual development. *Child Development, 64*(4), 1005–1021. https://doi.org/10.1111/j.1467-8624.1993.tb04184.x

Campos, J. J., Anderson, D. I., Barbu-Roth, M. A., Hubbard, E. M., Hertenstein, M. J., & Witherington, D. (2000). Travel broadens the mind. *Infancy, 1*(2), 149–219. https://doi.org/10.1207/S15327078IN0102_1

Carlisle, G. K., Johnson, R. A., Mazurek, M., Bibbo, J. L., Tocco, F., & Cameron, G. T. (2018). Companion animals in families of children with autism spectrum disorder: Lessons learned from caregivers. *Journal of Family Social Work, 21*(4-5), 294–312. https://doi.org/10.1080/10522158.2017.1394413

Caro, K., Tentori, M., Martinez-Garcia, A., & Alvelais, M. (2017). Using the FroggyBobby exergame to support eye-body coordination development of children with severe autism. *International Journal of Human Computer Studies, 105*, 12–27. https://doi.org/10.1016/j.ijhcs.2017.03.005

Caspersen, C. J., Powell, K. E., & Christenson, G. M. (1985). Physical activity, exercise, and physical fitness: Definitions and distinctions for health-related research. *Public Health Reports (Washington, D.C.: 1974), 100*(2), 126–131. https://www.ncbi.nlm.nih.gov/pmc/articles/PMC1424733/

Celiberti, D. A., Bobo, H. E., Kelly, K. S., Harris, S. L., & Handleman, J. S. (1997). The differential and temporal effects of antecedent exercise on the self-stimulatory behavior of a child with autism. *Research in Developmental Disabilities, 18*(2), 139–150. https://doi.org/10.1016/S0891-4222(96)00032-7

Charry-Sánchez, J. D., Pradilla, I., & Talero-Gutiérrez, C. (2018). Effectiveness of animal-assisted therapy in the pediatric population: Systematic review and meta-analysis of controlled studies. *Journal of Developmental & Behavioral Pediatrics, 39*(7), 580–590. http://doi.org/10.1097/DBP.0000000000000594

Chita-Tegmark, M. (2016). Social attention in ASD: A review and meta-analysis of eye-tracking studies. *Research in Developmental Disabilities, 48*, 79–93. https://doi.org/10.1016/j.ridd.2015.10.011

Chonchaiya, W., Nuntnarumit, P., & Pruksananonda, C. (2011). Comparison of television viewing between children with autism spectrum disorder and controls. *Acta Paediatrica, 100*(7), 1033–1037. https://doi.org/10.1111/j.1651-2227.2011.02166.x

Clearfield, M. W. (2011). Learning to walk changes infants' social interactions. *Infant Behavior and Development, 34*(1), 15–25. https://doi.org/10.1016/j.infbeh.2010.04.008

Cleffi, C., Su, W.-C., Srinivasan, S., & Bhat, A. (2022). Using telehealth to conduct family-centered, movement intervention research in children with autism spectrum disorder during the COVID-19 pandemic. *Pediatric Physical Therapy, 34*(2), 246–251. https://doi.org/10.1097/PEP.0000000000000872

Clevenger, K. A., Moore, R. W., Suton, D., Montoye, A. H., Trost, S. G., & Pfeiffer, K. A. (2018). Accelerometer responsiveness to change between structured and unstructured physical activity in children and adolescents. *Measurement in Physical Education and Exercise Science, 22*(3), 224–230. https://doi.org/10.1080/1091367X.2017.1419956

Cohen, J. (1988). Statistical power analysis for the behavioral sciences. Hillsdale: Lawrence Erlbaum Associates, Publishers. https://doi.org/10.4324/9780203771587

Cohen, K. E., Morgan, P. J., Plotnikoff, R. C., Barnett, L. M., & Lubans, D. R. (2015). Improvements in fundamental movement skill competency mediate the effect of the SCORES intervention on physical activity and cardiorespiratory fitness in children. *Journal of Sports Sciences, 33*(18), 1908–1918. https://doi.org/10.1080/02640414.2015.1017734

Courtney-Long, E. A., Carroll, D. D., Zhang, Q. C., Stevens, A. C., Griffin-Blake, S., Armour, B. S., & Campbell, V. A. (2015). Prevalence of disability and disability type among adults—united states, 2013. *MMWR.Morbidity and Mortality Weekly Report, 64*(29), 777–783. https://doi.org/10.15585/mmwr.mm6429a2

Craig, F., Margari, F., Legrottaglie, A. R., Palumbi, R., de Giambattista, C., & Margari, L. (2016). A review of executive function deficits in autism spectrum disorder and attention-deficit/hyperactivity disorder. *Neuropsychiatric Disease and Treatment, 12*, 1191–1202. https://doi.org/10.2147/NDT.S104620

Curtin, C., Anderson, S. E., Must, A., & Bandini, L. (2010). The prevalence of obesity in children with autism: A secondary data analysis using nationally representative data from the national survey of children's health. *BMC Pediatrics, 10*, 11. https://doi.org/10.1186/1471-2431-10-11

Davis, T. N., Scalzo, R., Butler, E., Stauffer, M., Farah, Y. N., Perez, S., Mainor, K., Clark, C., Miller, S., Kobylecky, A., & Coviello, L. (2015). Animal assisted interventions for children with autism spectrum disorder: A systematic review. *Education and Training in Autism and Developmental Disabilities, 50*(3), 316–329. https://www.jstor.org/stable/24827513

Degli Espinosa, F., Metko, A., Raimondi, M., Impenna, M., & Scognamiglio, E. (2020). A model of support for families of children with autism living in the COVID-19 lockdown: Lessons from Italy. *Behavior Analysis in Practice, 13*(3), 550–558. https://doi.org/10.1007/s40617-020-00438-7

Demetriou, E. A., Lampit, A., Quintana, D. S., Naismith, S. L., Song, Y. J., Pye, J. E., Hickie, I., & Guastella, E. A. (2018). Autism spectrum disorders: A meta-analysis of executive function. *Molecular Psychiatry, 23*(5), 1198–1204. https://doi.org/10.1038/mp.2017.75

Dewey, D. (1993). Error analysis of limb and orofacial praxis in children with developmental motor deficits. *Brain and Cognition, 23*, 203–221. https://doi.org/10.1006/brcg.1993.1055

Dewey, D. (1995). What is developmental dyspraxia. *Brain and Cognition, 29*(3), 254–274. https://doi.org/10.1006/brcg.1995.1281

Dewey, D., Cantell, M., & Crawford, S. G. (2007). Motor and gestural performance in children with autism spectrum disorders, developmental coordination disorder, and/ or attention deficit hyperactivity disorder. *Journal of the International Neuropsychological Society, 13*, 246–256. https://doi.org/10.1017/S1355617707070270

Diamond, A. (2000). Close interrelation of motor development and cognitive development and of the cerebellum and prefrontal cortex. *Child Development, 71*(1), 44–56. http://doi.org/10.1111/1467-8624.00117

Diamond, A., & Ling, D. S. (2016). Conclusions about interventions, programs, and approaches for improving executive functions that appear justified and those that, despite much hype, do not. *Developmental Cognitive Neuroscience, 18*, 34–48. http://doi.org/10.1016/j.dcn.2015.11.005

Dickinson, K., & Place, M. (2014). A randomised control trial of the impact of a computer-based activity programme upon the fitness of children with autism. *Autism Research and Treatment, 2014*, 419653. https://doi.org/10.1155/2014/419653

Dillon, S. R., Adams, D., Goudy, L., Bittner, M., & McNamara, S. (2017). Evaluating exercise as evidence-based practice for individuals with autism spectrum disorder. *Frontiers in Public Health, 4*(290), 1–9. https://doi.org/10.3389/fpubh.2016.00290

Downey, R., & Rapport, M. J. K. (2012). Motor activity in children with autism: A review of current literature. *Pediatric Physical Therapy, 24*(1), 2–20. https://doi.org/10.1097/PEP.0b013e31823db95f

Duffy, L., Baluch, B., Welland, S., & Raman, E. (2017). Effects of physical activity on debilitating behaviours in 13- to 20-year-old males with severe autism spectrum disorder. *Journal of Exercise Rehabilitation, 13*(3), 340–347. https://doi.org/10.12965/jer.1734960.480

Dykens, E. M., & Cohen, D. J. (1996). Effects of Special Olympics International on social competence in persons with mental retardation. *Journal of the American Academy of Child and Adolescent Psychiatry, 35*(2), 223–229. https://doi.org/10.1097/00004583-199602000-00016

Eaves, L. C., & Ho, H. H. (2008). Young adult outcome of autism spectrum disorders. *Journal of Autism and Developmental Disorders, 38*(4), 739–747. https://doi.org/10.1007/s10803-007-0441-x

Elliot, J., Connolly, K., & Doyle, A. (1988). Development of kinaesthetic sensitivity and motor performance in children. *Developmental Medicine & Child Neurology, 30*(1), 80–92. https://doi.org/10.1111/j.1469-8749.1988.tb04728.x

Engelhardt, C. R., Mazurek, M. O., & Hilgard, J. (2017). Pathological game use in adults with and without autism spectrum disorder. *PeerJ, 5*, e3393. https://doi.org/10.7717/peerj.3393

Epstein, L. H. (1998). Integrating theoretical approaches to promote physical activity. *American Journal of Preventive Medicine, 15*(4), 257–265. https://doi.org/10.1016/s0749-3797(98)00083-x

Fang, Q., Aiken, C. A., Fang, C., & Pan, Z. (2019). Effects of exergaming on physical and cognitive functions in individuals with autism spectrum disorder: A systematic review. *Games for Health Journal, 8*(2), 74–84. https://doi.org/10.1089/g4h.2018.0032

Ferguson, J., Craig, E. A., & Dounavi, K. (2019). Telehealth as a model for providing behaviour analytic interventions to individuals with autism spectrum disorder: A systematic review. *Journal of Autism and Developmental Disorders, 49*(2), 582–616. https://doi.org/10.1007/s10803-018-3724-5

Ferreira, J. P., Andrade Toscano, C. V., Rodrigues, A. M., Furtado, G. E., Barros, M. G., Wanderley, R. S., & Carvalho, H. M. (2018). Effects of a physical exercise program (PEP-aut) on autistic children's stereotyped behavior, metabolic and physical activity profiles, physical fitness, and health-related quality of life: A study protocol. *Frontiers in Public Health, 6*. https://doi.org/10.3389/fpubh.2018.00047

Ferreira, J. P., Ghiarone, T., Cabral Junior, C. R., Furtado, G. E., Moreira Carvalho, H., Machado-Rodrigues, A. M., & Andrade Toscano, C. V. (2019). Effects of physical exercise on the stereotyped behavior of children with autism spectrum disorders. *Medicina, 55*(10), 685. https://doi.org/10.3390/medicina55100685

Fine, A. H., Tedeschi, P., & Elvove, E. (2015). Forward thinking: The evolving field of human–animal interactions. In A. H. Fine (Ed.), *Handbook on animal-assisted therapy* (pp. 21–35). Amsterdam: Elsevier. https://doi.org/10.1016/B978-0-12-801292-5.00003-1

Flanagan, J. E., Landa, R., Bhat, A., & Bauman, M. (2012). Head lag in infants at risk for autism: A preliminary study. *The American Journal of Occupational Therapy, 66*(5), 577–585. https://doi.org/10.5014/ajot.2012.004192

Fletcher-Watson, S., Adams, J., Brook, K., Charman, T., Crane, L., Cusack, J., Leekam, S., Milton, D., Parr, J. R., & Pellicano, E. (2019). Making the future together: Shaping autism research through meaningful participation. *Autism, 23*(4), 943–953. https://doi.org10.1177/1362361318786721

Fontenelle, S. A., Kahrs, B. A., Neal, S. A., Newton, A. T., & Lockman, J. J. (2007). Infant manual exploration of composite substrates. *Journal of Experimental Child Psychology, 98*(3), 153–167. https://doi.org/10.1016/j.jecp.2007.07.001

Foran, A. C., & Cermak, S. A. (2013). Active and traditional videogame ownership and play patterns among youths with autism spectrum disorders and relationships to physical activity. *Palaestra, 27*(1). https://js.sagamorepub.com/palaestra/article/view/5049

Fournier, K. A., Hass, C. J., Naik, S. K., Lodha, N., & Cauraugh, J. H. (2010). Motor coordination in autism spectrum disorders: A synthesis and meta-analysis. *Journal of Autism and Developmental Disorders, 40*, 1227–1240. http://doi.org/10.1007/s10803-010-0981-3

Franchak, J. M., Kretch, K. S., Soska, K. C., & Adolph, K. E. (2011). Head-mounted eye tracking: A new method to describe infant looking. *Child Development, 82*(6), 1738–1750. https://doi.org/10.1111/j.1467-8624.2011.01670.x

Frey, G. C., Buchanan, A. M., & Rosser Sandt, D. D. (2005). "I'd rather watch TV": An examination of physical activity in adults with mental retardation. *Mental Retardation, 43*(4), 241–254. https://doi.org/10.1352/0047-6765(2005)43[241:IRWTAE]2.0.CO;2

Gabriels, R. L., Pan, Z., Dechant, B., Agnew, J. A., Brim, N., & Mesibov, G. (2015). Randomized controlled trial of therapeutic horseback riding in children and adolescents with autism spectrum disorder. *Journal of the American Academy of Child & Adolescent Psychiatry, 54*(7), 541–549. https://doi.org/10.1016/j.jaac.2015.04.007

Gandotra, A., Kotyuk, E., Szekely, A., Kasos, K., Csirmaz, L., & Cserjesi, R. (2020). Fundamental movement skills in children with autism spectrum disorder: A systematic review. *Research in Autism Spectrum Disorders, 78*, 101632. https://doi.org/10.1016/j.rasd.2020.101632

Garcia-Villamisar D, Dattilo J, & Muela, C. (2017). Effects of B-Active2 on balance, gait, stress, and well-being of adults with autism spectrum disorders and intellectual disability: A controlled trial. *Adapted Physical Activity Quarterly, 34*(2), 125–140. https://doi.org/10.1123/apaq.2015-0071

Garcia-Villamisar, D. A., & Dattilo, J. (2010). Effects of a leisure programme on quality of life and stress of individuals with ASD. *Journal of Intellectual Disability Research, 54*(7), 611–619. https://doi.org/10.1111/j.1365-2788.2010.01289.x

Gesell, A. (1946). The ontogenesis of infant behavior. In L. Carmichael (Ed.), *Manual of child psychology* (pp. 295–331). John Wiley & Sons, Inc. https://doi.org/10.1037/10756-006

Getchell, N., & Whitall, J. (2003). How do children coordinate simultaneous upper and lower extremity tasks? the development of dual motor task coordination. *Journal of Experimental Child Psychology, 85*(2), 120–140. https://doi.org/10.1016/S0022-0965(03)00059-6

Gibson, E. J. (1988). Exploratory behavior in the development of perceiving, acting, and the acquiring of knowledge. *Annual Review of Psychology, 39*, 1–42. https://doi.org/10.1146/annurev.ps.39.020188.000245

Gibson, E. J., & Walker, A. S. (1984). Development of knowledge of visual-tactual affordances of substance. *Child Development, 55*(2), 453–460. https://doi.org/10.2307/1129956

Gibson, J. J. (1979). *The ecological approach to visual perception*. Boston: Houghton Mifflin. https://doi.org/10.1002/bs.3830260313

Granic, I., Lobel, A., & Engels, R. C. (2014). The benefits of playing video games. *American Psychologist, 69*(1), 66. https://doi.org/10.1037/a0034857

Green, D., Charman, T., Pickles, A., Chandler, S., Loucas, T., Simonoff, E., & Baird, G. (2009). Impairment in movement skills of children with autistic spectrum disorders. *Developmental Medicine & Child Neurology, 51*(4), 311–316. https://doi.org/10.1111/j.1469-8749.2008.03242.x

Grondhuis, S., & Aman, M. (2014). Overweight and obesity in youth with developmental disabilities: A call to action. *Journal of Intellectual Disability Research, 58*(9), 787–799. https://doi.org/10.1111/jir.12090

Gunter, K. B., Almstedt, H. C., & Janz, K. F. (2012). Physical activity in childhood may be the key to optimizing lifespan skeletal health. *Exercise and Sport Sciences Reviews*, *40*(1), 13–21. https://doi.org/10.1097/JES.0b013e318236e5ee

Hadders-Algra, M., & Prechtl, H. (1992). Developmental course of general movements in early infancy. I. descriptive analysis of change in form. *Early Human Development*, *28*(3), 201–213. https://doi.org/10.1016/0378-3782(92)90167-f

Haibach, P. S., Reid, G., & Collier, D. H. (2011). *Motor learning and development*. Champaign, IL: Human Kinetics.

Hay, L., Bard, C., Ferrel, C., Olivier, I., & Fleury, M. (2005). Role of proprioceptive information in movement programming and control in 5 to 11-year old children. *Human Movement Science*, *24*(2), 139–154. https://doi.org/10.1016/j.humov.2005.05.002

Hayes, S. J., Hodges, N. J., Scott, M. A., Horn, R. R., & Williams, A. M. (2007). The efficacy of demonstrations in teaching children an unfamiliar movement skill: The effects of object-orientated actions and point-light demonstrations. *Journal of Sports Sciences*, *25*(5), 559–575. https://doi.org/10.1080/02640410600947074

Haywood, K. M., & Getchell, N. (2021). *Life span motor development* (4th ed.). Champaign, IL: Human Kinetics.

Healy, S., & Marchand, G. (2020). The feasibility of project CHASE: A facebook-delivered, parent-mediated physical activity intervention for children with autism. *International Journal of Disability, Development and Education*, *67*(2), 225–242. https://doi.org/10.1080/1034912X.2019.1597968

Healy, S., Nacario, A., Braithwaite, R. E., & Hopper, C. (2018). The effect of physical activity interventions on youth with autism spectrum disorder: A meta-analysis. *Autism Research: Official Journal of the International Society for Autism Research*, *11*(6), 818–833. https://doi.org/10.1002/aur.1955

Heller, T., Ying, G., Rimmer, J. H., & Marks, B. A. (2002). Determinants of exercise in adults with cerebral palsy. *Public Health Nursing*, *19*(3), 223–231. https://doi.org/10.1046/j.0737-1209.2002.19311.x

Heyn, P. (2003). The effect of a multisensory exercise program on engagement, behavior, and selected physiological indexes in persons with dementia. *American Journal of Alzheimer's Disease & Other Dementias*, *18*(4), 247–251. https://doi.org/10.1177/153331750301800409

Hildebrandt, M. K., Koch, S. C., & Fuchs, T. (2016). "We dance and find each other": Effects of dance/movement therapy on negative symptoms in autism spectrum disorder. *Behavioral Sciences (Basel, Switzerland)*, *6*(4). https://doi.org/10.3390/bs6040024

Hill, E. L. (2004). Executive dysfunction in autism. *Trends in Cognitive Sciences*, *8*(1), 26. https://doi.org/10.1016/j.tics.2003.11.003

Hillier, A., Murphy, D., & Ferrara, C. (2011). A pilot study: Short-term reduction in salivary cortisol following low level physical exercise and relaxation among adolescents and young adults on the autism spectrum. *Stress and Health: Journal of the International Society for the Investigation of Stress*, *27*(5), 395–402. https://doi.org/10.1002/smi.1391

Hilton, C., Attal, A., Best, J., Reistetter, T., Trapani, P., & Collins, D. (2015). Exergaming to improve physical and mental fitness in children and adolescents with autism spectrum disorders: Pilot study. *International Journal of Sports, Exercise, and Medicine*, *1*, 1–6. https://doi.org10.23937/2469-5718/1510017

Hilton, C. L., Cumpata, K., Klohr, C., Gaetke, S., Artner, A., Johnson, H., & Dobbs, S. (2014). Effects of exergaming on executive function and motor skills in children with autism spectrum disorder: A pilot study. *The American Journal of Occupational Therapy*, *68*(1), 57–65. https://doi.org/10.5014/ajot.2014.008664

Hind, K., & Burrows, M. (2007). Weight-bearing exercise and bone mineral accrual in children and adolescents: A review of controlled trials. *Bone*, *40*(1), 14–27. https://doi.org/10.1016/j.bone.2006.07.006

Von Hofsten, C. (1993). Prospective control: A basic aspect of action development. *Human Development*, *36*(5), 253–270. https://doi.org/10.1159/000278212

Howells, K., Sivaratnam, C., May, T., Lindor, E., McGillivray, J., & Rinehart, N. (2019). Efficacy of group-based organised physical activity participation for social outcomes in children with autism spectrum disorder: A systematic review and meta-analysis. *Journal of Autism and Developmental Disorders*, *49*(8), 3290–3308. https://doi.org/10.1007/s10803-019-04050-9

Hynes, J., & Block, M. (2022). Effects of physical activity on social, behavioral, and cognitive skills in children and young adults with autism spectrum disorder: A systematic review of the literature. *Review Journal of Autism and Developmental Disorders*, *10*(4), 1–22. https://doi.org/10.1007/s40489-022-00319-5

Iverson, J. M. (2010). Developing language in a developing body: The relationship between motor development and language development. *Journal of Child Language, 37*(2), 229–261. https://doi.org/10.1017/S0305000909990432

Iverson, J. M., Shic, F., Wall, C. A., Chawarska, K., Curtin, S., Estes, A., Gardner, J. M., Hutman, T., Landa, R. J., & Levin, A. R. (2019). Early motor abilities in infants at heightened versus low risk for ASD: A baby siblings research consortium (BSRC) study. *Journal of Abnormal Psychology, 128*(1), 69. https://doi.org/10.1037/abn0000390

Jenkins, S. R., & Reed, F. D. D. (2013). An experimental analysis of the effects of therapeutic horseback riding on the behavior of children with autism. *Research in Autism Spectrum Disorders, 7*(6), 721–740. https://doi.org/10.1016/j.rasd.2013.02.008

Jiménez-Muñoz, L., Peñuelas-Calvo, I., Calvo-Rivera, P., Díaz-Oliván, I., Moreno, M., Baca-García, E., & Porras-Segovia, A. (2022). Video games for the treatment of autism spectrum disorder: A systematic review. *Journal of Autism and Developmental Disorders, 52*(1), 169–188. https://doi.org/10.1007/s10803-021-04934-9

Jones, S. S. (2007). Imitation in infancy: The development of mimicry. *Psychological Science, 18*(7), 593–599. https://doi.org/10.1111/j.1467-9280.2007.01945.x

Jouen, F. (1990). Early visual-vestibular interactions and postural development. In H. Bloch & B. I. Bertenthal (Eds.), *Sensory-motor organizations and development in infancy and early childhood* (pp. 199–215). Cham: Springer. https://doi.org/10.1007/978-94-009-2071-2_15

Kappen, D. L., Mirza-Babaei, P., & Nacke, L. E. (2019). Older adults' physical activity and exergames: A systematic review. *International Journal of Human–Computer Interaction, 35*(2), 140–167. https://doi.org/10.1080/10447318.2018.1441253

Karasik, L. B., Tamis-LeMonda, C. S., & Adolph, K. E. (2011). Transition from crawling to walking and infants' actions with objects and people. *Child Development, 82*(4), 1199–1209. https://doi.org/10.1111/j.1467-8624.2011.01595.x

Karasik, L. B., Tamis-LeMonda, C. S., & Adolph, K. E. (2014). Crawling and walking infants elicit different verbal responses from mothers. *Developmental Science, 17*(3), 388–395. https://doi.org/10.1111/desc.12129

Katch, V. L. (1983). Physical conditioning of children. *Journal of Adolescent Health Care, 3*(4), 241–246. https://doi.org/10.1016/S0197-0070(83)80245-9

Kern, L., Koegel, R. L., & Dunlap, G. (1984). The influence of vigorous versus mild exercise on autistic stereotyped behaviors. *Journal of Autism and Developmental Disorders, 14*(1), 57–67. https://doi.org/10.1007/BF02408555

Kern, L., Koegel, R. L., Dyer, K., Blew, P. A., & Fenton, L. R. (1982). The effects of physical exercise on self-stimulation and appropriate responding in autistic children. *Journal of Autism and Developmental Disorders, 12*(4), 399–419. https://doi.org/10.1007/BF01538327

Keshavan, M. S., Vinogradov, S., Rumsey, J., Sherrill, J., & Wagner, A. (2014). Cognitive training in mental disorders: Update and future directions. *American Journal of Psychiatry, 171*(5), 510–522. https://doi.org/10.1176/appi.ajp.2013.13081075

Ketcheson, L., Hauck, J., & Ulrich, D. (2017). The effects of an early motor skill intervention on motor skills, levels of physical activity, and socialization in young children with autism spectrum disorder: A pilot study. *Autism: The International Journal of Research and Practice, 21*(4), 481–492. https://doi.org/10.1177/1362361316650611

Ketcheson, L. R., & Pitchford, E. A. (2021). Promoting physical activity participation and nutrition education through a telehealth intervention for children on the autism spectrum and their caregivers. *Contemporary Clinical Trials, 107*, 106496. https://doi.org/10.1016/j.cct.2021.106496

Kinder, C. J., Gaudreault, K. L., Jenkins, J. M., Wade, C. E., & Woods, A. M. (2019). At-risk youth in an after-school program: Structured vs. unstructured physical activity. *Physical Educator, 76*(5), 1157–1180. https://doi.org/10.18666/TPE-2019-V76-I5-9016

Kinder, C. J., Gaudreault, K. L., & Simonton, K. (2020). Structured and unstructured contexts in physical education: Promoting activity, learning and motivation. *Journal of Physical Education, Recreation & Dance, 91*(6), 30–35. https://doi.org/10.1080/07303084.2020.1768181

Kindregan, D., Gallagher, L., & Gormley, J. (2015). Gait deviations in children with autism spectrum disorders: A review. *Autism Research and Treatment, 2015*, 741480. https://doi.org/10.1155/2015/741480

Knutsen, J., Wolfe, A., Burke, B. L., Hepburn, S., Lindgren, S., & Coury, D. (2016). A systematic review of telemedicine in autism spectrum disorders. *Review Journal of Autism and Developmental Disorders, 3*(4), 330–344. https://doi.org/10.1007/s40489-016-0086-9

Koch, S. C., Mehl, L., Sobanski, E., Sieber, M., & Fuchs, T. (2015). Fixing the mirrors: A feasibility study of the effects of dance movement therapy on young adults with autism spectrum disorder. *Autism, 19*(3), 338–350. https://doi.org/10.1177/1362361314522353

Kools, J. A., & Tweedie, D. (1975). Development of praxis in children. *Perceptual and Motor Skills, 40*(1), 11–19. https://doi.org/10.2466/pms.1975.40.1.11

Kretch, K. S., Franchak, J. M., & Adolph, K. E. (2014). Crawling and walking infants see the world differently. *Child Development, 85*(4), 1503–1518. https://doi.org/10.1111/cdev.12206

Lang, R., Koegel, L. K., Ashbaugh, K., Regester, A., Ence, W., & Smith, W. (2010). Physical exercise and individuals with autism spectrum disorders: A systematic review. *Research in Autism Spectrum Disorders, 4*(4), 565–576. https://doi.org/10.1016/j.rasd.2010.01.006

Levinson, L. J., & Reid, G. (1993). The effects of exercise intensity on the stereotypic behaviors of individuals with autism. *Adapted Physical Activity Quarterly, 10*(3), 255–268. https://doi.org/10.1123/apaq.10.3.255

Liang, X., Li, R., Wong, S. H. S., Sum, R. K. W., Wang, P., Yang, B., & Sit, C. H. P. (2022). The effects of exercise interventions on executive functions in children and adolescents with autism spectrum disorder: A systematic review and meta-analysis. *Sports Medicine (Auckland, N.Z.), 52*(1), 75–88. https://doi.org/10.1007/s40279-021-01545-3

Lim, B. O., O'Sullivan, D., Choi, B. G., & Kim, M. Y. (2016). Comparative gait analysis between children with autism and age-matched controls: Analysis with temporal-spatial and foot pressure variables. *Journal of Physical Therapy Science, 28*(1), 286–292. https://doi.org/10.1589/jpts.28.286

Lima, J. L., Axt, G., Teixeira, D. S., Monteiro, D., Cid, L., Yamamoto, T., Murillo-Rodriguez, E., & Machado, S. (2020). Exergames for children and adolescents with autism spectrum disorder: An overview. *Clinical Practice and Epidemiology in Mental Health: CP & EMH, 16*, 1–6. https://doi.org/10.2174/1745017902016010001

Lloyd, M., MacDonald, M., & Lord, C. (2013). Motor skills of toddlers with autism spectrum disorders. *Autism: The International Journal of Research and Practice, 17*(2), 133–146. https://doi.org/10.1177/1362361311402230

Lovaas, O. I. (2003). *Teaching individuals with developmental delays: Basic intervention techniques.* PRO-ED.

Macdonald, M., Esposito, P., & Ulrich, D. (2011). The physical activity patterns of children with autism. *BMC Research Notes, 4*, 422. https://doi.org/10.1186/1756-0500-4-422

MacDonald, M., Lord, C., & Ulrich, D. (2013). The relationship of motor skills and adaptive behavior skills in young children with autism spectrum disorders. *Research in Autism Spectrum Disorders, 7*(11), 1383–1390. https://doi.org/10.1016/j.rasd.2013.07.020

Machado, S., Paes, F., Barbosa Ferreira Rocha, N., Yuan, T., Mura, G., Arias-Carrión, O., & Egidio Nardi, A. (2015). Neuroscience of exercise: Association among neurobiological mechanisms and mental health. *CNS & Neurological Disorders-Drug Targets (Formerly Current Drug Targets-CNS & Neurological Disorders), 14*(10), 1315–1316. https://doi.org/10.2174/1871527315999151119122238.

Mahy, J., Shields, N., Taylor, N., & Dodd, K. (2010). Identifying facilitators and barriers to physical activity for adults with Down syndrome. *Journal of Intellectual Disability Research, 54*(9), 795–805. https://doi.org/10.1111/j.1365-2788.2010.01308.x

Manicolo, O., Brotzmann, M., Hagmann-von Arx, P., Grob, A., & Weber, P. (2019). Gait in children with infantile/atypical autism: Age-dependent decrease in gait variability and associations with motor skills. *European Journal of Paediatric Neurology, 23*(1), 117–125. https://doi.org/10.1016/j.ejpn.2018.09.011

Marsh, K. L., Richardson, M. J., & Schmidt, R. (2009). Social connection through joint action and interpersonal coordination. *Topics in Cognitive Science, 1*(2), 320–339. https://doi.org/10.1111/j.1756-8765.2009.01022.x

Mastrominico, A., Fuchs, T., Manders, E., Steffinger, L., Hirjak, D., Sieber, M., Thomas, E., Holzinger, A., Konrad, A., Bopp, N., & Koch, S. C. (2018). Effects of dance movement therapy on adult patients with autism spectrum disorder: A randomized controlled trial. *Behavioral Sciences (Basel, Switzerland), 8*(7). https://doi.org/10.3390/bs8070061

Mazurek, M. O., Shattuck, P. T., Wagner, M., & Cooper, B. P. (2012). Prevalence and correlates of screen-based media use among youths with autism spectrum disorders. *Journal of Autism and Developmental Disorders, 42*(8), 1757–1767. https://doi.org/10.1007/s10803-011-1413-8

Mazurek, M. O., & Wenstrup, C. (2013). Television, video game and social media use among children with ASD and typically developing siblings. *Journal of Autism and Developmental Disorders, 43*(6), 1258–1271. https://doi.org/10.1007/s10803-012-1659-9

McCoy, S. M., Jakicic, J. M., & Gibbs, B. B. (2016). Comparison of obesity, physical activity, and sedentary behaviors between adolescents with autism spectrum disorders and without. *Journal of Autism and Developmental Disorders*, *46*(7), 2317–2326. https://doi.org/10.1007/s10803-016-2762-0

McCoy, S. M., & Morgan, K. (2020). Obesity, physical activity, and sedentary behaviors in adolescents with autism spectrum disorder compared with typically developing peers. *Autism*, *24*(2), 387–399. https://doi.org/10.1177/1362361319861579

McDonald, F., Robinson, K., Gallagher, A. L., & Pettigrew, J. (2021). Exploring the co-involvement of disabled adolescents in participatory action research; protocol for a critical interpretative synthesis. HRB Open Research, 4. https://doi.org/10.12688/hrbopenres.13343.1

McGraw, M. (1945). *Growth: A study of johnny and jimmy*. Crows Nest, NSW: Appleton-Century Company.

McLeroy, K. R., Bibeau, D., Steckler, A., & Glanz, K. (1988). An ecological perspective on health promotion programs. *Health Education Quarterly*, *15*(4), 351–377. https://doi.org/10.1177/109019818801500401

McNicholas, J., & Collis, G. M. (2006). Animals as social supports: Insights for understanding animal-assisted therapy. *Handbook on Animal-Assisted Therapy: Theoretical Foundations and Guidelines for Practice*, *2*, 49–72.

Van Der Meer, A., Holden, G., & van Der Weel, R. (2005). Coordination of sucking, swallowing, and breathing in healthy newborns. *Ped Neonatal*, *2*, 69–72. https://doi.org/10.1155/2015/741480

Menear, K. (2007). Parents' perceptions of health and physical activity needs of children with down syndrome. *Down Syndrome Research and Practice*, *12*(1), 60–68. https://doi.org/10.3104/reports.1996

Mesibov, G. B., Shea, V., Schopler, E., Adams, L., Merkler, E., Burgess, S., Mosconi, M., Chapman, S. M., Tanner, C., & Bourgondien, M. E. (2004). *The TEACCH approach to autism spectrum disorders*. Cham: Springer.

Mieres, A. C., Kirby, R. S., Armstrong, K. H., Murphy, T. K., & Grossman, L. (2012). Autism spectrum disorder: An emerging opportunity for physical therapy. *Pediatric Physical Therapy*, *24*(1), 31–37. https://doi.org/10.1097/PEP.0b013e31823e06d1

De Milander, M., Bradley, S., & Fourie, R. (2016). Equine-assisted therapy as intervention for motor proficiency in children with autism spectrum disorder: Case studies. *South African Journal for Research in Sport, Physical Education and Recreation*, *38*(3), 37–49. https://hdl.handle.net/10520/EJC199894

Minshew, N. J., Sung, K. B., Jones, B. L., & Furman, J. M. (2004). Underdevelopment of the postural control system in autism. *Neurology*, *63*(11), 2056–2061. https://doi.org/10.1212/01.WNL.0000145771.98657.62

Mooventhan, A., & Nivethitha, L. (2014). Scientific evidence-based effects of hydrotherapy on various systems of the body. *North American Journal of Medical Sciences*, *6*(5), 199. https://doi.org/10.4103/1947-2714.132935

Morris, P. O., Hope, E., & Mills, J. P. (2022). The non-fitness-related benefits of exergames for young individuals diagnosed with autism spectrum disorder: A systematic review. *Research in Autism Spectrum Disorders*, *94*. https://doi.org/10.1016/j.rasd.2022.101953

Morrison, H., Roscoe, E. M., & Atwell, A. (2011). An evaluation of antecedent exercise on behavior maintained by automatic reinforcement using a three-component multiple schedule. *Journal of Applied Behavior Analysis*, *44*(3), 523–541. https://doi.org/10.1901/jaba.2011.44-523

Mostofsky, S. H., Dubey, P., Jerath, V. K., Jansiewicz, E. M., Goldberg, M. C., & Denckla, M. B. (2006). Developmental dyspraxia is not limited to imitation in children with autism spectrum disorders. *Journal of the International Neuropsychological Society*, *12*, 314–326. https://doi.org/10.1017/s1355617706060437

Murata, N., & Tan, C. (2009). Collaborative teaching of motor skills for preschoolers with developmental delays. *Early Childhood Education Journal*, *36*, 483–489. https://doi.org/10.1007/s10643-007-0212-5

Nabors, L., Overstreet, A., Carnahan, C., & Ayers, K. (2021). Evaluation of a pilot healthy eating and exercise program for young adults with autism spectrum disorder and intellectual disabilities. *Advances in Neurodevelopmental Disorders*, *5*(4), 413–430. https://doi.org/10.1007/s41252-021-00214-w

Narzisi, A. (2020). Phase 2 and later of COVID-19 lockdown: Is it possible to perform remote diagnosis and intervention for autism spectrum disorder? An online-mediated approach. *Journal of Clinical Medicine*, *9*(6), 1850. https://doi.org/10.3390/jcm9061850

Needham, A., Barrett, T., & Peterman, K. (2002). A pick-me-up for infants' exploratory skills: Early simulated experiences reaching for objects using "sticky mittens" enhances young infants' object exploration skills. *Infant Behavior and Development, 25*(3), 279–295. https://doi.org/10.1016/S0163-6383(02)00097-8

Neely, L., Rispoli, M., Gerow, S., & Ninci, J. (2015). Effects of antecedent exercise on academic engagement and stereotypy during instruction. *Behavior Modification, 39*(1), 98–116. https://doi.org/10.1177/0145445514552891

Nichols, C., Block, M. E., Bishop, J. C., & McIntire, B. (2019). Physical activity in young adults with autism spectrum disorder: Parental perceptions of barriers and facilitators. *Autism, 23*(6), 1398–1407. https://doi.org/10.1177/1362361318810221

Nicholson, H. K., Bray, T. J., Heest, M. A., & Van, J. (2011). The effects of antecedent physical activity on the academic engagement of children with autism spectrum disorder. *Psychology in the Schools, 48*(2), 198–213. https://doi.org/10.1002/pits.20537

Nickel, L. R., Thatcher, A. R., Keller, F., Wozniak, R. H., & Iverson, J. M. (2013). Posture development in infants at heightened versus low risk for autism spectrum disorders. *Infancy, 18*(5), 639–661. https://doi.org/10.1111/infa.12025

Nieforth, L. O., Schwichtenberg, A., & O'Haire, M. E. (2021). Animal-assisted interventions for autism spectrum disorder: A systematic review of the literature from 2016 to 2020. *Review Journal of Autism and Developmental Disorders, 43*(7), 1602–1622. https://doi.org/10.1007/s40489-021-00291-6

de Nocker, Y. L., & Toolan, C. K. (2021). Using telehealth to provide interventions for children with ASD: A systematic review. *Review Journal of Autism and Developmental Disorders*, 1–31. https://doi.org/10.1007/s40489-021-00278-3

Nohelty, K., Bradford, C. B., Hirschfeld, L., Miyake, C., & Novack, M. N. (2021). Effectiveness of telehealth direct therapy for individuals with autism spectrum disorder. *Behavior Analysis in Practice*, 1–16. https://doi.org/10.1007/s40617-021-00603-6

O'Haire, M. E. (2013). Animal-assisted intervention for autism spectrum disorder: A systematic literature review. *Journal of Autism and Developmental Disorders, 43*(7), 1606–1622. https://doi.org/10.1007/s10803-012-1707-5

O'Haire, M. E. (2017). Research on animal-assisted intervention and autism spectrum disorder, 2012–2015. *Applied Developmental Science, 21*(3), 200–216. https://doi.org/10.1080/10888691.2016.1243988

O'Haire, M. E., McKenzie, S. J., McCune, S., & Slaughter, V. (2014). Effects of classroom animal-assisted activities on social functioning in children with autism spectrum disorder. *The Journal of Alternative and Complementary Medicine, 20*(3), 162–168. https://doi.org/10.1089/acm.2013.0165

Obrusnikova, I., & Miccinello, D. L. (2012). Parent perceptions of factors influencing after-school physical activity of children with autism spectrum disorders. *Adapted Physical Activity Quarterly, 29*(1), 63–80. https://doi.org/10.1123/apaq.29.1.63

Oh, Y., & Yang, S. (2010). Defining exergames and exergaming. In *Proceedings of International Conference on Meaningful Play* (pp. 21–23). https://meaningfulplay.msu.edu/proceedings2010/mp2010_paper_63.pdf

Olin, S. S., McFadden, B. A., Golem, D. L., Pellegrino, J. K., Walker, A. J., Sanders, D. J., & Arent, S. M. (2017). The effects of exercise dose on stereotypical behavior in children with autism. *Medicine and Science in Sports and Exercise, 49*(5), 983–990. https://doi.org/10.1249/MSS.0000000000001197

Oriel, K. N., George, C. L., Peckus, R., & Semon, A. (2011). The effects of aerobic exercise on academic engagement in young children with autism spectrum disorder. *Pediatric Physical Therapy: The Official Publication of the Section on Pediatrics of the American Physical Therapy Association, 23*(2), 187–193. https://doi.org/10.1097/PEP.0b013e318218f149

Özer, D., Baran, F., Aktop, A., Nalbant, S., Ağlamış, E., & Hutzler, Y. (2012). Effects of a special olympics unified sports soccer program on psycho-social attributes of youth with and without intellectual disability. *Research in Developmental Disabilities, 33*(1), 229–239. https://doi.org/10.1016/j.ridd.2011.09.011

Pan, C., Tsai, C., Chu, C., Sung, M., Ma, W., & Huang, C. (2016). Objectively measured physical activity and health-related physical fitness in secondary school-aged male students with autism spectrum disorders. *Physical Therapy, 96*(4), 511–520. https://doi.org/10.2522/ptj.20140353

Pan, C. -Y., Tsai, C. -L., & Hsieh, K. -W. (2011). Physical activity correlates for children with autism spectrum disorders in middle school physical education. *Research Quarterly for Exercise and Sport, 82*(3), 491–498. https://doi.org/10.1080/02701367.2011.10599782

Paquet, A., Olliac, B., Bouvard, M., Golse, B., & Vaivre-Douret, L. (2016). The semiology of motor disorders in autism spectrum disorders as highlighted from a standardized neuro-psychomotor assessment. *Frontiers in Psychology*, *7*. https://doi.org/10.3389/fpsyg.2016.01292

Peiper, A. (1963). *Cerebral function in infancy and childhood*. New York: Plenum.

Pennington, B. F., & Ozonoff, S. (1996). Executive functions and developmental psychopathology. *Journal of Child Psychology and Psychiatry*, *37*(1), 51–87. https://doi.org/10.1111/j.1469-7610.1996.tb01380.x

Petrus, C., Adamson, S. R., Block, L., Einarson, S. J., Sharifnejad, M., & Harris, S. R. (2008). Effects of exercise interventions on stereotypic behaviours in children with autism spectrum disorder. *Physiotherapy Canada*, *60*(2), 134–145. https://doi.org/10.3138/physio.60.2.134

Pickard, K. E., Wainer, A. L., Bailey, K. M., & Ingersoll, B. R. (2016). A mixed-method evaluation of the feasibility and acceptability of a telehealth-based parent-mediated intervention for children with autism spectrum disorder. *Autism*, *20*(7), 845–855. https://doi.org/10.1177/1362361315614496

Piercy, K. L., Troiano, R. P., Ballard, R. M., Carlson, S. A., Fulton, J. E., Galuska, D. A., George, S. M., & Olson, R. D. (2018). The physical activity guidelines for Americans. *JAMA*, *320*(19), 2020–2028. https://doi.org/10.1001/jama.2018.14854

Pitchford, E. A., Siebert, E., Hamm, J., & Yun, J. (2016). Parental perceptions of physical activity benefits for youth with developmental disabilities. *American Journal on Intellectual and Developmental Disabilities*, *121*(1), 25–32. https://doi.org/10.1352/1944-7558-121.1.25

Pitetti, K. H., Rendoff, A. D., Grover, T., & Beets, M. W. (2007). The efficacy of a 9-month treadmill walking program on the exercise capacity and weight reduction for adolescents with severe autism. *Journal of Autism and Developmental Disorders*, *37*(6), 997–1006. https://doi.org/10.1007/s10803-006-0238-3

Plavnick, J. B., & Hume, K. A. (2014). Observational learning by individuals with autism: A review of teaching strategies. *Autism*, *18*(4), 458–466. https://doi.org/10.1177/1362361312474373

Van der Ploeg, H. P., Van der Beek, A. J., Van der Woude, L. H. V., & van Mechelen, W. (2004). Physical activity for people with a disability. *Sports Medicine*, *34*(10), 639–649. https://doi.org/10.2165/00007256-200434100-00002

Powers, S., Thibadeau, S., & Rose, K. (1992). Antecedent exercise and its effects on self-stimulation. *Behavioral Interventions*, *7*(1), 15–22. https://doi.org/10.1002/bin.2360070103

Prechtl, H. (1986). Prenatal motor development. In M. G. Wade & H. T. A. Whiting (Eds.), *Motor development in children: Aspects of coordination and control* (pp. 53–64). Amsterdam: Martinus Nijhoff.

Prechtl, H. F. (1985). Ultrasound studies of human fetal behaviour. *Early Human Development*, *12*(2), 91–98. https://doi.org/10.1016/0378-3782(85)90173-2

Provost, B., Heimerl, S., & Lopez, B. R. (2007). Levels of gross and fine motor development in young children with autism spectrum disorder. *Physical & Occupational Therapy in Pediatrics*, *27*(3), 21–36. https://doi.org/10.1080/J006v27n03_03

Rapp, J. T., & Vollmer, T. R. (2005). Stereotypy I: A review of behavioral assessment and treatment. *Research in Developmental Disabilities*, *26*(6), 527–547. https://doi.org/10.1016/j.ridd.2004.11.005

Ratcliff, K., Hong, I., & Hilton, C. (2018). Leisure participation patterns for school age youth with autism spectrum disorders: Findings from the 2016 national survey of children's health. *Journal of Autism and Developmental Disorders*, *48*(11), 3783–3793. https://doi.org/10.1007/s10803-018-3643-5

Ratey, J. J., & Loehr, J. E. (2011). The positive impact of physical activity on cognition during adulthood: A review of underlying mechanisms, evidence and recommendations. *Reviews in the Neurosciences*, *22*(2), 171–185. https://doi.org/10.1515/rns.2011.017

Reiner, M., Niermann, C., Jekauc, D., & Woll, A. (2013). Long-term health benefits of physical activity–a systematic review of longitudinal studies. *BMC Public Health*, *13*(1), 1–9. https://doi.org/10.1186/1471-2458-13-813

Rimmer, J. H., Rowland, J. L., & Yamaki, K. (2007). Obesity and secondary conditions in adolescents with disabilities: Addressing the needs of an underserved population. *Journal of Adolescent Health*, *41*(3), 224–229. https://doi.org/10.1016/j.jadohealth.2007.05.005

Rinehart, N. J., Jeste, S., & Wilson, R. B. (2018). Organized physical activity programs: Improving motor and non-motor symptoms in neurodevelopmental disorders. *Developmental Medicine and Child Neurology*, *60*(9), 856–857. https://doi.org/10.1111/dmcn.13962

Rinehart, N. J., Tonge, B. J., Iansek, R., McGinley, J., Brereton, A. V., Enticott, P. G., & Bradshaw, J. L. (2006). Gait function in newly diagnosed children with autism: Cerebellar and basal ganglia related motor disorder. *Developmental Medicine and Child Neurology, 48*(10), 819–824. https://doi.org/10.1017/S0012162206001769

Robertson, C. E., & Baron-Cohen, S. (2017). Sensory perception in autism. *Nature Reviews Neuroscience, 18*(11), 671–684. https://doi.org/10.1038/nrn.2017.112

Rochat, P., & Goubet, N. (1995). Development of sitting and reaching in 5-to 6-month-old infants. *Infant Behavior and Development, 18*(1), 53–68. https://doi.org/10.1016/0163-6383(95)90007-1

Rose, S. A., & Ruff, H. A. (1987). Cross-modal abilities in human infants. In J. D. Osofsky (Ed.), *Handbook of infant development* (pp. 318–362). New York: John Wiley & Sons.

Rosenstock, I. M. (1974). The health belief model and preventive health behavior. *Health Education Monographs, 2*(4), 354–386. https://doi.org/10.1177/109019817400200405

Rosenthal, R., & Rosnow, R. L. (2008). *Essentials of behavioral research: Methods and data analysis* (3rd ed.). New York: McGraw-Hill. http://dx.doi.org/10.34944/dspace/66

Rosenthal-Malek, A., & Mitchell, S. (1997). Brief report: The effects of exercise on the self-stimulatory behaviors and positive responding of adolescents with autism. *Journal of Autism and Developmental Disorders, 27*(2), 193–202. https://doi.org/10.1023/a:1025848009248

Rowland, T. W. (1981). Physical fitness in children: Implications for the prevention of coronary artery disease. *Current Problems in Pediatrics, 11*(9), 5–54. https://doi.org/10.1016/0045-9380(81)90002-5

Ruggeri, A., Dancel, A., Johnson, R., & Sargent, B. (2020). The effect of motor and physical activity intervention on motor outcomes of children with autism spectrum disorder: A systematic review. *Autism, 24*(3), 544–568. https://doi.org/10.1177/1362361319885215

Russell, S. M. (2018). Hobby preferences and physical activity participation among children with and without autism spectrum disorder. *European Journal of Adapted Physical Activity, 11*(2), 8. https://doi.org/10.5507/euj.2018.008

Ryan, R. M., & Deci, E. L. (2000). Self-determination theory and the facilitation of intrinsic motivation, social development, and well-being. *American Psychologist, 55*(1), 68. https://doi.org/10.1037/0003-066X.55.1.68

Sallis, J. F., & Hovell, M. F. (1990). Determinants of exercise behavior. *Exercise and Sport Sciences Reviews, 18*(1), 307–330.

Sallis, J. F., Hovell, M. F., & Hofstetter, C. R. (1992). Predictors of adoption and maintenance of vigorous physical activity in men and women. *Preventive Medicine, 21*(2), 237–251. https://doi.org/10.1016/0091-7435(92)90022-A

Sallis, J. F., Patterson, T. L., Buono, M. J., & Nader, P. R. (1988). Relation of cardiovascular fitness and physical activity to cardiovascular disease risk factors in children and adults. *American Journal of Epidemiology, 127*(5), 933–941. https://doi.org/10.1093/oxfordjournals.aje.a114896

Sam, K., Chow, B., & Tong, K. (2015). Effectiveness of exercise-based interventions for children with autism: A systematic review and meta-analysis. *International Journal of Learning and Teaching, 1*(2), 98–103. https://doi.org10.18178/ijlt.1.2.98-103

Sams, M. J., Fortney, E. V., & Willenbring, S. (2006). Occupational therapy incorporating animals for children with autism: A pilot investigation. *The American Journal of Occupational Therapy, 60*(3), 268–274. https://doi.org/10.5014/ajot.60.3.268

Savage, M. N., Tomaszewski, B. T., & Hume, K. A. (2022). Step it up: Increasing physical activity for adults with autism spectrum disorder and intellectual disability using supported self-management and fitbit technology. *Focus on Autism and Other Developmental Disabilities, 37*(3), 146–157. https://doi.org/10.1177/10883576211073700

Schauder, K. B., & Bennetto, L. (2016). Toward an interdisciplinary understanding of sensory dysfunction in autism spectrum disorder: An integration of the neural and symptom literatures. *Frontiers in Neuroscience, 10*, 268. https://doi.org/10.3389/fnins.2016.00268

Shields, N., van den Bos, R., Buhlert-Smith, K., Prendergast, L., & Taylor, N. (2019). A community-based exercise program to increase participation in physical activities among youth with disability: A feasibility study. *Disability and Rehabilitation, 41*(10), 1152–1159. https://doi.org/10.1080/09638288.2017.1422034

Shields, N., Synnot, A. J., & Barr, M. (2012). Perceived barriers and facilitators to physical activity for children with disability: A systematic review. *British Journal of Sports Medicine, 46*(14), 989–997. http://dx.doi.org/10.1136/bjsports-2011-090236

Shirley, M. M. (1933). *The first two years: A study of twenty-five babies: Volume 1, postural and locomotor development*. Minneapolis: University of Minnesota Press.

Shumway-Cook, A., & Woollacott, M. (2007). *Motor control: Translating research in clinical practice* (3rd ed.). Philadelphia: Lippincott Williams & Wilkins.

Sigmundsson, H., Whiting, H., & Loftesnes, J. (2000). Development of proprioceptive sensitivity. *Experimental Brain Research, 135*(3), 348–352. https://doi.org/10.1007/s002210000531

Simacek, J., Elmquist, M., Dimian, A. F., & Reichle, J. (2020). Current trends in telehealth applications to deliver social communication interventions for young children with or at risk for autism spectrum disorder. *Current Developmental Disorders Reports, 8*(1), 15–23. https://doi.org/10.1007/s40474-020-00214-w

Sorensen, C., & Zarrett, N. (2014). Benefits of physical activity for adolescents with autism spectrum disorders: A comprehensive review. *Review Journal of Autism and Developmental Disorders, 1*(4), 344–353. https://doi.org/10.1007/s40489-014-0027-4

Soska, K. C., Adolph, K. E., & Johnson, S. P. (2010). Systems in development: Motor skill acquisition facilitates three-dimensional object completion. *Developmental Psychology, 46*(1), 129–138. https://doi.org/10.1037/a0014618

Sowa, M., & Meulenbroek, R. (2012). Effects of physical exercise on autism spectrum disorders: A meta-analysis. *Research in Autism Spectrum Disorders, 6*(1), 46–57. https://doi.org/10.1016/j.rasd.2011.09.001

Spelke, E. S. (1987) The development of intermodal perception. In P. Salapatek & L. Cohen (Eds.), *Handbook of infant perception, Vol. 2: From perception to cognition* (pp. 233–273). New York: Academic Press. https://www.harvardlds.org/wp-content/uploads/2017/01/the-development-of-intermodal-perception-1.pdf

Spencer, J. P., Vereijken, B., Diedrich, F. J., & Thelen, E. (2000). Posture and the emergence of manual skills. *Developmental Science, 3*(2), 216–233. https://doi.org/10.1111/1467-7687.00115

Srinivasan, S., Athreya, A., Kaba, M., Glenney, S., & Bubela, D. (2022, May 11–14). Perspectives of caregivers and youth with developmental disabilities on physical activity: A qualitative study [Poster presentation]. 2022 Annual Meeting of the International Society for Autism Research (INSAR). Austin, Texas. https://www.autism-insar.org/page/INSAR2022Archives

Srinivasan, S., Kaur, M., Park, I., Gifford, T., Marsh, K., & Bhat, A. (2015). The effects of rhythm and robotic interventions on the imitation/praxis, interpersonal synchrony, and motor performance of children with autism spectrum disorder (ASD): A pilot randomized controlled trial. *Autism Research and Treatment, 2015*:736516. https://doi.org/https://doi.org/10.1155/2015/736516

Srinivasan, S. M., & Bhat, A. N. (2013). A review of "music and movement" therapies for children with autism: Embodied interventions for multisystem development. *Frontiers in Integrative Neuroscience, 7.* https://doi.org/10.3389/fnint.2013.00022

Srinivasan, S. M., Cavagnino, D. T., & Bhat, A. N. (2018). Effects of equine therapy on individuals with autism spectrum disorder: A systematic review. *Review Journal of Autism and Developmental Disorders, 5*(2), 156–175. https://doi.org/10.1007/s40489-018-0130-z

Srinivasan, S. M., Eigsti, I., Neelly, L., & Bhat, A. N. (2016). The effects of embodied rhythm and robotic interventions on the spontaneous and responsive social attention patterns of children with autism spectrum disorder (ASD): A pilot randomized controlled trial. *Research in Autism Spectrum Disorders, 27*, 54–72. https://doi.org/10.1016/j.rasd.2016.01.004

Srinivasan, S. M., Eigsti, I. -M., Gifford, T., & Bhat, A. N. (2016). The effects of embodied rhythm and robotic interventions on the spontaneous and responsive verbal communication skills of children with autism spectrum disorder (ASD): A further outcome of a pilot randomized controlled trial. *Research in Autism Spectrum Disorders, 27*, 73–87. https://doi.org/10.1016/j.rasd.2016.04.001

Srinivasan, S. M., Park, I. K., Neelly, L. B., & Bhat, A. N. (2015). A comparison of the effects of rhythm and robotic interventions on repetitive behaviors and affective states of children with autism spectrum disorder (ASD). *Research in Autism Spectrum Disorders, 18*, 51–63. https://doi.org/10.1016/j.rasd.2015.07.004

Srinivasan, S. M., Pescatello, L. S., & Bhat, A. N. (2014). Current perspectives on physical activity and exercise recommendations for children and adolescents with autism spectrum disorders. *Physical Therapy, 94*(6), 875–889. https://doi.org/10.2522/ptj.20130157

Srinivasan, S. M., Su, W. -C., Cleffi, C., & Bhat, A. N. (2021). From social distancing to social connections: Insights from the delivery of a clinician-caregiver co-mediated telehealth-based intervention in young children with autism spectrum disorder. *Frontiers in Psychiatry, 12.* https://doi.org/10.3389/fpsyt.2021.700247

Staiano, A. E., & Calvert, S. L. (2011). Exergames for physical education courses: Physical, social, and cognitive benefits. *Child Development Perspectives, 5*(2), 93–98. https://doi.org/10.1111/j.1750-8606.2011.00162.x

Steiner, H., & Kertesz, Z. (2015). Effects of therapeutic horse riding on gait cycle parameters and some aspects of behavior of children with autism. *Acta Physiologica Hungarica, 102*(3), 324–335. https://doi.org/10.1556/036.102.2015.3.10

Tan, B. W., Pooley, J. A., & Speelman, C. P. (2016). A meta-analytic review of the efficacy of physical exercise interventions on cognition in individuals with autism spectrum disorder and ADHD. *Journal of Autism and Developmental Disorders, 46*(9), 3126–3143. https://doi.org/10.1007/s10803-016-2854-x

Tarr, C. W. (2019). *The effects of physical exercise on stereotypic behaviors in autism: A meta-analysis.* (Order No. 10984780). Available from ProQuest Dissertations & Theses Global; Publicly Available Content Database. (2099251527). https://ezproxy.lib.uconn.edu/login?url=https://www.proquest.com/dissertations-theses/effects-physical-exercise-on-stereotypic/docview/2099251527/se-2

Tarr, C. W., Rineer-Hershey, A., & Larwin, K. (2020). The effects of physical exercise on stereotypic behaviors in autism: Small-n meta-analyses. *Focus on Autism and Other Developmental Disabilities, 35*(1), 26–35. https://doi.org/10.1177/1088357619881220

Teh, E. J., Vijayakumar, R., Tan, T. X. J., & Yap, M. J. (2022). Effects of physical exercise interventions on stereotyped motor behaviours in children with ASD: A meta-analysis. *Journal of Autism and Developmental Disorders, 52*(7), 2934–2957. https://doi.org/10.1007/s10803-021-05152-z

Temple, V. A. (2009). Factors associated with high levels of physical activity among adults with intellectual disability. *International Journal of Rehabilitation Research, 32*(1), 89–92. https://doi.org/10.1097/MRR.0b013e328307f5a0

Temple, V. A., & Walkley, J. W. (2007). Perspectives of constraining and enabling factors for health-promoting physical activity by adults with intellectual disability. *Journal of Intellectual and Developmental Disability, 32*(1), 28–38. https://doi.org/10.1080/13668250701194034

Thelen, E. (1979). Rhythmical stereotypies in normal human infants. *Animal Behaviour, 27*, 699–715. https://doi.org/10.1016/0003-3472(79)90006-X

Thelen, E. (1981). Kicking, rocking, and waving: Contextual analysis of rhythmical stereotypies in normal human infants. *Animal Behaviour, 29*(1), 3–11. https://doi.org/10.1016/S0003-3472(81)80146-7

Thelen, E., & Smith, L. B. (1996). *A dynamic systems approach to the development of cognition and action*. Cambridge, MA: MIT Press.

Theobald, M., Danby, S., Einarsdóttir, J., Bourne, J., Jones, D., Ross, S., Knaggs, H., & Carter-Jones, C. (2015). Children's perspectives of play and learning for educational practice. *Education Sciences, 5*(4), 345–362. https://doi.org/10.3390/educsci5040345

Tint, A., Thomson, K., & Weiss, J. A. (2017). A systematic literature review of the physical and psychosocial correlates of Special Olympics participation among individuals with intellectual disability. *Journal of Intellectual Disability Research, 61*(4), 301–324. https://doi.org/10.1111/jir.12295

Todd, T., & Reid, G. (2006). Increasing physical activity in individuals with autism. *Focus on Autism and Other Developmental Disabilities, 21*(3), 167–176. https://doi.org/10.1177/10883576060210030501

Todd, T., Reid, G., & Butler-Kisber, L. (2010). Cycling for students with ASD: Self-regulation promotes sustained physical activity. *Adapted Physical Activity Quarterly, 27*(3), 226–241. https://doi.org/10.1123/apaq.27.3.226

Tohidast, S. A., Mansuri, B., Bagheri, R., & Azimi, H. (2020). Provision of speech-language pathology services for the treatment of speech and language disorders in children during the COVID-19 pandemic: Problems, concerns, and solutions. *International Journal of Pediatric Otorhinolaryngology, 138*. https://doi.org/10.1016/j.ijporl.2020.110262

Tomporowski, P. D., Lambourne, K., & Okumura, M. S. (2011). Physical activity interventions and children's mental function: An introduction and overview. *Preventive Medicine, 52*, S3–S9. https://doi.org/10.1016/j.ypmed.2011.01.028

Trevarthen, C., & Delafield-Butt, J. T. (2013). Autism as a developmental disorder in intentional movement and affective engagement. *Frontiers in Integrative Neuroscience, 7*, 49. https://doi.org/10.3389/fnint.2013.00049

Trost, S. G., Owen, N., Bauman, A. E., Sallis, J. F., & Brown, W. (2002). Correlates of adults' participation in physical activity: Review and update. *Medicine & Science in Sports & Exercise, 34*(12), 1996–2001. https://doi.org/10.1097/00005768-200212000-00020

Tudor-Locke, C., Lee, S. M., Morgan, C. F., Beighle, A., & Pangrazi, R. P. (2006). Children's pedometer-determined physical activity during the segmented school day. *Journal of the American College of Sports Medicine, 38*, 1732–1738. https://doi.org/10.1249/01.mss.0000230212.55119.98

Unholz-Bowden, E., McComas, J. J., McMaster, K. L., Girtler, S. N., Kolb, R. L., & Shipchandler, A. (2020). Caregiver training via telehealth on behavioral procedures: A systematic review. *Journal of Behavioral Education, 29*(2), 246–281. https://doi.org/10.1007/s10864-020-09381-7

Vanvuchelen, M., Roeyers, H., & De Weerdt, W. (2011). Do imitation problems reflect a core characteristic in autism? Evidence from a literature review. *Research in Autism Spectrum Disorders*, *5*(1), 89–95. https://doi.org/10.1016/j.rasd.2010.07.010

de Vinck-baroody, O., Shui, A., Macklin, E. A., Hyman, S. L., Leventhal, J. M., & Weitzman, C. (2015). Overweight and obesity in a sample of children with autism spectrum disorder. *Academic Pediatrics*, *15*(4), 396–404. https://doi.org/10.1016/j.acap.2015.03.008

Wainer, A. L., & Ingersoll, B. R. (2015). Increasing access to an ASD imitation intervention via a telehealth parent training program. *Journal of Autism and Developmental Disorders*, *45*(12), 3877–3890. https://doi.org/10.1007/s10803-014-2186-7

Warburton, D. E., & Bredin, S. S. (2017). Health benefits of physical activity: A systematic review of current systematic reviews. *Current Opinion in Cardiology*, *32*(5), 541–556. https://doi.org/10.1097/HCO.0000000000000437

Wass, S. V., & Porayska-Pomsta, K. (2014). The uses of cognitive training technologies in the treatment of autism spectrum disorders. *Autism*, *18*(8), 851–871. https://doi.org/10.1177/1362361313499827

Watters, R. G., & Watters, W. E. (1980). Decreasing self-stimulatory behavior with physical exercise in a group of autistic boys. *Journal of Autism and Developmental Disorders*, *10*(4), 379–387. https://doi.org/10.1007/BF02414814

Wegner, M., Helmich, I., Machado, S., E, Nardi, A., Arias-Carrion, O., & Budde, H. (2014). Effects of exercise on anxiety and depression disorders: Review of meta-analyses and neurobiological mechanisms. *CNS & Neurological Disorders-Drug Targets (Formerly Current Drug Targets-CNS & Neurological Disorders)*, *13*(6), 1002–1014. https://doi.org/10.2174/1871527313666140612102841

Weiss, J., Diamond, T., Demark, J., & Lovald, B. (2003). Involvement in Special Olympics and its relations to self-concept and actual competency in participants with developmental disabilities. *Research in Developmental Disabilities*, *24*(4), 281–305. https://doi.org/10.1016/s0891-4222(03)00043-x

Welk, G. J. (1999). The youth physical activity promotion model: A conceptual bridge between theory and practice. *Quest*, *51*(1), 5–23. https://doi.org/10.1080/00336297.1999.10484297

Whyatt, C. P., & Craig, C. M. (2012). Motor skills in children aged 7–10 years, diagnosed with autism spectrum disorder. *Journal of Autism and Developmental Disorders*, *42*(9), 1799–1809. https://doi.org/10.1007/s10803-011-1421-8

Wigal, S. B., Emmerson, N., Gehricke, J., & Galassetti, P. (2013). Exercise: Applications to childhood ADHD. *Journal of Attention Disorders*, *17*(4), 279–290. https://doi.org/10.1177/1087054712454192

Woods, A. M., Graber, K. C., Daum, D. N., & Gentry, C. (2015). Young school children's recess physical activity: Movement patterns and preferences. *Journal of Teaching in Physical Education*, *34*(3), 496–516. https://doi.org/10.1123/jtpe.2014-0048

Woollacott, M., Debû, B., & Mowatt, M. (1987). Neuromuscular control of posture in the infant and child: Is vision dominant? *Journal of Motor Behavior*, *19*(2), 167–186. https://doi.org/10.1080/00222895.1987.10735406

Yazdani, S., Yee, C. T., & Chung, P. J. (2013). Factors predicting physical activity among children with special needs. *Preventing Chronic Disease*, *10*, E119. https://doi.org/10.5888/pcd10.120283

Zeliadt, N. (2017). Autism in motion: Could motor problems trigger social ones. *Scientific American*. https://www.scientificamerican.com/article/autism-in-motion-could-motor-problems-trigger-social-ones/

26

Music Therapy

Marc J. Lanovaz and Ioulia Koniou
Université de Montréal, Centre de recherche l'Institut universitaire en santé mentale de Montréal

Eve-Marie Quintin
McGill University, Centre for Research on Brain, Language, and Music

26.1 Technical Abstract

Background: Music therapy may take on different forms and target various behaviors, but one commonality is that it systematically involves listening to or producing music. **Method:** To examine support for this treatment for persons on the autism spectrum, we conducted a literature search combining terms related to music therapy and autism. Then, the second author read the abstracts and full texts to identify empirical studies assessing the effects of music therapy for persons on the autism spectrum. The chapter provides a narrative review of the 42 studies meeting our inclusion criteria. **Results:** Three types of music therapy have sufficient support to warrant a favorable recommendation: background music to reduce engagement in repetitive vocalizations, singing instructions to promote engagement, and improvisational music therapy to support social development. **Discussion:** The main limitation of research on the treatment is that the parameters of music therapy (e.g., number of sessions, duration, activities) vary tremendously from one study to another, making it difficult for practitioners to identify the most promising strategies. Future research should conduct parametric and component analyses of music therapy. **Practitioner recommendations:** Practitioners may use music therapy to support the behavioral and social functioning of persons on the autism spectrum, but a rigorous and systematic process of ongoing assessment should be implemented to ensure that the treatment is producing the desired effects.

26.2 Layperson Summary

Music therapy does not refer to a single treatment, but rather to a group of different interventions that involve the use of music to support the behavioral and social development of persons on the autism spectrum. The treatment may

Marc J. Lanovaz, Ioulia Koniou, and Eve-Marie Quintin, *Music Therapy*. In: *Lifespan Treatment for Autistic Individuals*. Edited by: Peter Sturmey, Russell Lang, and James K. Luiselli, Oxford University Press. © Oxford University Press (2025).
DOI: 10.1093/oso/9780197635841.003.0026

improve behavior by motivating the person to engage in less challenging and more prosocial behaviors. If using background music as an intervention, practitioners with training in special education, behavior analysis, or psychology may supervise its implementation. In contrast, training in music therapy or education appears essential when implementing more active forms that involve teaching musical skills. Research supports some forms of music therapy such as playing background music to reduce specific challenging behaviors, singing instructions, and providing weekly intervention sessions that focus on musical improvisation. Depending on type, music therapy may reduce challenging behaviors or improve engagement and social responsiveness. The main risk of music therapy is its potential failure to produce any benefits for the person, which underlines the importance of a rigorous ongoing assessment process during implementation. For more information about music therapy for persons on the autism spectrum, we recommend consulting the website of the American Association of Music Therapy (https://www.musictherapy.org/), which contains information for both parents and professionals.

26.3 Treatment Summary Table

Treatment summary: Music Therapy

Treatment description: Music therapy refers to a group of interventions that involve listening to or producing music with a person on the autism spectrum. Examples include playing background music, singing the steps of a routine, and teaching persons to play musical instruments while encouraging social engagement.

Expected outcomes: Listening to music may reduce engagement in repetitive vocalizations, singing may promote engagement, and active music therapy may lead to improvements in social responsiveness.

Methods: Receptive music therapy involves selecting the music or the song that will be used to support the development of the person on the autism spectrum. The music is then played or the song sang during the implementation of treatment. In improvisational music therapy, a therapist designs activities to engage a person, or a group, in musical activities (e.g., singing, playing instruments, moving to the music) while promoting social engagement and encouraging improvisation. Albeit exceptions to this rule exist, the number and duration of standalone sessions generally range from 8 to 20, lasting between 30 and 60 minutes.

Expertise required to implement treatment: Using background music and simple singing requires training in managing behavior for persons on the autism spectrum (e.g., behavior analysis, special education, psychology), whereas interventions involving teaching how to play music necessitates formal training in musical education or therapy.

Risks and negative side effects: The main risk is that music therapy alone may be insufficient to bring about socially significant changes in the person's functioning.

Additional considerations and limitations: Given the heterogeneous nature of music therapy, its effects should be rigorously monitored by practitioners on an ongoing basis.

26.4 Introduction

26.4.1 Treatment Description

Music therapy does not refer to a single intervention, but rather encompasses a range of interventions that involve listening to music, producing music, or a combination thereof (Mayer-Banerous et al., 2021). To facilitate reviews and discussion about this group of interventions, researchers have proposed dividing music therapy into two broad categories: receptive and active music therapy (Gassner et al., 2022). Receptive music therapy does not require observable responding from the person on the autism spectrum. This category typically involves listening to music or songs while engaging in other activities (e.g., learning, playing). Behaviors targeted by the intervention have included vocal stereotypy (Gibbs et al., 2018), challenging behaviors (Lanovaz & Huxley, 2017), and learning vocabulary (Simpson et al., 2013). The duration of receptive music therapy is not fixed, but a strength of the intervention is that the effects may be observed in as little as a single session.

In contrast, active music therapy requires that the person participate in musical activities. Examples of activities conducted during active music therapy include singing (Sandiford et al., 2013), hand clapping (Sandiford et al., 2013), and playing instruments (Ghasemtabar et al., 2015; Yoo & Kim, 2018). Active music therapy typically aims to improve adaptive and prosocial behaviors such as social skills (Yoo & Kim, 2018), joint attention (Vaiouli et al., 2015), motor skills (Cibrian et al., 2020), and social communication (Carpente, 2017). The number of sessions of music therapy varies greatly, ranging from as few as seven sessions (e.g., Hillier et al., 2012) to weekly sessions over an entire year (e.g., Boso et al., 2007). In general, individual session durations range from 15 to 90 minutes for 1 to 4 times per week. During these sessions, the persons may participate in activities that focus on musical education, whereas others use music (e.g., a song) to teach specific skills or concepts. Regardless of type, music therapy may be useful across the lifespan ranging from young children who have recently received a diagnosis to adults over 100 years old (Gassner et al., 2022).

26.4.2 Rationale and Objectives

The association between autism and music goes back nearly a century when links were mentioned in the first written descriptions of what we now refer to as autism. Notably, three of the six children studied by Ssucharewa in 1926 (Wolff, 1996) and six of the eleven children studied by Kanner in 1943 showed a marked interest, ability, or excellent memory for music. Early reports also identified musical ability as a common special skill of autistic savants (Rimland, 1964, 1978). Case studies then went on to show that children on the autism spectrum could replicate pitches, short melodies, and rhythms as accurately as age-matched controls (Appelbaum et al., 1979), and that they could create or improvise music, a central component of improvisational music therapy (Frith, 1972). Given these musical strengths, music therapy quickly gained popularity and success with children on the autism spectrum (Alvin 1978; Gaston, 1968; Nordoff & Robbins, 1965, 1977) as a way to connect, interact, and communicate with the therapist and express emotions (Geretsegger et al., 2014).

More recent research also shows that children and adolescents on the autism spectrum demonstrate as much interest in music and spend as much time listening to music on a weekly basis as same-age peers without autism (Bhatara et al., 2013). Adults on the autism spectrum also report using music in everyday life much like the typical listener (e.g., while working out, to relax, to change their mood; Allen et al., 2009). Music is widely recognized as a powerful medium to communicate emotions (Juslin & Sloboda, 2001; Meyer, 1956), which seems to affect persons with autistic and neurotypical developments alike. Indeed, children, adolescents, and adults on the autism spectrum recognize music-evoked emotions as well as same-age peers (Allen et al., 2013; Heaton et al., 1999; Quintin et al., 2011; Stephenson et al., 2016), lending further support to the use of music therapy for this population.

The objectives of music therapy vary depending on type and implementation, as evidenced by the diversity of behaviors targeted by the treatment. Most studies of receptive music therapy have aimed to reduce engagement in challenging behaviors (most notably repetitive vocalizations) or in improving engagement, whereas active music therapy is often implemented to teach social responsiveness. The mechanisms that explain the observed behavior changes may thus differ based on the type of therapy and skills targeted by the intervention. The current chapter will focus on three of the most popular explanations from the behavior analytic, neurobiological, and cognitive perspectives.

In behavior analysis, reductions in repetitive and challenging behaviors brought about by receptive music therapy are typically explained in terms of changes in motivation (see Laraway et al., 2003, for a conceptualization of motivation). Specifically, music appears to function as an abolishing operation for engaging in repetitive or challenging behaviors. Background music reduces the value of the reinforcer associated with (or motivation to engage in) repetitive and challenging behaviors, which leads to a reduction in the frequency of the behavior itself. Changes in motivation may also explain increases in engagement during receptive music therapy. Singing instructions may increase the value of the reinforcer associated with the desired behavior evoked by singing. In this example, music would be referred to as an establishing operation.

When receptive and active music therapy lead to learning new behaviors, behavior analysts rely on teaching processes to explain the observed changes. For example, assume that a child learns a new social skill by participating in improvisational music therapy sessions. A behavior analyst may conclude that, during the activity, the therapist provided practice opportunities, models, and prompts to engage in the social skills. Finally, music itself may function as a reinforcer for the person's new social behaviors (Watson, 1979). Although providing a musical reinforcer in isolation is not typically considered as music therapy, its reinforcing properties may play a role in its effectiveness at both reducing undesirable and increasing desirable behaviors (Horrocks & Higbee, 2008; Lanovaz et al., 2012).

From a neurobiological perspective, persons on the autism spectrum show overall typical brain activation of areas associated with auditory processing and with reward and emotion processing when listening to music (Caria et al., 2011; Gebauer et al., 2014). As such, listening to music activates their dopaminergic reward response circuit, which is known to be associated with a pleasurable reaction to music in the typical population (Blood & Zatorre, 2001; Menon & Levitin, 2005; Salimpoor et al., 2011). Persons on the autism spectrum may thus be drawn to listening to or playing music, given its inherently rewarding and pleasurable nature (Quintin et al., 2019). Further, it is unsurprising that persons on the autism spectrum appreciate music, given their musical strengths, including enhanced or atypical ability to discriminate between pitches (Bonnel et al., 2003, 2010), to remember pitches and melodies (Heaton et al., 1998, 2003; Stanutz et al., 2014), and to process musical rhythms (Jamey et al., 2019).

From a cognitive perspective, the enhanced perceptual functioning theory (Mottron et al., 2006) may account for some of these musical strengths. The theory states that persons on the autism spectrum may show enhanced or atypical sensory and perceptual processing hindering their grasp of a global whole and may explain their unique cognitive style. Whether persons on the autism spectrum are drawn to music because of perceptual strengths and appreciation of its structure, repetitiveness, and organization, or due to its emotional content, remains unclear. Responding to this question seems nearly impossible at this point in time because the perceptual, structural, and emotional components of music are closely intertwined. Regardless, persons on the autism spectrum seem to benefit from music therapy, as discussed in the current chapter. Lense and Camarata (2020) propose that benefits accrue because "musical activities support key elements of evidence-based approaches for social engagement including predictability, reinforcement, emotion regulation, shared attention, and social play context, providing a platform for delivery and receipt of social and behavioral instruction" (p. 1).

26.4.3 Considerations for Implementation

As described in the research background section below, the three types of music therapy with the most empirical support are background music, singing instructions, and improvisational music therapy. First, background music simply involves playing music, ideally preferred by the person or group for whom the therapy is intended (i.e., not the therapist's personal preference), while the person on the autism spectrum engages in another activity (e.g., playing, learning). This intervention is most effective in reducing engagement in repetitive nonfunctional vocalizations, which are often referred to as vocal stereotypy. Note that we do not recommend reducing vocal stereotypy in all contexts of a person's life. Vocal stereotypy should only be targeted for reduction when it becomes disruptive and interferes with learning, mental health, or social inclusion due to its high intensity and duration. Practitioners may simply allow the person to listen to music over headphones in a context in which the repetitive vocalizations are disruptive. This approach may not only reduce vocal stereotypy, but it may also provide a functionally equivalent form of stimulation.

A second intervention with strong support involves having the therapist sing, rather than speak, instructions during learning activities. For example, practitioners may sing a song involving the steps of a daily routine or may sing novel words that a child has to learn. Singing appears to improve engagement in tasks and learning for persons on the autism spectrum. However, this increase in engagement does not necessarily lead to an increased rate of learning, which seems to limit the utility to situations where engagement (and not learning itself) is the issue that needs to be addressed. Singing songs related to what is being learned may produce better outcomes than unrelated songs. The main advantages of background music and singing are their low effort for implementation and simplicity. Practitioners and parents may implement these interventions with few modifications to the tasks and schedule. The drawback is that the gains may sometimes be short term, limited to the time the music or singing is ongoing.

Improvisational music therapy generally involves a therapist engaging a person, or a group, in musical activities such as singing, playing instruments, and moving to the music while promoting social engagement, communication, emotional expression, and improvisation (Geretsegger et al., 2014). The activities differ considerably during this type of therapy, but two commonalities among all exemplars are the involvement of music and improvisation. Albeit exceptions to this rule exist, the number and duration of standalone sessions generally range from 8 to 20 lasting between 30 and 60 minutes. In most of the exemplars in the research literature, the person is alone with a practitioner during therapy, although it is possible to deliver this type of intervention in small groups. The behaviors targeted by this therapy vary considerably from one study to another, but they generally involve some type of socially acceptable behavior (e.g., identifying emotions, joint attention, social skills). Improvisational music therapy is more disruptive to routine than receptive music therapy. However, the intervention may produce more long-term effects, particularly on teaching social responsiveness to persons on the autism spectrum, which may generalize to social situations in everyday life outside of the music therapy context.

26.5 Research Background

To provide a thorough overview of research on music therapy, we conducted a systematic review of the peer-reviewed literature. To be included in our review, a study had to evaluate the effects of an intervention involving music targeting persons on the autism spectrum within an empirical study (e.g., group design, randomized controlled trial, single-case design). Figure 26.1 presents a diagram of the results of our literature search. Our search involved the ERIC, MEDLINE, Embase, Health and Psychosocial instruments; Global Health, APA PsycInfo, and JBI EBP databases; and peer-reviewed studies published on or after January 1, 2000. On February 8, 2022, the second author searched the databases using the following keywords: [music therapy] AND [autism], [musical therapy] AND [autism], [musical intervention] AND [autism], [music intervention] AND [autism], and [noncontingent music] AND [autism].

Following the removal of duplicates, this search produced a total of 420 publications. Further removal of theses, dissertations, and conference abstracts reduced the number of articles to 400. Then, the second author assessed the abstracts and excluded (a) studies targeting populations characterized by a health condition or a mental health condition other than autism, (b) studies focusing on perceptions of music therapy, (c) studies on interventions other than music therapy, (d) studies focusing on assessment scales rather than treatment, and (e) studies investigating the neurophysiological and neurobiological effects of music efficiency. This initial screening resulted in a total of 171 articles, which were read in their entirety by the second author. During this phase, reviews, nonempirical article studies (including case reports), and studies that did not have a majority of participants on the autism spectrum were excluded, which left us with 34 articles. Lastly, we identified eight articles from other sources while reading and reviewing prior research. In the end, the search yielded 42 articles for the review. The next two sections provide a narrative review of the research on the use of receptive and active music therapy as treatments for persons on the autism spectrum.

26.5.1 Receptive Music Therapy

Our literature search found less research on receptive music therapy than on active music therapy. In total, 14 studies implemented some form of receptive music therapy and 10 of those studies used single-case experimental designs. In a series of four single-case studies, Lanovaz and colleagues (Lanovaz & Huxley, 2017; Lanovaz & Sladeczek, 2011; Lanovaz et al., 2011, 2012) examined the effects of background music on repetitive vocalizations and challenging behaviors. In their first two studies (Lanovaz & Sladeczek, 2011; Lanovaz et al., 2011), the researchers showed that background music reduced engagement in repetitive vocalizations in four of five children with autism spectrum disorder (ASD). In their subsequent study, Lanovaz

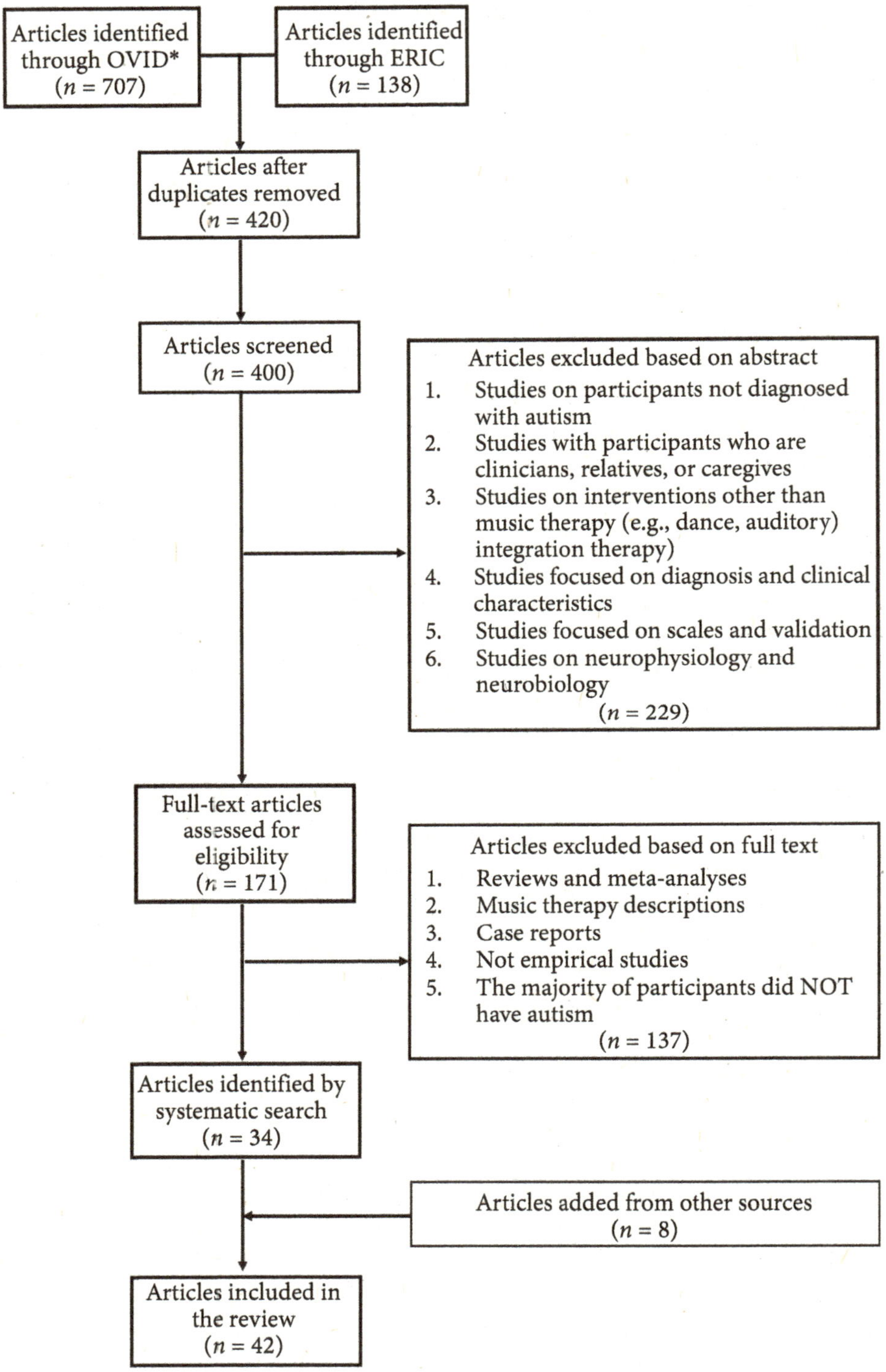

Figure 26.1 Diagram of our literature search
Note. We used OVID to search MEDLINE, Embase, Health and Psychosocial instruments, Global Health, APA PsycInfo, and JBI EBP.

et al. (2012) found that more preferred music produced lower levels of repetitive vocalizations than less preferred music in three of four participants, which underlines the potential importance of assessing musical preference. In their final study, Lanovaz and Huxley (2017) examined the effects of background music on other types of challenging behaviors (e.g., scratching, pinching, screaming, hitting, kicking, throwing) in three children with ASD. Background music produced reductions in challenging behaviors for two children.

Independent researchers have replicated the findings of Lanovaz and colleagues on repetitive vocalizations (e.g., Gibbs et al., 2018; Saylor et al., 2012). Saylor et al. (2012) found that music was the most effective form of auditory stimulation to reduce engagement in repetitive vocalizations in two children with ASD. Likewise, Gibbs et al. (2018) have observed that adding background music to a multiple-component intervention for two children on the autism spectrum suppressed repetitive vocalizations to a larger extent. As such, research supports the use of receptive music therapy to reduce engagement in repetitive vocalizations. Given that the results of Lanovaz and Huxley (2017) have not been replicated, we caution the reader against using background music to reduce engagement in other forms of challenging behaviors, unless it is part of a research study or of a rigorous clinical application with monitoring using single-case designs.

The remaining studies involved teaching or strengthening behavior using music and songs related to the concepts being taught (Finnigan & Starr, 2010; Kalas, 2012; Katagiri, 2009; Kern, Wakeford, & Aldridge, 2007; Kern, Wolery, & Aldridge, 2007; Lim & Draper, 2011; Paul et al., 2015; Simpson et al., 2013, 2015). As noted earlier, Lanovaz et al. (2012) reported that more preferred music may lead to larger reductions in vocal stereotypy than less preferred music. Hence, different types of music may produce differential effects. To address this issue, Kalas (2012) compared the effects of a simple melody with a complex melody on teaching joint-attention behaviors to 30 children on the autism spectrum. The therapist played the music immediately before making a bid for joint attention. Their results indicated that the complex music was more likely to evoke engagement in joint-attention responses in children with mild or moderate symptoms, whereas the simple music produced more bids for joint attention in children with more severe symptoms of autism. This study further supports the need to examine the effects of different types of music on the behavior of children on the autism spectrum.

In two studies by Kern and colleagues (Kern, Wakeford, & Aldridge, 2007; Kern, Wolery, & Aldridge, 2007), teachers sang songs describing the steps involved in greetings and self-care routines for three boys with ASD within single-case experimental designs. All boys completed more steps of the skill being taught when they were sung. In a cross-over group study, Lim and Draper (2011) compared the rate of learning verbal behaviors when using spoken and sung instructions in 22 children on the autism spectrum. Both the spoken and sung instructions led to similar rates of learning, suggesting that singing does not lead to more rapid acquisition. In a replication study, Simpson et al. (2013, 2015) implemented a cross-over design to examine the acquisition of vocabulary words in 22 children on the autism spectrum. On average, the children were more engaged when the words were sung than when they were simply spoken, but they did not learn faster in either condition.

In a study using an adapted alternating-treatment design, Paul et al. (2015) compared correct responses, social gestures, and eye contact during tasks that were spoken and sung in three children on the autism spectrum. All participants showed higher levels of social gestures and eye contact during sung sessions, and two of three participants also displayed better performance. In a similar example, Finnigan and Starr (2010) used a single-case design to examine the effects of music on turn taking, correct responding, and eye contact in a 3-year-old girl on the autism spectrum. As in Paul et al. (2015), background music increased engagement in these adaptive and prosocial behaviors in the participant. Katagiri (2009) conducted a cross-over study to examine the effects of background music on identifying emotions in 12 students with ASD. The results of the study indicated that playing background music referencing specific emotions led to better emotion identification. Taken together, the results of the prior studies suggest that singing instructions and novel concepts may increase appropriate engagement in children on the autism spectrum. The main limitation is that it remains unclear how to design the song and music most likely to support the development and maintenance of specific skills, but considering the child's personal musical preference seems to be a key ingredient of success.

26.5.2 Active Music Therapy

Our search found 28 studies examining the effects of active music therapy for persons on the autism spectrum, which is double the number of studies on receptive music therapy. Most of the interventions in this category contained multiple treatment components that encouraged active participation, or observable behaviors, of the persons on the autism spectrum. One of the most common active forms of treatment in the research literature is improvisational music therapy and other interventions containing an improvisational component (e.g., Carpente, 2017; Crawford et al., 2017; Kim et al., 2008; Latif et al., 2021; Mössler et al., 2020; Pasiali & Clark, 2018; Rabeyron et al., 2020; Sharda et al., 2018; Thompson et al., 2014; Vaiouli et al., 2015). The improvisational component typically involves the creation of novel lyrics, tunes, or music to support the development of novel skills, most often social.

In the largest randomized controlled trial to date, Crawford et al. (2017) and Bieleninik et al. (2017) compared the effects of low-frequency (one 30-minute session per week) and high-frequency (three 30-minute sessions per week) improvisational music therapy and enhanced standard care on social affect and responsiveness in 364 young children (4 to 7 years old) on the autism spectrum. After 5 months of therapy, the researchers observed no significant difference across conditions in their main outcomes. Mössler et al. (2020) conducted a follow-up study to explain the lack of observed effects. Specifically, the study examined the effects of attunement (or synchronization) between therapist and child on changes in the targeted outcomes, but failed to find significant changes. The choice of outcome measures (i.e., standardized measures typically used as part of autism diagnostic assessments; Bieleninik et al., 2017; Crawford et al., 2017; Mössler et al., 2020) may not have been optimal or sensitive enough to capture changes in social or communication skills (Quintin, 2019). As such, these studies raise questions concerning the effectiveness of improvisational music therapy in improving social responsiveness in children on the autism spectrum, and more importantly, how and if it should be measured as the main outcome.

Notably, smaller randomized controlled trials have found significant effects of improvisational music therapy on other components of social and communicative behaviors. For example, Sharda et al. (2018) conducted a randomized controlled trial with 51 elementary school-aged children on the autism spectrum. Their intervention consisted of 8 to 12 weeks of 45-minute one-to-one music interventions that included the "use of musical instruments, songs and rhythmic cues while targeting communication, turn-taking, sensorimotor integration, social appropriateness and musical interaction" (Sharda et al., 2018, p. 5). The children in the intervention group showed clear improvements in social communication skills when compared to the children in the waitlist control group. These improvements were associated with increased functional connectivity between auditory and subcortical brain areas, supporting the effectiveness and potential for lasting effects of the intervention due to brain plasticity. Subsequent analyses of the data from the same study indicated that the music intervention resulted in more joint engagement and more movement (Latif et al., 2021), which may explain some of the changes observed in the original study. In a randomized, repeated measures group study with 13 younger children (3 to 5 years old) on the autism spectrum, Kim et al. (2008) conducted 12 weekly 30-minute improvisational music therapy sessions targeting autistic symptoms and joint attention. The music therapy led to improvements in joint attention, and the children showed better turn taking and eye contact in music than in play-only sessions.

In an interesting variation, Thomson et al. (2014) examined the effects of a family-centered approach in which parents and their young children on the autism spectrum (N = 23) participated in a randomized controlled trial. The study identified improvements in emotional and social functioning of the children receiving 16 weekly 30- to 40-minute music therapy sessions. In the most recent randomized study of improvisational music therapy, Rabeyron et al. (2020) examined the effects of 25, 30-minute music improvisational sessions conducted over a period of 8 months with 4- to 7-year-old children on the autism spectrum. Their results showed that music therapy led to a reduction in symptoms of autism, most likely due to decreases in lethargy and stereotypy. Finally, one randomized controlled trial produced inconclusive results. Gattino et al. (2011) examined the effects of an improvisational music therapy consisting of 16 weekly 30-minute sessions in a small randomized controlled trial with 24 participants. There was no difference in autism symptoms between the music therapy and control groups, but a small subgroup (n = 5) of children on the autism spectrum showed improvements in nonverbal communication. Again, this study points to a need for future investigations with larger sample sizes, rigorous experimental designs, and careful choices of outcome measures related to the goals of music therapy (Gattino et al., 2011).

The prior randomized studies seem to partly support the use of improvisational music therapy with children, but the exact mechanisms responsible for the observed changes in behavior remain unclear due to the heterogeneity of the samples and treatment components. Further single-case (Vaiouli et al., 2015), repeated-measures, and small-scale pre-post designs (Bharathi et al., 2019; Dezfoolian et al., 2013; Ghasemtabar et al., 2015; Pasiali & Clark, 2018; Pasiali et al., 2014) also support the use of improvisational music therapy to teach social skills, joint attention, and attention skills. The problem with research on improvisational music therapy and its variations is that the intervention parameters, such as duration and number of sessions, often vary considerably across studies, making generalizations difficult to draw. The next step in research should thus involve a component analysis of improvisational music therapy to separate the essential ones from the nonessential ones (see Mössler et al., 2020; Latif et al., 2021) and better outcome measures consistent with the goals of music therapy (Quintin, 2019).

In a different form of active music therapy involving singing, Pasiali (2004) examined the effects of teaching three children on the autism spectrum to sing songs describing expected behavior using an ABAB reversal design. Even though initial reductions of repetitive behaviors were observed in each child, trends and lack of interparticipant replication prevent the drawing of clear conclusions from the data. In a second example with singing, Schmid et al. (2020) evaluated the effects of VOICSS (Vocal Interactive Communication and Social Strategies), a group-based music therapy program with a strong emphasis on singing to promote learning. Trained therapists implemented the program in nine self-contained classes containing a total of 64 children on the autism spectrum. Their pre-post design indicated that the program led to improvements in social communication. Similarly, Chiengchana and Trakarnrung (2014) implemented a program, Kodaly, that relies on singing, to promote joint attention in three children on the autism spectrum. The results indicated that the singing increased joint-attention responses in all their participants, but these conclusions are limited by a lack of return to baseline within their single-case designs.

In a randomized controlled trial with 12 participants, Sandiford et al. (2013) taught nonverbal children on the autism spectrum to melodically sing vocabulary words. Following the 5-week therapy, the children in the experimental group displayed more imitative attempts and produced more new words at home compared to the control group. Given the size of each group (five in the control group and seven in the experimental group), these results should be interpreted with caution as the participants seemed to differ at pretest. Although not captured by our literature search focusing on music, auditory-motor mapping training combines intonation and rhythm (i.e., singing and tapping) to teach vocabulary. It was associated with larger language gains than control treatments in studies of 23 (Chenausky et al., 2016) and 15 (Yan et al., 2021) minimally verbal children on the autism spectrum, with gains generalizing to untaught tones of a tonal language (Yan et al., 2021). In sum, these findings suggest that singing may be a promising avenue to improve language skills of children on the autism spectrum.

Another form of active music therapy involves an emphasis on drumming (Willemin et al., 2018; Yoo & Kim, 2018). In these studies, participation not only included drumming but also learning about rhythm. Yoo and Kim (2018) examined the effects of dyadic drum playing on the social skills of nine children on the autism spectrum in pre-post design. Dyadic drumming involves matching and synchronizing one's movements and rhythms to another person. Following eight, 30-minute sessions of rhythmic instructions, children showed better cooperation, self-control, and joint action. In another pre-post study, Willemin et al. (2018) implemented biweekly 60-minute dyadic drumming sessions with 14 participants ranging from 5 to 14 years old. After 5 weeks, the participants reported more enjoyment following the activity. Albeit still in its initial stages, research on dyadic drumming for autism seems encouraging. It will be important for future research to adopt experimental designs with a rigorous methodology, after which we may draw conclusions on the impact of dyadic drumming on social behaviors.

The research literature contains examples of other interventions that make use of music to support the development of persons on the autism spectrum. Despite a need for replication studies to draw stronger conclusions, we present some examples below to encourage research and for practitioners who may attempt to implement them using a rigorous monitoring system (e.g., single-case experimental designs). For example, Cibrian et al.'s (2020) intervention involved either using tambourines or an elastic-touch display designed to play sound while learning to press (or tap) harder or softer. The results of their randomized controlled trial suggested that all children improved their motor coordination and that the elastic-touch display may have produced better outcomes. This example is different as it focuses on motor rather than psychosocial skills as outcomes. In another study related to motor behaviors, Stephens (2008) examined the effects of imitating children playing musical instruments on evoking spontaneous motor imitation. Using single-case designs, their study showed that the therapist imitating the child's instrument play led to increases in spontaneous imitation in four children on the autism spectrum. This result is promising as some children on the autism spectrum struggle in initiating imitation, which can be difficult to evoke without physical prompting (Ross & Greer, 2003).

In a study of more traditional music therapy, LaGasse (2014) evaluated the effects of group music therapy involving listening, playing instruments, moving to musical cues, and practicing social skills during the activity. The results of the intervention indicated that the nine children who received therapy had higher changes in social responsiveness over time than the eight children in a social skills group. This study underlines how musical activities may be used to enhance the effects of interventions for social skills. Kern and Aldridge (2006) observed similar results in a study using peer mediation. Their intervention consisted of providing each child on the autism spectrum and a peer with an environment that involved musical instruments. The therapist provided prompting and reinforcers to the children for engaging with the instruments. Although the teacher-mediated intervention alone generally led to more positive interactions, the peer-mediated music intervention also increased positive peer interactions for the four participating children when compared to baseline within a multiple-baseline design. Their results also indicated that access to music alone was insufficient: The child on the autism spectrum and peer had to be prompted. Boso et al. (2007) also reported positive results for music therapy involving singing, piano playing, and drumming to promote social engagement in a long-term pre-post study. Specifically, their study found that, after 52 weekly 60-minute therapy sessions, eight adults on the autism spectrum showed fewer psychiatric symptoms.

26.6 Practice Implications

26.6.1 Treatment Outcomes

Most studies reported positive outcomes of music therapy on a variety of behaviors. However, what is referred to as "music therapy" varies tremendously from one study to another. A review of the literature indicates that only three types of music therapy have amassed considerable support. By far, the intervention with the most support is improvisational music therapy, an active therapy. Multiple randomized controlled trials have shown that improvisational music therapy may increase engagement in appropriate social responses. The limitation of this line of research is that most studies have implemented different treatment modalities. For example, the number, duration, frequency, and content of sessions vary widely; therefore, it is difficult to make specific recommendations involving the characteristics of treatment. In the same vein, outcome measures also vary widely across studies. In the future, researchers should include larger sample sizes within experimental designs while emphasizing parametric and component analyses (Latif et al., 2021; Mössler et al., 2020) and carefully selecting outcome measures in line with the goals of music therapy (Gattino et al., 2011; Quintin, 2019) to better guide practitioners in their selection of these modalities.

Background music has empirical support from numerous single-case experimental studies. Several independent teams of researchers (Lanovaz et al., 2011; Saylor et al., 2012) have reported reductions in vocal stereotypy of children on the autism spectrum with background music. The next step in research involves conducting group studies to examine the typical effect size of the treatment. Singing instructions has support from both group and single-case studies. Researchers have shown that singing instructions during routines or teaching tasks may improve engagement. However, the results of its effects on the pace of learning have been inconclusive: Increases in engagement are not necessarily associated with faster learning rates. Larger scale studies are needed to better isolate the unique contribution and interactions between music, engagement, and learning. Other interventions such as drumming, asking the child to sing, and using music to evoke imitation only have limited support in the research literature (e.g., one experimental study, two or three quasi-experiments). At this point in time, we cannot recommend them outside controlled research studies or evaluative clinical practices, but the evidence to date is promising and supports continued work in this area.

26.6.2 Practice Implication Guidelines

Because the effects of music appear to be idiosyncratic and the types of music may vary, implementation may vary tremendously from one practitioner to the next. Nevertheless, we can isolate four general guidelines to help practitioners in their implementation and caregivers in selecting appropriate service providers. First, practitioners should closely monitor the effects of music therapy with the person, regardless of the type or target behavior. Given the idiosyncratic effects of music, failure to closely monitor changes in behavior may lead to ineffective treatment being continued. To this end, we recommend using single-case designs to continuously monitor progress and make adaptations. Reviewing the literature on single-case designs goes beyond the scope of this paper, but we refer practitioners to Kazdin (2019) for a more thorough discussion.

A second guideline is to assess preference to music prior to beginning the intervention, especially when implementing receptive music therapy. For children who are able to communicate their needs, asking them what they prefer may be sufficient. However, practitioners may need to implement a more rigorous paired-choice preference to identify the best music choice to use during interventions (see Horrocks & Higbee, 2008). Listening to preferred music may produce more beneficial effects than less preferred music on behavior (Lanovaz et al., 2012), which underlines the importance of assessing preference.

Third, the target behavior may dictate the type of music therapy implemented with a person. For instance, nearly all research on reducing challenging behaviors has used receptive music therapy. Hence, we recommend receptive music therapy when the purpose of the intervention is to reduce repetitive and challenging behaviors. Alternatively, most research on active music therapy has focused on teaching social responsiveness (e.g., social skills, reciprocity, communication). When the purpose is to improve and increase socialization, our recommendation is to implement active music therapy. Minimally, the person on the autism spectrum should have the opportunity to practice and observe the targeted social skills during the music therapy sessions.

Finally, only qualified professionals should implement music therapy so that persons have access to best practices. As repeated throughout the chapter, music therapy may differ considerably depending on the target. Implementation by a qualified professional will ensure that the intervention truly meets the person's needs. If the intervention only involves simple musical components (e.g., listening to music, singing), a behavior analyst, a special education teacher, or a psychologist trained in behavior management may supervise the implementation of treatment. In this case, music is simply a medium provided to meet a specific goal. That said, practitioners with training in music education or therapy could implement interventions that involve teaching more complex musical skills (e.g., drumming, musical instruments, rhythms). Under ideal conditions, specialists in behavior management and music education should collaborate to take advantage of strengths and skills of each professional within an interdisciplinary framework to benefit the populations that they serve.

26.7 References

Allen, R., Davis, R., & Hill, E. (2013). The effects of autism and alexithymia on physiological and verbal responsiveness to music. *Journal of Autism and Developmental Disorders, 43*(2), 432–444. https://doi.org/10.1007/s10803-012-1587-8

Allen, R., Hill, E., & Heaton, P. (2009). "Hath charms to soothe ...": An exploratory study of how high-functioning adults with ASD experience music. *Autism, 13*(1), 21–41. https://doi.org/10.1177/1362361307098511

Alvin, J. (1978). *Music therapy for the autistic child.* Oxford: Oxford University Press.

Applebaum, E., Egel, A. L., Koegel, R. L., & Imhoff, B. (1979). Measuring musical abilities of autistic children. *Journal of Autism and Developmental Disorders, 9*(3), 279–285. https://doi.org/10.1007/BF01531742

Bharathi, G., Venugopal, A., & Vellingiri, B. (2019). Music therapy as a therapeutic tool in improving the social skills of autistic children. *The Egyptian Journal of Neurology, Psychiatry and Neurosurgery, 55*(1), 1–6. https://doi.org/10.1186/s41983-019-0091-x

Bhatara, A., Quintin, E. M., Fombonne, E., & Levitin, D. J. (2013). Early sensitivity to sound and musical preferences and enjoyment in adolescents with autism spectrum disorders. *Psychomusicology: Music, Mind, and Brain, 23*(2), 100–108. https://doi.org/10.1037/a0033754

Bieleninik, L., Geretsegger, M., Mössler, K., Assmus, J., Thompson, G., Gattino, G., Elefant, C., Gottfried, T., Igliozzi, R., Muratori, F., Suvini, F., Kim, J., Crawford, M., Odell-Miller, H., Oldfield, A., Casey, Ó., Finnemann, J., Carpente, J., Park, A-La, ... Gold, C. (2017). Effects of improvisational music therapy vs enhanced standard care on symptom severity among children with autism spectrum disorder: The TIME-A randomized clinical trial. *Journal of the American Medical Association, 318*, 525–535. https://doi.org/10.1001/jama.2017.9478

Blood, A. J., & Zatorre, R. J. (2001). Intensely pleasurable responses to music correlate with activity in brain regions implicated in reward and emotion. *Proceedings of the National Academy of Sciences of the United States of America*, 98(20), 11818–11823. https://doi.org/10.1073/pnas.191355898

Bonnel, A., McAdams, S., Smith, B., Berthiaume, C., Bertone, A., Ciocca, V., Burrack, J. A., & Mottron, L. (2010). Enhanced pure-tone pitch discrimination among persons with autism but not Asperger syndrome. *Neuropsychologia, 48*(9), 2465–2475. https://doi.org/10.1016/j.neuropsychologia.2010.04.020

Bonnel, A., Mottron, L., Peretz, I., Trudel, M., Gallun, E., & Bonnel, A. M. (2003). Enhanced pitch sensitivity in individuals with autism: A signal detection analysis. *Journal of Cognitive Neuroscience, 15*(2), 226–235. https://doi.org/10.1162/089892903321208169

Boso, M., Emanuele, E., Minazzi, V., Abbamonte, M., & Politi, P. (2007). Effect of long-term interactive music therapy on behavior profile and musical skills in young adults with severe autism. *Journal of Alternative and Complementary Medicine, 13*(7), 709–712. https://doi.org/10.1089/acm.2006.6334

Caria, A., Venuti, P., & de Falco, S. (2011). Functional and dysfunctional brain circuits underlying emotional processing of music in autism spectrum disorders. *Cerebral Cortex, 21*(12), 2838–2849. https://doi.org/10.1093/cercor/bhr084

Carpente, J. (2017). Investigating the effectiveness of a developmental, individual difference, relationship-based (DIR) improvisational music therapy program on social communication for children with autism spectrum disorder. *Music Therapy Perspectives, 35*(4), 160–174. https://doi.org/10.1093/mtp/miw013

Chenausky, K., Norton, A., Tager-Flusberg, H., & Schlaug, G. (2016). Auditory-motor mapping training: Comparing the effects of a novel speech treatment to a control treatment for minimally verbal children with Autism. *PLoS One, 11*(11), e0164930. https://doi.org/10.1371/journal.pone.0164930

Chiengchana, N., & Trakarnrung, S. (2014). The effect of Kodály-based music experiences on joint attention in children with autism spectrum disorders. *Asian Biomedicine, 8*(4), 547–555. https://doi.org/10.5372/1905-7415.0804.326

Cibrian, F. L., Madrigal, M., Avelais, M., & Tentori, M. (2020). Supporting coordination of children with ASD using neurological music therapy: A pilot randomized control trial comparing an elastic touch-display with tambourines. *Research in Developmental Disabilities, 106*, 103–741. https://doi.org/10.1016/j.ridd.2020.103741

Crawford, M. J., Gold, C., Odell-Miller, H., Thana, L., Faber, S., Assmus, J., Bieleninik, Ł., Geretsegger, M., Grant, C., Maratos, A., Sandford, S., Claringbold, A., McConachie, H., Maskey, M., Mössler, K. A., Ramchandani, P., & Hassiotis, A. (2017). International multicentre randomised controlled trial of improvisational music therapy for children with autism spectrum disorder: TIME-A study. *Health Technology Assessment, 21*(59), 1–40. https://doi.org/10.3310/hta21590

Dezfoolian, L., Zarei, M., Ashayeri, H., & Looyeh, M. Y. (2013). A pilot study on the effects of Orff-based therapeutic music in children with autism spectrum disorder. *Music and Medicine, 5*(3), 162–168. https://doi.org/10.47513/mmd.v5i3.325

Finnigan, E., & Starr, E. (2010). Increasing social responsiveness in a child with autism. A comparison of music and non-music interventions. *Autism: The International Journal of Research and Practice, 14*(4), 321–348. https://doi.org/10.1177/1362361309357747

Frith, U. (1972). Cognitive mechanisms in autism: Experiments with color and tone sequence production. *Journal of Autism and Childhood Schizophrenia, 2*(2), 160–173. https://doi.org/10.1007/BF01537569

Gassner, L., Geretsegger, M., & Mayer-Ferbas, J. (2022). Effectiveness of music therapy for autism spectrum disorder, dementia, depression, insomnia and schizophrenia: Update of systematic reviews. *European Journal of Public Health, 32*(1), 27–34. https://doi.org/10.1093/eurpub/ckab042

Gaston, E. T. (Ed.). (1968). *Music in therapy*. New York: Macmillan.

Gattino, G. S., Riesgo, R. D. S., Longo, D., Leite, J. C. L., & Faccini, L. S. (2011). Effects of relational music therapy on communication of children with autism: A randomized controlled study. *Nordic Journal of Music Therapy, 20*(2), 142–154. https://doi.org/10.1080/08098131.2011.566933

Gebauer, L., Skewes, J., Westphael, G., Heaton, P., & Vuust, P. (2014). Intact brain processing of musical emotions in autism spectrum disorder, but more cognitive load and arousal in happy vs. sad music. *Frontiers in Neuroscience, 8*, 192. https://doi.org/10.3389/fnins.2014.00192

Geretsegger, M., Elefant, C., Mossler, K. A., & Gold, C. (2014). Music therapy for people with autism spectrum disorder. *Cochrane Database of Systematic Reviews, 2014*(6). https://doi.org/10.1002/14651858.CD004381.pub3

Ghasemtabar, S. N., Hosseini, M., Fayyaz, I., Arab, S., Naghashian, H., & Poudineh, Z. (2015). Music therapy: An effective approach in improving social skills of children with autism. *Advanced Biomedical Research, 4*, 157. https://doi.org/10.4103/2277-9175.161584

Gibbs, A. R., Tullis, C. A., Thomas, R., & Elkins, B. (2018). The effects of noncontingent music and response interruption and redirection on vocal stereotypy. *Journal of Applied Behavior Analysis, 51*(4), 899–914. https://doi.org/10.1002/jaba.485

Heaton, P. (2003). Pitch memory, labelling and disembedding in autism. *Journal of Child Psychology and Psychiatry, 44*(4), 543–551. https://doi.org/10.1111/1469-7610.00143

Heaton, P., Hermelin, B., & Pring, L. (1998). Autism and pitch processing: A precursor for savant musical ability? *Music Perception, 15*(3), 291–305. https://doi.org/10.2307/40285769

Heaton, P., Hermelin, B., & Pring, L. (1999). Can children with autistic spectrum disorders perceive affect in music? An experimental investigation. *Psychological Medicine, 29*(6), 1405–1410. https://doi.org/10.1017/S0033291799001221

Hillier, A., Greher, G., Poto, N., & Dougherty, M. (2012). Positive outcomes following participation in a music intervention for adolescents and young adults on the autism spectrum. *Psychology of Music, 40*(2), 201–215. https://doi.org/10.1177/0305735610386837

Horrocks, E., & Higbee, T. S. (2008). An evaluation of a stimulus preference assessment of auditory stimuli for adolescents with developmental disabilities. *Research in Developmental Disabilities, 29*(1), 11–20. https://doi.org/10.1016/j.ridd.2006.09.003

Jamey, K., Foster, N. E., Sharda, M., Tuerk, C., Nadig, A., & Hyde, K. L. (2019). Evidence for intact melodic and rhythmic perception in children with autism spectrum disorder. *Research in Autism Spectrum Disorders, 64*, 1–12. https://doi.org/10.1016/j.rasd.2018.11.013

Juslin, P. N., & Sloboda, J.A. (2001). *Music and emotion: Theory and research.* New York: Oxford University Press.

Kalas, A. (2012). Joint attention responses of children with autism spectrum disorder to simple versus complex music. *Journal of Music Therapy, 49*(4), 430–452. https://doi.org/10.1093/jmt/49.4.430

Kanner, L. (1943). Autistic disturbances of affective contact. *Nervous Child, 2*, 217–250.

Katagiri, J. (2009). The effect of background music and song texts on the emotional understanding of children with autism. *Journal of Music Therapy, 46*(1), 15–31. https://doi.org/10.1093/jmt/46.1.15

Kazdin, A. E. (2019). Single-case experimental designs. Evaluating interventions in research and clinical practice. *Behaviour Research and Therapy, 117*, 3–17. https://doi.org/10.1016/j.brat.2018.11.015

Kern, P., & Aldridge, D. (2006). Using embedded music therapy interventions to support outdoor play of young children with autism in an inclusive community-based child care program. *Journal of Music Therapy, 43*(4), 270–294. https://doi.org/10.1093/jmt/43.4.270

Kern, P., Wakeford, L., & Aldridge, D. (2007). Improving the performance of a young child with autism during self-care tasks using embedded song interventions: A case study. *Music Therapy Perspectives, 25*(1), 43–51. https://doi.org/10.1093/mtp/25.1.43

Kern, P., Wolery, M., & Aldridge, D. (2007). Use of songs to promote independence in morning greeting routines for young children with autism. *Journal of Autism and Developmental Disorders, 37*(7), 1264–1271. https://doi.org/10.1007/s10803-006-0272-1

Kim, J., Wigram, T., & Gold, C. (2008). The effects of improvisational music therapy on joint attention behaviors in autistic children: A randomized controlled study. *Journal of Autism and Developmental Disorders, 38*(9), 1758–1766. https://doi.org/10.1007/s10803-008-0566-6

LaGasse, A. B. (2014). Effects of a music therapy group intervention on enhancing social skills in children with autism. *Journal of Music Therapy, 51*(3), 250–275. https://doi.org/10.1093/jmt/thu012

Lanovaz, M. J., & Huxley, S. C. (2017). Effects of background music on socially reinforced problem behaviors in children with autism spectrum disorders. *Psychology of Music, 45*(3), 450–456. https://doi.org/10.1177/0305735616657408

Lanovaz, M. J., Rapp, J. T., & Ferguson, S. (2012). The utility of assessing musical preference before implementation of noncontingent music to reduce vocal stereotypy. *Journal of Applied Behavior Analysis, 45*, 845–851. https://doi.org/10.1901/jaba.2012.45-845

Lanovaz, M. J., & Sladeczek, I. E. (2011). Vocal stereotypy in children with autism: Structural characteristics, variability, and effects of auditory stimulation. *Research in Autism Spectrum Disorders, 5*(3), 1159–1168. https://doi.org/10.1016/j.rasd.2011.01.001

Lanovaz, M. J., Sladeczek, I. E., & Rapp, J. T. (2011). Effects of music on vocal stereotypy in children with autism. *Journal of Applied Behavior Analysis, 44*(3), 647–651.https://doi.org/10.1901/jaba.2011.44-647

Laraway, S., Snycerski, S., Michael, J., & Poling, A. (2003). Motivating operations and terms to describe them: Some further refinements. *Journal of Applied Behavior Analysis, 36*(3), 407–414. https://doi.org/10.1901/jaba.2003.36-407

Latif, N., Di Francesco, C., Custo-Blanch, M., Hyde, K., Sharda, M., & Nadig, A. (2021). Joint engagement and movement: Active ingredients of a music-based intervention with school-age children with autism. *NeuroRehabilitation, 48*(2), 167–185. https://doi.org/10.3233/NRE-208012

Lense, M. D., & Camarata, S. (2020). PRESS-Play: Musical engagement as a motivating platform for social interaction and social play in young children with ASD. *Music & Science, 3*. https://doi.org/10.1177/2059204320933080

Lim, H. A., & Draper, E. (2011). The effects of music therapy incorporated with applied behavior analysis verbal behavior approach for children with autism spectrum disorders. *Journal of Music Therapy, 48*(4), 532–550. https://doi.org/10.1093/jmt/48.4.532

Mayer-Benarous, H., Benarous, X., Vonthron, F., & Cohen, D. (2021). Music therapy for children with autistic spectrum disorder and/or other neurodevelopmental disorders: A systematic review. *Frontiers in Psychiatry, 12*, 1–21. https://doi.org/10.3389/fpsyt.2021.643234

Menon, V., & Levitin, D. J. (2005). The rewards of music listening: Response and physiological connectivity of the mesolimbic system. *Neuroimage, 28*(1), 175–184. https://doi.org/10.1016/j.neuroimage.2005.05.053

Meyer, L. B. (1956). *Emotion and meaning in music.* Chicago: University of Chicago Press.

Mössler, K., Schmid, W., Aßmus, J., Fusar-Poli, L., & Gold, C. (2020). Attunement in music therapy for young children with autism: Revisiting qualities of relationship as mechanisms of change. *Journal of Autism and Developmental Disorders, 50*(11), 3921–3934. https://doi.org/10.1007/s10803-020-04448-w

Mottron, L., Dawson, M., Soulieres, I., Hubert, B., & Burack, J. (2006). Enhanced perceptual functioning in autism: An update, and eight principles of autistic perception. *Journal of Autism and Developmental Disorders, 36*(1), 27–43. https://doi.org/10.1007/s10803-005-0040-7

Nordoff, P., & Robbins, C. (1965). Improvised music for autistic children. *Music Journal, 23*(8), 35–67.

Nordoff, P., & Robbins, C. (1977). *Creative music therapy.* New York: The John Day Company.

Pasiali, V. (2004). The use of prescriptive therapeutic songs in a home-based environment to promote social skills acquisition by children with autism: Three case studies. *Music Therapy Perspectives, 22*(1), 11–20. https://doi.org/10.1093/mtp/22.1.11

Pasiali, V., & Clark, C. (2018). Evaluation of a music therapy social skills development program for youth with limited resources. *Journal of Music Therapy, 55*(3), 280–308. https://doi.org/10.1093/jmt/thy007

Pasiali, V., LaGasse, A. B., & Penn, S. L. (2014). The effect of musical attention control training (MACT) on attention skills of adolescents with neurodevelopmental delays: A pilot study. *Journal of Music Therapy, 51*(4), 333–354. https://doi.org/10.1093/jmt/thu030

Paul, A., Sharda, M., Menon, S., Arora, I., Kansal, N., Arora, K., & Singh, N. C. (2015). The effect of sung speech on socio-communicative responsiveness in children with autism spectrum disorders. *Frontiers in Human Neuroscience, 9*, 555. https://doi.org/10.3389/fnhum.2015.00555

Quintin, E. M. (2019). Music perception as a biomarker of social reward, cognition, and emotion for people with autism spectrum disorder. *Frontiers in Neural Circuits, 13*, 49. https://doi.org/10.3389/fncir.2019.00049

Quintin, E. M., Bhatara, A., Poissant, H., Fombonne, E., & Levitin, D. J. (2011). Emotion perception in music in high-functioning adolescents with autism spectrum disorders. *Journal of Autism and Developmental Disorder, 41*(9), 1240–1255. https://doi.org/10.1007/s10803-010-1146-0

Rabeyron, T., Robledo Del Canto, J. P., Carasco, E., Bisson, V., Bodeau, N., Vrait, F. X., Berna, F., & Bonnot, O. (2020). A randomized controlled trial of 25 sessions comparing music therapy and music listening for children with autism spectrum disorder. *Psychiatry Research, 293*(6), 113377. https://doi.org/10.1016/j.psychres.2020.113377

Rimland, B. (1964). *Infantile autism.* New York: Appleton-Century-Crofts.

Rimland, B. (1978). Inside the mind of the autistic savant. *Psychology Today, 12*(3), 68–80.

Ross, D. E., & Greer, R. D. (2003). Generalized imitation and the mand: Inducing first instances of speech in young children with autism. *Research in Developmental Disabilities, 24*(1), 58–74. https://doi.org/10.1016/S0891-4222(02)00167-1

Salimpoor, V. N., Benovoy, M., Larcher, K., Dagher, A., & Zatorre, R. J. (2011). Anatomically distinct dopamine release during anticipation and experience of peak emotion to music. *Nature Neuroscience, 14*(2), 257–262. https://doi.org/10.1038/nn.2726.

Sandiford, G. A., Mainess, K. J., & Daher, N. S. (2013). A pilot study on the efficacy of melodic based communication therapy for eliciting speech in nonverbal children with autism. *Journal of Autism and Developmental Disorders, 43*(6), 1298–1307. https://doi.org/10.1007/s10803-012-1672-z

Saylor, S., Sidener, T. M., Reeve, S. A., Fetherston, A., & Progar, P. R. (2012). Effects of three types of noncontingent auditory stimulation on vocal stereotypy in children with autism. *Journal of Applied Behavior Analysis, 45*(1), 185–190. https://doi.org/10.1901/jaba.2012.45-185

Schmid, L., DeMoss, L., Scarbrough, P., Ripple, C., White, Y., & Dawson, G. (2020). An investigation of a classroom-based specialized music therapy model for children with autism spectrum disorder: Voices together using the VOICSS^{TM} method. *Focus on Autism and Other Developmental Disabilities, 35*(3), 176–185. https://doi.org/10.1177/1088357620902505

Sharda, M., Tuerk, C., Chowdhury, R., Jamey, K., Foster, N., Custo-Blanch, M., Tan, M., Nadig, A., & Hyde, K. (2018). Music improves social communication and auditory-motor connectivity in children with autism. *Translational Psychiatry, 8*(1), 231. https://doi.org/10.1038/s41398-018-0287-3

Simpson, K., Keen, D., & Lamb, J. (2013). The use of music to engage children with autism in a receptive labelling task. *Research in Autism Spectrum Disorders, 7*(12), 1489–1496. https://doi.org/10.1016/j.rasd.2013.08.013

Simpson, K., Keen, D., & Lamb, J. (2015) Teaching receptive labelling to children with autism spectrum disorder: A comparative study using infant-directed song and infant-directed speech. *Journal of Intellectual & Developmental Disability, 40*(2), 126–136. https://doi.org/10.3109/13668250.2015.1014026

Stanutz, S., Wapnick, J., & Burack, J. A. (2014). Pitch discrimination and melodic memory in children with autism spectrum disorders. *Autism, 18*(2), 137–147. https://doi.org/10.1177/1362361312462905

Stephens, C. E. (2008). Spontaneous imitation by children with autism during a repetitive musical play routine. *Autism: The International Journal of Research and Practice, 12*(6), 645–671. https://doi.org/10.1177/1362361308097117

Stephenson, K. G., Quintin, E. M., & South, M. (2016). Age-related differences in response to music-evoked emotion among children and adolescents with autism spectrum disorders. *Journal of Autism and Developmental Disorders, 46*(4), 1142–1151. https://doi.org/10.1007/s10803-015-2624-1.

Thompson, G. A., McFerran, K. S., & Gold, C. (2014). Family-centred music therapy to promote social engagement in young children with severe autism spectrum disorder: A randomized controlled study. *Child: Care, Health and Development, 40*(6), 840–852. https://doi.org/10.1111/cch.12121

Vaiouli, P., Grimmet, K., & Ruich, L. J. (2015). Bill is now singing: Joint engagement and the emergence of social communication of three young children with autism. *Autism: The International Journal of Research and Practice, 19*(1), 73–83. https://doi.org/10.1177/1362361313511709

Watson, D. (1979). Music as reinforcement in increasing spontaneous speech among autistic children. *Missouri Journal of Research in Music Education, 4*(3), 8–20.

Willemin, T., Litchke, L. G., Liu, T., & Ekins, C. (2018). Social emotional effects of drumtastic: A dyadic within-group drumming pilot program for children with autism spectrum disorder. *International Journal of Special Education, 33*(1), 94–103. https://eric.ed.gov/?id=EJ1184084

Wolff, S. (1996). The first account of the syndrome Asperger described? Translation of a paper entitled "Die schizoiden Psychopathien im Kindesalter" by Dr. G. E., Ssucharewa. *European Child and Adolescent Psychiatry, 5*(3), 119–132. https://doi.org/10.1007/BF00571671

Yan, J., Chen, F., Gao, X., & Peng, G. (2021). Auditory-motor mapping training facilitates speech and word learning in tone language-speaking children with autism: An early efficacy study. *Journal of Speech, Language, and Hearing Research, 64*(12), 4664–4681. https://doi.org/10.1044/2021_JSLHR-21-00029

Yoo, G. E., & Kim, S. J. (2018). Dyadic drum playing and social skills: Implications for rhythm-mediated intervention for children with autism spectrum disorder. *Journal of Music Therapy, 55*(3), 340–375. https://doi.org/10.1093/jmt/thy013

27

Multisensory Environments

Jennifer Stephenson
Macquarie University

Mark Carter
University of Wollongong and MultiLit Research Unit, MultiLit Pty

27.1 Technical Abstract

Background: Multisensory environments (MSEs), including snoezelen rooms, are artificial environments designed to provide a range of sensory stimulation. The stimulation may be under the control of the participants or may be provided passively. The original purpose was to provide a leisure activity for people living in large institutions, but effects are now claimed to include reduction in challenging behavior and increases in engagement with tasks and people. MSEs have been employed with a wide variety of individuals, and those with autism spectrum disorder (ASD) are of particular interest, given sensitivities to sensory stimulation are commonly reported. **Method:** Searches of the databases ERIC, Cinahl, PubMed and Psychinfo using the terms (Autis* or ASD) AND (Snoezelen OR multisensory environment OR multisensory room OR multisensory therapy) and of the same databases using (Disbilit* OR handicap) instead of (Autis* or ASD) were carried out in November and December 2021. Studies were included if they were reported in a refereed journal article written in English, reported on an intervention that used an MSE, including snoezelen rooms, and included participants with ASD. Data were extracted on research design, participants, locations, interventionists, interventions, and outcomes. Study quality was also evaluated. **Results:** There is little solid evidence to support claims of therapeutic effects of MSEs. Study quality was generally poor. Group studies generally had small sample sizes, often lacked control groups, and allocation was not randomized. Only two single-case studies met the What Works Clearinghouse (WWC) (2022) standards. Studies measured a very wide range of variables, which suggests some uncertainty about expected effects, and generally reported mixed results. **Discussion:** There is little convincing evidence that MSEs provide any benefits to people with ASD, they but may be a leisure option for those who enjoy using them. Nevertheless, research is required to demonstrate that MSEs are better options than more normalized activities. Most research participants were adults or adolescents who also had intellectual disability, and there is little research on children with ASD and individuals without an

Jennifer Stephenson, and Mark Carter, *Multisensory Environments*. In: *Lifespan Treatment for Autistic Individuals*. Edited by: Peter Sturmey, Russell Lang, and James K. Luiselli, Oxford University Press. © Oxford University Press (2025).
DOI: 10.1093/oso/9780197635841.003.0027

intellectual disability. The poor quality of existing research, the wide variety of outcome measures, and variation in the way MSEs were used are all issues that need to be addressed. In particular, research comparing MSEs to other established interventions is needed. If claims are made for therapeutic benefits of MSEs, a clear, coherent theoretical underpinning needs to be developed that explains and predicts the benefits. **Practitioner recommendations:** At present, the use of MSEs other than for purposes of a leisure activity cannot be recommended. Practitioners should also consider whether more normalized leisure activities would be more appropriate and enjoyable than MSEs. If MSEs are to be used for therapeutic benefits, the expected effects should be clearly defined and closely monitored to determine the impact of any intervention.

27.2 Layperson Summary

MSEs, including snoezelen rooms, provide sensory stimulation through light, sound, aromas, and tactile experiences. They are claimed to have beneficial effects beyond their use as a leisure option for people with disabilities. In research studies, a range of persons have been used as implementers, and it appears no specific qualifications are required. Historically, the person accompanying the person with a disability was there to follow their lead, facilitate their use of the equipment, and build a relationship. The research relating to people with ASD, particularly for children and those without a cognitive disability, is sparse and of poor quality. Research results are mixed, with most indicting no clear effects, and no consistent outcomes appear to be targeted. Some persons with ASD have refused to use MSEs or have left sessions early. MSEs have been installed in a range of locations, and installation can be costly. There is currently no strong evidence to suggest that MSEs have any therapeutic benefit for individuals with ASD, and careful consideration should be given to whether other leisure experiences will offer greater benefit.

27.3 Treatment Summary Table

Treatment summary: Multisensory Environments (Including Snoezelen)

Treatment description: Users are exposed to a range of equipment that provides visual, auditory, and/or tactile stimulation and aromas. They may be accompanied by a care provider to facilitate their use of chosen equipment.

Expected outcomes: A wide range of outcomes such as decreased challenging behavior, stereotypy or self-injury, and increased engagement have been claimed.

Methods: Both group and single-case studies have been reported, but almost all are of poor quality.

Expertise required to implement treatment: A range of implementers have been reported, and it appears no specific qualifications are considered necessary.

Risks and negative side effects: Results have been mixed and need to be considered in the context of the poor quality of evidence. Some people with ASD refuse use, and increased problem behavior in the MSE has been reported in a few cases. The opportunity cost related to using MSEs as an alternative to evidence-based interventions and more normalized leisure activities needs to be considered. The usual risks associated with electrical equipment are present.

Additional considerations and limitations: Further quality research is needed, with clearly defined outcome measures and comparisons with interventions known to be effective in reducing problem behavior or promoting enjoyment and relaxation.

27.4 Introduction

27.4.1 Treatment Description

MSEs are artificial environments that contain electrical and other equipment intended to provide a range of sensory stimulation. The rooms are typically windowless, and walls and floors may be padded for safety. Equipment typically includes items such as bubble tubes, fiber optics, mirror balls, projectors providing various visual effects, sound systems, aroma diffusers, tactile equipment, and vibrating devices. Much of this equipment can be controlled by the user or interventionist by switches or other means, or it may be experienced passively. Interventionists can control the type and level of stimulation provided by the equipment to meet the perceived needs of individuals using the MSE (Cameron et al., 2020; Haegele & Porretta, 2014; ROMPA, 2021). Use of the room may be either individual or group and is typically supervised by a caregiver or therapist who may control the equipment and/or support users in accessing and controlling pieces of equipment.

MSEs, including snoezelen rooms (now a registered trademark of ROMPA who develop, design, and sell equipment for MSEs), were originally conceived as an environment to provide stimulation and relaxation to people with severe and multiple disabilities living in large institutions who had reduced opportunities to experience sensory stimulation and spent the majority of their time in wards (Hulsegge & Verheul, 1987; Mount & Cavet, 1995). The concept was developed in the Netherlands in the 1970s and 1980s and called snoezelen as a combination of the Dutch words *snuffelen*, meaning sniffing in the sense of exploring, and *doezelen*, meaning to doze (Hulsegge & Verheul, 1987). The snoezelen experience was to be an undirected one that placed no demands on the participants, but rather the caregiver or enabler supported the user to have an enjoyable experience and an opportunity to develop a relationship with the caregiver. There were no predetermined goals or intended therapeutic outcomes, and users were encouraged by the caregiver to engage with whatever equipment they preferred (Haggar & Hutchinson, 1991). The nondirective approach was stressed as an important characteristic of snoezelen with the outcomes being relaxation, enjoyment, and improved relationships (Hogg et al., 2001). Snoezelen was not regarded as a therapy, and thus any formal evaluation to demonstrate outcomes was not supported (Hutchinson & Haggar, 1994; Slevin & McClelland, 1999).

As MSEs became popular in schools and other settings, justifications for their use moved beyond the provision of stimulation and leisure, and they were recommended as an environment for assessment, therapy, and teaching with potential users now including people with a range of conditions, including ASD, brain injury, mental health problems, and dementia (Snoezelen Multi-Sensory Environments, 2022). Undirected use for leisure and relaxation may not always be fully compatible with use for educational or therapeutic interventions with predetermined outcomes (Lai, 2003). Pagliano (1998) suggested people needed to be more open to multiple uses of MSEs and that they could be "a dedicated space for relaxation and/or work" (p. 107) and stimulation could be controlled to meet the leisure or educational needs of the user.

27.4.2 Rationale and Objectives

As noted above, the original rationale in the 1970s for the use of snoezelen or multisensory rooms was simply for relaxation for people with severe disabilities in institutions who had extremely limited opportunities for experiences outside their residential wards. Care providers (enablers) were to be nondirective and support individual preferences. There was no intention for users to learn new skills (Bozic, 1997). By the 1990s, MSEs were being installed in schools serving students with severe disabilities, and the reasons for use began to extend beyond relaxation. Teachers took some control over the equipment to be used with specific aims in mind such as to promote concentration and to teach cause-and-effect relationships (Bozic, 1997). More recently, a range of uses have been suggested, including the use of the MSE for calming and helping users manage distress and self-regulate, building rapport, reducing self-injurious behavior, teaching self-regulation skills, and building parent–child relationships (Bergstrom et al., 2019). Some practitioners report using them to deliver structured teaching (Mey et al., 2015) and the use of switches to control equipment has also been explicitly taught in MSEs (Moir, 2010). The possibility of delivering different types of sensory stimulation within an MSE apart from other distractions has also allowed MSEs to be used for assessment of individual reactions to different stimuli (Munde & Vlaskamp, 2015; Munde et al., 2012).

As MSEs became "big business" (Cavet & Mount, 1995, p. 70), some individuals with a commercial interest in promoting MSEs made claims for benefits beyond relaxation, including changes in behavior, relaxation effects that continued outside the MSE, reductions in self-injury, stereotypy, and aggression and improvements in concentration and motivation (Botts et al., 2008). Installations could be costly. Mount and Cavet (1995) reported up to a quarter of a million sterling for large settings. MSEs became increasingly popular in a range of settings, including hospitals, schools, rehabilitation clinics, residential institutions, and homes. Several different professions could be involved, including occupational therapists, physiotherapists, and teachers, as well as other professionals and caregivers with no training (Castelhano et al., 2013). There has been debate about the desirability of MSEs as segregated settings unrelated to daily life and the danger that care providers and teachers might neglect the potential of sensory stimulation in regular everyday environments (Mount & Cavet, 1995).

There is little work examining the possible mechanisms producing the purported effects of MSEs (Breslin et al., 2020). Historically, and in relation to people with intellectual disability living in institutions, the viewpoint appeared to develop that the relaxed state resulting from the experience within the MSE would result in a decrease in challenging behavior, both within and beyond the MSE (Chan & Chien, 2017; Chan et al., 2010; Singh et al., 2004). Relaxation was also posited as possibly improving concentration and communication (Lindsay et al., 2001). This reasoning was applied to the early use of MSEs in schools for students with severe intellectual disability, and the perceived calming effect was believed to be beneficial (de Bunsen, 1992). The calm environment and the use of individualized sensory stimulation of an MSE resulting in optimal arousal was the rationale used by Lavie et al. (2005) for carrying out a hydrotherapy intervention in an MSE. Kaplan et al. (2006) suggested relaxation may reduce anxiety and thus reduce related problem behaviors. Toro (2019) also suggested that relaxation in the MSE which they likened to mindfulness meditation would reduce stress and anxiety, and this could improve short-term memory and balancing ability. Similarly, the provision of stimulation in an MSE was purported to reduce the need for stimulation provided by stereotypy or self-injurious behavior (Chan et al., 2005, 2010; Kwok et al., 2003; Martin et al., 1998). Breslin et al. (2020) suggested MSEs may act to calm the central nervous system or may distract the participant from unpleasant sensations.

Disentangling the effects of the equipment and the effects of the enabler may also be an issue (Martin et al. 1998). Pagliano (2006), when writing about MSEs and people with profound and severe disability, and usually a sensory impairment, emphasized the role of the facilitator in supporting the user's choices. He described the facilitator as "an immutable extension of the MSE" (p. 24), who also has a role in making detailed, systematic observations and collaborating with other professionals to provide appropriate support. Patterson (2004) also noted the importance of the caregiver in supporting the user and the potential for shared experiences to build relationships. The potential of MSEs for building relationships is supported by qualitative research with families of institutionalized people with severe and profound disabilities who report a sense of intimacy as well as relaxation as a result of family use of MSEs (Sachs & Nasser, 2009).

MSEs have been used with people with ASD who also had profound or severe intellectual disability from the 1990s onward (Hutchinson & Haggar, 1994), and by 2021, Unwin et al. (2021) claimed they were "widely used with autistic children" (p. 2). They are certainly marketed as beneficial for people with ASD by commercial firms promoting MSEs (see, for example, the Flaghounse/Rompa page: https://www.snoezelen.info/who-can-benefit/snoezelen-for-autism/). The majority of research studies including people with ASD as participants included people who had both intellectual disability, usually severe intellectual disability, and autism, and in about half these studies, participants were in residential institutions (Cuvo et al., 2001; Fava & Strauss 2010; Hill et al., 2012; Kwok et al., 2003; McKee et al., 2007; Mey et al., 2015; Slevin & McClelland, 1999; Toms et al., 2019).

There is often no theoretical underpinning offered in papers describing MSE use. Cameron et al. (2020) in a scoping review noted that the rationale for selecting specific equipment was not provided in the studies they reviewed. Some researchers have drawn on Ayres sensory integration theory (e.g., Shapiro et al., 1997; Toms et al. 2019). Mey et al. (2015) viewed sensory integration as a "conceptual framework" (p. 33) for using MSEs with people with ASD, and it was also part of the rationale for use in Novakovic et al. (2019). Toms et al. (2019), who worked with adults with ASD and intellectual disability, suggested that the sensory-motor activities in the MSE would develop sensory integration and thus improve behavior.

Sensitivity and other forms of unusual reactivity to sensory stimulation have been well documented in individuals with ASD (Kirby et al., 2022), and they now included in the *DSM-5* (American Psychiatric Association, 2013) diagnostic criteria. Given the sometimes intense forms of stimulation found in MSEs (e.g., mirror balls), it should not be assumed that such environments will necessary be pleasurable, or even tolerable, for some individuals with ASD. Thus, in evaluating the use of MSE, one important question relates to the degree to which exposure is terminated due to refusal or challenging behavior.

MSEs are typically constructed in specialized settings such as residential institutions (e.g., Cuvo et al., 2001; Toms et al., 2019). Comparison to "business as usual" activities in residential settings may not be very informative if the comparison conditions provide limited stimulation. If the aim of an MSE is to provide leisure and recreation, the question arises as to whether similar or greater benefits (enjoyment, relaxation) could be obtained with more normalized leisure activities in the community, which could potentially provide other advantages such as interaction with peers. Perhaps a more pressing question is whether when the claimed outcome relating to improvement in specific behaviors, such as challenging behavior or attention, could be obtained with more normalized community leisure activities. Answering such questions requires head-to-head comparison of MSEs to other normalized recreational activities.

27.5 Research Background

We examined the research base for the use of MSEs with people with ASD by first locating relevant refereed journal articles. The search was designed to locate all articles addressing use of MSEs that included participants with developmental disability. We could then, for the purpose of this chapter, identify articles including people with ASD from examination of the full text. Searches of the databases ERIC, Cinahl, PubMed, and Psychinfo using the terms (Autis* or ASD) AND (Snoezelen OR multisensory environment OR multisensory room OR multisensory therapy) and of the same databases using (Disbilit* OR handicap) instead of (Autis* or ASD) were carried out in November and December 2021. There were 175 hits and 77 remained when duplicates were removed. The abstracts and titles were screened independently by both authors, and studies were included if they were reported in a refereed journal, written in English, reported on an intervention that used an MSE (including snoezelen rooms), and included participants with a developmental disability (including ASD). If the title and abstract were unclear, the article was retained. After screening, 26 articles remained. Reliability for article inclusion calculated using the formula agreements divided by agreements plus disagreements multiplied by 100 was 97.4%.

An ancestral search of these 26 articles resulted in 11 additional articles. In addition, a search of the reference lists of previous reviews related to MSEs (Breslin et al., 2020; Chan et al., 2010; Haegele & Porretta, 2014; Hogg et al., 2001; Lai, 2003; Lancioni et al, 2002, 2005; Lotan & Gold, 2009) located one additional article.

Thirty-eight articles went forward for the next stage of data extraction and coding of the complete paper. Studies including participants with ASD were identified at this stage. Data extraction included (a) the research design (randomized controlled trial; pre-post single group; pre-post comparison group; post-only single group; AB design; multiple-baseline design; case study or other), (b) participant characteristics (number, gender, age, diagnosis), (c) intervention information (individual; group; number of sessions; frequency of sessions; length of sessions), (d) equipment used, (e) procedural reliability (presence and result if relevant), (f) interventionist (therapist; teacher; other), (g) location (school; residential, hospital; other), (h) comparison conditions, (i) other interventions, and (j) maintenance and generalization (any measure that was taken outside the MSE).

Where a study provided a description of a dependent variable and either inferential or descriptive numerical data related to that variable, we coded further details about that dependent variable and results. Where the nature of the dependent variable was unclear (e.g., conflicting information provided in the description or definition and what was measured and reported), we coded by consensus to identify the dependent variables and then coded each dependent variable independently.

Coding for the dependent variable included the type of target behavior categorized as challenging behavior (general, excluding other challenging behaviors coded separately); aggression; self-injurious behavior; stereotypy; physiological; communication; engagement; relaxation; alertness; and other (specify). Where specific behaviors such as screaming and arm biting were described, we classified them into one of these categories.

The measurement instrument used was noted where relevant, and (a) the type of measurement (direct observation; third party report not based on direct observation; formal assessment task; details of the assessment task where relevant), (b) when the assessment took place (during MSE session; immediately after MSE session; later), and (c) where the assessment occurred (in the MSE: outside the MSE; not stated). Whether observers were blinded, interrater reliability was recorded, and the results of interrater reliability were summarized, where relevant. We also coded whether the results reported for each dependent variable were positive (favored MSE) or negative. For single-case studies, given that interpretation of graphed results is usually based on researcher judgment, both authors examined graphic data using conventional criteria (Maggin et al., 2018) and summarized overall findings. These were subsequently compared, and any differences resolved by discussion.

Data extraction was completed independently by the two authors, apart from the consensus coding to identify some unclear dependent variables. At this stage, studies that included participants with ASD were identified, and those 13 articles are reviewed in detail in this chapter. Reliability of data extraction for those papers, including participants with ASD, was calculated using the formula agreements divided by agreements plus disagreements multiplied by 100 and was 95%. Disagreements were resolved by discussion.

We examined the quality of studies that included participants with ASD. Case studies and single-group studies cannot provide evidence of causal inference (Campbell & Stanley, 1963) so were not assessed for quality. Quality assessment for comparative group designs was based on the scheme described in Leong et al. (2015), which provides for assessment of key quality criteria of randomization, blinding, attrition, and establishing pretest equivalence. Two points were awarded for acceptable methods of randomization such as use of a random number table or generator or coin tossing. Two points were awarded if assessors were blind to group allocation on all measures, and one point was awarded if they were blinded on some measures. Two points were awarded if differential attrition was within 10% for all study groups. Two points were awarded if groups were demonstrated to be statistically equivalent at pretest on all measures (or if statistical adjustments were made for differences) and one point if this applied to some measures. Studies could obtain a maximum score of eight. There was one disagreement for quality assessment of group studies, and this was resolved by discussion.

For single-case designs, studies were evaluated independently by the two authors against the standards presented in WWC (2022). Studies had to meet the criterion for interobserver reliability (acceptable reliability for 20% or more of data points in each condition) and also provide the possibility of three demonstrations of control (have four total phases). For reversal designs, there needed to be five data points per phase or three or more data points with no within-phase variability and at least six data points in the baseline phase to meet the standard. For alternating treatment designs, there needed to be at least five data points per condition to meet the standard, or four data points per condition to meet the standard with reservation. Alternating treatment designs could only have a maximum of two sequential data points in the same condition to meet the standards. Agreement was 100% for whether or not single-case design studies met the WWC standards.

27.6 Results

Thirteen journal articles reporting on 15 studies that included participants with ASD were located. There were seven articles reporting nine single-case studies (Cuvo et al., 2001; Hill et al., 2012; Kaplan et al., 2006; Kim & Park, 2021; McKee et al., 2007; Slevin & McClelland, 1999; Toms et al., 2019, one case study (Mey et al., 2015), two single-group studies (Houghton et al., 1998; Kwok et al., 2003), one randomized controlled trial (Novakovic et al., 2019), one study that compared groups (Fava & Strauss, 2010), and one study that compared conditions for the same group (Unwin et al., 2021). See Table 27.1 for a summary of research designs.

27.6.1 Participants

A total of 113 participants with ASD were included. One participant was included in two studies reported Cuvo et al. (2001), and three participants were included in two studies reported in Kaplan et al. (2006). Of these participants, 56 were male, 19 were female, and in four studies, the gender of participants with ASD could not be determined (Fava & Strauss, 2010; Houghton et al., 1998; Kwok et al., 2003; Mey et al., 2015). Studies mostly included adolescents and adults, with a mean age of 24.4 years for studies where ages or mean age were provided. For some studies, ages of participants with ASD could not be determined (Fava & Strauss, 2010; Houghton et al., 1998; Kwok et al., 2003), and one study (Toms et al., 2019) gave an age range of early 20s to 40+ years. Only four studies clearly included children 12 years or under (Kim & Park, 2021; Mey et al., 2015; Unwin et al., 2021).

Most participants with ASD also had a diagnosis of intellectual disability with 49 with profound or severe intellectual disability and 16 with mild or moderate intellectual disability. The 10 participants in Kwok et al., 2003 had intellectual disability, but the level was not specified. Some of the participants in Unwin et al. (2021) had intellectual disability, but the numbers were not provided. The six participants in Mey et al. (2015) were described as having "delayed mental development" (p. 34).

Table 27.1 Study aims, research design, dependent variables, comparison conditions, and results

Study	Aim	Research Design	Dependent Variables	Comparison Conditions	Result
Cuvo et al. (2001), Experiment 1	Examined effect of MSE on stereotypic behavior and engagement during and after MSE sessions	Single-case, alternating treatments	Stereotypy, engagement	Institution living room with tables, chairs, couches, stereo, TV and cabinets with leisure materials and manipulative objects such as puzzles and games	Clear evidence that engagement was higher in MSE and equivocal evidence that rocking was lower. No difference in mouthing. No evidence of carryover of effects post session.
Cuvo et al., Experiment 2	Compared effect of MSE, living room, and outdoor activity on stereotypic behavior and engagement	Single-case, alternating treatments	Stereotypy, engagement	Institution living room as above. Outdoor condition involved a walk in the facility grounds with a researcher. Participant chose direction and could also sit in benches or the ground.	Outdoor condition was superior to MSE for all measured dependent variables. MSE was superior to living room for engagement only.
Fava & Strauss (2010)	Compared effect of MSE and stimulus preference environment on disruptive and prosocial behavior and carryover to living room	Pre-post comparison group	Aggression, stereotypy, communication, alertness	Control condition was the institution living room where participants could interact freely with objects or caregivers. Stimulus preference condition comprised preferred stimuli, and all sensory modalities were covered in each session.	Improvement for autism group for aggression and stereotypy but no significant difference for active behavior toward stimuli or prosocial behavior.

Hill et al. (2012)	Compared effect of MSE and living room in conditions of high and low attention on behavior maintained by automatic sensory reinforcement	Single-case, alternating treatments	Stereotypy, engagement, challenging behavior	Institution living room with chairs and sofas, TV, books, and puzzles. Other students and care workers may have been present.	Visual analysis indicated less stereotypy in MSE compared to living room regardless of care provider attention. Engagement results were mixed (although authors claimed higher engagement in high attention conditions) regardless of environment.
Houghton et al. (1998)	Explored if use of MSE resulted in skill achievement and generalization	Pre-post single-group	Number of foundation outcome statements not previously demonstrated	Baseline data collected in school classrooms. Generalization environment was a visit to a farm school.	For students with ASD, there was a very small pre to post increase in foundation outcome statement skills from 95.00 to 96.67. Eighteen instances of four previously unseen skills were exhibited by the three children with ASD in the generalization assessment.
Kaplan et al. (2006), Experiment 1	Determined the effect of MSE use on postsession engagement	Single-case BCBCB	Engagement	Occupational therapy session that did not use MSE.	Some evidence of higher task engagement for 2/3 participants following MSE condition.

continued

Table 27.1 *continued*

Study	Aim	Research Design	Dependent Variables	Comparison Conditions	Result
Kaplan et al., Experiment 2	Examined the effect of MSE use on challenging behavior	Single-case ABCBCB	Challenging behavior, self-injurious behavior, aggression	Baseline prior to experiment and any occupational therapy sessions. Alternating condition was the day program for the non-MSE portion of the participants' days.	Applying conventional visual analysis criteria, no convincing evidence of difference in favor of MSE condition.
Kim & Park (2021)	Examined the effect of MSE use and compared the effect of use of different MSE equipment on behaviors	Single-case ABCD	Stereotypy	Baseline was in a multipurpose room in a developmental center. Condition B was the MSE using visually focused equipment and C used auditory focused equipment. Condition D used both. Equipment varied for individuals depending on whether relaxing or stimulating conditions were needed.	Provided mixed evidence for improvement following introduction of MSE and, given research design (ABCD), limited evidence of differences between MSE conditions.
Kwok et al. (2003)	Evaluated the effectiveness of an MSE	Single-group, post only	Relaxation, motivation for learning, self-confidence, communication, leisure/enjoyment, engagement, aggression, self-injurious behavior	NA	Results for participants with ASD could not be separated.

McKee et al. (2007)	Examined the effect of MSE use on aggressive and destructive behaviors	Single-case ABAB	Challenging behavior, communication, physiological	General ward area with no MSE sessions	Time-series data revealed no clear evidence of improvement in either disruptive or prosocial behavior outside the MSE session.
Mey et al. (2015)	Explored the use of the MSE to meet the sensory needs of children with ASD	Case study			No numerical data were reported.
Novakovic et al. (2019)	Examined the effect of MSE use on CARS scale scores and stereotypic behavior	Randomized control trial	CARS total and subscale scores	Control conditions were normal daily activities in a daycare center: arrival, breakfast, music/occupational therapy, snack, speech, walking/gym, lunch, craft time/watering the plants, snack, going home.	Significant reduction in CARS total score and three examined subscales in MSE group but no change in control group.
Slevin & McClelland (1999)	Examine effect of MSE on relaxation	Single-case, alternating treatments	Relaxation, physiological, challenging behavior	Relaxation and physiological measures taken before and after MSE sessions. Behavior baseline was recorded on the ward in the 12 weeks prior to MSE use.	Greater relaxation and lower pulse immediately after MSE session but no evidence of change in challenging behavior outside sessions.

continued

Table 27.1 *continued*

Study	Aim	Research Design	Dependent Variables	Comparison Conditions	Result
Toms et al. (2019)	Explored the effects of an MSE with equipment turned on or off.	Single-case ABA	Stereotypy, self-injurious	Condition A was the MSE with all equipment turned off.	There was no consistent evidence that the MSE affected repetitive behavior for any participant.
Unwin et al. (2021)	Explored the effect of having control in the MSE on behavior, cognition and arousal.	Single-group, compare conditions	Stereotypy, sensory defensive and sensory seeking, speech, stereotyped communication, vocalization, social behavior, gestures, mimicry, rapport, anxiety, positive affect engagement, physiological	In the active condition, participants controlled the equipment in the MSE directly or with an iPad. In the passive condition, participants could not control the equipment.	Significant differences between conditions found for 14/27 comparisons (but nominated conservative alpha level often ignored in reporting results). Most differences favored active condition, but desired direction of change was not always clear.

ASD = autism spectrum disorder; CARS = Childhood Autism Rating Scale; MSE = multisensory environment.

Some of the participants in Kwok et al. (2003) may have had vision or hearing impairment, but there is insufficient information to know if these participants were those with ASD (see Table 27.2).

27.6.2 Intervention

Most studies explored the effect of MSE compared to conditions in an institutional living area or day program environment (Cuvo et al., 2001; Fava & Strauss, 2010; Hill et al., 2012; Kaplan et al., 2006; Novakovic et al., 2019; McKee et al., 2007; Slevin & McLelland, 1999). Houghton et al. (1998) recorded initial observations within segregated classrooms and generalization observations at a farm school. Slevin and McClelland (1999) compared relaxation and physiological measures immediately before and immediately after MSE sessions. Toms et al. (2019) compared the MSE with all equipment turned off to the MSE with equipment turned on. In addition to living room conditions, Cuvo et al. (2001) in Experiment 2 also compared the effects of the MSE to a walk outdoors. Two studies provided analysis of different conditions within the MSE. Kim and Park (2021) compared the effects of different equipment in the MSE selected to meet participant characteristics, and Unwin et al. (2021) compared the effect of the level of control provided to participants. Hill et al. (2012) also compared the effects of the level of attention provided by care providers in the MSE and the comparison condition. Procedural reliability was reported for only two studies. Hill et al. (2012) reported on the level of care provider attention provided, as attention was an independent variable across conditions. Unwin et al. (2021), who compared active versus passive choice conditions in the MSE, provided procedural reliability on equipment visited, time spent with each piece of equipment, and care provider utterances.

The MSE was located in a residential facility or hospital in six studies, and a range of other locations were reported (see Table 27.2). The equipment used in the MSEs typically provided light effects (e.g., projectors, mirror balls, bubble tubes, and fiber optics), tactile stimulation (vibrating equipment, rocking chair, waterbed), sound, and aromas. In 10 studies, the MSE was used as an individual intervention, in three studies intervention was provided to a group, and one study (Houghton et al., 1998) used both group and individual sessions. The number of sessions ranged from 2 to 62, frequency from twice a month to 5 times a week, and length of session from 15 minutes to 1 hour. A range of descriptions was given for the implementer, varying substantially in the degree of directiveness, with four described as therapists (see Table 27.2).

The original snoezelen approach of a supportive implementer who followed the participant's lead was used in four studies (Fava & Strauss, 2010; Kwok et al., 2003; McKee et al., 2007; Novakovic et al., 2019). Cuvo et al. (2001) used a similar approach in their two studies but prompted participants to engage with the equipment if they disengaged for more than 2 minutes in Study 1 or 1 minute in Study 2.

Table 27.2 Participants, intervention, location of MSE, role of implementer, and major limitations

Study	Participants With ASD	Intervention	Location of MSE	Role of Implementer	Major Limitations
Cuvo et al. (2001), Experiment 1	1 adult with severe/profound ID	Individual, 5X week, 20 minutes with researcher, 14 sessions	Residential	Introduced each piece of equipment by modeling, naming, and prompting use. After introduction, participant undirected but verbally prompted if disengaged for 2 minutes.	Design precluded counterbalancing of conditions.
Cuvo et al., Experiment 2	1 adult with severe/profound ID	Individual, 5X week, 20 minutes with researcher, 13 sessions	Residential	As above, but verbally prompted after 1 minute if disengaged	Only MSE and outdoor conditions counterbalanced.
Fava & Strauss (2010)	9 adults with severe/profound ID	Individual, 3X week for 25 minutes with caregiver, 20 sessions	Residential	Nondirective, followed preference of participant	Clinical significance of changes unclear. Only 3 participants in each treatment condition. No correction for familywise error across full study.
Hill et al. (2012)	2 adolescents with severe/profound ID	Individual, 2X week for 30 minutes with care provider, 20 sessions	Residential	Care provider controlled equipment.	Participants selected as functional assessment indicated stereotypic behavior was non-socially reinforced
Houghton et al. (1998)	Three (may have had either severe/profound ID or multiple disabilities	Group or individual, frequency and number not given, 30 to 40 minutes with a therapist teacher or teacher aide	School	Not clear; participants were allowed to interact with equipment.	Very weak research design. Compared 2-week baseline with 4–5-week MSE exposure.

Kaplan et al. (2006), Experiment 1	3 adults, 2 with severe/profound ID; 1 with mild/moderate ID	Individual, 2X week with occupational therapist for 30 minutes, 28 to 54 sessions	Day habilitation program	Adjusted equipment to effect arousal change	Number of prompts provided as a measure of task engagement for two participants at discretion of therapist.
Kaplan et al., Experiment 2	As above				
Kim & Park, (2021)	3 children with sensory sensitivities	Individual, 3X week with occupational therapist for 30 minutes, 18 sessions	Developmental center at a university	Therapist provided tailored intervention according to sensory characteristics of child.	Weak design for comparing conditions. Sequence related effects cannot be ruled out.
Kwok et al. (2003)	10 adolescents and adults with intellectual disability included, but results could not be separated from whole group.	Group, 1X week for 1 hour with therapist; 4 to 12 or more	Hospital (inpatient and outpatient)	Nondirective; participants free to explore the room	
McKee et al. (2007)	3 adults with mild/moderate ID	Individual, 5X week for 30–45 minutes with nurse trained in snoezelen; data collected on 20 sessions	Hospital	Nondirective; followed participant lead	Issues with continuity of data and extended B phases due to staff-related data collection issues. Breaks in data collection. Interrater reliability assessed only before baseline. Inappropriate use of ANOVA for nonindependent data.

continued

Study	Participants With ASD	Intervention	Location of MSE	Role of Implementer	Major Limitations
Mey et al. (2015)	6 children with delayed mental development	Group, 2X month for 1 hour with a facilitator and parents for 24 sessions	Service center	Explicit teaching of basic concepts; parents helped with behavior management	No numerical data were reported.
Novakovic et al. (2019)	40 adolescents and adults, 29 with severe/profound ID; 11 with mild/moderate ID	Group, 3X week for 30 minutes, with special educator/therapist; 36 scssions	Daycare center	Implementer named and demonstrated equipment, guided participants to use, and then took a nondirective approach, encouraging and supporting choice.	Examined pre-post change in each group rather than the appropriate direct comparisons between groups. Dropouts excluded from reporting. No control for attention.
Slevin & McClelland (1999)	1 adult with severe/profound ID;	Individual, 5X week with author for 20 minutes, 62 sessions	Not stated	Participant free to choose; no interaction with implementer who adjusted equipment as required.	Inappropriate use of t-test for nonindependent data. No correction for familywise error.
Toms et al. (2019)	3, adults, 2 with severe/profound ID and 1 with mil/moderate ID	Individual 2X week with staff member for 15 minutes, 2 to 4 sessions	Residential	Turned equipment on sequentially; participant choose which equipment to use	One participant declined to complete the A2 phase.
Unwin et al. (2021)	41 children, some with mild/moderate ID	Individual, with experimenter for 15 minutes, 2 sessions	Not stated	In active control condition, implementer activated equipment and then gave participants control of equipment, but then had to spend 3 minutes with each piece of equipment. In no control condition, participants could not control any equipment.	Compares active control MSE use and passive MSE use only so no direct implications for benefits of MSE. Large number of comparisons and many reported as significant when above conservative nominated alpha (0.01).

ASD = autism spectrum disorder; ID = intellectual disability; MSE = multisensory environment.

Slevin and McLelland (1999) allowed the participant free choice, but there was no interaction with the implementer. In the two Kaplan et al. (2006) studies and Kim and Park (2021), the implementer provided equipment to meet perceived participant needs. In Hill et al. (2012), Toms et al. (2019), and Mey et al. (2015), the implementer controlled the equipment, and in Mey et al. it was used for explicit teaching and parents were enlisted to help with managing the children. The role of the implementers in Houghton et al. (1998) was unclear. Unwin et al. (2021) additionally explored the effect of participant control and lack of control.

All studies, except Kwok et al. (2003) and Novakovic et al. (2019), which obtained reports from others, employed direct observation measures. A wide range of dependent variables were measured, and these have been categorized into broader classes (see Table 27.3). Between 1 and 19 variables were measured (*M* = 4). Stereotypic behaviors were the most frequently measured. Shaded cells in Table 27.3 indicate where results suggested that the MSE had a beneficial effect. As can be seen from Table 27.3, there were relatively few positive effects of MSEs. Note that Unwin et al. (2021) is not included in the table because this study compared two different MSE conditions and thus no conclusions about the effectiveness of MSEs generally can be drawn from the results. Kwok et al. (2003) is not included because results relating only to participants with ASD could not be isolated, and Mey et al. (2015) is also not included because no numerical data were reported.

The increased engagement reported in Cuvo et al. (2001) for one participant and Kaplan et al. (2006) for three participants was observed in tasks carried out immediately after an MSE session. There is no evidence of more prolonged effects on engagement. The decrease in aggression and increase in communication observed in Fava and Strauss (2010) was for three participants both within and immediately after an MSE session. An improvement in communication was also reported for McKee et al. (2007) and Unwin et al. (2021). Two participants in Hill et al. (2012) showed less stereotypy within MSE sessions than they did in the living room. The one participant in Slevin and McLelland (1999) was more relaxed and had a lower pulse rate immediately after an MSE session. Novakovic et al. (2019) reported a decrease in Childhood Autism Rating Scale (CARS) scores after 3 months of MSE treatment, but their analysis of the results is questionable because they compared pre to post changes in each group, rather than comparing groups directly (see Bland & Altman, 2011; Vorland et al., 2021). Houghton et al. (1998) reported very small increase in the number of foundation outcome skills observed after MSE use. Overall then, there were positive effects for 34 participants, 20 of whom were the MSE group in the Novakovic et al. study.

It should also be noted that some participants declined to complete sessions (Hill et al., 2012; McKee et al., 2007) and others refused to attend MSE sessions completely (Toms et al., 2019). There were also some results suggesting an increase in disruptive behavior in the MSE, although there was considerable overlap of data points for one participant in McKee et al. (2007) and also a higher rate of stereotypy in some sessions for some participants in Toms et al. (2019).

Table 27.3 Dependent variables measured in each study

Study	Aggression	Communication	Stereotypy	SIB	Challenging behaviors	Alertness	Relaxation	Physiological	Engagement	Other
Cuvo et al. (2001), Experiment 1			X						X	
Cuvo et al., Experiment 2			X						X	
Fava & Strauss (2010)	X	X	X			X				
Hill et al. (2012)			X						X	
Houghton et al. (1998)										X
Kaplan et al. (2006), Experiment 1									X	
Kaplan et al., Experiment 2	X			X	X					
Kim & Park (2021)			X							
McKee et al. (2007)		X			X			X	X	X
Mey et al. (2015)										
Novakovic et al. (2019)										X
Slevin & McClelland, (1999)					X		X	X		
Toms et al. (2019)			X	X						

Note. Shaded cells indicate positive results. SIB = self-injurious behavior.

The quality of the studies was generally poor. Three of the group studies (Houghton et al., 1998; Kwok et al., 2003; Unwin et al., 2021) were single-group studies that do not allow conclusions about the effects of MSEs to be drawn. Two group studies received a quality score of four out of eight (Fava & Strauss, 2010; Novakovic, 2019). Fava and Strauss did not randomize participants to groups, while Novakovic et al. had differential attrition of more than 10%, and for both there was no evidence of pretest equivalence or of adjustments for differences in their analyses. A number of other important methodological issues were evident in these two studies. Fava and Strauss (2010) had only three participants in each group, and it was unclear whether Novakovic et al. directly compared the performance of experimental and control groups, or rather looked at pre-to post-test changes in each group.

Only two of the eight single-case studies met the WWC standards (both experiments in Cuvo et al., 2001), with five others failing to report collection of interobserver reliability in all phases of the study with adequate levels (Hill et al., 2012; Kaplan et al., 2006, Experiment 2; McKee et al., 2007; Slevin & McLelland, 1999; Toms et al., 2019). Two experiments had acceptable reliability but failed to meet the WWC design standards on other criteria. One had insufficient data points in each phase (Kaplan et al., 2006, Experiment 1); and two had only one phase per condition in a reversal design (Kim & Park, 2021; Toms et al., 2019). In addition, two studies (McKee et al., 2007; Slevin & McClelland, 1999) employed inappropriate parametric inferential procedures for correlated data.

27.7 Discussion

The research on the use of MSEs with people with ASD has mostly involved adults with intellectual disability living in residential institutions. Only one study of poor quality examined the use of MSE in a school setting. There were no comparisons of MSE use with interventions shown to be effective and only one comparison with an alternative leisure option. Stereotypy and engagement were the variables most often addressed. Study results were mixed, but findings of no effect were more common than reports of benefits. The quality of the studies was, with one exception, poor, and inappropriate methods of analysis were used in some studies. Given the poor quality of studies, and very limited evidence for positive outcomes, conclusions about the length and number of MSE sessions cannot be offered. In practice most sessions were between 15 minutes and 1 hour, with 30 minutes being the most commonly reported. Frequency varied from 5 days a week to twice a month, with most studies providing sessions at least twice a week. Where the effects of MSE use were reported, the number of sessions provided varied considerably from 4 to 54, with 20 sessions the most common.

The results from this review of studies including participants with ASD are very similar to results from reviews of MSE use with people with developmental disability more generally, mostly those with moderate to profound intellectual disability.

Hogg et al. (2001), Chan et al. (2010), and Lai (2003) reported a similar range of dependent variables related to relaxation and challenging behavior such as stereotypy, self-injurious behavior, as well as affect, concentration, communication, and physiological measures, with Hogg et al. (2001) commenting that there needed to be more clarity around expected outcomes. All these more general reviews noted concerns with weak research designs (Chan et al., 2010; Hogg et al., 2001; Lai, 2003; Lancioni et al., 2002; Lotan & Gold, 2009).

Hogg et al. (2001) concluded that MSEs should not be the first choice intervention for challenging behavior, given the documented effectiveness of strategies derived from applied behavior analysis. Chan et al. (2010) concluded that MSEs may have a role as a leisure activity, but there was a "lack of evidence supporting multisensory therapy as a treatment" (p. 121). They also noted several cautions, including lack of evidence for generalization of changes observed within the MSE to other environments, lack of evidence for MSE conditions being superior to comparison conditions, and lack of long-term follow-up. Lancioni et al., (2002) also regarded the evidence then available as "rather preliminary and circumscribed" (p. 180). Lotan and Gold (2009), who completed a meta-analysis of 13 studies, suggested that the use of MSEs for recreation could be appropriate, but there was only preliminary support for use to increase adaptive behaviors.

We would endorse all these reservations for the research including participants with ASD. The overall quality of the research was poor with inadequate interobserver reliability in single-case designs and a lack of group studies that compared groups. For group studies that did compare groups, only one had random assignment, and group equivalence was neither established before analysis nor taken into account during analysis. A number of deviations for usual practice were present in analysis in the examined studies. These included inappropriate use of parametric statistics for correlated single-case data (McKee et al., 2007; Slevin & McClelland, 1999), failure to correct for familywise error (Fava & Strauss, 2010; Slevin & McClelland, 1999), conducting pre-post within-group comparisons rather than appropriate direct between-group comparisons (Novakovic et al., 2019), and failure to adhere to an experimenter nominated alpha value (Unwin et al., 2021).

Twenty years on from the Hogg et al. (2001) comment regarding the lack of clarity around expected outcomes, studies are still exploring a wide range of variables related to challenging behaviors, engagement, communication, and physiological measures. There is little evidence of a consistent and coherent rationale being used for the selection of outcome measures. Studies that used comparison conditions generally used an institution living room or the general ward environment, rather than another intervention. There have been no studies comparing MSE use as an intervention for challenging behavior (including stereotypy, aggression, self-injurious behavior) to interventions that have been shown to be effective in reducing these behaviors such as functional communication training and differential reinforcement of alternative, incompatible, or other behaviors (Steinbrenner et al., 2020). Only one study with one participant with ASD (Cuvo et al., 2001) compared the effects of MSE with an alternative leisure activity (a walk outdoors). In this instance, the walk was much more effective (and much less expensive) than the MSE in reducing stereotypy and increasing engagement, and this study met the WWC standards.

The effects of MSE use reported in the two high-quality experiments of Cuvo et al. (2001) are not impressive. They reported higher engagement during MSE sessions but no carryover after sessions, and as noted above, a walk outside was more effective than MSE use. Positive results from other studies must be treated with caution owing to the quality issues. For almost all positive reports, there are an equal number or more of studies reporting no effect for the same behaviors.

Most studies did not address generalization, and only four studies (including Cuvo et al., 2001) reported relevant results. In contrast to the Cuvo et al. (2001) study, the poorer quality Kaplan et al. (2006) reported postsession carryover for the engagement of two out of three participants. Houghton et al. (1998) reported a very small increase in the number of new foundation skills (such as eye tracking) that were observed in the MSE and then in the generalization setting post-MSE exposure. It is somewhat surprising that these skills were not observed in the classroom before MSE use, but there was no interobserver reliability data provided for the pre-MSE assessments which were carried out by teachers. The MSE data and generalization data, which were reported to have good interrater reliability, were collected from video recordings, not live observation. The group study by Novakovic et al. (2019), which reported improved CARS scores after MSE use, also implies generalization of improvements, but the groups in this study were very small, and there were other methodological problems.

Some studies compared different ways of using MSEs. Unwin et al. (2021) compared the effects on a wide range of variables of children actively controlling the equipment with passive use where changes to the equipment were preset. They reported that having control resulted in less stereotypy and an increase in attention, with no difference for other variables such as social behavior and anxiety. This finding, although from a poor-quality study, does offer some support to the original concept of participant-led choice in the use of the MSE being an important element. Unwin et al. suggested the better results in the control condition may be because children could choose predictable stimulation that met their sensory needs. However, the single-case study by Kim and Park (2021), where children were provided with stimulation designed to meet their sensory needs, showed no differences between the different MSE conditions for each of three participants. Regarding implementer behavior, Hill et al. (2012) reported less stereotypy in the MSE regardless of the level of attention provided, with the results for engagement mixed.

27.8 Practice Implications

27.8.1 Treatment Outcomes

Contrary to the assertion by Houghton et al (1998, p. 277) that "entry to the MSE is like accessing a 'cave of magic,'" the use of MSEs with people with ASD as an intervention to improve behavior cannot be endorsed due to the poor quality of research and because reports of no effect outnumber claimed improvements in behavior. There is no coherent and consistent rationale presented to inform choices for the nature and outcomes of treatment. The most examined variable, stereotypic behavior, was reduced in only one study. Since effective interventions, mostly based on the principles of applied behavior analysis, are available for behaviors such as stereotypy, aggression, and self-injurious behavior (Steinbrenner et al., 2020), these should be selected over MSE use as an intervention. There is an opportunity cost if MSE use is selected over interventions more likely to be effective. Use as a leisure option could be considered, but other leisure activities (such walking outdoors) are likely to have beneficial effects and are more cost-effective.

27.8.2 Practice Implication Guidelines

The use of MSEs with people with ASD as an intervention to improve behavior is not supported by research and cannot be recommended. Practitioners should treat the claims made by commercial firms selling installations and equipment for MSEs with considerable caution, given the research findings. Generally, alternate interventions with research support should be preferred. If practitioners choose to use an MSE, the expected changes in behavior should be clearly enunciated and carefully monitored. If MSEs are used as a leisure option, the research (given the reservations due to quality) suggests that the facilitator should provide the user with choice and control, as per the original concept of snoezelen. Again, more normalized leisure options should also be considered. There is no guidance in the literature as to appropriate qualifications for implementers, session length, frequency, or length of treatment.

There are general safety considerations for MSEs, given the use of electrical equipment. Circuit breaker sockets should be installed. Heat-generating equipment (such as projectors) should be kept away from fabrics and plastics. All equipment should be secured to prevent it falling or being pulled over during use. Careful supervision of users is required, especially if the room is dimly lit as is often recommended (Cavet & Mount, 1995).

In summary, the research on MSEs for people with ASD does not support effectiveness in reducing challenging behavior, improving engagement, or providing a leisure option. There is limited research that included children or people without intellectual disability, and most studies were conducted in institutions. We would recommend that practitioners look for alternative interventions and leisure activities and consider the high costs of creating a MSE.

27.9 References

American Psychiatric Association. (2013). *Diagnostic and statistical manual of mental disorders* (5th ed.). Washington, DC: Author.

Bergstrom, V. N. Z., O'Brien-Langer, A., & Marsh, R. (2019). Supporting children with fetal alcohol spectrum disorder: Potential applications of a Snoezelen multisensory room, *Journal of Occupational Therapy, Schools, & Early Intervention*, *12*(1), 98–114. https://doi.org/10.1080/19411243.2018.1496869

Bland, J. M., & Altman, D. G. (2011). Comparisons against baseline within randomised groups are often used and can be highly misleading. *Trials*, *12*, 264. https://doi.org/10.1186/1745-6215-12-264

Botts, B. H., Hershfeldt, P. A., & Christensen-Sandfort, R. J. (2008). Snoezelen: Empirical review of product representation. *Focus on Autism and Other Developmental Disabilities*, *23*(3), 138–147. https://doi.org/10.1177/1088357608318949

Bozic, N. (1997). Constructing the room: Multi-sensory rooms in educational contexts. *European Journal of Special Needs Education*, *12*(1), 54–70. https://doi.org/10.1080/0885625970120106

Breslin, L., Guerra, N., Ganz, L., & Ervin, D. (2020). Clinical utility of multisensory environments for people with intellectual and developmental disabilities: A scoping review. *American Journal of Occupational Therapy*, *74*(4), 1–12. https://doi.org/10.5014/ajot.2020.037267

de Bunsen, A. (1992) A study in the use and implications of the Snoezelen resource at Liminton House School. In R. Hutchinson & J. Kewin (Eds.), *Sensations and disability: Sensory environments for leisure, snoezelen, education and therapy* (pp. 139–162). Derbyshire, UK: ROMPA.

Cameron, A., Burns, P., Garner, A., Lau, S., Dixon, R., Pascoe, C., & Szafraniec, M. (2020). Making sense of multi-sensory environments: A scoping review. *International Journal of Disability, Development and Education*, *67*(6), 630–656. https://doi.org/10.1080/1034912X.2019.1634247

Campbell, D. T., & Stanley, J. C. (1963). *Experimental and quasi-experimental designs for research.* Chicago: Rand McNally.

Castelhano, N., Silva, F., Rezende, M., Roque, L., & Magalhaes, L. (2013). Ludic content in multisensory stimulation environments: An exploratory study about practice in Portugal. *Occupational Therapy International*, *20*(3), 134–143. https://onlinelibrary.wiley.com/doi/epdf/10.1002/oti.1347

Cavet, J., & Mount, H. (1995). Multisensory environments. In J. Hogg & J. Cavet (Eds.), *Making leisure provision for people with profound learning and multiple disabilities* (pp. 67–85). London: Chapman & Hall.

Chan, J., & Chien, W. (2017). A randomised controlled trial on evaluation of the clinical efficacy of massage therapy in a multisensory environment for residents with severe and profound intellectual disabilities: A pilot study. *Journal of Intellectual Disability Research*, *61*(6), 532–548. https://doi.org/10.1111/jir.12377

Chan, S., Fung, M. Y., Tong, C. W., & Thompson, D. (2005). The clinical effectiveness of a multisensory therapy on clients with developmental disability. *Research in Developmental Disabilities*, *26*(2), 131–142. http://dx.doi.org/10.1016/j.ridd.2004.02.002

Chan, S., Thompson, D., Chau, J. P. C., Tam, W. W. S., Chiu, I., W., S., & Lo, S. H. S. (2010). The effects of multisensory therapy in behaviour of adult clients with developmental disabilities - A systematic review. *International Journal of Nursing Studies*, *47*(1), 108–122. https://doi.org/10.1016/j.ijnurstu.2009.08.004

Cuvo, A. J., May, M. E., & Post, T. M., (2001). Effects of living room, Snoezelen room, and outdoor activities on stereotypic behavior and engagement by adults with profound mental retardation. *Research in Developmental Disabilities*, *22*(3), 183–204. https://doi.org/10.1016/S0891-4222(01)00067-1

Fava, L., & Strauss, K. (2010). Multi-sensory rooms: comparing effects of the snoezelen and the stimulus preference environment on the behavior of adults with profound mental retardation. *Research in Developmental Disabilities*, *31*(1), 160–171. http://dx.doi.org/10.1016/j.ridd.2009.08.006

Haegele, J. A., & Porretta, D. L. (2014). Snoezelen multisensory environment: An overview of research and practical implications. *Palaestra*, *28*(4), 29–32.

Haggar, L E., & Hutchinson, R. B. (1991). Snoezelen: An approach to the provision of a leisure resource for people with profound and multiple handicaps. *Mental Handicap, 19*(2), 51–55. https://doi.org/10.1111/j.1468-3156.1991.tb00620.x

Hill, L., Trusler, K., Furniss, F., & Lancioni, G. (2012). Effects of multisensory environment on stereotyped behaviours assessed as maintained by automatic reinforcement. *Journal of Applied Research in Intellectual Disabilities, 25*, 509–521. DOI: 10.1111/j.1468-3148.2012.00697

Hogg, J., Cavet, J., Lambe, L., & Smeddle, M. (2001). The use of "Snoezelen" as multisensory stimulation with people with intellectual disabilities: A review of the research. *Research in Developmental Disabilities, 22*(5), 353–372. https://doi.org/10.1016/S0891-4222(01)00077-4

Houghton, S., Douglas, G., Brigg, J., Langsford, S., Powell, L., West, J., Chapman, A., & Kellner, R. (1998). An empirical evaluation of an interactive multi-sensory environment for children with disability, *Journal of Intellectual and Developmental Disability, 23*(4), 267–278. https://doi.org/10.1080/13668259800033761

Hulsegge, J., & Verheul, A. (1987). *Snoezelen, another world: A practical book of sensory experience environments for the mentally handicapped.* Derbyshire, UK: ROMPA.

Hutchinson, R., & Hagger, L. (1994). The development and evaluation of s Snoezelen leisure resources for people with severe multiple disability. In R. Hutchinson R. & J. Kewin (Eds.), *Sensations and disability: Sensory environments for leisure, snoezelen, education and therapy* (pp. 18–55). Derbyshire, UK: ROMPA.

Kaplan, H., Clopton, M., Kaplan, M., Messbauer, L., & McPherson, K. (2006). Snoezelen multi-sensory environments: Task engagement and generalization. *Research in Developmental Disabilities, 27*(4), 443–455. http://dx.doi.org/10.1016/j.ridd.2005.05.007

Kim, M. K., & Park, N. K. (2021). Evaluating the impact of a multisensory environment on target behaviors of children with autism spectrum disorder. *HERD: Health Environments Research and Design Journal, 15*(2), 163–179. https://doi.org/10.1177/19375867211050686

Kirby, A. V., Bilder, D. A., Wiggins, L. D., Hughes, M. M., Davis, J., Hall-Lande, J. A., Lee, L., McMahon, W. M., Bakian, A. V. (2022). Sensory features in autism: Findings from a large population-based surveillance system. *Autism Research, 15*(4), 751–760.

Kwok, H. W. M., To, Y. F., & Sung, H. F. (2003). The application of a multisensory Snoezelen room for people with learning disabilities—Hong Kong experience. *Hong Kong Medical Journal, 9*(2), 122–126. https://www.hkmj.org/system/files/hkm0304p122.pdf

Lai, C. Y. (2003). The use of multisensory environments on children with disabilities: A literature review. *International Journal of Therapy and Rehabilitation, 10*(8). 358–363. https://doi.org/10.12968/bjtr.2003.10.8.13513

Lancioni, G. E., Cuvo, A. J., & O'Reilly, M. F. (2002). Snoezelen: An overview of research with people with developmental disabilities and dementia. *Disability and Rehabilitation, 24*(4), 175–184. https://doi.org/10.1080/09638280110074911

Lancioni, G. E., Singh, N. N., O'Reilly, M. F., Oliva, D., & G Basili, G.(2005) An overview of research on increasing indices of happiness of people with severe/profound intellectual and multiple disabilities. *Disability and Rehabilitation, 27*(3), 83–93. https://doi.org/10.1080/09638280400007406

Lavie, E., Shapiro, M., & Julius, M. (2005). Hydrotherapy combined with Snoezelen multi-sensory therapy. *International Journal of Adolescent Medicine & Health, 17*(1), 83–87. https://doi.org/10.1515/IJAMH.2005.17.1.83

Leong, H. M., Carter, M., & Stephenson, J. R. (2015). Meta-analysis of research on sensory integration therapy for individuals with developmental and learning disabilities. *Journal of Physical and Developmental Disabilities, 27*(2), 183–206. https://doi.org/10.1007/s10882-014-9408-y

Lindsay, W. R., Black, E., Broxholme, S., Pitcaithly, D., & Hornsby, N. (2001). Effects of four therapy procedures in communication in people with profound intellectual disabilities. *Journal of Applied Research in Intellectual Disabilities, 14*(2), 110–119. https://doi.org/10.1046/j.1468-3148.2001.00059.x

Lotan, M., & Gold, C. (2009). Meta-analysis of the effectiveness of individual intervention in the controlled multisensory environment (snoezelen) for individuals with intellectual disability. *Journal of Intellectual and Developmental Disability, 34*(3), 207–215. https://doi.org/10.1080/13668250903080106.

Maggin, D. M., Cook, B. G., & Cook, L. (2018). Using single-case research designs to examine the effects of interventions in special education. *Learning Disabilities Research and Practice, 33*, 182–191. https://doi.org/10.1111/ldrp.12184

Martin, N. T., Gaffan, E. A., & Williams, T. (1998). Behavioural effects of long-term multi-sensory stimulation. *British Journal of Clinical Psychology, 37*(1), 69–82. https://doi.org/10.1111/j.2044-8260.1998.tb01280.x

McKee, S. A., Harris, G. T., Rice, M. E., & Silk, L. (2007). Effects of a Snoezelen room on the behavior of three autistic clients. *Research in Developmental Disabilities, 28*(3), 304–316. https://doi.org/10.1016/j.ridd.2006.04.001

Mey, S. C., Cheng, L. M., & Ching, L. W. (2015). The effect of a multisensory program on children with autism. *International Journal of Child Development and Mental Health, 3*(2), 36–47. https://doaj.org/article/9bf9fc7c59d443119844279a797d1d89

Moir, L. (2010). Evaluating the effectiveness of different environments on the learning of switching skills in children with severe and profound multiple disabilities. *British Journal of Occupational Therapy, 73*(10), 446–456. https://doi.org/10.4276/030802210X12865330218186

Mount, H., & Cavet, J. (1995). Multi-sensory environments: An exploration of their potential for young people with profound and multiple learning difficulties. *British Journal of Special Education, 22*(2), 52–55. https://doi.org/10.1111/j.1467-8578.1995.tb01322.x

Munde, V., & Vlaskamp, C. (2015). Initiation of activities and alertness in individuals with profound intellectual and multiple disabilities. *Journal of Intellectual Disability Research, 59*(3), 284–292. https://doi.org/10.1111/jir.12138

Munde, V. S., Vlaskamp, C., Maees, B., & Ruijssenaars, A. J. J., M. (2012). Catch the wave! Time-window sequential analysis of alertness stimulation in individuals with profound intellectual and multiple disabilities. *Child: Care Health and Development, 41*(1), 95–105. https://doi.org/10.1111/j.1365-2214.2012.01415.x

Novakovic, N., Milovancevic, M. P., Dejanovic, S. D., & Aleksic, B. (2019). Effects of snoezelen-multisensory environment on CARS scale in adolescents and adults with autism spectrum disorder. *Research in Developmental Disabilities, 89*, 51–58. https://doi.org/10.1016/j.ridd.2019.03.007

Pagliano, P. (1998). The multi-sensory environment: An open-minded space. *British Journal of Visual Impairment, 16*(3), 105–109. https://doi.org/10.1177/026461969801600305

Pagliano, P. (2006). The multisensory environment: Providing a feeling of emotional closeness. *Journal of the South Pacific Educators in Vision Impairment, 3*(1), 23–25.

Patterson, I., (2004). Snoezelen as a casual leisure activity for people with a developmental disability. *Therapeutic Recreation Journal, 38*(3), 289–300. https://bctra.org/wp-content/uploads/tr_journals/993-3892-1-PB.pdf

ROMPA. (2021). *What is a Snoezelen sensory room?* https://www.rompa.com/interactive-sensory-room

Sachs, D., & Nasser, K., (2009). Facilitating family occupations: Family member perceptions of a specialized environment for children with mental retardation. *American Journal of Occupational Therapy, 63*(4), 453–462. https://doi.org/10.5014/ajot.63.4.453

Shapiro, M., Parush, S., Green, M., & Roth, D. (1997). The efficacy of the "snoezelen" in the management of children with mental retardation who exhibit maladaptive behaviours. *British Journal of Developmental Disabilities, 43*(85), 140–155. https://doi.org/10.1179/bjdd.1997.014

Singh, N. N., Lancioni, G. E., Winton, A. S. W., Molina, E. J., Sage, M., Brown, S., & Groeneweg, J., (2004). Effects of Snoezelen room, activities of daily living skills training, and vocational skills training on aggression and self-injury by adults with mental retardation and mental illness. *Research in Developmental Disabilities, 25*(3), 285–293. https://doi.org/10.1016/j.ridd.2003.08.003

Slevin, E., & McClelland, A., (1999). Multisensory environments: Are they therapeutic? A single-subject evaluation of the clinical effectiveness of a multisensory environment. *Journal of Clinical Nursing, 8*(1), 48–56. https://doi.org/10.1046/j.1365-2702.1999.00211.x

Snoezelen Multi-Sensory Environments. (2022). Benefits and applications. https://www.snoezelen.info/benefits-and-applications/

Steinbrenner, J. R., Hume, K., Odom, S. L., Morin, K. L., Nowell, S. W., Tomaszewski, B., Szendrey, S., McIntyre, N. S., Yücesoy-Özkan, S., & Savage, M. N. (2020). *Evidence-based practices for children, youth, and young adults with autism.* Chapel Hill: The University of North Carolina, Frank Porter Graham Child Development Institute, National Clearinghouse on Autism Evidence and Practice Review Team. https://ncaep.fpg.unc.edu/sites/ncaep.fpg.unc.edu/files/imce/documents/EBP%20Report%202020.pdf

Toms, B. S., Janke, M. C., Loy, D. P., & Watts, C. E. (2019). Research in recreational therapy practice: Findings and lessons learned from a study of a multisensory environment for adults with autism spectrum disorder. *Therapeutic Recreation Journal, 53*(4o, 381–401. https://doi.org/10.18666/TRJ-2018-V53-I4-9744

Toro, B. (2019). Memory and standing balance after multisensory stimulation in a snoezelen room in people with moderate learning disabilities. *British Journal of Learning Disabilities, 47*(4), 270–278. https://doi.org/10.1111/bld.12289

Unwin, K. L., Powell, G., & Jones, C. R. (2021). The use of multi-sensory environments with autistic children: Exploring the effect of having control of sensory changes. *Autism*. https://doi.org/10.1177/13623613211050176

Vorland, C. J., Brown, A. W., Dawson, J. A., Dickinson, S. L., Golzarri-Arroyo, L., Hannon, B. A., Heo, M., Heymsfield, S. B., Jayawardene, W. P., Kahathuduwa, C. N., Keith, S. W., Oakes, J. M., Tekwe, C. D., Thabane, L., & Allison, D. B. (2021). Errors in the implementation, analysis, and reporting of randomization within obesity and nutrition research: A guide to their avoidance. *International Journal of Obesity, 45*(11), 2335–2346. https://doi.org/10.1038/s41366-021-00909-z

What Works Clearinghouse. (2022). *What Works Clearinghouse procedures and standards handbook. Version 5.0*. Washington, DC: U.S. Department of Education, Institute of Education Sciences, National Center for Education Evaluation and Regional Assistance. https://iees.ed.gov/ncee/wwc/Handbooks

28

Alpha-2 Agonists in Autism Spectrum Disorder

Erin A. Henneberry
Cincinnati Children's Hospital, Department of Child and Adolescent Psychiatry

Craig A. Erickson
University of Wollongong and MultiLit Research Unit, MultiLit Pty

28.1 Technical Abstract

Background: Alpha-2 adrenergic agonists have been used to treat autism spectrum disorder (ASD) associated symptoms, including hyperactivity, self-injurious behavior, and sleep dysregulation, but benefit for core ASD symptoms is less clear. **Method:** A review of the literature was performed via the PubMed database. Based on prior literature reviews (Persico et al. 2021), the following string of search terms was used to identify sources: [autism OR autistic OR pervasive OR Asperger] AND [clonidine OR guanfacine OR alpha agonist]. Recent systematic reviews of ASD psychopharmacology literature were also searched for additional sources. Criteria for inclusion were as follows: English language; human subjects; ASD, Asperger's, or pervasive developmental disorder (PDD) diagnosis; and published in article format in a peer-reviewed journal. All standard study designs were included, and randomized controlled trials (RCTs) were prioritized. Sources were collated and summarized. **Results:** Evidence for guanfacine in treatment of hyperactivity in ASD is moderate strength, based on two RCTs and one open-label prospective study. Evidence for clonidine for hyperactivity in ASD is weak. Clonidine may improve sleep dysregulation based on one retrospective study. There is limited evidence that any alpha agonist improves core ASD symptoms; however, case reports and secondary data analysis suggest benefit for self-injurious and repetitive behaviors. **Discussion:** While the evidence for guanfacine is strong, it is limited to treatment of hyperactivity in ASD. The inclusion of participants with intellectual disability and aggressive behavior across studies allows broader applicability. Future directions include studies designed and powered to detect changes in core ASD symptoms and sleep disturbances and include objective measurements such as heart rate variability and polysomnography. **Practitioner recommendations:** Guanfacine should be considered a first-line pharmacological choice for hyperactivity in ASD. Guanfacine and clonidine can be considered for treatment of self-injurious behaviors, other disruptive repetitive behaviors, and

Erin A. Henneberry, and Craig A. Erickson, *Alpha-2 Agonists in Autism Spectrum Disorder*. In: *Lifespan Treatment for Autistic Individuals*. Edited by: Peter Sturmey, Russell Lang, and James K. Luiselli, Oxford University Press.
© Oxford University Press (2025). DOI: 10.1093/oso/9780197635841.003.0028

sleep dysregulation. Alpha agonists are generally well tolerated; however, patients should be monitored for sedation, hypotension, and increased irritability.

28.2 Layperson Summary

Clonidine and guanfacine are medications first developed to treat high blood pressure. They have been found to also improve some behavioral difficulties in youth with ASD. Guanfacine is the best studied. It has been shown to reduce hyperactivity for children and adolescents with ASD. Examples of hyperactivity can include difficulty sitting or staying still, running away frequently, and difficulty participating in activities due to being restless and easily distracted. Clonidine may be more helpful for individuals with ASD who have difficulty either falling or staying asleep. These medications are usually well-tolerated. There is low risk for serious side effects. Blood pressure does need to be monitored regularly at visits due to the risk of low blood pressure. The most common side effect for both medications is fatigue. Clonidine and guanfacine are both approved by the Food and Drug Administration (FDA) for treatment of attention-deficit/hyperactivity disorder (ADHD). They are not FDA approved for use in ASD. Patients with ASD can often also have a diagnosis for ADHD. If, however, they do not have a diagnosis of ADHD, these medications may still help reduce hyperactivity. Clonidine and guanfacine may be prescribed by a child or adult psychiatrist, developmental pediatrician, or general pediatrician or primary care physician. They are also sometimes prescribed by nurse practitioners or physician assistants who have additional training in psychiatric medication. They do so while working with physicians trained in use of these medications.

28.3 Treatment Summary Table

Treatment summary: Clonidine and Guanfacine

Treatment description: Alpha-2 adrenergic agonist medications. Both medications come in regular and extended-release oral formulations. Clonidine also comes in a transdermal patch.

Expected outcomes: There may be improvement in hyperactivity with guanfacine. There may also be improvement in repetitive behaviors and self-injurious behaviors. There may be improvement in sleep dysregulation with clonidine, but there is less evidence for benefit in hyperactivity or other symptoms.

Methods: Start with lowest dose and titrate slowly due to hypotension and sedation. See dosing recommendation in Table 28.1.

Expertise required to implement treatment: Treatment should be provided by a physician or other prescriber with additional training and expertise in youth and/or adults with neurodevelopmental disorders.

Risks and negative side effects: Risks and negative side effects include hypotension, sedation, irritability, and gastrointestinal effects. Rebound hypertension is a risk if medication is stopped abruptly.

Additional considerations and limitations: Screen for cardiac and vascular disease prior to starting, and monitor blood pressure and heart rate regularly. Screen for other sleep disorders (e. g., obstructive sleep apnea, restless leg syndrome) in patients with sleep dysregulation.

28.4 Introduction

28.4.1 Treatment Description

Clonidine and guanfacine are both alpha-2 adrenergic agonists which are increasingly used off-label in youth with ASD. They are often prescribed for ASD-associated symptoms, including dysregulated sleep and hyperactivity/hyperarousal. There is limited evidence for efficacy of these medications on the core symptoms of ASD (e. g., social deficits and restricted, repetitive behaviors). Both medications are FDA approved for the treatment of ADHD, and they are also commonly prescribed when there is comorbid ADHD and ASD.

28.4.2 Rationale and Objectives

Clonidine and guanfacine both act centrally on alpha-2 adrenergic receptors in the prefrontal cortex (PFC), an area of the brain involved in emotional regulation, cognitive flexibility, attention, and social cognition (Arnsten, 2010; Ferguson & Gao, 2018; Hiser & Koenigs, 2018; Park & Moghaddam, 2017). The alpha-2 receptor has multiple subtypes distributed throughout the central nervous system, and the alpha-2A subtype is widespread in the PFC and the locus coeruleus (Stahl, 2013). The mechanism of action of clonidine and guanfacine treating in ADHD is thought to be via binding at the postsynaptic alpha-2A receptor, which improves the "signal to noise ratio" and strengthens PFC connectivity (Arnsten, 2010; Xing et al., 2016). Guanfacine is 15–60 times more selective for the alpha-2A receptor than clonidine, which is relatively nonselective between the alpha-2 receptor subtypes (A, B, C). Clonidine also binds to imidazoline receptors and binds at a 10-fold higher rate to presynaptic alpha-2A receptors compared to guanfacine (Jasper et al., 1998; Stahl, 2013; Strange, 2008). This difference in selectivity for the alpha-2A receptor, including presynaptic versus postsynaptic alpha-2A, likely explains why clonidine has greater incidence of sedation, and it may explain why guanfacine appears to have greater efficacy in enhancing PFC function (Jäkälä et al., 1999). This may also explain why clonidine has been shown to improve sleep dysregulation in ASD, but guanfacine has not (Relia & Ekambaram, 2018).

The mechanism for how clonidine or guanfacine may benefit core ASD symptoms is less clear. Most of the research to date on use of alpha-2 agonists in ASD has focused on treating hyperactivity/hyperarousal in ASD, and patients in some of these studies may have had comorbid ADHD. The evidence regarding dysregulation of the noradrenergic system in ASD is mixed, with some studies potentially misattributing abnormal blood levels of catecholamines to ASD neuropathology (Beversdorf, 2020). There is evidence implicating the noradrenergic system in abnormal hippocampal functioning and consequently memory in ASD (Ring et al., 2020), as well as abnormal motor development (Yin et al., 2021). Most of the evidence implicating the noradrenergic system in ASD is indirect, and its applicability to treatment of core ASD symptoms is uncertain (London, 2018). As noted above, clonidine is active at multiple different receptors, which is thought to explain the greater sedation with clonidine.

28.4.3 Considerations for Implementation

This class of medications is indicated for ADHD comorbid with autism spectrum diorders. Guanfacine is the first choice agent. Medications should be prescribed with the lowest more effective dose. Contraindications include heart and vascular disorders. Practitioners should screen for sleep disorders and monitor for low blood pressure, fatigue, and sedation. See section 28.6 below.

28.5 Research Background

28.5.1 Clonidine

A recent systematic review of clonidine in ASD noted that there is currently not enough high-quality evidence to perform meta-analysis on, and that overall there is a significant risk for bias in the existing literature (Banas & Sawchuk, 2020). Clonidine has two small, placebo-controlled RCTs examining use in ASD, which both had a crossover study design, one of which used oral clonidine, and the other which used transdermal clonidine patch (Fankhauser et al., 1992; Jaselskis et al. 1992). In Fankhauser et al. (1992), nine male participants with ASD (per *DSM-III* criteria), ages 5–33 years, were treated with the transdermal clonidine patch versus placebo in crossover design. Participants were required to be medication-free for 2 weeks leading up to the study, and participants with schizophrenia, profound intellectual disability, or an "unstable medical condition" were excluded. All participants were described as exhibiting "hyperarousal behavior with stereotyped or rhythmic motions and self-stimulatory behavior." Participants were reported to have a range of impairment, with six having limited or no verbal skills, two having "good" verbal skills, and one of whom was deaf and used sign language. Intellectual ability ranged from moderate disability to no disability, and approximately half the participants had aggressive behaviors. The study used approximate weight-based dosing of clonidine patches, ranging from 0.1 to 0.3 mg, which were replaced every 7 days. Each treatment phase which compared placebo with active drug lasted 4 weeks, with a 2-week washout period between treatment phases. The primary outcomes of interest were the Ritvo-Freeman Real Life Rating Scale (RLRS) and the Clinical Global Impressions (CGI) scale, which were performed at weeks 0, 2, and 4 for each treatment phase. The RLRS has five subscales—sensory motor, social relationship to people, affectual responses, sensory responses, and language. The data were analyzed using one-way ANOVA for the seven different time/drug groups, and a multiple-range test was used to identify which pairs of data points were statistically different.

The study found improvement in the CGI scores in the clonidine and placebo phases and the washout period. The study also found improvement in three RLRS subscales ("social relationships to people," "affectual responses," and "sensory responses") via the multiple range test comparing clonidine versus the other two time periods. Only the "sensory responses" scores were also significant in the ANOVA test. The study had two dropouts, one for sedation from clonidine after 2 weeks, and one for moving out of town. Drowsiness and fatigue were the most common side effects; two subjects also developed redness and itching under the patch area. In terms of hemodynamic effects, the authors noted statistically significant lowering of systolic blood pressure with the clonidine versus final washout period (106.3 ± 6.0 mm Hg vs. 123.5 ± 5.8 mmHg, respectively), but no significant effects on diastolic BP and mixed effects on pulse.

In Jaselskis et al. (1992), eight male youths with ASD (per *DSM-III* criteria), ages 5–13 years, were treated with oral clonidine versus placebo in crossover design. Participant IQ ranges from 30 to 75. Six participants spoke in sentences, and the other two had only single words or utterances. All subjects were described as having "hyperactivity, distractibility, and impulsivity that impaired their function," and all of them had previously been treated with methylphenidate, neuroleptics, or desipramine before the study period, which were either ineffective or had intolerable side effects. Almost all participants (seven of eight) came from families with higher socioeconomic status. Participants were required to be medication-free for 1 month prior to the start of the study, and participants with medical or neurological illnesses were excluded. Participants were dosed to a goal range of 0.15 mg–0.2 mg of oral clonidine total per day, in three divided doses. Placebo and drug phases were 6 weeks each, with a 1-week taper in between, and a 1-week taper following the final treatment phase. The outcomes measured included weekly guardian-rated Conners Abbreviated Parent-Teacher Questionnaire, weekly teacher-rated Aberrant Behavior Checklist (ABC), and ADHD Comprehensive Teacher's Rating Scale (ACTeRs), all of which were averaged for each treatment period. Clinician ratings were based on 15-minute structured video recordings of participants at baseline, 6 weeks, and 13 weeks, using the Children's Global Assessment Scale, CGI scale, and Children's Psychiatric Rating Scale (CPRS). Ratings during placebo and drug treatment phases were compared using paired, two-tailed *t*-tests.

The mean weekly parent ratings on the Conners showed a 2.8 point greater reduction in score in the clonidine phase; likewise, the mean teacher ratings on ABC—irritability, hyperactivity, stereotypy, and inappropriate speech—all had a statistically significant greater improvement on clonidine versus placebo, with the greatest reduction being in the irritability subscale. However, none of the clinician ratings showed significant differences versus placebo. In terms of adverse effects, three participants required dose reduction due to hypotension (typically combined with somnolence/fatigue), with systolic blood pressure lowered 20–30 points for some participants. Somnolence and fatigue were the most common adverse effects. The authors noted that six of the participants were continued on oral clonidine in an open-label fashion after the end of the study, but that four of those began to lose treatment efficacy after 6–8 weeks, while the other two continued to benefit a year after study completion.

Aside from these two RCTs, there is one open-label prospective study, one open-label retrospective study, and seven case reports/series examining the use of clonidine in ASD. The open-label retrospective study included 19 youth with ASD, PDD, or Asperger's (4–16 years, 14 female, 5 male), and specifically focused the use of clonidine for sleep dysregulation in ASD, as well as behavioral disorders (Ming et al., 2008). This study included participants with and without intellectual disability (with a range of severity of intellectual disability). Seventeen participants had both sleep and behavioral disorders (ADHD, mood disorder, or aggression), and two participants had only behavioral disorders; most participants were also taking other psychotropic medication during the time of the study. Likewise, the reason for initiation of clonidine treatment for 17 participants was for impairment in sleep initiation and/or sleep maintenance. Clonidine doses were 0.05 mg–0.1 mg once at bedtime, with 8 participants ultimately taking additional daytime clonidine for behavioral symptoms. Initially, 12 children were prescribed oral clonidine and 7 were prescribed clonidine transdermal patch; however, 5 of them ultimately transitioned to oral clonidine due to issues with sensitivity to the patch. Clonidine was prescribed once daily in 17 of the participants and as needed in 2 of the participants. Participants were on clonidine between 6 months and 2 years. Data were dependent on caregiver estimation/recollection and examined average estimate of sleep onset time; number of nighttime awakenings with difficulty falling back asleep (defined as >30 minutes); and subjective rating of improvement in behavioral symptoms rated as no improvement (1), some improvement (2), or complete resolution (3) before and after at least 1 month initiation of clonidine. In terms of sleep, all 16 participants who had prolonged time to sleep onset (>1 hour) experience improvement, the range of sleep latency prior to clonidine was 2–5 hours, and following clonidine initiation, was 30 minutes to 2 hours, with only two participants still experiencing prolonged sleep latency (>1 hour). Out of 17 participants who had difficulty with sleep maintenance, 16 had reduction in the number of prolonged nighttime awakenings. Sleep typically improved quickly, within 1 week of starting clonidine; however, similar to the oral clonidine RTC, patients tended to develop tolerance and require higher doses after extended use (1 year and beyond). In terms of behavioral disturbances, there were no improvements in any particular behavior consistently between subjects, although four subjects were noted to have dramatic improvement in behavioral difficulties. The authors noted three potential participants were not included in the study due to being on clonidine only briefly before discontinuing, one for pallor and another for increased irritability.

Additionally, a case series also examined the use of clonidine for sleep dysregulation in a study of six youth (five male, one female, ages 6–14 years) who all had mild to severe intellectual disability, and one with PDD, one with ASD, and three with ADHD (Ingrassia & Turk, 2005). Similar to the retrospective study, they found improvement in sleep onset, sleep maintenance, and total sleep duration, as well as some reduction in aggressive behaviors.

Among the case reports, various benefits were reported for clonidine including reduced self-injurious behavior and aggression, reduced hyperactivity, and improved "social relatedness" (Cocchi, 1996; Dillon, 1990; Dowben et al., 2011; Ghaziuddin et al., 1992; Koshes & Rock, 1994). One case report of note reported major reduction in self-injurious behavior, maintained over a 2-year period, in a patient whose behavior had been severe and treatment resistant (Blew et al., 1999). Conversely, one case report noted an individual who had increased irritability and severe depression after treatment with clonidine (McCracken & Martin, 1997).

Overall, the existing literature on clonidine has several strengths. For instance, many studies included participants who were nonverbal and had significant intellectual disability, a population which may often be underrepresented in ASD research. Several of the studies also had long-term follow up (>6 months) and commented on issues with long-term treatment. Some limitations in these studies included a lack of consistent or well-validated outcomes measures, subjectivity of outcome measures, small sample sizes, lack of data on race/ethnicity, and cost of treatment.

28.5.2 Guanfacine

There were two double-blind RCTs examining the use of guanfacine in ASD. One was a small crossover study which used short-acting guanfacine; the other is a larger traditional RCT, which used extended-release guanfacine (Handen et al., 2008; Scahill et al., 2015). Both studies focus on hyperactivity and impulsivity in ASD as their primary outcome of interest, although other symptom areas were addressed. In the crossover trial, there were 11 participants (10 male, 1 female), ages 5 to 9 years, who had a diagnosis of intellectual disability and/or autism, who also had either a diagnosis of ADHD or significant hyperactivity/inattention symptoms (Handen et al., 2008). All participants had prior failed trials of a stimulant medication due to ineffectiveness or poor tolerance. Seven participants had concomitant psychotropic medication. Study duration was 6 weeks, with interim and terminal 6-day washout phases; the guanfacine phase was longer than the placebo phase to account for titration time. Dosing started at 0.5 mg/day of short-acting guanfacine and was gradually increased to a goal dose of 3 mg/day in three divided doses. Three participants could not tolerate the goal dose due to sedation, increased irritability, or enuresis and were continued on reduced doses. Primary outcomes of interest were the ABC-Hyperactivity subscale and the CGI. The authors found a statistically significant improvement on the ABC-Hyperactivity subscale and the CGI-Improvement scale between drug versus placebo, with five of the participants considered to be responders (based on 50% or greater reduction in ABC-Hyperactivity score). Drowsiness and lethargy were the most common side effects, and no significant difference was found in blood pressure, heart rate, or weight between groups.

The extended-release guanfacine RCT (Scahill et al., 2015) included 62 youth (5–14 years) with a diagnosis of ASD, PDD, or Asperger syndrome, who had a minimum score of 24 on the ABC-Hyperactivity subscale, and a CGI-Severity score of 4 or greater. There were 53 males and 9 females, and around 40% were non-White. Approximately two thirds of participants had intellectual disability; participants with well-controlled seizure disorders were also included. Children with obsessive-compulsive disorder or mood or psychotic disorders were excluded, and participants were required to be free of psychotropic medication (aside from antiepileptics) for 1–3 weeks prior to start of the study. Study duration was 8 weeks, with a subsequent open-label phase. Guanfacine extended-release dosing started at 1 mg and was titrated to a goal dose of 3 mg as tolerated. Primary outcomes of interest were the parent-rated ABC-Hyperactivity subscale, clinician rated CGI-I, and clinician-rated ADHD Rating Scale. The study showed a 43.6% decline in ABC-Hyperactivity subscale scores compared to a 13.2% decrease for placebo, and the rate of positive response (score of 1 or 2 on CGI-I) was 50.0% for guanfacine compared with 9.4% for placebo. An additional measure was a series of cognitive tasks targeted to working memory and motor planning; there was no difference found between groups on the cognitive tasks. The dropout rate was equivalent between placebo and treatment groups; one participant in the guanfacine did drop out following severe irritability and aggression requiring psychiatric hospitalization. Drowsiness, fatigue, and decreased appetite were the most common adverse effects. Nine participants in the guanfacine group required dose reduction versus five in the placebo group (due to drowsiness, irritability, and/or hypotension). The guanfacine group experienced a transient decrease in blood pressure noted at 4 weeks, which resolved by 8 weeks, and a decrease in heart rate that was persistent at 8 weeks.

A subsequent secondary analysis of the data from the extended-release guanfacine RCT found a reduction in repetitive behavior on the Children's Yale-Brown Obsessive-Compulsive Scale—modified for ASD (decline of 24% in the guanfacine group vs. <1% in placebo group), which, despite the name of the instrument, is not targeted to obsessive-compulsive disorder and has been validated for use in ASD (Politte et al., 2018). The authors also found a greater reduction in oppositional behavior in the guanfacine group (44%) compared to placebo (12%) on the Home Situation Questionnaire—ASD version. Limitations on this secondary analysis data are that the original study was not powered to evaluate these outcomes; therefore, the applicability of these results is unclear.

There is also an open-label prospective study, an open-label retrospective chart review, and several case reports on the use of guanfacine in ASD (Persico et al., 2021). The open-label prospective study was very similar in design to the crossover RCT, using short-acting guanfacine with the same dosing goals over 8 weeks, with the same primary outcome measures—ABC-Hyperactivity subscale and CGI-Improvement scale (Scahill et al., 2006). There were 25 participants, all with PDD and hyperactivity with prior failed treatment with methylphenidate. Like the RCT, there was significant improvement in the ABC-Hyperactivity scale scores, and 48% of participants were rated as "improved" or "much improved" on the CGI-Improvement scale. Common adverse effects included irritability, sedation, disrupted sleep, and constipation; of note, three participants discontinued treatment due to increased irritability. There were no significant changes in blood pressure or pulse.

The retrospective chart review (Posey et al., 2004) included 80 youths with PDD, ASD, or Asperger's treated with guanfacine, with age range 3–18 years; 70% had comorbid intellectual disability. Mean daily dose was 2.6 mg, with a range of 0.25–9 mg, and the mean duration of treatment was 334 days, with a range of 7–1,776 days. CGI-Improvement was the primary outcome of interest, although it was tied to varying different associated symptoms for different patients. The chart review found 23.8% of patients to be "responders" (score of much improved or very much improved on CGI-I), with greatest response rates in insomnia, hyperactivity, and inattention. The authors noted that there was no difference in response rate between patients who had or had not previously been treated with a stimulant; however, responders had fewer prior psychotropic drug trials overall than nonresponders. Transient sedation was by far the most common adverse effect (31.3%); other negative side effects were irritability (6.3%), constipation (3.8%), headache (2.5%), and nocturnal enuresis (2.5%). Several case reports note improvement in hyperactivity and inattention, as well as aggression, self-injurious behavior, and in one case, improvement in tics, although no improvements in core ASD symptoms were reported (Blankenship et al., 2011; Okazaki et al., 2019; Propper, 2018). Lastly, one case report of note documented guanfacine-induced lichenoid drug eruption, which appeared approximately 3 months after starting guanfacine and largely resolved within 3 months after drug cessation (Romanelli & Rhodes, 2014).

Overall, there is stronger evidence for use of guanfacine compared with clonidine in ASD due to the larger trials and more consistent outcome measures across studies. However, this evidence mainly supports use of guanfacine for treatment of hyperactivity in ASD; the evidence for addressing other ASD core or associated symptoms is more limited. Other strengths of these studies included high inclusion rates for patients with intellectual disabilities, and not excluding patients with seizure disorders, which as noted above are often underrepresented in ASD research. There were fewer studies with longer durations or follow-up periods, which makes it more difficult to predict to long-term efficacy. Some studies reported race/ethnicity and socioeconomic data, but not all. Cost of treatment was not discussed.

28.6 Practice Implications

28.6.1 Treatment Outcomes

The most evidence-based use of an alpha agonist in ASD is treatment of comorbid ADHD or significant hyperactivity, and generally, guanfacine is recommended as the first-line choice of pharmacological treatment if using an alpha agonist due to its greater selectivity at the alpha-2 receptor. Clonidine may be beneficial for sleep in patients with ASD who have difficulty with either sleep onset or maintenance. Outside of these uses, clonidine and guanfacine may be considered for self-injurious behavior, hyperarousal, or other functionally impairing repetitive behaviors in individuals with ASD. Although the evidence for these uses is generally lower quality, due to the relatively low risk side effect profile of the alpha agonists, they still may be considered first- or second-line choices of pharmacological treatment depending on overall patient presentation. Always use the lowest possible effective dose, and use small increments for dose increases, to minimize adverse effects and issues with developing tolerance. Prescribing clonidine for sleep dysregulation or behavioral disturbance on an as-needed basis, or having optional as-needed second dose, rather than scheduled, may also help reduce issues with developing tolerance and ultimately losing efficacy. When using as-needed dosing, however, be aware of the potential total daily maximum dose, to avoid hypotension from a patient suddenly getting a large total daily dose. Likewise, ensure caregivers are aware that if they are giving an alpha agonist regularly, particularly clonidine, it should not be stopped abruptly due to issues with rebound hypertension, and instead should be tapered down over 1–2 weeks.

Contraindications to treatment with alpha agonists are preexisting medical conditions, including heart and vascular disease where fluctuations in blood pressure or lowering of blood pressure place them at risk for vascular accidents, hypoperfusion, or provoked arrhythmia. In such cases, prescribers should collaborate with the patient's other physicians and medical team to ensure safety prior to initiation of an alpha agonist. All patients should also be screened for sleep disorders, including obstructive sleep apnea and restless leg syndrome, and referred to sleep medicine for polysomnography when there is a concern for a sleep disorder separate from ASD.

Most common side effects of alpha agonists are fatigue/sedation and dizziness; gastrointestinal side effects, such as headache, and irritability can also occur. Hypotension and sedation are the side effects which most commonly limit use and dose titration of alpha agonists; slow titration with small dose increases can help limit these adverse effects. While not documented as widely in the ASD-specific

Table 28.1 Drug dosing guidelines

Drug	Recommended Starting Dose	Titration Schedule	Recommended Max Dosing
Guanfacine (Tenex)	0.5 mg every night	0.5 mg every 3–4 days	2 to 4 mg daily 2–3 divided doses*
Guanfacine XR (Intuniv)	1 mg daily	No faster than 1 mg every week	0.05 to 0.12 mg/kg/day (1 to 7 mg/day)
Clonidine	0.025** to 0.05 mg every night	0.05 mg every 2–3 days	0.2 to 0.4 mg daily in 2–3 divided doses, or consolidated at night for sleep*
Clonidine XR (Kapvay)	0.1 mg daily	No faster than 0.1 mg every week	0.4 mg daily
Clonidine transdermal patch	0.1 mg patch changed every 5–7 days	0.1 mg every week	0.3 mg patch changed every 5–7 days

* Maximum dose ranges are approximately weight based; see lexicomp for more information. Consider higher maximum doses regardless of weight if medication is otherwise well tolerated.
** Smallest pill size is 0.1 mg; 0.025 mg requires cutting pills into quarters.

literature, gastrointestinal side effects can also be common with the alpha agonists (Lexicomp), including constipation, which some patients with ASD are already prone to at baseline (Alabaf et al., 2019). Lastly, the transdermal clonidine patch also commonly causes issues with skin irritation, which is often a reason for discontinuation or switch to oral formulation.

28.6.2 Practice Implication Guidelines

Oral clonidine and guanfacine both come in short-acting and extended-release formulations as (tablets and capsules); clonidine also comes in a transdermal patch. Dosing used in the studies is generally consistent with prescribing guidelines for ADHD, and it should at least initially be guided by patient weight. Clonidine and guanfacine both have relatively short half-lives, and often require twice or three times a day dosing (unless using only for sleep). Table 28.1 describes drug dosing guidelines.

Higher maximum doses than those listed in Table 28.1 are sometimes used and have been reported in the literature, but this should be done with significant caution. Initiation and management of these medications in youth with ASD is most ideally performed by child and adolescent psychiatrists or developmental pediatricians who have specific experience and/or training in working with patients with ASD. However, in many cases, this is not feasible due to either complete lack of access or prolonged wait-times for these physicians. General pediatricians and adult psychiatrists may both prescribe and manage these medications, again ideally with specific training or experience with this patient population. Adult psychiatrists may be a better fit for treating adolescents and, naturally adults with ASD. General pediatricians may be a better fit for younger children. Psychiatric nurse practitioners, physician assistants, and other appropriately licensed and supervised practitioners may also prescribe and manage these medications under supervision of a physician with the appropriate background and training as described above. Patients with complex medication regimens, complex medical comorbidities, and/or severe or treatment resistant presentations should if possible be managed by child psychiatrists or developmental pediatricians who are comfortable managing these presentations. For physicians and other providers caring for these patients who do not have specialized training or expertise, the use of state hotlines for child psychiatry recommendations, or other forms of collaborative care, may be helpful.

28.7 References

Alabaf, S., Gillberg, C., Lundström, S., Lichtenstein, P., Kerekes, N., Råstam, M., & Anckarsäter, H. (2019). Physical health in children with neurodevelopmental disorders. *Journal of Autism & Developmental Disorders, 49*, 83–95.

Arnsten, A. F. (2010). The use of alpha-2A adrenergic agonists for the treatment of attention-deficit/hyperactivity disorder. *Expert Reviews in Neurotheraeutics, 10*(10), 1595–1605.

Banas, K., & Sawchuk, B. (2020). Clonidine as a treatment of behavioural disturbances in autism spectrum disorder: A systematic literature review. *Journal of the Canadian Academy of Child & Adolescent Psychiatry, 29*(2), 110–120.

Beversdorf, D. Q. (2020). The role of the noradrenergic system in autism spectrum disorders: Implications for treatment. *Seminars in Pediatric Neurology, 25*, 185–175.

Blankenship, K., Erickson, C. A., Stigler, K. A., Posey, D. J., & McDougle, C. J. (2011). Guanfacine extended release in two patients with pervasive developmental disorders. *Journal of Child & Adolescent Psychopharmacology, 21*(3), 287–290.

Blew, P., Luiselli, J. K., & Thibadeau, S. (1999). Beneficial effects of clonidine on severe self- injurious behavior in a 9-year-old girl with pervasive developmental disorder. *Journal of Child & Adolescent Psychopharmacology, 9*(4), 285–291.

Cocchi, R. (1996). A work in progress on drug therapy of an autistic child aged three (at first consultation). 2. The second six-months' therapy. *Italian Journal of Intellective Impairment, 9*, 31–40.

Dillon, J. E. (1990). Self-injurious behavior associated with clonidine withdrawal in a child with Tourette's disorder. *Journal of Child Neurology, 5*(4), 308–310.

Dowben, J. S., Grant, J. S., & Keltner, N. L. (2011). Clonidine: Diverse use in pharmacologic management. *Perspectives in Psychiatric Care, 47*(2), 105–108.

Fankhauser, M. P., Karumanchi, V. C., German, M. L., Yates, A., & Karumanchi, S. D. (1992). A double-blind, placebo-controlled study of the efficacy of transdermal clonidine in autism. *Journal of Clinical Psychiatry, 53*(3), 77–82.

Ferguson, B. R., & Gao, W. J. (2018). PV interneurons: Critical regulators of E/I balance for prefrontal cortex-dependent behavior and psychiatric disorders. *Frontiers in Neural Circuits, 12*, 37.

Ghaziuddin, M., Tsai, L., & Ghaziuddin, N. (1992). Clonidine for autism. *Journal of Child and Adolescent Psychopharmacology, 2*(4), 239–240.

Handen, B. L., Sahl, R., & Hardan, A. Y (2008). Guanfacine in children with autism and/or intellectual disabilities. *Journal of Developmental & Behavioral Pediatrics, 29*(4), 303–308.

Hiser, J., & Koenigs, M. (2018). The multifaceted role of the ventromedial prefrontal cortex in emotion, decision making, social cognition, and psychopathology. *Biological Psychiatry, 83*(8), 638–647.

Ingrassia, A., & Turk, J. (2005). The use of clonidine for severe and intractable sleep problems in children with neurodevelopmental disorders—A case series. *European Child & Adolescent Psychiatry, 14*(1), 34–40.

Jäkälä, P., Riekkinen, M., Sirviö, J., Koivisto, E., Kejonen, K., Vanhanen, M., & Riekkinen, P. Jr. (1999). Guanfacine, but not clonidine, improves planning and working memory performance in humans. *Neuropsychopharmacology, 20*(5), 460–470.

Jaselskis, C. A., Cook, E. H. Jr., Fletcher, K. E., & Leventhal, B. L. (1992). Clonidine treatment of hyperactive and impulsive children with autistic disorder. *Journal of Clinical Psychopharmacology, 12*(5), 322–327.

Jasper, J. R., Lesnick, J. D. Chang, L. K. Yamanishi, S. S. Chang, T. K. Hsu, S. A. Daunt, D. A. Bonhaus D. W., & Eglen R. M. (1998). Ligand efficacy and potency at recombinant alpha2 adrenergic receptors: agonist-mediated [35S]GTPgammaS binding. *Biochemistry & Pharmacology, 55*(7), 1035–1043.

Koshes, R. J., & Rock, N. L. (1994). Use of clonidine for behavioral control in an adult patient with autism. *American Journal of Psychiatry, 151*(11), 1714.

London, E. B. (2018). Neuromodulation and a reconceptualization of autism spectrum disorders: Using the locus coeruleus functioning as an exemplar. *Frontiers in Neurology, 9*, 1120.

McCracken, J. T., & Martin W. (1997). Clonidine side effect. *Journal of the American Academy of Child & Adolescent Psychiatry, 36*(2), 160–161.

Ming, X., E., Kang, G. N., & Wagner, G. C. (2008). Use of clonidine in children with autism, spectrum disorders. *Brain Development, 30*(7), 454–460.

Okazaki, K., K. Yamamuro, J. I., & Kishimoto, T. (2019). Guanfacine monotherapy for ADHD/ASD comorbid with Tourette syndrome: A case report. *Annals of General Psychiatry, 18*, 2.

Park, J., & Moghaddam, B. (2017). Impact of anxiety on prefrontal cortex encoding of cognitive flexibility. *Neuroscience, 345*, 193–202.

Persico, A. M., Ricciardello, A., Lamberti, M., Turriziani, L., Cucinotta, F., Brogna, C., Vitiello, B., & Arango, C (2021). The pediatric psychopharmacology of autism spectrum disorder: A systematic review—Part I: The past and the present. *Progress in Neuropsychopharmacology & Biological Psychiatry, 110*, 110326.

Politte, L. C., Scahill, L., Figueroa, J., McCracken, J. T., King, B. & McDougle C. J. (2018). A randomized, placebo-controlled trial of extended-release guanfacine in children with autism spectrum disorder and ADHD symptoms: An analysis of secondary outcome measures. *Neuropsychopharmacology, 43*(8), 1772–1778.

Posey, D. J., Puntney, J. I., Sasher, T. M., Kem, D. L., & McDougle, C. J. (2004). Guanfacine treatment of hyperactivity and inattention in pervasive developmental disorders: A retrospective analysis of 80 cases. *Journal of Child & Adolescent Psychopharmacology, 14*(2), 233–241.

Propper, L. (2018). Managing disruptive behaviour in autism-spectrum disorder with guanfacine. *Journal of Psychiatry & Neuroscience, 43*(5), 359–360.

Relia, S., & Ekambaram, V. (2018). Pharmacological approach to sleep disturbances in autism spectrum disorders with psychiatric comorbidities: A literature review. *Medical Science (Basel), 6*(4), 95. DOI: 10.3390/medsci6040095.

Ring, M., Bowler, D. M., & Gaigg, S. B. (2020). A physiological marker of recognition memory in adults with autism spectrum disorder? The pupil old/new effect. *Autism Research, 13*(4), 627–640.

Romanelli, M., & Rhodes, A. (2014). Guanfacine-induced lichenoid drug eruption in a child with autism and attention deficit hyperactivity disorder. *Pediatric Dermatology, 31*(5), 614–615.

Scahill, L., Aman, M. G., McDougle, C. J., McCracken, J. T., Tierney, E. Dziura, J., Arnold, L. E., Posey, D., Young, C., Shah, B., Ghuman, J., Ritz, L., & Vitiello, B. (2006). A prospective open trial of guanfacine in children with pervasive developmental disorders. *Journal of Child & Adolescent Psychopharmacology, 16*(5), 589–598.

Scahill, L., McCracken, J. T., King, B. H., Rockhill, C., Shah, B. Politte, L., Sanders, R., Minjarez, M., Cowen, J., Mullet, J., Page, C., Ward, D., Deng, Y., Loo, S., dziura, J., & McDougle, C. J. (2015). Extended-release guanfacine for hyperactivity in children with autism spectrum disorder. *American Journal of Psychiatry, 172*(12), 1197–1206.

Stahl, S. M. (2013). *Stahl's essential psychopharmacology: Neuroscientific basis and practical applications*. Cambridge: Cambridge University Press.

Strange, B. C. (2008). Once-daily treatment of ADHD with guanfacine: Patient implications. *Neuropsychiatric Disease & Treatment, 4*(3), 499–506.

Xing, B., Li, Y. C., & Gao, W. J. (2016). Norepinephrine versus dopamine and their interaction in modulating synaptic function in the prefrontal cortex. *Brain Research, 1641*(Pt B), 217–233.
Yin, X., Jones, N., Yang, J., Asraoui, N., Mathieu, M. E., Cai, L., & Chen, S. X. (2021). Delayed motor learning in a 16p11.2 deletion mouse model of autism is rescued by locus coeruleus activation. *Nature Neuroscience, 24*(5), 646–657.

29

Mood Stabilizers and Antiepileptics

Shoumitro (Shoumi) Deb and Meera Roy
Hereford and Worcestershire Health and Care Trust

Bharati Limbu
Department of Brain Sciences, Faculty of Medicine, Imperial College London

29.1 Technical Abstract

Background: Despite the regular use of mood stabilizers in people with autism spectrum disorder (ASD), there is little evidence of their efficacy in treating ASD core symptoms or associated behaviors. In this chapter, we have reviewed the evidence of mood stabilizers' efficacy in people with ASD. **Method:** We have searched several relevant databases and journals to explore efficacy studies involving mood stabilizers, including lithium and some antiepileptic medications. **Results:** Apart from eight randomized controlled trials (RCTs), the rest of the evidence is based on case reports and retrospective chart reviews. These RCTs have methodological flaws and show conflicting results. Studies have assessed the efficacy of these medications on ASD core symptoms such as restrictive and repetitive behaviors, impaired communication, and associated behaviors, such as agitation and aggression. **Discussion:** Given the methodological flaws in the included studies and contradictory findings, it is difficult to draw any definitive conclusion about mood stabilizers' effectiveness in treating ASD core symptoms or associated behaviors. Robust, large-scale RCTs are needed in the future to address this issue. **Practitioner recommendations:** In the absence of any definitive evidence to support their use, practitioners should carefully weigh up the desired effect against the side effects of these medications before considering them for people with ASD.

29.2 Layperson Summary

Mood stabilizer medications are used to treat bipolar disorder. They include lithium and some antiepileptic medications. The latter is mainly used to treat epilepsy. Many psychiatric drugs, including mood stabilizers, are used regularly for people with autism. Their efficacy is not proven. We have reviewed the studies that assessed the efficacy of these medications in people with autism of all ages. We found only eight RCTs. RCTs are seen as the gold standard of evidence.

Shoumitro (Shoumi) Deb, Meera Roy, and Bharati Limbu, *Mood Stabilizers and Antiepileptics*. In: *Lifespan Treatment for Autistic Individuals*. Edited by: Peter Sturmey, Russell Lang, and James K. Luiselli, Oxford University Press.
© Oxford University Press (2025). DOI: 10.1093/oso/9780197635841.003.0029

These studies assessed the efficacy of these medications on autism core symptoms, such as restrictive and repetitive behavior, impaired communication, and other associated symptoms, such as irritability, agitation, and aggression. It is difficult to draw any definitive conclusion. This is because most of these RCTs did not show any superiority of these drugs over placebo (dummy pills). These studies often included a few participants and followed them up for a short period. Other studies had other design flaws. These studies did not look for the efficacy of these drugs on bipolar disorder for which they are indicated or any other psychiatric disorders. One antiepileptic drug, sodium valproate, is barred from use in women of childbearing age. This is because of its effect on the unborn child. Another mood stabilizer, lithium, can cause serious side effects. Regular blood tests are necessary to monitor this. However, regular blood tests may be challenging for many people with autism. Therefore, clinicians should use these medications with caution for psychological and behavioral symptoms in people with autism.

29.3 Treatment Summary Table

Treatment summary: Mood Stabilizers and Antiepileptics

Treatment description: Mood stabilizers, including some antiepileptic medications, are psychotropic medications. These medications can come as tablets, capsules, or liquids. Mood stabilizers are licensed to treat bipolar disorder, and antiepileptics are licensed to treat epilepsy.

Expected outcomes: They are sometimes prescribed to people with autism spectrum disorder (ASD) for ASD core symptoms or/and associated behaviors, such as restrictive and repetitive behaviors; mood disorders such as irritability, impulsivity, agitation, and aggression; and to treat any co-occurring epilepsy or seizures, but it is difficult to draw any definitive conclusion about mood stabilizers' effectiveness in treating ASD core symptoms or associated behaviors.

Methods: Mood stabilizers are a class of psychotropic medications. Practitioners should ensure that other interventions have been attempted first. Practitioners should start with a lower dose and titrate slowly.

Expertise required to implement treatment: Treatment should be provided by a physician, psychiatrist, or other licensed prescriber experienced in using these medications for people with ASD.

Risks and negative side effects: There can be many adverse events (negative side effects) associated with mood stabilizers and antiepileptics, such as sedation, nausea, stomach problems, thirst, dizziness, fatigue, headache, weight gain or loss, skin rash, and mild tremor.

Additional considerations and limitations: Sodium valproate is contraindicated in women of childbearing age. Depending on the type of medication prescribed, the prescriber will need to assess full blood count; renal, liver, and thyroid functions are monitored. Lithium needs regular blood tests to establish an optimum effective dose and assess its negative side effects. There is also no definite evidence of the effectiveness of mood stabilizers and antiepileptics in treating ASD core symptoms or associated behaviors.

29.4 Introduction

29.4.1 Treatment Description

Mood stabilizers and antiepileptics are psychotropic medications which are increasingly used off-label in people with ASD. Frequently used psychotropic medications in ASD include psychostimulants, antipsychotics (particularly risperidone), and mood stabilizers/antiepileptics. They are often prescribed for ASD core symptoms or/and associated behaviors, but there is limited evidence for their efficacy for the core symptoms of ASD or/and associated behaviors. None are approved for ASD core symptoms or/and associated behaviors. Antiepileptics, however, can be prescribed to treat any comorbid epilepsy.

29.4.2 Rationale and Objectives

Lithium is approved for treating bipolar disorder, and antiepileptic medications for epilepsy, but their use for treating ASD symptoms is not approved. These medications affect several neurotransmitters, including GABA (γ-aminobutyric acid), glutamate, serotonin, dopamine, and noradrenaline systems in the hippocampus, amygdala, prefrontal cortex, anterior cingulate cortex, and temporal lobes of the brain. Lithium is also known to act as a neuroprotector. Some antiepileptic medications induce the cytochrome P450 system and adversely affect bone, lipid, and gonadal steroid metabolism. Some antiepileptic medications work on sodium or calcium channels by blocking them. Some work by potentiating the GABA system or inhibiting the glutamatergic system through NMDA (N-methyl-D-aspartate) or AMPA receptors.

29.4.3 Considerations for Implementation

Due to contradictory findings and limited evidence supporting the use of mood stabilizers and antiepileptics in people with ASD to treat ASD core symptoms and associated behaviors, they should only be prescribed by practitioners and prescribers with expertise in this field and if the benefit of medication outweighs the harm and the cost. Nonpharmacological interventions should always be considered first.

29.5 Research Background

ASD is associated with an increased comorbidity of neurodevelopmental, medical, and psychiatric disorders (prevalence approximately 55–70%) (see Deb et al., 2022a). Comorbidities such as intellectual disabilities (ID) (prevalence approximately 38–45%), anxiety disorders (prevalence approximately 18–20%), attention-deficit/hyperactivity disorder (ADHD) (prevalence approximately 25–28%), schizophrenia spectrum disorder (prevalence approximately 4–12%), depression (prevalence approximately 11–19%), bipolar affective disorder (prevalence approximately 4%), and obsessive-compulsive disorder (prevalence approximately 7–10%) are common in people with ASD (Bertelli et al., 2022; Deb et al., 2022b; Lai et al., 2014, 2019; Lugo-Marín et al., 2019; Simonoff et al., 2008). Problem (challenging) behaviors, which may or may not be influenced by underlying anxiety, are also common in ASD (prevalence approximately 10–15%) (Lai et al., 2019).

A high proportion of children, adolescents, and adults with ASD receive psychotropic medication (prevalence approximately 33–44%) (Bachmann et al., 2013; Coury et al., 2012). The rate of psychotropic use for people with ASD has increased significantly over the years, from 57% in 1998 to 64% in 2014 ($p < .05$), according to one survey (Murray et al., 2014), and is also common in children as young as 2 years of age (Mandell et al., 2008). The prevalence of psychotropic use seems to increase with increasing age. For example, 11% of children aged 3–5 years, 46% of children aged 6–11 years, and 66% of children aged 12–17 years were reported to receive psychotropic medication (Coury et al., 2012). Frequently used psychotropics in ASD were psychostimulants (13%), followed by antipsychotics (particularly risperidone) (12%) and mood stabilizers/antiepileptics such as sodium valproate (9%), antidepressants (4%), and benzodiazepines (7%) (Bachmann et al., 2013).

Hirota et al. (2014) presented data from a systematic review and a meta-analysis on antiepileptic medications for ASD children and adolescents. Recently Limbu et al. (2022) published an updated systematic review and meta-analysis of mood stabilizers on people with ASD of all ages. None of these meta-analyses found any definitive evidence of the efficacy of mood stabilizers, including antiepileptics, in people with ASD.

Epilepsy may affect around 25–30% of people with ASD (Berney & Deb, 2012; Lai et al., 2014). However, EEG abnormalities in the absence of clinical seizures are also common in people with ASD (Chez et al., 2006; Spence & Schneider, 2009). The underlying EEG abnormalities may affect the emotion and behavior of some people with ASD leading to anxiety and problem behaviors (Hartley-McAndrew & Weinstock 2010; Kanemura et al., 2013 cited in Hirota et al., 2014). For that reason, mood stabilizers and antiepileptic medications may improve emotional and behavioral symptoms in people with ASD (Hirota et al., 2014). Therefore, this chapter reviewed mood stabilizers, including lithium, and some antiepileptics for people with ASD. Some antipsychotics and antidepressants are also used to treat bipolar disorders.

29.5.1 Mood Stabilizers

Divalproex sodium. Divalproex sodium treats bipolar disorder (Goodwin et al., 2016). Divalproex sodium and its active metabolites increase GABA transmission and inhibit histone deacetylases to protect chromatin structure (Logan et al., 2021).

In a recent systematic review and meta-analysis, Limbu et al. (2022) have found three RCTs on divalproex sodium that included people with ASD.

In a parallel design double-blind placebo controlled RCT, Hollander et al. (2006) included nine people with ASD in the divalproex sodium group and four in the placebo group who were followed up over 8 weeks. ASD was diagnosed using the *Diagnostic and Statistical Manual*, 4th edition (*DSM-IV*) (American Psychiatric Association, 1994), Autism Diagnostic Interview-Revised (ADI-R) (Lord et al., 1994), and Autism Diagnostic Observation Schedule (ADOS) (Lord et al., 1989). Participants' age varied between 5 and 17 years apart from one who was 40 years old. The participants' IQ ranged between 30 and 104 (mean IQ = 60). The gender of the participants was not described in the paper. The dose of medication ranged between 500 and 1,500 mg/day. The mean dose at the endpoint was 822.92 ± 326.21 mg/day. The mean trough serum level of divalproex sodium at the endpoint was 58.23 ± 21.63 μg/ml. The improvement in score in the primary outcome measure, the Children-Yale-Brown Obsessive Compulsive Scale (C-YBOCS) (Scahill et al., 1997), in the intervention group at follow-up was significantly better compared with the placebo group ($p = 0.037$; effect size: $d = 1.61$). However, the very small sample size may have caused a Type II error, and the follow-up period is too short for drawing any definitive conclusion from this study. Also, there was no statistically significant intergroup difference in the primary outcome measure when the data for one adult participant were excluded. Irritability, weight gain, anxiety, and aggression were reported in both groups, but the difference was not statistically significant.

In another small parallel design double-blind placebo-controlled RCT (Hollander et al., 2010), there were 16 children and adolescents in the divalproex sodium group and 11 in the placebo group (age 5–17 years; IQ: 30–89; 23 boys) who were followed up over 12 weeks using outcome measures such as Aberrant Behavior Checklist (ABC) (Aman et al., 1985), Overt Aggression Scale-Modified (OAS-M) (Kay et al., 1988), C-YBOCS (Scahill et al., 1997), Vineland Adaptive Behaviour Scale (VABS) (Sparrow et al., 1984), Young Mania Rating Scale (YMRS) (Young et al., 1978), and Clinical Global Impression Scale-Improvement (CGI–I) (National Institute of Mental Health, 1985). They used the same method to diagnose ASD as in their previous study (Hollander et al., 2006) but used a CGI-Severity (CGI-S) (NIMH, 1985) score of 4 or over to justify exposure to the medication. The medication dose was 125 mg/day–250 mg twice daily for those weighing <40 kg and 250 mg/day-500 mg twice daily for those weighing >40 kg. According to the CGI-Irritability score change at follow-up, the authors described 62.5% in the intervention group as opposed to 9% in the placebo group as responders (Odds ratio: 16.7; Fisher's exact $p = 0.008$). The authors also described marginally statistically significant improvement in the ABC-Irritability (ABC-I) subdomain (Aman et al., 1985) ($p = 0.048$). However, no statistically significant intergroup differences were observed in the VABS domains of communication and socialization or the YMRS (Young et al., 1978) scores. Neither was there any significant intergroup difference in the aggression score according to OAS-M (Kay et al., 1988) and repetitiveness score as per C-YBOCS (Scahill et al., 1997).

Controlling for IQ did not change these findings. There was a trend for responders to have higher valproate blood levels than nonresponders. Participants with an abnormal electroencephalogram (EEG) may have responded better on divalproex sodium than those without abnormality, but no definitive conclusion could be drawn because of the very small number involved. Overall, no definitive conclusion can be drawn from this study because of the small sample size and short study duration. Also, the findings were inconsistent depending on the outcome measures used. Whereas the primary outcome measure showed a significant difference, four secondary outcome measures failed to do so (although this may have been due to lack of statistical power). Insomnia, weight gain, headache, rash, polyuria, agitation, and infections were reported in both the intervention and the control groups without any statistically significant intergroup difference.

The third double-blind RCT on divalproex sodium is a noninferiority trial between divalproex sodium ($n = 43$) and risperidone ($n = 43$) among children with *DSM-IV* (American Psychiatric Association, 1994) and ADI-R (Lord et al., 1994) diagnosed ASD (age: 4.87 ± 0.41 years; gender and IQ of the participants were not reported in the paper) (Martsenkovsky, 2014). Divalproex sodium was dispensed in sprinkles and titrated to tolerance or serum valproate level between 50 and 100 pg/ml, and risperidone was administered at a dose of 0.01–0.07 mg/kg/day. The outcome was assessed in both groups using score changes from baseline to 16 weeks of follow-up on OAS-M (Kay et al., 1988), ABC (Aman et al., 1985), and CGI (NIMH, 1985). Risperidone was found to be statistically significantly better than divalproex sodium in improving aggression, impulsivity, hyperactivity and stereotype, and scores on CGI-I-Irritability ($p = 0.002$), OAS-M ($p = 0.005$), ABC-I (teacher rating) ($p = 0.04$). The study did not provide any information on the dropout rate or inclusion-exclusion criteria and was of poor quality as rated "0" on the Jadad risk of bias scale (Jadad et al., 1996). Both groups reported weight gain, autonomic symptoms, and sedation, but the difference was not statistically significant.

Sodium valproate. Sodium valproate is an antiepileptic medication used to treat bipolar disorder (Goodwin et al., 2016). Sodium valproate potentiates GABA, inhibits glutamate, and block sodium channel (Löscher et al., 2013). Sodium valproate and its derivatives are contraindicated in women of childbearing age because of their teratogenic effect (Logan et al., 2021). Limbu et al. (2022) found only one RCT on sodium valproate by Hellings et al. (2005). This is a parallel design placebo-controlled double-blind 8 weeks follow-up of sodium valproate (13 participants completed) at a dose of 250 mg/day to 20 mg/kg/day (mean trough serum level was 77.8 μg/ml at trial endpoint) versus placebo (12 participants completed the trial). Participants' age ranged from 6 to 20 years (11.2 ± 4.2 years). There were 20 males in the trial. Participants' IQs ranged from 20 to 137 (mean IQ was 54). Twenty-four had ID, two had borderline IQ, one each had average and above-average IQ, and for two participants, IQ data were missing. All participants had a diagnosis of *DSM-IV* ASD (American Psychiatric Association, 1994) confirmed by ADI-R (Lord et al., 1994) and ADOS (Lord et al., 1989). No statistically significant intergroup difference was reported on the scores of ABC-I (Aman et al., 1985), OAS (Yudofsky et al., 1986), CGI-I (NIMH, 1985), and CGI-S (NIMH, 1985). The same results were found when data on children with ID were analyzed separately. This study showed a negative finding, but the sample size was very small, which may have caused a Type II error. The study duration was short, the sample was heterogeneous, and the study showed a large placebo effect. Several gastrointestinal complaints were reported in both groups, but a raised serum level of ammonia was reported in the intervention group. This may damage the brain and cause neurological symptoms. One participant's parents reported cognitive slowing and slurred speech at times. The only adverse event reaching a significant level was increased appetite ($p = 0.03$). This was reported among 56% in the valproate group as opposed to 14% in the placebo group.

Lamotrigine. Lamotrigine is an antiepileptic, but it is also used as a mood stabilizer in treating bipolar disorder (Goodwin et al., 2016). Lamotrigine may inhibit voltage-gated sodium channels stabilizing presynaptic neuronal membranes and inhibit presynaptic glutamate and aspartate release (Coulter, 1997). Limbu et al. (2022) found only one RCT on lamotrigine by Belsito et al. (2001), who, in an 18-week parallel design double-blind placebo-controlled trial included 14 ADI-R confirmed (Lord et al., 1994) children with ASD in the lamotrigine group who received 0.5–5 mg/kg/day in two divided doses and another 14 children in the placebo group. Participants' age varied between 3 and 11 years (5.8 ± 1.75), 27 of whom were boys, but their IQ was not specified. No statistically significant intergroup differences were found on the scores of Autism Behavior Checklist (AUBC) (Krug et al., 1980), Aberrant Behavior Checklist—Community (ABC-C) (Aman et al., 1995), Vineland ABS (Sparrow et al., 1984) communication or daily living domains, ADOS (Lord et al., 1989), and Childhood Autism Rating Scale (CARS) (Schopler et al., 1980). No improvement was reported in stereotypies, lethargy, irritability, hyperactivity, emotional reciprocity, sharing pleasures, language and communication, socialization, and daily living skills. There was a marginally significant improvement in Vineland's social domain ($p = 0.045$) (score improved by 3.9% in the lamotrigine as opposed to 0.2% in the placebo group). For a small study like this, too many outcome measures have been used unnecessarily, which may have caused a Type I error for which no correction was undertaken. The study also showed a large placebo effect. Insomnia, skin rash, and hyperactivity were reported in both groups, but no statistically significant intergroup difference was observed in side effects.

Levetiracetam. Levetiracetam is an antiepileptic with neuroprotective properties, which may have a different mechanism of action than the other antiepileptic medications, binding to a presynaptic vesicle SV2A protein (Lynch et al., 2004). Levetiracetam is also used as a mood stabilizer in the treatment of bipolar disorder (Goodwin et al., 2016). Limbu et al. (2022) found only two RCTs on levetiracetam. In a parallel design placebo-controlled double-blind 10 weeks follow-up study, Wasserman et al. (2006) included 10 DSM-IV (American Psychiatric Association, 1994) diagnosed and ADI-R- (Lord et al., 1994), ADOS-confirmed (Lord et al.,

1989) children with ASD in the levetiracetam group (125 mg/day–250 mg/day or 20–30 mg/kg/day) and the same number of children in the placebo group. The mean age of participants in the intervention group was 7.62 years, and 9.82 years in the placebo group, of whom 17 were boys. Participants' IQ ranged from 29 to 107 (75.75 ± 33.4). No statistically significant intergroup difference was reported in the outcomes based on parent rating of ABC Irritability scale (Aman et al., 1985), CGI (NIMH, 1985), C-YBOCS (Scahill et al., 1997), and Conners' Parents Rating Scale-Revised (CPRS-R) (Conners et al., 1998), but the teachers' rating of ABC-I scale showed a statistically significant better outcome in the placebo group. The ABC-I score in the placebo group was reduced from 61.59 at baseline to 58.94 at follow-up, compared with an increase from 56.41 to 59.96 in the intervention group; these differences were not statistically significant. However, the very small sample size and short study duration make the interpretation of findings difficult. Agitation, aggression, hyperactivity, impulsivity, loss of appetite, self-injurious behavior, weight gain, weight loss, and enuresis were reported in both groups without any statistically significant intergroup difference.

The second RCT on levetiracetam is a non-placebo controlled single-blind, parallel design study of psychoeducation versus psychoeducation plus levetiracetam (60 mg/kg/day) by Wang et al. (2017). In this study, 35 children with ASD diagnosed with *DSM-V* criteria (American Psychiatric Association, 2013) received psychoeducation (age: 63.1 ± 12.7 months), and another 32 received levetiracetam over and above the psychoeducation (age: 61.6 ± 13.8 months), 57 of whom were boys. Participants' IQs were not specified. Both groups showed significant improvements in their behavioral and cognitive functions at 6 months follow-up, according to Psychoeducational Profile, 3rd ed. (PEP-3-Revised Chinese version) (Chen et al., 2011), CARS (Schopler et al., 1980), and ABC (Aman et al., 1985) scores, but all these outcomes were significantly better in the combined than the control group ($p < 0.05$). Subclinical EEG abnormalities improved significantly in the combined (75%) compared with the control group (14.3%) ($p < 0.05$). This study is not placebo-controlled and single-blind. Perhaps the outcome was expected, given that the combined group received both psychoeducation and medication. Anorexia, irritability, fatigue, and somnolence were reported in the levetiracetam-treated group, and no adverse events were assessed in the psychoeducation-alone group.

29.5.2 Topiramate

Topiramate is an antiepileptic medication that acts by inhibiting voltage-gated sodium and calcium channels and glutamate pathways while enhancing the inhibitory effects of GABA (Rosenfeld, 1997). Limbu et al. (2022) found only one RCT on topiramate by Rezaei et al. (2010), a double-blind placebo-controlled add-on study. In this study, 20 children and adolescents with ASD diagnosed by

DSM-IV-TR (American Psychiatric Association, 2000) and ADI-R (Lord et al., 1994) received risperidone (0.5–2 mg/day for children weighing up to 40 kg and 3 mg/day for children over 40 kg) (mean age: 7.85 years) and placebo. Another 20 children with ASD received risperidone at the same dose but in addition instead of receiving placebo received topiramate at 100 mg/day–200 mg/day dose (mean age: 8.17 years). All children scored ≥12 on the ABC-I score (Aman et al., 1985) at the study entry, 27 of whom were boys, and the participants' IQ was not specified. At 8 weeks follow-up, there was a significant improvement in the topiramate group compared with the control group in three, namely irritability, hyperactivity/ noncompliance, and stereotypy subdomains of ABC-C (Aman et al., 1995) (all *p*'s < 0.05) but not in lethargy/social withdrawal and inappropriate speech, which showed a nonsignificant intergroup difference. It is difficult to draw any definitive conclusion from this study because of its small sample size, short study duration, and contradictory findings according to the different ABC-C subdomain scores. A significantly higher rate of somnolence (35% vs 5%) and decreased appetite (35% vs. 5%) was reported in the topiramate and risperidone combined group compared with the topiramate and placebo combined group.

29.5.3 Lithium

Lithium is well-established prophylaxis for bipolar disorders (Goodwin et al., 2016) and may be neuroprotective (Wada et al., 2005). There is no RCT-based evidence of lithium for people with ASD. There are a small number of case studies and reports. For example, Siegel et al. (2014) carried out a retrospective case note review of 30 children and adolescents with ASD who were prescribed lithium for irritability or mood disorder across two inpatient settings. The mean age of participants was 13.6 years. Three fourths of them were male, and half of them had IDs. Using the CGI-I score, they found that mood symptoms, including mania and euphoria, improved in 71% of participants (NIMH, 1985). Forty-seven percent of participants reported at least one side effect, including vomiting, tremor, fatigue, irritability, and enuresis. Treatment with lithium requires regular blood tests, which may be difficult for many people with ASD, particularly those with a low IQ. Therefore, in the absence of RCT-based evidence to support its efficacy, lithium should only be used after a complete and detailed consideration of all options (Bertelli et al., 2022b; Deb et al., 2022a).

29.5.4 Carbamazepine and Oxcarbazepine

There is no RCT-based evidence on the efficacy of carbamazepine and oxcarbazepine in people with ASD. These antiepileptic medications also treat mood disorders and neuropathic pain (Goodwin et al., 2016). They induce cytochrome P450 enzymes and may increase the clearance of other medications and reduce their concentration (McLean et al., 1994). They act by inhibiting voltage-gated sodium channels (McLean et al., 1994).

A recent retrospective case study reported the effect of add-on carbamazepine on five consecutive patients with 15q duplication syndrome, autism, and mood disorder (four also had epilepsy) (Viamontes et al., 2022). Mood symptoms such as hyperactivity, irritability, impulsivity, intrusiveness, mood lability, and pressured speech responded better to carbamazepine. Anxiety symptoms also improved in three participants. Seizure control also improved in one of them. The report included a small number of participants and a retrospective data analysis, making this evidence unreliable.

In a letter to the editor, Kapetanovic (2007) reported improvement in problem behaviors such as aggression, self-injury, and hyperactivity in three children and adolescents with ASD (ages 13, 19, and 4.5 years, respectively) when treated with oxcarbazepine when other psychotropics failed or produced unacceptable side effects. In a retrospective case study of 30 ASD patients (mean age: 12 years; range: 5–21 years), Douglas et al. (2013) reported the effect of add-on treatment with oxcarbazepine on irritability and agitation. Fourteen patients scored "much improved" according to the CGI-I scale (NIMH, 1985), but only 10 (33%) showed improvement according to the CGI-S scale (NIMH, 1985). However, seven (23%) patients developed clinically significant side effects leading to the discontinuation of oxcarbazepine. The authors concluded that it is not possible to comment on oxcarbazepine's efficacy in improving agitation and aggression in people with ASD without a placebo group. They have also asked for caution while using this medication because of the high rate of clinically significant side effects.

29.5.5 Gabapentin and Tiagabine

Gabapentin is used primarily to treat focal seizures, neuropathic pain, and anxiety. It is a GABA derivative and binds to the voltage-gated calcium channels (Brodie et al., 2016; Löscher et al., 2013). There are no RCTs available on the efficacy of gabapentin in people with ASD. In one case report, a 27-year-old man with ASD and moderate ID whose aggression and repetitive behavior did not improve on several antipsychotics showed improvement after adding gabapentin according to the CGI scale. The improvement was observed within a couple of weeks of adding gabapentin and continued for 6 months, allowing some of the previously prescribed antipsychotics to be discontinued (Guglielmo et al., 2013).

Tiagabine is a GABA reuptake inhibitor licensed to treat epilepsy (Meldrum & Chapman, 1999). A prospective open-label study of add-on tiagabine on 14 ASD children and adolescents (mean age: 11.5 years; age range: 5–17 years), half of whom were boys, showed improvement in several of them on anxiety, aggression, and stereotypy (Chaleby & Zawawi, 2006). All children received other psychotropic medication as they had comorbid psychiatric disorders such as psychosis, bipolar disorder, ADHD, and obsessive-compulsive disorder. According to the CGI scale (NIMH, 1985), two did not improve, four were "improved," and eight were "much improved." One developed absence seizure status epilepticus after the initial response. No other significant side effects were reported.

In the absence of substantial evidence, it is impossible to draw any conclusion on the efficacy of either of these medications for people with ASD.

29.6 Practice Implications

29.6.1 Treatment Outcomes

Despite their common use in this population, there is very little good-quality evidence on mood stabilizers' efficacy in people with ASD. Only five mood stabilizers have RCT-based evidence (sodium valproate, divalproex sodium, lamotrigine, levetiracetam, and topiramate). Even in these RCTs, a small number of participants was often recruited, causing Type II error (only two included over 50 but less than 100 participants, *n*'s = 66 and 86, respectively) (Martsenkovsky, 2014; Wang et al., 2017). The overall quality of the RCTs, as measured by the Cochrane risk of bias tool and Jadad et al. (1996) score, was poor in a recent systematic review (Limbu et al., 2022). There is no RCT-based evidence for the rest of the mood stabilizers and antiepileptics (lithium, carbamazepine, oxcarbazepine, gabapentin, and tiagabine). Two recent reviews on the RCTs of mood stabilizers in people with ASD found no conclusive evidence of the efficacy of these medications (Hirota et al., 2014; Limbu et al., 2022).

Limbu et al. (2022) included eight RCTs on mood stabilizers involving 310 participants with ASD of any age (3–40 years) in their recent systematic review and meta-analysis. They included three RCTs on divalproex sodium, two on levetiracetam, and one each on lamotrigine, sodium valproate, and topiramate as an add-on to risperidone. However, in their systematic review, Hirota et al. (2014) included seven RCTs of antiepileptic medication in a total of 117 children with ASD. The justification for using RCTs on antiepileptic medications only is that Hirota et al. (2014) wanted to assess the effect of these medications on epilepsy or subclinical EEG changes that are common in people with ASD (Spence & Schneider, 2009). Their systematic review included two RCTs on divalproex sodium, one each on sodium valproate, lamotrigine, and levetiracetam, and one each combined topiramate and risperidone, and sodium valproate and fluoxetine.

Two of the three RCTs on divalproex sodium in this chapter were from the same authors (Hollander et al., 2006, 2010). Two of the RCTs on divalproex sodium used a placebo-controlled parallel design, but the third was a noninferiority comparison between divalproex sodium and risperidone rather than a placebo (Martsenkovsky, 2014). The two RCTs presented in this chapter on levetiracetam used parallel design, but one was placebo-controlled and double-blind (Wasserman et al., 2006), and the other one was a single-blind comparison of combined levetiracetam and psychoeducational program with psychoeducation alone (Wang et al., 2017). One RCT each on lamotrigine (Belsito et al., 2001) and sodium valproate (Hellings et al., 2005) presented in this chapter used a placebo-controlled parallel design. The single RCT on topiramate presented in this chapter compared two groups, both of which received risperidone but one with added topiramate and the other with added placebo (Rezaei et al., 2010). Most studies on mood stabilizers reported their effect on ASD core symptoms such as restrictive and repetitive behavior, and impaired communication measured by CYBOCS (Scahill et al., 1997), and associated behaviors such as aggression, agitation, and irritability measured by ABC (Aman et al., 1985) and OAS-M (Kay et al., 1988) but not on the symptoms of bipolar disorder for which these medications are indicated (Goodwin et al., 2016). Some studies have reported that autistic people do not want interventions to improve their ASD core symptoms unless this leads to improvement in their mental health or quality of life (Linden et al., 2023). No study has presented information on the person's quality of life (Bertelli et al., 2022).

Most studies included children and adolescents with ASD, except a couple of studies with a small number of young adults. Some RCTs included ASD participants with ID, but not all provided information on this. Even the studies that included participants with ID and ASD did not necessarily provide separate data on those with ID. Therefore, it is difficult to conclude about mood stabilizers' efficacy on ASD in the presence of ID.

Overall, the findings from the evidence presented in this chapter are far from conclusive. Only one study on levetiracetam showed a positive result, but this was not a placebo-controlled study. This study, not surprisingly, showed the superiority of combining levetiracetam with a psychoeducational program over the psychoeducational program alone (Wang et al., 2017). One study on lamotrigine showed a marginally significant result ($p = 0.045$) compared with placebo according to one outcome measure but failed to do so according to five other outcome measures (Belsito et al., 2001). Two studies on divalproex sodium carried out by the same group showed the superiority of the medication over the placebo, but the sample size in both was small (*n*'s = 13 and 27) (Hollander et al., 2006, 2010). Although one of these two studies showed a significantly better outcome from divalproex sodium over the placebo according to the primary outcome measure, it failed to show any significant intergroup difference according to four other secondary outcome measures (Hollander et al., 2010). The RCTs on sodium valproate (Hellings et al., 2005) and levetiracetam (Wasserman et al., 2006) showed negative findings. In one study, divalproex sodium was not superior to a combination with risperidone (Martsenkovsky, 2014). The only study on topiramate showed an equivocal result (Rezaei et al., 2010).

Limbu et al. (2022) carried out a meta-analysis by pooling data on ABC-I (four studies) and OAS-M and CGI-I scores (two each, respectively) of the mood stabilizer RCTs. None of these showed a significant intergroup difference. Similarly, Hirota et al.'s (2014) meta-analysis of antiepileptic medication in ASD found no significant intergroup difference. Although many side effects were reported among participants in both the intervention and the control group, they rarely showed any statistically significant intergroup difference.

Only one study followed up participants for 6 months, and this showed improvement in both groups of psychoeducation alone versus psychoeducation combined with levetiracetam (Wang et al., 2017). This study, however, was not a placebo-controlled double-blind study. The rest of the studies followed up participants for a short period, which may not be enough to see the effect of the intervention. The dosage of mood stabilizers used in the RCTs may not be adequate to detect a small effect size, although a balance has to be struck between the effective dose and the dose causing side effects. In some studies, different scales used to measure the same symptoms came up with inconsistent findings (Hollander et al., 2010). Similarly, inconsistent findings were reported in some studies based on the teacher and the parent scoring on the same scale (Wasserman et al., 2006). Some placebo-controlled RCTs have also shown a strong placebo effect (Belsito et al., 2001; Hellings et al., 2005), thus making the interpretation of data difficult. Despite the anticipated impact of underlying EEG abnormality on emotion and behavior in people with ASD, only one study looked into this (Hollander et al., 2010). According to this study, participants with an EEG abnormality may have responded better than those who did not have an EEG abnormality. However, because of the small number of participants included in this study, no definitive conclusion could be drawn on the effect of EEG abnormality on the behavior of people with ASD.

29.6.2 Practice Implication Guidelines

Despite common use, there is no definitive evidence to support the use of mood stabilizers, including lithium and some antiepileptic medications, in people with ASD to treat emotional and behavioral symptoms. There is very little RCT-based evidence available for these medications. Even the RCTs are small and prone to the risk of bias and show conflicting evidence. Most studies assessed the efficacy of these medications on ASD core symptoms such as restrictive and repetitive behavior, impaired communication, and associated behaviors such as agitation, irritability, and aggression. Despite the hypothesis that the underlying EEG abnormalities, which are not uncommon in people with ASD, even in the absence of clinical seizures, may predispose emotional and behavioral symptoms, no studies have presented data specifically on the effect of these medications on EEG and related behavioral symptoms. No RCT specifically assessed these medications' efficacy on bipolar disorder or other psychiatric disorders. Sodium valproate is contraindicated in women of childbearing age because of its teratogenic effect. Lithium can cause serious side effects, which may be difficult to investigate in some people with ASD. Practitioners should be aware of the side effects these medications can cause and ensure that people with ASD are monitored regularly. Therefore, practitioners should only use these medications with extreme caution and carefully weigh up the desired effect against the side effects of these medications before considering them for people with ASD. Practitioners should also be specialists with additional training and expertise in working with children, adolescents, and adults with ASD.

29.7 References

Aman, M. G., Burrow, W. H., & Wolford, P. L. (1995). The Aberrant Behavior Checklist- Community: Factor validity and effect of subject variables for adults in group homes. *American Journal on Mental Retardation, 100*(3), 293–292.

Aman, M. G., Singh, N. N., Stewart, A. W., & Field, C. J. (1985). The aberrant behaviour checklist: A behaviour rating scale for assessment of treatment effects. *American Journal of Mental Deficiency, 89*, 485–491.

American Psychiatric Association. (1994). *Diagnostic and statistical manual of mental disorders* (4th ed.). Washington, DC: Author.

American Psychiatric Association. (2000). *Diagnostic and statistical manual of mental disorders* (4th ed., text revision). Washington, DC: Author.

American Psychiatric Association. (2013). *Diagnostic and statistical manual of mental disorders* (5th ed.). Washington, DC: Author.

Bachmann, C. J., Manthey, T., Kamp-Becker, I., Glaeske, G., & Hoffmann, F. (2013). Psychopharmacological treatment in children and adolescents with autism spectrum disorders in Germany. *Research in Developmental Disabilities, 34*(9), 2551–2556.

Belsito, K. M., Law, P. A., Kirk, K. S., Landa, R. J., & Zimmerman, A. W. (2001). Lamotrigine therapy for autistic disorder: a randomized, double-blind, placebo- controlled trial. *Journal of Autism and Developmental Disorders, 31*(2), 175–181.

Berney, T., & Deb, S. (2012). Epilepsy in learning disability. In S. Shorvon, R. Guerrini, M. Cook, & S. Lahtoo (Eds.), *Oxford textbook of epilepsy and epileptic seizures: Oxford textbooks in clinical neurology* (pp. 195–199). Oxford: Oxford University Press.

Bertelli, M. O., Azeem, M. W., Underwood, L., Scattoni, M. L., Persico, A. M., Arianna Ricciardello, A., Sappok, T., Bergmann, T., Keller, R., Bianco, A., Corti, S., Miselli, G., Lassi, S., Croce, L., Bradley, E., & Munir, K. (2022). Autism spectrum disorder. In M. O. Bertelli, S. Deb, K. Munir, A. Hassiotis, & L. Salvador-Carulla (Eds.), *Textbook of psychiatry for intellectual disability and autism spectrum disorder* (pp. 369–456). Cham: Springer Nature.

Bertelli, M. O., Deb, S., & Bianco, A. (2022). Rational prescription of psychotropic medications. In M. O. Bertelli, S. Deb, K. Munir, A. Hassiotis, & L. Salvador-Carulla (Eds.), *Textbook of psychiatry for intellectual disability and autism spectrum disorder* (pp. 1121–1138). Cham: Springer Nature. https://doi.org/10.1007/978-3-030-88538-0_49

Brodie, M. J., Besag, F., Ettinger, A. B., Mula, M., Gobbi, G., Comai, S., Aldenkamp, A.P., & Steinhoff, B. J. (2016). Epilepsy, antiepileptic drugs, and aggression: An evidence-based review. *Pharmacological Review, 68*(3), 563–602.

Chaleby, K., & Zawawi, A. (2006). GABA reuptake inhibitor, tiagabine, in treatment of some anxiety symptoms of pervasive developmental disorder. *Arab Journal of Psychiatry, 17*(1), 40–51.

Chen, K. L., Chiang, F. M., Tseng, M. H., Fu, C. P., & Hsieh, C. L. (2011). Responsiveness of the psychoeducational profile-for children with autism spectrum disorders. *Journal of Autism and Developmental Disorders, 41*(12), 1658–1664.

Chez, M. G., Chang, M., Krasne, V., Coughlan, C., Kominsky, M., & Schwartz, A. (2006). Frequency of epileptiform EEG abnormalities in a sequential screening of autistic patients with no known clinical epilepsy from 1996 to 2005. *Epilepsy & Behavior, 8*, 267–271. DOI: 10.1016/j.yebeh.2005.11.001

Conners, C. K., Sitarenos, G., Parker, J. D., & Epstein, J. N. (1998). The revised Conners' Parent Rating Scale (CPRS-R): Factor structure, reliability, and criterion validity. *The Journal of Abnormal Child Psychology, 26*(4), 257–268.x

Coulter, D. A. (1997). Antiepileptic drug cellular mechanisms of action: Where does lamotrigine fit in? *Journal of Child Neurology, 12*(S1), S2–S9.

Coury, D. L., Anagnostou, E., Manning-Courtney, P., Reynolds, A., Cole, L., McCoy, R., Whitaker, A., & Perrin, J. M. (2012). Use of psychotropic medication in children and adolescents with autism spectrum disorders. *Pediatrics, 130*(Suppl. 2), S69–S76. DOI: 10.1542/peds.2012-0900D

Deb, S., Bertelli, M. O., & Rossi, M. (2022c). Psychopharmacology. In M. O. Bertelli, S. Deb, K. Munir, A. Hassiotis, L. Salvador-Carulla (Eds.), *Textbook of psychiatry for intellectual disability and autism spectrum disorder* (pp. 247–280). Cham: Springer Nature. https://doi.org/10.1007/978-3-319-95720-3_11

Deb, S., Farmah, B. K., Arshad, E., Deb, T., Roy, M., & Unwin, G. L. (2014). The effectiveness of aripiprazole in the management of problem behaviour in people with intellectual disabilities, developmental disabilities and/or autistic spectrum disorder: A systematic review. *Research in Developmental Disabilities, 35*(3), 711–725. DOI: 10.1016/j.ridd.2013.12.004.

Deb, S., Perera, B., Krysta, K., Ozer, M., Bertelli, M., Novell, R., Wieland, J., & Sappok, T. (2022a). The European guideline on the assessment and diagnosis of psychiatric disorders in adults with intellectual disabilities. *European Journal of Psychiatry, 36*, 11–25.

Deb, S., Roy, M., Lee, R., Majid, M., Limbu, B., Santambrogio, J., Roy, A., & Bertelli, M.O. (2021). Randomised controlled trials of antidepressant and anti-anxiety medications for people with autism spectrum disorder: Systematic review and meta-analysis. *British Journal of Psychiatry Open, 7*(6), e179, 1–15. DOI: 10.1192/bjo.2021.1003

Deb, S., Roy, M., & Limbu, B. (2022b) Psychopharmacological treatments for psychopathology in people with intellectual disabilities and/or autism spectrum disorder. *British Journal of Psychiatry Advances, 29*, 1–12. https://doi.org/10.1192/bja.2022.61.

Douglas, J. F., Sanders, K. B., Benneyworth, M. H., Smith, J. L., DeJean, V. M., McGrew, S. G., & Veenstra-VanderWeele, J. (2013). Brief report: Retrospective case series of oxcarbazepine for irritability/agitation symptoms in autism spectrum disorder. *Journal of Autism and Developmental Disorders, 43*(5), 1243–1247.

Goodwin, G. M., Haddad, P. M., Ferrier, I. N., Aronson, J. K., Barnes, T. R. H., Cipriani, A., et al. (2016). Evidence-based guidelines for treating bipolar disorder: Revised third edition recommendations from the British Association for Psychopharmacology. *Journal of Psychopharmacology, 30*(6), 495–553.

Guglielmo, R., Ioime, L., Grandinetti, P., & Janiri, L. (2013). Managing disruptive and compulsive behaviors in adult with autistic disorder with Gabapentin. *Journal of Clinical Psychopharmacology, 33*(2), 273–274.

Hartley-McAndrew, M., & Weinstock, A. (2010). Autism spectrum disorder: Correlation between aberrant behaviors, EEG abnormalities and seizures. *Neurology International, 2*, e10. DOI: 10.4081/ni.2010.e10

Hellings, J. A., Weckbaugh, M., Nickel, E. J., Cain, S. E., Zarcone, J. R., Reese, R. M., Hall, S., Ermer, D.J., Tsai, L.Y., Schroeder, S.R., & Cook, E.H. (2005). A double-blind, placebo-controlled study of valproate for aggression in youth with pervasive developmental disorders. *Journal of Child & Adolescent Psychopharmacology, 15*(4), 682–692.

Hirota, T., Veenstra-VanderWeele, J., Hollander, E., & Kishi, T. (2014). Antiepileptic medications in autism spectrum disorder: A systematic review and meta-analysis. *Journal of Autism & Developmental Disorders, 44*(4), 948–957.

Hollander, E., Chaplin, W., Soorya, L., Wasserman, S., Novotny, S., Rusoff, J., Feirsen, N., Pepa, L., & Anagnostou, E. (2010). Divalproex sodium vs placebo for the treatment of irritability in children and adolescents with autism spectrum disorders. *Neuropsychopharmacology, 35*(4), 990–998.

Hollander, E., Soorya, L., Wasserman, S., Esposito, K., Chaplin, W., & Anagnostou, E. (2006). Divalproex sodium vs. placebo in the treatment of repetitive behaviours in autism spectrum disorder. *International Journal of Neuropsychopharmacology, 9*(2), 209–213.

Jadad, A. R., Moore, R. A., Carroll, D., Jenkinson, C., Reynolds, D. J. M., Gavaghan, D. J., McQuay, H.J. (1996). Assessing the quality of reports of randomized clinical trials: Is blinding necessary? *Controlled Clinical Trials, 17*(1), 1–12.

Kanemura, H., Sano, F., Tando, T., Sugita, K., & Aihara, M. (2013). Can EEG characteristics predict development of epilepsy in autistic children? *European Journal of Paediatric Neurology, 17*, 232–237. DOI: 10.1016/j.ejpn.2012.10.002

Kapetanovic, S. (2007). Oxcarbazepine in youths with autistic disorder and significant disruptive behaviors. *American Journal of Psychiatry, 164*(5), 832–833.

Kay, S. R., Wolkenfeld, F., & Murrill, L. M. (1988). Profiles of aggression among psychiatric patients: I. Nature and prevalence. *Journal of Nervous and Mental Disease, 176*(9), 539–546. https://doi.org/10.1097/00005053-198809000-00007

Krug, D. A., Arick, J., & Almond, P. (1980). Behavior checklist for identifying severely handicapped individuals with high levels of autistic behavior. *The Journal of Child Psychology and Psychiatry, 21*, 221–229.

Lai, M. C., Kassee, C., Besney, R., Bonato, S., Hull, L., Mandy, W., Szatmari, P., & Ameis, S.H. (2019). Prevalence of co-occurring mental health diagnoses in the autism population: A systematic review and meta-analysis. *The Lancet Psychiatry, 6*(10), 819–829.

Lai, M. C., Lombardo, M. V., & Baron-Cohen, S. (2014). Autism. *Lancet, 383*, 896–910.

Limbu, B., Deb, S., Roy, M., Lee, R., Roy, A., & Taiwo, O. (2022). Randomised controlled trials of mood stabilisers for people with autism spectrum disorder: Systematic review and meta-analysis. *British Journal of Psychiatry Open, 8*, e52, 1–12. DOI: 10.1192/bjo.2022.18

Linden, A., Best, L., Elise, F., Roberts, D., Branagan, A., Tay, Y. B. E., Cusack, J., Davidson, B., Davidson, I., Hearst, C., Mandy, W., Rai, D., Smith, E., & Gurusamy, K. (2023). Benefits and harms of interventions to improve anxiety, depression, and other mental health outcomes for autistic people: A systematic review and network meta-analysis of randomised controlled trials. *Autism, 27*(1), 7–30. DOI: 10.1177/13623613221117931

Logan, R. W., Ozburn, A. R., Arey, R. N., Ketchesin, K. D., Winquist, A., Crain, A., Tobe, B. T. D., Becker-Krail, D., Jarpe, M. B., Xue, X., Zong, W., Huo, Z., Parekh, P. K., Zhu, X., Fitzgerald, E., Zhang, H., Oliver-Smith, J., DePoy, L. M., Hildebrand, M. A., . . . McClung, C. A. (2021). Valproate reverses mania-like behaviors in mice via preferential targeting of HDAC2. *Molecular Psychiatry, 26*(8), 4066–4084.

Lord, C., Rutter, M., Goode, S., Heemsbergen, J., Jordan, H., Mawhood, L., & Schopler, E. (1989). Autism diagnostic observation schedule: A standardized observation of communicative and social behavior. *Journal of Autism & Developmental Disorders, 19*(2), 185–212.

Lord, C., Rutter, M., & Le Couteur, A. (1994). Autism Diagnostic Interview-Revised: A revised version of a diagnostic interview for caregivers of individuals with possible pervasive developmental disorders. *Journal of Autism & Developmental Disorders, 24*(5), 659–685.

Löscher, W., Klitgaard, H., Roy, E., Twyman, R. E., & Schmidt, D. (2013). New avenues for antiepileptic drug discovery and development. *Nature Reviews, Drug Discovery, 12*, 757–776. DOI: 10.1038/nrd4126

Lugo-Marín, J., Magan-Maganto, M., Rivero-Santana, A., Cuellar-Pompa, L., Alviani, M., Jenaro-Rio, C., et al. (2019). Prevalence of psychiatric disorders in adults with autism spectrum disorder: A systematic review and meta-analysis. *Research in Autism Spectrum Disorders, 59*, 22–33.

Lynch, B. A., Lambeng, N., Nocka, K., PKensel-Hammes, P., Bajjalieh, S. M., Matagne, A., & Fuks, B. (2004). The synaptic vesicle protein SV2A is the binding site for the antiepileptic drug levetiracetam. *Proceedings of the National Academy of Sciences, 101*, 26, 9861–9866.

Mandell, D. S., Morales, K. H., Marcus, S. C., Stahmer, A. C., Doshi, J., & Polsky, D. E. (2008). Psychotropic medication use among Medicaid-enrolled children with autism spectrum disorders. *Pediatrics, 121*(3), e441–e448. DOI: 10.1542/peds.2007-0984

Martsenkovsky, I. (2014). Divalproex sodium and risperidone in the treatment of cognitive, behavioral and social dysfunction in preschool children with PDD and ADHD. *European Neuropsychopharmacology, 24*, S721– S722.

McLean, M. J., Schmutz, M., Wamil, A. W., Olpe, H-R., Portet, C., & Feldmann, K. F. (1994). Oxcarbazepine: Mechanisms of action. *Epilepsia, 35*(S3), S5–S9.

Meldrum, B. S., & Chapman, A. G. (1999). Basic mechanisms of gabitril (tiagabine) and future potential developments. *Epilepsia, 40*(S9), S2–S6.

Murray, M. L., Hsia, Y., Glaser, K., Simonoff, E., Murphy, D. G. M., Asherson, P. J., Eklund, H., & Wong, I.C. (2014). Pharmacological treatments prescribed to people with autism spectrum disorder (ASD) in primary health care. *Psychopharmacology, 231*(6), 1011–1021. DOI: 10.1007/s00213-013-3140

National Institute of Mental Health. (1985). CGI Clinical Global Impression Scale-NIMH. *Psychopharmacology Bulletin, 21*, 839–844.

Rezaei, V., Mohammadi, M. R., Ghanizadeh, A., Sahraian, A., Tabrizi, M., Rezazadeh, S. A., & Akhondzadeh, S. (2010). Double-blind, placebo-controlled trial of risperidone plus topiramate in children with autistic disorder. *Progress in Neuro-Psychopharmacology & Biological Psychiatry, 34*(7), 1269–1272.

Rosenfeld, W. E. (1997). Topiramate: A review of preclinicai, pharmacokinetic, and clinical data. *Clinical Therapeutics, 19*(6), 1294–1308.

Scahill, L., Riddle, M. A., McSwiggin-Hardin, M., Ort, S. I., King, R. A., Goodman, W. K., et al. (1997). Children's Yale-Brown obsessive compulsive scale: Reliability and validity. *Journal of the American Academy of Child & Adolescent Psychiatry, 36*(6), 844–852.

Schopler, E., Reichler, R. J., DeVellis, R. F., & Daly, K. (1980). Toward objective classification of childhood autism: Childhood Autism Rating Scale (CARS). *Journal of Autism & Developmental Disorders, 10*(1), 91–103.

Siegel, M., Beresford, C. A., Bunker, M., Verdi, M., Vishnevetsky, D., Karlsson, C., Teer, O., Stedman, A., & Smith, K.A. (2014). Preliminary investigation of lithium for mood disorder symptoms in children and adolescents with autism spectrum disorder. *Journal of Child & Adolescent Psychopharmacology, 24*(7), 399–402.

Simonoff, E., Pickles, A., Charman, T., Chandler, S., Loucas, T., & Baird, G. (2008). Psychiatric disorders in children with autism spectrum disorders: Prevalence, comorbidity, and associated factors in a population-derived sample. *Journal of the American Academy of Child & Adolescent Psychiatry, 47*(8), 921–929.

Sparrow, S. S., Balla, D., & Cicchetti, D. V. (1984). *Vineland adaptive behavior scales* (Survey ed.). Circle Pines, MN: American Guidance Service.

Spence, S. J., & Schneider, M. T. (2009). The role of epilepsy and epileptiform EEGs in autism spectrum disorders. *Pediatric Research, 65*, 599–606. DOI: 10.1203/PDR.0b013e31819e7168

Viamontes, C. G., Gonzalez, J. C., Najjar, F., & Cook, F. H. (2022). Maternal duplication 15q11-13 syndrome with autism spectrum disorder: Mood stabilization by carbamazepine. *Journal of Child & Adolescent Psychopharmacology, 32*(2), 122–126. DOI: 10.1089/cap.2021.0046

Wada, A., Yokoo, H., Yanagita, T., & Kobayashi, H. (2005). Lithium: Potential therapeutics against acute brain injuries and chronic neurodegenerative diseases. *Journal of Pharmacological Sciences, 99*, 307–321.

Wang, M., Jiang, L., & Tang, X. (2017). Levetiracetam is associated with decrease in subclinical epileptiform discharges and improved cognitive functions in pediatric patients with autism spectrum disorder. *Neuropsychiatric Disease & Treatment, 13*, 2321.

Wasserman, S., Iyengar, R., Chaplin, W. F., Watner, D., Waldoks, S. E., Anagnostou, E., Soorya, L., & Hollander, E. (2006). Levetiracetam versus placebo in childhood and adolescent autism: A double-blind placebo-controlled study. *International Clinical Psychopharmacology, 21*(6), 363–367.

Young, R. C., Biggs, J. T., Ziegler, V. E., & Meyer, D. A. (1978). A rating scale for mania: Reliability, validity and sensitivity. *The British Journal of Psychiatry, 133*(5), 429–435.

Yudofsky, S. C., Silver, J. M., Jackson, W., Endicott, J., & Williams, D. (1986). The Overt Aggression Scale for the objective rating of verbal and physical aggression. *The American Journal of Psychiatry, 143*(1), 35–39.

30

Melatonin for Sleep Problems

Camille Blouet
Faculté de Médecine, Pôle de Formation et de Recherche en Santé, Université de Caen Normandie, France

Edgar Moussaoui
Centre Ressources Autisme Calvados-Orne-Manche, Service de Psychiatrie de L'Enfant et de L'Adolescent du CHU de Caen, France

Fabian Guénolé
Service de Psychiatrie de L'Enfant et de L'Adolescent du CHU de Caen, France; Faculté de Médecine, Pôle de Formation et de Recherche en Santé, Université de Caen Normandie, France

30.1 Technical Abstract

Background: Melatonin is a neurohormone with circadian rhythm and hypnotic effects, whose secretion may be reduced in autism spectrum disorder (ASD). Exogenous melatonin has proved effective in several types of sleep disturbance in children and adults, and it has been proposed to treat sleep problems in ASD. It is administered orally, generally in the evening before bedtime, in the form of immediate-release (IR) melatonin, which is active during the first third of the night, or controlled-release (CR) melatonin, which is active during the whole night. **Method:** A review of efficacy and safety of melatonin for sleep problems in ASD was performed, on the basis of a Pubmed® documentary search, supplemented by manual review of references. **Results:** IR and CR melatonin are effective for treating idiopathic sleep initiation problems in children and adolescents with ASD; also, CR melatonin can be effective for treating sleep maintenance problems. Melatonin is safe and well tolerated. **Discussion:** Very few data exist in adults with ASD, and also for complex sleep disturbances. Also, a relapse of sleep problems when treatment is stopped may occur, and little is known about long-term treatment. **Practitioner recommendations:** Melatonin is effective and safe for treating common sleep problems in ASD, with adequate initial medical assessment.

30.2 Layperson Summary

Melatonin is a neurohormone. It is secreted by the pineal gland at the base of the brain. Melatonin helps sleep onset and continuity. It has been researched for

Camille Blouet, Edgar Moussaoui, and Fabian Guénolé, *Melatonin for Sleep Problems*. In: *Lifespan Treatment for Autistic Individuals*. Edited by: Peter Sturmey, Russell Lang, and James K. Luiselli, Oxford University Press. © Oxford University Press (2025). DOI: 10.1093/cso/9780197635841.003.0030 around 30 years for treating sleep problems. Sleep problems are very common in children and adults with ASD. Melatonin is taken by mouth in the evening before bedtime. This is done using IR melatonin. IR melatonin is active only during the first third of the night. It is also given as CR melatonin, which is active throughout the night. Melatonin is available over the counter in most countries. Its use for sleep problems in a person with ASD requires an indication by a physician. This is based on a comprehensive diagnosis. The comprehensive diagnosis must consider general medical causes. These include pain, anxiety, and gastrointestinal disturbances. The evaluation should also include specific medical causes, including sleep apnea, parasomnia, and sleep epilepsy. Sometimes further investigation may be needed. Only sleep problems which did not improve by nonpharmacological management require treatment with melatonin. Nonpharmacological treatments include sleep hygiene and behavioral interventions. Case reports, retrospective group studies, open-label clinical trials, and placebo-controlled trials have been published. They provide good insight into the effects of melatonin for common sleep problems in children and adolescents with ASD. IR and CR melatonin are good treatments for children and adolescents who have difficulty falling asleep. CR melatonin can also be a good treatment for awakenings and difficulty falling back to sleep during the night. Both are safe and well tolerated; only daytime somnolence and headache can sometimes occur as side effects. There are insufficient data for adults and for more complex sleep problems to be confident about effectiveness. A reappearance of sleep problems is possible when treatment is stopped, which can sometimes lead to its long-term prolongation.

30.3 Treatment Summary Table

Treatment summary: Melatonin

Treatment description: Melatonin is a neurohormone with circadian rhythm and hypnotic effects; its secretion may be reduced in individuals with ASD. Exogenous melatonin is administered orally, generally in the evening before bedtime, in the form of IR melatonin, which is active during the first third of the night, or CR melatonin, which covers a whole night.

Expected outcomes: IR and CR melatonin are effective for treating idiopathic sleep initiation problems in children and adolescents with ASD; also, CR melatonin can be effective for treating sleep maintenance problems.

Methods: After a comprehensive medical assessment, daily oral (30 minutes to 1 hour before desired bedtime) IR or CR melatonin can be used for idiopathic sleep initiation problems which have not responded to adequate nonpharmacological intervention such as sleep hygiene and behavioral interventions. In these cases, IR melatonin can be started at a dose of 0.5 mg, which can be doubled after at least 2 weeks, if necessary, up to 4 mg, or rarely more. CR melatonin, which is used also for sleep maintenance problems, can be started at a dose of 1 mg and progressively increased, if necessary, up to 10 mg/day at most.

Expertise required to implement treatment: Medical doctor.

Risks and negative side effects: Daytime sleepiness, headache.

Additional considerations and limitations: Very few data exist in adults, and also for complex sleep disturbances. Also, a reappearance of sleep problems when treatment is stopped is not excluded, and little is known about very long-term treatment.

30.4 Introduction

30.4.1 Treatment Description

Known since the late 1950s, melatonin (or 5-methoxy-N-acetyl-tryptamine) is a small endogenous hormone in vertebrates (Reiter & Tan, 2014); its name comes from the Greek μέλας, which means "black" (melatonin has a skin pigmentation effect in frogs), and from its chemical similarity to serotonin. Melatonin is a neurohormone, secreted mainly by an endocrine gland located at the base of the brain, the pineal gland.

In humans, the pineal secretion of melatonin begins in the first months of life and is inhibited by light (as in all diurnal vertebrates). It is also secreted in the gastrointestinal tract, in lungs, kidneys, and retina, but without being affected by light. The biosynthesis of melatonin starts from tryptophan, an essential amino acid provided by food, which is transformed into serotonin and then into melatonin through a series of enzymatic reactions. The enzymes involved in this synthesis are disinhibited when the activity of the retino-hypothalamic tract decreases with darkness, and pineal melatonin is then released into the bloodstream, at concentrations of the order of a few tens of pictograms per milliliter. Melatonin is metabolized in the liver (CYP1A2 and CYP2C19), mainly into 6-sulphatoxymelatoninare, which is excreted through the urine (Karasek & Winczyk, 2006).

Melatonin has a so-called chronobiotic effect on circadian rhythms, its nocturnal secretion peak being one of the components of the photic factor for synchronizing the endogenous circadian rhythm of the internal clock (Claustrat et al., 2005). This effect on the sleep/wake rhythm occurs via the strong affinity of melatonin for the membrane receptor MT1 (or Mel1A), the activation of which influences the intracellular activity of adenylate cyclase in the suprachiasmatic nuclei of the anterior hypothalamus (Ekmekcioglu, 2006). Melatonin also has a hypnotic effect; that is, it directly promotes sleep (Tzischinsky & Lavie, 1994) via the activation of the MT1 receptor again, and probably also that of the GABA-A receptor (Wang et al., 2003). Finally, melatonin has effects in other physiological domains, for instance on immune modulation, bone growth, or gastrointestinal motility (Slominskiet al., 2012).

The oral administration of exogenous melatonin has been studied for several decades, specifically for the treatment of various sleep disturbances (Tordjman et al., 2017). From a pharmacokinetic point of view, a fairly low absorption and a hepatic first-pass effect are observed, which means that the bioavailability of melatonin is considered to be low (around 10%); nevertheless, its administration at the usual doses (0.5 to 10 mg/day) produces plasma concentrations 10 to 100 times higher than the values of the endogenous peak.

There are two formulations available: immediate-release (IR) melatonin, which is the most common one, and sustained-release (SR) melatonin. IR melatonin reaches its plasma peak 30 to 45 minutes after administration, and it has a half-life just under an hour, so the product has no hypnotic effect beyond the first third of the night. SR melatonin is generally combined with the IR one, to form CR melatonin, whose precise pharmacokinetic properties depend on the proprietary medical product used; it generally has a slightly delayed peak of absorption compared to IR melatonin, followed by a plateau lasting several hours and possibly covering a whole night.

Melatonin has proved effective in several dyssomnias (disruption of sleep), parasomnias (abnormal behavior during sleep such as night terrors and sleepwalking), and sleep/wake rhythm disturbances of children and adults (Tordjman et al., 2017). It is usually taken within an hour before bedtime or during the day in certain sleep/wake rhythm disturbances (phase delay or advance). Its tolerability is generally very good, with adverse effects rarely reported. No clinically significant drug interaction is described, except the fact that enzymatic inductors and inhibitors may affect melatonin blood levels. People who are low CYP1A2/CYP2C19 metabolizers (~10% of people) may require lowered doses (Braam et al., 2010).

30.4.2 Rationale and Objectives

Sleep problems are common in individuals with ASD. Indeed, the prevalence rate of sleep problems in this population ranges from 43% to as high as 83% (Richdale & Schreck, 2009), and it is one of the most frequent management problems reported by parents (Konstantareas & Homatidis, 1989). As in typically developing children, poor sleep in ASD may lead to excessive daytime sleepiness, cognitive impairment, and impaired daytime functioning (Richdale & Schreck, 2009). Sleep problems in children with ASD also dramatically alter the sleep of their parents and are associated with family stress (Doo & Wing, 2006), possibly amplifying ASD symptoms and interfering with treatment (Glickman, 2009).

Several studies have aimed at characterizing sleep problems associated with ASD (Richdale & Schreck, 2009). The most frequently reported problems are settling difficulties, long sleep latencies, frequent/long nocturnal awakenings, and early-morning awakenings. It has been proposed that poor sleep in ASD is caused by a circadian rhythm disturbance (Richdale & Schreck, 2009). For example, settling and sleep onset difficulties could be linked to phase delay, early morning awakening to phase advance (Glickman, 2009), and nocturnal awakenings to an impaired nocturnal stability of the circadian clock.

Studies of melatonin in individuals with ASD showed reduced secretion (Lalanne et al., 2021). Also, Leu et al. (2010) found a positive correlation between urinary excretion rates of melatonin metabolites and proportions of NREM sleep stage 3, a deep stage of sleep, over total sleep time in children with ASD. These observations have led to the hypothesis that impaired quantities or patterns of melatonin secretion could be responsible for some of the sleep disturbances described in ASD. On this basis, and based also on its chronobiotic and hypnotic properties, exogenous melatonin has been proposed to treat sleep problems in ASD.

30.4.3 Considerations for Implementation

Although melatonin is listed among food supplements in some countries, and is generally available over the counter, its use for sleep problems in a person with ASD requires an indication by a physician, following a comprehensive diagnostic procedure. Indeed, as for any patient presenting with a sleep disturbance, various general (e.g., pain, anxiety, gastrointestinal disturbances) or specific medical causes (e.g., sleep apnea, parasomnia, morpheic epilepsy) must first be considered, and sometimes further investigated. Only cases of idiopathic dyssomnia with no behavioral cause found, and not sufficiently improved by sleep hygiene measures and other appropriate nonpharmacological management, constitute full and complete indications for treatment with melatonin.

Melatonin is taken orally, usually in the evening, up to an hour before bedtime. It can be IR, SR, or CR melatonin (or possibly a combination of two or all three of these forms). Some people with ASD often have difficulty accepting oral medications or swallowing them, especially children and when developmental disabilities are severe. IR melatonin is prepared in capsules, which can be opened and the contents put into food (such as yogurt or fruit juice). CR melatonin only exists in tablets, which are often quite large and can only be divided in halves without losing their pharmacokinetic properties (Chua et al., 2016), which may make it impossible to use in people with ASD. However, a miniature (3 mm) CR melatonin formulation has been developed in recent years (PedPRM; Slenyto® Neurim Pharmaceuticals Ltd.), which is well accepted in this population (Thomson et al., 2009).

30.5 Research Background

30.5.1 Case Reports and Single-Case Studies

The first data on the use of melatonin for sleep problems in ASD were brief single-case reports on children with treatment-resistant sleep problems, which showed sleep improvement for several months with IR melatonin, without side effects (Horrigan & Barnhill, 1997; Jan et al., 1994). Hayashi (2000) reported actigraphy data in a 14-year-old boy with autistic disorder and severe intellectual disability, whose sleep was characterized by a tendency toward phase delay with polyphasic sleep (two or more periods of sleep per day). After 1 month of IR melatonin 6 mg every evening at 9:00 p.m., sleep problems improved moderately. Melatonin was then given 2 hours later (11:00 p.m.) and sleep problems improved significantly, together with increased sleep duration, for the 4 follow-up months, with no reported side effects. Jan et al. reported the case of a 12-year-old boy with ASD without intellectual disability, who suffered from complex sleep disturbances, including chronic sleep phase delay and parasomnias (night terrors and sleepwalking). Treatment with CR melatonin 5 mg, given 30 minutes before desired bedtime, was associated with a normalization of the sleep/wake rhythm, disappearance of parasomnias, and no side effects for the complete follow-up period of 6 months (Jan et al., 2004).

More recently, Zucolo et al. (2017) studied another case of chronic phase delay in an 11-year-old boy with ASD without intellectual disability, whose sleep/wake rhythm disorder improved after 2 weeks of IR melatonin 3 mg, given 30 minutes before desired bedtime, with no reported side effect.

In summary, case reports and single-case studies suggested that melatonin in the evening may be useful in treating resistant sleep problems in children and adolescents with ASD, including problems due to phase delay and NREM parasomnias, with good tolerability in the short and medium term.

30.5.2 Retrospective Group Studies

In a short paper, Gupta and Hutchins (2005) reviewed nine cases of children with autistic disorder (2–11 years), who were treated for chronic sleep problems, using IR melatonin 2.5–5 mg per day, 45 minutes before desired bedtime. Parental reports indicated an improvement in total sleep duration in five of the cases (56%), without adverse effects.

Subsequently, Andersen et al. (2008) performed a retrospective review of melatonin use for sleep problems in 107 children and adolescents diagnosed with ASD. Patients were aged 2–18 years, and 45 of them (42%) were medication-free before melatonin was started. Melatonin (IR in 91% of the cases) was given 30–60 minutes before desired bedtime; the initial dose was 1–1.5 mg, and it was increased up to 6 mg when required. Sleep was evaluated for several months up to years (mean: 1.8 ± 1.4 years) via parental reports upon follow-up visits. A majority of parents reported an improvement in sleep: Twenty-five percent reported a full improvement, and 60% reported a partial one. In seven (6.5%) cases, the beneficial effects of melatonin were reported to stop after 3 to 12 months, despite the use of higher doses. According to parental reports, side effects were observed in three children (2.8%): morning sleepiness (n = 1), "fogginess" (n = 1), and increased nocturnal enuresis ($n = 1$). Though 25% of children had a history of epilepsy, no increases in seizures or new-onset seizures were reported.

Finally, Galli-Carminati et al. (2009) published a retrospective analysis on six adult patients (19–52 years old, mean = 39 years) diagnosed with autistic disorder and moderate to severe intellectual disability, who displayed sleep problems. IR melatonin 3 mg was taken 45 minutes before desired bedtime and increased to 6–9 mg after several weeks when clinically required. Sleep onset latency decreased in one case, sleep duration increased in three cases, nocturnal wanderings stopped in two cases, and early-morning awakening disappeared in two cases; no side effects were reported.

In summary, retrospective group studies confirmed that melatonin (1–9 mg) may durably improve sleep problems in patients with ASD—particularly children and adolescents and with few data in adults—with good tolerability.

30.5.3 Open-Label Clinical Trials

Paavonen et al. (2003) conducted the first prospective trial of melatonin for sleep problems in children and adolescents with ASD of mild to moderate intensity. This study involved 15 children aged 6–17 years presenting with severe sleep problems for at least 3 months. IR melatonin 3 mg was given for 14 consecutive days, 30 minutes before the children's desired bedtime. Patients did not receive any other psychotropic medication during the study. Sleep was assessed by wrist actigraphy for three continuous 72-hour periods: before treatment, 10 days after the beginning of medication, and 3 weeks after its discontinuation. Daytime sleepiness and behavior of the children were assessed using appropriate psychometric scales, their sleep was evaluated with actigraphy, and the sleep of parents was measured with diaries. Actigraphy results showed that melatonin treatment was associated with a significant decrease in sleep onset latency and mean nocturnal activity of the children, but number of awakenings significantly increased (without affecting total sleep time and sleep efficiency). Discontinuation of melatonin led to a significant decrease in sleep duration and more nocturnal activity. The parents' sleep did not change throughout the study. No significant difference was noted on daytime sleepiness during and after treatment; a significant but mild improvement of daytime behavior was observed. Potential side effects were reported for three children (20%). Two felt tired, one of whom complained of headaches during the first 2 days of treatment. The third child withdrew from the study because of severe daytime sleepiness, dizziness, and diarrhea, all of which stopped immediately after melatonin discontinuation.

A long-term clinical trial of melatonin in ASD was performed by Giannotti et al. (2006). Participants were 29 children aged 2–9 years, diagnosed with autistic disorder and presenting with current sleep problems. All were free from medication for at least 6 months, and none had ever received melatonin. Daily CR melatonin was initiated at 3 mg taken at 8:00 pm for 6 months. Doses were adjusted upon follow-up visits during the study, up to a maximum of 6 mg. Assessment of sleep included sleep diaries and the Children Sleep Habits Questionnaire, both completed by parents. Measures were taken at seven time points: at baseline; after 1, 3, and 6 months of treatment with melatonin; and 1, 12, and 24 months after melatonin was discontinued. Melatonin treatment could be reinstated 1 month after discontinuation if clinically required. Twenty patients (69%) completed the entire trial, and 25 patients (86%) were available at 6 initial months follow-up. Melatonin was associated with improvement on sleep onset latency, night wakings, and sleep duration as measured by the Children Sleep Habits Questionnaire. The diaries also showed significant increases in total sleep time and decreases in wake after sleep onset, but sleep onset latency was not examined. No side effects were noted. Sleep improvements generally vanished after melatonin was discontinued. Those children who maintained improved sleep without melatonin were found to be those with significantly lower baseline scores on the Children Sleep Habits Questionnaire, suggesting that the children needing longer-term melatonin treatment were those with the more severe sleep problems.

In another study, Malow et al. (2012) studied dose-response, using a dose-escalation paradigm. This study evaluated 24 children aged 3–10 years with ASD who displayed sleep initiation problems and were free of psychotropic medication. After several weeks of baseline assessment, during which a careful clinical assessment regarding sleep problems was conducted and parents received a session of structured sleep education, children received daily IR melatonin at 1 mg 30 minutes before desired bedtime for 3 weeks, which could be increased to 3, 6, and 9 mg in case of insufficient clinical response. This was done using 3-week intervals and for a total duration of 14 weeks. Effects on sleep were measured primarily by actigraphy; parental questionnaires were added as secondary measures. Results showed a significant and prolonged improvement in sleep latency from the first week of taking melatonin at optimal dose, which ranged from 1 to 6 mg for all participants, with a majority (87%) of children responding to 3 mg or less. Sleep duration, wake time after sleep onset, and sleep efficiency were not significantly different with melatonin treatment. Regarding secondary measures, the Withdrawn, Affective, and Attention Deficit Hyperactivity Disorder subscales of the Child Behavior Checklist, as well as the Stereotyped and Compulsive subscales of the Repetitive Behavior Scale, and the Difficult Child subscale of the Parenting Stress Index, improved significantly with treatment. Only one child exhibited possible mild adverse effects related to the melatonin preparation (loose stools).

Another long-term clinical trial was conducted by Yuge et al. (2020). Participants were 99 children and adolescents aged 6–15 years with neurodevelopmental disorders and chronic sleep onset insomnia. Seventy-four (75%) were diagnosed with ASD. Other patients displayed various other neurodevelopmental disorders, such as intellectual disability, attention-deficit/hyperactivity disorder, or learning disorders. IR melatonin 1 mg was given for 26 consecutive weeks, 45 minutes before desired bedtime; doses were adjusted upon follow-up visits during the study, up to a maximum of 4 mg. The main objective was to compare sleep onset latency before treatment and after 10 weeks of treatment, using sleep diaries. Ninety-three patients (94.9%) completed the entire study. A significant shortening of sleep onset latency (–36.8 minutes) was observed in ASD patients at 10 weeks. A similar improvement was seen for the whole sample as early as 2 weeks into treatment, and until its discontinuation. The tolerability and safety of melatonin were considered good, with only mild adverse events.

In summary, open-label clinical trials suggest that continuous daily intake of melatonin (1–6 mg) in the evening durably improves sleep initiation problems in children and adolescents with ASD, with good tolerability. CR melatonin (3–6 mg) may also be efficacious to improve sleep maintenance problems. It seems that sleep problems tend to reappear after melatonin discontinuation, particularly in severe cases. Finally, daytime behavior of children and adolescents could be more or less improved during treatment.

30.5.4 Placebo-Controlled Trials

Garstang and Wallis (2006) conducted the first placebo-controlled trial of melatonin for sleep problems in individuals with ASD. It was a randomized double-blind crossover trial, with patients receiving IR melatonin 5 mg or placebo for two periods of 4 weeks separated by 1 week of washout. Melatonin was given 1 hour before desired bedtime. Eleven children and adolescents (4–16 years) with ASD were recruited via community and hospital physicians, special schools, and a family association. All had chronic sleep problems resistant to behavioral treatment. While some of the participants were already taking sedative medication before entering the study, the regimen was the same for at least the previous 4 weeks, and no patient had received melatonin in the past. Sleep variables were collected before and during treatment using sleep diaries, completed by parents. Seven children (64%) completed the protocol. It was found that both melatonin and placebo were associated with shortened sleep latency, decreased nocturnal awakenings, and increased total sleep time, but results showed a significantly greater improvement under melatonin than placebo. No adverse effects were identified.

Wirojanan et al. (2009) performed a second placebo-controlled trial. Eighteen unmedicated children and adolescents aged 2–15 years, presenting unspecified sleep problems and with idiopathic ASD ($n = 8$), syndromic ASD associated with fragile X syndrome ($n = 4$), or fragile X syndrome without ASD ($n = 6$) entered a 4-week randomized double-blind crossover trial. After 1 week of baseline assessment, children received IR melatonin 3 mg or placebo 30 minutes before desired bedtime, for two consecutive blocks of 2 weeks, without any washout interval between crossovers. Sleep was continuously monitored with wrist actigraphy. Because of missing data, only 12 subjects (66%) were included in the analysis,

8 of whom (66%) received melatonin first, thus introducing the possibility of an order bias. Results showed a mild but significant increase in total sleep time (+21 minutes) during melatonin treatment, together with a significant decrease in sleep latency (−28 minutes) and advance of sleep onset time (−42 minutes). The number of nocturnal awakenings did not differ statistically between treatment conditions and total duration of wake after sleep onset was not investigated. Because of small sample sizes, results obtained in ASD participants were not analyzed separately. No side effects were observed during the study.

In another randomized controlled trial, Wright et al. (2010) studied 20 children and adolescents aged 4–16 years with ASD and presenting with chronic sleeplessness not amenable to behavioral management participated. Children were free of psychotropic medication and never received melatonin before entering the protocol. The study was a randomized double-blind crossover trial, with patients receiving IR melatonin 2 mg or placebo for two periods of 3 months separated by 1 month of washout. Melatonin was administered 30–40 minutes before desired bedtime and doses were increased according to clinical response, up to 10 mg/day. Sleep variables were measured before and during treatment using sleep diaries. Sixteen participants (80%) completed the protocol, a high rate relative to previous publications. Compared to placebo, melatonin was associated with a significantly shorter sleep latency (−52 versus −10 minutes) and longer sleep duration (+56 versus +8 minutes). The number of nocturnal awakenings was not decreased with melatonin as it could have been expected. It should however be noted that it is not the number of awakenings, but their durations that mostly interferes with sleep in ASD (Guénolé & Baleyte, 2011; Richdale & Schreck, 2009). Behavioral difficulties in the children and general health of the parents showed no significant differences between melatonin and placebo. The melatonin treatment phase showed no serious adverse events, and the tolerability profiles for melatonin and placebo were the same.

Cortesi et al. (2012) conducted the first randomized controlled trial of CR melatonin in ASD, among 160 children aged 4–10 years who displayed chronic sleep onset and maintenance insomnia and were free from psychotropic medication, 84% of whom completed the study. Participants were randomly assigned into four groups: (1) daily CR melatonin at 3 mg (1-mg IR and 2-mg SR melatonin; Armonia® Retard 3 mg; Nathura, Montecchio Emilia, Italy) at 9:00 p.m. (n = 34); (2) a four-session sleep-focused cognitive-behavior therapy (CBT; n = 33); (3) both treatments combined (n = 35); or (4) placebo (n = 32). Sleep was assessed principally by actigraphy, at baseline, and after 12 weeks of trial. Results showed significant improvements in sleep latency, total sleep time, wake after sleep onset, and sleep efficiency in the three treatment groups, compared to placebo. Greater improvements occurred in the combined melatonin-CBT group, which reached statistical significance for sleep latency only. Melatonin therapy alone was significantly more effective than CBT alone in increasing sleep latency. No adverse effects and biological abnormalities were observed.

The efficacy of pediatric prolonged-release melatonin (CR) for sleep problems in children with ASD was investigated in a multicenter, 13-week, randomized placebo-controlled trial, followed by a long-term, open-label treatment phase (Gringras et al., 2017). One hundred and twenty-five children and adolescents (2–17 years) were included in the study. All had significant chronic problems in sleep maintenance and/or initiation not amenable to nonpharmacological intervention. The starting dose was 2 mg daily 30–60 minutes before bedtime. Sleep was assessed after 3 weeks of treatment using a sleep diary, and the dose could be increased to 5 mg, if necessary. Sleep was then assessed with a sleep diary after the 13 weeks double-blind treatment period, after which all completers then entered a 90-week open-label pediatric prolonged-release melatonin phase (2 or 5 mg/day), including dose optimization after 13 weeks (2, 5, or 10 mg/day), with sleep diary assessment at several times of follow-up. Seventy-six percent of patients completed the placebo-controlled phase, and 84% of these participants also completed the open-label phase. Compared to placebo, sleep latency and duration significantly improved with pediatric prolonged-release melatonin during the first 3 months of treatment, which was maintained at 39 weeks follow-up (Maras et al., 2018). Children's behavioral problems according to the Strengths and Difficulties Questionnaire's score and subscores did not significantly improve; however, externalizing behavioral problems significantly improved in subpopulations with abnormal baseline scores on some subscales (Schroder et al., 2019). Parents' well-being (WHO-Five Well-Being Scale) significantly improved with pediatric prolonged-release melatonin versus placebo, and its change significantly correlated with the total Strengths and Difficulties Questionnaire score (Schroder et al., 2019). Somnolence and headache were significant adverse events of pediatric prolonged-release melatonin, but there were no unexpected safety issues reported (Malow et al., 2021).

Finally, Hayashi et al. (2022) recently reported on a multicenter, 14-day, randomized placebo-controlled trial of IR melatonin in children with ASD and chronic sleep initiation problems, followed by a medium-term open-label treatment phase. One hundred and ninety-six children aged 6–15 years were randomly assigned to three groups: (1) IR melatonin at 1 mg (n = 65); (2) IR melatonin at 4 mg (n = 65); or (3) placebo (n = 66). Each dose was administered daily, 45 minutes before bedtime. This initial phase was followed by a 42-day open-label phase, during which all children received IR melatonin, at 1, 2, or 4 mg, according to a weekly titration procedure. Efficacy was tested principally using the change in sleep latency on sleep diaries. Sleep latency significantly decreased for the two melatonin groups compared to placebo, without significant difference between both melatonin groups. Sleep latency also decreased during the open-label phase in the melatonin groups. Actigraphy measures during the placebo-controlled phase showed no effect of treatment on total sleep time or wake after sleep onset. Behavioral problems, assessed with the Aberrant Behavior Checklist, did not significantly change during the placebo-controlled phase but significantly improved during the open-label one. No serious adverse events were reported.

In summary, results of placebo-controlled trials confirm that IR melatonin durably improves sleep latency in children and adolescents with sleep initiation problems, with 1 to 4 mg being generally adequate doses. Research has also confirmed that only CR melatonin (2–10 mg) may have some effects on sleep maintenance problems, although this result seems less consistent. Another conclusion is that children and adolescents' daytime behavior can improve somewhat during treatment following improvement of sleep problems. Melatonin is well tolerated, and it did not pose any safety problem, either in the short or long term. The question remains, however, as to whether the sleep problems reappear when the treatment is stopped. Finally, it can be noted that no data from placebo-controlled trials currently exist for adult patients, and that parasomnia and sleep/wake rhythm disorders have not been specifically investigated.

30.6 Practice Implications

30.6.1 Treatment Outcomes

IR and CR melatonin are good treatments for idiopathic sleep initiation problems in children and adolescents with ASD, and CR melatonin can be an effective treatment for sleep maintenance problems. Melatonin is safe and well tolerated, with no important contraindications. Nevertheless, it is necessary that its use be established by a physician, in order not to overlook a cause requiring different treatment, and to ensure that appropriate nonpharmacological measures are tried beforehand. Limitations are that very few data exist in adults, and also for complex sleep disturbances (e.g., combed dyssomnia and parasomnia, sleep/wake rhythm disturbance, or nocturnal emotional/behavioral problems). Finally, the necessary duration of treatment is not well defined, and a reemergence of sleep problems when treatment is stopped is not excluded.

30.6.2 Practice Implication Guidelines

After a comprehensive medical assessment, daily oral (30 minutes to 1 hour before desired bedtime) IR or CR melatonin can be used for idiopathic sleep initiation problems not amenable to adequate nonpharmacological measures. In these cases, IR melatonin can be started at a dose of 0.5 mg, which can be doubled after at least 2 weeks, if necessary, up to 4 mg, or rarely a higher dose. CR melatonin, which is used also for sleep maintenance problems, can be started at a dose of 1 mg, and progressively increased, if necessary, up to 10 mg/day at most. Efficacy is monitored clinically, using a sleep diary, and tolerability by exploring the presence of daytime sleepiness and of headache. Given the indication for chronic problems, it seems reasonable to consider treatment at its optimal dose for about 3 months, after which tapering or discontinuation may be attempted. Though no withdrawal syndrome per se has been described, sleep problems can reappear when treatment is stopped; in such a case, its reinitiation, at the optimal prior dose, seems legitimate, for a longer period, which can be around 1 year as little is known to date about longer durations.

30.7 References

Andersen, I., Kaczmarska, J., McGrew, S., & Malow B. (2008). Melatonin for insomnia in children with autism spectrum disorders. *Journal of Child Neurology, 23*(5), 482–485.

Braam, W., Van Geijlswijk, I., Keijzer, H., Smits, M. G., Didden, R., & Curfs, L. M. (2010). Loss of response to melatonin treatment is associated with slow melatonin metabolism. *Journal of Intellectual Disability Research, 54*(6), 547–555.

Chua, H. M., Hauet Richer, N., Swedrowska, M., Ingham, S., Tomlin, S., & Forbes, B. (2016). Dissolution of intact, divided and crushed circadin tablets: Prolonged vs. immediate release of melatonin. *Pharmaceutics, 8*(1), 2.

Claustrat, B., Brun, J., & Chazot, G. (2005). The basic physiology and pathophysiology of melatonin. *Sleep Medicine Reviews, 9*(1), 11–24.

Cortesi, F., Giannotti, F., Sebastiani, T., Panunzi, S., & Valente, D. (2012). Controlled-release melatonin, singly and combined with cognitive behavioural therapy, for persistent insomnia in children with autism spectrum disorders: A randomized placebo-controlled trial. *Journal of Sleep Research, 21*(6), 700–709.

Doo, S., & Wing, Y. K. (2006). Sleep problems of children with pervasive developmental disorders: correlation with parental stress. *Developmental Medicine & Child Neurology, 48*(8), 650–655.

Ekmekcioglu, C. (2006). Melatonin receptors in humans: biological role and clinical relevance. *Biomedine Pharmacotherapy, 60*(3):97–108. doi: 10.1016/j.biopha.2006.01.002.

Galli-Carminati, G., Deriaz, N., & Bertschy, G. (2009). Melatonin in the treatment of chronic sleep disorders in adults with autism: A retrospective study. *Swiss Medical Weekly, 139*(19–20), 293–296.

Garstang, J., & Wallis, M. (2006). Randomized controlled trial of melatonin for children with autistic spectrum disorders and sleep problems. *Child: Care, Health & Development, 32*(5), 585–589.

Giannotti, F., Cortesi, F., Cerquiglini, A., & Bernabei, P. (2006). An open-label study of controlled-release melatonin in treatment of sleep disorders in children with autism. *Journal of Autism & Developmental Disorders, 36*, 741–752.

Glickman, G. (2009). Circadian rhythms and sleep in children with autism. *Neuroscience & Biobehavioral Reviews, 34*(5), 755–768.

Gringras, P., Nir, T., Breddy, J., Frydman-Marom, A., & Findling, R. L. (2017). Efficacy and safety of pediatric prolonged-release melatonin for insomnia in children with autism spectrum disorder. *Journal of the American Academy of Child & Adolescent Psychiatry, 56*(11), 948–957.

Guénolé, F., & Baleyte, J. M. (2011). Effectiveness of melatonin for sleep problems in autism spectrum disorders: Evidence grows but research is still needed. *Journal of Autism & Developmental Disorders, 41*, 974–975

Gupta, R., & Hutchins, J. (2005). Melatonin: A panacea for desperate parents? (Hype or truth). *Archives of Disease in Childhood, 90*(9), 986–987.

Hayashi, E. (2000). Effect of melatonin on sleep wake rhythm: The sleep diary of an autistic male. *Psychiatry & Clinical Neurosciences, 54*(3), 383–384.

Hayashi, M., Mishima, K., Fukumizu, M., Takahashi, H., Ishikawa, Y., Hamada, I., Sugioka, H., Yotsuya, O., & Yamashita, Y. (2022). Melatonin treatment and adequate sleep hygiene interventions in children with autism spectrum disorder: A randomized controlled trial. *Journal of Autism & Developmental Disorders, 52*, 2784–2793.

Horrigan, J. P., & Barnhill, L. J. (1997). More on melatonin. *Journal of the American Academy of Child & Adolescent Psychiatry, 36*, 1014.

Jan, J. E., Espezel, H., & Appleton, R. E. (1994). The treatment of sleep disorders with melatonin. *Developmental Medicine & Child Neurology, 36*(2), 97–107.

Jan, J. E., Freeman, R. D., Wasdell, M. B., & Bomben, M. M. (2004). A child with severe night terrors and sleepewaking responds to melatonin therapy. *Developmental Medicine & Child Neurology, 46*(11), 787–789.

Karasek, M., & Winczyk, K. (2006) Melatonin in humans. *Journal of Physiology & Pharmacology, 57*(5), 19–39.

Konstantareas, M. M., & Homatidis, S. (1989). Assessing child symptom severity and stress in parents of autistic children. *Journal of Child Psychology & Psychiatry, 30*(3), 459–470.

Lalanne, S., Fougerou-Leurent, C., Anderson, G. M., Schroder, C. M., Nir, T., Chokron, S., Delorme, R., Claustrat, B., Bellissant, E., Kermarrec, S., Franco, P., Denis, L., & Tordjman, S. (2021). Melatonin: From pharmacokinetics to clinical use in autism spectrum disorder. *International Journal of Molecular Sciences, 22*(3), 1490.

Leu, R. M., Beyderman, L., Botzolakis, E. J., Surdyka, K., Wang, L., & Malow, B. A. (2010). Relation of melatonin to sleep architecture in children with autism. *Journal of Autism & Developmental Disorders, 41*, 427–433.

Malow, B. A., Adkins, K. W., McGrew, S. G., Wang, L., Goldman, S. E., Fawkes, D., & Burnette, C. (2012). Melatonin for sleep in children with autism: A controlled trial examining dose, tolerability, and outcomes. *Journal of Autism & Developmental Disorders, 42*, 1729–1737.

Malow, B. A., Findling, R. L., Schroder, C. M., Maras, A., Breddy, J., Nir, T., Zisapel, N., & Gringras, P. (2021). Sleep, growth, and puberty after 2 years of rolonged-release melatonin in children with autism spectrum disorder. *Journal of the American Academy of Child & Adolescent Psychiatry, 60*(2), 252–261.

Maras, A., Schroder, C. M., Malow, B. A., Findling, R. L., Breddy, J., Nir, T., Shahmoon, S., Zisapel, N., & Gringras, P. (2018). Long-term efficacy and safety of pediatric prolonged-release melatonin for insomnia in children with autism spectrum disorder. *Journal of Child & Adolescent Psychopharmacology, 28*(10), 699–710.

Paavonen, E. J., Nieminen-von Wendt, T., Vanhala, R., Aronen, E. T., & von Wendt, L. (2003). Effectiveness of melatonin in the treatment of sleep disturbances in children with Asperger disorder. *Journal of Child & Adolescent Psychopharmacology, 13*(1), 83–95.

Reiter, R. J., Tan, D. X., & Galano, A. (2014). Melatonin. *Physiology, 29*(5), 325–333.

Richdale, A. L., & Schreck, K. A. (2009). Sleep problems in autism spectrum disorders: Prevalence, nature, and possible biopsychosocial aetiologies. *Sleep Medicine Reviews, 13*(6), 403–411.

Schroder, C. M., Malow, B. A., Maras, A., Melmed, R. D., Findling, R. L., Breddy, J., Nir, T., Shahmoon, S., Zisapel, N., & Gringras, P. (2019). Pediatric prolonged-release melatonin for sleep in children with autism spectrum disorder: Impact on child behavior and caregiver's quality of life. *Journal of Autism & Developmental Disorders, 49*, 3218–3230.

Slominski, R. M., Reiter, R. J., Schlabritz-Loutsevitch, N., Ostrom, R. S., & Slominski, A. T. (2012). Melatonin membrane receptors in peripheral tissues: Distribution and functions. *Molecular & Cellular Endocrinology, 351*(2), 152–166.

Thomson, S. A., Tuleu, C., Wong, I. C., Keady, S., Pitt, K. G., & Sutcliffe, A. G. (2009). Minitablets: New modality to deliver medicines to preschool-aged children. *Pediatrics, 123*(2), e235–e238.

Tordjman, S., Chokron, S., Delorme, R., Charrier, A., Bellissant, E., Jaafari, N., & Fougerou, C. (2017). Melatonin: Pharmacology, functions and therapeutic benefits. *Current Neuropharmacology, 15*(3), 434–443.

Tzischinsky, O., & Lavie, P. (1994). Melatonin possesses a time-dependent hypnotic effect. *Sleep, 17*(7), 638–645.

Wang, F., Li, J., Wu, C., Jang, J., Xu, F., & Zhao, Q. (2003). The GABA(A) receptor mediates the hypnotic activity of melatonin in rats. *Pharmacology, Biochemistry and Behavior, 74*(3), 573e8.

Wirojanan, J., Jacquemont, S., Diaz, R., Bacalman, S., Anders, T. F., Hagerman, R. J., & Goodlin-Jones, B. L. (2009). The efficacy of melatonin for sleep problems in children with autism, fragile X syndrome, or autism and fragile X syndrome. *Journal of Clinical Sleep Medicine, 5*(2), 145–150.

Wright, B., Sims, D., Smart, S., Alwazeer, A., Alderson-Day, B., Allgar, V., Whitton, C., Tomlinson, H., Bennett, S., Jardine, J., McCaffrey, N., Leyland, C., Jakeman, C., & Miles, J. (2010). Melatonin versus placebo in children with autism spectrum conditions and severe sleep problems not amenable to behaviour management strategies: A randomised controlled crossover trial. *Journal of Autism & Developmental Disorders, 41*, 175–184.

Yuge, K., Nagamitsu, S., Ishikawa, Y., Hamada, I., Takahashi, H., Sugioka, H., Yotsuya, O., Mishima, K., Hayashi, M., & Yamashita, Y. (2020). Long-term melatonin treatment for the sleep problems and aberrant behaviors of children with neurodevelopmental disorders. *BMC Psychiatry, 20*(1), 445.

Zuculo, G. M., Gonçalves, B. S. B., Brittes, C., Menna-Barreto, L., & Pinato L. (2017). Melatonin and circadian rhythms in autism: Case report. *Chronobiology International, 34*(4), 527–530.

31

Naltrexone and Self-Injury

Yesterday's Miracle Drug May Still Sometimes Be Helpful

Peter Sturmey
The Graduate Center and Queens College, City University of New York

31.1 Technical Abstract

Background: Naltrexone is an opioid agonist originally evaluated for treatment of nonsocial forms of self-injurious behavior (SIB). Most research took place between the mid-1980s and early 2000s, although individual case studies continue to be published. **Method:** The chapter is based on a search of Google Scholar using the terms "self-injurious behavior" and "naltrexone." The core literature is to be found in four review articles (Elchaar et al., 2006; Ricketts et al., 1992; Roy et al., 2015; Symons et al., 2004). **Results:** The effects of naltrexone on SIB are varied, ranging from complete abolition of SIB to increases in SIB. Both randomized controlled trials (RCTs) and small *N* experiments have produced a wide range of outcomes, but for some individuals the effects are very large. The evidence for the effects on other problem behavior and core autism spectrum disorder (ASD) symptoms is weak. Side effects such as sedation and weight loss are generally reported to be mild and tolerable. **Discussion:** The outcome literature is weak due to failures to replicate initial effectiveness, lack of experimental power, insensitive dependent variables, and failure to screen for nonsocial functions of SIB, but naltrexone may still have a role to play in the treatment of nonsocial forms of SIB in certain limited circumstances. **Practitioner recommendations:** Naltrexone is best considered a third-tier intervention for SIB to be used after behavioral and other pharmacological treatments have been given adequate trials.

31.2 Layperson Summary

Naltrexone is a medicine that blocks the effects of the body's naturally occurring opioids. It was originally evaluated for treatment of SIB. Specifically, it was evaluated for forms of SIB which result in excessive endogenous opioids. Perhaps SIB sometimes results in excessive internal opiates that create an internal state or provide stimulation experienced as a euphoric "rush." This may function as reinforcement for SIB that is not influenced by social consequences such as attention or

Peter Sturmey, *Naltrexone and Self-Injury*. In: *Lifespan Treatment for Autistic Individuals*. Edited by: Peter Sturmey, Russell Lang, and James K. Luiselli, Oxford University Press. © Oxford University Press (2025).
DOI: 10.1093/oso/9780197635841.003.0031

escape from unpleasant tasks. Although individual case studies are still occasionally published, most research took place between the mid-1980s and early 2000s. Core research is to be found in four review articles (Elchaar et al., 2006; Ricketts et al., 1993; Roy et al., 2015; Symons et al., 2004). Research includes several group experiments and experiments involving one to three participants. The outcomes of RCTs investigating the effects of naltrexone have varied. Some studies have demonstrated dramatic and large positive effects of naltrexone. Effects have varied across participants, ranging from complete cessation of SIB to an increase in SIB. The evidence for the effects on other problem behavior and core ASD symptoms is weak. Side effects are generally reported to be mild and tolerable. Side effects commonly include sedation and weight loss. Sometimes side effects include extinction bursts and rarely psychosis, and several empirical studies that have monitored the effects of naltrexone on learning have found that it does not inhibit ongoing learning as measured by discrimination training during a clinical trial (Campbell et al., 1993).

Naltrexone is best considered a third-choice intervention for SIB. This is because there are other behavioral and other pharmacological treatments which are often more effective. Some general advice for parents on psychotropic medication has been published by the American Psychiatric Association (2016).

31.3 Treatment Summary Table

Treatment summary: Naltrexone

Treatment description: Naltrexone is an opioid blocker taken as an oral pill.

Expected outcomes: In some cases, SIB may be abolished or greatly reduced. In other cases, there may be no effects on SIB or occasionally increases in SIB and other negative side effects, such as sedation and weight loss.

Methods: The medication is administered orally sometimes hidden inside of sweet food to mask its bitter taste.

Expertise required to implement treatment: A qualified mental health professional such as a psychiatrist or pediatric neurologist with appropriate training and experience with individuals with ASD and intellectual disability (ID) can administer and evaluate naltrexone. Additional team members such as psychologists and applied behavior analysts and others can play an important role in data collection and analysis as well as evaluation of alternative treatments.

Risks and negative side effects: The most common side effects are weight loss and sedation. Other negative side effects can include extinction bursts of SIB and psychosis (rarely).

Additional considerations and limitations: The place of naltrexone in the treatment of SIB among other treatment options is unclear. It is probably not usually a first-choice treatment. Practitioners should ensure that there have already been adequate trials of behavior analytic treatment and perhaps other psychotropic medication. In some cases of severe SIB, teams should consider adding and fading restraints where appropriate. Extensive staff and family training and support are usually indicated to ensure integrity of ongoing behavioral and other treatment.

31.4 Introduction

31.4.1 Treatment Description

Naltrexone is a psychotropic medication administered by a licensed physician. It is taken orally as a pill. It is administered at doses of either approximately 1–2 mg/kg body weight or 100 mg. It has a bitter taste and may be given with juice or pudding to mask its bitter flavor. It was originally developed for treatment of SIB, but subsequently was evaluated for use with a wider range of problem behavior, social behavior, and core symptoms of ASD. Prior to the development of naltrexone, naloxone was used. Naloxone was administered nasally or orally, but its short half-life made it impractical for long-term treatment of SIB. (Naloxone under the brand name Narcan is currently used to treat opioid overdoses rapidly.)

The basic rationale for the use of naltrexone is that nonsocial forms of SIB may result from a dysregulated opioid system in which SIB results in excessive endogenous opioids which result in what is sometimes described anecdotally as a reinforcing "rush." That is, SIB results in excessive endogenous opioids which create an internal state or provide stimulation that functions as reinforcement. Naltrexone is believed to block the release of endogenous opioids thereby removing or attenuating the reinforcing properties of SIB resulting in a decrease in SIB through operant extinction.

31.4.2 Rationale and Objectives

Humans have naturally occurring receptors for opioid substances that have many effects, including modulation of response to pain, anxiety, sleep regulation, diarrhea, and appetite suppression. Synthesis of opioid antagonists such as naltrexone block these receptors without activating their natural function and are used to both study opioid receptors and have the potential for treatment of drug abuse, including alcohol abuse, schizophrenia, and affective disorders (Singh et al., 1992). Naltrexone can be administered orally. Naltrexone and its metabolites can be active for up to approximately 100 hours after administration, and hence naltrexone can be administered practically and used for treatment with humans.

A clear rationale for the use of opioid blockers was provided by Sandman (1988, 1990/1991) and subsequent publications (Sandman & Kemp, 2011; Singh et al., 1992). The opioid hypothesis of SIB in autism proposes that individuals with ASD have a disturbed endogenous opioid system resulting in elevated levels of endogenous opioids. This results in insensitivity to pain and general hypoalgesia or general sensory depression. Singh et al. (1992) reviewed two hypotheses that provide a rationale for the use of naltrexone for SIB. The first is the *congenital opioid excess hypothesis*. This hypothesis suggests that high levels of opioids during development or early in life result in subsequent relative insensitivity to pain. This might reflect a sensitive period in which exposure to stress that elevates opioids results in later insensitivity to pain. The second hypothesis is the *addiction hypothesis*. This hypothesis suggests that SIB results in elevated levels of opioids as this is a kind of addictive behavior maintained by increases in endogenous opioids that result in a euphoric rush. The evidence for the second hypothesis includes the following: (1) some individuals with ASD and SIB have elevated levels of endogenous opioids both pre and post episodes of SIB; (2) levels of endogenous opioids predict response to treatment with naltrexone that blocks endogenous opioids, with higher baseline levels predicting better response to naltrexone; (3) treatment with opioid blockers such as naltrexone is effective, at least in some individuals; (4) previous environmentally based treatments and other pharmacological interventions that do not address the opioid system have been ineffective for those who may be responsive to naltrexone; (5) when access to SIB is blocked, for example through personal or mechanical restraints, some individuals vigorously attempt to escape or avoid those restraints in order to engage in SIB, suggesting that engaging in SIB is highly reinforcing, perhaps because it results in an opioid-mediated euphoria; and (6) there is at least one case report in which the individual reported that engaging in SIB resulted in a subjective rush and delay of onset of pain (Singh et al., 1992).

Sandman and Kemp (2011) suggested there are two types of SIB—socially mediated and non-socially mediated. They suggested that the opioid hypothesis applies to the non-socially mediated type of SIB that is not associated with caretaker interactions or other environmental variables. Thus, the use of naltrexone for SIB has a clearly stated and explicit rationale.

31.4.3 Considerations for Implementation

Because naltrexone is viewed as relatively safe and fast-acting, a trial of naltrexone can be conducted in a few weeks. It should be conducted by an appropriately qualified and experienced physician or other appropriately qualified progression. There should be adequate data collection such as observational data on SIB, standardized psychometric instruments, and careful monitoring of negative side effects, especially sedation, weight loss, and possible rare side effects such as a paradoxical increase in SIB which may be temporary.

For a trial to be meaningful, other interventions such as behavior treatment plans, other psychopharmacological interventions, and major programmatic changes should be held constant in order to be able to make strong conclusions about the efficacy of naltrexone. If an initial positive response to naltrexone is observed, then adequate monitoring of maintenance should be conducted to monitor for relapse or any long-term negative side effects.

There are other evidence-based practices for SIB, such as function-based behavior analytic interventions, behavior modification (Morano et al., 2017; Shawler et al., 2019), and other conventional pharmacological treatments, although evidence supporting psychopharmacology is generally poor quality and the outcomes are mixed to weak (Gormez et al., 2014). Hence, an important implementation consideration is where the use of naltrexone fits in within the range of other potentially effective treatment options such as in combination with behavioral treatments. This is considered in greater detail in section 31.6.2 below.

31.5 Research Background

Research on naltrexone and SIB was conducted mostly between the mid-1980s and 2010, and this research gave rise to great interest in both practice and research. There have been at least four systematic reviews of naltrexone and naloxone which have variously focused on SIB, core autism symptoms, broadly defined problem behavior, safety, and side effects. Data from the use of naltrexone in individuals with addictions (Carmen et al., 2004) and reports specifically from individuals with autism and related neurodevelopmental disabilities (Roy et al., 2015) both agree that naltrexone is quite safe and well tolerated. In individuals with neurodevelopmental disabilities, reports of sedation and weight loss are the most common negative side effects. There are also reports of other rare but significant negative side effects, including increases in SIB and rarely psychotic episodes. Thus, most reviews of safety have concurred that naltrexone is generally safe and well tolerated.

In an early review, Ricketts et al. (1993) identified nine empirical studies of naloxone and 18 of naltrexone. They concluded that 23 of the 27 studies reported positive outcomes using relatively broad criteria to define positive outcome. They noted that it was unclear if outcomes were due to the specific effects of naloxone and naltrexone or to its nonspecific effects, for example, due to its anxiolytic effects and mild sedation (Aman, 1991). Subsequently, Symons et al. (2004) conducted a quantitative analysis of published studies of short-term (i.e., 3-month maximum duration trials) of naltrexone. To compare outcomes from varied studies, the authors used the percentage change in behavior from baseline to treatment. They searched the literature published between 1983 and 2003. They retained articles that evaluated naltrexone hydrochloride to treat SIB in individuals reported to have ID that measured SIB in an English language, peer-refereed journal. The search yielded an initial pool of 48 articles of which 27 articles were retained. Data were extracted using standardized procedures. Dosing was coded as either absolute dose or dose per kilogram of body mass. Outcomes were coded as positive (decrease in SIB), negative (increase in SIB), or neutral (no change in SIB). Outcomes were further coded as level 1 (5–49% decrease) and level 2 (>50% reduction in SIB). Overall, agreement on data extraction was 93%. The 27 articles had 86 participants, 91% had severe/profound ID, and 35% had autism. Nine percent of studies were open label, 6% single blind, and 85% double blind. Forty-seven percent of participants improved by 50% or more over baseline. Doses of 50 mg and 100 mg were associated with larger reductions in SIB than other doses. Males were more likely to show a larger response to naltrexone than females. Outcomes were not associated with age, autism diagnosis, or SIB topography. The authors also reported a narrative description of four group design studies with 62 participants, 53% of whom had severe/profound ID. Two studies reported statistically significant reductions in SIB and two studies did not (Campbell et al., 1993; LeBoyer et al., 1992; Taylor et al., 1993). The authors concluded that "Forty-seven percent of the total pooled sample showed clinically significant reductions of 50% or greater during naltrexone treatment relative to baseline" (p. 197).

Two years later, Elchaar et al. (2006) also conducted an updated systematic review. They searched two databases and identified eight case series and 14 clinical studies, including eight double-blind RCTs. In a similar vein to Symons et al. (2004), the authors concluded that "the effects of naltrexone are most consistent in ameliorating SIB. Other possible behavioral improvements were noted for hyperactivity, agitation, aggression, irritability, temper tantrums, social withdrawal, attention, eye contact, and stereotyped behaviors" (p. 1093). Thus, this review suggested a potentially broader benefit of naltrexone beyond SIB. Subsequently, Roy et al. (2015) conducted a comprehensive systematic review of naltrexone in children with ASD. They searched four databases up to 2013, hand-searched six major ID journals from 2010 to 2012, and searched citations as well as articles that have cited those articles and searched databases of medication trials. They identified 10 RCTs with 155 children. These studies used a very wide range of outcomes measures, including standard psychometric measures of problem behavior, core ASD symptoms, broad symptoms of psychopathology, side effects, including measures of side effects specific to naltrexone, and direct measures of learning. Of the 128 participants who received naltrexone, 77% showed statistically significant improvements in irritability and hyperactivity. Five studies reported no negative side effects and two reported weight loss and two reported sedation. A small number of children showed paradoxical increases in aggression ($n = 2$) and stereotypy ($n = 4$). The authors concluded that there was insufficient data to conclude that naltrexone had improvements in core features of ASD.

These four systematic reviews present a developing overview of research on naltrexone and SIB from the 1980s through 2000s. The lack of subsequent meta-analyses and systematic reviews appears to reflect the general reduction in interest and publication from researchers in naltrexone and autism other than occasional case reports of very effective treatment of SIB in individual cases. Noting that the four studies review overlapping reports, all four systematic reviews are broadly consonant with one another in that (1) naltrexone sometimes produced large improvements in behavioral symptoms such as SIB for some individuals; (2) sometimes there may be other benefits such as reduction in hyperactivity and so on; (3) naltrexone does not impact the core features of autism; (4) naltrexone is relatively well tolerated as there are not excessive negative side effects or impairment in ongoing learning; (5) the effects on specific individuals are quite varied, ranging from complete abolition and large reductions in SIB in some cases, little or insignificant effects in others, and paradoxical increases and problematic negative side effects in a few individuals; and (6) the outcomes of both RCTs are highly varied with some reporting very positive effects and some reporting no effects of naltrexone. The possible reasons for the varied outcomes of naltrexone are unclear but might simply reflect lack of experimental power, small sample sizes, and/or insensitive dependent variables to detect positive effects; large individual differences in response to naltrexone; or other unknown factors. Nevertheless, it is reasonable to conclude that some individuals do indeed experience a large and clinically significant reduction in SIB, perhaps reductions in other problem behaviors, and perhaps other small benefits in some individuals with relatively low risks of negative side effects as reported in the literature. A further explanation for the mixed outcomes is that most studies did not explicitly describe if and how they determined if the forms of SIB were nonsocial. Rather, they usually described that a wide range of previous treatments, including behavioral treatments, had been attempted but did not describe how this was evaluated. Hence, a possible explanation for the varied outcomes might be that they included different proportions of individuals with socially mediated forms of SIB which might be nonresponsive to naltrexone. Some reports of naltrexone noted generally that many other behavioral and pharmacological treatments had been implemented, but only reported this anecdotally. Thus, it is unclear if trials of previous treatments were adequate. A final notable omission from these studies is that the issues of social validity, quality of life, and maintenance were not directly addressed by almost all of these studies.

31.5.1 Small *N* Experiments

Small *N* experiments have been used to evaluate the effectiveness of naltrexone within individuals by comparing placebo with various doses of naltrexone, typically collecting observational data on SIB and sometimes using experimental designs such as reversal designs (e.g., Luiselli et al., 1989). Small *N* experiments also permit more careful analysis of the effects of naltrexone on individual topographies of SIB which may respond differentially to naltrexone (Herman et al., 1987). Several small *N* experiments have also investigated the combined and potentially interactive effects of naltrexone and behavioral interventions. Since naltrexone may attenuate the reinforcing value of SIB, one might expect a variety of effects of naltrexone on SIB and other functionally related behavior.

An early example of a small *N* experiment comes from Symons et al. (1998), who compared the effectiveness of both naltrexone and functional communication training (FCT) in treatment of SIB in a 12-year-old boy with ASD severe ID with a history of SIB since the age of approximately 3½ years. He was nonverbal and communicated through pointing to pictures. He reportedly had multiple failed trials of both behavioral and pharmacological interventions for his SIB at the beginning of the study. The experiment used an ABCDC experimental design in which A denoted placebo, B naltrexone, C naltrexone plus FCT, and D placebo plus FCT. FCT consisted of teaching mands for attention, tangible items and breaks, among other mand training-related procedures. Naltrexone was delivered in a dose of 55 mg (1.45 mg/kg) hidden in his breakfast applesauce. Naltrexone resulted in an approximately 50% reduction in SIB, and the addition of FCT resulted in a further 50% reduction resulting in a large overall reduction in SIB. The effects of naltrexone and FCT appeared to be additive and independent of one another. His overall rates of communication responses increased with the implementation of FCT but did not increase further with the addition of naltrexone, perhaps due to a ceiling effect in the mand data. The authors also noted that naltrexone was helpful in reducing SIB during unstructured classroom times.

In a second small *N* experiment evaluating naltrexone for SIB, Johnson et al. (1994) evaluated the effects of behavioral intervention and naltrexone on high-rate SIB in a 7-year-old, African American boy with ASD and profound ID. He first engaged in SIB at around 2 years of age and had showed increases in SIB, aggression, and noncompliance over the last year resulting in severe injuries to himself, skill loss, and which resulted in admission to an inpatient unit for evaluation and treatment. At home, his parents managed his SIB by holding him in their laps more or less continuously. He also had at least two failed trials of psychotropic medications. Because of the severity of his SIB, splints were used after 48 hours of admission to prevent further injury. There were four phases in the experiment. In phase 1, splints were faded by taking him out of his splints for 15 minutes of structured play periods which involved differential reinforcement of other behavior (DRO) with edible reinforcers and praise and gradual increase in the DRO interval contingent upon the absence of SIB, and brief manual restraint (holding his hands down for 15 seconds) contingent upon SIB. In phase 2, the behavioral package was continued, and 50 mg of naltrexone was added. Restraints were reduced such that he remained out of splints for periods of 1–2 hours at various points during the day. In phase 3, naltrexone was replaced with placebo while the behavioral program continued. In phase 4, both splints, naltrexone and placebo, were discontinued and only the behavioral program was implemented. Finally, there was a 2-month follow-up phase in his classroom during which his teaching staff continued the behavioral program. The total frequencies of SIB were 544 (baseline), 197 (phase I), 424 (phase II), 226 (phase III), 34 (phase IV, with 0 incidents of SIB for the last 12 days), and 9.6 and 5.1 for the first and second month of follow-up. His parents and school staff reported anecdotally that these effects were maintained at 6- and 12-months follow-up and that there were a wide range of other behavioral benefits such as increased time in seat. The authors concluded that the behavioral program was highly effective, and that naltrexone was in fact iatrogenic for this young man. They also noted that this intervention involved extensive parent and staff training and that both groups were highly motivated to address the boy's SIB.

These two small *N*s confirm the results of the RCTs. Namely, the effects of naltrexone are quite idiosyncratic—Symons et al. (1998) found that naltrexone has an independent and additive effect on reducing SIB in addition to an effective behavioral intervention, whereas Johnson et al. (1994) observed an independent and iatrogenic effect of naltrexone on SIB.

31.6 Practice Implications

31.6.1 Treatment Outcomes

Research indicates that naltrexone is sometimes dramatically effective in treating SIB in individuals with ASD/ID, sometimes is ineffective, and sometimes is iatrogenic. Its reported side effects appear relatively modest and generally tolerable. The evidence that naltrexone is effective for core symptoms of autism, hyperactivity, or other outcomes is very limited and unconvincing at this time, and alternative potentially effective evidence-based treatment options exist. Thus, the practical question is where naltrexone fits within the array of treatment options for SIB. See Campbell (1996a, 1996b) and Harris (1996a, 1996b) for a discussion of the pros and cons of whether individuals with SIB must or must not have a trial of naltrexone.

31.6.2 Practice Implication Guidelines

SIB in individuals with ASD is amenable to behavioral treatments such as FCT, and effect sizes are generally larger when behavioral treatment based on a functional assessment and/or analysis and is conducted competently and with integrity (Morano et al., 2017; Shawler et al., 2019). In addition, there are several pharmacological alternatives to naltrexone, although the outcomes for pharmacological treatment of SIB are mixed and the evidence is weak (Gormez et al., 2014). Thus, there are alternative treatments which are more likely to be effective than naltrexone in many cases, and so naltrexone is not a first-choice treatment for SIB. The two common practical and ethical dilemmas that practitioners must resolve are to determine if there have already been adequate trials of alternative treatments prior to evaluating naltrexone, and if this is not the case, how to proceed. A common service challenge is that effective evidence-based practices (e.g., applied behavior analysis) may not be available in many service settings.

Another practice question involves identifying characteristics and other indicators that can be used to determine for whom naltrexone is particularly likely to be effective. So far, the only known possible predictors of response to this treatment are nonsocial function of SIB and abnormal opioid levels, although the latter is based only on correlational rather than direct evidence. Future research could assist practitioners in developing algorithms to identify best practices and to provide triage-like guidelines that practitioners could use to select appropriate treatments for SIB from the variety of available treatment options of which naltrexone is one option.

A final practice consideration is how to conduct adequate trials of naltrexone for SIB. There are several features of an adequate trial of naltrexone for practitioners to attend to. First, the evaluation of the trials should be based on objective and reliable data on SIB. Global ratings of overall response to treatment are inadequate and possibly insensitive and inaccurate. Thus, an adequate trial should include data on the rate of SIB, perhaps taking data only in high-risk situations to reduce the burden of data collection and to maximize the relevancy of the data. Second, an adequate trial should sample a full range of evaluated doses of naltrexone correcting for the individual's body mass. Third, all other programmatic features should be held constant as far as possible, including ongoing behavior support. Fourth, side effects should be monitored carefully and systematically, including possible negative effects on learning such as those related to sedation. Finally, it is good practice to evaluate the effects of SIB reduction more broadly using measures of quality of life and other relevant problem behavior.

31.7 References

Aman, M. G. (1991). Pharmacotherapy in the developmental disabilities: New developments. *Australia & New Zealand Journal of Developmental Disabilities, 17*, 183–199.

American Psychiatric Association. (2016). *Autism spectrum disorders: Parent's medication guide.* https://www.aacap.org/App_Themes/AACAP/Docs/resource_centers/autism/Autism_Spectrum_Disorder_Parents_Medication_Guide.pdf

Campbell, M. (1996a). Resolved: Autistic children should have a trial of naltrexone. *Journal of the American Academy of Child & Adolescent Psychiatry, 35*(2), 246–249.

Campbell, M. (1996b). Resolved: Autistic children should have a trial of naltrexone: Affirmative rebuttal. *Journal of the American Academy of Child & Adolescent Psychiatry, 35*(2), 249–250. DOI: 10.1097/00004583-199602000-00021

Campbell, M., Anderson, L. T., Small, A. M., Adams, P., Gonzalez, N. M., & Ernst, M. (1993). Naltrexone in autistic children: Behavioral symptoms and attentional learning. *Journal of the American Academy of Child & Adolescent Psychiatry, 32*(6), 1283–1291.

Carmen, B., Angeles, M., Ana, M., & María, A. J. (2004). Efficacy and safety of naltrexone and acamprosate in the treatment of alcohol dependence: A systematic review. *Addiction, 99*(7), 811–828.

Elchaar G. M., Maisch N. M., Augusto L. M. & Wehring, H. J. (2006) Efficacy and safety of naltrexone in paediatric patients with autistic disorder. *Annals of Pharmacotherapy, 40*, 1086–1095.

Gormez, A., Rana, F., & Varghese, S. (2014). Pharmacological interventions for self-injurious behaviour in adults with intellectual disabilities: Abridged republication of a Cochrane systematic review. *Journal of Psychopharmacology, 28*(7), 624–632.

Harris, J. C. (1996a). Resolved: Autistic children should have a trial of naltrexone: Negative. *Journal of the American Academy of Child & Adolescent Psychiatry, 35* (2), 248–249. DOI: 10.1097/00004583-199602000-00020

Harris, J. C. (1996b). Resolved: Autistic children should have a trial of naltrexone: Negative rebuttal. *Journal of the American Academy of Child & Adolescent Psychiatry, 35*(2): 250–251. DOI: 10.1097/00004583-199602000-00022

Herman, B. H., Kathryn Hammock, M., Egan, J., Chatoor, I., Werner, A., & Zelnik, N. (1987). Naltrexone decreases self-injurious behavior. *Annals of Neurology, 22*(4), 550–552.

Johnson, K., Johnson, C. R., & Sahl, R. A. (1994). Behavioral and naltrexone treatment of self- injurious behavior. *Journal of Developmental & Physical Disabilities, 6*(2), 193–202. https://doi.org/10.1007/BF02579359

Leboyer, M., Bouvard, M. P., Launay, J. M., Tabuteau, F., Waller, D., Dugas, M., Kerdelhue, B., Lensing, P., & Panksepp, J. (1992). Brief report: A double-blind study of naltrexone in infantile autism. *Journal of Autism & Developmental Disorders, 22*, 309–319.

Luiselli, J. K., Beltis, J. A., & Bass, J. (1989). Clinical analysis of naltrexone in the treatment of self-injurious behavior. *Journal of the Multihandicapped Person, 2*, 43–50. https://doi.org/10.1007/BF01098757

Morano, S., Ruiz, S., Hwang, J., Wertalik, J. L., Moeller, J., Karal, M. A., & Mulloy, A. (2017). Meta-analysis of single-case treatment effects on self-injurious behavior for individuals with autism and intellectual disabilities. *Autism & Developmental Language Impairments, 2*, 2396941516688399.

Ricketts, R. W., Goza, A. B., & Matese, M. (1992). Effects of naltrexone and SIBIS on self-injury. *Behavioral Residential Treatment, 7*(4), 315–326. https://doi.org/10.1002/bin.2360070406

Roy, A., Roy, M., Deb, S., Unwin, G., & Roy, A. (2015). Are opioid antagonists effective in attenuating the core symptoms of autism spectrum conditions in children: A systematic review. *Journal of Intellectual Disability Research, 59*(4), 293–306.

Sandman, C. A. (1988). B-endorphin disregulation in autistic and self-injurious behavior: A neurodevelopmental hypothesis. *Synapse*, 2, 193–199.

Sandman, C. A. (1990/1991). The opiate hypothesis in autism and self-injury. *Journal of Child & Adolescent Psychopharmacology, 1*, 237–248.

Sandman, C. A., & Kemp, A. S. (2011). Opioid antagonists may reverse endogenous opiate "dependence" in the treatment of self-injurious behavior. *Pharmaceuticals, 4*(2), 366–381.

Shawler, L. A., Russo, S. R., Hilton, J. L., Kahng, S., Davis, C. J., & Dorsey, M. F. (2019). Behavioral treatment of self-injury: 2001 to 2016. *American Journal on Intellectual & Developmental Disabilities, 124*(5), 450–469.

Singh, Y. N., Ricketts, R. W., Ellis, C. R., & Singh, N. N. (1992). Opiate antagonists. I.: Pharmacology and rationale for use in treating self-injury. *Journal of Developmental & Physical Disabilities, 5*, 5–15.

Symons, F. J., Fox, N. D., & Thompson, T. (1998). Functional communication training and naltrexone treatment of self-injurious behaviour: An experimental case report. *Journal of Applied Research in Intellectual Disabilities, 11*(3), 273–292.

Symons, F. J., Thompson, A., & Rodriguez, M. C. (2004). Self-injurious behavior and the efficacy of naltrexone treatment: A quantitative synthesis. *Mental Retardation and Developmental Disabilities Research Reviews, 10*(3), 193–200.

Taylor, D. V., Sandman, C. A., Touchette, P., Hetrick, W. P., & Barron, J. L. (1993). Naltrexone improves learning and attention in self-injurious individuals with developmental disabilities. *Journal of Developmental & Physical Disabilities, 5*, 29–42.

32

Secretin

The Unfulfilled Promise

Beth Johnson, Mark Bellgrove, and Katrina Williams
Monash University

32.1 Technical Abstract

Background: Secretin is a gastrointestinal hormone and neuropeptide, with pleiotropic effects in a range of biological systems. In the late 1990s, secretin was reported to improve language and social skills in three autistic children. This initial case report was followed by a dramatic uptake of secretin as a therapeutic agent for autistic children, despite no clinical trials having been undertaken. A meta-analysis (Williams et al., 2012) examined the use of intravenous secretin for autistic children from 16 randomized, placebo-controlled trials (n = 900 children) and found no evidence to support its continued use. **Method:** We reviewed the literature from the year 2000 to find publications about secretin to assess biological plausibility in neurodevelopmental conditions and evidence of effectiveness in autism. **Results:** Secretin is highly conserved among mammalian species, with new evidence from animal and molecular studies showing that secretin modulates multiple behaviors, including social interaction, spatial and motor learning, and water and food intake, via multiple molecular pathways. There is no evidence from clinical trials to support secretin's therapeutic role in autism or other neurodevelopmental conditions. **Discussion:** There is biological plausibility for secretin to have a role in brain function, with the possibility of changing abilities or behavior. However, the role of secretin as a therapeutic agent for specific abilities or behavior associated with autism or other neurodevelopmental conditions is not supported. **Practitioner recommendations:** There is currently no evidence that single- or multiple-dose intravenous secretin is an effective therapy for autism, and as such it should not be recommended or administered as a treatment for autistic children or adults.

32.2 Layperson Summary

Secretin is a gastrointestinal hormone and neuropeptide. It was first studied in 1998 in three autistic children with intellectual disability. The authors reported that following gastrointestinal investigation that included administration of intravenous

Beth Johnson, Mark Bellgrove, and Katrina Williams, *Secretin*. In: *Lifespan Treatment for Autistic Individuals*.
Edited by: Peter Sturmey, Russell Lang, and James K. Luiselli, Oxford University Press. © Oxford University Press (2025).
DOI: 10.1093/oso/9780197635841.003.0032

secretin, the children's language and eye contact improved. Following this report, many families sought treatment with intravenous secretin, even though secretin was not a proven, effective treatment. Randomized controlled trials (RCTs) with a placebo group were conducted internationally. There were 16 RCTs involving over 900 children. There has also been a systematic review. This review found no evidence for single- or multiple-dose intravenous secretin improving symptoms of autism. There were no effects on social interaction, communication, and restrictive, repetitive behavior and routines. Since that time, no further clinical research has been undertaken. While there is new laboratory evidence that secretin influences brain function, there is no clinical evidence to support the role of secretin as a therapeutic agent. Currently there is no evidence to support the use of single or multiple doses of intravenous secretin. Therefore, it is not currently recommended for use.

32.3 Treatment Summary Table

Treatment summary: Intravenous Secretin

Treatment description: Secretin is an endogenous gastrointestinal peptide that stimulates the release of bicarbonate and water into the intestine. Secretin is typically administered intravenously, as a single dose, primarily to assess pancreatic and intestinal function, and to aid diagnoses of pancreatic conditions. More recent laboratory evidence has shown that secretin also acts as a neuropeptide, although the clinical relevance of this is yet to be investigated.

Expected outcomes: Early case studies reported improvement in social interaction or communication and restrictive, repetitive behavior and routines in autistic children with intellectual disability undergoing investigation for gastrointestinal difficulties. However, multiple RCTs and a systematic review and meta-analysis have failed to demonstrate the effectiveness of secretin for autistic children.

Methods: The patient fasts for 12 hours prior to receiving secretin. Single or multidoses of secretin are administered by a doctor in a healthcare environment via intravenous infusion over a 1-minute period, with monitoring over the next hour for adverse events. Synthetic secretin has a short half-life (~2–4 minutes) and therefore needs to be intravenously administered.

Expertise required to implement treatment: Healthcare setting with an emergency response team to ensure safety during intravenous administration

Risks and negative side effects: Secretin has a low toxicity profile when administered in the usual diagnostic dose. However, there is limited understanding of the relationship of age to the effects of secretin injection in children, and safety and efficacy have not been well established for pediatric populations. Adverse reactions include abdominal discomfort and nausea, a burning sensation in the stomach, diaphoresis, bradycardia, and hypotension. There is also risk of trauma for autistic children because of the experience of attending hospital environments to receive intravenous injections and clinical monitoring.

Additional considerations and limitations: Currently there is no evidence to support the use of single or multiple doses of intravenous secretin as an effective therapy for autistic children.

32.4 Introduction

32.4.1 Treatment Description

Secretin is an endogenous gastrointestinal peptide that stimulates the release of bicarbonate and water into the intestine. Secretin is typically administered intravenously as a single dose to assess pancreatic and intestinal function, and diagnose patients with pancreatic conditions. Although more recently it has been understood to act as a neuropeptide (Wang et al., 2019), its role and clinical relevance as a neuromodulator remain poorly understood.

Synthetic secretin preparations have a short half-life of 2–4 minutes and thus must be administered intravenously (Dengler et al., 2021). Secretin is administered by a doctor in a healthcare setting with availability to an emergency response team. The patient will typically fast for 12 hours prior to receiving secretin. Single or multidoses of secretin are administered via intravenous infusion over a period of 1 minute, with monitoring over the next hour for adverse events.

32.4.2 Rationale and Objectives

Secretin was first proposed as a potential treatment for autism spectrum disorders (autism) after a report that three autistic and intellectually disabled children, who had secretin administered for an evaluation of their pancreatic function, had improvements in eye contact, alertness, and language (Horvath et al., 1998). Intravenous secretin was rapidly adopted as a therapy for autistic children, despite a lack of evidence from clinical trials to support its use.

Autistic children are more likely to report gastrointestinal symptoms but with inconsistent associations with co-occurring conditions reported (Leader et al., 2022). Consequently, there have been several hypotheses around the role of the gut-brain axis on brain development and symptoms for autism spectrum disorder (Leader et al., 2022). However, there has been no new clinical evidence to support the utility of secretin in the treatment of autism following the publication in the early 2010s of two systematic reviews, one including a meta-analysis (Krishnaswami et al., 2011; Williams et al., 2012). We evaluated studies undertaken over the past decade relating to secretin's neurobiological, molecular, and genetic mechanisms from animal models, to evaluate whether any advances have been made in the field since that time.

32.4.3 Considerations for Implementation

Following multiple randomized, placebo-controlled studies of intravenous secretin in autistic children, no supporting evidence for improvement in autistic symptoms, or other associated symptoms, was found. The first negative clinical trial results were published in 1999 (Sandler et al., 1999) and the first systematic review of RCTs examining the efficacy of secretin in autism, published in 2005, did not show improvements in the diagnostic features of autism (Williams et al., 2005). Two early reviews (Esch & Carr 2004; Sturmey, 2005) and two updated systematic reviews (Krishnaswami et al., 2011, 2012), one with a meta-analysis which included 16 randomized controlled trials and over 900 participants (Williams et al., 2012), found no evidence to support its continued use among autistic children, and research into the use of intravenous secretin as a therapeutic agent ceased. Whether secretin improves other specific neurodevelopmental abilities or behaviors that are associated with autism is uncertain because effectiveness has not been measured in an adequate sample size. Therefore, based on current clinical evidence, the use of single or multiple doses of intravenous secretin as an effective therapy for autistic children is not supported.

Although there is new emerging evidence from animal studies demonstrating the role of secretin in modulating multiple behaviors, including social interaction, spatial and motor learning, and water and food intake, this evidence has not translated to meaningful clinical outcomes for intravenous secretin as a therapeutic support for autistic children or adults.

32.5 Research Background

Autistic children have inconsistently been reported to experience gastrointestinal symptoms, such as constipation, abdominal pain, bloating, chronic diarrhea, gastroesophageal reflux, or inflammatory bowel disease (Leader et al., 2022). This, along with long-standing hypotheses around the impact of the gut-brain axis on brain development and behaviors through the neuroendocrine, neuroimmune, and autonomic nervous systems, has led to a range of supplements, vitamins, and peptides being proposed as possible therapies for autism (Kryszak & Mulick, 2022). However, these therapies often have poorly understood mechanisms. Nonetheless, use of such therapies can become widespread before double-blinded studies have been undertaken. Secretin is one such example where uptake in clinical practice outstripped the objective evidence.

Secretin is widely recognized as an endogenous gastrointestinal peptide hormone. It was first described over a century ago for its role in facilitating exocrine secretion of digestive fluids from the pancreas. Secretin is a polypeptide comprising 27 amino acids produced in the duodenal mucosa; it stimulates the release of bicarbonate and water into the intestine. Secretin is typically administered intravenously, as a single dose, to diagnose patients with pancreatic conditions.

The use of intravenous secretin among autistic children rose in popularity following a case series by Horvath et al., (1998). This case series included 12 autistic children with intellectual disability and co-occurring gastrointestinal problems sufficient to warrant investigation. They were administered porcine secretin during endoscopy to assess pancreatic function, and a subgroup of 4 of the 12 cases were reported at a conference to show improved eye contact, alertness, and language after the investigation. A significant increase in blood serotonin levels after secretin injection was also reported in several children (Horvath et al., 1998). A follow-up publication by the same authors provided detailed information about three autistic children aged 3–5 years that showed clinical improvement (Horvath et al., 1998). It was not stated in either publication and is unknown whether the three participants in the peer-reviewed publication overlapped with participants reported in the conference abstract. All three participants in this uncontrolled, nonblinded study were reported to have had an increased pancreaticobiliary secretory response, and within 5 weeks of the secretin infusion, gastrointestinal symptoms were resolved (Sokolski et al., 1998). More typical eye contact, overall alertness, and improved expressive language abilities were also qualitatively reported (Sokolski et al., 1998). In a letter to the editor of the *New England Journal of Medicine* (Horvath, 2000), the authors comment on a separate study (Horvath et al., 1999), which had focused on autistic children ($n = 36$) receiving secretin specifically for investigation and treatment of gastrointestinal abnormalities, and in their letter noted that "The majority of these patients had gradual improvements in social and behavioral skills after repeated injections," which they had not reported in their peer-reviewed study (Horvath et al., 1999); it was not indicated how improvements in social or behavioral skills had been measured, how many injections had been administered, or over what time period. Horvath (2000) did note that further randomized, double-blind, placebo-controlled studies should be conducted in order to support the use of secretin for autism.

Shortly thereafter, even in the absence of randomized, double-blind, placebo-controlled studies, the use of secretin became widespread in the treatment of autism and was dispensed in many different forms and in countries where it was not licensed. It was estimated that thousands of children might have received intramuscular and intravenous secretin prior to any double-blinded studies having been completed to assess its efficacy (Sandler et al., 1999), with attendant implications for the financial expenditure by families, in addition to the medical and emotional impact on the child (Kastner et al., 2016). The product development and dissemination that followed this single report reflects the high level of unmet need of autistic children and their families, the power of market forces, and the way we function as a global community.

The initial case report (Sokolski et al., 1998) was followed by the first double-blind trial (Sandler et al., 1999), which found no effect of a single dose of intravenous secretin compared to placebo, on any of the 16 psychometric outcome measures used. Sandler et al. (1999) used standardized behavioral measures of the primary and secondary features of autism to evaluate change in autistic symptoms at baseline and over the course of a 4-week period post treatment. While there was a significant improvement reported in both the placebo and secretin groups on 6 of 16 measures over time, there was no difference between treatment groups.

This spurred the publication of a further 16 randomized, placebo-controlled trials over the next 10 years, providing evidence to aid the decision-making of families, clinicians, pharmaceutical companies, and health services. Two early reviews showed no support for use of secretin for autistic children or adults (Esch & Carr 2004; Sturmey, 2005); however, critics noted that a single dose might be insufficient, the type of secretin used must be specified (human, porcine, or synthetic), and that the psychometric measures used may not adequately capture the effects of secretin; therefore, preliminary negative results should not preclude further research (Sturmey, 2005).

Williams et al. (2005) published the first systematic review of RCTs examining the efficacy of secretin in autism, which did not show improvements in the diagnostic features of autism. In a report commissioned by the Agency for Healthcare Research and Quality (Krishnaswami et al., 2011), which reviewed eight publications examining the use of human, porcine, or biologic secretin in autistic children, no publications reported changes in autistic symptoms, language, or cognition when compared with placebo. Shortly after this publication, Williams et al. (2012) undertook a meta-analysis examining the use of intravenous secretin for autistic children from 16 clinical trials (n = 900 children) and also found no evidence to support its continued use. There was neither supporting evidence of symptom improvement in diagnostic autistic symptoms nor other nondiagnostic domains such as visuospatial skills (Krishnaswami et al., 2011; Williams et al., 2012). The cumulative evidence was so convincing that, since that time, there have been no further clinical trials of secretin as a therapy for autistic children. Moreover, use of secretin in the community was dramatically reduced; a large 2014 study of complementary medicine utilization showed that only 0.2% of parents reported having used secretin (Akins et al., 2014; Kryszak & Mulick, 2022).

32.5.1 Understanding the Role of Secretin in the Brain

At the time intravenous secretin was being investigated for possible therapeutic use in autistic children, results from animal studies showed preliminary evidence for the role of secretin as a neuropeptide, but its role in neuromodulation was poorly understood (Horvath et al., 1998; Krishnaswami et al., 2011). Studies have continued because secretin is highly conserved among mammalian species, which has made it an ideal candidate for studying its expression and role in the central nervous system. Over the past two decades, animal studies have provided an increased understanding of the function of secretin in the brain with attention drawn to its potential roles in brain development, brain function, and neurodegeneration. Evidence for a role for secretin in modulating multiple behaviors, including social interaction, spatial and motor learning, and water and food intake in animal studies is now available (Wang et al., 2019).

Mouse and rat studies have revealed that secretin and its receptor (SCTR) are expressed throughout the hippocampus, amygdala, striatum, cerebellum, brainstem, and cortical pyramidal cells. Secretin has been found to be involved in a range of cellular functions spanning neurotransmission, gene expression regulation, neurogenesis, and neural protection (Wang et al., 2014). Secretin can also activate the vasoactive intestinal polypeptide receptors (VPAC1) and related oxytocin receptors, at lower affinity (Welch et al., 2010). SCTR is a member of the type II G-protein-coupled receptor family, and in addition to binding secretin, it will also bind glucagon and vasointestinal polypeptide (VIP) but with lower affinity. Synthetic secretin represents the only clinically utilized SCTR ligand for diagnostic purposes, due to its short half-life (~2–4 minutes) and the need for intravenous administration (Lee et al., 2014).

In mouse models, secretin and the secretin receptor gene show age-dependent expression patterns (Wang et al., 2014). Secretin is postulated to play a role in the embryonic development of the serotonergic (5-HT) system. Transient expression of secretin in serotonergic mesencephalic neurons, specifically the dorsal raphe, raphe magnus, and lateral paragigantocellularis nucleus, has been found in embryonic stage 14 to birth, but not adult brain development (Lossi et al., 2004). The dorsal raphe is the largest source of serotonergic neurons in the brain, and the raphe magnus and lateral paragigantocellularis nucleus modulate endogenous pain inhibition and blood pressure, respectively (Myers et al., 2004). No study has directly examined serotonin levels in secretin or secretin receptor knockout mouse models (Wang et al., 2014). However, one clinical single-blind, placebo-controlled crossover study of intravenous secretin in children with autism provided putative evidence that secretin increases tetrahydrobiopterin, a cofactor involved in the synthesis and potentiation of dopamine, serotonin, and nitric oxide (Toda et al., 2006). Within this study (n = 12 children with autism with co-occurring intellectual disability), autistic symptoms diminished following intravenous secretin in 7 of the 12 participants. However, symptoms in the restricted and repetitive behavior domain became elevated in two of the participants, as measured by the Autism Diagnostic Interview-Revised. Among children whose symptoms diminished, both tetrahydrobiopterin and homovanillic acid, a major catecholamine metabolite, were elevated in cerebrospinal fluid (Toda et al., 2006).

There is evidence from mouse secretin knockout models for the role of secretin in a range of learning behaviors, including motor and spatial learning, linked to modulation of neurogenesis, neural protection, and synaptic plasticity in the cerebellum and hippocampus, respectively (Wang et al., 2014). For example, it has been shown that secretin helps to regulate cerebellar motor and learning functions by maintaining synaptic transmission and modulating lamination of cerebellar cortical neurons (Wang et al., 2014). Mouse secretin knockout models also show altered migration of cerebellar granular precursor cells, diminished Purkinje cell formation and dendritic arborization, and higher apoptosis levels at the early postnatal stage (Zhang & Chow, 2014). Secretin has also been shown to modulate the sensitivity of Purkinje neurons to the neurotransmitter GABA (Myers et al., 2004). Secretin-deficient mice have exhibited accelerated apoptosis of neural progenitor cells in the dentate gyrus (DG) during the early postnatal period, leading to smaller dentate gyrus volumes (Jukkola et al., 2011). In adult secretin-deficient mice, reduced long-term potentiation and impaired spatial learning ability have also been reported (Jukkola et al., 2011).

Gastrointestinal symptoms have been inconsistently reported as being frequent among autistic children with co-occurring intellectual disability (Leader et al., 2022). There have been ongoing hypotheses around the role of secretin in the bidirectional signaling in gut-brain behavior, with mouse models showing interactions are mediated in part by systemic secretin and oxytocin (Velmurugan et al., 2010; Welch et al., 2010). In mouse model studies, secretin has acted on oxytocin receptors to both directly and indirectly stimulate the release of oxytocin within the brain and in the gut. Secretin increases the firing rate of oxytocin neurons (as measured in the supraoptic nucleus) and increases plasma oxytocin concentration in a dose-dependent way (Velmurugan et al., 2010). Secretin has a predominantly excitatory effect, with noradrenergic pathways mediating the excitation of oxytocin neurons via α1-adrenoceptors when stimulated by systemic secretin (Velmurugan et al., 2010). Within the brain, oxytocin administration was shown to restore social recognition abilities in secretin receptor–deficient mice (Takayanagi et al., 2017). One mouse study showed chronic intestinal inflammation reportedly activated forebrain neurons, with systemically administered secretin and oxytocin ameliorating this colitis-associated activation (Welch et al., 2010).

32.5.2 Potential Future Research Directions

Autism is a broad neurodevelopmental condition that arises from multiple etiological factors. Given both the phenotypic and etiological heterogeneity of autism and other neurodevelopmental and psychiatric conditions, and the pleiotropic effects of secretin in a range of molecular pathways and organ systems, emerging technologies such as pharmacogenetics could potentially identify candidate individuals who may benefit, or respond adversely, to therapies such as secretin. However, a study investigating the effectiveness of secretin in schizophrenia (Sheitman et al., 2004) showed that following intravenous secretin infusions in 22 patients with treatment-resistant schizophrenia, only three individuals experienced clinical improvements in symptoms, and this improvement was transient, lasting only 1–5 days; there was no statistically significant difference from placebo treatment over the 4-week study period (Cáceda et al., 2007; Sheitman et al., 2004). A similar pattern of brief, transient response was reported in a separate single-case study of a patient with co-occurring schizophrenia and autism (Alamy et al., 2004). These findings, taken together with the emerging laboratory study outcomes, leads us to speculate that even if a subpopulation of initial responders to intravenous secretin therapy were identified, there is no evidence that secretin would provide any sustained or clinically meaningful outcomes for individuals over time.

32.6 Practice Implications

32.6.1 Treatment Outcomes

There is currently insufficient evidence to suggest that intravenous secretin is an effective therapy for autistic children or adults.

32.6.2 Practice Implication Guidelines

Whether secretin is effective for some specific abilities or behaviors associated with autism and other neurodevelopmental conditions is uncertain. Further explorations of the use of secretin for children with autism should only be undertaken if there is biological plausibility for effectiveness in the children who participate and the findings can be translated into practice. New personalized medicine techniques, such as pharmacogenetics, could potentially allow the field to identify targets that might, in turn, assist identifying individuals who could benefit from secretin. Any such research would also need to provide valid evidence about improvements in outcomes that are of value to autistic individuals and their families.

In summary, although there is now evidence from animal models for the role of secretin in brain development and behavior, there is currently no evidence that single- or multiple-dose intravenous secretin is an effective therapy, and as such it should not currently be recommended or administered as a treatment for autistic children.

32.7 References

Akins, R. S., Krakowiak, P., Angkustsiri, K., Hertz-Picciotto, I., Hansen, R. L. (2014). Utilization patterns of conventional and complementary/alternative treatments in children with autism spectrum disorders and developmental disabilities in a population-based study. *Journal Developmental & Behavioral Pediatrics, 35*(1):1-10. doi:10.1097/DBP.0000000000000013.

Alamy, S. S., Jarskog, L. F., Sheitman, B. B., & Lieberman, J. A. (2004). Secretin in a patient with treatment-resistant schizophrenia and prominent autistic features. *Schizophrenia Research, 66*(2–3), 183–186.

Cáceda, R., Kinkead, B., & Nemeroff, C. B. (2007). Involvement of neuropeptide systems in schizophrenia: Human studies. *International Review of Neurobiology, 78*, 327–376.

Dengler, D. G., Sun, Q., Holleran, J., Pollari, S., Beutel, J., Brown, B. T., Iwaya, A. S., Ardecky, R., Harikumar, K. G., Miller, L. J., & Sergienko, E. A. (2021). Development of a testing funnel for identification of small-molecule modulators targeting secretin receptors. *SLAS DISCOVERY: Advancing the Science of Drug Discovery, 26*(1), 1–16.

Esch, B. E., & Carr, J. E. (2004). Secretin as a treatment for autism: A review of the evidence. *Journal of Autism & Developmental Disorders, 34*(5), 543–556.

Horvath, K. (2000). Secretin treatment for autism. *The New England Journal of Medicine, 342*, 1216-1218. DOI: 10.1056/NEJM200004203421614

Horvath, K., Cataldo, M., Wachtel, R., Spurrier, A., Papadimitriou, J., & Tildon, J. T. (1998). Gastrointestinal findings in autistic children: Hypersecretory response to secretin predicts behavioural improvement. *Journal of Pediatric Gastroenterology and Nutrition, 26*(5), 549.

Horvath, K., Papadimitriou, J. C., Rabsztyn, A., Drachenberg, C., & Tildon, J. T. (1999) Gastrointestinal abnormalities in children with autistic disorder. *Journal of Pediatrics, 135*, 559–563

Horvath, K., Stefanatos, G., Sokolski, K. N., Wachtel, R., Nabors, L., & Tildon, J. T. (1998), Improved social and language skills after secretin administration in patients with autistic spectrum disorders. *Journal of the Association for Academic Minority Physicians, 9*(1), 9–15.

Jukkola, P. I., Rogers, J. T., Kaspar, B. K., Weeber, E. J., & Nishijima, I. (2011). Secretin deficiency causes impairment in survival of neural progenitor cells in mice. *Human Molecular Genetics, 20*(5), 1000–1007.

Kastner, T., Walsh, K., Shulman, L., Alam, F., & Flood, S. (2016). Ketamine and the core symptoms of autism. *International Journal on Disability and Human Development, 15*(1), 121–123.

Krishnaswami, S., McPheeters, M. L., & Veenstra-Vanderweele, J. (2011). A systematic review of secretin for children with autism spectrum disorders. *Pediatrics, 127*(5), e1322–e1325. https://doi.org/10.1542/peds.2011-0428

Kryszak, E. M., & Mulick, J. A. (2022). History of non-evidence-based practices for individuals diagnosed with ASD. In J. B. Leaf, J. H. Cihon, J. L. Ferguson, J. L., & M. J. Weiss (Eds.), *Handbook of applied behavior analysis interventions for autism: Integrating research into practice* (pp. 23–45). Cham: Springer.

Leader, G., Abberton, C., Cunningham, S., Gilmartin, K., Grudzien, M., Higgins, E., Joshi, L., Whelan, S., & Mannion, A. (2022). Gastrointestinal symptoms in autism spectrum disorder: A systematic review. *Nutrients, 14*(7), 1471. DOI: 10.3390/nu14071471

Lee, Y. J., Oh, S. H., Park, C., Hong, M., Lee, A. R., Yoo, H. J., Shin, Y. S., Cheon, K., & Bahn, G. H. (2014). Advanced pharmacotherapy evidenced by pathogenesis of autism spectrum disorder. *Clinical Psychopharmacology & Neuroscience, 12*(1), 19–30. https://doi.org/10.9758/cpn.2014.12.1.19

Lossi, L., Bottarelli, L., Candusso, M. E., Leiter, A. B., Rindi, G., & Merighi, A. (2004). Transient expression of secretin in serotoninergic neurons of mouse brain during development. *European Journal of Neuroscience, 20*, 3259–3269. doi: 10.1111/j.1460-9568.2004.03816.x

Myers, K., Goulet, M., Rusche, J., Boismenu, R., & Davis, M. (2004). Inhibition of fear potentiated startle in rats following peripheral administration of secretin. *Psychopharmacology, 172*, 94–99. https://doi.org/10.1007/s00213-003-1633-5

Sandler, A. D., Sutton, K. A., DeWeese, J., Girardi, M. A., Sheppard, V., & Bodfish, J. W. (1999). Lack of benefit of a single dose of synthetic human secretin in the treatment of autism and pervasive developmental disorder. *New England Journal of Medicine, 341*(24), 1801–1806.

Sheitman, B. B., Knable, M. B., Jarskog, L. F., Chakos, M., Boyce, L. H., Early, J., & Lieberman, J. A. (2004) Secretin for refractory schizophrenia. *Schizophrenia Research, 66*, 177–181. doi: 10.1016/S0920-9964(03)00068-9.

Sturmey, P. (2005). Secretin is an ineffective treatment for pervasive developmental disabilities: A review of 15 double-blind randomized controlled trials. *Research in Developmental Disabilities, 26*(1), 87–97.

Takayanagi, Y., Yoshida, M., Takashima, A., Takanami, K., Yoshida, S., Nishimori, K., Nishijima, I., Sakamoto, H., Yamagata, T. & Onaka, T. (2017). Activation of supraoptic oxytocin neurons by secretin facilitates social recognition. *Biological Psychiatry, 81*(3), 243–251.

Toda, Y., Mori, K., Hashimoto, T., Miyazaki, M., Nozaki, S., Watanabe, Y., Kuroda, Y. & Kagami, S. (2006). Administration of secretin for autism alters dopamine metabolism in the central nervous system. *Brain and Development, 28*(2), 99–103.

Velmurugan, S., Brunton, P. J., Leng, G., & Russell, J. A. (2010). Circulating secretin activates supraoptic nucleus oxytocin and vasopressin neurons via noradrenergic pathways in the rat. *Endocrinology, 151*(6), 2681–2688.

Wang, R., Chow, B. K. C., & Zhang, L. (2019) Distribution and functional implication of Secretin in multiple brain regions. *Journal of Molecular Neuroscience, 68*, 485–493. https://doi.org/10.1007/s12031-018-1089-z

Welch, M. G., Anwar, M., Chang, C. Y., Gross, K. J., Ruggiero, D. A., Tamir, H., & Gershon, M. D. (2010). Combined administration of secretin and oxytocin inhibits chronic colitis and associated activation of forebrain neurons. *Neurogastroenterology & Motility*, *22*(6), 654–e202.

Williams, K. J., Wray, J. J., & Wheeler, D. M. (2005). Intravenous secretin for autism spectrum disorder. *Cochrane Database of Systematic Reviews*, (3), CD003495. doi: 10.1002/14651858.CD003495.pub2

Williams, K., Wray, J. A., & Wheeler, D. M. (2012). Intravenous secretin for autism spectrum disorders (ASD). *Cochrane Database of Systematic Reviews*, (4): doi: 10.1002/14651858.CD003495.pub2.

Zhang, L., & Chow, B. K. (2014). The central mechanisms of secretin in regulating multiple behaviors. *Frontiers in Endocrinology*, 5, 77.

33
Cannabis

Laura Fusar-Poli, Cecilia Guiot, Davide Marisca, Udi Yehuda Levi, Pierluigi Politi, and Natascia Brondino
Department of Brain and Behavioral Sciences, University of Pavia

33.1 Technical Abstract

Background: The interest in medical cannabis has been growing over the last few years. Cannabis interacts with the endocannabinoid system and may modulate different aspects related to cognition, socioemotional responses, susceptibility to seizures, nociception, and neuronal plasticity, which are often altered in autism spectrum disorder (ASD). **Method:** We searched PubMed and PsycInfo and identified 13 papers reporting the results of 12 studies evaluating the efficacy and/or safety of medical cannabis for autistic people. **Results:** Medical cannabis and related compounds appeared to improve some autism-associated symptoms, such as sleep disturbances and behavioral problems. The main adverse event was sedation, while reported cardiac and metabolic side effects were limited. Findings were mainly based on open-label studies; only one randomized placebo-controlled trial has been conducted so far. **Discussion:** Research on the use of medical cannabis for ASD is insufficient to provide clinical guidance on the efficacy, safety, composition, and dosage. However, medical cannabis might represent a promising treatment for ASD-associated symptoms based on the results of one randomized controlled trial (RCT). Future research should develop rigorously designed studies to compare the efficacy and safety of medical cannabis alone or in combination with antipsychotics to other treatments. **Practitioner recommendations:** Medical cannabis and cannabis-derived products may be used to manage some ASD-associated symptoms on an individual basis in case other evidence-based treatments have failed, after a comprehensive assessment and under medical surveillance.

33.2 Layperson Summary

Cannabis is a recreational drug. Its use has been approved in several countries to treat some medical conditions. For ASD, it is typically administered in the form of an oil, which may contain different concentrations of active compounds, not always accurately reported on labels. Some cannabis compounds interact with

Laura Fusar-Poli et al., *Cannabis*. In: *Lifespan Treatment for Autistic Individuals*. Edited by: Peter Sturmey, Russell Lang, and James K. Luiselli, Oxford University Press. © Oxford University Press (2025).
DOI: 10.1093/oso/9780197635841.003.0033

the endocannabinoid system, which is a signaling system naturally present in the human body. That system may be altered in people with ASD. This interaction could modulate some behaviors or symptoms associated with ASD. We searched two important databases. We found 13 articles reporting the results of 12 studies. There was only one true experiment that compared the efficacy of medical cannabis to placebo. Medical cannabis can be effective in managing some symptoms, such as sleep problems, irritability, self-injury, and hyperactivity. However, it is unclear whether these effects were caused by medical cannabis itself or other medications taken by the participants. Also, medical cannabis could improve seizures in people with associated epilepsy. However, the measures used to evaluate the efficacy were frequently not standardized. The most important side effects of medical cannabis were related to sleepiness and increased appetite. Given the limited and sparse evidence, it is difficult to develop guidelines. Pharmaceutical compounds based on medical cannabis could be prescribed by a licensed physician. That licensed physician should be thoroughly informed on the history and current conditions of the person with ASD. The use of medical cannabis should be monitored constantly.

33.3 Treatment Summary Table

Treatment summary: Cannabis

Treatment description: Medical cannabis is composed of cannabinoids derived from the cannabis plant, including Δ9-tetrahydrocannabinol (THC), cannabidiol (CBD), or a combination of THC and CBD. It may be supplied as oil, capsules, dried cannabis, or prescription liquid solution.

Expected outcomes: Cannabis may improve sleep disturbances and behavioral problems.

Methods: Medical cannabis may be administered by various routes. In individuals with ASD, it is usually administered orally in the form of an oil.

Expertise required to implement treatment: Medical expertise is required, as typically shown by a licensed physician.

Risks and negative side effects: Sleep disturbances, appetite changes, and restlessness are some possible side effects.

Additional considerations and limitations: There are no specific indications on the optimal dosage and CBD:THC ratio. The choice of cannabis to manage sleep should be taken in the context of alternate treatments such as behavioral interventions, sleep hygiene, and alternate medications such as melatonin.

33.4 Introduction

33.4.1 Treatment Description

Cannabis is one of the most widely used recreational drugs today. It derives from the genus of a flowering plant in the family *Cannabaceae*. Various strains of cannabis exist, but there is no consensus on taxonomy. *Sativa*, *indica*, and *ruderalis* might be three separate species or subspecies of *Cannabis sativa*. Cannabis contains more than 500 known active compounds, such as cannabinoids, flavonoids, and terpenes, and fatty acids (Gould, 2015; Rock & Parker, 2021).

Cannabinoids that naturally occur in the cannabis plant are also called phytocannabinoids and bind to the endocannabinoid system receptors in humans and animals (Gould, 2015). Hundreds of phytocannabinoids have been isolated from cannabis, of which the most important are delta-9-tetrahydrocannabinol (THC) and cannabidiol (CBD). THC is the primary intoxicating compound in cannabis and appears to be responsible for the psychoactive effects of cannabis. Endocannabinoids are derivatives of integral components of cellular membranes and act as hydrophobic lipid messengers in the endocannabinoid system. N-arachidonoylethanolamine (anandamide) and 2-arachidonoyl glycerol (2-AG) are the major endocannabinoids. Despite similarities in chemical structure, 2-AG and anandamide are synthesized and degraded by distinct enzymatic pathways, which impart fundamentally different physiological and pathophysiological roles to these two endocannabinoids (Lu & Mackie, 2021). Synthetic cannabinoids are a class of designer drug molecules that bind to the same receptors of phytocannabinoids and endocannabinoids (Alves et al., 2020).

Cannabis has been cultivated in many parts of the world and used as medicine since ancient times. In ancient China, it was used to target malaria, rheumatism, constipation, gout, and menstrual cramps, and it was used as a remedy for earache, edema, and inflammation by the ancient Greeks. Since medieval times, practitioners in the West have used cannabis for pain, depression, epilepsy, nausea, and vomiting. Recent years have seen renewed research interest, and further evidence has accumulated on the therapeutic potential of cannabis—the whole plant extract, and some of its individual active constituents and their synthetic mimics—in many different conditions (Crocq, 2020).

Research on the therapeutic potential of cannabis parallels increasing legalization of both medical and recreational cannabis. Currently, evidence on the efficacy of medicinal cannabis is limited to a few conditions, including chronic pain, nausea and vomiting from chemotherapy, spasticity due to multiple sclerosis or spinal cord injury, Tourette's syndrome, and sleep disorders (Whiting et al., 2015).

33.4.2 Rationale and Objectives

Medical cannabis and cannabinoids act on the endocannabinoid system (ECS), a widespread neuromodulatory system that plays important roles in central nervous system development, synaptic plasticity, and the response to endogenous and environmental insults. The ECS comprises cannabinoid receptors, endocannabinoids, and the enzymes responsible for the synthesis and degradation of the endocannabinoids (Lu & Mackie, 2021).

The effects of cannabinoids are mediated by cannabinoid receptors type 1 (CB1) and type 2 (CB2). CB1 and CB2 are G protein–coupled receptors, primarily coupling to inhibitory G proteins. They inhibit adenylyl cyclase and certain voltage-sensitive calcium channels, stimulate mitogen-activated protein kinases and inwardly rectifying potassium channels, and recruit beta-arrestins, among other actions.

CB1 receptors are particularly enriched in the nervous system but are also present in diverse organs, including the liver, adipose tissue, and skin. In the adult central nervous system neurons, the CB1 receptor is most abundant on certain gamma-aminobutyric acidergic interneurons. However, CB1 receptors are found on a wide range of other neurons, including glutamatergic, cholinergic, glycinergic, and serotonergic neurons. CB2 receptors are primarily expressed in cells of immune origin, including microglia, though they may also be expressed in neurons, particularly in pathological states. CB1 receptor stimulation is responsible for the cannabis effects, while activation of the CB2 receptor leads to attenuated inflammation, decreased tissue damage, and accelerated regeneration in several disease states (Kendall & Yudowski, 2016).

CBD has a low affinity for CB1 and CB2 receptors, where it may act as a negative allosteric modulator of CB1 activity and a weak inverse agonist or partial agonist of CB2 receptors. CBD also has indirect effects on endocannabinoid signaling, such as increasing levels of the endocannabinoid ligand anandamide by decreasing its cellular reuptake by fatty acid binding proteins, and decreasing endocannabinoid hydrolysis by fatty acid amide hydrolase. Beyond the endocannabinoid system, CBD may modulate serotonin 5-HT1A receptors, G protein–coupled receptors, and transient receptor potential cation channel subfamily V, member 1 receptors, as well as μ- and δ-opioid receptors, and may modulate opioid actions and addiction vulnerability. The exact mechanisms of CBD are not yet clear, and the relevance of the numerous proposed targets needs to be further investigated (Mandolini et al., 2018).

Imbalances in the ECS neurotransmission have been found in animal models of ASD (Kerr et al., 2013; Zamberletti et al., 2017). Additionally, lower serum levels of endocannabinoids were detected in children with ASD compared to typically developing peers (Aran, Eylon, et al., 2019). Notably, the ECS seems to regulate some of the functions typically impaired in ASD, such as social interaction and emotional responses. Recent findings indicate that anandamide-mediated signaling at CB1 receptors modulates oxytocin-dependent social reward, suggesting that deficits in the signaling mechanism of anandamide may contribute to social impairment in ASD (Wei et al., 2015). In fact, enhancement of ECS in mouse models may correct some aspects of social impairment (Servadio et al., 2016; Wei et al., 2016).

As of 2022, the US Food and Drug Administration (FDA) has approved Epidiolex, a purified CBD-based oral solution, for the treatment of refractory epilepsy in patients with Dravet syndrome, Lennox-Gastaut syndrome, and tuberous sclerosis complex (Talwar et al., 2023). Epilepsy is one of the most frequent co-occurring conditions of ASD (Frye, 2016); the presence of seizures or nonepileptic abnormalities in EEG patterns might be partially responsible for the challenging behaviors in autistic individuals (Austin & Dunn, 2002).

33.4.3 Considerations for Implementation

The legality of medical cannabis varies by country, in terms of how it can be consumed and which conditions it can be used for. Medical cannabis and analog products (excluding CBD) must be prescribed by a doctor included in the register of specialist medical practitioners.

Medical cannabis can be taken internally in multiple ways, including by inhaling cannabis smoke or vapor, by taking it orally, and by administering it as an aerosol spray into the cheek. More frequently, in ASD it may be supplied as CBD oil containing only CBD as the active ingredient (excluding THC), CBD-dominant hemp extract oil, capsules, dried cannabis, or prescription liquid solution (Baratta et al., 2021; VanDolah et al., 2019).

33.5 Research Background

33.5.1 Search Strategy

In November 2022, we searched the Web of Science database using the following search terms: (cannab*) AND (autis* OR asperger OR "neurodevelop* disorder*"). We selected all original studies written in English and published in peer-reviewed journals without time restrictions, evaluating the efficacy and/or safety of medical cannabis in autistic individuals. Dissertations, master and doctoral theses, conference abstracts, and articles written in languages other than English were excluded from the present selection. Studies evaluating the acute effect or cannabis-based compound to understand the functioning mechanisms were also excluded.

33.5.2 Characteristics of the Included Studies

Overall, we retrieved 13 papers reporting the data from 12 studies, as Aran et al. (2021) and Schnapp et al. (2022) reported different outcome measures from the same RCT. Study characteristics are summarized in Table 33.1. Most studies (6 out of 12 studies) were conducted in Israel, with the second most represented nation being Canada (2 studies). The other studies were conducted in Brazil, Austria,

Table 33.1 *Study characteristics*

Study (Year)	Country	Design	Sample Characteristics	Treatment Characteristics
Aran et al. (2021)	Israel	Randomized controlled trial	N = 150, mean age: 11.8 years, age range: 5.1–20.8 years, 80% males. 78.7% severe symptoms	Group (1) was given a whole-plant cannabis extract with a 20:1 CBD:THC ratio. Group (2) was given purified CBD and THC with a 20:1 ratio. Group (3) was given placebo. Sublingual administration was divided into three daily doses. Starting dose was 1 mg/kg/day CBD + 0.05 mg/kg/day THC, titrated up to 10 mg/kg/day bodyweight CBD + 0.5 mg/kg/day THC for children weighing 20–40 kg, or 7.5 mg/kg/day CBD + 0.375 mg/kg/day THC for weight >40 kg (maximum 420 mg CBD and 21 mg THC per day).
Aran et al. (2019)	Israel	Retrospective cohort study	N = 60, mean age: 11.8, age range: 5–17.5, 77% low functioning	Cannabinoid oil solution at a 20:1 ratio of CBD and THC. Sublingual assumption 2 or 3 times/daily with CBD doses started at 1 mg/kg/day and titrated up to 10 mg/kg/day.
Barchel et al. (2019)	Israel	Prospective cohort study	N = 53, mean age:11, age range: 4–22	Cannabinoid oil solution at a concentration of 30% and 20:1 ratio of CBD and THC. CBD: 16 mg/kg (maximal daily dose 600 mg), THC: 0.8 mg/kg (maximal daily dose of 40 mg).
Bar-Lev Schleider et al. (2019)	Israel	Prospective cohort study	N = 188, mean age: 12.9, age range: <5–18	Most patients consumed oil with 30% CBD and 1.5% THC. Insomnia was treated with an evening dose of 3% THC oil. On average 79.5 ± 61.5 mg CBD and 4.0 ± 3.0 mg THC, three times a day. Average additional 5.0 ± 4.5 mg THC daily for insomnia.

continued

Table 33.1 *continued*

Study (Year)	Country	Design	Sample Characteristics	Treatment Characteristics
Bilge et al. (2021)	Turkey	Prospective cohort study	N = 33, 27 males, mean age: 7.7 ± 5.5 years. 15 mild autism, 18 severe autism	Two brands of full-spectrum CBD were used that had similar available forms of drops of 500, 1,000, and 2,500 mg/30 ml and contained full-spectrum CBD and trace THC of less than 3%. Starting dosage was calculated according to bodyweight, with one sublingual drop twice a day and one drop every 3 days. Average daily dosage of CBD was 0.7 mg/kg/day (0.3–2 mg/kg/day), maximum dosage was 40 mg/day. The median duration of treatment was 6.5 months (3–28 months).
Erridge et al. (2022)	United King-dom	Retrospective cohort study	N = 74, mean age 32.7 (±11.6) years old	Heterogeneous formulations were used: the median prescribed CBD dose per day at the date of extraction was 10.0 mg, while the median THC dose was 112.5 mg per day. Patients were treated for a minimum of 1 month up to 6 months.
Fleury-Teixeira et al. (2019)	Brazil	Prospective cohort study	N = 18 (15 analyzed), mean age: 10.9, age range: 6–17	Cannabis sativa extract containing a 75:1 CBD:THC ratio. CBD: mean 175 mg/day (100–350); THC: 2.33 mg/day (1.33–2.33).
Hacohen et al. (2022)	Israel	Prospective cohort study	N = 110 (82 analyzed), 65 male, mean age: 9.2 years old, range: 5–25 years old (53 completed all assessments and 29 completed partial assessments)	Cannabis whole-plant extract infused in oil with a CBD:THC ratio of 20:1 for a period of 6 months. Starting with one drop daily (each drop contains: 0.3 mg THC and 5.7 mg CBD) increasing the dosage until perceived improvement, up to 10 mg/kg/day of CBD and 0.5 mg/kg/day of THC.
Kurz and Blaas (2010)	Austria	Case report	N = 1, 6 years old	Dronabinol (delta-9-THC) dissolved in sesame oil. Initial dosage was one drop (0.62 mg) in the morning which was increased up to 3.62 mg/die.

Study (Year)	Country	Design	Sample Characteristics	Treatment Characteristics
Ma et al. (2022)	Canada	Case report	N = 1, male, 9 years old, diagnosed with nonverbal ASD	CBD and THC oil formulation, with each milliliter containing 20 mg of CBD and <1 mg of THC. Starting dose was 0.1 ml twice daily, increased every 3–4 days to 0.5 ml twice daily.
Ponton et al. (2020)	Canada	Case report	N = 1, male, 15 years old	CBE (1:20 CBE—0.001% THC and 0.02% CBD), 0.1 ml twice a day (2 mg CBD and 0.1 mg THC) increasing by 0.1 ml per dose if no effects were shown up to 0.5 ml per dose. Patient used 0.1 ml twice a day for 3 months and then 0.2 ml twice a day for 9 months.
Schnapp et al. (2022)	Israel	Randomized controlled trial	N = 150, mean age: 11.8, age range: 5.1–20.8, 78.7% severe symptoms	Group (1) was given a whole-plant cannabis extract with a 20:1 CBD:THC ratio. Group (2) was given purified CBD and THC with a 20:1 ratio. Group (3) was given placebo. Sublingual administration was divided into three daily doses. Starting dose was 1 mg/kg/day CBD + 0.05 mg/kg/day THC, titrated up to 10 mg/kg/day bodyweight CBD + 0.5 mg/kg/day THC for children weighing 20–40 kg, or 7.5 mg/kg/day CBD + 0.375 mg/kg/day THC for weight >40 kg (maximum 420 mg CBD and 21 mg THC per day).
Stolar et al. (2022)	Israel	Prospective cohort phase 3 study	N = 59; 85% male and 15% female); mean age: 10.7 years old; range: 5–25 years old	Cannabis extract infused in MCT oil with a CBD:THC ratio of 20:1 for 6 months. Starting with one oral drop daily (each drop contains: 0.3 mg THC and 5.7 mg CBD), increasing gradually until perceived improvements, up to 10 mg/kg/day (or total of 400 mg/day) of CBD and 0.5 mg/kg/day (or total of 20 mg/day) of THC.

CBD = Cannabidiol; CBE = Cannabidiol-based extract; MCT = Medium-chain triglycerides; THC = Tetrahydrocannabinol.

Turkey, and the United Kingdom. As for study design, three were case reports, one was an RCT, and the remaining eight were retrospective or prospective cohort studies. Apart from one case report (Kurz & Blaas, 2010), all papers were published within the last 3 years. The number of participants for studies that were not case reports ranged from 18 to 150 participants. Mean age of participants was between 6 and 11.8 years, with the exception of Erridge et al. (2022), who reported a mean age of 32.7 years. Male gender was more represented in most studies. Interestingly, autism severity was reported only in a minority of studies. Many participants were taking concurrent medications.

Treatment regimens and formulations of cannabinoid solution were heterogeneous between studies. A CBD:THC ratio of approximately 20:1 was reported in eight studies, while one study reported a CBD:THC ratio of 75:1; the remaining studies did not report a CBD:THC ratio. Cannabinoid concentration varied across studies. Concerning treatment dosage, no uniform strategy was used; however, all studies started from a minimum dosage and then titrated up to a maximum dosage monitoring symptom improvement and onset of side effects.

33.5.3 Summary of Findings

Efficacy and safety results are summarized in Table 33.2. Studies typically had multiple outcomes, the most investigated being problem behaviors and sleep problems. There is overall preliminary evidence showing that cannabinoid compounds might exert beneficial effects on some ASD-associated symptoms and that treatment with cannabinoids reduced the number of prescribed medications with a higher number of metabolic and neurological side effects.

Problem behaviors represented the most frequently evaluated outcome category. This outcome was assessed in 10 studies using the Aberrant Behavior Checklist (ABC), the Caregiver Global Impression (CaGI-C), the Home Situation Questionnaire (HSQ), or by means of ad hoc interviews on self-injurious behavior, behavioral disorder symptoms, or stereotypies. Most studies found some degree of improvement in problem behaviors. One study found no significant change in the HSQ.

The second most frequent category concerned sleep problems, which were assessed in seven studies by means of the Children's Sleep Habits Questionnaire (CSHQ), the Single-Item Sleep Quality Scale (SQS), or ad hoc questions concerning sleep-related symptomatology. Most studies found improvement in sleep problems, except one study that found no significant differences in any CSHQ subscale. Two of these studies (Ma et al., 2022; Ponton et al., 2020) were case reports in which daily dose was increased when no effects were detected. However, it is important to note that, although the majority of studies found some degree of improvement, the only RCT which evaluated sleep problems as an outcome

Table 33.2 *Efficacy and safety*

Study (Year)	Efficacy	Adverse Events
Aran et al. (2021)	Home Situation Questionnaire (HSQ-ASD) scores did not differ significantly between participants who received cannabinoids and participants who received placebo. CGI-I: 49% of participants receiving the whole-plant extract treatment responded versus 21% on placebo. SRS-2: significant improvement in participants receiving the whole-plant extract treatment versus those on placebo. No clear advantages for the whole-plant extract over pure cannabinoids were found.	Somnolence (27% whole-plant extract, 24% pure cannabinoids); decreased appetite (24% whole-plant extract, 22% pure cannabinoids); weight loss (12% whole-plant extract, 13% pure cannabinoids); tiredness (25% whole-plant extract, 34% pure cannabinoids); euphoria (20% whole-plant extract, 19% pure cannabinoids); anxiety (20% whole-plant extract, 27% pure cannabinoids)
Aran et al. (2019)	HSQ: improved by 29%. APSI: improved by 33%. CaGI-C: Behavior improved in 61%; anxiety improved in 39%; communication improved in 47% of the children. Following the cannabis treatment, 33% received fewer medications or lower dosage, 24% stopped taking medications, and 8% received more medications or higher dose.	Any adverse event (51%), sleep disturbances (14%), restlessness (9%), nervousness (9%), loss of appetite (9%), gastrointestinal symptoms (7%), unexplained laugh (7%), mood changes (5%), fatigue (5%), nocturnal enuresis (3.5%), gain of appetite (3.5%), weight loss (3.5%), weight gain (3.5%), dry mouth (3.5%), tremor (3.5%), sleepiness (2%), anxiety (2%), confusion (2%), cough (2%), psychotic event (2%)
Barchel et al. (2019)	Hyperactivity: improvement: 68.4%; no change: 28.9%; worsening: 2.6% Self-Injury: improvement: 67.6%; no change: 23.5%; worsening: 8.8% Sleep problems: improvement: 71.4%; no change: 23.8%; worsening: 4.7% Anxiety: improvement: 47.1%; no change: 29.4%; worsening: 23.5% Overall: improvement: 74.5%; no change: 21.6%; worsening: 3.9%	Somnolence (22.6%), appetite decrease (11.3%), appetite increase (7.5%), Insomnia (3.7%), sense abnormality response (to temperature) (3.7%), eyes blinking (3.7%), diarrhea (3.7%), hair loss (1.8%), nausea (1.8%), confusion (1.8%), acne (1.8%), palpitations (1.8%), urinary (1.8%), incontinence (1.8%), rye redness (1.8%), constipation (1.8%)
Bar-Lev Schleider et al. (2019)	Quality of life: 66.8% improvement Mood: 63.5% improvement Adaptive abilities: 42.9% improvement Sleep: 24.7% improvement Concentration: 14% improvement	Restlessness (6.6%), sleepiness (3.2%), psychoactive effect (3.2%), increased appetite (3.2%), digestion problems (3.2%), dry mouth (2.2%), lack of appetite (2.2%)

continued

Table 33.2 *continued*

Study (Year)	Efficacy	Adverse Events
Bilge & Ekici (2021)	Clinical interviews: No change in daily life activity in 6 (19.35%) patients Decrease in behavioral problems in 10 patients (32.2%) Increase in expressive language in 7 patients (22.5%) Improved cognition in 4 patients (12.9%) Increase in social interaction in 3 patients (9.6%) Decrease in stereotypies in 1 patient (3.2%) Antipsychotic drug could be stopped in one patient who showed mild ASD symptoms	Generalized seizures in one patient, persisting after drug discontinuation, treated with valproic acid Significant increase in stereotypies in one patient Restlessness in 7 (22%) out of 31 patients who continued treatment for at least 3 months; restlessness decreased as dosage was reduced
Erridge et al. (2022)	General health-related quality of life (EQ-5D-5L): Improvement at 1, 3, and 6 months Sleep (SQS): improvement at 1, 3, and 6 months Anxiety severity: General anxiety disorder-7 reduction at 1 and 3 months, but no change at 6 months	Fourteen (18.9%) participants reported 180 total adverse events. Adverse events were commonly mild (n = 58; 78.4%) or moderate (n = 81; 109.5%), rather than severe (n = 41; 55.4%). There were no (0.0%) life-threatening or disabling adverse events. Abdominal pain (4.1%), agitation (4.1%), amnesia (6.8%), anorexia (8.1%), anxiety (1.4%), ataxia (6.8%), blurred vision (8.1%), cognitive disturbance (6.8%), concentration impairment (13.5%), confusion (2.7%), constipation (1.4%), delirium (2.7%), depression (5.4%), diarrhea (1.4%), dizziness (6.8%), dry mouth (14.9%), dysgeusia (5.4%), dyspepsia (8.1%), fall (2.7%), fatigue (13.5%), fasciculations (1.4%), generalized muscle weakness (6.8%), headache (10.8%), increased seizure frequency (4.1%), insomnia (17.6%), lethargy (14.9%), nausea (8.1%), pharyngitis (4.1%), pyrexia (1.4%), rash (2.7%), somnolence (12.2%), spasticity (8.1%), tremor (9.5%), vertigo (5.4%), vomiting (2.7%), weight loss (5.4%), upper respiratory tract infection (4.1%)

Study (Year)	Efficacy	Adverse Events
Fleury-Teixeira et al. (2019)	Attention deficit/hyperactivity disorder (ADHD): median perception of improvement: 30% Behavioral disorders (BD): median perception of improvement 20% Motor deficits (MD): median perception of improvement 20% Autonomy deficits (AD): median perception of improvement 10% Communication and social interaction deficits (CSID): median perception of improvement 25% Cognitive deficits (CD): median perception of improvement 20% Sleep disorders (SD): median perception of improvement 40% Seizures (SZ): three participants reported ≥50% of improvement; two participants reported 100% of improvement. Concomitant medication: complete withdrawal (n = 3), partial withdrawal (n = 1), partial withdrawal + dosage reduction (n = 3), dosage reduction (n = 2), no changes in medication use (n = 1)	Sleepiness, moderate irritability (n = 3); diarrhea, increased appetite, conjunctival hyperemia, and increased body temperature (n = 1). All these side effects were mild and/or transient. Nocturia (n = 2) in one case appeared concomitantly to an improvement in sleep quality.
Hacohen et al. (2022)	ASD symptom severity (ADOS-2 CSS): improvement; participants with more severe initial symptoms exhibited larger improvements. Age and final dosage were not significantly associated with changes. Social affect (ADOS Social Affect domain CSS): improvement Restricted and repetitive behavior (ADOS RRB domain CSS): no significant impact Cognitive abilities (Block design, Matrix, Vocabulary, Similarities & Information, coding processing speed of Wechsler Intelligence Scale; Wechsler Preschool and Primary Scale of Intelligence, Wechsler Intelligence Scale for Children or Wechsler Adult Intelligence Scale): no significant impact of treatment on any of the cognitive subtests: Adaptive behavior (Vineland 3): improvement in total scores; apparent in the communication, daily living, and socialization subscales. Social responsiveness (SRS-2): improvement; participants with more severe initial symptoms exhibited larger improvements. Age and final dosage were not significantly associated with changes.	Not assessed 12 dropout (11% of the initial sample) because of increased aggression (5), increased anxiety (3), weight gain (1), abdominal pain (1), increased hyperactivity (1), decrease in communication (1)
Kurz and Blaas (2010)	Problem behaviors (ABC): Significant improvement in all subscales (irritability, agitation, & crying; lethargy/social withdrawal; stereotypic behavior; hyperactivity/noncompliance; and inappropriate speech)	None reported

continued

Table 33.2 *continued*

Study (Year)	Efficacy	Adverse Events
Ma et al. (2022)	Reduction in negative behaviors (including violent outbursts and self-injurious behaviors) Improved sleep time and quality Improvement in social interactions and communication (followed simple instructions) Improvement in concentration (with better academic performance) and emotional stability	No side effects reported
Ponton et al. (2020)	At 0.2 ml twice a day for almost 9 months: Overall anxiety, social anxiety and irritability (VAS): improved 7 points Aggressiveness (VAS): improved 6 points Talkativeness (VAS): improved 4 points Concentration (VAS): improved 2 points Sleep disturbances (CSHQ): he slept 7 hours and only had trouble falling asleep in his own bed as he resists going to bed	No side effects were reported (nausea/vomiting, diarrhea, headaches, euphoria, feeling high, anxiety, panic attacks, palpitations, somnolence during the day or drowsiness)
Schnapp et al. (2022)	Sleep disturbances (CSHQ): no significant differences were found in no CSHQ subscale between groups	Not assessed
Stolar et al. (2022)	Not assessed	No significant differences were found between baseline levels and levels after 3 months of treatment of complete blood count, glucose, urea, creatinine, electrolytes, liver enzymes (AST, ALT, gamma GT), bilirubin, lipid profile, thyroid antibodies, prolactin, and testosterone. A few statistically significant changes were observed in the level of LDH and thyroid hormones (TSH, fT4); however, these changes have no clinical significance. No differences in safety test results were identified between children taking or not taking antipsychotic medications together with CBD-rich cannabis oil, nor between those receiving high or low dose of medical cannabis.

ABC = Aberrant Behavior Checklist; ADOS-2-CSS = Autism Diagnostic Observation Schedule—Calibrated Severity Score; APSI = Autism Parenting Stress Index; CaGI = Caregiver Global Impression; CSHQ = Children's Sleep Habits Questionnaire; HSQ = Home Situation Questionnaire; SQS = Single-Item Sleep Quality Scale; SRS-2 = Social Responsiveness Scale-2nd edition; VAS = Visual Analog Scale.

(Schnapp et al., 2022) found no significant differences in the CSHQ subscale among the three groups, one of which was a placebo group. However, sleepiness was reported as an adverse effect in four studies (Aran, Eylon, et al., 2019; Barchel et al., 2019; Bar-Lev Schleider et al., 2019; Fleury-Teixeira et al., 2019).

Regarding ASD core symptoms, a prospective cohort study (Hacohen et al., 2022) with a sample of 82 participants reported improvement in both overall Autism Diagnostic Observation Schedule-Second Edition (ADOS-2) Calibrated Severity Scores (CSS) and the Social Affect domain. Notably, participants with more severe initial symptoms exhibited larger improvements while age and final dosage were not significantly associated with changes; improvement in the Social Responsiveness Schedule-Second Edition (SRS-2) also supported these findings. However, this study found no significant impact on the Restricted and Repetitive Behavior domain of the ADOS-2. Changes in communication and social interaction were specifically assessed in four other studies. Aran and colleagues (2019) reported improvement of communication as measured by CaGI-C in 47% of participants. Bilge and Ekici (2021) conducted clinical interviews that assessed some degree of improvement in both expressive language and social interaction. A prospective cohort study (Fleury-Teixeira et al., 2019) and a case report (Ma et al., 2022) also identified improvement in communication and social interaction. Two studies specifically investigated the effect of cannabinoids on repetitive behaviors or restricted interests, one finding decreased stereotypies in 1 participant out of 33, and a case report (Kurz & Blaas, 2010) reporting significant improvement in the Stereotypic Behavior subscale of the ABC.

Four studies targeted *adaptive abilities and daily life activities*. In one study (Bilge & Ekici, 2021), parents reported no change in daily life activity in 19.35% of participants. Another study (Hacohen et al., 2022) found improvement in both total scores of the Vineland 3 scale and in communication, daily living, and socialization subscales. Two more studies (Bar-Lev Schleider et al., 2019; Fleury-Teixeira et al., 2019) reported improvement in autonomy and adaptive abilities. Four other studies focused on changes in concentration. Two case reports (Ma et al., 2022; Ponton et al., 2020) and a prospective cohort study (Bar-Lev Schleider et al., 2019) found an improvement in concentration, while Erridge et al. (2022) reported concentration impairment as an adverse effect in 10 out of 74 participants (13.5% of the sample). Impact on anxiety was assessed by four studies. One retrospective cohort study (Erridge et al., 2022) found reduction of anxiety measured using the General Anxiety Disorder-7 scale at 1 and 3 months, but not at the 6-months follow-up. A case report (Ponton et al., 2020) reported a 7-point improvement in the Visual Analogue Scale (VAS) for overall anxiety, social anxiety, and irritability when treatment was titrated at 0.2 ml twice a day. In a prospective cohort study (Barchel et al., 2019), anxiety improved in 47.1% of participants; however, no change was found for 29.4%, and anxiety even worsened in 23.5% of participants.

Cognition was evaluated in three studies. Two of these studies (Bilge & Ekici, 2021; Fleury-Teixeira et al., 2019) reported an improvement in cognitive abilities through clinical interview and perception of improvement. The only prospective study using standardized tests such as Wechsler Preschool and Primary Scale of Intelligence, Wechsler Intelligence Scale for Children, or Wechsler Adult Intelligence Scale found no significant impact of the treatment on any of the cognitive subtests. Erridge et al. (2022) reported cognitive disturbance as an adverse effect in a small percentage of the participants. Reduction of hyperactivity was reported in three studies (Barchel et al., 2019; Fleury-Teixeira et al., 2019; Kurz & Blaas, 2010).

Two studies (Bar-Lev Schleider et al., 2019; Erridge et al., 2022) also assessed a general improvement in the quality of life. Other outcomes were motor development, autism parenting stress index, seizures, and mood. Of note, one study (Fleury-Teixeira et al., 2019) reported that in individuals with comorbid epilepsy, the use of cannabinoids significantly reduced the frequency and intensity of seizures. However, Erridge et al. (2022) reported an increase in seizures frequency in a small proportion of participants, and in another study (Bilge & Ekici, 2021) generalized seizures occurred in one patient, persisting after drug discontinuation, which was subsequently treated with valproic acid.

Three studies (Aran, Cassuto, et al., 2019; Bilge & Ekici, 2021; Fleury-Teixeira et al., 2019) measured changes in medications reporting that the number and dosage of used medications were reduced after the treatment with cannabinoids. In some cases, following cannabis treatment, the antipsychotic drugs could be stopped. This is a secondary, but extremely important finding. In fact, pharmacological therapies commonly prescribed to individuals with ASD can be burdened by negative side effects, such as weight gain, dyslipidemia, diabetes, and metabolic syndrome. According to a phase 3 cohort study (Barchel et al., 2019), the treatment with a cannabis extract infused in medium-chain triglycerides (MCT) oil with a CBD:THC ratio of 20:1 for 6 months produced no significant differences between baseline levels and levels after 3 months of treatment of various biochemical values such as complete blood count, glucose, lipid profile, thyroid antibodies, and prolactin.

The most common side effects of cannabinoids reported in these 13 papers were somnolence, increased appetite, and irritability. As many patients were taking concomitant medications, it is not possible to determine if these adverse events were caused by the cannabinoids, by other drugs, or their interactions. Only Aran et al. (2019) reported a severe adverse event (a psychotic episode) that resolved after stopping the cannabinoid oil solution and treating the patient with an antipsychotic (i.e., ziprasidone). None of the included studies reported cardiac adverse events (i.e., QTc prolongation) or severe metabolic side effects (i.e., hyperlipidemia, diabetes, hyperprolactinemia).

33.6 Practice Implications

33.6.1 Treatment Outcomes

Based on currently available literature, medical cannabis might be effective for treating sleep disorders and behavioral problems, such as irritability, aggressiveness, or self-injurious behaviors in people with ASD. Also, medical cannabis could be useful in reducing the number of seizures in patients with ASD and comorbid epilepsy. Conversely, the efficacy on core symptoms has yet to be proven. It is worth underlying that, to date, only one RCT has been conducted; thus, evidence is substantially based on observational studies. Additionally, in most of the studies, participants were taking concomitant medications. Psychotropic medications, particularly antipsychotics, are frequently prescribed in the ASD population, and may be utilized for their sedative effects. Therefore, it is difficult to establish whether the efficacy of medical cannabis on certain symptoms, such as sleep disorders or behavioral problems, is actually due to the sedative effects given by psychotropic medications or by medical cannabis itself. Moreover, it is difficult to determine whether the positive effect on autistic core symptoms and problem behaviors found in some studies may be the result of a general sedative effect expressed by medical cannabis. In addition, the most commonly reported adverse events of medical cannabis were somnolence, increased appetite, and irritability. Only one study (Aran, Eylon, et al., 2019) reported the onset of a psychotic episode as a side effect, which resolved after stopping the cannabinoid oil solution and treating the patient with an antipsychotic. None of the included studies reported cardiac adverse events or severe metabolic side effects that could suggest a better safety profile in medical cannabis than antipsychotics.

33.6.2 Practice Implication Guidelines

At present, scientific evidence is insufficient to inform clear clinical guidance regarding the use of medical cannabis in terms of composition and dosage to treat core and associated symptoms of ASD. Results from one RCT have shown that medical cannabis may represent a promising treatment for some ASD-associated symptoms, such as sleep disorders and behavioral problems. However, there is no evidence that medical cannabis might be more effective than other treatments suggested by current guidelines, such as sleep hygiene, behavioral treatment of sleep problems, and melatonin. Therefore, medical cannabis should be considered on a case-by-case basis, in association with other psychotropic medications or alone, weighing up risks and possible benefits, after the other treatment options have failed.

Published studies have used predominant-CBD oil, with no or minimal THC, starting with low doses (i.e., 1–2 mg/kg/day) and titrated up slowly according to tolerance and response. As with any medication, it should only be prescribed after a comprehensive clinical assessment, and only if adverse events can be monitored closely by the prescriber.

In the future, randomized placebo-controlled trials should be developed to evaluate the efficacy of medical cannabis and related compounds and to determine which are the optimal dosage and composition. However, it is worth acknowledging that the physical effects provoked by medical cannabis (e.g., drowsiness, dry mouth) might be in some cases too evident to guarantee a real double blindness and objectivity in outcome evaluation. Head-to-head clinical studies are thus essential to establish whether medical cannabis is superior to other treatments (i.e., sleep hygiene, behavioral interventions, melatonin) in terms of efficacy in order to implement evidence-based guidelines.

Studies should provide a detailed clinical characterization of participants in terms of severity and psychiatric co-occurrent conditions, as well as medical comorbidities, particularly seizures. Moreover, concomitant pharmacological therapy should be reported and possibly harmonized to determine whether the effect is determined by medical cannabis or by psychotropic medications. Finally, the use of selected standardized outcome tool instead of ad hoc measures (i.e., percentage of participants improved) is warranted to allow a clear interpretation and comparison of results (Provenzani et al., 2020).

33.7 References

Alves, Vera L, Gonçalves, João L, Aguiar, Joselin, Teixeira, Helena M, & Câmara, José S. (2020). The synthetic cannabinoids phenomenon: From structure to toxicological properties. A review. *Critical Reviews in Toxicology*, *50*(5), 359–382.

Aran, A., Cassuto, H., Lubotzky, A., Wattad, N., & Hazan, E. (2019). Brief report: Cannabidiol-rich cannabis in children with autism spectrum disorder and severe behavioral problems—A retrospective feasibility study. *Journal of Autism and Developmental Disorders*, *49*(3), 1284–1288. DOI: 10.1007/s10803-018-3808-2

Aran, A., Eylon, M., Harel, M., Polianski, L., Nemirovski, A., Tepper, S., Schnapp, A., Cassuto, H., Wattad, N. & Tam, J. (2019). Lower circulating endocannabinoid levels in children with autism spectrum disorder. *Molecular Autism*, *10*. DOI: 10.1186/s13229-019-0256-6

Aran, A., Harel, M., Cassuto, H., Polyansky, L., Schnapp, A., Wattad, N., Shmueli, D., Golan, D., & Castellanos, F. X. (2021). Cannabinoid treatment for autism: A proof-of-concept randomized trial. *Molecular Autism*, *12*(1). DOI: 10.1186/s13229-021-00420-2

Austin, J. K., & Dunn, D. W. (2002). Progressive behavioral changes in children with epilepsy. *Progress in Brain Research*, *135*, 419–427. DOI: 10.1016/s0079-6123(02)35039-8

Baratta, F., Simiele, M., Pignata, I., Ravetto Enri, L., D'Avolio, A., Torta, R., Luca, A. D., Collino, M., & Brusa, P. (2021). Cannabis-based oral formulations for medical purposes: Preparation, quality and stability. *Pharmaceuticals (Basel)*, *14*(2). DOI: 10.3390/ph14020171

Barchel, D., Stolar, O., De-Haan, T., Ziv-Baran, T., Saban, N., Fuchs, D. O., Koren, G., & Berkovitch, M. (2019). Oral cannabidiol use in children with autism spectrum disorder to treat related symptoms and co-morbidities. *Frontiers in Pharmacology*, *9*. DOI: 10.3389/fphar.2018.01521

Bar-Lev Schleider, L., Mechoulam, R., Saban, N., Meiri, G., & Novack, V. (2019). Real life experience of medical cannabis treatment in autism: Analysis of safety and efficacy. *Scientific Reports*, *9*. DOI: 10.1038/s41598-018-37570-y

Bilge, S., & Ekici, B. (2021). CBD-enriched cannabis for autism spectrum disorder: an experience of a single center in Turkey and reviews of the literature. *Journal of Cannabis Research, 3*(1). DOI: 10.1186/s42238-021-00108-7

Crocq, M. A. (2020). History of cannabis and the endocannabinoid system. *Dialogues Clinical Neuroscience, 22*(3), 223–228. DOI: 10.31887/DCNS.2020.22.3/mcrocq

Erridge, S., Kerr-Gaffney, J., Holvey, C., Coomber, R., Barros, D. A. R., Bhoskar, U., Mwimba, G., Praveen, K., Symeon, C., Sachdeva-Mohan, S., Sodergren, M. H., & Rucker, J. J. (2022). Clinical outcome analysis of patients with autism spectrum disorder: Analysis from the UK Medical Cannabis Registry. *Therapeutic Advances in Psychopharmacology, 12*. DOI: 10.1177/20451253221116240

Fleury-Teixeira, P., Caixeta, F. V., da Silva, L. C. R., Brasil-Neto, J. P., & Malcher-Lopes, R. (2019). Effects of CBD-enriched cannabis sativa extract on autism spectrum disorder symptoms: An observational study of 18 participants undergoing compassionate use. *Frontiers in Neurology, 10*. DOI: 10.3389/fneur.2019.01145

Frye, R. E. (2016). Prevalence, significance and clinical characteristics of seizures, epilepsy and subclinical electrical activity in autism. *North American Journal of Medicine and Science, 8*(3), 113–122.

Gould, J. (2015). The cannabis crop. *Nature, 525*(7570), S2–S3. DOI: 10.1038/525S2a

Hacohen, M., Stolar, O. E., Berkovitch, M., Elkana, O., Kohn, E., Hazan, A., Heyman, E., Sobol, Y., Waissengreen, D., Gal, E. & Dinstein, I. (2022). Children and adolescents with ASD treated with CBD-rich cannabis exhibit significant improvements particularly in social symptoms: An open label study. *Translational Psychiatry, 12*(1). DOI: 10.1038/s41398-022-02104-8

Lu, H.-C., & Mackie, K. (2021). Review of the endocannabinoid system. *Biological Psychiatry: Cognitive Neuroscience and Neuroimaging, 6*(6), 607–615.

Kendall, D. A., & Yudowski, G. A. (2016). Cannabinoid receptors in the central nervous system: Their signaling and roles in disease. *Frontiers in Cell Neuroscience, 10*, 294. DOI: 10.3389/fncel.2016.00294

Kerr, D. M., Downey, L., Conboy, M., Finn, D. P., & Roche, M. (2013). Alterations in the endocannabinoid system in the rat valproic acid model of autism. *Behavioural Brain Research, 249*, 124–132. DOI: 10.1016/j.bbr.2013.04.043

Kurz, R., & Blaas, K. (2010). Use of dronabinol (delta-9-THC) in autism: a prospective single-case-study with an early infantile autistic child. *Cannabinoids, 5*(4), 4–6.

Ma, L., Platnick, S., & Platnick, H. (2022). Cannabidiol in treatment of autism spectrum disorder: A case study. *Cureus Journal of Medical Science, 14*(8). DOI: 10.7759/cureus.28442

Mandolini, G. M., Lazzaretti, M., Pigoni, A., Oldani, L., Delvecchio, G., & Brambilla, P. (2018). Pharmacological properties of cannabidiol in the treatment of psychiatric disorders: A critical overview. *Epidemiology and Psychiatric Sciences, 27*(4), 327–335.

Ponton, J. A., Smyth, K., Soumbasis, E., Llanos, S. A., Lewis, M., Meerholz, W. A., & Tanguay, R. L. (2020). A pediatric patient with autism spectrum disorder and epilepsy using cannabinoid extracts as complementary therapy: A case report. *Journal of Medical Case Reports, 14*(1), 162. DOI: 10.1186/s13256-020-02478-7

Provenzani, U., Fusar-Poli, L., Brondino, N., Damiani, S., Vercesi, M., Meyer, N., Rocchetti, M., & Politi, P. (2020). What are we targeting when we treat autism spectrum disorder? A systematic review of 406 clinical trials. *Autism, 24*(2), 274–284.

Rock, E. M., & Parker, L. A. (2021). Constituents of cannabis sativa. *Advances in Experimental Medicine and Biology, 1264*, 1–13. DOI: 10.1007/978-3-030-57369-0_1

Schnapp, A., Harel, M., Cayam-Rand, D., Cassuto, H., Polyansky, L., & Aran, A. (2022). A placebo-controlled trial of cannabinoid treatment for disruptive behavior in children and adolescents with autism spectrum disorder: Effects on sleep parameters as measured by the CSHQ. *Biomedicines, 10*(7). DOI: 10.3390/biomedicines10071685

Servadio, M., Melancia, F., Manduca, A., Di Masi, A., Schiavi, S., Cartocci, V., Pallottini, V., Campolongo, P., Ascenzi, P., & Trezza, V. (2016). Targeting anandamide metabolism rescues core and associated autistic-like symptoms in rats prenatally exposed to valproic acid. *Translational Psychiatry, 6*. DOI: 10.1038/tp.2016.182

Stolar, O., Hazan, A., Vissoker, R. E., Kishk, I. A., Barchel, D., Lezinger, M., Dagan, A., Treves, N., Meiri, D., Berkovitch, M., Kohn, E., & Heyman, E. (2022). Medical cannabis for the treatment of comorbid symptoms in children with autism spectrum disorder: An interim analysis of biochemical safety. *Frontiers in Pharmacology, 29*, 1–8. doi: 10.3389/fphar.2022.977484.

Talwar, A., Estes, E., Aparasu, R., & Reddy, D. S. (2023). Clinical efficacy and safety of cannabidiol for pediatric refractory epilepsy indications: A systematic review and meta-analysis. *Experimental Neurology, 359*, 114238. DOI: 10.1016/j.expneurol.2022.114238

VanDolah, H. J., Bauer, B. A., & Mauck, K. F. (2019). Clinicians' guide to cannabidiol and hemp oils. *Mayo Clinic Proceedings, 94*, 1840–1851 DOI: 10.1016/j.mayocp.2019.01.003

Wei, D., Dinh, D., Lee, D., Li, D. D., Anguren, A., Moreno-Sanz, G., Gall, C. M., & Piomelli, D. (2016). Enhancement of anandamide-mediated endocannabinoid signaling corrects autism-related social impairment. *Cannabis and Cannabinoid Research, 1*(1), 81–89. DOI: 10.1089/can.2015.0008

Wei, D., Lee, D., Cox, C. D., Karsten, C. A., Penagarikano, O., Geschwind, D. H., Gall, C. M., & Piomelli, D. (2015). Endocannabinoid signaling mediates oxytocin-driven social reward. *Proceedings of the National Academy of Sciences of the United States of America, 112*(45), 14084–14089. DOI: 10.1073/pnas.1509795112

Whiting, P. F., Wolff, R. F., Deshpande, S., Di Nisio, M., Duffy, S., Hernandez, A. V., Keurentjes, J. C., Lang, S., Misso, K., Ryder, S., Schmidlkofer, S., & Kleijnen, J. (2015). Cannabinoids for medical use: A systematic review and meta-analysis. *JAMA, 313*(24), 2456–2473. DOI:10.1001/jama.2015.6358

Zamberletti, E., Gabaglio, M., & Parolaro, D. (2017). The endocannabinoid system and autism spectrum disorders: Insights from animal models. *International Journal of Molecular Sciences, 18*(9). DOI: 10.3390/ijms18091916

34

Dietary Interventions for Treating Symptoms Associated With Autism Spectrum Disorder

Haifa Batarseh, Suhad Abumweis, and Janet DeLany
Towson University

34.1 Technical Abstract

Background: The research has indicated that some disorders can be treated partially or totally using dietary interventions. The objective of this chapter is to critique the current evidence regarding the efficacy of dietary interventions for individuals with autism spectrum disorder (ASD). Included are summaries of the rationale supporting the commonly used dietary interventions and procedures to follow when implementing the interventions. Also included are analyses of the strengths and limitations of the existing research so that healthcare professionals, families, and the general public can assess the options and prioritize the directions of future research about dietary interventions for people with ASD. Gluten-free and casein-free (GFCF) diets are the primary dietary interventions that are explored in this chapter. General information about the ketogenic diet (KD) and probiotic interventions as promising dietary strategies for individuals with ASD also are discussed. **Method:** PubMed and Cochrane library search and a hand search were conducted to identify and critique the results of randomized control trials (RCTs), systematic reviews, and meta-analyses regarding the efficacy of dietary interventions for individuals with ASD, specifically GFCF diets, the KD, and the probiotic intervention. Also, information published in a book and book chapters were analyzed to provide a comprehensive review of the evidence regarding the aforementioned dietary interventions for managing some of the core symptoms associated with ASD. **Results:** To date, the research does not yield solid evidence about the efficacy of GFCF diets to manage or treat symptoms associated with ASD. Similarly, because there is only limited research about the KD and probiotic supplements, their benefits for individuals with ASD remain speculative. The studies varied in their use of methods and measurement tools, resulted in conflicting data and outcomes about the benefits of GFCF diets and KD probiotics to ameliorate the symptoms associated with ASD. However, data collected across a number of studies

Haifa Batarseh, Suhad Abumweis, and Janet DeLany, *Dietary Interventions for Treating Symptoms Associated With Autism Spectrum Disorder*. In: *Lifespan Treatment for Autistic Individuals*. Edited by: Peter Sturmey, Russell Lang, and James K. Luiselli, Oxford University Press. © Oxford University Press (2025). DOI: 10.1093/oso/9780197635841.003.0034 provided evidence that all three methods help to alleviate gastrointestinal (GI) symptoms. **Discussion:** The rigor of most of the GFCF, KD, and probiotics intervention studies was limited by their small sample size and methodological drawbacks. In addition, these studies were conducted for a short period, so that their long-term effect was not assessed. **Practitioner recommendations:** Currently, evidence supporting the use of GF and/or CF diets, the KD, and probiotics as effective dietary interventions for individuals with ASD remains inconclusive.

34.2 Layperson Summary

Since ASD is a lifelong disorder, it is crucial to identify the most appropriate interventions that have been proven effective at decreasing bizarre behaviors and improving adaptive behaviors. Parents of individuals with ASD might have heard anecdotal stories about dietary interventions. These stories report that diets minimize or alleviate behavioral challenges associated with ASD. Examples of these dietary interventions involve eliminating some food elements. There are three common diets. The first is eliminating gluten and casein proteins as in GFCF diets. The second is controlling the amount of carbohydrates and fats as in a KD diet. The third is increasing the amount of probiotics in the diet. It is the responsibility of the healthcare professionals to provide parents of individuals with ASD with recommendations about these interventions. The recommendations should be based on evidence of their efficacy. They should also support parents' choice to pick what suits their situation and fits the needs of their children. Parenting children with ASD requires sustained effort, time, and financial input. Several studies claim that dietary interventions have a positive effect on the behavioral problems of individuals with ASD. Yet, most reviews and RCTs find no relationship between dietary interventions and the improvement of behaviors associated with ASD. Some studies find conflicting evidence, which is limited in scope. Thus, there is not strong scientific evidence that diets are effective. The goal of the authors of this chapter is to provide parents with a clear, useful analysis about the current empirical evidence. In that way, parents can make informed decisions about the healthcare of their children.

Implementing dietary interventions requires parental dedication and consistency. It includes time and money to prepare often more costly specialized foods at scheduled times. In addition, the parents should assess the potential negative side effects of diets. Parents need to weigh whether such diets alleviate or exacerbate ASD symptoms. They also need to evaluate GI difficulties such as abdominal pain, vomiting, constipation, gastroesophageal reflux, inflammatory bowel diseases, and the loss of essential food elements.

34.3 Treatment Summary Table

34.3.1 Gluten- and Casein-Free Diet

Treatment summary: Gluten-Free and Casein-Free Diets

Treatment description: Provide individuals with ASD with eating regimens that contain no gluten and/or casein components. The proposed treatment depends on elimination of those proteins from the diets of individuals with ASD.

Expected outcomes: Evidence suggests that the GFCF diet may reduce GI inflammation by limiting the amount of opioid peptide release by inhibiting the amino acids cysteine (CYS) expression and improving the levels of glutathione (GSH) in the body, which is essential for regulating the cell cycle and protecting cells against oxidative damage (Lázaro et al., 2016). However, evidence of using the GFCF diet to ameliorate the symptoms associated with ASD, such as social communication, language delay, maladaptive behaviors, cognition, and sleep, is inconclusive. There is no wide-scale evidence of positive findings that can be generalized (Batarseh et al., 2022).

Methods: The release of neurotransmitters and peptides with opioid action into the intestines is connected to the most common theory of using GFCF diets with individuals with ASD. Exogenous neuropeptides such as gluteomorphin and casomorphin, which are opioid peptide species, are produced by hydrolyzing milk and grain proteins. In children diagnosed with ASD, partially digested peptides pass through the intestinal mucosa of the permeable intestines (Mari-Bauset et al., 2014). Once these peptides cross the blood-brain barrier through the bloodstream and reach the central nervous system (Navarro et al., 2015), they negatively affect learning, brain maturation, attention, and social communication. The higher the levels of peptide, the more severe the symptoms such as loss of eye contact, learning impairment, hyperactivity, stereotypic movement, and self-mutilation (Knivsberg et al., 2001).

Expertise required to implement treatment: Recommendations regarding who is responsible for overseeing the administration of the GF and/or CF diets to people with ASD could not be found in the literature. However, the authors recommend that dietitians should guide families about the implementation of GF and/or CF diets to ensure that the food does not contain gluten and/or casein. Pediatricians or general physicians should provide medical oversight to monitor how the body functions and responds biologically, chemically, and physiologically to this dietary intervention.

Risks and negative side effects: Several gluten-free (GF) foods are not often supplemented and may be lacking in a number of nutrients, including dietary fiber, folate, iron, niacin, riboflavin, and thiamine (Thompson, 1999, 2000). Also, in comparison to items containing gluten, processed GF nutritional products have higher levels of lipids, trans fats, and salt (Caponio et al., 2008; Polito et al., 1992; Rea et al., 1996). Significantly lowering or removing gluten-containing items from the diet may have negative consequences on health (Niland & Cash, 2018). In regards to the CF diet, given that calcium is very crucial element for bone development, suitable dietary support should be implemented to counteract the elimination of dairy products, a core source of calcium (Adams et al., 2008; Cornish, 2002). The additional cost of GF and/or CF dietary interventions should also be considered. Some families may struggle with this extra financial burden. According to several studies, GF foods cost more than their gluten-containing counterparts (MacCulloch & Rashid, 2014; Singh & Whelan, 2011; Stevens & Rashid, 2008). In their 2019 study, Lee et al. (2019) found that some GF foods cost up to 183% more than their gluten counterparts. A study by Myhrstad et al. (2021) found that the cost of the GF items was 46% to 443% more expensive than the cost of the products containing gluten.

GF diets also demand constant commitment and adherence to a restricted diet and way of life, which might lead to social isolation and have a detrimental psychological impact (Niland & Cash, 2018). It may be difficult for those individuals with ASD who tolerate only a narrow range of foods to further limit their dietary intake to comply with GFCF food requirements.

Additional considerations and limitations: Because there is poor evidence for the usefulness of GFCF diets in children with ASD, health professionals should not advocate them as evidence-based interventions (Baspinar & Yardimci, 2020; Batarseh et al., 2022). Rather, if parents want to try these diets with their children, they should do so under the supervision of the child's physician and dietitian and collect data recording the daily effect on the child's behaviors, health, and GI system. The measurement of clinical versus statistical significance, which entails examining how individuals perform on a diet on a day-to-day basis to see what (if any) positive changes are present that improve their quality of life and overall daily functioning rather than just providing statistical evidence of the effect (Whiteley et al., 2013), is another crucial issue that has not yet been adequately addressed by many of the dietary studies completed to date.

34.3.2 Ketogenic Diet

Treatment summary: Ketogenic Diet

Treatment description: The KD, which is high in fat, low in protein, and low in carbohydrates, was primarily created to help children who frequently experience epileptic fits. It resembles the body's fasting condition where most of the energy comes from fat and the remaining comes from protein and carbohydrates (Neal et al., 2008; Rho, 2017).

Expected outcomes: The studies that investigated the KD on humans are few (Karhu et al., 2020), especially studies that investigated the effect of the KD with individuals with ASD. But, in the recent review about using the KD with individuals with ASD, the authors found some evidence that a KD may improve social behavior in children with ASD. Furthermore, the authors stated that the effects vary widely among individuals adhering to the KD and further high-quality studies are need (Li et al., 2021; Taha & Abdalhai, 2021).

Methods: The KD's underlying working mechanisms are unknown (Li et al., 2021). In addition, the effects of KD vary greatly among individuals with ASD (Li et al., 2021). The KD works by restoring normal g-aminobutyric acid (GABA) levels, enhancing mitochondrial function, reducing oxidative stress and inflammatory activity in the brain, blocking the mammalian target of rapamycin (mTOR) signaling pathway, and regulating gut microbiota (Li et al., 2021). However, there is a dearth of clinical research to support KD as an effective dietary intervention for individuals with ASD (Karhu et al., 2020; Li et al., 2021).

Expertise required to implement treatment: It has not been suggested in the literature who is responsible for implementing the KD with individuals with ASD. Based on the risk factors and negative side effects that are stated in the literature, the authors recommend that a physician and a nutritionist provide medical and dietary supervision when implementing the KD for individuals with ASD.

Risks and negative side effects: It can be challenging to introduce a KD to individuals with ASD. Individuals with ASD who have selective, routinized eating habits and behavioral rigidity may reject KD meals (Karhu et al. 2020; Li et al., 2021). In a cohort study, 23% of the children with ASD could not handle and stick to the KD regimen (Evangeliou et al., 2003).

According to Fujiwara et al. (2016), children with ASD have vitamin D and folic acid deficiencies (Ballaban-Gil et al., 1998; Napoli et al., 2014). The KD creates additional challenges, such as an increased risk of inflammation and mitochondrial dysfunction, constipation, reflux, and other comorbidities. Consequently, Li et al. (2021) stated that a KD long-term therapy is likely to cause a nutritional deficiency.

Additional considerations and limitations: There were no studies that investigated the long-term effect of using KD as a dietary intervention. Consequently, the long-term effects of the KD for individuals with ASD are not yet known; its efficacy is not yet substantiated.

34.3.3 Probiotics

Treatment summary: Probiotics

Treatment description: This diet focuses on providing probiotic supplements and foods for individuals with ASD. Probiotics are living microorganisms that have been shown to improve health when taken or administered to the body. Many of the bacteria found in probiotic supplements are the same or comparable to those found naturally the human bodies (National Center for Complementary and Integrative Health, 2019).

Expected outcomes: Overall, there is a dearth of RCTs investigating the use of probiotics in children with ASD (Ng et al., 2019). A recent study conducted by Zhang et al. (2022) provided a protocol for an RCT study to use probiotics with individuals with ASD. According to a recent literature review, there is little evidence to support the function of prebiotics or probiotics in reducing GI or behavioral symptoms in children with ASD. Few open-label trials found significant improvements in GI symptoms, ameliorating the behaviors associated with ASD (Kałużna-Czaplińska & Błaszczyk, 2012; Shaaban et al., 2018; West et al., 2013). Two double-blind RCTs, on the contrary, found no significant improvement in the GI symptoms or in ASD behaviors (Parracho et al., 2010; Slykerman et al., 2018).

Methods: GI inflammation and intestinal permeability can be regulated by the interaction between the probiotics and gut microbiota (Doenyas, 2018b). The effects of probiotics are based on opioid-excess theory, which contends that probiotics may aid in processing gluten products without seriously impairing intestinal permeability while guarding against peptide leakage and enhancing the blood–brain barrier (Anderson et al., 2010; De Angelis et al., 2006; Doenyas, 2018a; Zareie et al., 2006). Another theory explaining the mechanism of using probiotic is dietary protein intolerance. According to this notion, probiotics' anti-inflammatory qualities might help treat behavioral issues associated with ASD by reducing inflammatory immune responses in people with ASD (Rachmilewitz et al., 2004; West et al., 2013). Last, probiotics are being used to treat gut dysbiosis and reduce endotoxin generation, which would then decrease gut inflammation and permeability and stop these endotoxins from having an impact on the central nervous system (Doenyas, 2018a).

Expertise required to implement treatment: Probiotic supplementation is much more risk-free than medications (Zhang et al., 2022). Until there is robust evidence of the safety and usefulness of using probiotics with individuals with ASD, the authors of this chapter recommend that implementing probiotic supplementation with individuals with ASD should be used under the provision and supervision of the physician and nutritionist.

Risks and negative side effects: In 2011, the Agency for Healthcare Research and Quality published a report that came to the conclusion that while the probiotic clinical trials that have been conducted so far have not shown any evidence of an increased risk, the current body of literature is not sufficient to confidently address concerns about the safety of probiotics in intervention studies (Hempel et al., 2011).

Additional considerations and limitations: Evidence about the efficacy of probiotics as a dietary intervention for ameliorating the symptoms associated with ASD has not been substantiated in the literature. Findings are contradictory and range from no clear effect of using oral probiotics, to recommending probiotics as an adjunctive therapy, to the need for further research to determine the role of probiotics as a dietary intervention for ASD (Karhu et al., 2020). In addition, there are no established probiotics regimens, and this has resulted in a use of a variety of probiotic strains, dosages, and treatment durations when using probiotics as an intervention (Ng et al., 2019).

34.4 Introduction

ASD is a neurodevelopmental disorder characterized by deficits and limitations in communication and social participation combined with restrictive repetitive interests and behaviors (American Psychiatric Association, 2013). The prevalence of ASD worldwide and in the United States has been increasing year by year. Worldwide, it has been estimated that 1 in 100 children have ASD (World Health Organization, 2022); in the United States, it is estimated that 1 in 44 children have ASD (Maenner et al., 2021). The etiology of ASD may be influenced by genetic and environmental factors. The heritability of ASD is estimated to be around 80%, meaning that inherited genetics account for the majority of the prevalence of ASD (Bai et al., 2019). There is no cure for ASD. However, there are various treatment options for individuals with ASD. Those treatment approaches may typically be divided into behavioral, developmental, educational, social-relational, pharmacological, psychological, and complementary and alternative therapies (Centers for Disease Control and Prevention, 2022). Treating individuals with ASD utilizing dietary protocols such as GF and/or CF, KD, and probiotics is considered a complementary and alternative treatment option. There has been an increase in research on how diet and nutrition can reduce GI challenges and minimize or eliminate behavioral challenges related with ASD. The following provides an overview of the more promising dietary interventions and their associated concepts and terminologies.

34.4.1 Treatment Descriptions

34.4.1.1 Gluten-Free and Casein-Free Diets

The GF and CF diets are two of the most well-used dietary interventions. The CFCF diet refers to both interventions used concurrently. Gluten and casein are proteins found in foods. In a GF diet, foods that contain gluten proteins are excluded. The gluten protein is found in grains such as wheat, oat, barley, and rye. Food such as bread, candies, cakes, pies, palatable doughs, cereals, cookies, crackers, bulgur, beer, pastas, chips, and salad dressings often contain gluten proteins. The protein casein is found in milk and dairy products such as ice cream, pudding, cream, butter, cheese, half and half, yogurt, and sour cream. A number of studies have investigated if and how GF, CF, and CFCF diets ameliorate the symptoms associated with ASD.

34.4.1.2 Ketogenic Diet

The KD is high in fat, low in carbohydrates, and high in protein, causing the body to use fat metabolism as its major fuel source (Karhu et al., 2020). In a KD diet, foods that contain carbohydrates are excluded. Certain acceptable KD foods include fish, seafood, meat, pork, poultry, and nonstarchy vegetables, including asparagus, bell peppers, broccoli, spinach, zucchini, cauliflower, avocados, berries, nuts and seeds, eggs, high-fat dairy products, olive oil and other oils such as avocado oil, and high-cocoa chocolate.

34.4.1.3 Probiotics

This dietary intervention relies on providing individuals with ASD with probiotic supplements. Probiotics are live microorganisms. The human body has 38 trillion microorganisms, which comprise microbiota and help to keep human bodies healthy. Probiotics can be beneficial in these processes. Probiotic bacteria may be found in a range of foods, including yogurt, baby formula, and nutritional supplements (Prebiotics, 2020). Kefir, sauerkraut, kimchi, and miso are examples of other foods that also contain probiotics. Probiotics may alter the balance of microbiota in the body. It is speculated that this altered balance may reduce some of the symptoms associated with ASD (Zhang et al., 2022).

34.4.2 Rationale and Objectives

This section provides a discussion about the premise that GF and/or CF, KD, and probiotic diets may reduce some of the symptoms associated with ASD. Currently, such findings remain controversial, and there is no scientific consensus of the efficacy of the proposed dietary interventions.

34.4.2.1 Gluten-Free and Casein-Free Diets

The advantage of avoiding foods containing gluten or casein is based on the idea that children with autism may be allergic or have a high sensitivity to them. According to this idea, children with autism digest peptides and proteins in meals that include gluten and casein differently than children who are not sensitive to gluten and casein. This processing discrepancy hypothetically may make autistic symptoms worse (Reichelt & Knivsberg, 2009). The digestive benefits resulting from the decrease in opioid peptides when gluten and casein are eliminated from the diet are the main justification for the use of GFCF diets for individuals with ASD. Using the GFCF diet is intended to ameliorate the digestive difficulties and the associated ASD symptoms such as social, communicational, cognitive, and behavioral challenges. According to Edler et al. (2015), individuals with ASD may suffer from untreated GI disorders and sensitivities that are brought on by or made worse by consuming casein and gluten. Due to the associated pain, discomfort, or even severe pain in certain situations, externalizing behaviors (such as tantrums, yelling, and violence) and inattention may show up on individuals with ASD. It is thought that opioid peptides generated by the digestive system in response to the digestion of gluten and casein can cross the blood-brain barrier, pass through the mucosa, and enter the central nervous system, where they might influence brain function and contribute to the associated features of ASD (Jarmołowska et al., 2019; Lázaro et al., 2016).

34.4.2.2 Ketogenic Diet

Using the KD as a dietary intervention is based upon the premise that a KD may reduce core symptoms as well as comorbidities such as seizures (Qian et al., 2020). Dr. Russel Wilder first proposed the notion of the KD in 1921 for the treatment of refractory seizures with children (Kim, 2017). The KD as administered and reported by parents were thought to significantly result in notable improvements in several parameters of symptoms associated with ASD and in accordance with the Childhood Autism Rating Scale in a cohort study of children with ASD (Evangeliou et al., 2003).

34.4.2.3 Probiotics

Using exogenous probiotics has been shown to boost the host's health when provided in sufficient levels. Also, a well-balanced diet that includes prebiotic dietary components can help to modify the makeup and function of the gut microbiota (Qian et al., 2020). Probiotics can help in preventing peptide leakage and strengthening the blood-brain barrier as represented by opioid-access theory (Anderson et al., 2010; De Angelis et al., 2006; Doenyas, 2018b; Zareie et al., 2006). These reasons and those discussed in the Methods section have been used to justify the use of probiotics with individuals with ASD.

34.4.3 Considerations for Implementation

To determine the successful and a proper implementation of the dietary intervention with individual with ASD, one needs to evaluate the implications, side effects, and contraindicating factors. Therefore, the aim of this section is to present a comprehensive picture of crucial considerations while administering such chosen dietary interventions.

34.4.3.1 Gluten-Free and Casein-Free Diets

In contrast to the perceived benefits of a GFCF diet, challenges also exist. Significantly decreasing or eliminating gluten-containing foods from the diet may have detrimental effects on both health and finances (Niland & Cash, 2018). Foods containing gluten are an important part of many diets, particularly the Western diet. These meals are widely available and inexpensive solutions for meeting the caloric needs of a large population. They are also reasonably simple to grow and prepare. Due to its physical characteristics and flavor, gluten is also a frequently used food additive. With the rise in popularity of GF diets, it is crucial to evaluate the impact on nutritional value and food availability that eliminating gluten may have on the general populace and food sector (Niland & Cash, 2018).

A study in Austria compared 63 GF items to 126 of their gluten-containing counterparts based on nutrient composition, nutritional information, and price. The study evaluated seven categories of foods. In more than half of all food categories, the authors discovered a greater than twofold reduction in the protein content of GF goods. Most GF goods have higher levels of fiber and less salt (Missbach et al., 2015). Overall, adults following the GF diet did not eat enough nutrient-rich meals to comply with all dietary recommendations (Niland & Cash, 2018). Several studies have indicated that alternatives made without gluten are more expensive than those made with gluten (Burden et al., 2015; Lee et al., 2019; MacCulloch & Rashid, 2014; Singh & Whelan, 2011; Stevens & Rashid, 2008).

There also are sociopsychological implications to adhering to a GFCF diet. People often hold strong, ingrained views about the enjoyability and social elements of food. GFCF diets necessitate steadfast commitment to a restricted diet, which could contribute to social isolation and other unhealthy psychosocial behaviors. An individual may become frustrated with trying to adhere to a GF or CF diet, particularly when it is difficult to find or prepare GF and CF foods. Individuals with ASD frequently are hypersensitive to food textures and tastes and thus tolerate eating only a narrow range of foods (Cermak et al., 2010). Such hypersensitivity may complicate the ability of these individuals to adhere to GF, CF, and GFCF diets.

34.4.3.2 Ketogenic Diet

Low blood pressure, kidney stones, constipation, vitamin shortages, and an increased risk of heart disease may result from implementing a KD. Strict diets, such as the KD, may also result in social isolation or disordered eating. The KD is not recommended for people who have pancreas, liver, thyroid, or gallbladder problems (University of Chicago Medicine, 2023).

By using the KD for extended periods of time, more than 12 months, an increase in low-density lipoprotein-cholesterol and very-low-density lipoproteins may enhance the risk of cardiovascular disease. Moreover, the dietary limitations necessary to maintain ketosis may actually contribute to its low sustainability (Batch et al., 2020).

34.4.3.3 Probiotics

Some probiotic strains are extremely delicate and must be kept away from heat, oxygen, light, and humidity. If the probiotics are exposed to these factors, they may begin to degrade or die (Cleveland Clinic, 2020); therefore, storing probiotics could be an issue and must be taken into account. Providers of probiotic supplements should exercise caution when implementing it to individuals with immune system weakness (e.g., chemotherapy), a serious illness, and/or recently undergone surgical procedures. Unlikely but possible risks include acquiring an infection, developing antibiotic resistance, and producing toxic byproducts from the probiotic supplement (Cleveland Clinic, 2020). Individuals with ASD are at a higher risk when associated with such risk factors.

34.5 Research Background

This section discusses the literature pertinent to three promising and controversial dietary interventions: the GFCF diet, the KD, and probiotic supplements. The current guidelines of autism therapies do not include dietary intervention for children and individuals with ASD. Recent systematic reviews and meta-analyses of RCTs investigating the efficacy of dietary interventions, including the GF and/or CF diet, the KD, and probiotics on autism symptoms will be used to reach evidence-based recommendations. The systematic reviews and meta-analyses included in this section were conducted according to the Preferred Reporting Items for Systematic reviews and Meta-Analyses (PRISMA) guidelines. The PRISMA guidelines ensure that the reviews are transparently reported in terms of the method and findings (Page et al., 2021). RCTs are considered the gold standard to test the efficacy of dietary factors in the treatment of diseases and health conditions (Lichtenstein et al., 2021). Yet, exclusive reliance on them to formulate guidelines is limited as their methodological procedures reduce their quality and thus internal validity (Lichtenstein et al., 2021). To date, RCTs addressing questions concerning different dietary interventions to treat symptoms of autism have certain design flaws, as will be discussed below.

In total, four systematic reviews were used to evaluate the evidence surrounding the efficacy of the GFCF diet in improving a wide range of outcomes, including language delays, social-communication difficulties, aloofness, and maladaptive behaviors (Batarseh et al., 2022; Piwowarczyk et al., 2018; Quan et al., 2022; Yu et al. 2022). Piwowarczyk et al. (2018) reviewed six trials with 214 children between 2 and 16 years of age who were diagnosed with ASD using criteria described in the *Diagnostic and Statistical Manual of Mental Disorders-IV* (*DSM-IV*), *DSM-IV—Text Revision* (*DSM-IV-TR*), or *Manual of the International Statistical Classification of Diseases and Related Health Problems* (ICD-10).

The studies included in the review by Piwowarczyk et al. (2018) varied in their treatment duration (ranged from 7 days to 18 months), the amount of gluten and/

or casein in the intervention or the control diet, and the ways by which diets were provided (controlled feeding vs. instructions to follow GFCF or regular diets). In addition, these RCTs used different scales to assess the changes in ASD behavior. Piwowarczyk et al. (2018) concluded that the available evidence does not support the use of GFCF diets to improve the symptoms of children with ASD. Similarly, Batarseh et al. (2022) reviewed 11 trials and reached the same conclusion as Piwowarczyk et al. (2018). The majority of studies included in the previous reviews were of small sample size with a wide age range of children and adolescents (ages ranging from 2 to 18 years) and conducted for varied periods of time (from 1 to 52 weeks). Moreover, the dietary intervention was provided in different ways. Some studies provided GFCF food products and instructions to follow a GFCF diet, while others provided only instructions on how to follow a GFCF diet. One study was conducted as controlled-feeding trials, meaning that full GFCF diets were given to the children according to their recommended dietary intakes. Ideally, full controlled-feeding trials where investigators provide participants with all food and drink items robustly investigate the cause-effect relationship between a certain diet and disease outcomes (Davy & Davy, 2019). Another major limitation of RCTs conducted to evaluate the effect GFCF diets on ASD symptoms is how participants' adherence to the diet was assessed. Adherence to dietary intervention can be monitored in many ways (Lichtenstein et al., 2021), including consumption of food under the supervision of the study investigators, dietary intake assessment on regular basis by 24-hour recall or food records, and use of blood or urinary biomarkers. Seven trials on the GFCF diet in individuals with ASD assessed adherence by dietary assessment. Other trials did not report the method of monitoring dietary adherence, and one trial measured a urinary biomarker, beta-casomorphin, which is derived from the digestion of casein. Usually, participants who fail to adhere to the dietary intervention of interest should be excluded from efficacy trials (Lichtenstein et al., 2021). It is worth mentioning that not all studies assessed changes in GI symptoms that could be associated with following the GFCF diet. Some studies did not find any changes in GI symptoms between the dietary intervention group and the control group. Some studies reported improvement in GI symptoms post-treatment compared to pre-treatment.

Clinical trials that were reviewed assessed various ASD symptoms and outcomes such as language delays, social-communication difficulties, aloofness, maladaptive behaviors, sensorimotor issues, cognition, sleep, or anxiety using more than 20 different standardized scales such as *Gilliam Autism Rating Scale*; *Autism Children's Behavior Checklist*; *Autism Treatment Evaluation Checklist*; *DIPAB*, a standardized Danish scheme to evaluate behavior; and the *Autism Diagnostic Observation Schedule.*

Despite the large heterogeneity between trials on GFCF diet and symptoms of ASD, Quan et al. (2022) and Yu et al. (2022) performed quantitative analysis on these trials and concluded that a GFCF diet can improve some behaviors of children with ASD. This conclusion comes from analyzing heterogeneous studies.

Ideally, it is recommended that quantitative analysis on groups of studies that are homogenous in terms of participants' characteristics and study design be performed. Moreover, Quan et al. (2022) and Yu et al. (2022) included some studies that were previously rigorously assessed for methodological qualities by two independent reviews and were found to have a high risk of bias. As discussed in depth by Piwowarczyk et al. (2018) and Batarseh et al. (2022), these studies were at high risk of bias. Briefly, the majority of studies suffered from selection bias because allocation concealment was not clear, and performance bias because blinding was not appropriate. In addition, similar results were based on a review where no effect of using GFCF dietary intervention on core symptoms of ASD was found (Keller et al., 2021). Despite the conclusion of Quan et al. (2022) and Yu et al. (2022) and given the fact that heterogeneity and low quality of studies were included in their reviews, similar to Piwowarczyk et al. (2018) and Batarseh et al. (2022), they recommended that more studies are needed before conclusive evidence can be drawn.

Concerning the KD and ASD symptoms, one systematic review summarized the RCT that was carried out to test the efficacy of the KD as a modulator for ASD symptoms (Yu et al., 2022). El-Rashidy et al. (2017) studied a KD—a modified Atkins diet for 6 months. Fifteen children participated, although five later dropped out. They observed improvement in the *Autism Treatment Evaluation Test* and the *Childhood Autism Rating Scale* scores compared to the baseline values and not to the control group. The diet in El-Rashidy et al. study (2017) was composed of 60% of the calories from fat sources, 30% from proteins, and 10% from carbohydrates. However, typically a KD consists of 90% of calories from fat. Thus, the modified Atkins diet and the atypical KD limited this study. Also, comparisons were made to baseline values and not to the control group. Thus, a time effect cannot be excluded. In addition, the dropout rate was high—about 30% dropped out due to compliance issues with the diet.

In another study, Lee et al. (2018) investigated the effects of instructing the families to follow a modified ketogenic GF diet regimen with supplemental medium-chain triglycerides. Twenty-seven children aged 2–17 years participated, although only 15 children adhered to the diet as recorded by the authors. After 3 months there was some improvement in total *Autism Diagnostic Observation-2* scores and *Childhood Autism Rating Scale-2*. However, these improvements were in comparison to baseline values and not to a control group, and they were associated with an increase in cholesterol levels. In addition, the observed improvement due to the KD in the Lee study cannot be separated from the effect of a GF diet as it was administrated as a cointervention. Again, adherence to the KD was an issue in the Lee study, as in the El-Rashidy study, which raises concerns about the effectiveness of a long-term KD.

Last, a systematic review summarized eight studies of the potential effects of prebiotics/probiotics on ASD and its symptoms, including the GI ones; it was conducted by Ng et al. (2019). The eight studies involved children with ages ranging from birth to 16 years; thus, not all studies involved children with autism diagnosed according to standardized criteria. One study was carried out on pregnant women and their infants (Slykerman et al., 2018). Pregnant women were randomly assigned to receive probiotics or a placebo daily from 35 weeks to 6 months, if nursing, and their babies received the same therapy from birth to 2 years. When the children were 11 years old, they were tested for intelligence, executive function, attention, depression, and anxiety, where there was no significant effect. Five out of the eight studies did not have a control group; in one study the control group was the siblings of the children with ASD. The lack of a control group or the use of an inappropriate one in clinical trials is a major defect as any changes in the outcomes of interest cannot solely be attributed to the intervention itself. The clinical trials supplemented different probiotic strains at different frequencies (1 to 3 times daily) for duration ranges from 3 to 16 weeks. Although some clinical trials, mainly the open-labeled ones, have shown improvement in some GI symptoms or some behaviors (irritability scores, stereotype, ability to concentrate), the effect of probiotic supplementation should be examined in future studies using the same probiotic strain with more robust selection criteria, appropriate control group, and implementation of a strategy to measure compliance to the dietary intervention.

34.6 Practice Implications

34.6.1 Treatment Outcomes

Generalized outcomes, contraindications, and side effects of using dietary interventions, including GF, CF, GFCF, KD, and probiotic supplementations, with individuals with ASD to treat or decrease the associated ASD symptoms cannot be asserted because of the controversial findings of using these diets, as mentioned in the above sections. Though few studies indicated promising results of using the above-mentioned diets with individuals with ASD, they suffered from methodological drawbacks and very small sample sizes. Thus, health professionals cannot confidently recommend their use. As a result, parents and caregivers are left with the responsibility of determining whether to use nutritional treatments, especially since some anecdotal reports have shown clinical gains when utilizing diet as an intervention strategy.

34.6.2 Practice Implication Guidelines

To the extent empowered by the evidence-based research under review and critique of using GF, CF, GFCF, KD, and probiotic supplementations the following guidelines will be recommended:

- Dietary interventions for individual with ASD are not considered a viable treatment by the Center for Disease Control and Prevention (CDC) and American Academy for Pediatrics (AAP) for individual with ASD.
- Robust evidence about using GFCF, GF, CF, KD, and probiotics dietary interventions cannot be found.
- Methodological flaws and small sample sizes were indicated in the majority of the RCT research that studies the effect of above-mentioned dietary interventions.
- Longitudinal studies are needed to explore the long-term effects of using dietary interventions with individuals with ASD.
- All proposed dietary interventions have their own advantages, disadvantages, and risk factors.
- Consultation with a healthcare specialist is recommended before implementing any dietary interventions.
- Close supervision by a physician while implementing dietary interventions is recommended to track biological signs.
- A pertinent interdisciplinary team should be involved in utilizing and administering such dietary therapies with individuals with ASD.
- Social and economic factors of the individuals with ASD and their families should be taken into account and discussed before implementing the dietary interventions.
- The ability of the individuals with ASD and their families to adhere to the proposed dietary interventions should be considered prior to implementing such approaches.
- If a dietary intervention is chosen to be administered to individuals with ASD, families and involved healthcare professionals can help enhance compliance.

Despite all the effort that has been made to reach a robust and generalized conclusion about the effectiveness of utilizing dietary interventions for individuals with ASD, the findings remain inconclusive. No single dietary intervention or combination of dietary interventions has been proven to treat the symptoms and maladaptive behaviors associated with ASD. Research findings remain inconclusive. Future research is needed to further investigate the effectiveness of such intervention with a strong methodological procedure.

The goal of this chapter is to provide a practical guidance for dietary therapies to address fundamental symptoms associated with ASD based on clinical and scientific research. We believe that this chapter will aid healthcare professionals in providing educated, evidence-based guidance to caregivers and families of persons with ASD. We believe it is the most probable approach to accomplish major improvements that will improve the quality of life of individuals with ASD.

34.7 References

Adams, S., Burton, N., Cutress, A., Adamson, A., McColl, E., O'Hare, A., Baird, G., & Le Couteur, A. (2008). Development of double blind gluten and casein free test foods for use in an autism dietary trial. *Journal of Human Nutrition and Dietetics, 21*(4), 374–374.

American Pychiatric Association. (2013). *Diagnostic and statistical manual of mental disorders: DSM-5*. Washington, DC: Author.

Anderson, R. C., Cookson, A. L., McNabb, W. C., Kelly, W. J., & Roy, N. C. (2010). Lactobacillus plantarum DSM 2648 is a potential probiotic that enhances intestinal barrier function. *FEMS Microbiology Letters, 309*(2), 184–192.

De Angelis, M., Rizzello, C. G., Fasano, A., Clemente, M. G., De Simone, C., Silano, M., De Vincenzi, M., Losito, I., & Gobbetti, M. (2006). VSL# 3 probiotic preparation has the capacity to hydrolyze gliadin polypeptides responsible for Celiac sprue probiotics and gluten intolerance. *Biochimica et Biophysica Acta (BBA)-Molecular Basis of Disease, 1762*(1), 80–93.

Bai, D., Yip, B. H. K., Windham, G. C., Sourander, A., Francis, R., Yoffe, R., Glasson, E., Mahjani, B., Suominen, A., & Leonard, H. (2019). Association of genetic and environmental factors with autism in a 5-country cohort. *JAMA Psychiatry, 76*(10), 1035–1043.

Ballaban-Gil, K., Callahan, C., O'dell, C., Pappo, M., Moshé, S., & Shinnar, S. (1998). Complications of the ketogenic diet. *Epilepsia, 39*(7), 744–748.

Baspinar, B., & Yardimci, H. (2020). Gluten-free casein-free diet for autism spectrum disorders: Can it be effective in solving behavioural and gastrointestinal problems? *The Eurasian Journal of Medicine, 52*(3), 292.

Batarseh, H., AbuMweis, S., Almakanin, H. A., & Anderson, C. (2022). Gluten-free and casein-free diet for children with autism spectrum disorder: A systematic review. *Advances in Neurodevelopmental Disorders, 6*, 280–289.

Batch, J. T., Lamsal, S. P., Adkins, M., Sultan, S., & Ramirez, M. N. (2020). Advantages and disadvantages of the ketogenic diet: A review article. *Cureus, 12*(8), 1–8.

Burden, M., Mooney, P. D., Blanshard, R. J., White, W. L., Cambray-Deakin, D. R., & Sanders, D. S. (2015). Cost and availability of gluten-free food in the UK: In store and online. *Postgraduate Medical Journal, 91*(1081), 622–626.

Caponio, F., Summo, C., Clodoveo, M. L., & Pasqualone, A. (2008). Evaluation of the nutritional quality of the lipid fraction of gluten-free biscuits. *European Food Research and Technology, 227*(1), 135–139.

Centers for Disease Control and Prevention. (2022). Treatment and intervention services for autism spectrum disorder. https://www.cdc.gov/ncbddd/autism/treatment.html

Cermak, S. A., Curtin, C., & Bandini, L. G. (2010). Food selectivity and sensory sensitivity in children with autism spectrum disorders. *Journal of the American Dietetic Association, 110*(2), 238–246.

Cleveland Clinic. (2020). Probiotics. https://my.clevelandclinic.org/health/articles/14598-probiotics

Cornish, E. (2002). Gluten and casein free diets in autism: A study of the effects on food choice and nutrition. *Journal of Human Nutrition and Dietetics, 15*(4), 261–269.

Davy, K. P., & Davy, B. M. (2019). Advances in nutrition science and integrative physiology: Insights from controlled feeding studies. *Frontiers in Physiology, 10*, 1341.

Doenyas, C. (2018a). Dietary interventions for autism spectrum disorder: New perspectives from the gut-brain axis. *Physiology & Behavior, 194*, 577–582.

Doenyas, C. (2018b). Gut microbiota, inflammation, and probiotics on neural development in autism spectrum disorder. *Neuroscience, 374*, 271–286.

Elder, J. H., Kreider, C. M., Schaefer, N. M., & de Laosa, M. B. (2015). A review of gluten- and casein-free diets for treatment of autism: 2005–2015. *Nutrition and Dietary Supplements, 7*, 87–101. https://doi.org/10.2147/NDS.S74718

El-Rashidy, O., El-Baz, F., El-Gendy, Y., Khalaf, R., Reda, D., & Saad, K. (2017). Ketogenic diet versus gluten free casein free diet in autistic children: a case-control study. *Metabolic Brain Disorders, 32*, 1935-1941. doi: 10.1007/s11011-017-0088-z.

Evangeliou, A., Vlachonikolis, I., Mihailidou, H., Spilioti, M., Skarpalezou, A., Makaronas, N., Prokopiou, A., Christodoulou, P., Liapi-Adamidou, G., & Helidonis, E. (2003). Application of a ketogenic diet in children with autistic behavior: Pilot study. *Journal of Child Neurology, 18*(2), 113–118.

Fujiwara, T., Morisaki, N., Honda, Y., Sampei, M. &Tani, Y. (2016) Chemicals, Nutrition, and Autism Spectrum Disorder: A Mini-Review. *Frontiers in Neuroscience, 10*, 174. doi: 10.3389/fnins.2016.00174

Hempel, S., Newberry, S., Ruelaz, A., Wang, Z., Miles, J., Suttorp, M. J., Johnsen, B., Shanman, R., Slusser, W., & Fu, N. (2011). Safety of probiotics used to reduce risk and prevent or treat disease. *Evidence Report/Technology* Assessment, *200*, 1–645.

Jarmołowska, B., Bukało, M., Fiedorowicz, E., Cieślińska, A., Kordulewska, N. K., Moszyńska, M., Świątecki, A., & Kostyra, E. (2019). Role of milk-derived opioid peptides and proline dipeptidyl peptidase-4 in autism spectrum disorders. *Nutrients, 11*(1), 87.

Kałużna-Czaplińska, J., & Błaszczyk, S. (2012). The level of arabinitol in autistic children after probiotic therapy. *Nutrition, 28*(2), 124–126.

Karhu, E., Zukerman, R., Eshraghi, R. S., Mittal, J., Deth, R. C., Castejon, A. M., Trivedi, M., Mittal, R., & Eshraghi, A. A. (2020). Nutritional interventions for autism spectrum disorder. *Nutrition Reviews, 78*(7), 515–531.

Keller, A., Rimestad, M. L., Friis Rohde, J., Holm Petersen, B., Bruun Korfitsen, C., Tarp, S., Briciet Lauritsen, M., & Händel, M. N. (2021). The effect of a combined gluten-and casein-free diet on children and adolescents with autism spectrum disorders: A systematic review and meta-analysis. *Nutrients, 13*(2), 470.

Kim, J.-M. (2017). Ketogenic diet: Old treatment, new beginning. *Clinical Neurophysiology Practice, 2*, 161.

Knivsberg, A., Reichelt, K., & Nødland, M. (2001). Reports on dietary intervention in autistic disorders. *Nutritional Neuroscience, 4*(1), 25–37.

Lázaro, C. P., Pondé, M. P., & Rodrigues, L. E. (2016). Opioid peptides and gastrointestinal symptoms in autism spectrum disorders. *Brazilian Journal of Psychiatry, 38*, 243–246.

Lee, A. R., Wolf, R. L., Lebwohl, B., Ciaccio, E. J., & Green, P. H. (2019). Persistent economic burden of the gluten free diet. *Nutrients, 11*(2), 399.

Lee, R. W., Corley, M. J., Pang, A., Arakaki, G., Abbott, L., Nishimoto, M., Miyamoto, R., Lee, E., Yamamoto, S., & Maunakea, A. K. (2018). A modified ketogenic gluten-free diet with MCT improves behavior in children with autism spectrum disorder. *Physiology & Behavior, 188*, 205–211.

Li, Q., Liang, J., Fu, N., Han, Y., & Qin, J. (2021). A ketogenic diet and the treatment of autism spectrum disorder. *Frontiers in Pediatrics, 9*, 1–7.

Lichtenstein, A. H., Petersen, K., Barger, K., Hansen, K. E., Anderson, C. A., Baer, D. J., Lampe, J. W., Rasmussen, H., & Matthan, N. R. (2021). Perspective: Design and conduct of human nutrition randomized controlled trials. *Advances in Nutrition, 12*(1), 4–20.

MacCulloch, K., & Rashid, M. (2014). Factors affecting adherence to a gluten-free diet in children with Celiac disease. *Paediatrics & Child Health, 19*(6), 305–309.

Maenner, M. J., Shaw, K. A., Bakian, A. V., Bilder, D. A., Durkin, M. S., Esler, A., Furnier, S. M., Hallas, L., Hall-Lande, J., & Hudson, A. (2021). Prevalence and characteristics of autism spectrum disorder among children aged 8 years—Autism and developmental disabilities monitoring network, 11 sites, United States, 2018. *MMWR Surveillance Summaries, 70*(11), 1.

Mari-Bauset, S., Zazpe, I., Mari-Sanchis, A., Llopis-González, A., & Morales-Suarez-Varela, M. (2014). Evidence of the gluten-free and casein-free diet in autism spectrum disorders: A systematic review. *Journal of Child Neurology, 29*(12), 1718–1727.

Missbach, B., Schwingshackl, L., Billmann, A., Mystek, A., Hickelsberger, M., Bauer, G., & König, J. (2015). Gluten-free food database: The nutritional quality and cost of packaged gluten-free foods. *PeerJ, 3*, e1337.

Myhrstad, M. C. W., Slydahl, M., Hellmann, M., Garnweidner-Holme, L., Lundin, K. E. A., Henriksen, C., & Telle-Hansen, V. H. (2021) Nutritional quality and costs of gluten-free products: a case-control study of food products on the Norwegian marked. *Food and Nutrition Research, 65*, 1–10. doi: 10.29219/fnr.v65.6121.

Napoli, E., Dueñas, N., & Giulivi, C. (2014). Potential therapeutic use of the ketogenic diet in autism spectrum disorders. *Frontiers in Pediatrics, 2*, 69.

National Center for Complementary and Integrative Health. (2019). Probiotics: What you need to know. https://www.nccih.nih.gov/health/probiotics-what-you-need-to-know#hed1

Navarro, F., Pearson, D. A., Fatheree, N., Mansour, R., Hashmi, S. S., & Rhoads, J. M. (2015). Are "leaky gut"and behavior associated with gluten and dairy containing diet in children with autism spectrum disorders? *Nutritional Neuroscience, 18*(4), 177–185.

Neal, E. G., Chaffe, H. M., Edwards, N., Lawson, M. S., Schwartz, R. H., & Cross, J. H. (2008). Growth of children on classical and medium-chain triglyceride ketogenic diets. *Pediatrics, 122*(2), e334–e340.

Ng, Q. X., Loke, W., Venkatanarayanan, N., Lim, D. Y., Soh, A. Y. S., & Yeo, W. S. (2019). A systematic review of the role of prebiotics and probiotics in autism spectrum disorders. *Medicina, 55*(5), 129.

Niland, B., & Cash, B. D. (2018). Health benefits and adverse effects of a gluten-free diet in non–Celiac disease patients. *Gastroenterology & Hepatology, 14*(2), 82.

Page, M. J., McKenzie, J. E., Bossuyt, P. M., Boutron, I., Hoffmann, T. C., Mulrow, C. D., Shamseer, L., Tetzlaff, J. M., Akl, E. A., & Brennan, S. E. (2021). The PRISMA 2020 statement: An updated guideline for reporting systematic reviews. *Systematic Reviews, 10*(1), 1–11.

Parracho, H. M., Gibson, G. R., Knott, F., Bosscher, D., Kleerebezem, M., & McCartney, A. L. (2010). A double-blind, placebo-controlled, crossover-designed probiotic feeding study in children diagnosed with autistic spectrum disorders. *International Journal of Probiotics & Prebiotics, 5*(2), 69.

Piwowarczyk, A., Horvath, A., Łukasik, J., Pisula, E., & Szajewska, H. (2018). Gluten- and casein-free diet and autism spectrum disorders in children: a systematic review. *European Journal of Nutrition, 57*(2), 433–440. doi: 10.1007/s00394-017-1483-2.

Polito, C., Olivieri, A. N., Marchese, L., Desiderio, G., Pullano, F., & Rea, F. (1992). Weight overgrowth of coeliac children on gluten-free diet. *Nutrition Research, 12*(3), 353–358.

International Scientific Association for Probibiotics and Prebiotics (2020). *Probiotics: The science of what they are and how they work.* https://isappscience.org/for-consumers/learn/probiotics/

Qian, L., Huang, J., & Qin, H. (2020). Probiotics and dietary intervention modulate the colonic mucosa-associated microbiota in high-fat diet populations. *Turkish Journal of Gastroenterology, 31*(4), 295.

Quan, L., Xu, X., Cui, Y., Han, H., Hendren, R. L., Zhao, L., You, X. (2022). A systematic review and meta-analysis of the benefits of a gluten-free diet and/or casein-free diet for children with autism spectrum disorder. *Nutrition Reviews, 80*(5), 1237–1246. doi: 10.1093/nutrit/nuab073.

Rachmilewitz, D., Katakura, K., Karmeli, F., Hayashi, T., Reinus, C., Rudensky, B., Akira, S., Takeda, K., Lee, J., & Takabayashi, K. (2004). Toll-like receptor 9 signaling mediates the anti-inflammatory effects of probiotics in murine experimental colitis. *Gastroenterology, 126*(2), 520–528.

Rea, F., Polito, C., Marotta, A., Di Toro, A., Iovene, A., Collini, R., Rea, L., & Sessa, G. (1996). Restoration of body composition in Celiac children after one year of gluten-free diet. *Journal of Pediatric Gastroenterology and Nutrition, 23*(4), 408–412.

Reichelt, K., & Knivsberg, A. (2009). The possibility and probability of a gut-to-brain connection in autism. *Annals of Clinical Psychiatry, 21*(4), 205–211.

Rho, J. M. (2017). How does the ketogenic diet induce anti-seizure effects? *Neuroscience Letters, 637*, 4–10.

Shaaban, S. Y., El Gendy, Y. G., Mehanna, N. S., El-Senousy, W. M., El-Feki, H. S., Saad, K., & El-Asheer, O. M. (2018). The role of probiotics in children with autism spectrum disorder: A prospective, open-label study. *Nutritional Neuroscience, 21*(9), 676–681.

Singh, J., & Whelan, K. (2011). Limited availability and higher cost of gluten-free foods. *Journal of Human Nutrition and Dietetics, 24*(5), 479–486.

Slykerman, R., Kang, J., Van Zyl, N., Barthow, C., Wickens, K., Stanley, T., Coomarasamy, C., Purdie, G., Murphy, R., & Crane, J. (2018). Effect of early probiotic supplementation on childhood cognition, behaviour and mood a randomised, placebo-controlled trial. *Acta Paediatrica, 107*(12), 2172–2178.

Stevens, L., & Rashid, M. (2008). Gluten-free and regular foods: A cost comparison. *Canadian Journal of Dietetic Practice and Research, 69*(3), 147–150.

Taha, Z., & Abdalhai, K. A. (2021). A review of the efficacy of the dietary intervention in autism spectrum disorder. *Open Access Macedonian Journal of Medical Sciences, 9*, 88.

Thompson, T. (1999). Thiamin, riboflavin, and niacin contents of the gluten-free diet: Is there cause for concern? *Journal of the Academy of Nutrition and Dietetics, 99*(7), 858.

Thompson, T. (2000). Folate, iron, and dietary fiber contents of the gluten-free diet. *Journal of the Academy of Nutrition and Dietetics, 100*(11), 1389.

University of Chicago Medicine. (2023). Ketogenic diet: What are the risks? https://www.uchicagomedicine.org/forefront/health-and-wellness-articles/ketogenic-diet-what-are-the-risks

West, R., Roberts, E., Sichel, L., & Sichel, J. (2013). Improvements in gastrointestinal symptoms among children with autism spectrum disorder receiving the Delpro® probiotic and immunomodulator formulation. *Journal of Probiotics & Health, 1*(1), 1–6.

Whiteley, P., Shattock, P., Knivsberg, A.-M., Seim, A., Reichelt, K. L., Todd, L., Carr, K., & Hooper, M. (2013). Gluten-and casein-free dietary intervention for autism spectrum conditions. *Frontiers in Human Neuroscience, 6*, 344.

World Health Organization. (2022). Autism. https://www.who.int/news-room/fact-sheets/detail/autism-spectrum-disorders#:~:text=The%20level%20of%20intellectual%20functioning,profoun d%20impairment%20to%20superior%20levels.&text=It%20is%20estimated%20tat%20worldwide,prevalence%20varies%20substantially%20across%20studies

Yu, Y., Huang, J., Chen, X., Fu, J., Wang, X., Pu, L., Gu, C., & Cai, C. (2022). Efficacy and safety of diet therapies in children with autism spectrum disorder: A systematic literature review and meta-analysis. *Frontiers in Neurology, 13*.

Zareie, M., Johnson-Henry, K., Jury, J., Yang, P.-C., Ngan, B.-Y., McKay, D. M., Soderholm, J. D., Perdue, M. H., & Sherman, P. M. (2006). Probiotics prevent bacterial translocation and improve intestinal barrier function in rats following chronic psychological stress. *Gut, 55*(11), 1553–1560.

Zhang, L., Xu, Y., Li, H., Li, B., Duan, G., & Zhu, C. (2022). The role of probiotics in children with autism spectrum disorders: A study protocol for a randomised controlled trial. *PloS One, 17*(2), e0263109.

35

Electroconvulsive Therapy

Lee E. Wachtel
Johns Hopkins School of Medicine, Kennedy Krieger Institute

James K. Luiselli
Melmark New England

35.1 Technical Abstract

Background: Electroconvulsive therapy (ECT) is a commonly administered treatment for persons with severe major depression, bipolar disorder, schizophrenia, catatonia, and neuroleptic malignant syndrome. Children and adults diagnosed with autism spectrum disorder (ASD) and co-occurring catatonic symptoms, affective and psychotic disorders, and severe challenging behavior such as self-injury and aggression also have been treated successfully with ECT. Usual indications for ECT are patients who have not responded successfully to previous treatment modalities or require immediate intervention due to the severity of their condition that at times can be life-threatening. During ECT, a patient receives general anesthesia and a muscle relaxant, the brain is stimulated briefly with electrical pulses via two electrodes placed bi-temporally or a right unilateral electrode, causing a seizure that lasts approximately 60 to 90 seconds. Treatment sessions run 5–10 minutes scheduled 2 to 3 times per week for 10–12 sessions depending on symptom severity and therapeutic response. Maintenance ECT (m-ECT) in which sessions are tapered gradually typically is prescribed to prevent relapse. The most common side effect from ECT is headache but may include temporary short-term memory loss, transient cognitive impairment, nausea, muscle aches, and fatigue. **Method:** For this chapter, we reviewed published studies in peer-reviewed journals from an Internet search using the keywords "autism spectrum disorder, self-injury, catatonia, electroconvulsive therapy." Participant characteristics, clinical presentation, previous interventions (behavioral, psychosocial, pharmacological), course of ECT, treatment outcomes, side effects, and evaluation criteria in studies guided the review process. **Results:** There is supporting evidence that ECT is a safely tolerated and effective treatment for persons with ASD, catatonia, self-injury, and affective and psychotic comorbidities. A positive response to ECT has been associated with restoration of self-care, daily living, communication, and social skills; reduced challenging behavior; and return to normative service settings. Negative side effects from ECT were rarely reported, and m-ECT was

Lee E. Wachtel and James K. Luiselli, *Electroconvulsive Therapy*. In: *Lifespan Treatment for Autistic Individuals*. Edited by: Peter Sturmey, Russell Lang, and James K. Luiselli, Oxford University Press. © Oxford University Press (2025).
DOI: 10.1093/oso/9780197635841.003.0035

provided in every published case given the status of ECT as a treatment rather than a cure. Most patients continued with pharmacotherapy during and following ECT. **Discussion:** The reported efficacy of ECT in persons with ASD notwithstanding, evaluation methodology in the current literature is almost exclusively case report lacking single-case research design (SCRD) experimental control and many times based on narrative descriptions of patient outcomes without representative behavior data. Symptom presentation among patients and the types of treatments they received preceding ECT also varied extensively and should be considered when interpreting findings. **Practitioner recommendations:** Safe and effective delivery of ECT is dependent on a skilled medical team comprised of psychiatrists, anesthesiologists, nurses, and other hospital staff. Multidisciplinary practitioners for persons with ASD in outpatient clinical, school, residential, rehabilitation, and community settings must coordinate support services with and report treatment outcomes to the ECT team.

35.2 Layperson Summary

Some persons with ASD are diagnosed with co-occurring catatonia that is comprised of motor, vocal, and behavioral symptoms. Catatonia also may include markedly slow movement or frenetic and purposeless psychomotor agitation, mutism, echolalia, speech abnormalities, body rigidity, posturing or waxy flexibility, negativism and slowing, and vital sign instability in the most dangerous cases. Further, catatonia in ASD is characterized by diminished motivation, prompt dependence, and loss of skills needed to communicate and interact socially with other people. A catatonic state can emerge suddenly without evidence of earlier symptoms, possibly influenced by a mood or psychotic illness, genetic susceptibility, biological factors, and occurrence of a traumatic event. Catatonia is estimated to occur in 12–20% of persons with ASD.

Self-injurious behavior (SIB) also can be present in persons with ASD and catatonia. There are multiple forms of SIB, including but not limited to hitting face, head, and torso with hands; biting parts of the body; striking head against hard surfaces; and poking eyes. Such behavior often occurs at high frequency and an intensity that produces tissue damage, concussions, open wounds, detached retinas, traumatic cataracts, and broken bones. In the most severe cases, SIB can be life-threatening. Persons who engage in such volatile SIB often are fitted with restrictive protective equipment (e.g., helmets, arm pads) and may have to be restrained by care providers to ensure health safety.

There are effective behavioral and medication treatments for persons who have ASD and are self-injurious. However, catatonia associated with SIB in autism as well as intellectual disability poses a complex problem, and conventional interventions may not be successful. Over several decades, evidence has emerged that ECT can be effective in such cases and with lasting positive results when continued for many years. ECT is administered to a patient who is sedated through anesthesia and also receives a muscle relaxant with ongoing oxygenation and medical monitoring in a surgical suite. During sessions lasting approximately 10 minutes, electrical pulses produce stimulation to the brain via electrodes attached to the patient's scalp. The stimulation causes a brief seizure that usually lasts between 30 and 90 seconds. It is common for ECT sessions to be scheduled 2 to 3 times per week on an outpatient basis for several weeks depending on the severity of symptoms and how rapidly the patient responds to treatment with the acute course continuing until the patient's symptoms remit or plateau.

Studies with persons who have ASD, catatonia, self-injury, and additional mental health problems indicate that ECT can restore functional life skills, cognitive functioning, and communication abilities; eliminate health-threatening and other challenging behavior; and improve quality of life. Following an initial course of ECT, patients typically continue with treatment on a reduced schedule to avoid relapse, that is, symptoms that reappear or an unanticipated worsening condition. Medications usually are prescribed with m-ECT in conjunction with other services and therapies such as applied behavior analysis (ABA) programs. Experienced medical teams headed by psychiatrists, anesthesiologists, and nurses administer ECT and coordinate treatment with a patient's family and other health providers. Access to and availability of ECT varies widely in the United States and internationally depending on the existence of reputable hospital centers, regulatory guidelines, and insurance reimbursement policies.

ECT is a safe and generally well-tolerated treatment. Some patients may experience a period of short-term memory loss and cognitive confusion that quickly resolves over hours to days. Rapidly overcome side effects caused by anesthesia include nausea, fatigue, and headache. Persons with preexisting heart disease are at increased risk for complication, and as with any procedure, preevaluation by anesthesiology is required. Otherwise, the recovery profile for persons receiving ECT is good and therapeutic benefit to persons with ASD, catatonia, and self-injury is evident.

35.3 Treatment Summary Table

Treatment summary: Electroconvulsive Therapy

Treatment description: ECT involves stimulation of the brain through quickly administered electrical pulses that produce a seizure while a person is sedated, relaxed, and closely monitored by a medical team. A typical course of ECT includes multiple weekly treatment sessions (5–10-minute duration), 10 to 12 sessions on average, which are scheduled based on symptom severity and therapeutic responsiveness. Treatment usually occurs on an outpatient basis with follow-up (maintenance) sessions arranged at a reduced schedule.

continued

Expected outcomes: ECT is intended to alleviate impairment and treat problems associated with major depression, bipolar disorder, schizophrenia, catatonia, and affective dysregulation. In persons with ASD, catatonia, and self-injury, the expected outcomes from ECT are recovery of functional life skills, communication abilities, socialization, and harmonious quality of life, as well as elimination of self-injury and offending behavior. For individuals with comorbid affective and/or psychotic illness, marked reduction in these symptoms also is expected.

Methods: ECT is a medical treatment used in conjunction with psychosocial modalities, behavioral intervention, and pharmacotherapy.

Expertise required to implement treatment: Psychiatrists, anesthesiologists, nurses, and other medical specialists administer ECT in specialized hospital centers. Considerable expertise is demanded in order to administer ECT safely, effectively, and with lasting positive results.

Risks and negative side effects: Side effects from ECT can include anesthesia-induced nausea, headaches, and fatigue on the day of treatment. Temporary short-term memory loss and transient cognitive confusion are encountered in some instances. Potential cardiovascular risks must be considered in patients with preexisting conditions and longer-term gaps of memory have been reported. As a cautionary note, some patients with ASD may be unable to self-assess ECT side effects; thus, detection through practitioner administered ratings scales and direct observation would apply.

Additional considerations and limitations: A still persistent and negative opinion of ECT exists in some corners of the professional community and by the lay public despite documented treatment effectiveness in the general population and among persons with ASD and intellectual disability. Access to ECT is not uniform and may be limited due to a number of factors which impact who is eligible for treatment and the locations where treatment is provided. More research with autistic individuals referred for ECT is needed to broaden the current evidence support and inform best practices.

35.4 Introduction

This chapter reviews ECT for the treatment of severe catatonic, affective, and psychotic pathology that occurs more readily in ASD and intellectual disability than in the general population (Collins et al., 2012; Dhossche & Wachtel, 2013; Wachtel et al., 2018). The recent recognition of some forms of repetitive SIB along the catatonic spectrum and the life-changing role of ECT in amelioration also is addressed. Notably, Wachtel and Dhossche (2010) posited that "A clear distinction should be made between self-injury found through formal behavior analyses to be under operant control and therefore amenable to applied behavioral interventions, as compared to self-injury that is likely internally maintained and representative of a neurobiological disturbance, particularly catatonia" (p. 112). However, ECT does not treat the core symptoms of autism nor is it a cure for associated language delay and/or intellectual disability. Rather, ECT is a medical and symptom-focused intervention directed at global psychopathology and externalizing behavior. As presented in the chapter, much has been learned about ECT and its contribution to autism treatment, but more inquiry is required on a clinical level and from a research framework.

The utility of convulsions in the treatment of severe psychopathology was first demonstrated in 1934 by Meduna, who successfully used camphor-in-oil injection to induce seizures in psychotic patients, many of whom were discharged after years of hospitalization. Four years later in 1938, Bini and Cerletti introduced the usage of electricity for seizure induction. Subsequent modalities to produce a seizure included pentylenetetrazole injection and fluorothyl inhalation that were largely abandoned by the 1970s in favor of electricity, leading to the development of the modern field of ECT. Since its inception, ECT has repeatedly demonstrated high efficacy rates in the treatment of multiple psychiatric conditions, including major depression, acute mania and bipolar disorder, schizophrenia spectrum disorders, catatonia, and neuroleptic malignant syndrome (Shorter & Healy, 2013). Neurological indications for ECT include Parkinson's disease and status epilepticus (Abrams, 2002; Fink, 2009).

In adults, ECT is most commonly used for treatment-refractory depression, where its efficacy is unparalleled and far exceeds the effects from psychotropic medications. For adult major depressive disorder, the multisite Columbia University Consortium (CUC) and Consortium for Research in ECT (CORE) studies demonstrated robust and rapid remission rates of 54.8% and 86.5% for right unilateral (RUL) and bilateral (BL) ECT with the average number of treatments to remission at 10.6 and 7.3, respectively (Fink, 2014; Husain et al., 2004). The CORE studies further demonstrated equal efficacy of ECT in unipolar and bipolar depression and confirmed an even higher remission rate of 95% in psychotic depression (Bailine et al., 2010; Petrides et al., 2001). The subsequent Prolonging Remission in Depressed Elderly (PRIDE) study of RUL ECT showed 61% remission and 70% response rates with a substantial average reduction of 24.7 points on the Hamilton Depression Index (HAM-D) (Kellner et al., 2016).

A literature review of ECT usage in mania from 1942 to 1992 reported that 80% of 589 patients "showed substantial clinical improvement of remission," and a subsequent literature review of the last three decades found similar efficacy for both medication-refractory and delirious mania (Elias et al., 2021; Mukherjee et al., 1994). Research on ECT in schizophrenia is less extensive, but meta-analyses of available data report benefit in patients who do not respond sufficiently to antipsychotic medications such as clozapine and especially those with positive symptoms of schizophrenia and comorbid catatonia (Grover et al., 2019; Sanghani et al., 2018). ECT is exquisitely efficacious in catatonia, with responses rates ranging from 80 to 100% when first-line benzodiazepine intervention is insufficient (Bush et al., 1996b; Caroff et al., 2004; Fink & Taylor, 2006). Similarly, neuroleptic malignant syndrome, a potentially fatal condition best conceptualized as malignant catatonia induced by antipsychotic medication, is highly responsive to ECT (Abrams, 2002; Caroff et al., 2004; Fink, 1996, 2009).

ECT was used in children and adolescents shortly after its advent by Heuyer et al. (1943) in Paris and Bender (1947) at Bellevue Hospital in New York. Many of the children described as schizophrenic in the Bender report may have qualified for a modern diagnosis of autism or intellectual disability. There has been increased interest in the utility of ECT for affective, psychotic, and catatonic presentation in youth over the past three decades, and evidence supports similar robust efficacy in pediatrics. For example, Rey and Walter (1997) reviewed 50 years of ECT use in youth, reporting efficacy rates of 60–80% for depression, 80–100% for mania, 80% for catatonia, and 20–50% for schizophrenia. Reported side effects from ECT were few, the most common complaint among patients being headache. A more recent review of 51 youth who received ECT between 1991 to 2013 for affective, psychotic, and catatonic illness documented that 77% of subjects were rated as "much" or "very much" improved on the Clinical Global Impression (CGI) scale after completion of an acute course of ECT (Puffer et al., 2016). The American Academy of Child and Adolescent Psychiatry established a three-criteria, best-practice parameter for usage of ECT in which youth must (a) have an ECT-responsive diagnosis, (b) sufficient symptom severity to warrant ECT, and (c) failed at least two full psychotropic medication trials (Ghaziuddin et al., 2004).

Persons with ASD and intellectual disability have increased susceptibility to psychiatric illness. Substantive literature supports the heightened incidence of a range of potentially ECT-responsive psychiatric diagnoses in autism with many children and adults carrying more than one comorbid diagnostic classification. The risk of psychiatric comorbidity in autism is likely higher than for other psychiatric diagnoses—for example, one study found that 57.5% of autistic subjects had at least one diagnosis from the *Diagnostic and Statistical Manual of Mental Disorders*, 5th ed. (*DSM-5*: American Psychiatric Association, 2013) compared to only 40% of attention-deficit/hyperactivity disorder (ADHD) subjects (van Steensel et al., 2013). A meta-analysis of prevalence of psychosis and bipolar disorder in autistic adults by Varcin et al. (2022) reviewed 53 studies from which the pooled prevalence of psychosis was 9.4% and that of bipolar disorder was 7.5%. Catatonia is known to occur in 12–20% of individuals with autism (Billstedt et al., 2005; Breen & Hare, 2017; Ghaziuddin et al., 2012; Wing & Shah, 2000), and this important condition will be expanded upon below. Note that multiple diagnoses are often the rule of thumb—Mosner et al. (2019) reported that 91% of autistic children and 31% of autistic adults received at least one *DSM-5* diagnosis, and 70–95% of ASD youth have at least one *DSM-5* diagnosis, 41–60% carry two or more diagnoses, and 24% had three or more diagnoses.

Further, intellectual disability is a common comorbidity of ASD. A Centers for Disease Control and Prevention (CDC) study on trends in developmental disability from 2009 to 2017 indicated that 35.2% of children with ASD in the United States qualified for a diagnosis of intellectual disability and 23.1% had borderline intellectual functioning (Maenner et al., 2021). A half century ago, the Isle of Wight studies established that the prevalence of psychiatric illness was increased three- to fivefold in youth with intellectual disability, a finding repeatedly documented in the international literature (Harris, 1998; Rutter et al., 1970). Among 438 youth in the United Kingdom, 39% with intellectual disability met criteria for an anxiety, behavior, or conduct disorder, compared to only 8% without intellectual disability (Emerson, 2003). From Scotland, Hughes-McCormack et al. (2017) evaluated 26,349 subjects with intellectual disability from a total sample of 5,295,403 children and adults and found that the presence of intellectual disability predicted psychiatric disorders with an *odds ratio of 7.1*. The study revealed that 12.8% of children, 23.4% of adults, and 27.2% of older adults with intellectual disability had comorbid psychiatric conditions as compared to 0.3%, 5.3%, and 4.5%, respectively, of those without intellectual disability in the same age classes.

In the United States, Platt et al. (2019) reported that 65.1% of persons with intellectual disability (IQ < 76) met criteria for a psychiatric disorder, and in Australia, a meta-analysis of 19 studies including 6,151 subjects revealed prevalence of mental health disorders at 38% using the Developmental Behavioral Checklist and 38% using the Child Behavior Checklist (Buckley et al., 2020). These are significant numbers that clearly establish intellectual disability as a major risk factor for comorbid psychopathology. The implications for ECT in a patient population of individuals with ASD, intellectual disability alone, or both conditions simultaneously are obvious in that the same ECT-responsive affective, psychotic, and catatonic illnesses that occur in the neurotypical patient population are *more likely to occur in autistic individuals.*

Catatonia deserves specific attention in any discussion of ECT in ASD (DeJong et al., 2014; Vaqueizo-Serrano et al., 2022; Wing & Shah, 2006). Wing and Shah (2000) first reported a population-based study of 506 children and adults with autism in which 17% met criteria for catatonia. Onset in these cases most commonly occurred in late adolescence to early adulthood, possibly attributed to genetic susceptibility (Dhossche & Bouman, 1997), biological influences (Rasmussen et al., 2016), and traumatic life events (Shorter & Fink, 2018). In addition to (a) the classic motor, vocal, and behavioral symptoms of catatonia as originally delineated by Kalhbaum, (b) later crystallized in formal rating scales like the Bush-Francis Catatonia Rating Scale (Bush et al., 1996a; Sienaert et al., 2011), and (c) currently included in the *DSM-5* (American Psychiatric Association, 2013), Wing and Shah (2000) commented upon increased slowness, difficulty with initiation and completion of tasks, poor motivation, and prompt dependence as common catatonic symptoms in ASD. Billstedt et al. (2005) evaluated a smaller group of 120 patients with ASD diagnosed in childhood who had been followed for 13 to 22 years, finding that 12% were diagnosed with catatonia. Notably, 50% of these individuals also presented with SIB, 19% with "extreme violence," and 23% with tics. A retrospective study of 101 inpatients under 18 years old with hospital diagnoses of pervasive developmental disorder, intellectual disability, intermittent explosive disorder, psychosis NOS, and neuroleptic malignant syndrome revealed that 17.8% met criteria for catatonia, although only two had been correctly diagnosed at time of admission (Ghaziuddin et al., 2012). Finally, Breen and Hare (2017) sought to validate an "attenuated behavior questionnaire" in 87 persons with ASD and found that 20.2% already had a formal catatonia diagnosis, with 48.3% having three or more core "attenuated" motor, vocal, or behavioral symptoms on their questionnaire.

The impact of catatonia in all patient populations is replete with multiple somatic complications that can compound baseline psychiatric compromise. Catatonic patients are at risk for contractures, skin ulceration and breakdown, malnutrition, dehydration, aspiration from tube feeding, electrolyte abnormalities, severe localized and/or diffuse tissue injury, and hemodynamic and thermoregulatory instability. The latter presentation of malignant catatonia carries a 10–20% fatality rate untreated, a presentation first poignantly detailed by Stauder (1934) of subsequent global organ system collapse (Caroff et al., 2004; Fink, 2013; Fink & Taylor, 2006). Catatonia can be life-threatening, and any potentially lethal condition in ASD should be on the radar of families and care providers. Since the late 1990s, the literature has featured case reports and case series of individuals with ASD who have experienced catatonia with a wide range of symptoms and marked overall skill regression. Many of them showed profound positive response to ECT after failure of other treatment initiatives such as first-line benzodiazepine therapy (Consoli et al., 2013; Dhossche, 1998; Dhossche et al., 2009; Ghaziuddin et al., 2021; Wachtel et al., 2008, 2009). These patients had become mute, immobile, stuporous, and unable to maintain sufficient oral intake or void, some confined to 24-hour restrictive full-body protective equipment subsequent to dramatic deterioration from baseline functioning. Malignant catatonia also has been reported in multiple individuals with ASD who required ECT for symptom remission, typically after intensive care admission (Ghaziuddin et al., 2017; Wachtel, Crawford, et al., 2010, 2015). A review by Wachtel (2018) of 22 autistic patients described the range of catatonic symptomology, noting stereotypy, posturing, negativism, mutism, and stupor as the most common catatonic signs. Twenty of the 22 patients in this descriptive study also displayed repetitive SIB apparently devoid of operant function.

The anti-catatonia treatment paradigms were first concretized by Bush et al. (1996b) and include (a) benzodiazepines in increasing dosages, (b) discontinuation of potentially offending agents such as antipsychotic medications, and (c) ECT if benzodiazepines are insufficient or clinical morbidity demands more immediate response. This model subsequently has been adopted as the gold standard of catatonia care (Caroff et al., 2004; Fink & Taylor, 2006). The same algorithms are supported in ASD, and adjunctive supportive psychological measures for prompting and engagement are endorsed as well to bolster imperative biological interventions (Dhossche et al., 2006; Fink et al., 2006). The case reports and case series over the past two decades, summarized below, have documented the safety and efficacy of both acute and m-ECT in individuals with catatonia in the context of ASD and other forms of neurodevelopmental disability (Consoli et al., 2010; Ghaziuddin & Walter, 2013; Wachtel, 2019; Wachtel, Crawford, et al., 2010; Wachtel, Griffin, Dhossche, et al., 2010; Wachtel, Griffin, & Reti, 2010).

In illustration, Wachtel et al. (2008) reported the case of an 18-year-old girl with ASD and intellectual disability who presented with classic catatonic posturing affecting multiple limbs, mutism, stupor, food refusal requiring gastrostomy tube placement, and immobility. With ECT, she experienced marked reduction in all of these classically recognized catatonic symptoms accompanied by significantly less frequent SIB that had caused bilateral retinal detachment and traumatic cataract formation, heterotopic ossifications (formation of bone in extraskeletal soft tissue), and localized wounds throughout her body. ECT afforded this young woman dramatic medical and behavioral stabilization, and the case subsequently opened exploration of repetitive SIB as possibly within the catatonia spectrum. Further case reports detailed a similar reduction of SIB in several autistic youth who had previously exhausted extensive behavioral and psychotropic medication interventions and were often confined to a life of physical and chemical restraint (Wachtel et al., 2009, 2011). The later literature explored the range of catatonic symptomology, including both psychomotor impaired and agitated signs. A preliminary hypothesis from this work was that repetitive self-injury could be a defining symptom of the catatonia diagnosis. Of course, clinicians-researchers emphasized early on that this profile only applied to repetitive treatment-refractory SIB without confirmed behavior function (Wachtel & Dhossche, 2010).

Another critical distinction made with the nascent usage of ECT for repetitive SIB in autism was that between ECT and contingent electric shock (CES) in which a painful stimulus is delivered as a form of punishment (Linscheid et al., 1994; Linscheid & Reichenbach, 2002).This type of aversive conditioning essentially has been abandoned in autism due to myriad ethical concerns. Thus, CES bears no similarity to ECT other than the usage of electricity, and even then, CES uses standard sine wave electrical current, whereas all modern ECT devices use the alternating brief pulse currents developed nearly 40 years ago to more closely mimic brain activity (Fink, 1979). It is also of utmost importance to recognize that the usage of electricity in ECT is a method of seizure induction, and it is the convulsion that is at the crux of the therapeutic benefit of ECT. Finally, whereas CES is a punishment procedure involving painful stimuli, ECT is a medical intervention that can bring about immediate and long-term changes in the brain that alleviate severe affective, psychotic, and catatonic pathology (Abrams, 2002; Fink, 2009).

35.5 Research Background

We relied on a clinical review of ECT studies by Luiselli et al. (2021) and additional publications appearing thereafter through 2022. Studies extracted from Internet searches were included if they reported ECT implemented with one or more persons diagnosed with ASD, self-injury, and catatonia, and were published in a peer-reviewed journal. Additional inclusion criteria were that publications could be categorized by one of five evaluation methodologies. A *narrative case report* described the course of ECT but without supporting outcome data. *Case report with outcome data* included measures such as the frequency of challenging behavior or metrics taken from rating scales. Publications qualified as a *single-case baseline-treatment (A-B) design* if data were recorded before a patient received and during administration of ECT. In a *single-case replication design*, ECT with recorded outcome data had to be temporarily removed and reinstated (reversal design) or introduced sequentially and time-staggered with two or more patients (multiple-baseline design). Finally, *a group-comparison design* compared patients treated with ECT against no-treatment or alternative treatment cohorts.

Table 35.1 presents the 19 studies reviewed herein, totaling 21 persons (male = 76.1%, female = 23.8%) between 8 and 33 years old (children = 52.3%, adults = 47.6%). All of the persons treated with ECT had comorbid conditions such as major depression, bipolar disorder, intellectual disability, Tourette's disorder, and neuroleptic malignant syndrome. In virtually every case, ECT followed a course of debilitating instability of adaptive living, communication, social, and self-care skills, accompanied by mood dysregulation, serious externalizing behavior, and self-injury leading to physical trauma and body disfigurement on many occasions. Common treatments preceding ECT were behavioral intervention (e.g., differential positive reinforcement, extinction, functional communication training, response interruption and redirection) and pharmacotherapy while children and adults attended schools, were enrolled in residential care facilities, and lived at home. Many patients were fitted with personal protective equipment to minimize the effects from self-harming behavior and/or required physical restraint from care providers to further guard against injury to self and others.

ECT commonly started at one to three sessions per week for 3–4 weeks, although the duration of acute treatment was variable with many more sessions sometimes scheduled weeks apart (Haq & Ghaziuddin, 2014). Reports uniformly described positive treatment effects from ECT, and time-attenuated side effects were limited to headache, fatigue, and mild delirium (Bird et al., 2021; Dhossche, 2014; Wachtel, Griffin, & Reti, 2010). Notable outcomes across studies were (a) decreased challenging behavior and catatonic symptoms, (b) improved skills, (c) return to baseline functioning, and (d) reintegration within school, home, and community settings. ECT-induced changes often were immediate but also gradual and sensitive to treatment withdrawal. Most studies reported sustained therapeutic response with m-ECT administered to persons months and years following initial treatment (Bird et al., 2022; Gonzalez-Romero et al., 2019; Wachtel, Crawford, et al., 2010; Wachtel, Hermida, & Dhossche, 2010), though relapse remained a concern even with multiyear follow-up.

All but one of the studies were in the format of a narrative case report (44.4%), narrative case report with outcome data (16.6%), and single-case baseline-treatment (A-B) design (33.3%). In the studies with data recording, the period of evaluation varied greatly from 12 to 15 ECT sessions across 4 to 5 weeks of acute treatment (Wachtel et al., 2008, 2009) to 726 days of continuous outcome

Table 35.1 ECT studies included in research review

Publication Citation
Adiguzel Akman et al. (2021)
Bird et al. (2021)
Bird et al. (2022)
Burns et al. (2021)
Dhossche (2014)
Gonzalez-Romero et al. (2019)
Hau & Ghaziuddin (2014)
Machado et al. (2019)
Sajith et al. (2017)
Smith et al. (2022)
Triplett et al. (2020)
Wachtel et al. (2008)
Wachtel et al. (2009)
Wachtel, Crawford, et al. (2010)
Wachtel, Griffin, Dhossche, et al. (2010)
Wachtel, Griffin, & Reti (2010)
Wachtel et al. (2011)
Wachtel et al. (2014)
Withane & Dhossche (2018)

ECT = electroconvulsive therapy.

measurement (Bird et al., 2021). The only exception to case report and single-case, baseline-treatment studies was a retrospective analysis of group data by Smith et al. (2022). This study compared symptom presentation following ECT among individuals who had ASD and intellectual disability (N = 12), ASD without intellectual disability (N = 7), and solely intellectual disability (N = 13). To be expected, the vast majority of reviewed studies were published in medical journals (psychiatry, neurology, pharmacology) and only occasionally in sources more generally devoted to ASD and intellectual disability.

35.6 Practice Implications

ECT can benefit children and adults with ASD who are impaired by affective, psychotic, and catatonic processes. Such pathology can lead to devastating health effects and unstable psychosocial functioning combined with unremitting self-injury that often is extreme and life-threatening. Many persons referred for ECT have been unresponsive to conventional treatments for many years without signs of symptom remission and indications of therapeutic improvement. In this chapter, we surveyed the ECT literature with this population, summarized findings, and derived practice implications from the available evidence. It is acknowledged that our review may have overlooked other publications but nonetheless represents a reasonable summary of the evidence accumulated thus far.

We would be remiss not to conclude that since inception in 1938, ECT has been plagued throughout medicine by insufficient knowledge, misinformation, and stigma that adversely impact patients, families, and practitioners, and often delays timely referral to ECT. The media, in both international film and television, has largely succeeded in portraying ECT as an aversive treatment modality devoid of therapeutic benefit and replete with devastating lifelong cognitive impairments not supported by either psychiatric research or literature over the past 80 years (Matthews et al., 2016; McDonald & Walter, 2009). Similar issues have surfaced with the usage of ECT in youth, particularly those with autism and intellectual disability. There are erroneous comparisons of ECT to contingent electric shock as a punishment procedure and alleged claims of "brain damage" to the developing mind (Wachtel & Dhossche, 2012). In light of our review, ECT can be endorsed as a potentially effective treatment for children and adults with ASD, catatonia, and self-injury, but must be qualified by the small number of studies that are exclusively case-based, frequently narratively reported without supporting outcome data, and none with single-case design experimental rigor (Kazdin, 2011). Direct comparison of ECT against other treatment modalities also is missing from the extant literature, for example, ABA interventions that have been shown to increase verbal and daily living skills in adolescent women diagnosed with catatonia and ASD (Vener et al., 2019, 2021). And yet the reports reviewed in this chapter detailed exceptional treatment responsiveness from ECT among children and adults who required life-sustaining intervention. We believe these powerful findings are persuasive and should be considered by persons on the autism spectrum, their families, and the professional community.

Concerning practice implications, we reiterate that ECT is a treatment rather than a cure, and as such, many individuals who respond favorably to acute ECT will also require m-ECT, possibly indefinitely. This standard applies to both autistic and neurotypical individuals. Ideally, m-ECT schedules should be optimized based on patient response and symptom recurrence, with patients, families, and providers working together to monitor ongoing remission and rapidly detect any signs of recidivism (Frederikse et al., 2006; Kellner et al., 2006; Lisanby et al., 2008). The COVID-19 pandemic, in particular, illustrates the detrimental sequelae in persons whose access to ECT was interrupted or terminated altogether. Wachtel (2021) described a 27-year-old man with ASD and intellectual disability who had received monthly m-ECT successfully for 2 years preceding COVID-19 and then deteriorated significantly during a 7-week suspension of sessions before ECT was reinstated with good effect. In a sample of nine adolescent and young-adult patients with ASD, intellectual disability, and catatonia, Ghaziuddin et al. (2021) detailed "a significant clinical decline over a 14-week period after ECT was either reduced or discontinued due to COVID-19 related capacity in service and/or caregiver preference" (p. 2). Four of the nine cases were severe enough to require hospitalization from loss of speech and food intake, aggressive behavior, paranoid symptoms, and safety concerns at home. The anticipation of future pandemics heightens the awareness of preventing prolonged treatment pauses in persons needing and responding favorably to m-ECT.

Regrettably, practice is not uniform because availability of ECT differs greatly in the United States and other countries. Some jurisdictions have additional restrictions based on age, disability, and capacity to consent. These barriers can hinder ECT access for autistic individuals, especially those with serious challenging behavior (Livingston et al., 2017). Appraisals of ECT have found that the practice meets the applicable ethical standards of beneficence, nonmaleficence, and "do not harm" but not justice, given lack of universal availability (Ottosson & Fink, 2004). The contemporary landscape suggests a clinical inequity that absolutely must be remedied in the interest of all patients whose diagnostic profile suggests they should be assessed for and could benefit from ECT.

A third practice implication gleaned from ECT research is to include data-based outcome measurement as a standard for evaluating treatment effectiveness. For example, in Bird et al. (2021), the participant was a 30-year-old man diagnosed with ASD, intellectual disability, and catatonia who was referred for ECT following a multiyear period of deteriorating skills, social isolation, prompt dependency, behavior outbursts, and self-injury. Care providers at his residential school conducted daily data recording of self-injurious episodes, incidents of aggression, and percentage of meals he consumed successfully. These data were plotted each day in time-series graphs that documented decreasing trends in self-injury and aggression with increased consumption at meals throughout the course of ECT. Direct measurement of clinical indices in this case provided vital empirical evidence to the medical team that supported continuation of ECT, further revealed in a 4-year maintenance evaluation report (Bird et al., 2022).

Finally, increased reports of effective treatment with ECT will advance practice in ASD, particularly through single-case studies, repeated case series, and experimental replication designs whenever possible. Group comparison studies are unlikely to be conducted, given the heterogeneity of persons with ASD under clinical study, small sample sizes, and the ethical concern of withholding treatment with some research participants. Studies which feature controlled evaluations of ECT schedule effects and the optimal combination of complimentary educational, behavior support, rehabilitation, and medication interventions also will fortify practice across the lifespan. A last consideration is that many professionals outside of medicine are unfamiliar with ECT among autistic individuals. Therefore, publishing studies that reach nonmedical practitioners within the larger neurodevelopmental and intellectual disabilities literature would be of value.

35.7 References

Abrams, R. (2002). *Electroconvulsive therapy* (4th ed.). New York: Oxford University Press.

Adıgüzel Akman, Ö., Kahraman Girgeç, S., Çelik, S., Çakır Kardeş, V., & Atasoy, N. (2021). Maintenance electroconvulsive therapy for agitation and self-injurious behaviors in autism spectrum disorder. *Turkish Journal of Psychiatry, 32*(1), 65–69. https://doi.org/10.5080/u23768

American Psychiatric Association. (2013). *Diagnostic and statistical manual of mental disorders* (5th ed.). Washington, DC: Author.

Bailine, S., Fink, M., Knapp, R., Pertrides, G., Husain, M. M., Rasmussen, K., Sampson, S., Mueller, M., McClintock, S. M., Tobias, K. G., & Kellner, C. H. (2010). Electroconvulsive therapy is equally effective in unipolar and bipolar depression. *Acta Psychiatr Scand, 121*, 431–436. https://doi.org/10.1111/j.1600-0447.2009.01493.x

Bender, L. (1947). One hundred cases of childhood schizophrenia treated with electric shock. *Transactions of the American Neurological Society, 72*, 165–169. https://doi.org/10.1111/j.1939-0025.1947.tb04975.x

Billstedt, E., Gillberg, C., & Gillberg, C. (2005). Autism after adolescence population-based 13- to 22-year follow-up study of 120 individuals with autism diagnosed in childhood. *Journal of Autism and Developmental Disorders, 35*(3), 351–360. https://doi.org/10.1007/s10803-005-3302-5

Bird, F., Shah, R., Williams, S., Shlesinger, A., Luiselli, J. K., & Wachtel, L. E. (2022). Multiyear evaluation of electroconvulsive therapy in an adult with autism spectrum disorder, catatonia, and challenging behavior. *Journal of ECT, 39*, 53–55. https://doi.org/10.1097/yct.0000000000000856

Bird, F., Wachtel, L. E., Henry, M., Gold, J., Fernandez-Robles, C., Orchanian, S., Shlesinger, A., & Luiselli, J. K. (2021). Treatment and maintenance effects of behavioral intervention and electroconvulsive therapy (ECT) in a man with catatonia, life-threatening self-injury, and autism spectrum disorder. *Advances in Neurodevelopmental Disorders, 5*, 135–143 https://doi.org/10.1007/s41252-020-00189-03

Breen, J., & Hare, D. J. (2017). The nature and prevalence of catatonic symptoms in young children with autism. *Journal of Intellectual Disability Research, 61*(6), 580–593. https://doi.org/10.1111/jir.12362

Buckley, N., Glasson, E. J., Chen, W., Epstein, A., Leonard, H., Skoss, R., Jacoby, P., Blackmore, A. M. Srinivasjois, R., Bourke, J., Sanders, R. J., & Downs, J. (2020). Prevalence estimates of mental health problems in children and adolescents with intellectual disability: A systematic review and meta-analysis. *Australian and New Zealand Journal of Psychiatry, 54*, 970–984. https://doi.org/10.1177/0004867420924101

Burns, N. K., Grissett, K., Macaluso, M., Raza, M., & Gracious, B. (2021). Excited catatonia in autism spectrum disorder: A case series. *Frontiers in Psychiatry, 12*. https://doi.org/10.3389%2Ffpsyt.2021.674335

Bush, G., Fink, M., Petrides, G., Dowling, F., & Francis, A. (1996a). Catatonia: I: Rating scale and standardized examination. *Acta Psychiatrica Scandinavica, 93*, 129–136. https://doi.org/10.1111/j.1600-0447.1996.tb09814.x

Bush, G., Fink, M., Petrides, G., Dowling, F., & Francis, A. (1996b). Catatonia: II. Treatment with lorazepam and electroconvulsive therapy. *Acta Psychiatrica Scandinavica, 93*, 137–143. https://doi.org/10.1111/j.1600-0447.1996.tb09814.x

Caroff, S., Mann, S. C., Francis, A., & Fricchione, G. L. (2004). *Catatonia: From psychopathology to neurobiology*. Washington, DC: American Psychiatric Press.

Collins, C., Halder, N., & Chaudhry, N. (2012). Use of ECT in patients with intellectual disability: Review. *Psychiatrist, 36*, 55–60. https://doi.org/10.1192/pb.bp.110.033811

Consoli, A., Benmiloud, M., Wachtel, L. E., Dhossche, D. M., Cohen, D., & Bonnot, O. (2010). Electroconvulsive therapy in adolescents with the catatonia syndrome: Efficacy and ethics. *Journal of ECT, 26*, 259–265. https://doi.org/10.1111/j.1600-0447.2009.01493.x

Consoli, A., Cohen, J., Bodeau, N., Guinchat, V., Wachtel, L., & Cohen, D. (2013). Electroconvulsive therapy in adolescents with intellectual disability and severe self-injurious behavior and aggression: A retrospective study. *European Child and Adolescent Psychiatry, 22*(1), 55–62. https://doi.org/10.1007/s00787-012-0320-7

DeJong, H., Bunton, P., & Hare, D. J. A. (2014). Systematic review of interventions used to treat catatonic symptoms in people with autism spectrum disorders. *Journal of Autism and Developmental Disorders, 44*(9), 2127–2136. https://doi.org/10.1007/s10803-014-2085-y.

Dhossche, D. (1998). Brief report: Catatonia in autistic disorders. *Journal of Autism and Developmental Disorders, 28*, 329–331. https://doi.org/10.1023/a:1026064720287

Dhossche, D. M. (2014). Decalogue of catatonia in autism spectrum disorders. *Frontiers in Psychiatry, 5*, 1–4. https://doi.org/10.3389/fpsyt.2014.00157

Dhossche, D. M., & Bouman, N. (1997). Catatonia in an adolescent with Prader-Willi syndrome. *Annals of Psychiatry, 4*, 247–253. https://doi.org/10.1023/a:1022308511313

Dhossche, D. M., Reti, I. M., & Wachtel, L. E. (2009). Catatonia and autism: A historical review with implications for electroconvulsive therapy. *Journal of ECT, 25*, 19–22. https://doi.org/10.1097/YCT.0b013e3181957363

Dhossche, D. M., Shah, A., & Wing, L. (2006). Blueprints for the assessment, treatment, and future study of catatonia in autism spectrum disorders. *International Review of Neurobiology, 72*, 267–284. https://doi.org/10.1016/s0074-7742(05)72016-x

Dhossche, D. M., & Wachtel, L. E. (2013). ECT for catatonia in autism. In M. Ghaziuddin, & G. Walter (Eds.), *Electroconvulsive therapy for children and adolescents* (pp. 217–246). New York: Oxford University Press.

Elias, A. N., Thomas, N., & Sackeim, H. A. (2021). Electroconvulsive therapy in mania: A review of 80 years of clinical experience. *American Journal of Psychiatry, 178*, 229–239. https://doi.org/10.1176/appi.ajp.2020.20030238

Emerson, E. (2003). Prevalence of psychiatric disorders in children and adolescents with and without intellectual disability. *Journal of Intellectual Disability Research, 47*, 51–58. https://doi.org/10.1046/j.1365-2788.2003.00464.x

Fink, M. (1979). *Convulsive therapy: Theory and practice.* New York: Raven Press.

Fink, M. (1996). Neuroleptic malignant syndrome and catatonia: One entity or two? *Biological Psychiatry, 39*, 1–4. https://doi.org/10.1016/0006-3223(96)82518-2

Fink, M. (2009). Catatonia: A syndrome appears, disappears, and is rediscovered. *Canadian Journal of Psychiatry, 54*, 437–445. https://doi.org/10.1177/070674370905400704

Fink, M. (2013). Rediscovering catatonia: The biography of a treatable syndrome. *Acta Psychiatrica Scandinavica, 127*, 1–50. https://doi.org/10.1111/acps.12038

Fink, M. (2014). What was learned: Studies by the consortium for research in ECT (CORE) 1977–2011. *Acta Psychiatry Scandanavia, 129*, 417–426.

Fink, M., & Taylor, M. (2006). *Catatonia: A clinician's guide to diagnosis and treatment.* New York: Oxford University Press.

Fink, M., Taylor, M. A., & Ghaziuddin, N. (2006). Catatonia in autism spectrum disorders: A medical treatment algorithm. *International Review of Neurobiology, 72*, 267–284. https://doi.org/10.1016/s0074-7742(05)72014-6

Frederikse, M. G., Petrides, G., & Kellner, C. (2006). Continuation and maintenance electroconvulsive therapy for the treatment of depressive illness: A response to the National Institute for Clinical Excellence report. *Journal of ECT, 22*, 13–17. https://doi.org/10.1097/00124509-200603000-00003

Ghaziuddin, N., Dhossche, D., & Marcotte, K. (2012). Retrospective chart review of catatonia in child and adolescent psychiatric patients. *Acta Psychiatrica Scandinavica, 125*, 33–38. https://doi.org/10.1111/j.1600-0447.2011.01778.x

Ghaziuddin, N., Hendriks, M., Patel, P., Wachtel, L. E., & Dhossche, D. D. (2017). Neuroleptic malignant syndrome/malignant catatonia in child psychiatry: Literature review and a case series. *Journal of Child and Adolescent Psychopharmacology, 27*, 359–365. https://doi.org/10.1089/cap.2016.0180

Ghaziuddin, N., Kutcher, S. P., & Knapp, P. (2004). Summary of the practice parameter for the use of electroconvulsive therapy with adolescents. *Journal of the American Academy of Child and Adolescent Psychiatry, 43*, 119–122. https://doi.org/10.1097/00004583-200401000-00028

Ghaziuddin, N., & Walter, G. (Eds.) (2013). *Electroconvulsive therapy in children and adolescents.* New York: Oxford University Press.

Ghaziuddin, N., Yaqub, T., Shamseddeen, W., Reddy, P., Reynard, H., & Maixner, D. (2021). Maintenance electroconvulsive therapy is an essential medical treatment for patients with catatonia: A COVID-19 related experience. *Frontiers in Psychiatry, 12*. https://doi.org/10.3389/fpsyt.2021.670476

Gonzalez-Romero, M. F., Avina-Galind, A. M., Elbe, D., Friedlander, R., & Vila-Rodriguez, F. (2019). Lifesaving electroconvulsive therapy for a child with autism spectrum disorder, severe self-injurious behavior, and neuroleptic malignant syndrome. *Journal of ECT, 35*, 55–56. https://doi.org/10.1097/yct.0000000000000598

Grover, S., Sahoo, S., Rabha, A., & Koirala, R. (2019). ECT in schizophrenia: A review of the evidence. *Acta Neuropsychiatr, 31*, 115–127. https://doi.org/10.1017/neu.2018.32

Haq, A. U., & Ghaziuddin, N. (2014). Maintenance electroconvulsive therapy for aggression and self-injurious behavior in two adolescents with autism and catatonia. *Journal of Neuropsychiatry and Clinical Neurosciences, 26*(1), 64–72. https://doi.org/10.1176/appi.neuropsych.12110284

Harris, J. (1998). *Developmental neuropsychiatry.* New York: Oxford University Press.

Heuyer, G., Bour, T., & Leroy, R. (1943). L'electrochoc chez les enfants. *Annals of Medical Psychology, 2*, 402–407.

Hughes-McCormack, L. A., Rydzewska, E., Henderson, A., MacIntyre, C., Rintoul, J., & Cooper, S. A. (2017). Prevalence of mental health conditions and relationship with general health in a whole-country population of people with intellectual disabilities compared with the general population. *BJPsych Open, 3*, 243–248. https://doi.org/10.1192/bjpo.bp.117.005462

Husain, M. M., Rush, A. J., Fink, M., Knapp, R., Petrides, G., Rummans, T., Biggs, M. M., O'Connor, K., Rasmussen, K., Litle, M., Zhao, W., Bernstein, H. J., Smith, G., Mueller, M., McClintock, S. M., Bailine, S. H., & Kellner, C. H. (2004). Speed of response and remission in major depressive disorder with acute electroconvulsive therapy (ECT): A consortium for research in ECT (CORE) report. *Journal of Clinical Psychiatry, 65*, 485–491. https://doi.org/10.4088/jcp.v65n0406

Kazdin, A. E. (2011). *Single-case research designs: Methods for clinical and applied settings* (2nd ed.). New York: Oxford University Press.

Kellner, C. H., Husain, M. M., Knapp, R. G., McCall, W. V., Petrides, G. P., Rudorfer, M. V., Young, R. C., Sampson, S., McClintock, S. M., Mueller. M., Prudic, J., Greenberg, R. M., Weiner, R. D., Bailine, S. H., Rosenquist, P. B., Raza, A., Kaliora, S., Latoussakis, V., Tobias, K. G ... Lisanby, S. H. (2016). Right unilateral ultra-brief pulse ECT in geriatric depression: Phase 1 of the PRIDE study. *American Journal of Psychiatry, 173*, 1101–1109.

Kellner, C. H., Knapp, R. G., Petrides, G., Rummans, T. A., Husain, M. M., Rasmussen, K., Mueller, M., Bernstein, H. J., O'Connor, K., Smith, G., Biggs, M., Bailine, S. H., Malur, C., Yim, E., McClintock, S., Sampson, S., & Fink, M. (2006). Continuation electroconvulsive therapy vs pharmacotherapy for relapse prevention in major depression: A multisite study from the Consortium for Research in Electroconvulsive Therapy (CORE). *Archives of General Psychiatry, 63*, 1337–1344. https://doi.org/10.1001/archpsyc.63.12.1337

Linscheid, T., Pejeau, C., Cohen, S., & Footo-Lenz, M. (1994). Positive side effects in the treatment of SIB using the self-injurious behavior inhibiting system (SIBIS): Implications for operant and biochemical explanations of SIB. *Research in Developmental Disabilities, 15*, 81–90. https://doi.org/10.1016/0891-4222(94)90040-x

Linscheid, T., & Reichenbach, H. (2002). Multiple factors in the long-term effectiveness of contingent electric shock treatment for self-injurious behavior: A case example. *Research in Developmental Disabilities, 23*, 161–177. https://doi.org/10.1016/s0891-4222(02)00093-8

Lisanby, S. H., Sampson, S. M., Husain, M. M., & Petrides, G. (2008). Toward individualized post-electroconvulsive therapy care: Piloting the symptom-titrated, algorithm longitudinal ECT (STABLE) intervention. *Journal of ECT, 24*, 179–182. https://www.researchgate.net/deref/http%3A%2F%2Fdx.doi.org%2F10.1097%2FYCT.0b013e318185fa6b

Livingston, R., Wu, C., Mu, K., & Coffey, M. J. (2017). Regulation of electroconvulsive therapy: A systematic review of US state laws. *Journal of ECT, 34*, 60–68. https://doi.org/10.1097/yct.0000000000000460

Luiselli, J. K., Bird, F., & Wachtel, L. E. (2021). Electroconvulsive therapy (ECT) for autism spectrum disorder associated with catatonia and self-injury: A clinical review. *Advances in Neurodevelopmental Disabilities, 5*, 117–125. https://doi.org/10.1007/s41252-021-00202-0

Machado, A. F., de Marigny, R. F., & Schlitter, L. X. (2019). Satisfactory response to electroconvulsive therapy in an autistic patient with severe self-injurious behavior. *Brazilian Journal of Psychiatry, 41*, 458–459. https://doi.org/10.1590%2F1516-4446-2019-0534

Maenner, M. J., Shaw, K. A., Bakian, A. V., Bilder, D. A., Durkin, M. S., Esler, A., Furnier, S. M., Hallas, L., Hall-Lande, J., Hudson, A., Hughes, M. H., Patrick, M., Pierce, K., Poynter, J. N., Salinas, A., Shenouda, J., Vehorn, A., Warren, Z., Constantino, J. N. ... Cogswell, M. E. (2021). Prevalence and characteristics of autism spectrum disorder among children aged 8 years-Autism and developmental disabilities monitoring network, 11 sites, United States, 2018. *MMWR Surveillance Summit, 70*, 1–16. https://doi.org/10.15585/MMWR.SS7011A1

Matthews, A. M., Rosenquist, P. B., & McCall, W. V. (2016). Representations of ECT in English-language film and television in the new millennium. *Journal of ECT, 32*, 187–191. https://doi.org/10.1097/yct.0000000000000312

McDonald, A., & Walter, G. (2009). Hollywood and ECT. *International Review of Psychiatry, 21*, 200–206. https://doi.org/10.1080/09540260902747888

Mosner, M. G., Kinard, J. L., Shah, J. S., McWeeny, S., Greene, R. K., Lowery, S. C., Mazefsky, C. A., & Dichter, G. S. (2019). Rates of co-occurring psychiatric disorders in autism spectrum disorder using the Mini International Neuropsychiatric Interview. *Journal of Autism and Developmental Disorders, 49*, 3819–3832. https://doi.org/10.1007/s10803-019-04090-1

Mukherjee, S., Sackeim, H. A., & Schnur, D. B. (1994). Electroconvulsive therapy of acute manic episodes: A review of 50 years' experience. *American Journal of Psychiatry, 151*, 169–176. https://doi.org/10.1176/ajp.151.2.169

Ottosson, J. O., & Fink, M. (2004). *Ethics of electroconvulsive therapy.* New York: Brunner-Routledge.

Pertrides, G., Fink, M., Husain, M. M., Knapp, R. J., Rush, A. J., Mueller, M., Rummans, T. A., O'Connor, K. M., Rasmussen, K. G., Bernstein, H. J., Biggs, M., Bailine, S. H., Kellner, C. H. (2001).

ECT remission rates in psychotic versus non-psychotic depressed patients: A report from CORE. *Journal of ECT, 17*, 244–253. https://doi.org/10.1097/00124509-200112000-00003
Platt, J. M., Keyes, K. M., McLaughlin, K. A., & Kaufman, A. S. (2019). Intellectual disability and mental disorders in a US population representative sample of adolescents. *Psychology and Medicine, 49*, 952–961. https://doi.org/10.1017/s0033291718001605
Puffer, C. C., Wall, C. A., Huxsahl, J. E., & Frye, M. A. (2016). A 20 year practice review of electroconvulsive therapy for adolescents. *Journal of Child and Adolescent Psychopharmacology, 26*, 632–636. https://doi.org/10.1089/cap.2015.0139
Rasmussen, S. A., Mazurek, M. F., & Rosebush, P. I. (2016). Catatonia: Out current understanding of its diagnosis, treatment, and pathophysiology. *World Journal of Psychiatry, 6*(4), 391–398. https://doi.org/10.5498/wjp.v6.i4.391.
Rey, J., & Walter, G. (1997). Half a century of ECT use in young people. *American Journal of Psychiatry, 154*, 595–602. https://doi.org/10.1176/ajp.154.5.595
Rutter, M., Graham, P., & Yule, W. (1970). A neuropsychiatric study in childhood. In *Clinics in Developmental Medicine, 35 & 36*. London: MacKeith Press.
Sajith, S. G., Liew, S. F., & Phern, C. (2017). Response to electroconvulsive therapy in patients with autism spectrum disorder and intractable challenging behavior associated with symptoms of catatonia. *Journal of ECT, 33*, 63–67. https://doi.org/10.1097/yct.0000000000000338
Sanghani, S. N., Petrides, G., & Kellner, C. H. (2018). Electroconvulsive therapy (ECT) in schizophrenia: A review of recent literature. *Current Opinion in Psychiatry, 31*, 213–222. https://doi.org/10.1097/yco.0000000000000418
Shorter, E., & Fink, M. (2018). *The madness of fear: A history of catatonia*. New York: Oxford University Press.
Shorter, E., & Healy, D. (2013). *Shock therapy: A history of electroconvulsive treatment in mental illness*. New Brunswick, NJ: Rutgers University Press.
Sienaert, P., Rooseleer, J., & De Fruyt, J. (2011). Measuring catatonia: A systematic review of rating scales. *Journal of Affective Disorders, 135*, 1–9. https://doi.org/10.1016/j.jad.2011.02.012
Smith, J. R., Hopkins, C. E., Xiong, J., Luccarelli, J., Shultz, E., & Vandekar, S. (2022). Use of ECT in autism spectrum disorder and/or intellectual disability: A single site retrospective analysis. *Journal of Autism and Developmental Disorders*. https://doi.org/10.1007/s10803-022-05868-6
Stauder, K. (1934). Die todliche katatonie. *Archives of Psychiatry Nervenkrank, 102*, 614–634.
van Steensel, F. J., Bogels, S. M., & de Bruin, E. I. (2013). Psychiatric comorbidity in children with autism spectrum disorders: A comparison with children with ADHD. *Journal of Child and Family Studies, 22*, 368–376. https://doi.org/10.1007/s10826-012-9587-z
Triplett, P., Gerstenblith, A., Reti, I. M., & Wachtel, L. E. (2020). Treatment of catatonic symptoms in a patient with autism spectrum disorder and Addison disease: A case report. *Journal of ECT, 36*, 10–11. https://doi.org/10.1097/YCT.0000000000000670
Vaquerizo-Serrano, J., Salazar De Pablo, G., Singh, J., & Santosh, P. (2022). Catatonia in autism spectrum disorders: a systematic review and meta-analysis. *European Psychiatry, 65*(1), 1–10. https://doi.org/10.1192/j.eurpsy.2021.2259
Varcin, K. J., Hernimann, S. E., Lin, A., Chen, Y., Perry, Y., Pugh, C., Chisholm, K., Whitehouse, A. J. O., & Wood, S. J. (2022). Occurrence of psychosis and bipolar disorder in adults with autism: A systematic review and meta-analysis. *Neuroscience and Biobehavioral Review, 134*, 1–14. https://doi.org/10.1016/j.neubiorev.2022.104543
Vener, S. M., Gillis, A. M., & Poulson, C. L. (2021). Increasing verbal behavior in a young adolescent girl with catatonia and ASD. *Journal of Autism and Developmental Disorders, 51*, 3857–3867. https://doi.org/10.1007/s10803-020-04843-3
Vener, S. M., Wichnick-Gillis, A. M., Badala, D. F., & Poulson, C. L. (2019). Increasing behavior incompatible with catatonia in a young adolescent girl with autism spectrum disorder. *Research in Autism Spectrum Disorder, 57*, 7–18. https://doi.org/10.1007/s10803-020-04843-3
Wachtel, L. E. (2018). The multiple faces of catatonia in autism spectrum disorders: descriptive clinical experience of 22 patients over 12 years. *European Child & Adolescent Psychiatry, 28*, 471–480. https://doi.org/10.1007/s00787-018-1210-4
Wachtel, L. E. (2019). Treatment of catatonia in autism spectrum disorder. *Acta Psychiatricia Scandinavica, 139*(1), 46–55. https://doi.org/10.1111/acps.12980
Wachtel, L. E. (2021). Far from an elective procedure: Electroconvulsive therapy and autism in the era of COVID-19. *Journal of ECT, 37*, 10–12. https://doi.org/10.1097/yct.0000000000000720
Wachtel, L. E., Commins, E., Park, M., Rolider, N., Stephens, R., & Reti, I. (2015). Neuroleptic malignant syndrome and delirious mania as malignant catatonia in autism: Prompt relief with

electroconvulsive therapy. *Acta Psychiatricia Scandinavica, 132*, 319–320. https://doi.org/10.1111/acps.12441

Wachtel, L. E., Contrucci-Kuhn, S. A., Griffin, M., Thompson, A., Dhossche, D. M., & Reti, I. M. (2009). ECT for self-injury in an autistic boy. *European Child and Adolescent Psychiatry, 18*(7), 458–463. https://doi.org/10.1007/s00787-009-0754-8.

Wachtel, L. E., Crawford, T. O., Dhossche, D. M., & Reti, I. M. (2010). Electroconvulsive therapy for pediatric malignant catatonia with cerebellar dysgenesis. *Pediatric Neurology, 43*, 427–430. https://doi.org/10.1016/j.pediatrneurol.2010.06.009

Wachtel, L. E., & Dhossche, D. M. (2010). Self-injury in autism as an alternative sign of catatonia: Implications for electroconvulsive therapy. *Medical Hypotheses, 75*(1), 111–114. https://doi.org/10.1016/j.mehy.2010.02.001.

Wachtel, L. E., & Dhossche, D. M. (2012). Challenges of electroconvulsive therapy for catatonia in youth with intellectual disabilities: Another tomato effect? *Journal of ECT, 28*, 151–153. https://doi.org/10.1097/YCT.0b013e31825692e2

Wachtel, L. E., Griffin, M. M., Dhossche, D., & Reti, I. (2010). Brief report: Electroconvulsive therapy for malignant catatonia in an autistic adolescent. *Autism, 14*, 449–358. https://www.researchgate.net/deref/http%3A%2F%2Fdx.doi.org%2F10.1177%2F1362361309350135

Wachtel, L. E., Griffin, M., & Reti, I. M. (2010). Electroconvulsive therapy in a man with autism experiencing severe depression, catatonia, and self-injury. *Journal of ECT, 26*, 70–73. https://doi.org/10.1097/YCT.0b013e3181a744ec

Wachtel, L. E., Hermida, A., & Dhossche, D. M. (2010d). Maintenance electroconvulsive therapy in autistic catatonia: A case series review. *Progressive Neuropsychopharmacology and Biological Psychiatry, 34*(4), 581–587. https://doi.otg/10.1016/j.pnpbp.2010.03.012.

Wachtel, L. E., Jaffe, R., & Kellner, C. H. (2011). Electroconvulsive therapy for psychotropic-refractory bipolar affective disorder and severe self-injury and aggression in an 11-year-old autistic boy. *European Child and Adolescent Psychiatry, 20*, 147–152. https://doi.org/10.1007/s00787-010-0155-z

Wachtel, L. E., Kahng, S. W., Dhossche, D. M., Cascella, N., & Reti, I. M. (2008). ECT for catatonia in an autistic girl. *American Journal of Psychiatry, 165*(3), 329–333. https://doi.org/10.1176/appi.ajp.2007.07081246.

Wachtel, L. E., Reti, I. M., & Ying, H. (2014). Stability of intraocular pressure after retinal reattachment surgery during electroconvulsive therapy for intractable self-injury in a 12-year-old autistic boy. *Journal of ECT, 30*, 73–76. https://doi.org/10.1097/yct.0b013e31829b2d61

Wachtel, L. E., Shorter, E., & Fink, M. (2018). Electroconvulsive therapy for self-injurious behavior in autism spectrum disorders: Recognizing catatonia is the key. *Current Opinion in Psychiatry, 31*, 116–122. https://doi.org/10.1097/YCO.0000000000000393

Wing, L., & Shah, A. A. (2000). Catatonia in autistic spectrum disorders. *British Journal of Psychiatry, 176*, 357–362. https://doi.org/10.1192/bjp.176.4.357

Wing, L., & Shah, A. A. (2006). A systematic examination of catatonic-like clinical pictures in autism spectrum disorders. *International Review of Neurobiology, 72*, 21–39. https://doi.org/10.1016/S0074-7742(05)72002-X.

Withane, N., & Dhossche, D. M. (2018). Electroconvulsive treatment for catatonia in autism spectrum disorders. *Child and adolescent psychiatric clinics of North America, 28*, 101– 110. https://doi.org/10.1016/j.chc.2018.07.006

36

Research-Based Professional Development for Educators Who Teach Students on the Autism Spectrum

Matthew E. Brock
Crane Center for Early Childhood Research and Practice, Ohio State University

36.1 Technical Abstract

Background: The best way to improve outcomes for students on the autism spectrum is through evidence-based practices, but evidence-based practices are only effective if they are used with fidelity by educators. Traditional approaches for professional development are not up to the task of closing the research-to-practice gap, but research-based principles of professional development offer a promising path forward. **Method:** This chapter focuses on research-based principles grounded in comprehensive meta-analyses of the educator training literature. These meta-analyses included any experimental studies (i.e., single-case design or randomized controlled trials) in which teachers, paraeducators, or related service personnel were trained to implement interventions for students with disabilities, including students on the autism spectrum. **Results:** This chapter focuses on three research-based principles: effective training strategies (i.e., written directions, didactic instruction, modeling, practice, and performance feedback), professional development that is sustained over time, and supporting educators to generalize their implementation to unique students and situations. While these principles apply to training for all educators, additional considerations for training paraeducators are also discussed. Finally, innovations are discussed, such as tiered training models and virtual delivery, which have the potential to improve the feasibility of research-based professional development. **Discussion:** While there is clear evidence to support basic principles of effective professional development, more research is needed on how to make delivery efficient, feasible, and widely adopted. **Practitioner recommendations:** Traditional approaches to professional development, such as "sit and get" or "one-shot" workshops, are unlikely to result in educators making meaningful changes to their teaching. Administrators and trainers should ensure that professional development includes effective strategies, is sustained over time, and supports educators to generalize their implementation to unique students and situations.

Matthew E. Brock, *Research-Based Professional Development for Educators Who Teach Students on the Autism Spectrum*. In: *Lifespan Treatment for Autistic Individuals*. Edited by: Peter Sturmey, Russell Lang, and James K. Luiselli, Oxford University Press. © Oxford University Press (2025). DOI: 10.1093/oso/9780197635841.003.0036

36.2 Layperson Summary

Students on the autism spectrum learn best when educators use strategies that have been tested and proven to work. However, these strategies are only effective when educators use them as designed. There are three ways that educators should be supported to use teaching strategies as designed. First, educator training should include written directions, clear instructions from a trainer, and feedback about how they are doing. Second, training should include follow-up to make sure educators are successful with the new strategies. Third, training should focus on how educators can use the strategies with different students and in different situations. In addition to these three principles, this chapter discusses special considerations for training paraprofessionals who usually lack any formal training in special education. Finally, this chapter discusses promising new approaches designed to make training more effective while keeping costs low. One example is tiered training, where all educators get the same training at first, but educators who struggle get extra help. Another example is online training. The ideas in this chapter can help educators use strategies that are proven to help students learn. Resources that can help to design research-based professional development can be found at the Autism Focused Intervention Resources and Modules (https://afirm.fpg.unc.edu/afirm-modules; Sam et al., 2020) as well as the Autism Internet Modules (https://autisminternetmodules.org/; Ohio Center for Autism and Low Incidence, 2020).

36.3 Treatment Summary Table

Treatment summary: Research-Based Principles

Treatment description: This chapter focuses on research-based principles for helping educators implement evidence-based practices for students with autism. These principles include (1) effective training strategies (i.e., written directions, didactic instruction, modeling, practice, and performance feedback), (2) professional development that is sustained over time, and (3) supporting educators to generalize their implementation to unique students and situations.

Expected outcomes: The research-based principles of professional development discussed in this chapter enable educators to (1) implement evidence-based practices with fidelity and (2) generalize their implementation to unique students and situations. They may also result in increased adaptive behavior and decreased problem behavior in individuals with autism.

Methods: The research-based principles discussed in this chapter are grounded in comprehensive meta-analyses of the educator training literature. These meta-analyses included any experimental studies (i.e., single-case design or randomized controlled trials) in which teachers, paraeducators, or related service personnel were trained to implement interventions for students with disabilities, including students on the autism spectrum.

Expertise required to implement treatment: Before using the principles discussed in this chapter to train educators, trainers should (1) demonstrate the ability to implement the targeted evidence-based practice with fidelity; (2) have adequate experience working in school classrooms to understand the context for implementation; and (3) be skilled to providing feedback that is constructive and goal-directed.

Risks and negative side effects: There are no known risks or negative side effects to delivering research-based professional development to educators.

Additional considerations and limitations: Much of the research on professional development involves researcher-delivered training. More work needs to be done to identify the most feasible and efficient methods for how administrators and other school-based trainers can deliver research-based professional development under real-world conditions.

36.4 Introduction

36.4.1 Treatment Description

This chapter focuses on research-based professional development than enables educators to implement evidence-based practices with fidelity. Professional development involves any training or support provided to in-service practitioners who serve students on the autism spectrum. Evidence-based practices include educational practices for students on the autism spectrum that are supported by multiple rigorous scientific research studies, including well-designed randomized controlled trials and single-case design studies. Implementing a practice with fidelity involves an educator using the practice in a way that is consistent with how it was originally designed and implemented in research studies.

36.4.2 Rationale and Objectives

Like all students, students on the autism spectrum deserve to receive instruction and support that are grounded in evidence-based practice. Today, we know more than ever about which interventions are supported by research evidence, the types of outcomes they can improve, and the conditions under which they are most effective. In their recent exhaustive review of the research literature, the National Clearinghouse on Autism Evidence and Practice identified 28 focused interventions that met criteria as evidence-based practices based on the standards established by the What Works Clearinghouse (Hume et al., 2021; WWC, 2020). Among these evidence-based practices, there are proven pathways to promote a wide range of improved outcomes for students on the autism spectrum, including social, communication, adaptive, behavioral, and vocational outcomes. Collectively, these practices provide a clear blueprint for how schools can provide the education and support that students on the autism spectrum need and deserve.

The degree to which students benefit from these evidence-based practices hinges entirely on the degree to which educators—including teachers, paraeducators, and related service personnel—implement these practices as intended. Based on surveys of educators and observational studies in schools, a wide gap continues to separate research and practice in special education for students on the autism spectrum. Many educators describe approaches to teaching that are devoid of evidence-based practices (Brock et al., 2020). Some report utilizing practices without an evidence base more often than those that are evidence-based (Hess et al., 2008). Others report employing evidence-based practices frequently, but the quality of their implementation is variable (Odom et al., 2013). Educators frequently report a lack of confidence in using evidence-based practices for students on the autism spectrum and express a desire for further training and support (Brock et al., 2014). Indeed, a wide gap separates cutting-edge research from the reality of everyday practice in schools.

The research-to-practice gap is not a new problem. Scholars have raised concerns about this gap for decades (e.g., Carnine, 1997), and there has been a movement in recent years to focus on implementation science—or research-based methods for ensuring that evidence-based practices are routinely implemented with fidelity by educators (Odom et al., 2020). This chapter focuses on what scholars have learned from implementation science research. It is divided into four sections that focus on why current professional development efforts fall short of closing the research-to-practice gap, promising research-based strategies that represent a better path forward, special considerations for better supporting paraeducators, and efforts to make research-based professional development more efficient and feasible.

A clear lesson from the research literature is that the most common approaches to in-service training do not produce optimal results. Professional development for educators commonly includes three ineffective features (see Table 36.1). First, trainers often use strategies that are unlikely to enable educators to work toward proficient implementation of evidence-based practices. Specifically, training opportunities often involve a lecture to a passive audience (Colbert et al., 2008). Colloquially dubbed "sit and get" trainings, educators are expected to absorb the content of the lecture and translate it into action in their classrooms. Unsurprisingly, this style of professional development rarely results in educators frequently or skillfully implementing evidence-based practices (Odom, 2009). Second, most professional development for educators involves a single training event without any follow-up. Often called a "one-and-done," this type of training fits neatly into a half or full-day that has been designated for professional development. While it might allow for convenient scheduling, single training events are unlikely to result in long-term behavior change (Joyce & Showers, 2002). Third, trainers often put the onus on educators to figure out how to apply the evidence-based practice to their own unique students and situations. Given that the autism spectrum encompasses people with an enormous range of abilities, characteristics, and support needs, it is unsurprising that educators might struggle to independently envision how to successfully generalize an evidence-based practice to their own students (Brock et al., 2018). Collectively, these three features—overreliance on lectures with passive participation, single-event training without follow-up, and lack of focus on generalization to authentic contexts—are a recipe for limited change and maintaining the status quo.

Table 36.1 Common features of ineffective professional development practices versus research-based approaches

Features of Professional Development	Common Ineffective Approaches	Research-Based Approaches
Strategies	Overreliance on verbal description of a practice Passive participation	Includes detailed written directions, didactic instruction that aligns with the written directions, and models of correct implementation Participants have opportunities to practice and receive feedback on what they did well and how they could improve.
Format	Single event without follow-up	Sustained professional development that includes feedback on classroom implementation
Generalization	Without any guidance or support, teachers are expected to figure out how to apply a practice to unique students and situations.	Emphasis on guiding and supporting teachers to apply a practice to unique students and situations

To promote more effective professional development practices, this chapter provides a more promising path forward that is grounded in research evidence. Specifically, the objectives of this chapter are to:

1. identify and describe research-based principles of professional development for educators,
2. identify and describe research-based principles specifically for supporting paraeducators who typically have no formal training in special education, and
3. discuss promising innovations such as tiered training models and virtual delivery that have the potential to improve the feasibility of research-based professional development.

36.4.3 Considerations for Implementation

This chapter focused on three research-based principles: effective training strategies (i.e., written directions, didactic instruction, modeling, practice, and performance feedback), professional development that is sustained over time, and supporting educators to generalize their implementation to unique students and situations. While these principles apply to training for all educators, additional considerations for training paraeducators are also discussed. Specially, administrators and teachers should ensure that paraeducator responsibilities are appropriate and clearly defined, that paraeducators are provided with background knowledge and a rationale to understand why they are being asked to use certain practices, and that there is adequate administrative support for teachers to be effective coaches for paraeducators. These concepts, as well as the research that supports them, are described in detail in the subsequent section.

36.5 Research Background

Researchers have worked to develop and test professional development strategies that are designed to enable educators to implement evidence-based practices with fidelity and improve student outcomes. Based on two meta-analyses that summarize effects across the research literature, there are clear trends in what features make professional development most effective (Brock et al., 2017; Brock & Carter, 2017).

In the first meta-analysis, Brock and Carter (2017) conduct an exhaustive review of group design studies that tested the impact of educator training on fidelity of interventions for students with disabilities. The authors found that high-quality training can produce large changes in how well educators implement evidence-based practices, and that a combination of specific training strategies—modeling and performance feedback—were associated with the largest improvements. Furthermore, they found that professional development was most effective when it was sustained over time, but that longer training was only effective when the training featured modeling and performance feedback.

In the second meta-analysis, Brock et al. (2017) reviewed 118 single-case design studies focused on training for educators who serve students with disabilities. Findings from this review confirmed and extended the findings from the earlier meta-analysis on group design studies. Specifically, the authors found that behavioral skills training (BST) that included didactic instruction, modeling, and performance feedback produced the most consistent improvement in educator implementation. BST was sustained over time, and it was focused on enabling educators to generalize to the classroom or setting where they would ultimately be using a new intervention. Modeling, written instructions for implementation, and oral description of implementation steps were the strongest individual predicators of how much educator implementation improved. Furthermore, analysis of student outcomes showed that when research-based professional development was focused on evidence-based practices, improved educator implementation led directly to improved student outcomes.

In sum, these two rigorous meta-analyses coalesce around three principles of effective professional development. These principles include (1) utilizing a collection of effective training strategies, (2) sustaining professional development

Table 36.2 Research-based professional development strategies

Strategy	What Is It?	Variations
Written directions	Clear description of all implementation behaviors associated with an evidence-based practice	• Implementation checklists of practices with sequential steps • Detailed descriptions of discrete behaviors
Didactic instruction	Guidance from a trainer on how to implement the practice that aligns with the written directions	• Oral instruction from a trainer • Video of trainer • Intervention manual or textbook
Modeling	Exemplars of implementation	• In-person live models • Video models
Practice	Opportunities for trainees to attempt implementation of the practice	• Role play with the trainer • Role play with a peer • Implementation with at student
Performance Feedback	After observing the trainee, a trainer provides feedback about what was done well and what could be improved.	• In-person observations • Video-based observations • Oral feedback • Written feedback • Visual feedback

beyond a one-time training, and (3) supporting educators to generalize implementation to their own unique students and situations (see Table 36.1). Each of these principles is discussed in detail in the sections below.

36.5.1 Effective Strategies

Across research studies on professional development, a collection of five strategies have emerged that are associated with effective professional development (see Table 36.2). These strategies include written directions, didactic instruction, modeling, practice, and performance feedback (Brock et al., 2017; Brock & Carter, 2017). When used together, the combination of didactic instruction, modeling, practice, and performance feedback is called BST (Kirkpatrick et al., 2019). In research studies, training that involves BST led to the most consistent improvement in educator implementation fidelity (Brock et al., 2017).

When one considers how these strategies fit together, it is unsurprising that they would be highly effective when used in combination (Brock & Carter, 2015). First, educators benefit from someone explaining how a practice is implemented and providing written directions so that they can both follow along during the training and refer back to them later. Second, once educators are familiar with directions for implementation, they benefit from watching exemplars that enable them to visualize what they just learned. Third, educators need opportunities to practice and learn from feedback. Having just reviewed the practice and watching exemplars of implementation, educators are likely to implement many aspects of the practice correctly the first time. If mistakes are made, a trainer who is experienced in the practice can help them identify their errors and fix them. Each of these individual strategies is defined and reviewed in detail below.

36.5.1.1 Written Directions

Written directions involve a clear description of all behaviors associated with an evidence-based practice. For practices that have sequential steps such as discrete trial training or video prompting, written directions can take the form of an implementation checklist that lists each step in chronological order. For examples of implementation checklists of evidence-based practices for students on the autism spectrum, visit the Autism Focused Intervention Resources and Modules (Sam et al., 2020). In other cases, practices like pivotal response treatment (Koegel & Koegel, 2019) may involve principles for implementation instead of sequential steps. These principles can still be included in a checklist, but without the expectation that they will be followed as sequential steps. In still other cases, the targeted practice might consist of a single behavior such as behavior-specific praise or providing an opportunity for students to respond. In this case, a checklist would not make sense because there is only a single implementation step. Instead, written directions can describe the target behavior and provide multiple examples of what the behavior might look like in different contexts.

36.5.1.2 Didactic Instruction

Didactic instruction involves providing additional detail and guidance about the written directions. A trainer describes each implementation step or principle of implementation, provides explanation, and addresses common misunderstandings or misconceptions. While didactic instruction often involves oral instruction from a trainer, it can also take the form of a video or a detailed intervention manual or textbook.

36.5.1.3 Modeling

Modeling involves showing educators exemplars of implementation. This strategy helps educators envision what implementation should look like. It is critical that models are aligned with the written directions so that educators can match what they learned from the didactic instruction to the model. The degree to which a model is helpful depends on how closely it resembles the context in which the educator will use the practice (Brock et al., 2018). When providing models to educators who serve students with a wide array of profiles or in different types of settings, it can be helpful to use multiple exemplars that represent this spectrum. This is especially important with highly versatile evidence-based practices such as response prompting that could be used to address a variety of goals for students across the autism spectrum (Shawbitz & Brock, 2022). Furthermore, it is important to include exemplars that include students with different profiles, including students who communicate in different ways such as speech and augmentative and alternative communication, those who do and do not exhibit challenging behavior, and those who need varying amounts of support in order to be successful.

36.5.1.4 Practice

Practice involves educators attempting implementation of the evidence-based practice. Often the most practical way for educators to get immediate practice is to engage in role play during a training session. This might involve partnering with another participant at the training or with the trainer. One person pretends to be a student receiving instruction, while the other plays the teacher delivering the instruction. Role play has some clear advantages over jumping straight to implementing with a student. First, it is possible to carefully design and control the role-play situations. This can aid in helping an educator be successful with implementing a new practice in a relatively easy situation before increasing the difficulty. This also can help with training across a broader range of student profiles and goals. Second, role play lends itself well to immediate feedback. In contrast to implementation with real students, it is not a problem to interrupt a session, provide feedback, and then direct the educator to jump right back in where they left off.

Another option is to attempt implementation with a student. There are some advantages to engaging in role play before jumping straight to implementing with students. For example, role play during a training session provides an opportunity to practice while the directions are still fresh in the minds of educators, and while the trainer is already present to observe and provide feedback. Role play also can provide an opportunity to practice many times in a row until the educators achieve mastery, whereas a student might not have the stamina or tolerance for this repetition. In addition, if the teacher realizes they made a mistake, it is easier in a role-play situation to stop, regroup, and start over. Also, some students on the autism spectrum may have challenging behaviors and managing these behaviors may demand some of a teacher's focus. In this situation, it might be easier to implement the evidence practice with the student after already achieving initial mastery through role play.

36.5.1.5 Performance Feedback

As educators practice, it is important that they are implementing the evidence-based practice correctly so that they avoid practicing mistakes that might develop into bad habits. The best way to ensure that educators avoid practicing mistakes is through performance feedback. Performance feedback involves an experienced implementer observing the educator and providing feedback about what they did well and how they could improve. Performance feedback should be tied directly to the written directions for implementation. This way, the trainer can direct the educator's attention to the aspects of implementation that they did well, or a step that was missed or needs improvement. Scholars have suggested that performance feedback might be the most powerful individual training strategy, and it has adequate research support to be considered a standalone evidence-based practice (Fallon et al., 2015).

Both the observation and the performance feedback can be completed in multiple ways. Observations can be delivered both in person and by watching a video recording. In-person observations involve the trainer watching the educator practice implementation in real time. This is very feasible in a training context, but it is sometimes less feasible when an educator is working with a student in the classroom. There are some advantages to in-person observations. First, if the trainer observes an error, they have the opportunity to interject and help the educator fix the error immediately before moving on. Second, there may be opportunities for the trainer to model implementation steps that the educator is finding difficult. Especially when working with students in the classroom, an educator may find it helpful to see an expert model implementation with the same student that they will be teaching. Similarly, there can be some advantages to the trainer watching a video recording of the educator practicing implementation. In some cases, the trainer might be an administrator or another teacher at the school who has other responsibilities that make it difficult for them to observe classroom implementation in real time. Watching a video recording offers much more flexibility with timing. Second, watching a video together can be a helpful tool for feedback. Sometimes, an educator can recognize their own mistakes when watching a video recording. Other times, it is helpful for a trainer to pause the video and replay a short clip so the educator can better understand the aspect of implementation the trainer is describing.

The feedback itself can also take a number of different forms. The most common form of feedback is verbal feedback, in which the trainer talks about what went well and what could be improved. Verbal feedback can be delivered after an observation is complete, or it can be delivered during the observation. One way to deliver verbal feedback during a classroom observation without distracting the student is to use bug-in-ear technology, where the teacher hears verbal feedback from the trainer through an earpiece (Horn & Rock, 2022). An advantage of verbal feedback is that it can be delivered quickly and easily, while a disadvantage is that without any record of the feedback the educator may not remember pertinent information. Therefore, it may be helpful to use written feedback either as a standalone method or as a supplement to verbal feedback. Written feedback might involve notes that are handed to the educator, an email, or a text message.

A third method of feedback is visual, in which a trainer shares a visual representation of data such as a chart or a graph. This kind of feedback is most common when the goal is to increase the frequency of a discrete behavior such as behavior-specific praise or opportunities to respond (Criss et al., 2022). For example, it can be helpful to have an educator set a goal for how many times they will provide students with opportunities to respond during a lesson and then graph how many opportunities were observed so that the educator can track their progress toward the goal. Researchers have combined methods of feedback to simultaneously leverage the advantages of different approaches. For example, it might be helpful to provide verbal feedback immediately after on observation and then to provide a text message summarizing key points immediately before the next observation (Barton et al., 2019). In this way, the trainer is able to immediately provide feedback in the moment and also ensure that the educator references a record of the feedback just before the next observation.

Some scholars have recommended trainers provide performance feedback during or immediately after the observation (Scheeler et al., 2004). Their theory is that immediate feedback prevents educators from continuing to make the same mistakes and building bad habits. While this theory makes sense, there are many situations in which immediate feedback might not be practical. For example, if an administrator is using video-based feedback because they are not available to conduct an in-person observation, it may be a few days before feedback is delivered. Researchers have found that feedback delayed several days can still enable educators to make progress toward implementing an evidence-based practice with fidelity (Brock et al., 2021). When considering whether immediate feedback is important, a trainer might consider how many times the educators will be attempting implementation while they are waiting for feedback. For example, if the educator will be attempting implementation many times, then immediate feedback to prevent practiced errors might be a consideration. However, if the evidence-based practice is only used occasionally, such as a preference assessment or a functional analysis of behavior, there is unlikely to be much practice between observations and the immediacy of feedback may be less of a concern.

36.5.2 Sustained Professional Development

In addition to the use of effective training strategies, another feature of research-based professional development is sustaining support beyond a single-event training. There are a variety of ways to accomplish this goal. One of the most common is a group training with follow-up coaching. This involves an initial workshop that features written directions, didactic instruction, modeling, role play, and performance feedback. Then after the workshop is over, a trainer visits educators in their classrooms to observe them and provide feedback (Brock & Carter, 2015). Alternatively, educators might video record their implementation with students and bring it back to a second group meeting where they share the video recording and receive feedback from the trainer and from their peers (Brock et al., 2021). How long professional development should be sustained depends on the complexity of the evidence-based practice and the speed with which the educators acquire implementation fidelity. For simple evidence-based practices such as constant time delay, a single follow-up session might be sufficient to enable educators to implement with fidelity (Brock & Carter, 2015). But for more complex practices, such as peer-mediated interventions, additional follow-up sessions may be required (Brock & Carter, 2016).

36.5.3 Promoting Generalization to the Classroom

The final key feature of research-based professional development is a focus on supporting educators to generalize implementation of evidence-based practices to their unique students and situations. Although it is typically discussed in the context of student learning, generalization is a ubiquitous concept that applies to all learners, including educators. The need for supporting generalization is clear: Students on the autism spectrum have a wide range of characteristics and support needs, and many evidence-based practices are highly versatile and can be used in very different situations. For example, a teacher could use constant time delay to teach a student to button a jacket, login to a computer, or solve an algebra problem. If educators were only to observe and practice constant time delay in one context, they understandably might have a hard time applying it to a completely different context.

There are four different approaches that have most commonly been used in research studies to promote generalization: focusing training on authentic situations, multiple exemplars, linking to student outcomes, and self-monitoring (see Table 36.3). The first three of these approaches align with categories identified by Stokes and Baer (1977) in their seminal paper on generalization.

36.5.3.1 Training on Authentic Situations

The most common form of promoting generalization is to train on authentic situations (Brock et al., 2017). This approach aligns with Stokes and Baer's (1977) category of "sequential modification" and involves providing training or feedback that is specific to the student and situation in which the practice will be generalized. This approach is not technically training for generalization, because the trainer is removing the need for the educators to generalize by directly targeting the authentic situation.

This approach would involve the trainer supporting the educator to develop an instructional plan, providing a model of instruction, and/or observing and providing feedback that is specific to the student and situation. In most cases in the existing literature, this approach is used in the context of coaching in which all training is embedded in the classroom to which the educator will be generalizing implementation.

Table 36.3 Approaches for promoting generalization to unique students and situations

Approach	What Is It?	Examples
Training on authentic situations	The trainer provides training or feedback that is specific to the student and situation to which the practice will be generalized.	• The trainer supports the educator to develop an instruction plan that is specific to the student and situation. • The trainer models implementation with the student, or creates a video model that is specific to the student and situation. • The trainer observes the educators implementing with the student and provides feedback.
Multiple exemplars	The trainer provides exemplars that show optimal implementation across a range of outcomes and students with different profiles.	• Through role play, the trainer models how a practice could be used to target a range of outcomes for students with different learning profiles. • Providing access to a library of video models that show exemplars of implementation across a range of students and situations
Linking to student performance	The trainer helps the educators to make a direct connection between their implementation and improvement of student outcomes.	• Collecting student data prior to attempting implementation and after implementation and then comparing rates of progress
Self-monitoring	The trainer helps the educator to monitor their own implementation fidelity when attempting generalization to a new student or situation.	• Education completes a checklist as they implement with the student. • Educator video records their own implementation with a student and fills out an implementation checklist as they review their implementation. • Educator audio records a lesson, listens to a 5-minute sample, and counts the number of times they provided opportunities to respond.

36.5.3.2 Multiple Exemplars

This approach, similar to Stokes and Baer's category of "training sufficient exemplars," involves showing the educator exemplars of implementation across a range of outcomes and students with different profiles. There should be a sufficient number and variety of exemplars so that at least one is likely to resemble the student and situation to which the educator will be generalizing. Options for providing multiple exemplars include the trainer providing models in-person or providing access to a library of video models of implementation. Video models may have some advantages over in-person models, as the educators can revisit the models later and can focus their attention on the model that most closely resembles the student and goal they are targeting (Brock et al., 2018).

When designing multiple exemplars, it is wise to thoughtfully select a range of students and situations. For example, varied student profiles might include both students who use speech and those who use alternative and augmentative communication, students who engage in challenging behavior, students who have varying support needs, and students who have varying levels of engagement. In addition, exemplars should illustrate the full range of outcomes that can be effectively targeted with the intervention. For a versatile intervention like systematic prompting, exemplars could include academic, self-help, communication, social, play, vocational, and motor skills (Hume et al., 2021; Shawbitz & Brock, 2022).

36.5.3.3 Linking to Student Outcomes

This approach, similar to Stokes and Baer's "introduce to natural contingencies," involves guiding educators to collect student data before and after implementation of the evidence-based practice. In this way, the educators can see for themselves that the evidence-based practice has a positive impact on student progress. The idea is that educators will see the student progress as rewarding and therefore will be more motivated to continue to implement the practice with fidelity in the future to ensure continued student progress.

36.5.3.4 Self-Monitoring

Self-monitoring involves guiding the educator to collect data on their own implementation fidelity when implementing in the classroom. This might involve the educator completing a checklist at the same time as they are implementing with the student or video recording their implementation and completing a checklist at a later time. Self-monitoring is a good way for educators to self-assess what they are doing well and to identify steps of the intervention that are absent or need improvement. A prerequisite for self-monitoring is that the educator is able to accurately assess the implementation fidelity of others. Therefore, if a trainer plans to have an educator self-monitor, they should provide opportunities for the educator to practice and become proficient assessors of implementation fidelity.

36.6 Special Considerations for Paraeducators

While the aforementioned principles apply to professional development for all educators, there are additional special considerations for training paraeducators. Paraeducators, who are not required to have any formal training in special education, outnumber special education teachers (Rispoli et al., 2011). Given their prevalence and the degree to which special education programs depend on them, paraeducators have a substantial impact on the quality of education for students on the autism spectrum. For students with more extensive support needs, the role of the paraeducators is even more pronounced. On average, self-contained classrooms have more than three paraeducators for every special education teacher (Suter & Giangreco, 2009). When students with extensive support needs are included in regular education classrooms, they often receive the bulk of their support from individually assigned paraeducators.

Given their prevalence and their lack of formal training in special education, there are several important concepts to keep in mind when designing training for paraeducators. This section discusses three key concepts to consider: clearly defined and appropriate responsibilities, providing background information and a rationale for practices, and administrative support.

36.6.1 Clearly Defined and Appropriate Responsibilities

A critical precondition to designing training for paraeducators is ensuring that their responsibilities are clearly defined and fall within those that are permitted under the law. Federal law requires that all instruction for students with disabilities be planned and directed by licensed teachers, and that paraeducators may provide services under their direction and supervision (IDEIA, 2004). Therefore, it is inappropriate to put paraeducators in a position where they are being asked to make instructional decisions or implement instruction outside of the supervision of a licensed teacher.

Apart from ensuring that a paraeducator's responsibilities fall under the law, it is equally important to ensure that they are well defined. Without a clearly defined role, it is not possible to design training opportunities that align with that role. Role ambiguity has long been a problem, with both teachers and paraeducators reporting that they are not always clear on where a paraeducator's responsibilities begin and end (Biggs et al., 2019; Mason et al., 2021). In the absence of clearly defined roles and responsibilities, paraeducators are left to themselves to infer what they should be doing—despite having no formal training in special education. Unsurprisingly, this can lead to paraeducators taking on inappropriate roles or supporting students in ways that are inconsistent with evidence-based practice (Carter et al., 2008). In sum, the principles discussed in this chapter for training educators cannot be appropriately applied to paraeducators until their roles have been appropriately and unambiguously defined.

36.6.2 Background Knowledge and Rationale

Another important consideration is that paraeducators might lack the background knowledge to understand *why* they are being asked to use a given evidence-based practice. For example, for teachers or related service personnel who have a background in applied behavior analysis, it seems intuitive that reducing a challenging behavior might involve teaching a replacement behavior that meets the same function. But for a paraeducator with no background knowledge in applied behavior analysis, this might not make any sense at all.

Like any educator, paraeducators are more likely to be willing and motivated to adopt a new practice when they understand why the practice was selected and how it will benefit students. This is why providing a rationale for the training topic is a common feature of effective paraeducator training (Brock & Anderson, 2021). With the previous example regarding an alternative replacement behavior, a trainer could first teach the concept that all behavior has a function, that these functions typically fall into one of several categories, and that through a process called functional analysis the function of the student's behavior has been identified. Then the trainer could explain that one way to reduce the challenging behavior is to give the student a new way to achieve the same function without engaging in the challenging behavior, and therefore they are teaching the replacement behavior. Once the paraeducator understands these concepts, they are more likely to enthusiastically support implementation of differential reinforcement that promotes use of the replacement behavior.

36.6.3 Administrative Support

An additional challenge related to paraeducators is a basic foundation for training and supervision. Many teachers report that their teacher preparation programs were designed to teach them how to implement instructional strategies but did little to prepare them to train and supervise paraeducators (Biggs et al., 2019). Similarly, some paraeducators report frustration over unclear expectations and a lack of feedback from their supervising teachers (Mason et al., 2021). Indeed, the field of teacher preparation has not fully transitioned to training teachers to be good managers. Often, there are other factors that exacerbate this problem. For example, some schools only pay paraeducators to work during the hours that children are at school, making it impossible to have before or after-school meetings during paid time. In other cases, teachers are asked to supervise large numbers of paraeducators who are serving students in different classrooms throughout a school building.

To be successful supervisors of paraeducators, teachers need administrative support in multiple areas. First, they need mentoring in how to manage a team of paraeducators. Second, they need help from administrators to identify times during the day that they can meet with paraeducators while still maintaining appropriate staffing levels with students. Third, they need administrators to help build a community where paraeducators respect teachers as leaders of instructional teams and are responsive to their direction and feedback. Without this support, teachers do not have a basic foundation to leverage the principles of research-based training for paraeducators.

36.7 Future Directions: Increasing Efficiency and Feasibility

Through research, scholars have accumulated substantial evidence to support the research-based principles of professional development discussed in this chapter—effective strategies, sustaining training over time, and supporting generalization of practices to unique students and situations. However, relatively few school districts implement professional development that is consistent with these strategies (Brock & Anderson, 2021). One reason for this reluctance may be the perceived cost and intensity of research-based professional development. A criticism of the research literature is that it largely focuses on professional development in the context of one-to-one coaching (Brock et al., 2017), and it is not practical or feasible to deliver all professional development in this format (Russo, 2004).

Therefore, the next major frontier in professional development research might be identifying effective ways to leverage research-based principles in ways that are practical and feasible. To date, researchers have focused on two major innovations to achieve this goal: tiered models of professional development and virtual delivery of training. In the sections below, research findings related to both innovations are discussed, as well as opportunities for further research.

36.7.1 Tiered Models

For students, tiered intervention models such as response to intervention (RtI) were developed based on the premise that different children need different levels of support in order to be successful. With RtI, all students receive high-quality instruction in a group format, and students who might be at risk for not making adequate progress on targeted learning skills are identified through progress monitoring. At-risk students who do not make progress given supplemental group instruction receive targeted interventions characterized by increased intensity and smaller instructional groupings (e.g., small group or one-to-one). Just as RtI provides an efficient and effective means to support all students, multitier professional development systems could provide an efficient and effective means to support all educators to implement evidence-based practices.

Two different research groups have developed and tested multitier professional development with encouraging results. Gage et al. (2017) showed that when school-wide professional development was provided to teachers, the majority of teachers were successful with increasing their behavior-specific praise after only a didactic training while the remaining teachers made progress after receiving individualized feedback. Similarly, Brock et al. (2021) found that most paraeducators could master systematic prompting strategies after group training alone, while a subset required follow-up coaching that featured observation and performance feedback. In both cases, researchers measured the degree to which educators were implementing the practice as intended, and they only provided the most intensive professional development with the practitioners who were not yet implementing with fidelity.

While these findings are encouraging, more research is needed in this area. Given that only these two research groups have focused on tiered models of professional development, more replication is needed to validate their findings. In addition, existing research only focuses on a few evidence-based practices, and it is not clear whether tiered systems would be well suited for all practices. Also, more research is required to identify empirically based criterion levels at which to designate educators for more intensive professional development.

36.7.2 Virtual Delivery

In addition to tiered models, virtual delivery of training is also a promising avenue for improving the feasibility of research-based professional development. These virtual methods leverage the same research-based principles that are described in this chapter but are delivered in ways that are designed to decrease costs associated with in-person training.

One well-established form of virtual professional development is Web-based modules. When well-designed, online modules provide educators with written directions, didactic instruction, and video exemplars of evidence-based practices. In research studies, Web-based modules have been situated within a larger model of professional development that also included observation and feedback. This combination of practices has been shown to promote improved implementation of evidence-based practices for teachers, related service personnel, and paraeducators (Sam et al., 2021, 2022). The same modules described in these research studies are also freely available to anyone (Sam et al., 2020). Because there are high-quality modules available for free and they can be accessed at any time, this approach can help decrease the cost and increase the flexibility of research-based professional development.

Another promising approach involves virtual observations and feedback. Researchers have studied several variations of this approach. The first involves real-time feedback with virtual bug-in-ear training (Rock et al., 2009). Pre-service teachers used a webcam to broadcast live video footage of their teaching to a trainer. The trainer watched their teaching and provided real-time feedback through a wireless earpiece. The second variation involves real-time observations that are streamed to the trainer, with feedback delivered after the observation is complete. A third variation involves educators video recording their teaching, uploading their video so that it can be viewed by a trainer, and the trainer providing written or oral feedback through teleconference (Billingsley & Sheuermann, 2014). All three variations offer opportunities to provide observations and feedback without the expense of paying for the expert to travel to the school to conduct observations. This approach might be especially appealing to schools in rural areas where there is limited access to trainers who have expertise in a given evidence-based practice.

Although virtual delivery of professional development has become more common during and after the COVID-19 pandemic, research on these approaches is very limited compared to in-person training. Future research is needed to better understand the degree to which virtual training produces optimal implementation fidelity, if and how these approaches should be paired with in-person training, and the degree to which these approaches are more cost-effective than in-person training.

36.8 Practice Implications

36.8.1 Treatment Outcomes

The research-based principles of professional development discussed in this chapter have the potential to support educators to adopt and implement evidence-based practices with fidelity, which will in turn improve critical outcomes for students on the autism spectrum.

36.8.2 Practice Implication Guidelines

Resources that can help to design research-based professional development can be found at Autism Focused Intervention Resources and Modules (https://afirm.fpg.unc.edu/afirm-modules; Sam et al., 2020) as well as the Autism Internet Modules (https://autisminternetmodules.org/; Ohio Center for Autism and Low Incidence, 2020).

36.9 References

Barton, E. E., Rigor, M. N., Pokorski, E. A., Velez, M., & Domingo, M. (2019). Using text messaging to deliver performance feedback to preservice early childhood teachers. *Topics in Early Childhood Special Education*, *39*(2), 88–102. https://doi.org/10.1177/027112141880001

Biggs, E. E., Gilson, C. B., & Carter, E. W. (2019). "Developing that balance": Preparing and supporting special education teachers to work with paraprofessionals. *Teacher Education and Special Education*, *42*(2), 117–131. https://doi.org/10.1177/0888406418765611

Billingsley, G. M., & Scheuermann, B. K. (2014). Using virtual technology to enhance field experiences for pre-service special education teachers. *Teacher Education and Special Education*, *37*(3), 255–272. https://doi.org/10.1177/0888406414530413

Brock, M. E., & Anderson, E. J. (2021). Training paraprofessionals who work with students with intellectual and developmental disabilities: What does the research say? *Psychology in the Schools*, *58*(4), 702–722. https://doi.org/10.1002/pits.22386

Brock, M. E., Barczak, M. A., Anderson, E. J., & Bordner-Williams, N. M. (2021). Efficacy of tiered training on paraeducator implementation of systematic instructional practices for students with severe disabilities. *Exceptional Children*, *87*(2), 217–235. https://doi.org/10.1177/0014402920947641

Brock, M. E., Cannella-Malone, H. I., Seaman, R. L., Andzik, N. R., Schaefer, J. M., Page, E. J., Barczak, M. A., & Dueker, S. A. (2017). Findings across practitioner training studies in special education: A comprehensive review and meta-analysis. *Exceptional Children*, *84*(1), 7–26. https://doi.org/10.1177/0014402917698008

Brock, M. E., & Carter, E. W. (2015). Effects of a professional development package to prepare special education paraprofessionals to implement evidence-based practice. *The Journal of Special Education, 49*(1), 39–51. https://doi.org/10.1177/0022466913501882

Brock, M. E., & Carter, E. W. (2016). Efficacy of teachers training paraprofessionals to implement peer support arrangements. *Exceptional Children, 82*(3), 354–371. https://doi.org/10.1177/0014402915585564

Brock, M. E., & Carter, E. W. (2017). A meta-analysis of educator training to improve implementation of interventions for students with disabilities. *Remedial and Special Education, 38*(3), 131–144. https://doi.org/10.1177/0741932516653477

Brock, M. E., Dynia, J. M., Dueker, S., & Barczak, M. (2020). Teacher-reported priorities and practices for students with autism: Characterizing the research-to-practice gap. *Focus on Autism and Other Developmental Disabilities, 35*, 67–78. https://doi.org/10.1177/1088357619881217

Brock, M. E., Huber, H. B., Carter, E. W., Juarez, A. P., & Warren, Z. E. (2014). Statewide assessment of professional development needs related to educating students with autism spectrum disorder. *Focus on Autism and Other Developmental Disabilities, 29*, 67–79. https://doi:10.1177/1088357614522290

Brock, M. E., Seaman, R. L., & Gatsch, A. L. (2018). Efficacy of video modeling and brief coaching on teacher implementation of an evidence-based practice for students with severe disabilities. *Journal of Special Education Technology, 33*(4), 259–269. https://doi.org/10.1177/0162643418770639

Carnine, D. (1997). Bridging the research-to-practice gap. *Exceptional Children, 63*(4), 513–521. https://doi.org/10.1177/0014402914551738

Carter, E. W., Sisco, L. G., Brown, L., Brickham, D., & Al-Khabbaz, Z. A. (2008). Peer interactions and academic engagement of youth with developmental disabilities in inclusive middle and high school classrooms. *American Journal on Mental Retardation, 113*(6), 479–494. https://doi.org/10.1352/2008.113:479-494

Colbert, J. A., Brown, R. S., Choi, S., & Thomas, S. (2008). An investigation of the impacts of teacher-driven professional development on pedagogy and student learning. *Teacher Education Quarterly, 35*(2), 135–154.

Criss, C. J., Konrad, M., Alber-Morgan, S. R., & Brock, M. E. (2022). A systematic review of goal setting and performance feedback to improve teacher practice. *Journal of Behavioral Education.* https://doi.org/10.1007/s10864-022-09494-1

Fallon, L. M., Collier-Meek, M. A., Maggin, D. M., Sanetti, L. M., & Johnson, A. H. (2015). Is performance feedback for educators an evidence-based practice? A systematic review and evaluation based on single-case research. *Exceptional Children, 81*(2), 227–246. https://doi.org/10.1177/0014402914551738

Gage, N. A., MacSuga-Gage, A. S., & Crews, E. (2017). Increasing teachers' use of behavior-specific praise using a multitiered system for professional development. *Journal of Positive Behavior Interventions, 19*(4), 239–251. https://doi.org/10.1177/1098300717693568

Hess, K. L., Morrier, M. J., Heflin, L. J., & Ivey, M. L. (2008). Autism treatment survey: Services received by children with aut-ism spectrum disorders in public school classrooms. *Journal of Autism and Developmental Disorders, 38*(5), 961–971. https://doi.org/10.1007/s10803-007-0470-5

Horn, A. L., & Rock, M. L. (2022). Practice with feedback makes permanent: eCoaching through online bug-in-ear during clinical experiences. *Journal of Special Education Preparation, 2*(1), 58–69. https://doi.org/10.33043/JOSEP.2.1.58-69

Hume, K., Steinbrenner, J. R., Odom, S. L., Morin, K. L., Nowell, S. W., Tomaszewski, B., Szendrey, S., McIntyre, N. S., Yucesoy-Ozkan, S., & Savage, M. N. (2021). Evidence-based practices for children, youth, and young adults with autism: Third generation review. *Journal of Autism and Developmental Disorders, 51*(11), 4013–4032. https://doi.org/10.1007/s10803-022-05438-w

Individuals with Disabilities Education Improvement Act, U.S.C. § 1400 (2004).

Joyce, B. R., & Showers, B. (2002). *Student achievement through staff development* (Vol. 3). Alexandria, VA: Association for Supervision and Curriculum Development.

Kirkpatrick, M., Akers, J., & Rivera, G. (2019). Use of behavioral skills training with teachers: A systematic review. *Journal of Behavioral Education, 28*(3), 344–361. https://doi.org/10.1007/s10864-019-09322-z

Koegel, R. L., & Koegel, L. K. (2019). *Pivotal response treatment for autism spectrum disorders.* Towson, MD: Brookes.

Mason, R. A., Gunersel, A. B., Irvin, D. W., Wills, H. P., Gregori, E., An, Z. G., & Ingram, P. B. (2021). From the frontlines: Perceptions of paraprofessionals' roles and responsibilities. *Teacher Education and Special Education, 44*(2), 97–116. https://doi.org/10.1177/0888406419896627

Odom, S. L. (2009). The tie that binds: Evidence-based practice, implementation science, and outcomes for children. *Topics in Early Childhood Special Education, 29*(1), 53–61. https://doi.org/10.1177/0271121408329171

Odom, S. L., Cox, A. W., & Brock, M. E., and the National Professional Development Center. (2013). Implementation science, professional development, and autism spectrum disorders. *Exceptional Children, 79*(2), 233–251. https://doi.org/10.1177/001440291307900207

Odom, S. L., Hall, L. J., & Steinbrenner, J. R. (2020). Implementation science research and special education. *Exceptional Children, 86*(2), 117–119. https://doi.org/10.1177/0014402919889888

Ohio Center for Autism and Low Incidence. (2020). *Autism Internet modules.* www.autisminternetmodules.org.

Rispoli, M., Neely, L., Lang, R., & Ganz, J. (2011). Training paraprofessionals to implement interventions for people with autism spectrum disorders: A systematic review. *Developmental Neurorehabilitation, 14*, 378–388. https://doi.org/10.3109/17518423.2011.620577

Rock, M. L., Gregg, M., Thead, B. K., Acker, S. E., Gable, R. A., & Zigmond, N. P. (2009). Can you hear me now? Evaluation of an online wireless technology to provide real-time feedback to special education teachers-in-training. *Teacher Education and Special Education, 32*(1), 64–82. https://doi.org/10.1177/0888406414525048

Russo, A. (2004). School-based coaching. *Harvard Education Letter, 20*(4), 1–4.

Sam, A. M., Cox, A. W., Savage, M. N., Waters, V., & Odom, S. L. (2020). Disseminating information on evidence-based practices for children and youth with autism spectrum disorder: AFIRM. *Journal of Autism and Developmental Disorders, 50*(6), 1931–1940. https://doi.org/10.1007/s10803-019-03945-x

Sam, A. M., Odom, S. L., Tomaszewski, B., Perkins, Y., & Cox, A. W. (2021). Employing evidence-based practices for children with autism in elementary schools. *Journal of Autism and Developmental Disorders, 51*(7), 2308–2323.

Sam, A. M., Steinbrenner, J. R., Odom, S. L., Nowell, S. W., Waters, V., Perkins, Y., White, M., Swaminathan, H., & Rogers, H. J. (2022). Promoting paraeducators' use of evidence-based practices for students with autism. *Exceptional Children, 89*, 314–331. https://doi.org/10.1177/00144029221135572

Scheeler, M. C., Ruhl, K. L., & McAfee, J. K. (2004). Providing performance feedback to teachers: A Review. *Teacher Education and Special Education, 27*(4), 396–407. https://doi.org/10.1177/088840640402700407

Shawbitz, K. N., & Brock, M. E. (2022). A systematic review of training educators to implement response prompting. *Teacher Education and Special Education*46, 127–145. https://doi.org/10.1177/08884064221114130

Stokes, T. F., & Baer, D. M. (1977). An implicit technology of generalization. *Journal of Applied Behavior Analysis, 10*(2), 349–367. https://doi.org/10.1901/jaba.1977.10-349

Suter, J. C., & Giangreco, M. F. (2009). Numbers that count: Exploring special education and paraprofessional service delivery in inclusion-oriented schools. *The Journal of Special Education, 43*(2), 81–93. https://doi.org/10.1177/0022466907313353

What Works Clearinghouse (WWC). (2020). *What Works Clearinghouse standards handbook, version 4.1.* Washington, DC: US Department of Education, Institute of Education Sciences, National Center for Education Evaluation and Regional Assistance. https://ies.ed.gov/ncee/wwc/handbooks

37

Parent Training and Family Support

Kelly M. Schieltz and Matthew J. O'Brien
The University of Iowa, Carver College of Medicine, Stead Family Department of Pediatrics

Jessica E. Graber
Nationwide Children's Hospital, Center for Autism Spectrum Disorders

Alyssa N. Suess
Milestone Health Partners

37.1 Technical Abstract

Background: Parent training teaches parents and other caregivers skills to increase their child's engagement in adaptive behaviors and positive interactions with others, and to decrease their child's engagement in disruptive behaviors. Parent training is a process that is not specific to one particular procedure. Rather, it includes a continuum of evidence-based treatments that range from manualized to individualized programs with each program requiring different levels of parent and child involvement. **Method:** A nonsystematic review of the extant parent training literature is summarized across three broad types of parent training: care coordination, psychoeducation, and parent-mediated interventions. **Results:** Across all types of parent training, research shows positive effects on parent and child variables with parent-mediated interventions having the strongest support. The research is limited for care coordination and psychoeducation. **Discussion:** Parent training is evidence-based and essential for effective treatment programs across the care continuum. However, parent training is underutilized, with providers lacking expertise in its delivery being one major contributing factor. **Practitioner recommendations:** Each parent training model may be appropriate depending on various factors such as program goals, provider characteristics and qualifications, and parent and child characteristics. Thus, a comprehensive parent training approach is likely to include all three parent training models at different points in time and dosages.

37.2 Layperson Summary

Parent training is a process that teaches parents and other caregivers a variety of skills. These skills are used to increase their child's engagement in adaptive

Kelly M. Schieltz et al., *Parent Training and Family Support*. In: *Lifespan Treatment for Autistic Individuals*.
Edited by: Peter Sturmey, Russell Lang, and James K. Luiselli, Oxford University Press. © Oxford University Press (2025).
DOI: 10.1093/oso/9780197635841.003.0037

behavior and positive interactions with others, and to decrease their child's engagement in disruptive behavior. Parent training is a process that is not specific to one procedure. Rather, it is a continuum of evidence-based treatments. It includes family-centered care, including care coordination, psychoeducation, and parent-mediated interventions. Each of these types of parent training requires different levels of parent and child involvement. Care coordination makes organizing healthcare services easier. Psychoeducation shares knowledge. Parent-mediated interventions involve training on how to implement treatment procedures. Several factors contribute to the use of each parent training approach. These factors include program goals, provider characteristics and qualifications, and parent and child characteristics. Across all types of parent training approaches, research has shown positive outcomes related to increases in child appropriate behaviors. These child outcomes include increases in social communication and decreases in child disruptive behavior. There are also sometimes improvements in parenting stress. However, research support for parent training is limited. This is especially true for care coordination and psychoeducation models. Research support for parent-mediated interventions is stronger and more extensive. Parent training is evidence-based. It is an essential component of treatment programs. Unfortunately, it is underused in practice. This may be because providers lack expertise in delivering it. To further support their children's gains in the areas of adaptive behavior, parents and other caregivers should advocate for parent training across the continuum of approaches.

37.3 Treatment Summary Table

Treatment summary: Parent Training and Family Support

Treatment description: Parent training teaches parents and other caregivers a variety of skills to increase their child's engagement in adaptive behaviors and positive interactions with others, and to decrease their child's engagement in disruptive behaviors. Parent training is a process that is not specific to one particular procedure. Rather, it includes a continuum of evidence-based treatments that range from manualized to individualized programs with each program requiring different levels of parent and child involvement.

Expected outcomes: These include increased parent self-efficacy, decreased parenting stress, and gains in child outcomes (e.g., increased social communication, decreased disruptive behavior).

Methods: Three broad types of parent training include care coordination, psychoeducation, and parent-mediated interventions. A nonsystematic summary of the extant literature on these parent training approaches is provided. Descriptive methods are the most widely used when evaluating care coordination models. Results of these demonstrations show that care coordination models increase access to and satisfaction with care and improve relationships. Direct child outcomes are not reported. Psychoeducation models are rarely evaluated in isolation, and when they are studied, evaluation methods differ. Randomized controlled trials (RCTs) have been conducted on psychoeducation models on a limited basis. Results have been mixed by demonstrating variations in outcomes on parental stress and mental health, and child behavior. Parent-mediated interventions have been the most widely studied parent training model across methodologies, including RCTs and single-case designs. Overall, results are robust relative to parent–child interactions, modest relative to improvements in autism symptoms and social communication, and mixed relative to parent well-being and child outcomes.

Expertise required to implement treatment: Providers are trained to engage in effective parent training across the continuum (i.e., care coordination, psychoeducation, parent-mediated interventions).

Risks and negative side effects: Providers lacking experience in delivering parent training may result in suboptimal outcomes.

Additional considerations and limitations: Each parent training approach may be appropriate depending on a variety of factors, including program goals, provider characteristics and qualifications, and parent and child characteristics. The three parent training models do not have to occur independently. Rather, a comprehensive parent training approach is likely to include all three parent training models at different times and dosages, depending on the needs of the family.

37.4 Introduction

37.4.1 Treatment Description

Parent training is an evidence-based treatment for increasing child skills and decreasing disruptive behaviors that encompasses a variety of structured programs including, but not limited to, The Incredible Years (Webster-Stratton, 2006), parent management training (Kazdin, 2005), and parent-child interaction therapy (PCIT; Eyberg & Robinson, 1982; McNeil & Hembree-Kigin, 2011). Across these parent training programs, parents and other caregivers are taught a variety of skills through didactic instruction, modeling, role playing, coaching, feedback, and homework to increase positive interactions with their children, promote the occurrence of positive and adaptive behaviors from their children, and decrease the occurrence of disruptive behaviors displayed by their children (Centers for Disease Control and Prevention, 2009). Historically, these particular parent training programs were developed to address the disruptive behaviors displayed by typically developing children and adolescents. In the area of autism spectrum disorder (ASD), parent training targets the same general goals and utilizes similar strategies to train parents in these skills. However, the evidence-based treatment programs are more varied and nuanced, including the terms used to describe them (e.g., parent training, parent education, parent-mediated intervention). These variations and nuances reflect the idea that parent training is a process that is not specific to one particular procedure, resulting in a continuum of evidence-based treatments that range from manualized to individualized programs, with each varying its levels of involvement of the parents and their children.

37.4.2 Rationale and Objectives

Over the past century, the roles and relation between the family and the professional in autism care services have transformed (Bennett et al., 2019; Eyal, 2013). For example, in just about the span of one lifetime, our understanding of the etiology of autism has been reconstructed from that of the emotionally distant "refrigerator mother" myth (Bennett et al., 2019; Eyal, 2013) to an understanding of autism as a neurodevelopmental disorder rooted in genetics (Abrahams & Geschwind, 2008; de la Torre-Ubieta et al., 2016). At the same time, the context for support has evolved from one of institutionalization to community-based care (Brookman-Frazee et al., 2010; Eyal, 2013; Silberman, 2015), and from expert-centered to family-centered care (Arango, 2011; Coogle & Hanline, 2016; Kuhlthau et al., 2011; Ngui & Flores, 2006). Further, the formation of national advocacy organizations, aimed at partnering parents and professionals in support of children with autism, were developed (Bennett et al., 2019; Silberman, 2015). Such paradigmatic shifts have made for a complex and continually evolving landscape in terms of professionally provided family support and parent training services in autism care. Importantly, parents themselves have been a driving force in this evolution (Eyal, 2013; Silberman, 2015), which is exemplified by the creation and destruction of the "refrigerator mother" myth.

As parents have taken the lead in advocacy and policy initiatives surrounding autism care services, the profound and complex challenges experienced by families and children with autism have been increasingly illuminated (Eyal, 2013), including financial stress (Karst & Van Hecke, 2012; Serrata, 2012), emotional stress (e.g., Hayes & Watson, 2013; Karst & Van Hecke, 2012), disruptive and dangerous behaviors (e.g., Davis & Carter, 2008), and concerns related to core differences associated with autism, including difficulties with reciprocal social engagement and shared play between a parent and their child with autism (Bebko et al., 1987; Davis & Carter, 2008; Ekas et al., 2010; Hayes & Watson, 2013).

From a behavior analytic perspective, a child's behavior is the result of person–environment interactions (Bijou & Baer, 1961; Skinner, 1938, 1945). Insofar as the family is the most central environment in which a child learns, a behavior analytic approach requires that learning be interwoven within the family system. Specifically, the ethical and practical guidelines within behavior analysis define *effective* and *generalized* outcomes as central to the goals of therapy, with long-term maintenance of treatment effects and successful generalization of learning across contexts (Behavior Analyst Certification Board, 2020; Stokes & Baer, 1977). In this way, a behaviorally based approach to family support and parent training requires careful planning and responsive implementation within the family context.

37.4.3 Considerations for Implementation

Parent training models for autism have been discussed and categorized into three broad types that include care coordination, psychoeducation, and parent-mediated interventions (Bearss, Burrell, et al., 2015). These categories involve varying levels and types of participation from both the child and parent. Because each type of parent training model has its own distinct goals, levels of involvement for the parent and child, and procedures, we define and describe each type of parent training model in the sections below.

37.4.3.1 Care Coordination

Care coordination is the "deliberate organization of patient care activities between two or more participants involved in a patient's care to facilitate the appropriate delivery of health care services" (Agency for Healthcare Research and Quality, 2014, para. 1). It can involve the provider describing the types of services (e.g., speech therapy, medication management, special education services) available, discussing the importance of and need for each service, providing information on how the parent can establish services, and coordinating treatment plans (e.g., therapy goals and behavior intervention strategies) with other service providers (American Academy of Pediatrics [AAP] Committee on Children with Disabilities, 1999). Because children with ASD have complex medical, behavioral, social, and educational needs and they are at higher risk of having unmet healthcare needs (Farmer et al., 2014), the AAP considers care coordination a key component in treatment for children with ASD as it facilitates partnerships across healthcare settings, education, childcare, social services, and community organizations (AAP Council on Children with Disabilities, 2005). Without care coordination, the process of understanding which services are needed and how to establish care can be overwhelming to parents of children with ASD, leading to delays in receiving critical intervention services that will potentially impact their daily functioning and long-term development (Farmer et al., 2014).

In general, care coordination is a parent training model that involves relatively low levels of parent involvement and little to no child involvement. At the onset of services, the service provider, often a licensed social worker or professional counselor, meets with the family to gather information about the needs of the child and identify other intervention services that child is currently receiving. If the needs of the child are narrow in scope (e.g., seeking treatment for one topography of disruptive behavior), the need for the service provider to offer care coordination is more limited. In contrast, a child with broader needs (e.g., significant deficits with communication skills, high levels of disruptive behavior, and complex medical needs) may require more extensive supports, wherein the service provider spends more time in care coordination with the family to assist them in getting other intervention services established (e.g., speech therapy) and/or discussing treatment goals and programming with other interventionists or medical specialists.

In addition to the general scope of care coordination practice that is individualized and based on the needs of the child and family, a variety of factors further influence this practice. First, the timing with which services are sought may influence the extent to which services for the child and family are coordinated. For example, if a child is newly diagnosed with ASD and has not established intervention services, the provider may assist the family in establishing more global intervention services (e.g., speech therapy, occupational therapy, and special education services) and offering suggestions on interventionists to provide care. However, if a family has established care with other interventionists, then the current service provider may only offer care coordination by communicating treatment goals and programming with others on the child's intervention team. Additionally, care coordination may be sought out as the child moves along various developmental (e.g., early childhood to school age to young adult) and life stages (e.g., transitioning to employment or independent living). It should be noted that the focus of care coordination is also influenced by the provider's general scope of practice and knowledge regarding related services.

Second, the intensity of care coordination is likely to be brief or time-limited (e.g., one-time appointment) and can also occur intermittently and in combination with other family guidance models. However, other family factors may further influence the timing and dose of this service. For example, care coordination may need to be intermittent and narrowly focused on one target at a time because the family's access to insurance coverage can affect the type of services available to them (Karpur et al., 2019), the cost of interventions for autistic children can be of significant hardship for the family, and/or time allocation for participating in multiple services may be limited, given restrictions with employment time off. Any and all of these factors may result in the family's need to limit the number of services in which they participate. In contrast, care coordination may need to be more consistent and extensive because parents of children with autism spend significantly more time coordinating intervention services than parents of children with other special healthcare needs (Kogan et al., 2008).

Third, care coordination can vary greatly across geographical locations, given the differences in resources available to families (Bearss, Burrell, et al., 2015). A service provider may engage in more care coordination with a family in more populated areas where there are likely more options for services compared to a service provider located in a more rural area.

37.4.3.2 Psychoeducation

Psychoeducation is a therapeutic process of sharing knowledge between a professional and a client for the purpose of improving the client's short- and long-term well-being, relative to the specific condition for which the client is seeking services and their goals for treatment (Lukens & McFarlane, 2004; Sarkhel et al., 2020). The focus is on providing education relative to etiological factors of a condition, clarifying myths and misconceptions related to the condition, identifying common differences and difficulties associated with the condition, coping with and problem-solving common challenges (including when and how to seek professional support), and building skills for self-advocacy (Sarkhel et al., 2020).

Specific to autism, psychoeducation programs may serve several important functions. Most psychoeducation programs are designed for the parent(s) of a child with autism, with the goal of increasing parents' knowledge about ASD, including its etiology, prognosis, and effective interventions. These areas may be especially important at the time of a child receiving an ASD diagnosis (Bearss, Johnson, et al., 2015). Parents are likely to feel more empowered with their newly acquired knowledge and may be better equipped to apply what they have learned to make evidence-informed decisions, within the context of their unique, individual family circumstances (Bearss, Johnson, et al., 2015; Farmer & Reupert, 2013). Another common benefit of psychoeducation is increased parental support. Parents of children with ASD experience higher levels of mental health concerns (Hayes & Watson, 2013; Schnabel et al., 2020) and isolation (Farrugia, 2009; Samsell et al., 2022) than parents of non-ASD children. Psychoeducation, and particularly group-based models, may provide formal and informal social support, which in turn lead to increased mental well-being (Pottie et al., 2009) and decreased social isolation (Karst & Van Hecke, 2012).

Psychoeducation generally involves high levels of parent involvement and little to no child involvement. To be successful, psychoeducation must be provided skillfully to be appropriately matched to the client's prior knowledge, abilities, needs, values, and priorities (Magaña et al., 2017). These client characteristics inform the timing, dosage, and focus of the psychoeducation provided. For example, the needs of a parent with a young autistic child entering the school system may include education on special education law (including individualized education plans) and information on navigating decisions about various types of educational and therapeutic options available to the child and family. In contrast, psychoeducation may also be narrowly focused, such as when families seek psychoeducation on developmental signs of puberty and sex education for their prepubertal adolescent with ASD.

Psychoeducation programs for parents of autistic children vary across several dimensions. For example, psychoeducation may be a formal or informal process (Bearss, Burrell, et al., 2015; Lukens & McFarlane, 2004). Informal psychoeducation may include independent parent readings of books and Web content, as well as general parent support groups, while formal methods may include attending virtual or in-person classes, usually with a predetermined number of sessions and sequence (Bearss, Burrell, et al., 2015). Thus, formal psychoeducation programs commonly utilize a manualized approach whereby the education is provided in a highly systematic manner by a professional or through a Web-based program.

Another dimension of psychoeducation is the delivery format. More specifically, psychoeducation can be delivered in an individual or group format (Bearss, Burrell, et al., 2015; Farmer & Reupert, 2013). The individual format typically involves a provider and the parent(s) of a single child with ASD. The benefit of this approach is that it can be tailored to the individual education needs of the parent. For example, as a family navigates the various stages of their child's development, there may be a need for education specific to puberty, graduation from high school, independent living, and opportunities for employment. The group format is often conducted between a provider and a small group of parents. Although this may include more general information than an individual format, the provider is able to reach a larger number of parents, thus making it a more efficient model for the provider aiming to serve multiple families (Brookman-Frazee et al., 2006). An additional benefit of the group format is that parents are able to connect to, and learn from, other parents of children with ASD (Bearss, Burrell, et al., 2015; Farmer & Reupert, 2013).

Although psychoeducation may be more accessible than other forms of parent training, it is rarely provided as a stand-alone treatment. Often, parent training programs offer psychoeducation as an adjunctive component to parent training programs focused on behavioral or social communication interventions (Bearss, Johnson, et al., 2015). Although the line between parent education (i.e., skill-based training to implement effective practices) and psychoeducation is not always clear, parent-mediated interventions, which are described in the next section, often include psychoeducation components.

37.4.3.3 Parent-Mediated Interventions

In care coordination and psychoeducation programs, a provider offers parents the knowledge and support to prepare for challenges they may face in raising a child with ASD and guidance regarding the best intervention options for their children. By contrast, parent-mediated interventions entail a provider training parents to deliver interventions directly to their child, often targeting social communication difficulties or disruptive behaviors (Bearss, Burrell, et al., 2015). Thus, the goal of the parent-mediated approach is to move away from the traditional provider-driven intervention model to a model where the parent serves as the primary interventionist. This transfer of intervention control offers many benefits over a provider-driven model. Access to clinic-based services is very limited and when accessed the timing and dosage may be far less than a child's needs warrant. However, parents are present in a child's life more than anyone else, resulting in substantially more opportunities to implement intervention strategies. Moreover, unlike a clinic setting, parents can implement these strategies in natural contexts (e.g., home, restaurant) throughout natural everyday routines (e.g., bedtime, dinner, play), which is likely to promote generalization (O'Brien et al., 2021). Although there are costs to the family during the initial stages of parent training, the potential for long-term cost savings when travel and ongoing therapist-delivered treatment is circumvented is high.

The degree of parent involvement in parent-mediated interventions may range from the parent functioning as the sole interventionist to serving as one member of an intervention team. When the parent role is the primary interventionist, it is considered a parent-mediated primary intervention (Bearss, Burrell, et al., 2015). In this model, the parent is trained to deliver the intervention without any direct service to the child by the provider. Interventions using this approach can involve a provider training the parent both with and without the child present. During sessions where the child is present, the provider can offer immediate feedback to the parent.

Parent-mediated complementary interventions involve professionals providing intervention services directly to the child, with periodic and/or increasingly more opportunities for parent involvement (Bearss, Burrell, et al., 2015). For example, a child might work directly with a provider in a clinic setting, often accumulating a large number of intervention hours each week, with periodic meetings between the child's provider and the parent to discuss the child's progress, provide instruction on how to deliver the targeted intervention, and provide feedback on the parent's performance. In this scenario, the child may be present during the parent–provider training sessions. Another example of a complementary parent-mediated approach is often seen in clinics providing services for children with severe and challenging behavior (e.g., intensive day treatment). In this example, a parent may be involved to varying degrees in both the initial behavioral assessment (e.g., functional analysis) and the subsequent treatment. Even when the parent is minimally involved in the assessment and the initial treatment sessions, they are often trained on the procedures and asked to implement those procedures during the generalization phase of the intervention.

Although parent training has been a part of ASD research and practice dating back to the 1970s (Lovaas et al., 1973), over the past couple of decades a substantial shift toward more family-centered care (Arango et al., 2011; Coogle & Hanline, 2016; Kuhlthau et al., 2011; Ngui & Flores, 2006) has occurred. In this parent-mediated model, the goal is to provide care that is based on the unique family's needs, including cultural and socioeconomic considerations, such that the family is set up for success. In this way, the provider is responsible for more than implementation of a set protocol and is instead expected to be able to augment and adjust procedures and techniques based on each unique family's needs and circumstances. Thus, considerable flexibility and fluidity with various options for service delivery are often indicated.

37.5 Research Background

Because the parent training models of care coordination, psychoeducation, and parent-mediated interventions have unique goals and foci, we continue to maintain these categorizations when describing and summarizing the extant research literature below.

37.5.1 Care Coordination

Empirically based models of care coordination, in general and specific to ASD, are sparse, in part because of the vast array of regional differences in the availability of services and the need for services to cover both developmental and severity spectrums (Bearss, Burrell, et al., 2015). However, existing models demonstrate success with their overarching purpose of coordinating care. Specific to ASD, the Comprehensive Medical Care for Autism Spectrum Disorders (AMITEA) program was developed in Madrid, Spain, to coordinate and provide care to address the specialty needs of autistic individuals (Parellada et al., 2013). In this model, the needs and preferences of the individual with ASD and/or their family are evaluated following a referral to the AMITEA program. Next, a psychiatrist conducts a comprehensive assessment to determine the individual's needs related to development, healthcare, and behavior. This information then guides specific referrals to specialists and other follow-up care that is coordinated by a case manager who also attends appointments when needed to provide additional support and communication. During the initial 18 months of the AMITEA program, 513 children and adults with ASD were served, resulting in over 1,500 psychiatric visits, 1,000 specialty clinic visits, and 300 medical tests. These results demonstrated achievement of the program's aim, which was to coordinate care for the spectrum of needs for autistic individuals, and although direct benefits to these ASD individuals were not reported, it is possible that benefits included increased access to specialty care that was not otherwise triaged or provided prior to a referral to this care coordination program.

In addition to the AMITEA program that targeted coordination of care for individuals with ASD, there is empirical support for care coordination models for children with special healthcare needs (McNally Keehn et al., 2020), which include children on the autism spectrum. For example, the Riley Care Coordination program (McAllister, 2014) offers a care coordination model for service providers across many disciplines to implement in practice with children with neurodevelopmental disabilities. This program was developed on the overarching idea that an individualized shared plan of care (SPoC) is needed to coordinate high-quality care across professionals. The two main components of the SPoC include a "medical summary" that describes historical information (e.g., history of diagnostic evaluations, current treatment services, relevant medical information, and family composition and idiosyncratic needs) and "negotiated actions" that describes the treatment plan (e.g., family and child goals, timeframe to meet goals, and interventions to be implemented) (McAllister, 2014; McNally Keehn et al., 2020). The care planning process involves four steps, including: (a) identifying the needs and strengths of the child and family, (b) identifying the need for partnerships with other service providers, (c) developing the SPoC, and (4) implementing the SPoC. Ongoing oversight and management of the SPoC is required, whereby goals are updated or added as the child and family progresses through intervention services (McAllister, 2014; McNally Keehn et al., 2020). The results of the Riley Care Coordination program have been shown to improve access to care coordination, meet individual and family intervention goals, and empower parents to be an advocate for their child (McAllister et al., 2018a, 2018b), which suggests that the child benefited from these specialty services and advocacy even though not directly evaluated.

The care coordination models developed for individuals with ASD (Parellada et al., 2013) and developmental disabilities, including ASD (McAllister et al., 2018a, 2019b; McNally Keehn et al., 2020), are consistent with the medical home model which seeks to facilitate partnerships among patients, families, and providers across services that include, but are not limited to, medical specialty care, educational services, and family support (AAP Medical Home Initiatives for Children With Special Needs Project Advisory Committee, 2002; Hyman & Johnson, 2012). Taken together, care coordination has been shown to be an important component in the treatment of children with special healthcare needs (Turchi et al., 2009). More specifically, families receiving care coordination have shown greater satisfaction with intervention services (Farmer et al., 2011), improvements in relationships with professionals (Turchi et al., 2009), improvements in shared decision-making (Golnik et al., 2012), more consistent attendance to appointments (Moeenuddin et al., 2019), and reduction in financial and time burdens (Turchi et al., 2009). One limitation of care coordination models that should be studied is the lack of evaluation on the direct benefits of increased access on child outcomes.

37.5.2 Psychoeducation

Parent training in the form of psychoeducation is rarely studied in isolation. It is often included as one component of parent training programs, and when it is studied in isolation, it often serves as a control condition with which to compare the effectiveness of another intervention. Thus, the research on psychoeducation as a stand-alone intervention is limited to only a few studies. Among the studies that have evaluated parent psychoeducation, determination of program effectiveness has been partly dependent on the outcomes being measured. Although the ultimate goal of any parent training program is to improve the lives of children with ASD, unlike most parent training approaches, parent psychoeducation attempts to improve child outcomes indirectly by increasing parent knowledge regarding the diagnosis of ASD and strategies for parenting a child with ASD. Research on parent psychoeducation has largely focused on outcomes related to parent knowledge gained, parent stress, and parent program satisfaction, with only a few studies measuring child outcomes (Kalalo et al., 2021; Magaña et al., 2017).

Studies on parent psychoeducation programs as a stand-alone intervention have yielded mixed results, which may be due in part to the varied methodologies employed in these studies (e.g., content, dosage, and format). Pilot studies have demonstrated positive outcomes related to parent stress (Kalalo et al., 2021; Patra et al., 2015), anxiety (Farmer & Reupert, 2013; Zhou et al., 2019), self-efficacy and empowerment (Farmer & Reupert, 2013; Kaiser et al., 2022; Magaña et al., 2017; Zhou et al., 2019), knowledge regarding ASD (Farmer & Reupert, 2013; Magaña et al., 2017; Mukhtar et al., 2018; Patra et al., 2015), and child autism symptoms (Kalalo et al., 2021). Despite many positive outcomes, several of these same studies showed no significant improvement in a variety of parent and child outcomes, including caregiver burden (Magaña et al., 2017), daily stress (Mukhtar et al., 2018), stress from daily care of an ASD child (Patra et al., 2015), child ASD symptoms (Magaña et al., 2017), and child behavior problems (Kalalo et al., 2021).

Only two RCTs have been conducted to evaluate parent psychoeducation in isolation. Suzuki et al. (2014) evaluated a brief (i.e., four, 120-minute sessions every other week) group parent psychoeducation intervention versus treatment-as-usual control with 72 mothers of preschool children with autism. No differences were observed between the treatment and control group post intervention on measures of maternal mental health (e.g., anxiety, depression, social dysfunction), caregiver burden, or child disruptive behavior. In the other RCT, DaWalt et al. (2018) evaluated a multifamily group psychoeducation program with 41 adolescents with ASD and their parents. Using parallel programming for parents and their children, this 60-minute weekly program lasted a total of 8 weeks and was compared to a waitlist control group. In comparison to a waitlist control group following intervention, significant improvements were observed for parent depressive symptoms and problem-solving skills, and child social interactions; however, no statistically significant differences were found with regard to parent stress, parent–child relationships, and child ASD symptoms.

Overall, a limited number of studies have evaluated psychoeducational programs for parents of children with ASD in isolation. Findings from several pilot studies, as well as two RCTs, were mixed. Although some benefit from psychoeducation seems likely, research has yet to scientifically validate a psychoeducation program resulting in global improvements in parent well-being or child ASD symptoms. If parent psychoeducation programs have the potential to yield such improvements, high-quality RCTs must be conducted to establish their effectiveness and research is also needed to determine the optimal educational content, intervention timing and dosage, and format for delivery.

37.5.3 Parent-Mediated Interventions

In comparison to parent psychoeducation programs, appreciably more research has been conducted on parent-mediated interventions. In fact, at least 30 RCTs have been conducted on parent-mediated interventions for children and adolescents with ASD (Conrad et al., 2021) with most interventions targeting skill deficits (e.g., social communication; Green et al., 2010) in young children with autism.

However, RCTs have also been conducted on interventions targeting behavioral excesses (e.g., disruptive behavior; Bearss, Johnson, et al., 2015) and a combination of skill deficits and behavioral excesses (Iadorola et al., 2018) across childhood and adolescence. As a result, the types of outcomes used to evaluate these programs have ranged from child adaptive behavior, ASD symptom severity, and level of disruptive behavior to parent well-being and quality of parent–child interactions.

In terms of overall effectiveness, several meta-analyses have been conducted on parent-mediated interventions for children with ASD and have shown modest support for their effectiveness in improving ASD symptoms, social communication, and cognition (Conrad et al., 2021; Nevill et al., 2018; Ratliff-Black & Therrien, 2021). Improvements in parent–child interactions (e.g., shared or joint attention) appear to be a robust finding (Oono et al., 2013), while there is less support for benefits to parent well-being (e.g., stress, self-efficacy; Conrad et al., 2021). Interestingly, treatment effects related to child outcomes (e.g., adaptive behavior, social communication) often vary based on the informant. For example, across a variety of child outcomes, parent ratings are more likely to show significant effects (Conrad et al., 2021; Nevill et al., 2018), while clinician ratings are more likely to show small to no effects (Conrad et al., 2021; Nevill et al., 2018). Despite modest results overall, one area that parent-mediated interventions appear to be well-suited for is child disruptive behavior (Nevill et al., 2018; Ratliff-Black & Therrien, 2021). In fact, large effect sizes have routinely been reported for parent-mediated programs targeting disruptive behavior (Cheng et al., 2022; Conrad et al., 2021; Postorino et al., 2017; Ratliff-Black & Therrien, 2021).

Notwithstanding the large number of studies on parent-mediated interventions, there is still a need for higher quality research and replication studies, especially in light of some of the mixed findings. Furthermore, there is still much that is unknown about parent-mediated approaches. For example, little research has been conducted on parent-mediated interventions for older children or adolescents with ASD. In fact, of the 32 RCTs included in a meta-analysis by Conrad and colleagues (2021), only two RCTs targeted children 5 years of age or older, and the majority of studies targeting social communication focused on very young children.

37.5.3.1 Parent-Mediated Delivery of Early Intensive Behavioral Intervention

The earliest forms of applied behavior analysis (ABA) intervention for children with ASD were based on the work of Ivar Lovaas and the UCLA Young Autism Project. This intervention is now often referred to as early intensive behavioral intervention (EIBI). EIBI programs are often focused on language development, reducing interfering behaviors, socialization, and early academic skills for children who are often no older than 6 years of age. These programs are characterized by their discrete trial teaching methods, one-on-one instruction, and 20 to 40 hours of weekly teaching within the home and/or school settings (Smith & Lovaas, 1998). In addition to one-on-one instruction between the child and therapist, EIBI programs often include parent training whereby the parent provides similar instruction under the supervision of the therapist. Despite being one of the oldest interventions for children with ASD, only a handful of large-scale RCTs have evaluated its effectiveness. Among studies employing a control group (e.g., treatment as usual, parent education), EIBI has consistently demonstrated greater positive effects than the control on measures of child adaptive behavior (Cohen et al., 2006; Howard et al., 2014; Magiati et al., 2007; Remington et al., 2007), language development (Howard et al., 2014; Remington et al., 2007; Smith et al., 2000), and cognition (Cohen et al., 2006; Howard et al., 2014; Remington et al., 2007; Smith et al., 2000); however, there is less evidence that EIBI improves ASD severity (Magiati et al., 2007; Remington et al., 2007), reduces disruptive behavior (Smith et al., 2000), or improves parental well-being (Remington et al., 2007).

37.5.3.2 Parent-Mediated Interventions for Social Communication

Primary parent-mediated interventions have been developed with a focus on social skills and social communication. Among these are Program for the Education and Enrichment of Relational Skills (PEERS) for preschoolers (Park et al., 2022) and Project ImPACT (Improving Parents as Communication Teachers; Ingersoll & Wainer, 2013). Project ImPACT teaches parents intervention techniques in social engagement, language, imitation, and play, which a trainer first models for the parent and then provides feedback as the parent demonstrates the strategies with their child (Ingersoll & Wainer, 2013). Studies have found many positive outcomes from Project ImPACT, including improved child imitation, social communication, and expressive language (Ingersoll & Wainer, 2013; Yoder et al., 2021), and positive parent–child interactions (Stahmer et al., 2019). There is also preliminary evidence that Project ImPACT may decrease parent stress and increase parents' perception of self-competence (Li et al., 2022). Although initially developed for clinical implementation, Project ImPACT has expanded delivery into community settings (Stadnick et al., 2015; Stahmer et al., 2020) and via telehealth (Ingersoll et al., 2016; Li et al., 2022).

37.5.3.3 Parent-Mediated Interventions for Joint Attention

Several parent-mediated interventions have explicitly targeted joint attention based on research that suggests that the development of language skills in young children relies heavily on precursor joint attention (Adamson et al., 2009). Examples include the Joint Attention Mediated Learning intervention (Schertz et al., 2013) and the Joint Attention, Symbolic Play, Engagement, and Regulation program (JASPER; Kasari et al., 2010). JASPER is one of the earliest parent-mediated interventions for children with autism to be evaluated in an RCT (Kasari et al., 2010). This intervention involves caregiver coaching during play routines to develop child engagement with the parent and play activities. Studies of parent-mediated JASPER have shown positive outcomes for several child behaviors, including initiation of and responsiveness to joint attention (Kasari et al., 2010,

2015), play diversity (Kasari et al., 2010, 2015), and social communication (Kasari et al., 2014). However, only a few studies on parent-mediated JASPER have assessed the effects of intervention on ASD core characteristics, and those studies have failed to show improvements relative to a control group (Harrop et al., 2017; Nordahl-Hansen et al., 2016). Limited research has also been done on parent outcomes, but in one study (Kasari et al., 2015), a brief version of parent-mediated JASPER did not result in reduced parent stress for parents considered low-resourced.

37.5.3.4 Parent-Mediated Interventions for Disruptive Behavior

As noted previously, there is strong research support for parent-mediated interventions for children with ASD who exhibit disruptive behavior. These programs draw largely on the vast research on principles and procedures used in ABA. Among the most well-known interventions with strong research support are Stepping Stones Triple P (Whittingham et al., 2009), Research Units in Behavioral Intervention (RUBI; Research Units on Pediatric Psychopharmacology Autism Network, 2007), and PCIT (Eyberg & Robinson, 1982). While Stepping Stones Triple P and PCIT were initially scientifically validated on non-ASD children before being modified for children with ASD, RUBI is one of only a few parent-mediated programs that were developed solely for parents of children with ASD. The manualized version of RUBI includes parent education and training related to understanding the function of disruptive behavior and strategies for preventing disruptive behavior and reinforcing more appropriate behaviors. Studies of RUBI have used a combination of parent rating scales (e.g., Aberrant Behavior Checklist; Home Situations Questionnaire) and clinician ratings on the Clinical Global Impression scale. Significant positive effects from RUBI have been demonstrated with regard to child adaptive behavior (Bearss et al., 2013; Bearss, Johnson, et al., 2015) and noncompliant and disruptive behavior (Bearss et al., 2013, 2018; Bearss, Johnson, et al., 2015; Burrell et al., 2020). Similar findings on child disruptive behaviors have been shown in both telehealth (Graucher et al., 2022) and group-delivered formats (Burrell et al., 2020; Edwards et al., 2019; Graucher et al., 2022). Additionally, long-term maintenance of treatment effects has been shown for up to 24 weeks post intervention (Bearss, Johnson, et al., 2015). Lecavalier et al. (2017) analyzed possible moderator variables in an RCT of RUBI and found that positive effects of RUBI on disruptive behavior was significantly affected by the severity of attention-deficit/hyperactivity disorder (ADHD) and anxiety, and to some extent household income. Despite positive research outcomes on child behavior, there is only limited research showing support for improvement on selected measures of parent stress (Iadarola et al., 2018).

37.5.3.5 Comprehensive Interventions Modified for Parent Implementation

Several highly effective comprehensive treatment approaches that were initially developed without a parent-mediated component have since been adapted to be fully or partially parent-mediated. The most well-known of these approaches are the Early Start Denver model (ESDM; Dawson et al., 2010) and pivotal response treatment (PRT; Koegel et al., 1999). ESDM is one of the most well-researched comprehensive early development interventions for children with ASD and was modified to include a parent-mediated component (P-ESDM; Rogers et al., 2012). Like its predecessor, multiple studies of the P-ESDM have demonstrated significant improvements in child behaviors, such as adaptive functioning (Rogers et al., 2012, 2019; Vismara et al., 2013, 2019), and social interaction and communication (Vismara et al., 2012, 2019; Waddington et al., 2021; Zhou et al., 2019), and positive parent outcomes, such as reduced stress (Estes et al., 2014; Vismara et al., 2018) and engagement (Vismara et al., 2012, 2018, 2019). Despite overall positive findings, it should be noted that three studies of P-ESDM evaluated child ASD severity and found no significant improvement in that child outcome (Rogers et al., 2012, 2019; Zhou et al., 2019).

Numerous large RCTs have been conducted on PRT that have demonstrated its effectiveness (Barrett et al., 2020; Gengoux et al., 2019; de Korte et al., 2022; Mohammadzaheri et al., 2014, 2015; Vernon et al., 2019). Most of these studies have utilized a partially parent-mediated approach where clinicians deliver much of the therapy with an added parent training component (Gengoux et al., 2019). Among the studies where PRT is more fully parent-mediated, the results have shown improvement on measures of child adaptive behavior (de Korte et al., 2022; Hardan et al., 2015), affect (McGarry et al., 2020), and communication (Hardan et al., 2015; McGarry et al., 2020). Additionally, there is support for parent-mediated PRT when delivered in individual (Bradshaw et al., 2017), group (Hardan et al., 2015), and telehealth (McGarry et al., 2020) formats. Outside of parent fidelity, studies with fully parent-mediated PRT have not evaluated parent behaviors (e.g., stress).

37.5.3.6 Parent-Mediated Interventions Using Single-Case Design

Most systematic literature reviews and meta-analyses have focused solely on the dozens of primary parent-mediated interventions evaluated using group designs and usually only those conducted as an RCT (e.g., Conrad et al., 2021). However, there exists a long history of parent-mediated approaches for children with ASD that have been evaluated using rigorous single-case experimental designs (SCDs). Like many of the approaches evaluated using group designs, approaches using SCDs are based on the operant learning model. Parent-mediated intervention research employing SCDs has targeted a broad range of skill deficits and behavioral excesses, including social skills (Dogan et al., 2017), social communication (Charlop-Christy & Carpenter, 2000), food refusal (Cosbey & Muldoon, 2017), restricted and repetitive behaviors (Lanovaz et al., 2016), and disruptive behaviors (Koegel et al., 1998).

Perhaps the most studied parent-mediated intervention for children with autism within the SCD literature is functional communication training (FCT; Carr & Durand, 1985). FCT is an intervention targeting disruptive behavior that involves teaching an individual to use an appropriate communicative alternative rather than disruptive behavior to access reinforcement (Tiger et al., 2008). Dozens of studies using SCD have demonstrated positive effects of parent-mediated FCT on disruptive behavior and communication for children with ASD (Gerow et al., 2018). A smaller number of studies have evaluated generalization and maintenance of parent-mediated FCT, showing that positive effects generalized to other child behaviors, settings, work tasks, and implementers (Berg et al., 2007; Moes & Frea, 2002; O'Brien et al., 2021; Schieltz et al., 2011; Wacker et al., 2005), with maintenance of effects ranging from months (Wacker et al., 2017) to years (Lucyshyn et al., 2007). In an attempt to validate FCT using a group design, Lindgren and colleagues (2020) conducted an RCT of parent-mediated FCT for young children with autism. In this study, behavior therapists coached parents of young children with autism via telehealth to conduct behavioral assessments and FCT with their child in their own home. The results showed that parent-mediated FCT led to statistically significant reductions in child disruptive behavior and increases in functional communication when compared to a treatment-as-usual control group.

37.6 Practice Implications

37.6.1 Treatment Outcomes

Various forms of parent training are considered evidence-based and may be essential for effective ASD treatment programs (National Autism Center, 2015; National Research Council, 2001; Wong et al., 2015). Their use has resulted in gains in social communication (Ferguson et al., 2022), reductions in disruptive behavior (Bearss, Johnson, et al., 2015), and improvements in parent self-efficacy and parenting stress (Zhou et al., 2019). Despite the research support for a variety of parent training programs, they are underutilized in ASD treatment programs (Hume et al., 2005; Thomas et al., 2007). Underutilization may be attributed to a variety of factors, including limited parent time and resources, low family engagement, and limited organizational support or recognition (Sanders et al., 2009; Shapiro et al., 2012). Care coordination (i.e., access to services to address unmet specialty care needs) is less likely to be a part of a child's treatment program when a child with ASD does not have a medical home (Farmer et al., 2014), and psychoeducation and/or parent-mediated interventions are less likely to be utilized by providers who have fewer training experiences (Ingersoll et al., 2020; McClain et al., 2020). To illustrate this latter point, Ingersoll et al. (2020) surveyed more than 1,000 Board-Certified Behavior Analysts (BCBAs) and found that fewer professional training experiences in parent training programs and larger client caseloads were associated with less use and engagement in parent training. Thus, the promotion of parent training programs for children with ASD must rely on several structural improvements, including increasing family resources, and an emphasis on training providers to effectively deliver scientifically validated parent training programs and do so in a manner that is efficient enough such that it does not preclude providers serving large client caseloads.

37.6.2 Practice Implication Guidelines

As noted previously, not all forms of parent training have strong research support. While research on care coordination models and psychoeducation is limited, with modest outcomes, parent-mediated interventions have stronger research support, especially for those targeting disruptive behavior. Nonetheless, each approach to parent training may be appropriate depending on a variety of factors, including intervention or program goals, provider characteristics and qualifications, and parent and child characteristics. Additionally, care coordination, psychoeducation, and parent-mediated interventions do not have to occur independently. In fact, a comprehensive parent training approach that is compassionate, observant, responsive, and empirical is likely to include all three parent training models. In the remaining sections of this chapter, we describe considerations across program, provider, and parent/child factors to inform guidelines for incorporating these parent training models in practice.

37.6.2.1 Program Considerations

With regard to intervention goals, care coordination is often an important first step for children newly diagnosed with ASD whose goals may not yet be fully established. Thus, care coordination is often a preintervention process to develop goals and triage to services based on those goals. Once intervention goals have been determined, the care coordination process continues, but it will be impacted by the types of services offered by the provider and any other providers for whom the child and parent may be referred. For example, if a behavior analyst provides brief, consultative services (e.g., one 90-minute appointment), the behavior analyst might provide the family with a list of resources of other interventionists that could be helpful in implementing the proposed intervention plan. This contrasts with a behavior analyst who provides EIBI services (e.g., 40 hours per week), wherein the behavior analyst might provide care coordination through more ongoing discussions with other interventionists to ensure consistency in treatment programming. The provider will need to assess how care coordination can be incorporated into the child's plan of care to meet treatment goals developed by the provider.

It is important that the service provider be aware of other services available and that the appropriateness of those services be based on the child's needs. In more geographically isolated regions, care coordination could be warranted but limited due to the lack of availability of services or service providers. As telehealth is becoming a more widely used platform to deliver services, care coordination could involve the service provider connecting a family to other interventionists located many miles from the family. Service providers should be knowledgeable about the types of services available to families through a telehealth model.

For service providers offering care coordination, there are numerous care coordination tools and organizations available to the broader healthcare community. For example, the Care Coordination Curriculum (Antonelli et al., 2019), funded by the US Maternal and Child Health Bureau, is a robust curriculum to be implemented in various training programs to support service providers who have responsibilities of care coordination in their practice. Furthermore, the National Resource Center for Patient/Family-Centered Medical Home developed by the AAP (n.d.) provides a list of resources and templates for providers to use when providing care coordination. Service providers should compile a list of resources to assist them in providing more streamlined care coordination that is matched to the child and family's needs.

Like care coordination, psychoeducation may be an important intervention for parents of children newly diagnosed with ASD. Despite increasing public awareness of ASD, the general population is still undereducated when it comes to the signs and symptoms of ASD, its etiology, and effective treatments (Golson et al., 2022), and some international populations may have even less knowledge related to ASD (Yu et al., 2020). Thus, psychoeducation may serve a critical role for parents when the goals include increasing parents' basic understanding of ASD, dispelling common ASD myths (e.g., vaccinations cause autism), and educating parents on effective and scientifically validated treatments. For parents who are already well-educated on ASD, psychoeducation may still be an important training component, particularly regarding education on effective intervention strategies.

When the parent-provider team's goal is to address social communication deficits or disruptive behaviors, parent-mediated intervention should be considered. In addition to the strong research support for outcomes ranging from improvements in parent–child interactions (Oono et al., 2013) to reductions in child disruptive behavior (Nevill et al., 2018; Ratliff-Black & Therrien, 2021), parent engagement is likely to produce additional benefits that have yet to be studied thoroughly. For example, it seems reasonable that by incorporating parents into the interventions there would be greater resulting parent "buy in," further promoting attendance and intervention maintenance (Haine-Schlagel & Walsh, 2015).

37.6.2.2 Provider Considerations: Skills and Qualifications

Despite the benefits of parent training programs described in this chapter, not all providers who serve children with ASD are likely to be successful using these approaches. As noted previously, provider training and experiences in delivering parent training programs are essential; however, parent training is not a common focus of graduate school instruction in psychology or behavior analysis and obtaining training or certification in many of the commercially available parent training programs may be costly. Nonetheless, providers interested in delivering parent-mediated interventions should do so only after receiving adequate training in the interventions they plan to deliver. Thus, providers should have both the content knowledge (i.e., conceptual understanding of the approach) and the procedural skills (i.e., high procedural fidelity) required to implement the program effectively. For interventions originally developed without a primary parent-mediated delivery format, such as the ESDM or FCT, providers should first be proficient in delivering the intervention before offering a parent-mediated version. More specifically, providers should be able to successfully implement an intervention directly with a client prior to offering a parent-mediated version. By delivering the intervention directly, the provider has the opportunity to experience implementation challenges and develop strategies to overcome those challenges. This is likely to enhance the provider's empathy when working with a parent experiencing the same challenges but also effectively draw upon his or her experiences to offer solutions.

Even the most skilled therapists may find parent training challenging. Unlike direct services, in parent training the provider serves as more of a coach than a therapist (Larsen et al., 2022). Thus, there is a heavy emphasis on the coach's vocal behaviors, such as instruction and performance feedback. Indeed, a therapist's ability to effectively coach and provide in vivo feedback is necessary for positive outcomes in parent-mediated approaches (Shanley & Niec, 2010). Larsen et al. (2022) conducted a study of therapists' coaching behaviors in a parent-mediated FCT intervention provided via telehealth and showed that much of the therapists' behavior included procedural comments (i.e., describing specific intervention procedures and the parents' roles in those procedures) and process comments (i.e., communicating the reasons for the procedures and how they result in beneficial outcomes). Interestingly, over time therapists shifted their coaching behaviors from more procedural comments (i.e., the "what") to process comments (i.e., the "why"), seemingly to promote more parent understanding and ultimately independence.

As a starting point, providers must be able to instruct parents in a clear and concise manner that is not filled with technical jargon; however, these skills must also be accompanied by good interpersonal or relational skills. In Larsen et al.'s (2022) study, a third class of coaching behaviors called "social engagement behaviors" also occurred at a high level. This class was primarily comprised of conversational comments (e.g., "Did you have a nice weekend?") and attentive listening (i.e., vocal and nonvocal behaviors to indicate listening). In parent training programs, the parent–provider relationship is built upon rapport, similar to the therapeutic alliance in psychotherapy. In fact, in an attempt to build a provider–parent bond, therapists delivering parent training should emulate a psychotherapist building therapeutic alliance by showing responsiveness to parent and child thoughts and feelings, establishing a collaborative relationship (as opposed to a hierarchy), displaying warmth and positivity, and maintaining flexibility in the interactions and procedural approach (Ryan et al., 2021).

37.6.2.3 Parent and Child Considerations

The characteristics of parents involved in parent training and their relationship to positive outcomes has garnered little research (Shalev et al., 2020). However, there are likely parent characteristics that may enhance or diminish the possibility of effective parent training outcomes. For example, while it may sound commonsense that a parent should be ready and comfortable with a parent training program before initiating it, intervention success requires that the parent hold both a positive view of the intervention and a commitment to carrying it out. Throughout parent training, parents are guaranteed to experience everyday barriers to their investment in treatment (e.g., sicknesses, unexpected competing events); however, for a parent who is not fully committed at the outset, such barriers will often result in failure. Thus, parents and providers considering a parent training program should discuss the parent's commitment to intervention prior to commencement of the intervention and periodically revisit the parent's feelings and preferences toward the intervention and their commitment to continue.

Even when a parent expresses a strong commitment to a parent training program, there may be parent characteristics that will make implementation more challenging or may even preclude parent involvement. Parents of children with ASD, like other parents, experience a variety of learning or intellectual disabilities and mental health conditions commonly observed in the general public. Whether these conditions reduce the capability of the parent to participate in parent training is dependent, in part, on the type of the parent training program and the severity of the condition or disability. Shalev et al. (2020) conducted a systematic review related to parent characteristics and their effects on parent-mediated interventions for children with ASD. They found that parent characteristics, such as stress, anxiety, and autistic traits (i.e., broader autism phenotype), may serve to moderate child outcomes, although not always in a negative manner. Rather than exclude families where a parent exhibits a learning, intellectual, or mental health condition, it may be possible for a provider to include intervention components that specifically target the parent's condition. For example, Reaven et al. (2015) implemented a group cognitive-behavioral therapy program for children with ASD experiencing anxiety and included a component targeting parent anxiety that led to significant reductions in parent anxiety post treatment. With regard to learning disabilities, parents with dyslexia or comprehension difficulties may require instruction in various formats (e.g., vocally, written, visually) that allows them to still participate in parent training.

When interventions targeting disruptive behavior are implemented, it is not uncommon for there to be an initial exacerbation of those disruptive behaviors (i.e., extinction bursts; Lerman et al., 2020). In parent-mediated intervention, there is a heavy onus on the parent to work through the exacerbation and ensure the child and other family members are safe. Parents prone to emotional responding, such as screaming, crying, or using excessive physical force when stressful events occur, may not be good candidates for delivering this type of intervention. Even when a parent has demonstrated the ability to remain calm and implement the intervention with good fidelity in the face of intense behavioral episodes, parent-mediated approaches targeting challenging behavior are best delivered with close provider supervision and, when possible, additional in-person adult support (e.g., another caregiver is present). Additionally, the provider should always prepare a parent fully for the possibility of exacerbation of disruptive behavior and gauge the parent's emotional condition when they do occur.

A number of studies have evaluated the relationship between baseline child characteristics and positive outcomes in parent-mediated interventions (Dawson et al., 2010; Harden et al., 2015). Although it does not appear that a child's cognitive abilities, language skills, or ASD severity significantly impact outcomes, research studies have not found consensus as to what makes a child a good candidate for parent-mediated approaches. Nonetheless, there are several child factors that should be considered prior to enrolling a parent–child dyad in a parent training program. To begin, it is not uncommon in clinical settings to observe a child perform better or show less disruptive behavior for a therapist than for his or her parent. The opposite may sometimes be true, but in the former situation, it would be wise for the therapist and parent to consider whether a parent-delivered intervention would produce the same positive outcomes as a therapist-delivered approach. One solution to this challenge would include the therapist conducting direct therapy with the child, followed by generalization sessions with parents.

A second child factor to consider is whether disruptive behavior exists and its corresponding topographies and severity. Most studies on parent training, and particularly those using parent-mediated interventions, have specifically excluded individuals with severe and challenging behavior. Moreover, studies targeting severe and challenging behavior in children with ASD have largely focused on young children (i.e., below the age of 7 years). Parent-mediated interventions often place the parent in close proximity to the child during procedures that may be upsetting to the child, which could make the parent a target for physical aggression. This is especially true when implementing treatments targeting disruptive behavior. Many treatments targeting disruptive behavior utilize extinction, which entails withholding reinforcement previously associated with the disruptive behavior. One side effect of extinction is a rapid increase in the frequency of the targeted behavior, called an extinction burst (Catania, 2013), or the emergence of new disruptive behaviors. Providers and parents should consider the likelihood of such events and whether parent and child safety would be too compromised for a parent-mediated approach. Parent implementation may still be practical if the intervention is being delivered with the therapist, in the presence of additional adult support, or with the inclusion of protective equipment; however, delivery using telehealth would not be advised, given the inability of the therapist to provide support. Although the same risks for extinction bursts and the emergence of new disruptive behaviors exists when a therapist delivers the intervention, most therapists who work with severe and challenging behavior have extensive safety training and experience with such episodes.

An important third child factor is the age of the child. Although there is no research to suggest that older children and adolescents would not benefit from parent training, there is also a paucity of research to suggest that they are likely to benefit. Consistent with the previous point about disruptive behavior, a particular challenge inherent in working with an older, larger child or adolescent is the potential for injury if the intervention is targeting disruptive behavior. Additionally, as a child reaches school age, a large portion of each child's day is spent in the school setting, leaving much less time for intervention, parent-mediated or otherwise. As a child progresses into adolescence and preadulthood, new stressors associated with puberty, peer relationships, and educational transitions may increase the difficulty of utilizing parent-mediated approaches, although this is purely speculation because little research has been done on parent-mediated interventions with this age range.

The fourth and final child factor to consider is the presence of co-occurring psychiatric conditions. Children with ASD are at high risk for other psychiatric conditions, including ADHD, mood disorders, anxiety disorders, and seizure disorders (Shoaib et al., 2022), and many of these co-occurring conditions may require treatment separate from those targeting ASD symptoms. Thus, time in other behavioral therapies may reduce the opportunity for parent training and may increase the level of parent and child stress when the expectations to implement multiple therapies are in place. Moreover, some psychiatric conditions may make delivery of the parent training more challenging. For example, children with ASD and co-occurring ADHD symptoms may be less responsive to common ASD interventions than children without co-occurring ADHD (Leitner, 2014). Child impairments in attention and impulse control require a parent delivering an intervention to understand how to capture that child's attention and remain patient when they cannot.

37.7 References

Abrahams, B. S. & Geschwind, D. H. (2008) Advances in autism genetics: on the threshold of a new neurobiology. *Nature Reviews Genetics, 9*, 341–355. doi: 10.1038/nrg2346.

Adamson, L. B., Bakeman, R., Deckner, D. F., & Romski, M. (2009). Joint engagement and the emergence of language in children with autism and Down syndrome. *Journal of Autism and Developmental Disorders, 39*(1), 84–96. https://doi.org/10.1007/s10803-008-0601-7

Agency for Healthcare Research and Quality. (2014). What is care coordination? In *Care coordination measures atlas update*. Rockville, MD: Agency for Healthcare Research and Quality. http://www.ahrq.gov/professionals/prevention-chronic-care/improve/coordination/atlas2014/chapter2.html

American Academy of Pediatrics Committee on Children with Disabilities. (1999). Care coordination: Integrating health and related systems of care for children with special health care needs. *Pediatrics, 104*(4), 978–981. https://doi.org/10.1542/peds.104.4.978

American Academy of Pediatrics Council on Children with Disabilities. (2005). Care coordination in the medical home: Integrating health and related systems of care for children with special health care needs. *Pediatrics, 116*(5), 1238–1244. https://doi.org/10.1542/peds.2005-2070

American Academy of Pediatrics Medical Home Initiatives for Children with Special Needs Project Advisory Committee. (2002). The medical home: Medical home initiatives for children with special needs project advisory committee. *Pediatrics, 110*(1), 184–186. https://doi.org/10.1542/peds.110.1.184

American Academy of Pediatrics National Resource Center for Patient/Family-Centered Medical Home. (n.d.). Medical home. https://www.aap.org/en/practice-management/medical-home

Antonelli, R. C., Bottino, C. J., Coleman, C. L., Frank, B., Fleegler, E., Hassan, A., Huntington, N., Huth, K., Sprague Martinez, L., McAllister, J., Rosenberg, H., Turchi, R., Wilkinson, G. W., Ziniel, S., Bailey, D., Gagnon, N., & Slater, D. H. (2019). *Pediatric care coordination curriculum: An interprofessional resource to effectively engage patients and families in achieving optimal child health outcomes* (2nd ed.). Boston: Boston Children's Hospital.

Arango, P. (2011). Family-centered care. *Academic Pediatrics, 11*(2), 97–99. https://doi.org/10.1016/j.acap.2010.12.004

Barrett, A. C., Vernon, T. W., McGarry, E. S., Holden, A. N., Bradshaw, J., Ko, J. A., Horowitz, E. J., & German, T. C. (2020). Social responsiveness and language use associated with an enhanced PRT approach for young children with ASD: Results from a pilot RCT of the PRISM model. *Research in Autism Spectrum Disorders, 71*, 1–11. https://doi.org/10.1016/j.rASD.2019.101497

Bearss, K., Burrell, T. L., Challa, S. A., Postorino, V., Gillespie, S. E., Crooks, C., & Scahill, L. (2018). Feasibility of parent training via telehealth for children with autism spectrum disorder and disruptive behavior: A demonstration pilot. *Journal of Autism and Developmental Disorders, 48*(4), 1020–1030. https://doi.org/10.1007/s10803-017-3363-2

Bearss, K., Burrell, T. L., Stewart, L., & Scahill, L. (2015). Parent training in autism spectrum disorder: What's in a name? *Clinical Child and Family Psychology Review, 18*(2), 170–182. https://doi.org/10.1007/s10567-015-0179-5

Bearss, K., Johnson, C., Handen, B., Smith, T., & Scahill, L. (2013). A pilot study of parent training in young children with autism spectrum disorders and disruptive behavior. *Journal of Autism and Developmental Disorders, 43*(4), 829–840. https://doi.org/10.1007/s10803-012-1624-7

Bearss, K., Johnson, C., Smith, T., Lecavalier, L., Swiezy, N., Aman, M., McAdam, D. B., Butter, E., Stillitano, C., Minshawi, N., Sukhodolsky, D. G., Mruzek, D. W., Turner, K., Neal, T., Hallett, V., Mulick, J. A., Green, B., Handen, B., Deng, Y., ... Scahill, L. (2015). Effect of parent training vs parent education on behavioral problems in children with autism spectrum disorder: A randomized clinical trial. *Journal of the American Medical Association, 313*(15), 1524–1533. https://doi.org/10.1001/jama.2015.3150

Bebko, J. M., Konstantareas, M. M., & Springer, J. (1987). Parent and professional evaluations of family stress associated with characteristics of autism. *Journal of Autism and Developmental Disorders, 17*(4), 565–576. https://doi.org/10.1007/BF01486971

Behavior Analyst Certification Board. (2020). Ethics code for behavior analysts. https://www.bacb.com/wp-content/uploads/2022/01/Ethics-Code-for-Behavior-Analysts-220316-2.pdf

Bennett, M., Webster, A. A., Goodall, E., & Rowland, S. (2019). *Life on the autism spectrum: Translating myths and misconceptions into positive futures.* Cham: Springer.

Berg, W. K., Wacker, D. P., Harding, J. W., Ganzer, J., & Barretto, A. (2007). An evaluation of multiple dependent variables across distinct classes of antecedent stimuli pre and post functional communication training. *Journal of Early and Intensive Behavior Intervention, 4*(1), 305. https://doi.org/10.1037/h0100346

Bijou, S. W., & Baer, D. M. (1961). *Child development.* New York: Appleton-Century-Crofts.

Bradshaw, J., Koegel, L. K., & Koegel, R. L. (2017). Improving functional language and social motivation with a parent-mediated intervention for toddlers with autism spectrum disorder. *Journal of Autism and Developmental Disorders, 47*(8), 2443–2458. https://doi.org/10.1007/s10803-017-3155-8

Brookman-Frazee, L., Stahmer, A., Baker-Ericzen, M. J., & Tsai, K. (2006). Parenting interventions for children with autism spectrum and disruptive behavior disorders: Opportunities for cross-fertilization. *Clinical Child and Family Psychology Review, 9*(3), 181–200. DOI: 10.1007/s10567-006-0010-4

Brookman-Frazee, L. I., Taylor, R., & Garland, A. F. (2010). Characterizing community-based mental health services for children with autism spectrum disorders and disruptive behavior problems. *Journal of Autism and Developmental Disorders, 40*(10), 1188–1201. https://doi.org/10.1007/s10803-010-0976-0

Burrell, T. L., Postorino, V., Scahill, L., Rea, H. M., Gillespie, S., Evans, A. N., & Bearss, K. (2020). Feasibility of group parent training for children with autism spectrum disorder and disruptive behavior: A demonstration pilot. *Journal of Autism and Developmental Disorders, 50*(11), 3883–3894. https://doi.org/10.1007/s10803-020-04427-1

Carr, E. G., & Durand, V. M. (1985). Reducing behavior problems through functional communication training. *Journal of Applied Behavior Analysis, 18*(2), 111–126. https://doi.org/10.1901/jaba.1985.18-111

Catania, A. C. (2013). *Learning* (5th ed.). Hudson, NY: Sloan.

Centers for Disease Control and Prevention. (2009). *Parent training programs: Insight for practitioners.* Atlanta, GA: Author.

Charlop-Christy, M. H., & Carpenter, M. H. (2000). Modified incidental teaching sessions: A procedure for parents to increase spontaneous speech in their children with autism. *Journal of Positive Behavior Interventions, 2*(2), 98–112. https://doi.org/10.1177/109830070000200203

Cheng, W. M., Smith, T. B., Butler, M., Taylor, T. M., & Clayton, D. (2022). Effects of parent-implemented interventions on outcomes of children with autism: A meta-analysis. *Journal of Autism and Developmental Disorders*, 53, 4147–4163. https://doi.org/10.1007/s10803-022-05688-8

Cohen, H., Amerine-Dickens, M., & Smith, T. (2006). Early intensive behavioral treatment: Replication of the UCLA model in a community setting. *Journal of Developmental and Behavioral Pediatrics, 27*(2 Suppl.), S145–155. https://doi.org/10.1097/00004703-200604002-00013

Conrad, C. E., Rimestad, M. L., Rohde, J. F., Petersen, B. H., Korfitsen, C. B., Tarp, S., Cantio, C., Lauritsen, M. B., & Händel, M. N. (2021). Parent-mediated interventions for children and adolescents with autism spectrum disorders: A systematic review and meta-analysis. *Frontiers in Psychiatry, 12.* https://doi.org/10.3389/fpsyt.2021.773604

Coogle, C. G., & Hanline, M. F. (2016). An exploratory study of family-centred help-giving practices in early intervention: Families of young children with autism spectrum disorder. *Child & Family Social Work, 21*(2), 249–260. https://doi.org/10.1111/cfs.12148

Cosbey, J., & Muldoon, D. (2017). Eat-up™ family-centered feeding intervention to promote food acceptance and decrease challenging behaviors: A single-case experimental design replicated across three families of children with autism spectrum disorder. *Journal of Autism and Developmental Disorders, 47*(3), 564–578. https://doi.org/10.1007/s10803-016-2977-0

Davis, N. O., & Carter, A. S. (2008). Parenting stress in mothers and fathers of toddlers with autism spectrum disorders: Associations with child characteristics. *Journal of Autism and Developmental Disorders, 38*(7), 1278–1291. https://doi.org/10.1007/s10803-007-0512-z

DaWalt, L. S., Greenberg, J. S., & Mailick, M. R. (2018). Transitioning together: A multi-family group psychoeducation program for adolescents with ASD and their parents. *Journal of Autism and Developmental Disorders, 48*(1), 251–263. https://doi.org/10.1007/s10803-017-3307-x

Dawson, G., Rogers, S., Munson, J., Smith, M., Winter, J., Greenson, J., Donaldson, A., & Varley, J. (2010). Randomized, controlled trial of an intervention for toddlers with autism: The Early Start Denver model. *Pediatrics, 125*(1), e17–23. https://doi.org/10.1542/peds.2009-0958

de la Torre-Ubieta, L., Won, H., Stein, J. L., & Geschwind, D. H. (2016). Advancing the understanding of autism disease mechanisms through genetics. *Nature Medicine, 22*(4), 345–361. https://doi.org/10.1038/nm.4071

Dogan, R. K., King, M. L., Fischetti, A. T., Lake, C. M., Mathews, T. L., & Warzak, W. J. (2017). Parent-implemented behavioral skills training of social skills. *Journal of Applied Behavior Analysis, 50*(4), 805–818. https://doi.org/10.1002/jaba.411

Edwards, G. S., Zlomke, K. R., & Greathouse, A. D. (2019). RUBI parent training as a group intervention for children with autism: A community pilot study. *Research in Autism Spectrum Disorders, 66,* 1–10. https://doi.org/10.1016/j.rASD.2019.101409

Ekas, N. V., Lickenbrock, D. M., & Whitman, T. L. (2010). Optimism, social support, and well-being in mothers of children with autism spectrum disorder. *Journal of Autism and Developmental Disorders, 40*(10), 1274–1284. https://doi.org/10.1007/s10803-010-0986-y

Estes, A., Vismara, L., Mercado, C., Fitzpatrick, A., Elder, L., Greenson, J., Lord, C., Munson, J., Winter, J., Young, G., Dawson, G., & Rogers, S. (2014). The impact of parent-delivered intervention on parents of very young children with autism. *Journal of Autism and Developmental Disorders, 44*(2), 353–365. https://doi.org/10.1007/s10803-013-1874-z

Eyal, G. (2013). For a sociology of expertise: The social origins of the autism epidemic. *American Journal of Sociology, 118*(4), 863–907. https://doi.org/10.1086/668448

Eyberg, S. M., & Robinson, E. A. (1982). Parent–child interaction training: Effects on family functioning. *Journal of Clinical Child Psychology, 11*, 130–137. https://doi.org/10.1080/15374418209533076

Farmer, J., & Reupert, A. (2013). Understanding autism and understanding my child with autism: An evaluation of a group parent education program in rural Australia. *The Australian Journal of Rural Health, 21*(1), 20–27. https://doi.org/10.1111/ajr.12004

Farmer, J. E., Clark, M. J., Drewwl, E. H., Swenson, T. M., & Ge, B. (2011). Consultative care coordination through the medical home for CSHCN: A randomized controlled trial. *Maternal and Child Health Journal, 15*, 1110–1118. https://doi.org/10.1007/s10995-010-0658-8

Farmer, J. E., Clark, M. J., Mayfield, W. A., Cheak-Zamora, N., Marvin, A. R., Law, J. K., & Law, P. A. (2014). The relationship between the medical home and unmet needs for children with autism spectrum disorders. *Maternal and Child Health Journal, 18*, 672–680. https://doi.org/10.1007/s10995-013-1292-z

Farrugia, D. (2009). Exploring stigma: Medical knowledge and the stigmatisation of parents of children diagnosed with autism spectrum disorder. *Sociology of Health & Illness, 31*(7), 1011–1027. https://doi.org/10.1111/j.1467-9566.2009.01174.x

Ferguson, J., Dounavi, K., & Craig, E. A. (2022). The efficacy of using telehealth to coach parents of children with autism spectrum disorder on how to use naturalistic teaching to increase mands, tacts and intraverbals. *Journal of Developmental and Physical Disabilities*, 35, 417–447. https://doi.org/10.1007/s10882-022-09859-4

Gengoux, G. W., Abrams, D. A., Schuck, R., Millan, M. E., Libove, R., Ardel, C. M., Phillips, J. M., Fox, M., Frazier, T. W., & Hardan, A. Y. (2019). A pivotal response treatment package for children with autism spectrum disorder: An RCT. *Pediatrics, 144*(3), e20190178. https://doi.org/10.1542/peds.2019-0178

Gerow, S., Hagan-Burke, S., Rispoli, M., Gregori, E., Mason, R., & Ninci, J. (2018). A systematic review of parent-implemented functional communication training for children with ASD. *Behavior Modification, 42*(3), 335–363. https://doi.org/10.1177/0145445517740872

Golnik, A., Scal, P., Wey, A., & Gaillard, P. (2012). Autism-specific primary care medical home intervention. *Journal of Autism and Developmental Disorders, 42*, 1087–1093. https://doi.org/10.1007/s10803-011-1351-5

Golson, M. E., Benallie, K. J., Benney, C. M., Schwartz, S. E., McClain, M. B., & Harris, B. (2022). Current state of autism knowledge in the general population of the United States. *Research in Autism Spectrum Disorders, 90*, 1–8.https://doi.org/10.1016/j.rASD.2021.101886

Graucher, T., Sinai-Gavrilov, Y., Mor, Y., Netzer, S., Cohen, E. Y., Levi, L., Avtalion, T. B., & Koller, J. (2022). From clinic room to zoom: Delivery of an evidence-based, parent-mediated intervention in the community before and during the pandemic. *Journal of Autism and Developmental Disorders, 52*, 5222–5231. https://doi.org/10.1007/s10803-022-05592-1

Green, J., Charman, T., McConachie, H., Aldred, C., Slonims, V., Howlin, P., Le Couteur, A., Leadbitter, K., Hudry, K., Byford, S., Barrett, B., Temple, K., Macdonald, W., Pickles, A., & PACT Consortium. (2010). Parent-mediated communication-focused treatment in children with autism (PACT): A randomised controlled trial. *Lancet, 375*(9732), 2152–2160. https://doi.org/10.1016/S0140-6736(10)60587-9

Haine-Schlagel, R., & Walsh, N. E. (2015). A review of parent participation engagement in child and family mental health treatment. *Clinical Child and Family Psychology Review, 18*(2), 133–150. https://doi.org/10.1007/s10567-015-0182-x

Hardan, A. Y., Gengoux, G. W., Berquist, K. L., Libove, R. A., Ardel, C. M., Phillips, J., Frazier, T. W., & Minjarez, M. B. (2015). A randomized controlled trial of pivotal response treatment group for parents of children with autism. *Journal of Child Psychology and Psychiatry, and Allied Disciplines, 56*(8), 884–892. https://doi.org/10.1111/jcpp.12354

Harrop, C., Gulsrud, A., Shih, W., Hovsepyan, L., & Kasari, C. (2017). The impact of caregiver-mediated JASPER on child restricted and repetitive behaviors and caregiver responses: Caregiver-Mediated JASPER and RRBs. *Autism Research, 10*(5), 983–992. https://doi.org/10.1002/aur.1732

Hayes, S. A., & Watson, S. L. (2013). The impact of parenting stress: A meta-analysis of studies comparing the experience of parenting stress in parents of children with and without autism spectrum disorder. *Journal of Autism and Developmental Disorders, 43*(3), 629–642. https://doi.org/10.1007/s10803-012-1604-y

Howard, J. S., Stanislaw, H., Green, G., Sparkman, C. R., & Cohen, H. G. (2014). Comparison of behavior analytic and eclectic early interventions for young children with autism after three years. *Research in Developmental Disabilities, 35*(12), 3326–3344. https://doi.org/10.1016/j.ridd.2014.08.021

Hume, K., Bellini, S., & Pratt, C. (2005). The usage and perceived outcomes of early intervention and early childhood programs for young children with autism spectrum disorder. *Topics in Early Childhood Special Education, 25*(4), 195–207. https://doi.org/10.1177/02711214050250040101

Hyman, S. L., & Johnson, J. K. (2012). Autism and pediatric practice: Toward a medical home. *Journal of Autism and Developmental Disorders, 42*, 1156–1164. https://doi.org/10.1007/s10803-012-1474-3

Iadarola, S., Levato, L., Harrison, B., Smith, T., Lecavalier, L., Johnson, C., Swiezy, N., Bearss, K., & Scahill, L. (2018). Teaching parents behavioral strategies for autism spectrum disorder (ASD): Effects on stress, strain, and competence. *Journal of Autism and Developmental Disorders, 48*(4), 1031–1040. https://doi.org/10.1007/s10803-017-3339-2

Ingersoll, B., Straiton, D., & Rivera Caquias N. (2020). The role of professional training experiences and manualized programs in ABA providers' use of parent training with children with autism. *Behavior Therapy, 51*(4), 588–600. https://doi.org/10.1016/j.beth.2019.09.004

Ingersoll, B., & Wainer, A. (2013). Initial efficacy of project ImPACT: A parent-mediated social communication intervention for young children with ASD. *Journal of Autism and Developmental Disorders, 43*(12), 2943–2952. https://doi.org/10.1007/s10803-013-1840-9

Ingersoll, B., Wainer, A. L., Berger, N. I., Pickard, K. E., & Bonter, N. (2016). Comparison of a self-directed and therapist-assisted telehealth parent-mediated intervention for children with ASD: A pilot RCT. *Journal of Autism and Developmental Disorders, 46*(7), 2275–2284. https://doi.org/10.1007/s10803-016-2755-z

Kaiser, K., Villalobos, M. E., Locke, J., Iruka, I. U., Proctor, C., & Boyd, B. (2022). A culturally grounded autism parent training program with Black parents. *Autism, 26*(3), 716–726. https://doi.org/10.1177/13623613211073373

Kalalo, R. T., Yuniar, S., & Ariyanto, F. C. (2021). Effect of parental skills-based psychoeducation intervention on parental stress index and severity of children with autism spectrum disorders: A pilot study. *Annals of Medicine and Surgery, 70*, 1–6. https://doi.org/10.1016/j.amsu.2021.102873

Karpur, A., Lello, A., Frazier, T., Dixon, P. J., & Shih, A. J. (2019). Health disparities among children with autism spectrum disorders: Analysis of the national survey of children's health 2016. *Journal of Autism and Developmental Disorders, 49*, 1652–1664. https://doi.org/10.1007/s10803-018-3862-9

Karst, J. S., & Van Hecke, A. V. (2012). Parent and family impact of autism spectrum disorders: A review and proposed model for intervention evaluation. *Clinical Child and Family Psychology Review, 15*(3), 247–277. https://doi.org/10.1007/s10567-012-0119-6

Kasari, C., Gulsrud, A., Paparella, T., Hellemann, G., & Berry, K. (2015). Randomized comparative efficacy study of parent-mediated interventions for toddlers with autism. *Journal of Consulting and Clinical Psychology, 83*(3), 554–563. https://doi.org/10.1037/a0039080

Kasari, C., Gulsrud, A. C., Wong, C., Kwon, S., & Locke, J. (2010). Randomized controlled caregiver mediated joint engagement intervention for toddlers with autism. *Journal of Autism and Developmental Disorders, 40*(9), 1045–1056. https://doi.org/10.1007/s10803-010-0955-5

Kasari, C., Lawton, K., Shih, W., Barker, T. V., Landa, R., Lord, C., Orlich, F., King, B., Wetherby, A., & Senturk, D. (2014). Caregiver-mediated intervention for low-resourced preschoolers with autism: An RCT. *Pediatrics, 134*(1), e72–79. https://doi.org/10.1542/peds.2013-3229

Kazdin, A. E. (2005). *Parent management training: Treatment for oppositional, aggressive, and antisocial behavior in children and adolescents.* New York: Oxford University Press.

Koegel, L. K., Koegel, R. L., Harrower, J. K., & Carter, C. M. (1999). Pivotal response intervention I: Overview of approach. *Journal of the Association for Persons with Severe Handicaps, 24*(3), 174–185. https://doi.org/10.2511/rpsd.24.3.174

Koegel, L. K., Stiebel, D., & Koegel, R. L. (1998). Reducing aggression in children with autism toward infant or toddler siblings. *Journal of the Association for Persons with Severe Handicaps, 23*(2), 111–118. https://doi.org/10.2511/rpsd.23.2.111

Kogan, M. D., Strickland, B. B., Blumberg, S. J., Singh, G. K., Perrin, J. M., & van Dyck, P. C. (2008). A national profile of the health care experiences and family impact of autism spectrum disorder among children in the United States, 2005-2006. *Pediatrics, 122*(6), e1149–e1158. https://doi.org/10.1542/peds.2008-1057

de Korte, M. W. P., van Dongen-boomsma, M., Oosterling, I. J., Buitelaar, J. K., & Staal, W. G. (2022). Pivotal response treatment (PRT) parent group training for young children with autism spectrum disorder: A pilot study. *Scientific Reports, 12*(1), Article 1. https://doi.org/10.1038/s41598-022-10602

Kuhlthau, K. A., Bloom, S., Van Cleave, J., Knapp, A. A., Romm, D., Klatka, K., Homer, C. J., Newacheck, P. W., & Perrin, J. M. (2011). Evidence for family-centered care for children with special health care needs: A systematic review. *Academic Pediatrics*, *11*(2), 136–143. https://doi.org/10.1016/j.acap.2010.12.014

Lanovaz, M. J., Rapp, J. T., Maciw, I., Dorion, C., & Prégent-Pelletier, É. (2016). Preliminary effects of parent-implemented behavioural interventions for stereotypy. *Developmental Neurorehabilitation*, *19*(3), 193–196. https://doi.org/10.3109/17518423.2014.986821

Larsen, A., Schieltz, K. M., Barrett, A., & O'Brien, M. J. (2022). A retrospective analysis of therapists' coaching behavior when directing parents to conduct behavioral assessments and treatments via telehealth. *Behavior Modification*, *47*(1), 154–184. https://doi.org/10.1177/01454455221106127

Lecavalier, L., Smith, T., Johnson, C., Bearss, K., Swiezy, N., Aman, M. G., Sukhodolsky, D. G., Deng, Y., Dziura, J., & Scahill, L. (2017). Moderators of parent training for disruptive behaviors in young children with autism spectrum disorder. *Journal of Abnormal Child Psychology*, *45*(6), 1235–1245. https://doi.org/10.1007/s10802-016-0233-x

Leitner, Y. (2014). The co-occurrence of autism and attention deficit hyperactivity disorder in children - what do we know? *Frontiers in Human Neuroscience*, *8*, 268. https://doi.org/10.3389/fnhum.2014.00268

Lerman, D. C., O'Brien, M. J., Neely, L., Call, N. A., Tsami, L., Schieltz, K. M., Berg, W. K., Graber, J., Huang, P., Kopelman, T., & Cooper-Brown, L. J. (2020). Remote coaching of caregivers via telehealth: Challenges and potential solutions. *Journal of Behavioral Education*, *29*, 195–221. https://doi.org/10.1007/s10864-020-09378-2

Li, F., Wu, D., Ren, F., Shen, L., Xue, M., Yu, J., Zhang, L., Tang, Y., Liu, X., Tao, M., Zhou, L., Jiang, L., Xu, M., & Li, F. (2022). Effectiveness of online-delivered Project ImPACT for children with ASD and their parents: A pilot study during the covid-19 pandemic. *Frontiers in Psychiatry*, *13*. https://doi.org/10.3389/fpsyt.2022.806149

Lindgren, S., Wacker, D., Schieltz, K., Suess, A., Pelzel, K., Kopelman, T., Lee, J., Romani, P., & O'Brien, M. (2020). A randomized controlled trial of functional communication training via telehealth for young children with autism spectrum disorder. *Journal of Autism and Developmental Disorders*, *50*, 4449–4462. https://doi.org/10.1007/s10803-020-04451-1

Lovaas, O. I., Koegel, R. L., Simmons, J. Q., & Long, J. (1973). Some generalization and follow-up measures on autistic children in behavior therapy. *Journal of Applied Behavior Analysis*, *6*(1), 131–166. https://doi.org/10.1901/jaba.1973.6-131

Lucyshyn, J. M., Albin, R. W., Horner, R. H., Mann, J. C., Mann, J. A., & Wadsworth, G. (2007). Family implementation of positive behavior support for a child with autism: Longitudinal, single-case, experimental, and descriptive replication and extension. *Journal of Positive Behavior Interventions*, 9(3), 131–150. https://doi.org/10.1177/10983007070090030201

Lukens, E. P., & McFarlane, W. R. (2004). Psychoeducation as evidence-based practice: Considerations for practice, research, and policy. *Brief Treatment & Crisis Intervention*, *4*(3), 205–225. https://doi.org/10.1093/brief-treatment/mhh019

Magaña, S., Lopez, K., & Machalicek, W. (2017). Parents taking action: A psycho-educational intervention for Latino parents of children with autism spectrum disorder. *Family Process*, *56*(1), 59–74. https://doi.org/10.1111/famp.12169

Magiati, I., Charman, T., & Howlin, P. (2007). A two-year prospective follow-up study of community-based early intensive behavioural intervention and specialist nursery provision for children with autism spectrum disorders. *Journal of Child Psychology and Psychiatry*, *48*(8), 803–812. https://doi.org/10.1111/j.1469-7610.2007.01756.x

McAllister, J. W. (2014). *Achieving a shared plan of care with children and youth with special health care needs.* Palo Alto, CA: Lucile Packard Foundation for Children's Healthcare.

McAllister, J. W., McNally Keehn, R., Rodgers, R., & Lock, T. M. (2018a). Care coordination using a shared plan of care approach: From model to practice. *Journal of Pediatric Nursing*, *43*, 88–96. https://doi.org/10.1016/j.pedn.2018.09.009

McAllister, J. W., McNally Keehn, R., Rodgers, R., Mpofu, P. B., Monahan, P. O., & Lock, T. M. (2018b). Effects of a care coordination intervention with children with neurodevelopmental disabilities and their families. *Journal of Developmental & Behavioral Pediatrics*, *39*(6), 471–480. https://doi.org/10.1097/DBP.0000000000000576

McClain, M. B., Shahidullah, J. D., Mexher, K. R., Haverkamp, C. R., Benallie, K. J., & Schwartz, S. E. (2020). School-clinic care coordination for youth with ASD: A national survey of school psychologists. *Journal of Autism and Developmental Disorders, 50*, 3081–3091. https://doi.org/10.1007/s10803-019-03985-3

McGarry, E., Vernon, T., & Baktha, A. (2020). Brief report: A pilot online pivotal response treatment training program for parents of toddlers with autism spectrum disorder. *Journal of Autism and Developmental Disorders, 50*(9), 3424–3431. https://doi.org/10.1007/s10803-019-04100-2

McNally Keehn, R., Enneking, B., Ramaker, M., Goings, M., Yang, Z., Carroll, A., & Ciiccarellli, M. (2020). Family-centered care coordination in an interdisciplinary neurodevelopmental evaluation clinic: Outcomes from care coordinator and caregiver reports. *Frontiers in Pediatrics, 8*. https://doi.org/10.3389/fped.2020.538633

McNeil, C. B., & Hembree-Kigin, T. L. (2011). *Parent-child interaction therapy* (2nd ed.). Cham: Springer.

Moeenuddin, Z., Kim-Kupfer, C., Owchar, E., Baker, J., Duffield, A., & Santoro, T. (2019). The influence of care coordination on patients with special health care needs in a pediatric residency continuity clinic. *Global Pediatric Health, 6*, 1–6. https://doi.org/10.1177/2333794XI9848677

Moes, D. R., & Frea, W. D. (2002). Contextualized behavioral support in early intervention for children with autism and their families. *Journal of Autism and Developmental Disorders, 32*(6), 519–533. https://doi.org/10.1023/a:1021298729297

Mohammadzaheri, F., Koegel, L. K., Rezaee, M., & Rafiee, S. M. (2014). A randomized clinical trial comparison between pivotal response treatment (PRT) and structured applied behavior analysis (ABA) intervention for children with autism. *Journal of Autism and Developmental Disorders, 44*(11), 2769–2777. https://doi.org/10.1007/s10803-014-2137-3

Mohammadzaheri, F., Koegel, L. K., Rezaei, M., & Bakhshi, E. (2015). A randomized clinical trial comparison between pivotal response treatment (PRT) and adult-driven applied behavior analysis (ABA) intervention on disruptive behaviors in public school children with autism. *Journal of Autism and Developmental Disorders, 45*(9), 2899–2907. https://doi.org/10.1007/s10803-015-2451-4

Mukhtar, D., Hastjarjo, T., Kumara, A., & Adiyanti, M. (2018). Psychoeducation group for parents who raise a child with autism spectrum disorder. *COUNS-EDU: The International Journal of Counseling and Education, 3*. https://doi.org/10.23916/0020180311210

National Autism Center. (2015). *Findings and conclusions: National standards project, phase 2*. Randolph, MA: Author.

National Research Council. (2001). *Educating children with autism*. Washington, DC: The National Academies Press. https://doi.org/10.17226/10017

Nevill, R. E., Lecavalier, L., & Stratis, E. A. (2018). Meta-analysis of parent-mediated interventions for young children with autism spectrum disorder. *Autism: The International Journal of Research and Practice, 22*(2), 84–98. https://doi.org/10.1177/1362361316677838

Ngui, E. M., & Flores, G. (2006). Satisfaction with care and ease of using health care services among parents of children with special health care needs: The roles of race/ethnicity, insurance, language, and adequacy of family-centered care. *Pediatrics, 117*(4), 1184–1196. https://doi.org/10.1542/peds.2005-1088

Nordahl-Hansen, A., Fletcher-Watson, S., McConachie, H., & Kaale, A. (2016). Relations between specific and global outcome measures in a social-communication intervention for children with autism spectrum disorder. *Research in Autism Spectrum Disorders, 29–30*, 19–29. https://doi.org/10.1016/j.rasd.2016.05.005

O'Brien, M. J., Pelzel, K. E., Hendrix, N. M., Schieltz, K. M., Miller, K., Call, N. A., Tsami, L., Lerman, D. C., Berg, W. K., Kopelman, T. G., Wacker, D. P., & Lindgren, S. D. (2021). Parent ratings of generalized and indirect effects of functional communication training for children with autism spectrum disorder. *Behavior Modification, 46*(5), 971–1001. https://doi.org/10.1177/01454455211018815

Oono, I. P., Honey, E. J., & McConachie, H. (2013). Parent-mediated early intervention for young children with autism spectrum disorders (ASD). *Cochrane Database of Systematic Reviews, 4*. https://doi.org/10.1002/14651858.CD009774.pub2

Parellada, M., Boada, L., Moreno, C., Llorente, C., Romo, J., Muela, C., & Arango, C. (2013). Specialty care programme for autism spectrum disorders in an urban population: A case-management model for health care delivery in an ASD population. *European Psychiatry, 28*, 102–109. https://doi.org/10.1016/j.eurpsy.2011.06.004

Park, M. N., Moulton, E. E., & Laugeson, E. A. (2022). Parent-assisted social skills training for children with autism spectrum disorder: PEERS for preschoolers. *Focus on Autism and Other Developmental Disabilities*, 38, 80–89. https://doi.org/10.1177/10883576221110158

Patra, S., Arun, P., & Chavan, B. S. (2015). Impact of psychoeducation intervention module on parents of children with autism spectrum disorders: A preliminary study. *Journal of Neurosciences in Rural Practice*, *6*(4), 529–535. https://doi.org/10.4103/0976-3147.165422

Postorino, V., Sharp, W. G., McCracken, C. E., Bearss, K., Burrell, T. L., Evans, A. N., & Scahill, L. (2017). A systematic review and meta-analysis of parent training for disruptive behavior in children with autism spectrum disorder. *Clinical Child and Family Psychology Review*, *20*(4), 391–402. https://doi.org/10.1007/s10567-017-0237-2

Pottie, C. G., Cohen-Filipic, J., & Ingram, K. M. (2009). Parenting a child with autism: Contextual factors associated with enhanced daily parental mood. *Journal of Pediatric Psychology*, *34*(4), 419–429. https://doi.org/10.1093/jpepsy/jsn094

Ratliff-Black, M., & Therrien, W. (2021). Parent-mediated interventions for school-age children with ASD: A meta-analysis. *Focus on Autism and Other Developmental Disabilities*, *36*(1), 3–13. https://doi.org/10.1177/1088357620956904

Reaven, J., Washington, L., Moody, E. J., Stern, J. A., Hepburn, S. L., & Blakeley-Smith, A. (2015). Examining the relationship between parental anxiety and treatment response in children and adolescents with autism spectrum disorder and anxiety. *Journal of Autism and Developmental Disorders*, *45*(8), 2464–2473. https://doi.org/10.1007/s10803-015-2410-0

Remington, B., Hastings, R. P., Kovshoff, H., Degli Espinosa, F., Jahr, E., Brown, T., Alsford, P., Lemaic, M., & Ward, N. (2007). Early intensive behavioral intervention: Outcomes for children with autism and their parents after two years. *American Journal of Mental Retardation*, *112*(6), 418–438. https://doi.org/10.1352/0895-8017(2007)112[418:EIBIOF]2.0.CO;2

Research Units on Pediatric Psychopharmacology [RUPP] Autism Network. (2007). Parent training for children with pervasive developmental disorders: A multisite feasibility trial. *Behavioral Interventions*, *22*, 179–199. https://doi.org/10.1002/bin.236

Rogers, S. J., Estes, A., Lord, C., Vismara, L., Winter, J., Fitzpatrick, A., Guo, M., & Dawson, G. (2012). Effects of a brief Early Start Denver model (ESDM)-based parent intervention on toddlers at risk for autism spectrum disorders: A randomized controlled trial. *Journal of the American Academy of Child and Adolescent Psychiatry*, *51*(10), 1052–1065. https://doi.org/10.1016/j.jaac.2012.08.003

Rogers, S. J., Estes, A., Vismara, L., Munson, J., Zierhut, C., Greenson, J., Dawson, G., Rocha, M., Sugar, C., Senturk, D., Whelan, F., & Talbott, M. (2019). Enhancing low-intensity coaching in parent implemented Early Start Denver model intervention for early autism: A randomized comparison treatment trial. *Journal of Autism and Developmental Disorders*, *49*(2), 632–646. https://doi.org/10.1007/s10803-018-3740-5

Ryan, R., Berry, K., & Hartley, S. (2021). Review: Therapist factors and their impact on therapeutic alliance and outcomes in child and adolescent mental health—A systematic review. *Child and Adolescent Mental Health*, *28*, 195–211. https://doi.org/10.1111/camh.12518

Samsell, B., Lothman, K., Samsell, E. E., & Ideishi, R. I. (2022). Parents' experiences of caring for a child with autism spectrum disorder in the United States: A systematic review and metasynthesis of qualitative evidence. *Families, Systems, & Health*, *40*(1), 93–104. https://doi.org/10.1037/fsh0000654

Sanders, M. R., Prinz, R. J., & Shapiro, C. J. (2009). Predicting utilization of evidence-based parenting interventions with organizational, service-provider and client variables. *Administration and Policy in Mental Health and Mental Health Services Research*, *36*, 133–143. https://doi.org/10.1007/s10488-009-0205-3

Sarkhel, S., Singh, O. P., & Arora, M. (2020). Clinical practice guidelines for psychoeducation in psychiatric disorders general principles of psychoeducation. *Indian Journal of Psychiatry*, *62*(Suppl. 2), S319–S323. https://doi.org/10.4103/psychiatry.IndianJPsychiatry_780_19

Schertz, H. H., Odom, S. L., Baggett, K. M., & Sideris, J. H. (2013). Effects of joint attention mediated learning for toddlers with autism spectrum disorders: An initial randomized controlled study. *Early Childhood Research Quarterly*, *28*(2), 249–258. https://doi.org/10.1016/j.ecresq.2012.06.006

Schieltz, K. M., Wacker, D. P., Harding, J. W., Berg, W. K., Lee, J. F., Padilla Dalmau, Y. C., Mews, J., & Ibrahimović, M. (2011). Indirect effects of functional communication training on non-targetetd disruptive behavior. *Journal of Behavioral Education*, *20*(1), 15–32. https://doi.org/10.1007/s10864-011-9119-8

Schnabel, A., Youssef, G. J., Hallford, D. J., Hartley, E. J., McGillivray, J. A., Stewart, M., Forbes, D., & Austin, D. W. (2020). Psychopathology in parents of children with autism spectrum disorder: A systematic review and meta-analysis of prevalence. *Autism*, *24*(1), 26–40. https://doi.org/10.1177/1362361319844636

Serrata, C. A. (2012). Psychosocial aspects of parenting a child with autism. *Journal of Applied Rehabilitation Counseling, 43*(4), 29–35. https://doi.org/10.1891/0047-2220.43.4.29

Shalev, R. A., Lavine, C., & Di Martino, A. (2020). A systematic review of the role of parent characteristics in parent-mediated interventions for children with autism spectrum disorder. *Journal of Developmental and Physical Disabilities, 32*, 1–21. https://doi.org/10.1007/s10882-018-9641-x

Shanley, J. R., & Niec, L. N. (2010). Coaching parents to change: The impact of in vivo feedback on parents' acquisition of skills. *Journal of Clinical Child and Adolescent Psychology, 39*(2), 282–287. https://doi.org/10.1080/15374410903532627

Shapiro, C. J., Prinz, R. J., & Sanders, M. R. (2012). Facilitators and barriers to implementation of an evidence-based parenting intervention to prevent child maltreatment: The Triple P-positive parenting program. *Child Maltreatment, 17*(1), 86–95. https://doi.org/10.1177/1077559511424774

Shoaib, A., Cepeda, M. S., Murray, G., & Ochs-Ross, R. (2022). Autism: Comorbidities and treatment patterns in the real world, a retrospective cohort study among children, adolescents and adults newly diagnosed with autism. *Journal of Autism and Developmental Disorders, 52*(10), 4311–4320. https://doi.org/10.1007/s10803-021-05289-x

Silberman, S. (2015). *Neurotribes: The legacy of autism and the future of neurodiversity*/Steve Silberman. New York: Avery.

Skinner, B. F. (1938). *The behavior of organisms: An experimental analysis.* Cambridge, MA: B.F. Skinner Foundation.

Skinner, B. F. (1945). The operational analysis of psychological terms. *Psychological Review, 52*, 270–277. https://doi.org/10.1037/h0062535

Smith, T., Groen, A. D., & Wynn, J. W. (2000). Randomized trial of intensive early intervention for children with pervasive developmental disorder. *American Journal of Mental Retardation, 105*(4), 269–285. https://doi.org/10.1352/0895-8017(2000)105<0269:RTOIEI>2.0.CO;2

Smith, T., & Lovaas, O. I. (1998). Intensive and early behavioral intervention with autism: The UCLA Young Autism Project. *Infants and Young Children, 10*(3), 67–78. https://doi.org/10.1097/00001163-199810030-00010

Stadnick, N. A., Stahmer, A., & Brookman-Frazee, L. (2015). Preliminary effectiveness of Project ImPACT: A parent-mediated intervention for children with autism spectrum disorder delivered in a community program. *Journal of Autism and Developmental Disorders, 45*(7), 2092–2104. https://doi.org/10.1007/s10803-015-2376-y

Stahmer, A. C., Rieth, S. R., Dickson, K. S., Feder, J., Burgeson, M., Searcy, K., & Brookman-Frazee, L. (2020). Project ImPACT for Toddlers: Pilot outcomes of a community adaptation of an intervention for autism risk. *Autism: The International Journal of Research and Practice, 24*(3), 617–632. https://doi.org/10.1177/1362361319878080

Stahmer, A. C., Suhrheinrich, J., Roesch, S., Zeedyk, S. M., Wang, T., Chan, N., & Lee, H. S. (2019). Examining relationships between child skills and potential key components of an evidence-based practice in ASD. *Research in Developmental Disabilities, 90*, 101–112. https://doi.org/10.1016/j.ridd.2019.04.003

Stokes, T. F., & Baer, D. M. (1977). An implicit technology of generalization. *Journal of Applied Behavior Analysis, 10*(2), 349–367. https://doi.org/10.1901/jaba.1977.10-349

Suzuki, M., Yamada, A., Watanabe, N., Akechi, T., Katsuki, F., Nishiyama, T., Imaeda, M., Miyachi, T., Otaki, K., Mitsuda, Y., Ota, A., & Furukawa, T. A. (2014). A failure to confirm the effectiveness of a brief group psychoeducational program for mothers of children with high-functioning pervasive developmental disorders: A randomized controlled pilot trial. *Neuropsychiatric Disease and Treatment, 10*, 1141–1153. https://doi.org/10.2147/NDT.S60058

Thomas, K. C., Ellis, A. R., McLaurin, C., Daniels, J., & Morrissey, J. P. (2007). Access to care for autism-related services. *Journal of Autism and Developmental Disorders, 37*(10), 1902–1912. https://doi.org/10.1007/s10803-006-0323-7

Tiger, J. H., Hanley, G. P., & Bruzek, J. (2008). Funnctional communication training: A review and practical guide. *Behavior Analysis in Practice, 1*(1), 16–23. https://doi.org/10.1007/BF03391716

Turchi, R. M., Berhane, Z., Bethell, C., Pomponio, A., Antonelli, R., & Minkovitz, C. S. (2009). Care coordination for CSHCN: Associations with family-provider relaattions and family/child outcomes. *Pediatrics, 124*(Suppl. 4), S428–S434. https://doi.org/10.1542/peds.2009-12550

Vernon, T. W., Holden, A. N., Barrett, A. C., Bradshaw, J., Ko, J. A., McGarry, E. S., Horowitz, E. J., Tagavi, D. M., & German, T. C. (2019). A pilot randomized clinical trial of an enhanced pivotal response treatment approach for young children with autism: The PRISM model. *Journal of Autism and Developmental Disorders, 49*(6), 2358–2373. https://doi.org/10.1007/s10803-019-03909-1

Vismara, L. A., McCormick, C., Young, G. S., Nadhan, A., & Monlux, K. (2013). Preliminary findings of a telehealth approach to parent training in autism. *Journal of Autism and Developmental Disorders, 43*(12), 2953–2969. https://doi.org/10.1007/s10803-013-1841-8

Vismara, L. A., McCormick, C. E. B., Shields, R., & Hessl, D. (2019). Extending the parent-delivered Early Start Denver Model to young children with fragile X syndrome. *Journal of Autism and Developmental Disorders, 49*(3), 1250–1266. https://doi.org/10.1007/s10803-018-3833-1

Vismara, L. A., McCormick, C. E. B., Wagner, A. L., Monlux, K., Nadhan, A., & Young, G. S. (2018). Telehealth parent training in the Early Start Denver model: Results from a randomized controlled study. *Focus on Autism and Other Developmental Disabilities, 33*(2), 67–79. https://doi.org/10.1177/1088357616651064

Vismara, L. A., Young, G. S., & Rogers, S. J. (2012). Telehealth for expanding the reach of early autism training to parents. *Autism Research and Treatment, 2012*, 121878. https://doi.org/10.1155/2012/121878

Wacker, D. P., Berg, W. K., Harding, J. W., Barretto, A., Rankin, B., & Ganzer, J. (2005). Treatment effectiveness, stimulus generalization, and acceptability to parents of functional communication training. *Educational Psychology, 25*(2–3), 233–256. https://doi.org/10.1080/0144341042000301184

Wacker, D. P., Schieltz, K. M., Berg, W. K., Harding, J. W., Dalmau, Y. C. P., & Lee, J. F. (2017). The long-term effects of functional communication training conducted in young children's home settings. *Education and Treatment of Children, 40*(1), 43–56.

Waddington, H., Reynolds, J. E., Macaskill, E., Curtis, S., Taylor, L. J., & Whitehouse, A. J. (2021). The effects of JASPER intervention for children with autism spectrum disorder: A systematic review. *Autism, 25*(8), 2370–2385. https://doi.org/10.1177/13623613211019162

Webster-Stratton, C. (2006). *The Incredible Years: A trouble-shooting guide for parents of children aged 3–8.* Seattle, WA: Incredible Years Press.

Whittingham, K., Sofronoff, K., Sheffield, J., & Sanders, M. R. (2009). Stepping Stones Triple P: An RCT of a parenting program with parents of a child diagnosed with an autism spectrum disorder. *Journal of Abnormal Child Psychology, 37*(4), 469–480. https://doi.org/10.1007/s10802-008-9285-x

Wong, C., Odom, S. L., Hume, K. A., Cox, A. W., Fettig, A., Kucharczyk, S., Brock, M. E., Plavnick, J. B., Fleury, V. P., & Schultz, T. R. (2015). Evidence-based practices for children, youth, and young adults with autism spectrum disorder: A comprehensive review. *Journal of Autism and Developmental Disorders, 45*(7), 1951–1966. https://doi.org/10.1007/s10803-014-2351-z

Yoder, P. J., Stone, W. L., & Edmunds, S. R. (2021). Parent utilization of ImPACT intervention strategies is a mediator of proximal then distal social communication outcomes in younger siblings of children with ASD. *Autism, 25*(1), 44–57. https://doi.org/10.1177/1362361320946883

Yu, L., Stronach, S., & Harrison, A. J. (2020). Public knowledge and stigma of autism spectrum disorder: Comparing China with the United States. *Autism, 24*(6), 1531–1545. https://doi.org/10.1177/1362361319900839

Zhou, Y., Yin, H., Wang, M., & Wang, J. (2019). The effect of family-focused psychoeducational therapy for autism spectrum disorder children's parents on parenting self-efficacy and emotion. *Archives of Psychiatric Nursing, 33*(1), 17–22. https://doi.org/10.1016/j.apnu.2018.08.002

38

Ineffective and Harmful Treatments

Elizabeth M. Kryszak
Nationwide Children's Hospital and The Ohio State University

James A. Mulick
The Ohio State University

This chapter is different from most of the others in this book. It addresses the many incorrect notions and ineffective treatments that continue to be offered to individuals and families seeking to deal with autism spectrum disorder (ASD). There have been so many such false starts and treatment blind alleys that we have had to be selective. Our examples have been chosen to illustrate the problem and to provide a conceptual approach to recognizing the difference between a well-supported approach and an approach that might not be.

ASD is a neurodevelopmental disorder characterized by differences in communication and social interaction that vary along a dimension of severity of impact on social functioning. Such differences first manifest in early childhood and are thought to have a biological basis but are then expressed in behavior as a function of how altered neurological function leads to altered learning and adaptation to the demands of the environment. This biological influence on development and behavior continues as the individual matures and gains experiences. Because learning is continuous and depends on opportunities, long-term outcomes differ depending on the severity of biological impairment and specific life history. Human development occurs over many years, and settings differ in terms of the complexity of the demands they impose and the extent to which they require communication and social skills. For example, social avoidance sometimes seen in young children with ASD discourages early learning of language skills. Subsequently, delayed language learning can lead to avoidance of activities that require speech and related learning opportunities. Behavioral and medical research has yielded both educational and pharmaceutical intervention strategies that can partly compensate for the altered developmental influence of ASD during development. These effective intervention strategies are discussed elsewhere in this book.

Why, then, are there ineffective and pseudoscientific approaches competing for time and resources with verifiably effective alternatives? Why are they adopted by some despite their detrimental effects? The answer is human nature. People make decisions in two ways, either based on objective evidence gathered in a logical and

Elizabeth M. Kryszak, and James A. Mulick, *Ineffective and Harmful Treatments*. In: *Lifespan Treatment for Autistic Individuals*. Edited by: Peter Sturmey, Russell Lang, and James K. Luiselli, Oxford University Press. © Oxford University Press (2025). DOI: 10.1093/oso/9780197635841.003.0038 systematic manner, or based on what feels right at the time of the decision. The latter approach is likely to be strongly influenced by what has been referred to as cognitive bias, first described and characterized by Kahneman and Tversky (1972). Each person comes to interpret the world based on their perception and experience within limits imposed by how the nervous system processes information. These limitations have come to be called cognitive biases, including those related to which events are remembered and how an individual selectively pays attention to the world around them. Memory and attention, in turn, sort the world and what we do according to an orienting brain process that represents motivation and emotion. Thus, what we see, hear, understand, and act on sorts the world according to the dominant state of our fears, desires, fatigue or state of rest, hungers, thirsts, and many other biological or acquired motivational filters.

Psychologists have characterized dozens of cognitive biases as they have examined human decision-making and choice in various situations. They represent an irrational approach to decision-making that often functions to increase efficiency in the short term, but that can result in costly mistakes. For example, the *framing effect* describes how the effect of how things are presented affects decision-making (Tversky & Kahneman, 1981). This is why advertisers emphasize attractive aspects of the option they hope you will select. The flip side is that potential loss is perceived as more impactful than potential gain, a point not lost on political advertisers who hope to convince voters that the opposition will take away what voters value most. *Recency bias* makes recent events both easier to remember and to influence decisions more than past experience with similar circumstances, otherwise known as "What have you done for me lately?" (Tversky & Kahneman, 1973). Perhaps most relevant to the present discussion, *outcome bias* occurs when hearing about the success of other people makes the approach they took look more desirable than other options (Baron & Hershey, 1988). This is especially dangerous when their success was improperly understood, inapplicable to a different situation, or simply untrue. Finally, *confirmation bias* occurs when information supports what a person already believes whether or not it is relevant or applicable to the realities of the present decision-making context (World Health Organization, 2017). Many dozens of cognitive biases affecting decision-making have been described (see de Backer, 2022 for an exhaustive list), but they all boil down to relying on how things feel rather than logic and evidence to make important decisions. Scientific approaches are more likely to help selecting useful treatments than relying on feelings and intuition.

38.1 Supported Versus Unsupported Treatments

Supported treatments for ASD are characterized by a body of evidence based on sound scientific methodology. As treatments are designed and tested, they can be classified based on what evidence is available. *Well-established treatments*

(Chambless & Ollendick, 2001) have previously been defined as those that either have (1) two quality between-group design experiments demonstrating that the treatment in question is better than a placebo or other treatment, or is shown to be equivalent to an already established treatment; or (2) a large series of well-controlled single-case design experiments demonstrating efficacy. These experiments must also be conducted with well-defined treatment protocols, the characteristics of the sample must be well defined, and an independent group of researchers must be able to replicate the effects. More recently there has been discussion that this definition may not be rigorous enough (Tackett et al., 2017; Tolin et al., 2015), because it does not consider published evidence that does not support the treatment. Tolin et al. (2015) outlines a more rigorous set of criteria for determining when a treatment should be considered truly well established, which focuses on considering the entire body of evidence for an intervention, including evidence not in support of the intervention, as well as consideration of the quality of outcomes (i.e., Is the evidence only for specific symptom reduction or is there also evidence on broader improvement of functioning and quality of life?). Other chapters in this book focus on describing the current body of *well-established* treatments for ASD in detail.

Science done well is difficult. It can take significant time, money, and effort to complete a quality scientific trial that controls for other possible explanations and uses outcome measures that show a meaningful and lasting change in behavior. These results then need to be replicated by an independent group, which presents its own challenges. Therefore, testing a new intervention does not typically start with a full-fledged, double-blind randomized controlled trial (RCT) or a long series of single-case design studies. Instead, initial evidence is often gathered through case studies, pilot studies to determine if methods are feasible, or pre- or quasi-experimental studies (e.g., studies that have no control group, include a rater or evaluator who is not blinded to the participants' condition, or the outcome measure is not objective or representative of a long-term meaningful change). These are valid and important steps to determine if more investment of resources is warranted to further study the treatment. *Experimental* treatments are such interventions that are still under study (Chambless & Ollendick, 2001). Potential treatments typically start as experimental. In an ideal world, all experimental treatment would then go through a rigorous process of scientific examination that would allow them to be clearly identified as well-established or discarded as unsupported, despite any initial sign of promise. Unfortunately, as preliminary results are published, the treatment often begins to be implemented before quality experimental studies are complete, if they ever are. Many treatments will continue to live in this experimental zone for years, building a larger and larger following without garnering further evidence that what is being done works, or by continuing to publish nonexperimental or poor-quality experimental evidence leading to the appearance of a large quantity of "support" without improving the quality of the evidence. Even when some of these treatments are finally shown to be ineffective, widespread use often continues due to an established following.

The primary focus of this chapter is those treatments which eventually go on to be shown through rigorously controlled study to be *unsupported*. For the purposes of this chapter, "perpetually experimental" treatments will also be included as *unsupported*. We define interventions as "perpetually experimental" when no studies have been done with the scientific rigor needed to determine whether the treatment is safe and effective despite enough time having passed to allow for such studies to have been completed. As several examples in this chapter will show, often no further evidence is published, or a series of lower quality studies or meta-analyses continue to conclude that there is "potential" for benefit and that "further study is needed." When that further rigorous study does not occur, these ineffective treatments go on being used, leading to wasted time, money, and energy.

38.2 A Review of Unsupported Treatments

The following section describes several unsupported treatments for ASD. Due to the multitude that exists, the list is not exhaustive. Instead, we choose examples based on their popularity, now or in the past, as well as examples that illustrate particular processes that allow for these unsupported interventions to rise in popularity and continue to persist despite a lack of evidence showing they work. For each treatment, the pseudoscience theory or mechanism describing why it is *supposed* to work is provided. These theories often sound plausible on the surface, but break down upon more detailed examination. Examples chosen also illustrate how the same poor theory can underlie multiple interventions and can lead new provider groups to repackage the same ineffective mechanisms in new ways, leading unsupported interventions to find new life long after the scientific community assumed they were dead and gone. For each intervention, we also lay out the evidence for why it is classified as unsupported, often highlighting how quantity of evidence means little without quality science. Finally, we discuss how the intervention is currently being employed, how available it is, and how widely it is still used, despite the lack of support and, quite often, the associated risks.

38.2.1 Psychoanalytic Approaches

38.2.1.1 Pseudoscience Theory/Mechanism

When Leo Kanner first described autism in the 1940s, he laid out the possibility that the etiology for these symptoms could be either biological or psychogenic (Silverman, 2011). He noted that many of the symptoms seemed to have been present from an early age, suggesting biological origins, but also that many of the parents of these children seemed emotionally cold. While Bernard Rimland and others completed work in the 1960s that concluded that the origins of autism were biological, early psychodynamic theories put the onus on bad parenting (Silverman, 2011).

The social and emotional deficits associated with autism were misattributed to children coping with cold and emotionally distant parents, particularly mothers, by withdrawing from the world (Baker, 2010). These "refrigerator mothers" were described as incapable of providing emotional warmth to their children due to their own unconscious motivations supposedly caused by their own flawed upbringing. Bruno Bettelheim, who did much to popularize this theory, posited that the goal of treatment then was to rescue these children from parents who he likened to guards in a concentration camp (Cook & Willmerdinger, 2015).

38.2.1.2 Description of the Therapy

If emotionally unavailable parenting was causing autism, then it made sense that the treatment was to remove children with autism from these parents and put them in schools and institutions where they could supposedly receive needed care and emotional warmth through psychoanalytic and milieu play therapy therapeutic approaches (Cook & Willmerdinger, 2015). Parents would also often go through years of their own psychoanalytic therapy to attempt to discover how they had somehow unconsciously rejected their child, causing their child to withdraw from the world (Baker, 2010). If parents made "sufficient progress" (which was never well defined) in overcoming these unconscious predispositions, their children might be able to return home. If not, these children were institutionalized for many years, if not for the rest of their lives.

38.2.1.3 Review of Evidence Indicating That the Treatment Is Unsupported

Bettlehiem's initial accounts of miraculous progress of the children in his care have long been discredited (Severson et al., 2008). Investigation into his life and practice revealed that he did not have a degree in psychology and it is likely that many of the children he treated did not have ASD in the first place. Former patients also described the "care" they received as often physically and emotionally abusive. In the 1960s and 1970s, research regarding etiology in autism indicated that parents of children with autism did not differ in any important way from those without autism (Silverman, 2011). Instead, it became increasingly clear within the research community that autism likely had biological origins, although it would take many more years for psychogenic theories to completely lose their hold. Parent advocates, clinicians, educators, and researchers banded together to create advocacy groups, such as the National Society for Autistic Children (now the Autism Society of America), which worked to educate the public that institutionalization was ineffective and harmful (Baker, 2010). It has also been shown that children institutionalized at a young age have an increased rate of social communication difficulties and an increased risk of developing ASD (Levin et al., 2015), indicating that long-term early institutionalization would not be an effective treatment for delayed development. It should be noted that there are instances of dangerous behavior (i.e., self-injury and aggression) and psychiatric symptoms (i.e., severe depression, suicidal ideation, and psychotic symptoms) in which specialized inpatient treatment may be indicated for the safety of the individual and others and can have beneficial effects (Siegel, 2018).

38.2.1.4 Current Use of the Intervention

Institutionalization is no longer recommended as a first-line treatment for ASD. Inpatient treatment for dangerous behavior, self-injury, and psychiatric symptoms is still relatively common with approximately 11% of children with ASD being hospitalized at least once before the age of 21 (Siegel, 2018). It should be noted that the majority of these stays are short term, although some individuals may need to be in a highly supported living environment for several years, if not for the rest of their life, if the behavior is too dangerous to manage safely in an outpatient setting.

38.2.2 Holding Therapy

38.2.2.1 Pseudoscience Theory/Mechanisms

Also born from psychoanalytical roots, the theory behind holding therapy posited that the lack of bond between mothers and their autistic children created an emotional imbalance, which stopped the child being able to learn from interactions with others and led to social withdrawal (Barth et al., 2005). Holding therapy seeks to repair the mother–child bond by forcing a new emotional connection by provoking distress in the child, which then allows the mother to provide the needed comfort (Mercer, 2013).

38.2.2.2 Description of the Therapy

Early iterations of this therapy provoked child distress in a number of inhumane and dangerous ways, including having multiple people forcibly hold a child down, wrapping the child in blankets or other material, and withholding food and access to bathroom facilities (Mercer, 2013). The holding is the therapy, without specifically addressing other habilitative strategies. Following several deaths and reports of lasting trauma, this form of holding therapy unsurprisingly fell out of favor. The next iterations of the therapy advocated for the holding to be carried out by parents with a therapist coaching the parent. Parents were instructed to either hold the face of young children or to lie on older children to encourage prolonged and direct eye contact.

38.2.2.3 Review of Evidence Indicating That the Treatment Is Unsupported

There is no scientific evidence to support the use of any type of holding therapy, beyond a few case studies. Reports of child emotional distress continue even for this "gentler" form of forced eye contact (Koocher & Gill, 2015). Several studies have shown that, despite deficits in social skills, children with autism typically show a strong attachment to their parents (Rutgers et al., 2004). This research discounts the underlying theory behind holding therapy and other psychodynamic-based interventions.

38.2.2.4 Current Use of the Intervention

Given the documented physical and psychological dangers of using holding therapy, the American Psychological Association, the American Psychiatric Association, the National Association of Social Workers, and other groups have formally stated that they do not support its use (Mercer, 2013). Despite this united opposition, low levels of use continue to be reported (0.2%; Jonkman et al., 2022).

38.2.3 Gentle Teaching

38.2.3.1 Pseudoscience Theory/Mechanisms

Gentle teaching was developed in the 1980s by Dr. John McGee as a possible alternative to more traditional behavior therapy models. It is described as a nonaversive strategy to reduce challenging behavior by focusing on making individuals feel safe, loved, and connected to their caretakers, and not on changing maladaptive behavior or teaching new skills (McGee et al., 2009). It is purported that just through creating strong bonds with others in safe environments, individuals will be motivated to naturally make better choices, so more direct behavior intervention is not needed.

38.2.3.2 Description of the Therapy

Despite its description, gentle teaching does still attempt to employ a number of behavioral techniques, including errorless teaching, task analysis, environmental management, prompting, choice making, and fading assistance, but these strategies are described within this framework of "bonding with" and "valuing" the individual rather than described in more straightforward terms. The suggested benefit is that this language makes these behavior techniques more palatable to those who find the language describing behavior analytic methods to be too harsh (Arnold-Saritepe et al., 2015). Unfortunately, because the focus is more on promoting a bond and less on clear outcomes of increasing or decreasing specific forms of behavior, the behavioral principles are not taught with the level of clarity and detail needed to apply them with the fidelity and consistency needed to lead to actual behavior change.

38.2.3.3 Review of Evidence Indicating That the Treatment Is Unsupported

The 1992 review by Jones and McCaughey lays out how gentle teaching appears to repackage behavior analytic techniques under a philosophical structure that is more appealing to the wider community who care for individuals with developmental disabilities. In particular, gentle teaching explicitly highlights a need to take a wider ecological approach when considering which behaviors to change, consider how the caregivers and individuals with developmental disabilities influence each other's behaviors, and makes clear that individuals with developmental disabilities are valued. As pointed out by Bailey in his critique of this review (1992), these tenets are also embraced by behavior analysts, although they are often not well articulated to the public. With a primary focus on philosophical approach instead of operationally defined techniques, gentle teaching is difficult to study in a systematic way, particularly as definitions and emphasis on particular principles of gentle teaching shifted over time with no clear explanation or evidence to explain why (Jones & McCaughey, 1992). Reviews of the several single-case design studies assessing the effectiveness of gentle teaching concluded that this approach produces little positive change in behavior, particularly as compared to behavior analytic techniques (Arnold-Saritepe et al., 2015; Bailey, 1992; Jones & McCaughy, 1992).

38.2.3.4 Current Use of the Intervention

While few scientific studies of gentle teaching have been published in the 21st century, use of the method continues, with a few organizations continuing to promote use and provide training including Gentle Teaching International (https://gentleteaching.com/us/) and the Center for Education and Caregiving (https://www.gentleteaching.nl/gentle/en/).

38.2.4 Facilitated Communication

38.2.4.1 Pseudoscience Theory/Mechanisms

Facilitated communication (FC) began in the 1980s based on the reasonable idea that all people, including those with autism, want to communicate (Crossley et al., 1980). Somehow, proponents of FC extended this to mean that all children with autism have intact internal verbal capabilities but that they suffer from some sort of physical ailment that prevents them from being able to express themselves to their full potential either using verbal or sign language. The underlying mechanism of this physical "praxis" that autistic individuals purportedly suffer from has never been fully described or measured (Biklen, 1990; Jacobson et al., 1995). Unfortunately, this did not stop the proponents of FC from creating an intervention to address the praxis that has since become one of the most well-known unsupported treatments for autism.

38.2.4.2 Description of the Intervention

To address the purported physical praxis preventing communication, a therapist "facilitates" communication by taking the hand or arm of the individual with autism and guiding them to spell out what they want to say on a keyboard, letterboard, or adapted communication device. The facilitator is supposedly not purposefully moving the individual or cuing them in any way, even though the individual has often previously never been taught letters or learned how to spell and often is not even looking at the board or device. Somehow, just by "supporting" the person's hand or wrist or touching them on the shoulder, the often nonverbal or minimally verbal autistic person suddenly has the ability to type out their thoughts in full sentences. Despite no prior learning history or relevant exposure, these individuals are said suddenly to be able to do a range of skills that typically take years of learning and practice, including college-level academic work and writing profound poems expressing their inner emotional state (Biklen, 1990). Its advocates also stress that FC only works if the facilitator has an unshakable core belief that the individual with autism can communicate using this method. Therefore, it only works for those who have faith that it works, and simply questioning FC makes it stop working.

38.2.4.3 Review of Evidence Indicating That the Treatment Is Unsupported

FC was introduced to the world through a set of papers describing compelling and emotional accounts of individuals experiencing miraculous results and finding a voice for how awful their lives were before FC came along (Biklen, 1990, 1992; Biklen et al., 1992, 1995). Unsurprisingly, those who worked with individuals with autism asked for actual evidence that the facilitators were not just moving the person with autism's hand (Jacobson & Mulick, 1994). Several tidy experiments were completed asking autistic individuals to name pictures that their facilitator could not see or showing the person with ASD and the facilitator a series of picture sets that sometimes matched and sometimes did not (Jacobson et al., 1995; Wheeler et al., 1993). Results from these initial experiments showed undeniably that facilitators were unknowingly determining what was being typed (Jacobson et al., 1995; Wheeler et al., 1993), and a review of all FC studies from 1995 to 2000 (Mostert, 2001) comes to the firm conclusion that there is no valid evidence to support FC. Given the clarity of these results, no further valid qualitative research has been completed as there was no valid reason to continue this line of study on a clearly unproven and dangerous intervention (Beals, 2022).

It would seem like with such clear evidence that this is an unsupported treatment with a huge potential for harm and that this story should end here with FC never being used again. Unfortunately, proponents of FC disputed these results by countering that the supposed "confrontational naming" tasks used in quantitative studies violated the core tenant of FC, that FC only works if you believe FC works. Some went even further to suggest that participants only typed what their facilitator saw because they were reading the minds of their facilitators at the same time as they were attempting to type (Haskew & Donnellan, 1993). More recently, proponents of FC have claimed that the dismissal of FC as pseudoscience is "ableist" (Heyworth et al., 2022). They instead cite the body of publications that include language analysis (Saloviita, 2018), case studies using technology such as eye tracking and acceletronomy to try to show individuals are anticipating what letter the facilitators are going to put their finger on (Faure et al., 2021), facilitator opinion that FC seems real (Sipilä & Määttä, 2011), and the *facilitated* testimonials by the people with ASD that they are not being manipulated by the people facilitating them (McKee & Gomez, 2020) as evidence that the continued study of FC is valid. The many flaws in these studies aside, the larger concern is that they continue to fail to provide any experimental evidence of the underlying tenet of FC, that messages provided by autistic individuals using FC are authored by the autistic individuals themselves (Beals, 2022).

38.2.4.4 Current Use of the Intervention

A large majority of those working with autistic individuals understand that FC is not supported. Several large organizations, including the American Psychological Association (1994), American Academy of Child and Adolescent Psychiatry (2008), American Psychiatric Association, and the American Speech-Language-Hearing Association (2018), have all put out clear statements condemning the use of FC. Despite clear evidence indicating it is not a real treatment, FC continues to live on. A recent study indicated that 0.7% of participants had used FC (Jonkman et al., 2022). The Inclusion and Communication Initiatives (formerly the Institute on Communication and Inclusion, which was formerly the Facilitated Communication Institute), housed in the Syracuse University's Center on Disability and Inclusion, continues to provide training for those who would like to be facilitators of FC (https://disabilityinclusioncenter.syr.edu/). FC also continues to crop up in popular culture. A recent article in *Autism Parenting Magazine* describes the possible pros and cons of FC, including that there does not seem to be any research supporting it, and yet still the article somehow concludes: "With all this in mind, is FC beneficial? It depends on the person" (Ansell Efler, 2022).

38.2.5 Animal-Assisted Intervention

38.2.5.1 Pseudoscience Theory/Mechanisms

Animal-assisted intervention (AAI) is a broad term to refer to any intervention using an animal to provide therapeutic benefit based on a positive relationship between the client and the animal. Many people, including many people with ASD, like animals. There is some research available showing that interacting with animals can have a small to medium effect on stress reduction (Crossman, 2017), including decreasing cortisol levels (Crossman et al., 2020). There is also documentation in popular media of individual autistic children who have developed strong relationships with an animal that seem to have contributed to decrease in behavior concerns associated with ASD and helped to encourage social relationships (Grandin et al., 2015). This led to a theory that perhaps using animals in a therapeutic context could systematically aid in improving social interaction skills for a larger group of children with autism. There are several proposed mechanisms for how AAI supposedly can accomplish improved social interactions (Grandin et al., 2015). First, animals may be "social catalysts" and serve as a transitional relationship (i.e., first the child builds relationships with animals and then they can do so with others). Second, they may reduce general stress, allowing the child to feel more comfortable engaging in stressful activities like social interactions. Third, it has been suggested that both animals and autistic individuals are "sensory-based thinkers" in that they process information in sensory terms (e.g., pictures, smells, sounds) rather than as words. As such, perhaps people with ASD can communicate more easily with animals than with other people, although it is unclear then how this would lead to improved social interactions with people. Although these various generalized mechanisms have been suggested for why AAI may be beneficial, the field of AAI appears to lack one unifying empirically supported theoretic framework on which interventions are based (Davis et al., 2015), which likely explains why there is very little consistency in what constitutes AAI.

38.2.5.2 Description of the Intervention

AAI is difficult to describe as a unified treatment due to the large amount of variation in practice (Davis et al., 2015). It includes both animal-assisted therapy, where an animal is employed in a treatment protocol with set therapeutic goals, and animal-assisted activities, which involve pairing an animal with a person with the goal of general positive benefit with no set activities or goals. AAI is provided by a range of both clinicians (e.g., psychologists, occupational therapists, speech therapist) and nonclinicians (e.g., animal trainers, riding instructors, "dog guides") using a plethora of animals, most often dogs and horses, but also dolphins, guinea pigs, llamas, and rabbits. How often the therapy takes place varies widely, with durations varying from a few weeks to several years. What activities are done also varies with some AAI's pairing other interventions (i.e., social skills training) with time spent with the animal, others focusing more on building skills with the animal (i.e., learning to care for and ride a horse), and still others with no set activities other than to spend time with the animal.

38.2.5.3 Review of Evidence Indicating That the Treatment Is Unsupported

Reviews of the literature report some positive and many mixed findings (Davis et al., 2015; Hardy & Weston, 2020, Marino & Lilienfeld, 2007; O'Haire, 2013, 2017; Rehn et al., 2023; Trzmiel et al., 2019). More importantly, the vast majority of studies reviewed were found to have a host of methodological flaws. These include nonexperimental designs, small sample sizes, use of anecdotal evidence, nonstandard outcome measures designed for the specific intervention, outcome measures only completed by parents or clinicians who were not blinded to the treatment condition, lack of control for the effect of other concurrent interventions, comparing intervention only to waitlist controls (particularly problematic when attempting to determine if the animal is the key component of the intervention), no measurements of treatment fidelity, and lack of detail describing the independent variables. Concerns were also noted for safety risks to both participants and animals. Therefore, there is no current convincing evidence that AAI leads to any *objective* changes in social or communication variables related to ASD.

AAI is an excellent example of a "perpetually experimental" intervention. Despite decades' worth of research resulting in no conclusive evidence showing that AAI leads to meaningful long-term changes in skills or behavior for autistic individuals, many reviews and meta-analyses somehow concluded that AAI was at least partially supported (Davis et al., 2015 and Marino & Lilienfeld, 2007 are noted exceptions). While noting the significant flaws in the available research, reviewers often describe AAI as "may be useful" (Trzmiel et al., 2019), "promising" (O'Haire, 2013), "may have positive effects" (Rehn et al., 2023), and "supported but in need of more evidence" (Hardy & Weston, 2020; O'Haire, 2017; Sissons, 2022), seemingly because there are also no well-done published experimental studies showing firmly that AAI does not work. Despite this lack of firm evidence, many clinicians and medical staff (Marino & Lilienfeld, 2007; Yap et al., 2017), autistic adults (Benevides et al., 2020), and parents of children with ASD (London et al., 2020) support AAI. This persistence likely is related to how much people generally seem to like interacting with animals. Therefore, the idea of being able to intervene with ASD using activities with animals has good face validity, despite no firm evidence of it improving the social functioning of children with ASD.

38.2.5.4 Current Use of the Intervention

AAI remains a widely available intervention with equine therapy being the most commonly available and canine-assisted therapy coming in second (Sissons, 2022). A recent study indicated that use of AAI ranged from around 5% with horses, 2% with dogs, 0.3% with dolphins, and 0.4% with other animals (Jonkman et al., 2022).

38.2.6 Sensory integration Therapy

38.2.6.1 Pseudoscience Theory/Mechanisms

Sensory integration therapy proposes that the core difficulty underlying ASD and other psychiatric disorders like attention-deficit/hyperactivity disorder, and learning disabilities is disordered "sensory processing." This is explained vaguely as disordered neurobiological organization and interpretation of sensory stimuli coming from the body and the environment (Borkowska, 2017). These sensory processing disorders supposedly involve a lack of ability to use information received by the senses to efficiently function in everyday life. While sensory differences and/or an unusual interest in sensory aspects of the environment is one of the four categories of restricted and repetitive behavior associated with ASD (American Psychiatric Association, 2013), there is no evidence that a lack of sensory integration is what is interfering with higher order social, cognitive, or adaptive functioning for these individuals (Smith et al., 2015). The nervous system is not a linear pathway where dysfunction in a lower order system would prevent the functioning of a higher order system, but instead it is a network of co-occurring systems. This is why individuals with other sensory impairments (e.g., blindness, deafness, motor impairment) are still often capable of average cognitive functioning (Smith et al., 2015). Sensory processing disorders also include a list of possible symptoms so long it is difficult to imagine that this describes a solitary syndrome: over- or undersensitivity to touch, movement, sights, or sounds; being easily distracted; having social and/or emotional problems; having an activity level that is unusually high or unusually low; showing physical clumsiness or apparent carelessness; being impulsive and lacking in self-control; having difficulty making transitions from one situation to another; having the inability to unwind or calm oneself; having a poor self-concept; or having delays in speech, language, or motor skills (Jacobson et al., 2015). As is likely apparent when reviewing this list, there is a strong overlap between this supposed disorder and other well-recognized disorders such as ASD, attention-deficit/hyperactivity disorder, and anxiety disorders, and it has been shown that sensory processing disorders are rarely diagnosed independently of another disorder (Borkowska, 2017). There is also no empirical evidence to suggest that most of these behaviors are "sensory" in nature, and even for those that do have a sensory component, there is no evidence that addressing these sensory integration problems will lead to any meaningful outcomes in learning or adaptive functioning (Jacobson et al., 2015). While still common in the field of occupational therapy, sensory processing disorders remain unrecognized in the most well-known and widely used medical, psychiatric, or psychological nomenclatures, including the *Diagnostic and Statistical Manual*, 5th edition (*DSM-5*; American Psychiatric Association, 2013) and the *International Classification of Diseases*, 10th edition (ICD-10, World Health Organization, 2019).

38.2.6.2 Description of the Intervention

Sensory integration therapy (SIT) was first described in the 1960s (Ayres, 1963) and has continued to be a popular intervention among occupational therapists in school and outpatient settings. SIT involves creating a specific, individualized "sensory diet" of different physical activities and exercises that the child practices. Specific interventions include proprioceptive stimulation (e.g., providing deep pressure by squeezing the child in gym pads, brushing the child's body, joint compression, weighted vests, weighted blankets, and playing with textured toys) and vestibular stimulation activities (e.g., swinging, rolling, jumping on a trampoline) (Smith et al., 2015). The Ayres SIT method also emphasizes an "active collaboration" between the child and therapist, including a solid therapeutic relationship, engaging the child through play, regularly assessing progress on individualized goals, and adjusting the intervention as needed (Schoen et al., 2019).

38.2.6.3 Review of Evidence Indicating That the Treatment Is Unsupported

A large body of published research spanning the last several decades has attempted in every which way to show the effectiveness of SIT therapies. Unfortunately, systematic reviews also continue to be published concluding that there is little to no evidence supporting actual changes in behavior that would meaningfully improve a child's quality of life (Hyatt et al., 2009; Lang et al., 2012; Smith et al., 2015; Weitlauf et al., 2017). A recent review (Schoen et al., 2019) concluded that there was support for SIT, although several concerns should be noted with this review. Although 19 studies were identified as possible candidates, only 3 studies were determined to be appropriate for detailed analysis. This therefore excluded several studies included in previous reviews. The authors explained that they only wanted to include studies that accurately adhered to the Ayres SIT method, but this meant that they had to exclude studies that included children with an IQ below 65, as SIT would have to be modified too much for these children. Since a large number of children, especially young children with ASD, have significantly delayed cognitive functioning, this would bias the sample for whom SIT was supposedly beneficial. The review also excluded ABAB reversal designs because the removal of SIT "is not expected to produce a return to baseline" (Schoen et al., 2019, p. 9). They did not address that many of the ABAB studies excluded actually showed no significant change in baseline levels of behavior following the introduction of the sensory intervention (see Smith et al., 2015 for a summary). They also glossed over the methodological flaws included in the three studies they did review, including one that did not randomize the sample, standardized measures that were completed by individuals not fully blinded, and that outcome measures were often individualized to the child and therefore problematic to compare in group analyses. There are also few studies comparing the components of SIT to determine if it is truly the *sensory* part of the intervention that leads to any perceived change. Children with and without ASD enjoy many of the activities employed by SIT. As noted previously, SIT involves using these activities to actively engage and interact with children, which is comparable to how applied behavior analysts use preferred activities to motivate children to engage in the learning communication and social skills. Therefore, it is very possible that gains in communication and social skills noted by parents and teachers in studies such as those outlined by Schoen et al. (2019) are not caused by some sort of unproven sensory integration, but by the unintended direct practice of social and communication skills while engaging in an enjoyable activity (Smith et al., 2015). A recent RCT was completed comparing SIT to treatment as usual (i.e., occupational therapists giving advice orally or through written materials on how to use sensory strategies to increase behavior regulation) (Randell et al., 2022). This study showed no significant improvement in the primary outcome of decreased irritability and secondary outcomes of adaptive functioning and socialization for children who received SIT over those who received treatment as usual. While it was shown that caregivers and therapists initially perceived general positive changes related to SIT, no changes in standardized measures was found. It was also shown that SIT was more expensive, therefore indicating a waste of resources compared to treatment as usual. While there are no studies comparing SIT to behavior interventions focused on skill acquisition, direct comparisons of SIT and behavior therapy focused on addressing challenging behavior show that behavioral interventions reliably decrease challenging behavior, while SIT has no demonstrable effects on the same behaviors (Addison et al., 2012; Cox et al., 2009; Devlin et al., 2009, 2011; Lydon et al., 2017).

38.2.6.4 Current Use of the Intervention

Despite a vast body of evidence showing little effect, sensory integration remains one of the most frequently used interventions available for children with ASD, with an estimated 95% of occupational therapist using this intervention (Schaaf et al., 2018). This is likely related to several factors, including that it is widely available and far easier to access than applied behavior analysis (ABA). Like many pseudoscience interventions, the theory behind it also sounds simple and plausible to families, oversimplifying a complex neurodevelopmental disorder into one core, although vaguely defined, deficit that can be addressed through simple often enjoyable activities (Smith et al., 2015). Unfortunately, this leads families investing valuable resources into an unproven intervention, often at the expense of delaying or missing out on far more helpful behavior interventions. Promisingly, a recent study indicated that 9% of participants reported accessing SIT (Jonkman et al., 2022), indicating its use may be on the decline.

38.2.7 Audio Integration Treatments

38.2.7.1 Pseudoscience Theory/Mechanisms

Audio integration treatment (AIT) is another group of therapies that overextend the importance of sensory differences seen in autism (Sinha et al., 2011), particularly that many children with ASD experience sensitivity to certain sounds. AIT was first developed in France in the 1960s and became popular in the United States for the treatment of ASD in the 1990s (Mudford & Cullen, 2015). Similar to SIT, the founders of AIT suggested that sensitivity to sound somehow more broadly limits people's ability to learn and pay attention. "By re-educating the hearing process," individuals would be able to better integrate and process auditory information which would translate into improved learning and behavior associated with a variety of disorders, including ASD (Sinha et al., 2011, p. 1), a theory which has no basis in what is currently known about auditory functioning.

38.2.7.2 Description of the Intervention

AIT is an example of an unsupported treatment that continues to be repackaged under different names. The original AIT method uses exposure to recorded music played at loud volumes, from which the sound frequencies supposedly identified as being associated with "hyperacuity" have been removed (Sinha et al., 2011). The Tomatis Method attempts to achieve the same aim using a device called the "electronic ear" to deliver an electrically modified human voice (Sinha et al., 2011). Samonas sound therapy uses a combination of modified human voices, music, and sounds of nature to reduce sensory difficulties (Sinha et al., 2011). The most recent iteration, integrated listening systems, combines modified sounds with other movement-based sensory interventions (Schoen et al., 2015). There is a large amount of variability in implementation of all AIT variations, including no uniform lengths of sessions or volumes, complicating evaluation attempts.

38.2.7.3 Review of Evidence Indicating That the Treatment Is Unsupported

AIT was popularized, like many pseudoscience treatments, through a compelling narrative. *The Sound of a Miracle: A Child's Triumph Over Autism* describes an unbelievable story of a child completely recovering from both autism and schizophrenia following just 10 hours of AIT (Stehli, 1991). Since this initial emotional account, a few other case studies reported changes in language and behavior functioning following AIT, although there was no control to account for other concurrent therapies or maturation (Gerritsen, 2010). A few controlled studies were attempted to illustrate therapeutic benefits from the use of AIT (Edelson et al., 1999; Edelson & Rimland, 2001), although outcome measures have been primarily behavior checklists completed by parents or therapists. Comprehensive reviews taking into account the numerous methodological flaws of current research concluded that there is no evidence that AIT leads to meaningful change in language, cognitive skills, or behavior (Sinha et al., 2011; Villasenor et al., 2018). Furthermore, there are concerns that the therapy could actually harm hearing if done inappropriately (Sinha et al., 2011).

38.2.7.4 Current Use of the Intervention

With these safety concerns and lack of evidence to support this method, use appears to be relatively low (0.4–0.2%; Jonkman et al., 2022). Like many unsupported therapies, however, AIT continues to be repackaged and presented as something new. While only one uncontrolled pilot study has been published looking at initial feasibility of using the newest iteration of integrated listening systems for ASD (Schoen et al., 2015), the treatment has already been widely marketed to families as a possible intervention.

38.2.8 Craniosacral Therapy and Chiropractic Care

38.2.8.1 Pseudoscience Theory/Mechanisms

Craniosacral therapy (CST) traces its roots back to the early 19th century to the introduction of cranial osteopathy (Kratz et al., 2017). Cranial osteopathy proposed that the root of various brain and body dysfunctions was related to the placement of cranial bones and sutures. In the 1970s, Upledger and colleagues extended this theory specifically to ASD, proposing that ASD symptoms were the result of "restrictions" in the meningeal tissues and the cerebral spinal fluid that make up the craniosacral system. Proponents of CST claim to be able to restore the "rhythm" of cerebral spinal fluid by gently touching, massaging, and manipulating the bones of the skull. Studies investigating the underpinnings of this claim found no movement of bony sutures or alteration of cerebral spinal fluid pressure could be demonstrated in a laboratory model or in humans (Levy & Hyman, 2008).

Proponents of chiropractic care similarly suggest that autism symptoms can somehow be relieved through proper spine alignment and the reduction of pressure on spinal nerves. Little detail is given about why poor spinal alignment would cause these symptoms in the first place, other than vague suggestions that the pressure on nerves from poor spinal alignment causes poor brain functioning (Jennings & Barker, 2006). Some chiropractors have gone so far as to suggest that chiropractic care should be a primary treatment for ASD, aligning with the anti-vaccine and anti-behavior treatment communities (Gleberzon, 2006).

38.2.8.2 Description of the Intervention

CST uses gentle force of no greater than 5 grams, or the weight of a nickel, to release restrictions in the nervous system (Upledger Institute International, https://www.upledger.com/therapies/index.php). The therapy involves a 10-step process that allows the therapist to become familiar with each client's various tensions, vibrations, and natural rhythms through touching and massaging the person's head (Kratz et al., 2017). The protocol also allows plenty of room for improvisation, as the therapist becomes familiar with the client's "energy." In fact, Upledger claimed that those in touch with their creative side were particularly good at the therapy, while those skeptical of the therapy were far less likely to be able to feel these subtle natural rhythms (Upledger, 1995).

Chiropractic care involves applying various amounts of pressure on various parts of the spine to realign vertebrae into proper alignment. Which parts of the spine are addressed with what movements appear to vary based on the individual (Alcantara et al., 2011).

38.2.8.3 Review of Evidence Indicating That the Treatment Is Unsupported

Upledger reportedly did research on using CST with children with ASD from 1978 to 1980, but unfortunately, he and his team were "too busy doing the work to summarize it" (Upledger, 1995, p. 23). He also reported that they were unable to document their remarkable findings because they "could find no independent specialist who seemed able to objectively rate the behavior of autistic children in any way that would lend itself to statistical analysis" (Upledger, 1995, p. 23). Like many pseudoscience therapies, the majority of support that has followed consists of emotionally charged case studies and testimonials, which unsurprisingly indicate that families and practitioners who invest their money and energy into doing the therapy like it, despite the lack of evidence of objective behavior change (Kratz et al., 2017). There continues to be no RCTs or quality single subject research studies showing any definitive support for this treatment reducing symptoms related to autism (Kratz et al., 2017; Levy & Hyman, 2008).

Chiropractic care also remains unsupported for treating symptoms of ASD. While there are several case studies, cohort studies, and even a supposed "randomized control" study stating that chiropractic care led to positive changes in children with ASD (Alcantara et al., 2011), these studies were all methodologically flawed. The primary outcome measure in the majority of studies was parent or clinician *unblinded* report, and none of the studies included a control group. Therefore, there was no way of accounting for the effect of other interventions that the child may have been receiving during the time each study was conducted or even the effects of natural maturation. Even in the RCT, the only groups compared were two different chiropractic treatments, and there was no objective measure of behavior change. Other chiropractors note concern about the suggestion of using chiropractic care as a frontline treatment for ASD, citing the lack of evidence along with the existence of behavior therapies with strong research support (Gleberzon, 2006).

38.2.8.4 Current Use of the Intervention

This lack of scientific evidence supporting CST did not stopped Upledger and many others from using and widely marketing the therapy for the last 4 decades with an incredible wide range of difficulties and disorders, including autism. Current use appears to be low but still present, with almost 3% of participants in a current study reporting using CST (Jonkman et al., 2022). The Upledger Institute also continues to offer trainings and to sell a variety of products to potential clients and therapists (https://www.upledger.com). Chiropractic care also continues to be used regularly, with just over 5% of families in a recent study indicating they had accessed this intervention (Owen-Smith et al., 2015).

38.2.9 Hypobaric Oxygen Therapy

38.2.9.1 Pseudoscience Theory/Mechanisms

Hyperbaric oxygen therapy (HBOT) has its roots in the purported neuroinflammation theory of ASD. Neuroinflammation of the central nervous system refers to a proliferation and increase in sustained functioning of the glial cells, which typically occurs after injury, infection, or disease (Matta et al., 2019). It has been proposed that autism might be caused by such inflammation affecting brain functioning and development. Support for this theory remains slim at this time, with proponents primarily relying on data from case studies, postmortem studies in people with autism, and animal models (Goldfarb et al., 2016; Matta et al., 2019). HBOT is legitimately used to treat inflammation related to decompression sickness, a disorder resulting from the formation of inert gas bubbles in the body in response to rapidly declining partial pressures (e.g., ascending too quickly to the surface when scuba diving), as well as inflammatory conditions such as chronic diabetic ulcers. Therefore, proponents theorize that if ASD is caused by inflammation, HBOT could also be used to decrease this inflammation and therefore reduce symptoms of ASD. This is a dangerous theory to test, given the risks of the treatment.

38.2.9.2 Description of Intervention

HBOT involves enclosing an individual in a pressurized chamber, which allows the person to inhale up to 100% oxygen at a pressure greater than one atmosphere. This process allows high concentrations of oxygen to be delivered more deeply into tissues than would normally occur (Goldfarb et al., 2016). Treatment can vary based on the level of oxygen (20–100%), amount of pressure used (up to 1.5 is purported to be "safe" for children with ASD; Rossignol et al., 2012, how long the individual is in the chamber (sessions typically were an hour for studies reviewed; Goldfarb et al., 2016), and how often the treatment is administered (sessions ranged from 10 to 80 minutes for studies reviewed; Goldfarb et al., 2016; Podgórska-Bednarz & Perenc, 2021). Common side effects include barotrauma, which is physical damage to body tissue due to changes in air pressure (2% incidence), sinus squeeze, serous otitis, claustrophobia, reversible myopia, and new-onset seizure (Rossignol et al., 2012).

38.2.9.3 Review of Evidence Indicating That the Treatment Is Unsupported

HBOT is validated for use in treating a variety of medical conditions, but ASD is not one of them. Several initial case studies and uncontrolled pilot studies indicated some possible benefits (Rossignol et al., 2012), but as with many pseudoscience treatments, these benefits did not hold up in more rigorous studies. Multiple RCTs have shown no indication that HBOT significantly reduces symptoms of ASD or improves functioning for these individuals (Goldfarb et al., 2016; Podgórska-Bednarz & Perenc, 2021).

38.2.9.4 Current Use of the Intervention

Given the clear dangers present with this therapy, consumer warnings have been issued by the US governmental agencies that HBOT is not approved for treating autism and could be potentially harmful (United States Department of Health and Human Services, Food and Drug Administration, 2019). The treatment is also costly ($250–$600 per session) and is not typically covered by insurance since the use of HBOT for autism is considered off-label (Katz, 2022). Despite the lack of evidence, concern for harm, and high cost, some promotion of HBOT as a treatment for autism continues, as shown by a recent article in an autism parenting magazine concluding that "Multiple studies show that hyperbaric oxygen therapy can help to alleviate the symptoms of autism in children and adults" (Andersen, 2022). Fortunately, current use is very low, with only one participant (0.1%) in a recent study endorsing use of this therapy (Jonkman et al., 2022).

38.2.10 Dietary Interventions

38.2.10.1 Pseudoscience Theory/Mechanisms

Children with ASD do appear to have a high prevalence of gastrointestinal concerns, with almost half of autistic individuals experiencing some level of gastrointestinal distress (Holingue et al., 2018). This has led many to look for a connection among ASD, gut health, and brain functioning. One example that has become particularly popular is the opioid excess theory, which posits that ASD is supposedly caused by digestion problems with certain foods containing proteins related to opioid activity (Mari-Bauset et al., 2014). While these proteins do exist in the intestines, where this pseudoscience theory differs from accepted knowledge on digestive health is the idea that the intestinal mucosa in autistic people is somehow more permeable. This "leaky gut" is then purported to allow proteins associated with opioid activity to move intact into the bloodstream and across the blood-brain barrier, where they reportedly affect brain functioning. Multiple studies have shown no support for this theory by highlighting that people with ASD do not have a higher concentration of opioid peptides in blood plasma, the nervous system, or urinary excretion (Mari-Bauset et al., 2014). Unfortunately, lack of support for the underlying mechanisms of opioid excess theory and other brain-gut theories of ASD has not prevented the wide implementation of multiple popular dietary interventions.

38.2.10.2 Descriptions of the Intervention

Dietary interventions consist of changing the diet by either systematically removing or adding a substance. Elimination diets involve removing one particular food type or ingredient from a person's diet that is thought to be causing physical difficulties. Two of the most popular elimination diets for ASD involve (1) eliminating the intake of dairy products, which all contain casein, and (2) not eating any food containing gluten (e.g., wheat, oats, barley, and rye flours, bread, cereals, pasta). This is because gluten and casein are thought to be sources of "exorphins," which are the peptides implicated by the opioid excess theory (Mari-Bauset et al., 2014).

Digestive enzymes, vitamins, and supplements are common dietary interventions for ASD that involve adding a substance. Particular digestive enzymes are thought to improve the digestion of proteins like gluten and casein by breaking down the exorphins into smaller peptides that do not have opioid activity (Saad et al., 2015). This in turn will supposedly reduce the characteristics of autism. Several vitamins and dietary supplements, including secretin (Sokolski & Wachtel, 1998); omega 3 fatty acids (James et al., 2011; Li et al., 2018); vitamin D, vitamin B6, and magnesium (Li et al., 2018; Nye & Brice, 2005); antifungal agents; and probiotics (Ng et al., 2019), have also been put forth as possible treatments for ASD under vague claims that they will improve digestive health and therefore brain functioning.

38.2.10.3 Review of Evidence Indicating That the Treatment Is Unsupported

It should be noted that gluten- and casein-free diets are supported interventions for certain medical conditions such as Celiac disease and lactose intolerance. These interventions remain unsupported, however, for treating symptoms related to ASD (Mulloy et al., 2010). While there is plenty of testimonial evidence from families and providers purporting changes in children after the introduction of such diets, these diets remain unsupported following several RCTs using objective measures of behavioral change (Mari-Bauset et al., 2014; Millward et al., 2008; Piwowarczyk et al., 2018, 2020). A recent review of all available research also concluded that there is no support for these diets (Keller et al., 2021).

Digestive enzymes similarly have been found to have little support for the treatment of ASD. Of the only two RCTs completed to assess the effectiveness of digestive enzyme therapy, the first found no evidence of improvement in symptoms and skills related to ASD (Munasinghe et al., 2010), while the second did find a very small but significant improvement in scores on the Childhood Autism Rating Scale (Saad et al., 2015). It should be noted that both articles were found to have a moderate risk for bias (Sathe et al., 2017). Therefore, there is no evidence as of yet to support the wide use of digestive enzymes to treat ASD. A similar lack of support for treating ASD symptoms was found through systematic reviews of the use of probiotics (Ng et al., 2019), vitamin B6 and magnesium (Li et al., 2018; Nye & Brice, 2005), and omega 3 fatty acids (James et al., 2011; Li et al., 2018).

All three of these types of treatments have followed a cycle often seen in non-evidence-based interventions. A few initial studies, often case studies done by the same group of authors, document miraculous results. Use of the intervention then becomes widespread, long before quality studies can be completed. This is particularly the case with dietary interventions as they are easy to access over the counter without the need to wait for specialty care. By the time controlled, double-blinded research studies with quality outcome measures showing no support are published, it is difficult to counter the flood of testimonial evidence lauding the intervention as a miracle cure.

Secretin supplementation to treat ASD provides a particularly clear example of his cycle. Secretin stimulates the secretion of digestive fluids from the pancreas and can be used by gastroenterologists during diagnostic tests to determine the etiology of intestinal complaints. A case study was published in 1998 documenting large improvements in the language and social skills of three children with ASD after they received secretin injections as part of routine gastrointestinal diagnostic tests (Sokolski & Wachtel, 1998). Sokolski and Wachtel (1998) theorized that these improvements could be related to a brain-gut interaction involving the secretin receptors in the brain, although they did indicate that more research was needed to better understand this mechanism as the function of these receptors is not understood. Before such research could be done, however, secretin supplementation became widespread, with estimates indicating that thousands of children were receiving secretin just 1 year later (Esch & Carr, 2004). Then several years later, multiple RCTs were completed showing no evidence of improvement across several areas of deficits related to ASD (Krishnaswami et al., 2011; Williams et al., 2012). The evidence was so compelling that reviewers stated that further study of secretin as a treatment for ASD was not recommended barring any drastically new evidence. This example does also show that good science can lead to a decrease in the use of unsupported treatments, as a later survey found only one family (0.2% of the sample) still using the treatment (Akins et al., 2014).

Vitamin D supplementation is currently going through this same cycle. One small group of researchers first published highly promising results for an increase in functioning through a case study (Jia et al., 2015) and further studies using parent report and unblinded clinician ratings of behavior (Jia et al., 2018). This same group then attempted to publish a randomized control study; however, several inconsistencies in the results led to an examination of the data by the journal's editors. The article was retracted after results found in the paper were unable to be replicated by the editors (Saad et al., 2019). Unfortunately, this retraction came after publication of a review by the same group discussing the connection between vitamin D and ASD, citing the retracted article as key support for this intervention (Jia et al., 2018). This shows how bad science can often continue to proliferate and confuse those seeking supported treatments, even when steps are taken to correct it.

38.2.10.4 Current Use of the Intervention

Dietary interventions continue to be widely used to treat ASD. Previous studies indicated that 16–20% of families with a child with ASD were employing alternative diets and 25–56% were using some sort of dietary supplement to attempt to treat their child's autism symptoms (Akins et al., 2014; Owen-Smith et al., 2015). A more recent study indicates possibly lower use of dietary interventions (3% using alternative diets; 5% using dietary supplements), indicating a promising downward trend. Continued use of dietary interventions, despite a lack of support, may be explained by ease of access. Diet is something families may feel more in control of and there is no waitlist for changing diet. Therefore, there is likely a feeling of "what is the harm in trying?" Unfortunately, while there may be no waitlist, these interventions are not cost-free. Costs include expense of specialty foods and supplements, further dietary restriction leading to risk of malnutrition for children who are often already extremely picky eaters, gastrointestinal irritation, and even possible limitation on certain social opportunities and further stigmatization by peers (Keller et al., 2021; Mari-Bauset et al., 2014; Millward et al., 2008).

38.2.11 Chelation

38.2.11.1 Pseudoscience Theory/Mechanisms

The pseudoscience theory that autism could somehow be caused by vaccines remains one of the most insidious, leading families to forgo well-studied preventive treatment as well as to seek out outrageous and at times dangerous treatments. This theory entraps many due to the timing of certain vaccines with the presentation of ASD symptoms. A subgroup of children with ASD goes through a period of apparently typical development and then loses skills such as language and eye contact around 18 months of age, which happens to be when the measles, mumps, and rubella (MMR) vaccine is given. Andrew Wakefield capitalized on this unfortunate coincidence by proposing an extension of the opioid excess theory, suggesting that the measles part of the MMR vaccine created a "leaky gut" for some children, leading to autism (Wakefield et al., 2010). The data he used to support this theory were largely falsified, and the original article was retracted due to severe methodological flaws, including not having approval of an institutional review board (Caplan, 2009). Unfortunately, instead of ending the proliferation of the idea that autism was caused by vaccines, Wakefield and his group turned to thimerosal, a preservative contained in several common childhood vaccines, proposing that autism was caused by mercury poisoning from the thimerosal in vaccines (Davis et al., 2013). While there have been several studies done showing clearly that vaccines do not cause autism (Davis et al., 2013; Madsen et al., 2003), this fear has led many families to choose not to give lifesaving vaccines, resulting in multiple outbreaks of measles, which can lead to lifelong cognitive disabilities in children (Phadke et al., 2020). It also has led families to look for ways to get rid of these supposedly toxic heavy metals. Chelation is one such treatment.

38.2.11.2 Description of the Intervention

Chelation is purported to remove specific metals from the body by injecting various chemical substances into the bloodstream that bind with these metals and then are excreted in the urine (Davis et al., 2013; James et al., 2015). The chemical substances used in chelation are unfortunately associated with several potential serious side effects, including fever, vomiting, diarrhea, loss of appetite, hypertension, hemorrhoid symptoms, metallic taste, hypotension, cardiac arrhythmias, and hypocalcemia, the latter of which can in turn cause fatal cardiac arrest (Davis et al., 2013).

38.2.11.3 Review of Evidence Indicating That the Treatment Is Unsupported

The use of chelation for treating symptoms related to ASD remains unsupported. Following the common pattern illustrated several times in this chapter, the research body consists of a few case studies and poorly designed experimental studies (i.e., no control group, no control for additional interventions such as behavior therapy), which primarily used anecdotal parent report as an outcome measure, although even the majority of these poorly designed studies showed mixed results at best (Davis et al., 2013; James et al., 2015). While quality randomized control studies have not yet been done, given the danger of this treatment and lack of clear results in preliminary studies, further study does not seem warranted.

38.2.11.4 Current Use of the Intervention

The Food and Drug Administration has issued statements warning consumers away from using chelation to treat autism, given the high risk for harm and lack of support (United States Department of Health and Human Services, Food and Drug Administration, 2019). Use of chelation is low, with only 0.3–4% of families endorsing using this treatment for their child with autism (Akins et al., 2014; Owen-Smith et al., 2015), although this still seems too high, given the dangers.

38.3 Why Is ASD a Target for Unsupported Treatments?

While unsupported treatments abound for almost all disorders and concerns, autism has become a particular magnet for unsupported or fad treatments. Of the over 400 different treatments that exist for ASD, most have little to no support (Frame & Casey, 2019; Matson et al., 2013), and less than half of families with a child with ASD choose a research-supported treatment (Miller et al., 2012). Research suggests that parents from a wide variety of financial, educational, and familial backgrounds are all equally likely to choose unsupported treatment options (Miller et al., 2012). Why is this population such a good target for unsupported treatments?

While much progress has been made in understanding ASD and how best to help individuals with autism, there is still much that is unknown. ASD is considered a lifelong condition that leads to significant deficits in functioning for many individuals (Steinhausen et al., 2016), and, so far, the interventions that work best are primarily learning and behavior based and come with a heavy cost in resources, including time, effort, and money. Good treatment is also difficult to obtain, and outcomes are incremental, long-term, and sometimes limited by the underlying physiological nature of the disability profile (Smith & MacDonald, 2017). Families and individuals can feel hopeless or overwhelmed when faced with possible dire prognoses and recommendations for difficult-to-access interventions. These gaps in knowledge and absence of "rapid cures" provide openings for the inception of false theories about the mechanisms of ASD and how to best address these symptoms. This leads to the creation and proliferation of unsupported treatments.

Those who develop and promote unsupported interventions do so for varying motivations. At times, profit is the primary motivator and those behind the treatment appear to have a clear intent to scam unsuspecting families out of their money. ASD has no cure and families are often desperate for a miracle, making them more susceptible to those offering to sell one. Many times, though, those perpetuating these unsupported interventions start with good intentions, truly hoping to create an intervention that helps others. At times, bad science perpetuates when these individuals succumb to pressure to publish in order to advance in their careers, leading to a focus on quantity versus quality of studies and articles. Evidence of a current "replication crisis" suggests that a large number of published results of positive treatment outcomes cannot be replicated by independent groups, which seems related to a series of questionable research practices that lead to an increase in type 1 errors or mistakenly finding support for a hypothesis (Tackett et al., 2017). This phenomenon is made more difficult to study due to a publication bias that leads editors and publishers to be less likely to publish results that show no effect of a treatment.

Still others appear to become "true believers" of the theories behind their treatments. They "know" their intervention works, as it is based on their strong beliefs about ASD and how best to treat it. This can often lead to cognitive biases that further the use of questionable research practices to find the evidence to support their intervention that they "know" is there. They deny challenges to their beliefs and often begin to build a following of other believers. Instead of being deterred by criticism from scientific peers, they see their isolation as "the indication of their intellectual courage against the dominant orthodoxy and the accompanying political correctness" (Diethelm & McKee, 2009, p. 3). No matter what the motivation is, once such misinformation is out there, it is difficult to combat.

38.4 The (Mis)information Age: The Internet, Social Media, and the Spread of Misinformation

The amount of information on autism and related interventions is overwhelming and often conflicting (Frame & Casey, 2019), and the average person does not have the time, resources, or expertise to review all available information to make evidence-based decisions on whether interventions are supported (Matson et al., 2013). Further adding to the confusion for families trying to make the right decision, professionals, including physicians, educators, psychologists, and speech, occupational, and physical therapists, often recommend unsupported treatments (Frame & Casey, 2019; McCormack et al., 2020; Miller et al., 2012). Families and individuals with autism weigh information differently than clinicians or researchers due to the cognitive biases discussed previously. Since families frequently rely on testimonials and recommendations from other parents and parent support groups more than scientific sources (Matson et al., 2013; Miller et al., 2012), they are particularly susceptible to the narrative bias, which states that personal stories are far more compelling to the human brain than scientific evidence (World Health Organization, 2017). The Internet will further play into this misinformation by showing more and more similar information and filtering out information that might counter this belief, invoking the confirmation bias, which suggests that people tend to seek information that confirms beliefs already held (World Health Organization, 2017). Algorithms of social medical platforms and Internet search engines are designed to support confirmation biases by allowing people to more easily only see information that is aligned with their beliefs. This is because the purpose of those algorithms is to reinforce maintenance of attention and additional clicks on the website. Unfortunately, it also prevents individuals from seeing a third thinking error that allows for the easy spread of misinformation is the illusory truth effect, meaning the more we hear the same information (even false information), the more likely we are to believe it is true (van der Linden, 2022). Social media platforms play into this error, as they become echo chambers where the same misinformation is repeated over and over until it falsely feels like a large body of evidence exists.

Take, for example, a family who hears about ABA from their doctor and then attempts to further "research" it through an Internet search. This search will bring up a range of information, including testimonials from many parents and autistic adults that ABA traumatizes children and turns them into robots. The fear a single article or video evokes will lead this parent to look at others, which will increase the likelihood that similar videos and testimony will pop up in their feed, playing into the effect of familiarity. These Internet search algorithms will also start to bring in other possible interventions for ASD that similar consumers have "liked" and soon the parent is seeing videos promoting a miracle supplement that "cures" autism in weeks. Given the information available to the parent at this point, it becomes easier to understand why they would be at least tempted to try such unsupported treatments.

38.4.1 How to Stop the Spread of Misinformation

Any professional who works with families of children with autism will eventually encounter a family who is considering or even already using one or more of these pseudoscience interventions. It is the ethical responsibility of all scientist-practitioners to help families make informed decisions based on sound information and to correct misinformation whenever possible to avoid wasted time and resources. Unfortunately, correcting misinformation is more complex than just telling a family that their information is wrong and providing the right information. The continued influence effect is a phenomenon where people continue to rely on misinformation in their thinking and decision-making even when they understand, believe, and later remember the correction (Paynter et al., 2019). Well-intentioned, but ineffective corrections can lead to inadvertently strengthening a person's belief in the misinformation. This typically happens due to one of four reasons (Paynter et al., 2019). First, simply retracting the information without sufficient explanation can strengthen the belief through repetition of the belief.

Second, experts often speak in an offputting authoritative manner that can lead others to resist the correction. Third, emotive manipulations (e.g., use of images of sick children when correcting vaccine myth) can backfire, potentially because of a misattribution of the evoked fear. Finally, if the misinformation is related to a strongly held worldview, the correction can be interpreted as an attack on one's core beliefs and thus be ineffective or backfire by strengthening the person's desire to defend the misbelief.

Framing the corrective message with these biases in mind can increase its acceptability. It is important to avoid arguing with families or presenting messages in an overly authoritarian fashion that leaves little room for discussion. Putting families in a position where they are arguing in support of misinformation, whether aloud or internally, can inadvertently strengthen their belief in that information. Instead, reaffirm the family's values and beliefs (e.g., "You are working so hard to find the most effective interventions to help your child be happy and achieve their full potential"). Then provide a counternarrative consistent with those beliefs (e.g., "While on the surface it sounds amazing, this intervention does not have any true support to show it is worth your valuable time and resources"; Finn, 2019). Present the correction using clear, informative language that avoids jargon, along with well-designed visuals (e.g., pictures, videos, graphs, charts, handouts) when appropriate (Paynter et al., 2019). Avoid repeating the untrue claims of the intervention as learning involves repetition, so the more false claims are repeated, in any context, the more likely they are to be remembered (Finn, 2019). Corrections tend to be most effective when they go beyond just saying that a piece of information is wrong but focus also on why it is wrong and how people came to believe this information in the first place (Paynter et al., 2019). This frame can help avoid making a family feel stupid or silly for bringing up the intervention and inoculate them against further arguments in favor of the intervention by showing them how the pseudoscience explanation was created. It is then key to end by filling the gap in knowledge by giving correct information (Paynter et al., 2019). The credibility of the source of the information can make a correction more effective, with trustworthiness being more salient than expertise information (Paynter et al., 2019). This can help explain why families can be more willing to take advice from a well-known teacher or early intervention therapist over that of a doctor with a specialty in autism. This supports the need for continuing education on effective treatment for all individuals working with families of children with autism in order to maximize the chances that families will hear correct information from those they trust.

It may also be possible to inoculate families before they come in contact with misinformation about unsupported treatments (van der Linden, 2022). This can be a particularly important role for any individuals involved in the early identification and initial diagnosis of autism. This initial set of professionals can go beyond providing information on supported interventions, by helping families understand how to evaluate any intervention they come across. Professionals can outline what they look for when judging a new intervention (e.g., "I want to see a study where they had two groups of children with autism. One group got the intervention, one did not, and then someone who did not know which intervention the children received evaluates them on a meaningful measure of change such as did their language increase"). Further, professionals can explain that many unsupported interventions will provide information that might look like "evidence," such as parent testimonials or where the person evaluating the treatment new who got which intervention, which can lead to unconsciously false results (e.g., "Any time someone puts a lot of time, energy, and money into something, they can be biased to seeing the results they want to, even if those results are not truly present"). This inoculation method can protect families from misinformation by helping foster a healthy distrust of pseudoscience from the beginning (Finn, 2019). If it sounds too good to be true, it likely is.

38.5 References

Addison, L. R., Piazza, C. C., Patel, M. R., Bachmeyer, M. H., Rivas, K. M., Milnes, S. M., & Oddo, J. (2012). A comparison of sensory integrative and behavioral therapies as treatment for pediatric feeding disorders. *Journal of Applied Behavior Analysis, 45*(3), 455–471. DOI: 10.1901/jaba.2012.45-455

Akins, C. R. S., Krakowiak, P., Angkustsiri, K., Hertz-Picciotto, I., & Hansen, R. L. (2014). Utilization patterns of conventional and complementary/alternative treatments in children with autism spectrum disorders and developmental disabilities in a population-based study. *Journal of Developmental & Behavioral Pediatrics: JDBP, 35*(1), 1. DOI: 10.1097/DBP.0000000000000013

Alcantara, J., Alcantara, J. D., & Alcantara, J. (2011). A systematic review of the literature on the chiropractic care of patients with autism spectrum disorder. *Explore, 7*(6), 384–390. DOI: 10.1016/j.explore.2011.08.00

American Psychiatric Association. (2013). *Diagnostic and statistical manual of mental disorders* (5th ed.). https://doi.org/10.1176/appi.books.9780890425596.

American Academy of Child & Adolescent Psychiatry (2008). Facilitated communication. Retrieved from https://www.aacap.org/AACAP/Policy_Statements/2008/Facilitated_Communication.aspx

American Psychological Association. (1994). Chapter XI: Scientific affairs: Facilitated communication. Retrieved from https://www.apa.org/about/policy/chapter-11

American Speech-Language-Hearing Association. (2018). Facilitated communication [Position Statement]. www.asha.org/policy/

Andersen, R. (2022, March 9). Hyperbaric oxygen therapy for autism. *Autism Parenting Magazine.* https://www.autismparentingmagazine.com/autism-hyperbaric-oxygen-therapy/

Ansell Efler, E. (2022, February 1). Facilitated communication for children with autism. *Autism Parenting Magazine.* https://www.autismparentingmagazine.com/autism-children-facilitated-communication/

Arnold-Saritepe, A. M., Mudford, O. C., & Cullen, C. (2015). Gentle teaching. In R. M. Foxx & J. A. Mulick (Eds.), *Controversial therapies for autism and intellectual disabilities* (2nd ed., pp. 65–90). London: Routledge. DOI: 10.4324/9781315754345

Ayres, A. J. (1963). The development of perceptual-motor abilities: A theoretical basis for treatment of dysfunction. *American Journal of Occupational Therapy, 17*(6), 221–225.

de Backer, G. (2022, April 22). Cognitive biases (2023): Complete list of 151 biases. https://gustdebacker.com/cognitive-biases/

Bailey, J. S. (1992). Gentle teaching: Trying to win friends and influence people with euphemism, metaphor, smoke, and mirrors. *Journal of Applied Behavior Analysis, 25*(4), 879. DOI: 10.1901/jaba.1992.25-879

Baker, J. P. (2010). Autism in 1959: Joey the mechanical boy. *Pediatrics, 125*(6), 1101–1103. DOI: 10.1542/peds.2010-084

Baron, J., & Hershey, J. C. (1988). Outcome bias in decision evaluation. *Journal of Personality & Social Psychology, 54*(4), 569. DOI: 10.1037/0022-3514.54.4.569

Barth, R. P., Crea, T. M., John, K., Thoburn, J., & Quinton, D. (2005). Beyond attachment theory and therapy: Towards sensitive and evidence-based interventions with foster and adoptive families in distress. *Child & Family Social Work, 10*(4), 257–268. DOI: 10.1111/j.1365-2206.2005.00380.x

Beals, K. P. (2022). Why we should not presume competence and reframe facilitated communication: a critique of Heyworth, Chan & Lawson. *Evidence-Based Communication Assessment and Intervention, 16*(2), 66–76. DOI: 10.1080/17489539.2022.2097872

Benevides, T. W., Shore, S. M., Palmer, K., Duncan, P., Plank, A., Andresen, M. L., Caplan, R., Cook, B., Gassner, D., Hector, B. L., Morgan, L., Nebeker, L., Purkis, Y., Rankowski, B., Wittig, K., & Coughlin, S. S. (2020). Listening to the autistic voice: Mental health priorities to guide research and practice in autism from a stakeholder-driven project. *Autism, 24*(4), 822–833. DOI: 10.1177/1362361320908410

Biklen, D. (1990). Communication unbound: Autism and praxis. *Harvard Educational Review, 60*(3), 291–315. DOI: 10.17763/haer.60.3.013h5022862vu732

Biklen, D. (1992). Typing to talk: Facilitated communication. *American Journal of Speech-Language Pathology, 1*(2), 15–17. DOI: 10.1044/1058-0360.0102.15

Biklen, D., Morton, M. W., Gold, D., Berrigan, C., & Swaminathan, S. (1992). Facilitated communication: Implications for individuals with autism. *Topics in Language Disorders, 12*(4), 1–28.

Biklen, D., Saha, N., & Kliewer, C. (1995). How teachers confirm the authorship of facilitated communication: A portfolio approach. *Journal of the Association for Persons with Severe Handicaps, 20*(1), 45–56. DOI: 10.1177/154079699502000105

Borkowska, A. R. (2017). Sensory processing disorders: Diagnostic and therapeutic controversies. *Current Issues in Personality Psychology, 5*(3), 196–205. DOI: 10.5114/cipp.2017.70140

Caplan, A. L. (2009). Retraction—Ileal-lymphoid-nodular hyperplasia, non-specific colitis, and pervasive developmental disorder in children. *The Weekly Epidemiological Record, 84*, 301–308. DOI: 10.1016/S0140-6736(97)11096-0

Chambless, D. L., & Ollendick, T. H. (2001). Empirically supported psychological interventions: Controversies and evidence. *Annual Review of Psychology, 52*(1), 685–716. DOI: 10.1146/annurev.psych.52.1.685

Cook, K. A., & Willmerdinger, A. N. (2015). The history of autism. *Narrative Documents*. 1. https://scholarexchange.furman.edu/schopler-about/1

Cox, A. L., Gast, D. L., Luscre, D., & Ayres, K. M. (2009). The effects of weighted vests on appropriate in-seat behaviors of elementary-age students with autism and severe to profound intellectual disabilities. *Focus on Autism and Other Developmental Disabilities, 24*(1), 17–26. DOI: 10.1177/108835760833075

Crossley, R., McDonald, A., & Molloy, S. P. A. (1980). *Annie's coming out*. New York: Penguin.

Crossman, M. K. (2017). Effects of interactions with animals on human psychological distress. *Journal of Clinical Psychology, 73*(7), 761–784. DOI: doi.org/10.1002/jclp.22410

Crossman, M. K., Kazdin, A. E., Matijczak, A., Kitt, E. R., & Santos, L. R. (2020). The influence of interactions with dogs on affect, anxiety, and arousal in children. *Journal of Clinical Child & Adolescent Psychology, 49*(4), 535–548. DOI: 10.1080/15374416.2018.1520119

Davis, T. N., O'Reilly, M., Kang, S., Lang, R., Rispoli, M., Sigafoos, J., Lancioni, G., Copeland, D., Attai, S., & Mulloy, A. (2013). Chelation treatment for autism spectrum disorders: A systematic review. *Research in Autism Spectrum Disorders, 7*(1), 49–55. DOI: 10.1016/j.rasd.2012.06.005

Davis, T. N., Scalzo, R., Butler, E., Stauffer, M., Farah, Y. N., Perez, S., Mainor, K., Clark, C., Miller, S., Kobylecky, A., & Kobylecky, A. (2015). Animal assisted interventions for children with autism spectrum disorder: A systematic review. *Education and Training in Autism & Developmental Disabilities, 50*(3), 316–329. DOI: http://www.jstor.org/stable/24827513

Devlin, S., Healy, O., Leader, G., & Hughes, B. M. (2011). Comparison of behavioral intervention and sensory-integration therapy in the treatment of challenging behavior. *Journal of Autism and Developmental Disorders, 41*(10), 1303–1320. DOI: 10.1007/s10803-010-1149-x

Devlin, S., Leader, G., & Healy, O. (2009). Comparison of behavioral intervention and sensory-integration therapy in the treatment of self-injurious behavior. *Research in Autism Spectrum Disorders, 3*(1), 223–231. DOI: 10.1016/j.rasd.2008.06.004

Diethelm, P., & McKee, M. (2009). Denialism: What is it and how should scientists respond? *The European Journal of Public Health, 19*(1), 2–4. DOI: 10.1093/eurpub/ckn139

Edelson, S., & Rimland, B. (2001). The efficacy of auditory integration training: Summaries and critiques of 28 reports (January, 1993—May, 2001). www.up-to-date.com/saitwebsite/aitsummary.html.

Edelson, S. M., Arin, D., Bauman, M., Lukas, S. E., Rudy, J. H., Sholar, M., & Rimland, B. (1999). Auditory integration training: A double-blind study of behavioral and electrophysiological effects in people with autism. *Focus on Autism and Other Developmental Disabilities, 14*(2), 73–81. DOI: 10.1177/108835769901400202

Esch, B. E., & Carr, J. E. (2004). Secretin as a treatment for autism: A review of the evidence. *Journal of Autism & Developmental Disorders, 34*(5), 543–556. DOI: 10.1007/s10803-004-2549-6

Faure, P., Legou, T., & Gepner, B. (2021). Evidence of authorship on messages in Facilitated Communication: A case report using accelerometry. *Frontiers in Psychiatry, 11*, 1560. DOI: ARTN 543385.10.3389/fpsyt.2020.543385

Finn, P. (2019). Countering the false promise of pseudoscience in schools. *Leader, 24*(7), 36–37. DOI: 10.1044/leader.SCM.24072019.36

Frame, K. N., & Casey, L. B. (2019). Variables influencing parental treatment selection for children with autism spectrum disorder. *Children & Youth Services Review, 106*, 1–9. DOI: 10.1016/j.childyouth.2019.104464

Gerritsen, J. (2010). The effect of Tomatis therapy on children with autism: Eleven case studies. *The International Journal of Listening, 24*(1), 50–68. DOI: 10.1080/10904010903466378

Gleberzon, B. J. (2006). Chiropractic and the management of children with autism. *Clinical Chiropractic, 9*(4), 176–181. doi.org/10.1016/j.clch.2006.06.001

Goldfarb, C., Genore, L., Hunt, C., Flanagan, J., Handley-Derry, M., Jethwa, A., Jones-Stokreef, N., Kirkpatrick, S. M. L., Richards, A., Rojnica, L., Schwartz, C., Shawn, D., Superina-Bell, D., Young, E., & Anagnostou, E. (2016). Hyperbaric oxygen therapy for the treatment of children and youth with autism spectrum disorders: An evidence-based systematic review. *Research in Autism Spectrum Disorders, 29–30*, 1–7. DOI: 10.1016/j.rasd.2016.05.004

Grandin, T., Fine, A. H., O'Haire, M. E., Carlisle, G., & Bowers, C. M. (2015). The roles of animals for individuals with autism spectrum disorder. In A. H. Fine (Ed.), *Handbook on animal-assisted therapy* (pp. 225–236). New York: Academic Press. https://doi.org/10.1016/B978-0-12-801292-5.00016-X

Hardy, K. K., & Weston, R. N. (2020). Canine-assisted therapy for children with autism spectrum disorder: A systematic review. *Review Journal of Autism and Developmental Disorders, 7*(2), 197–204. DOI: 10.1007/s40489-019-00188-5

Haskew, P., & Donnellan, A. M. (1993). *Emotional maturity and well-being: Psychological lessons of facilitated communication*. Saint Paul, MN: DRI Press.

Heyworth, M., Chan, T., & Lawson, W. (2022). Perspective: Presuming autistic communication competence and reframing facilitated communication. *Frontiers in Psychology, 13*, 938. DOI: 10.3389/fpsyg.2022.864991

Holingue, C., Newill, C., Lee, L.-C., Pasricha, P. J., & Daniele Fallin, M. (2018). Gastrointestinal symptoms in autism spectrum disorder: A review of the literature on ascertainment and prevalence. *Autism Research, 11*(1), 24–36. DOI: 10.1002/aur.1854

Hyatt, K. J., Stephenson, J., & Carter, M. (2009). A review of three controversial educational practices: Perceptual motor programs, sensory integration, and tinted lenses. *Education and Treatment of Children*, 313–342. http://www.jstor.org/stable/42900024

Jacobson, J. W., & Mulick, J. A. (1994). Facilitated communication: Better education through applied ideology. *Journal of Behavioral Education, 4*(1), 93–105. DOI: 10.1007/BF01560511

Jacobson, J. W., Mulick, J. A., Foxx, R. M., & Kryszak, E. (2015). History of fad, pseudoscientific, and dubious treatments in intellectual disabilities: From the 1800s to today. In R. M. Foxx & J. A. Mulick (Eds.). *Controversial therapies for autism and intellectual disabilities* (2nd ed., pp. 65–90). London: Routledge. DOI: 10.4324/9781315754345

Jacobson, J. W., Mulick, J. A., & Schwartz, A. A. (1995). A history of facilitated communication: Science, pseudoscience, and antiscience science working group on facilitated communication. *American Psychologist, 50*(9), 750. DOI: 10.1037/0003-066X.50.9.750

James, S., Montgomery, P., & Williams, K. (2011). Omega-3 fatty acids supplementation for autism spectrum disorders (ASD). *Cochrane Database of Systematic Reviews, 11*, CD007992. DOI: 10.1002/14651858.CD007992.pub2

James, S., Stevenson, S. W., Silove, N., & Williams, K. (2015). Chelation for autism spectrum disorder (ASD). *Cochrane Database of Systematic Reviews, 5*. DOI: 10.1002/14651858.CD010766.pub2

Jennings, J., & Barker, M. (2006). Autism: A chiropractic perspective. *Clinical Chiropractic, 9*(1), 6–10. DOI: 10.1016/j.clch.2005.08.001

Jia, F., Shan, L., Wang, B., Li, H., Miao, C., Xu, Z., Lin, C., & Saad, K. (2018). Bench to bedside review: Possible role of vitamin D in autism spectrum disorder. *Psychiatry Research, 260*, 360–365. DOI: 10.1016/j.psychres.2017.12.005

Jia, F., Wang, B., Shan, L., Xu, Z., Staal, W. G., & Du, L. (2015). Core symptoms of autism improved after vitamin D supplementation. *Pediatrics, 135*(1), e196–e198. DOI: 10.1542/peds.2014-2121

Jones, R. S., & McCaughey, R. E. (1992). Gentle teaching and applied behavior analysis: A critical review. *Journal of Applied Behavior Analysis, 25*(4), 853–867. DOI: 10.1901/jaba.1992.25-853

Jonkman, K. M., Back, E., Staal, W. G., Benard, L., van der Doelen, D. M., & Begeer, S. (2022). Alternative treatments for autism: Prevalence and predictors. *Research in Autism Spectrum Disorders, 98*, 1–11. DOI: 10.1016/j.rasd.2022.102046.

Kahneman, D., & Tversky, A. (1972). Subjective probability: A judgment of representativeness. *Cognitive Psychology, 3*(3), 430–454. DOI: 10.1016/0010-0285(72)90016-3

Katz, A. (2022, September 1). How much does hyperbaric oxygen therapy cost? Hyperbaric Medical Solutions. https://www.hyperbaricmedicalsolutions.com/blog/how-much-does-hyperbaric-oxygen-therapy-cost

Keller, A., Rimestad, M. L., Friis Rohde, J., Holm Petersen, B., Bruun Korfitsen, C., Tarp, S., Lauritsen, M. B., & Händel, M. N. (2021). The effect of a combined gluten-and casein-free diet on children and adolescents with autism spectrum disorders: A systematic review and meta-analysis. *Nutrients, 13*(2), 470. DOI: 10.3390/nu13020470

Koocher, G. P., & Gill, E. (2015). Pet me, sniff me, squeeze me: Quack treatment for autism. In R. M. Foxx & J. A. Mulick (Eds.), *Controversial therapies for autism and intellectual disabilities* (2nd ed., pp. 65–90). London: Routledge. DOI: 10.4324/9781315754345

Kratz, S. V., Kerr, J., & Porter, L. (2017). The use of craniosacral therapy for autism spectrum disorders: Benefits from the viewpoints of parents, clients, and therapists. *Journal of Bodywork & Movement Therapies, 21*(1), 19–29. DOI: 10.1016/j.jbmt.2016.06.006

Krishnaswami, S., McPheeters, M. L., & Veenstra-vanderweele, J. (2011). A systematic review of secretin for children with autism spectrum disorders. *Pediatrics, 127*(5), e1322–e1325. DOI: 10.1542/peds.2011-0428

Lang, R., O'Reilly, M., Healy, O., Rispoli, M., Lydon, H., Streusand, W., Davis, T., Kang, S., Sigafoos, J., Lancioni, G., Didden, R., & Giesbers, S. (2012). Sensory integration therapy for autism spectrum disorders: A systematic review. *Research in Autism Spectrum Disorders, 6*(3), 1004–1018. DOI: 10.1016/j.rasd.2012.01.006

Levin, A. R., Fox, N. A., Zeanah Jr, C. H., & Nelson, C. A. (2015). Social communication difficulties and autism in previously institutionalized children. *Journal of the American Academy of Child & Adolescent Psychiatry, 54*(2), 108–115. DOI: 10.1016/j.jaac.2014.11.011

Levy, S. E., & Hyman, S. L. (2008). Complementary and alternative medicine treatments for children with autism spectrum disorders. *Child and Adolescent Psychiatric Clinics of North America, 17*(4), 803–820. DOI: 10.1016/j.chc.2008.06.004

Li, Y.-J., Li, Y.-M., & Xiang, D.-X. (2018). Supplement intervention associated with nutritional deficiencies in autism spectrum disorders: A systematic review. *European Journal of Nutrition, 57*(7), 2571–2582. DOI: 10.1007/s00394-017-1528-6

Mulloy, A., Lang, R., O'Reilly, M., Sigafoos, J., Lancioni, G., & Rispoli, M. (2010). Gluten-free and casein-free diets in the treatment of autism spectrum disorders: a systematic review. *Research in Autism Spectrum Disorders, 4*, 328–339. https://doi.org/10.1016/j.rasd.2009.10.008

van der Linden, S. (2022). Misinformation: susceptibility, spread, and interventions to immunize the public. *Nature Medicine, 28*(3), 460–467. DOI: 10.1038/s41591-022-01713-6

London, M. D., Mackenzie, L., Lovarini, M., Dickson, C., & Alvarez-Campos, A. (2020). Animal assisted therapy for children and adolescents with autism spectrum disorder: Parent perspectives. *Journal of Autism & Developmental Disorders, 50*(12), 4492–4503. DOI: 10.1007/s10803-020-04512-5

Lydon, H., Healy, O., & Grey, I. (2017). Comparison of behavioral intervention and sensory integration therapy on challenging behavior of children with autism. *Behavioral Interventions, 32*(4), 297–310. DOI: 10.1002/bin.1490

Madsen, K. M., Lauritsen, M. B., Pedersen, C. B., Thorsen, P., Plesner, A.-M., Andersen, P. H., & Mortensen, P. B. (2003). Thimerosal and the occurrence of autism: negative ecological evidence from Danish population-based data. *Pediatrics, 112*(3), 604–606. DOI: 10.1542/peds.112.3.604

Mari-Bauset, S., Zazpe, I., Mari-Sanchis, A., Llopis-González, A., & Morales-Suarez-Varela, M. (2014). Evidence of the gluten-free and casein-free diet in autism spectrum disorders: A systematic review. *Journal of Child Neurology, 29*(12), 1718–1727. DOI: 10.1177/0883073814531330

Marino, L., & Lilienfeld, S. O. (2007). Dolphin-assisted therapy: More flawed data and more flawed conclusions. *Anthrozoös, 20*(3), 239–249. DOI: 10.2752/089279307x224782

Matson, J. L., Adams, H. L., Williams, L. W., & Rieske, R. D. (2013). Why are there so many unsubstantiated treatments in autism? *Research in Autism Spectrum Disorders, 7*(3), 466–474. DOI: 10.1016/j.rasd.2012.11.006

Matta, S. M., Hill-Yardin, E. L., & Crack, P. J. (2019). The influence of neuroinflammation in autism spectrum disorder. *Brain, Behavior, and Immunity, 79*, 75–90. DOI: 10.1016/j.bbi.2019.04.037

McCormack, G., Dillon, A. C., Healy, O., Walsh, C., & Lydon, S. (2020). Primary care physicians' knowledge of autism and evidence-based interventions for autism: A systematic review. *Review Journal of Autism & Developmental Disorders, 7*(3), 226–241. DOI: https://doi.org/10.1007/s40489-019-00189-4

McGee, J., Menolascino, F., Hobbs, D., & Menousek, P. (2009). *Gentle teaching*. Abbotsford, Canada: Gentle Teaching International.

McKee, A., & Gomez, A. S. (2020). The voices of typers: Examining the educational experiences of individuals who use facilitated communication. *Disability Studies Quarterly, 40*(4). DOI: 10.18061/dsq.v40i4.6981

Mercer, J. (2013). International concerns about holding therapy. *Research on Social Work Practice, 24*(2), 188–191. DOI: 10.1177/1049731513497518

Miller, V. A., Schreck, K. A., Mulick, J. A., & Butter, E. (2012). Factors related to parents' choices of treatments for their children with autism spectrum disorders. *Research in Autism Spectrum Disorders, 6*(1), 87–95. DOI: 10.1016/j.rasd.2011.03.008

Millward, C., Ferriter, M., Calver, S. J., & Connell-Jones, G. G. (2008). Gluten- and casein-free diets for autistic spectrum disorder. *Cochrane Database of Systematic Reviews, 2*, CD003498. DOI: 10.1002/14651858.CD003498.pub3

Mostert, M. P. (2001). Facilitated communication since 1995: A review of published studies. *Journal of Autism & Developmental Disorders, 31*(3), 287–313. DOI: 10.1023/A:1010795219886

Mudford, O. C., & Cullen, C. (2015). Auditory integration training. In R. M. Foxx & J. A. Mulick (Eds.), *Controversial therapies for autism and intellectual disabilities* (2nd ed., pp. 65–90). London: Routledge. DOI: 10.4324/9781315754345

Munasinghe, S. A., Oliff, C., Finn, J., & Wray, J. A. (2010). Digestive enzyme supplementation for autism spectrum disorders: a double-blind randomized controlled trial. *Journal of Autism and Developmental Disorders, 40*(9), 1131–1138. DOI: 10.1007/s10803-010-0974-2

Ng, Q. X., Loke, W., Venkatanarayanan, N., Lim, D. Y., Soh, A. Y. S., & Yeo, W. S. (2019). A systematic review of the role of prebiotics and probiotics in autism spectrum disorders. *Medicina, 55*(5), 129. DOI: 10.3390/medicina55050129

Nye, C., & Brice, A. (2005). Combined vitamin B6-magnesium treatment in autism spectrum disorder. *Cochrane Database of Systematic Reviews, 4*, CD003497. DOI: 10.1002/14651858.CD003497.pub2

O'Haire, M. E. (2013). Animal-assisted intervention for autism spectrum disorder: A systematic literature review. *Journal of Autism & Developmental Disorders, 43*(7), 1606–1622. DOI: 10.1007/s10803-012-1707-5

O'Haire, M. E. (2017). Research on animal-assisted intervention and autism spectrum disorder, 2012–2015. *Applied Developmental Science, 21*(3), 200–216. doi.org/10.1080/10888691.2016.1243988

Owen-Smith, A. A., Bent, S., Lynch, F. L., Coleman, K. J., Yau, V. M., Pearson, K. A., Massolo, M. L., Quinn, V., & Croen, L. A. (2015). Prevalence and predictors of complementary and alternative medicine use in a large insured sample of children with autism spectrum disorders. *Research in Autism Spectrum Disorders, 17*, 40–51. DOI: 10.1016/j.rasd.2015.05.002

Paynter, J., Luskin-Saxby, S., Keen, D., Fordyce, K., Frost, G., Imms, C., Miller, S., Trembath, D., Tucker, M., & Ecker, U. (2019). Evaluation of a template for countering misinformation—Real-world autism treatment myth debunking. *PloS One, 14*(1), 1–13. DOI: 10.1371/journal.pone.0210746

Phadke, V. K., Bednarczyk, R. A., & Omer, S. B. (2020). Vaccine refusal and measles outbreaks in the US. *JAMA, 324*(13), 1344–1345. DOI: 10.1001/jama.2020.14828

Piwowarczyk, A., Horvath, A., Łukasik, J., Pisula, E., & Szajewska, H. (2018). Gluten-and casein-free diet and autism spectrum disorders in children: A systematic review. *European Journal of Nutrition, 57*(2), 433–440. DOI: 10.1007/s00394-017-1483-2

Piwowarczyk, A., Horvath, A., Pisula, E., Kawa, R., & Szajewska, H. (2020). Gluten-free diet in children with autism spectrum disorders: A randomized, controlled, single-blinded trial. *Journal of Autism & Developmental Disorders, 50*, 482–490. DOI: 10.1007/s10803-019-04266-9

Podgórska-Bednarz, J., & Perenc, L. (2021). Hyperbaric oxygen therapy for children and youth with autism spectrum disorder: A review. *Brain Sciences, 11*(7), 916. DOI: 10.3390/brainsci11070916

Randell, E., Wright, M., Milosevic, S., Gillespie, D., Brookes-Howell, L., Busse-Morris, M., Hastings, R., Maboshe, W., Williams-Thomas, R., Mills, L., Romeo, R., Yaziji, N., McKigney, A. M., Ahuja, A., Warren, G., Glarou, E., Delport, S., & McNamara, R. (2022). Sensory integration therapy for children with autism and sensory processing difficulties: The SenITA RCT. *Health Technology Assessment, 26*(29). DOI: 10.3310/TQGE0020

Rehn, A. K., Caruso, V. R., & Kumar, S. (2023). The effectiveness of animal-assisted therapy for children and adolescents with autism spectrum disorder: A systematic review. *Complementary Therapies in Clinical Practice, 50*, 101719. DOI: 10.1016/j.ctcp.2022.101719

Rossignol, D. A., Bradstreet, J. J., Van Dyke, K., Schneider, C., Freedenfeld, S. H., O'Hara, N., Cave, S., Buckley, J. A., Mumper, E. A., & Frye, R. E. (2012). Hyperbaric oxygen treatment in autism spectrum disorders. *Medical Gas Research, 2*(1), 1–13. DOI: 10.1186/2045-9912-2-16

Rutgers, A. H., Bakermans-Kranenburg, M. J., van Ijzendoorn, M. H., & van Berckelaer-onnes, I. A. (2004). Autism and attachment: A meta-analytic review. *Journal of Child Psychology and Psychiatry, 45*(6), 1123–1134. DOI: 10.1111/j.1469-7610.2004.t01-1-00305.x

Saad, K., Abdel-Rahman, A., Elserogy, Y., Al-Atram, A., El-Houfey, A., Othman, H., ... Abdel-Salam, A. (2019). Retraction: Randomized controlled trial of vitamin D supplementation in children with autism spectrum disorder. *Journal of Child Psychology and Psychiatry, 60*(6), 711–711. DOI: 10.1111/jcpp.13076

Saad, K., Eltayeb, A. A., Mohamad, I. L., Al-Atram, A. A., Elserogy, Y., Bjørklund, G., El-Houfey, A., & Nicholson, B. (2015). A randomized, placebo-controlled trial of digestive enzymes in children with autism spectrum disorders. *Clinical Psychopharmacology & Neuroscience, 13*(2), 188. DOI: 10.9758/cpn.2015.13.2.188

Saloviita, T. (2018). Does linguistic analysis confirm the validity of facilitated communication? *Focus on Autism and Other Developmental Disabilities, 33*(2), 91–99. DOI: 10.1177/1088357616646075

Sathe, N., Andrews, J. C., McPheeters, M. L., & Warren, Z. E. (2017). Nutritional and dietary interventions for autism spectrum disorder: A systematic review. *Pediatrics, 139*(6), 1–8. DOI: 10.1542/peds.2017-0346

Schaaf, R. C., Dumont, R. L., Arbesman, M., & May-Benson, T. A. (2018). Efficacy of occupational therapy using Ayres Sensory Integration®: A systematic review. *American Journal of Occupational Therapy, 72*(1). DOI: 10.5014/ajot.2018.028431

Schoen, S.A., Lane, S.J., Mailloux, Z., May-Benson, T., Parham, L.D., Smith Roley, S. and Schaaf, R.C. (2019), A systematic review of Ayres sensory integration intervention for children with autism. *Autism Research, 12*(1), 6–19. DOI: 10.1002/aur.2046

Schoen, S. A., Miller, L. J., & Sullivan, J. (2015). A pilot study of integrated listening systems for children with sensory processing problems. *Journal of Occupational Therapy, Schools, & Early Intervention, 8*(3), 256–276. DOI: 10.1080/19411243.2015.1055418

Severson, K., Aune, J., & Jodlowski, D. (2008). Bruno Bettelheim, autism, and the rhetoric of scientific authority. In M. Osteen (Ed.), *Autism and representation* (1st ed., pp. 65–77). London: Routledge.

Siegel, M. (2018). The severe end of the spectrum: Insights and opportunities from the autism inpatient collection (AIC). *Journal of Autism & Developmental Disorders, 48*(11), 3641–3646. DOI: 10.1007/s10803-018-3731-6

Silverman, C. (2011). *Understanding autism: Parents, doctors, and the history of a disorder.* Princeton, NJ: Princeton University Press. https://doi.org/10.1515/9781400840397

Sinha, Y., Silove, N., Hayen, A., & Williams, K. (2011). Auditory integration training and other sound therapies for autism spectrum disorders (ASD). *Cochrane Database of Systematic Reviews, 12*, 1–43. CD003681. DOI: 10.1002/14651858.CD003681.pub3

Sipilä, A.-K., & Määttä, K. (2011). Can the facilitated communication method support autistic people, according to facilitators' opinions? *Psychology of Language and Communication, 15*(1), 1. DOI: 10.2478/v10057-011-0001-5

Sissons, J. H., Blakemore, E., Shafi, H., Skotny, N., & Lloyd, D. M. (2022). Calm with horses? A systematic review of animal-assisted interventions for improving social functioning in children with autism. *Autism, 26*(6), 1320–1340. DOI: 10.1177/13623613221085338

Smith, I. M., & MacDonald, N. E. (2017). Countering evidence denial and the promotion of pseudoscience in autism spectrum disorder. *Autism Research, 10*(8), 1334–1337. DOI: 10.1002/aur.1810

Smith, T., Mruzek, D. W., & Mozingo, D. (2015). Sensory integration therapy. In R. M. Foxx & J. A. Mulick (Eds.), *Controversial therapies for autism and intellectual disabilities* (2nd ed., pp. 267–289). London: Routledge. DOI: 10.4324/9781315754345

Sokolski, K. N., & Wachtel, R. (1998). Improved social and language skills after secretin administration in patients with autistic spectrum disorders. *Journal of the Association for Academic Minority Physicians*, *9*(1), 9–15

Stehli, A. (1991). *The sound of a miracle: A child's triumph over autism*. New York: Doubleday.

Steinhausen, H. C., Mohr Jensen, C., & Lauritsen, M. (2016). A systematic review and meta-analysis of the long-term overall outcome of autism spectrum disorders in adolescence and adulthood. *Acta Psychiatrica Scandinavica*, *133*(6), 445–452. DOI: https://doi.org/10.1111/acps.12559

Tackett, J. L., Lilienfeld, S. O., Patrick, C. J., Johnson, S. L., Krueger, R. F., Miller, J. D., Oltmanns, T. F., & Shrout, P. E. (2017). It's time to broaden the replicability conversation: Thoughts for and from clinical psychological science. *Perspectives on Psychological Science*, *12*(5), 742–756. https://doi.org/10.1177/1745691617690042

Tolin, D. F., McKay, D., Forman, E. M., Klonsky, E. D., & Thombs, B. D. (2015). Empirically supported treatment: Recommendations for a new model. *Clinical Psychology: Science and Practice*, *22*(4), 317–338. DOI: 10.1037/h0101729

Trzmiel, T., Purandare, B., Michalak, M., Zasadzka, E., & Pawlaczyk, M. (2019). Equine assisted activities and therapies in children with autism spectrum disorder: A systematic review and a meta-analysis. *Complementary Therapies in Medicine*, *42*, 104–113. DOI: 10.1016/j.ctim.2018.11.004

Tversky, A., & Kahneman, D. (1973). Availability: A heuristic for judging frequency and probability. *Cognitive Psychology*, *5*(2), 207–232. DOI: 10.1016/0010-0285(73)90033-9

Tversky, A., & Kahneman, D. (1981). The framing of decisions and the psychology of choice. *Science*, *211*(4481), 453–458.

United States Department of Health and Human Services, Food and Drug Administration. (2019). Be aware of potentially dangerous products and therapies that claim to treat autism. https://www.fda.gov/consumers/consumer-updates/be-aware-potentially-dangerous-products-and-therapies-claim-treat-autism

Upledger, J. E. (1995). Craniosacral therapy Part I: Its origins and development. *Subtle Energies & Energy Medicine Journal Archives*, *6*(1), 1–53.

Villasenor, R. F., Smith, S. L., & Jewell, V. D. (2018). A systematic review of sound-based intervention programs to improve participation in education for children with sensory processing and integration challenges. *Journal of Occupational Therapy, Schools, & Early Intervention*, *11*(2), 172–191. DOI: 10.1080/19411243.2018.1432444

Wakefield, A. J., Murch, S. H., & Anthony, A. (2010). Ileal-lymphoid-nodular hyperplasia, non-specific colitis, and pervasive developmental disorder in children (Retraction of vol 351, pg 637, 1998). *Lancet*, *375*(9713), 445–445. DOI: 10.1016/S0140-6736(10)60175-4

Weitlauf, A. S., Sathe, N., McPheeters, M. L., & Warren, Z. E. (2017). Interventions targeting sensory challenges in autism spectrum disorder: A systematic review. *Pediatrics*, *139*(6). DOI: 10.1542/peds.2017-0347

Wheeler, D. L., Jacobson, J. W., Paglieri, R. A., & Schwartz, A. A. (1993). An experimental assessment of facilitated communication. *Mental Retardation*, *31*(1), 49–59.

Williams, K., Wray, J. A., & Wheeler, D. M. (2012). Intravenous secretin for autism spectrum disorders (ASD). *Cochrane Database of Systematic Reviews*, *4*, CD003495. DOI: 10.1002/14651858.CD003495.pub3

World Health Organization. (2017). *How to respond to vocal vaccine deniers in public: best practice guidance* (No. WHO/EURO: 2017-2899-42657-59427). Geneva: World Health Organization Regional Office for Europe.

World Health Organization. (2019). *International statistical classification of diseases and related health problems* (11th ed.). https://icd.who.int/

Yap, E., Scheinberg, A., & Williams, K. (2017). Attitudes to and beliefs about animal assisted therapy for children with disabilities. *Complementary Therapies in Clinical Practice*, *26*, 47–52. DOI: 10.1016/j.ctcp.2016.11.009

Index

For the benefit of digital users, indexed terms that span two pages (e.g., 52–53) may, on occasion, appear on only one of those pages.

Tables and figures are indicated by an italic *t* and *f* following the page number.

N

O

P